a LANGE medical book

Pathophysiology of Disease

An Introduction to Clinical Medicine

first edition

Edited By

Stephen J. McPhee, MD
Professor of Medicine,
University of California,
San Francisco

Vishwanath R. Lingappa, MD, PhD
Professor of Physiology and Medicine,
University of California, San Francisco

William F. Ganong, MD
Jack and DeLoris Lange Professor
of Physiology Emeritus,
University of California, San Francisco

Jack D. Lange, MD
Clinical Professor of Medicine Emeritus,
University of California, San Francisco

Appleton & Lange
Stamford, Connecticut

95 96 97 98 99 / 10 9 8 7 6 5 4 3 2

Prentice Hall International (UK) Limited, *London*
Prentice Hall of Australia Pty. Limited, *Sydney*
Prentice Hall Canada, Inc., *Toronto*
Prentice Hall Hispanoamericana, S.A., *Mexico*
Prentice Hall of India Private Limited, *New Delhi*
Prentice Hall of Japan, Inc., *Tokyo*
Simon and Schuster Asia Pte. Ltd., *Singapore*
Editora Prentice Hall do Brasil Ltda., *Rio de Janeiro*
Prentice Hall, *Englewood Cliffs, New Jersey*

ISSN: 1079-6185
ISBN: 0-8385-7815-2

Illustrators: Teshin Associates
Art Coordinator: Becky Hainz-Baxter
Acquisitions Editor: John J. Dolan

PRINTED IN THE UNITED STATES OF AMERICA

ISBN 0-8385-7815

90000

9 780838 578155

Table of Contents

Preface

WHAT THE BOOK IS

This is a text designed to present an orientation to disease as disordered physiology. It is intended to enable the student and practitioner to understand how and why the symptoms and signs of various conditions appear. In approaching disease as disordered physiology, this text analyzes the mechanism of production of the symptoms and signs of different disease syndromes. In so doing, it recognizes the student's and practitioner's need to understand the mechanisms underlying the disease and its clinical manifestations so that rational therapies can be devised.

WHAT THE BOOK IS NOT

We do not offer a standard textbook of medicine, proceeding in conventional sequence from etiology, pathology, symptoms and signs, laboratory findings, diagnosis, and differential diagnosis to treatment and prognosis. Nor is *Pathophysiology of Disease* intended to serve as a standard textbook of physiology, pathology, or physical diagnosis. Furthermore, the text is not intended to be all-encompassing in the disordered physiologic mechanisms or disease states described. Rather, the authors have selected those examples of disordered physiology and those disease states which seemed most relevant to the clinical practice of medicine.

INTENDED AUDIENCE

Medical students in basic pathophysiology courses will find in this text a concise and useful contribution to their understanding of how disordered physiology produces common disease syndromes. Medical students in the Introduction to Clinical Medicine courses who are in transition from preclinical to clinical training will find this a useful reference in understanding how and why the symptoms and signs of various disease states appear. House officers will find the concise, up-to-date descriptions of disease mechanisms, with citations to the current literature, of usefulness in devising proper patient management. Practitioners (internists, family physicians, and other specialists who provide generalist care) will find *Pathophysiology of Disease* useful as a refresher text, designed to update their understanding of the mechanisms underlying disease. Nurses and other health practitioners will find that the concise format and broad scope of the book facilitate their understanding of basic disease entities.

ORGANIZATION OF THE BOOK

Pathophysiology of Disease is divided into 20 chapters, developed chiefly by organ system. Each chapter is divided into sections emphasizing normal structure and function, pathology and disordered physiology, common clinical presentations, and mechanisms underlying consequent symptoms and signs. A list of pertinent recent references is provided at the end of each chapter as suggestions for further reading.

Stephen J. McPhee, MD
Vishwanath R. Lingappa, MD, PhD
William F. Ganong, MD
Jack D. Lange, MD

San Francisco, California
February, 1995

Authors

Daniel C. Adelman, MD
Assistant Professor of Clinical Medicine; Director, Clinical Programs in Allergy and Immunology, Department of Medicine, University of California, San Francisco.

Tomás J. Aragón, MD, MPH
Fellow, Infectious Disease Epidemiology and Center for AIDS Prevention Studies, University of California, San Francisco.

Gregory Barsh, MD, PhD
Assistant Professor of Pediatrics and Genetics, Stanford University School of Medicine, Stanford.

Kenneth R. Feingold, MD
Professor of Medicine and Dermatology, University of California, San Francisco; Chief, Metabolism Clinic, Veterans Affairs Medical Center, San Francisco.

Janet L. Funk, MD
Assistant Professor of Medicine, University of California, San Francisco.

William F. Ganong, MD
Jack and DeLoris Lange, Professor of Physiology Emeritus, University of California, San Francisco.

Fred Kusumoto, MD
Director, Electrophysiology and Pacing, Lovelace Medical Center, Albuquerque, New Mexico.

Jack D. Lange, MD
Clinical Professor of Medicine Emeritus, University of California, San Francisco.

Vishwanath R. Lingappa, MD, PhD
Professor of Physiology and Medicine, University of California, San Francisco.

Stephen J. McPhee, MD
Professor of Medicine, University of California, San Francisco.

Robert O. Messing, MD
Assistant Professor, Department of Neurology, San Francisco General Hospital, San Francisco.

Thomas J. Prendergast, MD
Postdoctoral Fellow in Pulmonary and Critical Care Medicine, University of California, San Francisco.

Stephen J. Ruoss, MD
Assistant Professor of Medicine, Division of Pulmonary and Critical Care Medicine, Stanford University Medical Center, Stanford.

Richard S. Shames, MD
Assistant Clinical Professor of Pediatrics and Director, Pediatric Allergy, University of California, San Francisco.

Dolores M. Shoback, MD
Associate Professor of Medicine, Veterans Affairs Medical Center, San Francisco.

Gordon J. Strewler, MD
Professor of Medicine and Chief, Endocrine Unit, Veterans Affairs Medical Center, San Francisco.

Debasish Tripathy, MD
Assistant Clinical Professor of Medicine, Division of Hematology and Oncology, University of California, San Francisco.

Introduction 1

Jack D. Lange, MD

WHAT IS PATHOPHYSIOLOGY?

Pathophysiology may be defined as the physiology of disease, of disordered function, or derangement of function seen in disease that is produced by the action of an etiologic agent (eg, bacteria) on susceptible tissues or organs. The term "pathophysiology" emphasizes alterations in function, as distinguished from structural changes (pathology). Pathophysiology also includes the study of the mechanisms underlying disease. The study of pathophysiology is an essential introduction to clinical medicine and serves as a bridge between the basic sciences and the clinic.

Pathophysiology differs from pathogenesis. Pathogenesis is the mode of origin or development of any disease process (eg, development of autoimmunity to the thyroid-stimulating hormone receptor). Pathophysiology describes the resulting disordered physiology and clinical consequences (eg, release of excess thyroid hormone, producing the syndrome of hyperthyroidism).

WHY IS PATHOPHYSIOLOGY IMPORTANT?

An orientation to disease as disordered physiology can enable the student and practitioner to understand how and why the symptoms and signs of various conditions appear. A pathophysiologic approach to disease as disordered physiology enables the clinician to analyze the mechanism of production of the symptoms and signs of different disease syndromes. In so doing, it recognizes the student's and practitioner's need to understand the mechanisms underlying the disease and its clinical manifestations so that rational therapies can be devised.

This book was written with the principles described above in mind. It summarizes the normal structure and function of each organ system, then discusses a number of the major diseases of each system, showing how symptoms and signs of the selected diseases are produced by disordered physiology. It also provides an introduction to clinical medicine by analyzing in the same way the broad topics of genetic abnormalities, neoplasia, and infectious disease.

2 Genetic Disease

Gregory Barsh, MD, PhD

Mechanisms of cellular and tissue dysfunction in genetic diseases are as varied as the organs they affect. To some extent, these mechanisms are similar to those that occur in nonheritable disorders. For example, a fracture caused by decreased bone density in osteoporosis heals in the same fashion as one caused by a defective collagen gene in osteogenesis imperfecta, and the response to coronary atherosclerosis in most individuals does not depend on whether they have inherited a defective LDL receptor. Thus, the pathophysiologic principles of genetic disease are not so much those of the affected organ system as they are mechanisms of mutation, inheritance, and molecular pathways from genotype to phenotype.

This chapter will begin with a discussion of the terminology used to describe inherited conditions, the prevalence of genetic disease, and some important principles and considerations in clinical genetics. Important terms and keywords used throughout the chapter are defined in Table 2–1.

Next, a group of disorders caused by mutations in collagen genes will be discussed, ie, **osteogenesis imperfecta.** Though osteogenesis imperfecta is often considered a single entity, different mutations and different genes subject to mutation lead to a wide spectrum of clinical phenotypes. The different types of osteogenesis imperfecta exhibit typical patterns of autosomal dominant or autosomal recessive inheritance and are therefore examples of so-called **mendelian conditions.**

Recently, several genetic conditions have been found to depend not only on the gene being inherited but also on the phenotype or the sex of the parent. As an example of a condition that exhibits nonclassic inheritance, the **fragile X-associated mental retardation syndrome** will be discussed. This syndrome is not only the most common cause of inherited mental retardation but also illustrates a recently discovered principle of molecular and cellular biology.

One of the most common types of human genetic disease that does not affect DNA structure per se is **aneuploidy,** or a change in the normal chromosome content per cell. The example that will be considered, **Down's syndrome,** has had a major impact on reproductive medicine and reproductive decision making and serves to illustrate general principles that apply to many aneuploid conditions.

Finally, to show how environmental factors can influence the relationship between genotype and phenotype, we will discusss **phenylketonuria,** which serves as the paradigm for newborn screening programs and treatment of genetic disease.

UNIQUE ASPECTS OF GENETIC PATHOPHYSIOLOGY

Although the phenotypes of genetic diseases are diverse, their causes are not. The primary cause of any genetic disease can be defined as a discrete event that affects gene expression in a group of cells related to each other by lineage. Most genetic diseases are caused by an alteration in DNA sequence that alters the synthesis of a single gene product. However, some genetic diseases are caused (1) by chromosome rearrangements that result in deletion or duplication of a group of closely linked genes or (2) by mistakes during mitosis or meiosis that result in an abnormal number of chromosomes per cell. In most genetic diseases, every cell in an affected individual carries the mutated gene or genes as a consequence of its inheritance via a mutant egg or sperm **(gamete).** However, mutation of the gametic cell may have arisen during its development, in which case somatic cells of the parent do not carry the mutation and the affected individual is said to have a "new mutation." In addition, some mutations may arise in somatic cells during early embryogenesis, in which case tissues of the affected individual contain a mixture, or **mosaic,** of mutant and nonmutant cells (Figure 2–1).

It is important to remember the distinctions between gene, locus, and allele and between mutation, polymorphism, and phenotype, since confusion about the terminology of genetics and genetic diseases can have unfortunate consequences for patients and their families. Although genes were recognized and studied long before the structure of DNA was known, it has become common usage to regard a **gene** as a

Table 2–1. Glossary of terms and keywords.

Term	Definition
Acrocentric	Pertaining to the terminal location of the centromere on chromosomes 13, 14, 15, 21, and 22, which contain so-called satellite DNA on their short arms that encodes for ribosomal RNA genes.
Allele	Alternative forms of a gene that occupy the same locus on a specific chromosome.
Allelic heterogeneity	The state in which multiple alleles at a single locus can produce a disease phenotype or phenotypes.
Amorphic	Refers to a mutation that results in a complete loss of function.
Aneuploidy	A general term used to denote any unbalanced chromosome complement.
Antimorphic	Refers to a mutation which, when present in heterozygous form opposite a nonmutant allele, results in a phenotype similar to homozygosity for loss-of-function alleles.
Ascertainment bias	The problem that arises when individuals or families in a genetic study are not representative of the general population because of the way in which they are identified.
Autosomal	Located on chromosomes 1–22 rather than X or Y.
CpG island	A segment of DNA that contains a relatively high density of 5′-CG-3′ dinucleotides. Such segments are frequently unmethylated and located close to ubiquitously expressed genes.
Dictyotene	The end of prophase during female meiosis I in which fetal oocytes are arrested prior to ovulation.
Dominant	A pattern of inheritance or mechanism of gene action in which the effects of a variant allele can be observed in the presence of a nonmutant allele.
Dominant negative	Mutant alleles that give rise to structurally abnormal proteins that interfere with the normal function of the nonmutant gene products.
Dosage compensation	Mechanism by which a difference in gene dosage between two cells is equalized; for XX cells, decreased expression from one of the two X chromosomes results in a concentration of gene product similar to that of an XY cell.
End product deficiency	A pathologic mechanism in which absence or reduction in the product of a particular enzymatic reaction leads to disease.
Epigenetic	Refers to a phenotypic effect that does not depend on genotype. DNA methylation that occurs during gametogenesis can affect gene expression in zygotic cells, but the pattern of methylation can also be reversed in subsequent generations and thus does not affect genotype.
Expressivity	The extent to which a mutant genotype affects phenotype. A quantitative measure of a disease state that may vary from mild to severe but is never completely absent.
Fitness	The likelihood that an individual who carries a particular mutant allele will produce progeny that also carry the allele.
Founder effect	One of several possible explanations for an unexpectedly high frequency of a deleterious gene in a population. If the population was founded by a small ancestral group, it may have, by chance, contained a large number of carriers for the deleterious gene.
Gamete	The egg or sperm cell that represents a potential reproductive contribution to the next generation. Gametes have undergone meiosis and so contain half the normal number of chromosomes found in zygotic cells.
Gene dosage	The principle that the amount of product expressed for a particular gene is proportionate to the number of gene copies present per cell.
Genetic anticipation	A clinical phenomenon that occurs when the phenotype observed in individuals carrying a deleterious gene appears more severe in successive generations. Possible explanations include ascertainment bias or a multistep mutational mechanism such as expansion of triplet repeats.
Genetic heterogeneity	A situation in which mutations of different genes produce similar or identical phenotypes. Also referred to as locus heterogeneity.
Haplotype	A set of closely linked alleles that are not easily separated by recombination. Often refers to DNA sequence alterations such as restriction fragment length polymorphisms.
Heterochromatin	One of two alternative forms of chromosomal material (the other is euchromatin) as determined by the way in which chromosomal DNA is bound to proteins and condensed. Heterochromatin is highly condensed and usually does not contain genes that are actively transcribed.
Heterozygote advantage	One way to explain an unexpectedly high frequency of a recessively inherited mutation in a particular population. During recent evolution, carriers (ie, heterozygotes) are postulated to have had a higher fitness than homozygous nonmutant individuals.
Hypermorphic	Refers to a mutation that has an effect similar to increasing the number of normal gene copies per cell.
Hypomorphic	Refers to a mutation that reduces but does not eliminate the activity of a particular gene product.

(*continued*)

Table 2–1. Glossary of terms and keywords. (continued)

Term	Definition
Imprinting	As applied most commonly, the process whereby expression of a gene depends on whether it is transmitted through a female or male gamete.
Linkage disequilibrium	The situation occurring when certain combinations of closely linked alleles are present in a population at frequencies not predicted by their individual frequencies.
Monosomy	A reduction In zygotic cells from two to one in the number of copies for a particular chromosomal segment or chromosome.
Mosaicism	A situation in which a genetic alteration is present in some but not all cells of a single individual. In germline or gonadal mosaicism, the alteration is present in germ cells but not in somatic cells. In somatic mosaicism, the genetic alteration is present in some but not all of the somatic cells (and is generally not present in the germ cells).
Neomorphic	Refers to a mutation that imparts a novel function to its gene product and thus results in a phenotype distinct from an alteration in gene dosage.
Nondisjunction	Failure of two homologous chromosomes to separate, or disjoin, at metaphase of meiosis I; or the failure of two sister chromatids to disjoin at metaphase of meiosis II or mitosis.
Penetrance	In a single individual of a variant genotype, penetrance is an all-or-none phenomenon determined by the absence or presence of defined phenotopic criteria. In a population, reduced penetrance implies that an individual of a variant genotype is less likely to be recognized according to the same phenotypic criteria.
Phenotypic heterogeneity	The situation occurring when mutations of a single gene produce multiple different phenotypes.
Polymorphism	An allele that is present in 1% or more of the population.
Postzygotic	Refers to a mutational event that occurs after fertilization, and that commonly gives rise to mosaicism.
Premutation	A genetic change that does not itself result in a phenotype but has a high probability of developing a second alteration—a full mutation—that does cause a phenotype.
Primordial germ cells	The group of diploid cells set aside early in development that go on to give rise to gametes.
Recessive	A pattern of inheritance or mechanism of gene action in which a particular mutant allele gives rise to a phenotype only in the absence of a nonmutant allele. Thus, for autosomal conditions, the variant or disease phenotype is manifest when two copies of the mutant allele are present. For X-linked conditions, the variant or disease phenotype is manifest in cells, tissues, or individuals in which the nonmutant allele is either inactivated (a heterozygous female) or not present (a hemizygous male).
RFLP	Restriction fragment length polymorphism, a type of DNA-based allele variation in which different alleles at a single locus are recognized and followed through pedigrees based on the size of a restriction fragment. The locus is defined by the segment of DNA that gives rise to the restriction fragment; the different alleles are generally (not always) caused by a single change in DNA sequence that creates or abolishes a site of restriction enzyme cleavage.
Robertsonian translocation	A type of translocation in which two acrocentric chromosomes are fused together with a single functional centromere. A carrier of a Robertsonian translocation with 45 chromosomes has a normal amount of chromosomal material and is said to be euploid.
Substrate accumulation	A pathogenetic mechanism in which deficiency of a particular enzyme causes disease because the substrate of that enzyme accumulates in tissue or blood.
Triplet repeat	A three-nucleotide sequence that is tandemly repeated many times, ie, $(XYZ)_n$. Alterations in length of such simple types of repeats (dinucleotide and tetranucleotide as well) occur much more frequently than most other kinds of mutations; however, alterations in the length of trinucleotide repeats is the molecular basis for several heritable disorders.
Trisomy	An abnormal situation in which there are three instead of two copies of a chromosomal segment or chromosome per cell.

short stretch of DNA (usually but not always < 100 kb in length) that encodes a product (usually protein) responsible for a measurable trait. The word **locus** refers to the place where a particular gene lies on its chromosome. A gene's DNA sequence nearly always shows slight differences when many unrelated individuals are compared, and the variant sequences are described as **alleles. Mutation** refers to a biochemical event such as a nucleotide change, deletion, or insertion that has produced a new allele. Many changes in the DNA sequence of a gene, such as those within introns or at the third "wobble" position of codons for particular amino acids, do not affect the structure or expression of the gene product; therefore, although all mutations result in a biochemical phenotype, only some result in a clinically abnormal phenotype. The word **polymorphism** denotes an allele that is present in 1% or more of the population. At

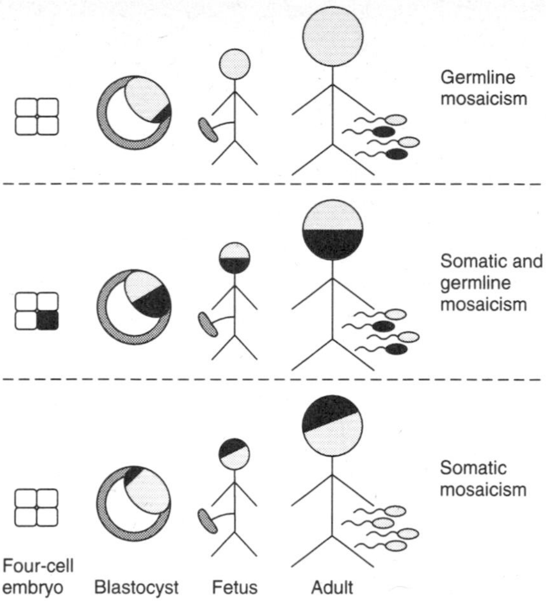

Figure 2–1. Cellular origin of mutations can lead to somatic mosaicism, germline mosaicism, or both. The effects of a mutation on mosaicism depend on the cell and the developmental stage in which the mutation occurs. The early blastocyst is composed of two different tissues: the inner cell mass (light hatching), which mostly gives rise to embryonic tissues, including somatic and germ cells; and the trophoblast (dark hatching), which gives rise to extraembryonic tissue cells such as the placenta. If a mutation (black) occurs in a portion of the inner cell mass whose daughter cells contribute exclusively to the germline, the adult will not exhibit phenotypic features of the mutation in somatic tissues but may produce germ cells both with and without the mutation (germline mosaicism; upper panel). However, if a mutation occurs in the four-cell embryo, the adult may also exhibit phenotypic features of the mutation in some but not all somatic tissues (somatic and germline mosaicism; middle panel). Finally, a mutation that occurs in a portion of the blastocyst or fetus that does not give rise to germ cells results only in somatic mosaicism (lower panel).

the biochemical level, polymorphic alleles are usually recognized by their effect on the size of a restriction fragment (**restriction *f*ragment *l*ength *p*olymorphism [RFLP]),** or the length of a short but highly repetitive region of DNA. On the other hand, at the clinical level, polymorphic alleles are recognized by their effect on a phenotype such as HLA type or eye color. These latter two traits are examples in which each gene has many polymorphic alleles; therefore, the chances are good that a single individual will carry two different alleles.

Finally, this discussion helps to illustrate the use of the word **phenotype,** which refers simply to any characteristic that can be described by an observer, regardless of the nature of that observation. RFLPs and eye color differences are both phenotypes, but only the former requires a biochemical measurement.

PENETRANCE & EXPRESSIVITY

It is an important principle of human genetics that two individuals with the same mutated gene may have different phenotypes. For example, in the autosomal dominant condition type I osteogenesis imperfecta, pedigrees may occur in which there is both an affected grandparent and an affected grandchild yet the obligate carrier parent is asymptomatic (Figure 2–2). Given a set of defined criteria, recognition of the condition in individuals known to carry the mutated gene is described as **penetrance.** In other words, if seven out of ten individuals over age 40 with the type I osteogenesis imperfecta mutation have an abnormal bone density scan, the condition is said to be 70% penetrant by these criteria. Penetrance may vary both with age and according to the set of criteria being used; for example, type I osteogenesis imperfecta may be 90% penetrant at age 40 when the conclusion is based on a bone density scan in conjunction with laboratory tests for abnormal collagen synthesis. **Reduced penetrance** or **age-dependent penetrance** is a common feature of dominantly inherited conditions that have a relatively high **fitness** (likelihood of reproduction by the individual with the mutant allele), such as Huntington's disease or polycystic kidney disease.

Although the presence of a mutated gene can be diagnosed in many individuals, their phenotypes may still be different. For example, blue scleras and slightly reduced height may be the only manifestations of type I osteogenesis imperfecta in a particular individual, while a sibling that carries the identical mutation may be confined to a wheelchair as a result of multiple fractures and deformities. The phenomenon of different phenotypes in these individuals is referred to as **variable expressivity.** Both reduced penetrance and variable expressivity occur when the relevant individuals carry the same mutated gene; therefore, phenotypic differences must be due to the effects of other "modifier" genes, to environmental interactions, or to chance.

MECHANISMS OF MUTATION & INHERITANCE PATTERNS

Mutations can be characterized both by their molecular nature, ie, deletion, insertion, substitution, or by their effects on the gene product, ie, no effect (neutral), complete loss of function (amorphic), partial loss of function (hypomorphic), gain of function (hypermorphic), or acquisition of a new property (neomorphic). Geneticists who study experimental organisms frequently use specific deletions to ensure that a

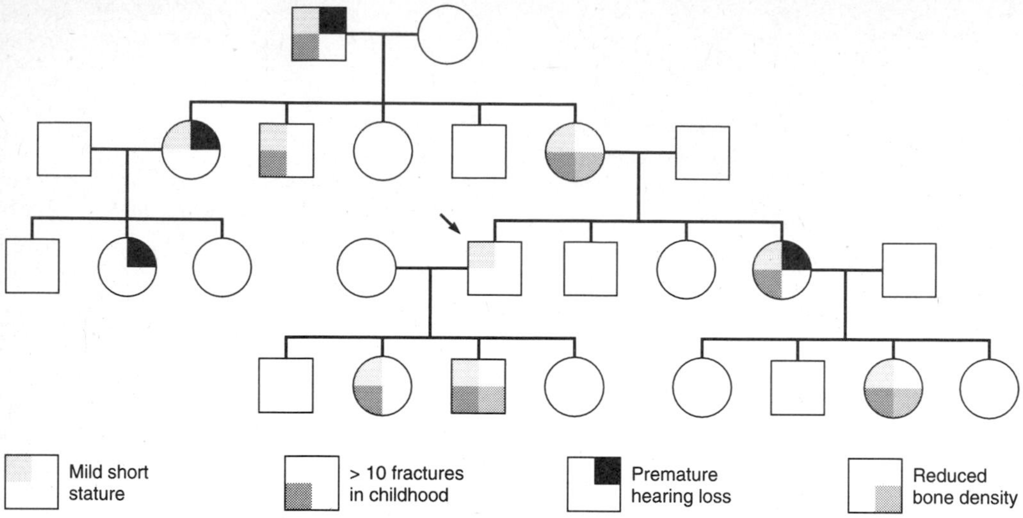

Figure 2–2. Penetrance and expressivity in type I osteogenesis imperfecta. In this schematic pedigree of the autosomal dominant condition type I osteogenesis imperfecta, nearly all of the affected individuals exhibit different phenotypic features that vary in severity (variable expressivity). As is shown, type I osteogenesis imperfecta is fully penetrant, since every individual who transmits the mutation is phenotypically affected to some degree. However, if mild short stature in the individual indicated with the arrow had been considered to be a normal variant, then the condition would have been nonpenetrant in this individual. Thus, in this example, judgments about penetrance or nonpenetrance depend on the criteria for normal and abnormal stature.

mutated allele causes a loss of function, but human geneticists rely on biochemical or cell culture studies. Amorphic and hypomorphic mutations are probably the most frequent type of mutation in human genetic disease because there are many ways to interfere with a protein's function.

For autosomal genes (those that lie on chromosomes 1–22), the fundamental difference between dominant and recessive inheritance is that with dominant inheritance, the disease state or trait being measured is apparent to the observer when one copy of the mutated allele and one copy of the normal allele are present. With recessive inheritance, however, two copies of the mutated allele must be present for the disease state or trait to be apparent. For genes that lie on the X chromosome, the same definitions apply to females (with two X chromosomes): A phenotype caused by one copy of a mutant gene is dominant; a phenotype caused by two copies is recessive. Because most mutations are amorphic or hypomorphic, however, one copy of an X-linked mutant allele in males is not "balanced" with a nonmutant allele, as it would be in females; therefore, One copy of an X-linked recessive gene is sufficient to produce a mutant phenotype in males.

Recessive Inheritance & Loss-of-Function Mutations

As mentioned above, most recessive mutations are due to a loss of function of the mutated allele, which can occur by a variety of different pathways, including failure of the gene to be transcribed or translated or failure of the translated gene product to function correctly. There are two general principles to keep in mind when considering loss-of-function mutations. First, because expression from the nonmutant allele usually does not change (ie, there is no **dosage compensation**), gene expression in a heterozygous carrier of a loss-of-function allele is reduced to 50% of normal. Second, for most biochemical pathways, a 50% reduction in enzyme concentration is not sufficient to produce a disease state. Thus, most diseases due to enzyme deficiencies such as phenylketonuria (Table 2–2) are inherited in a recessive fashion.

Dominant Inheritance & Loss-of-Function Mutations

If a loss-of-function mutation produces a dominantly inherited phenotype, this implies that 50% of the normal gene product is insufficient to sustain the nonmutant phenotype. Such mutations usually occur in structural proteins; the example we will consider below is type I osteogenesis imperfecta. In semidominant inheritance, two copies of the mutant allele produce a phenotype more severe than one mutant and one normal copy. Note that most dominantly inherited human conditions are probably semidominant but that the homozygous mutant individual is rarely observed. For example, inheritance of achondroplasia, the most common genetic cause of very short

Table 2–2. Phenotype, genetic mechanism, and prevalence of selected genetic disorders.

Disorder	Phenotype	Genetic Mechanism	Prevalence
Down's syndrome	Mental and growth retardation, dysmorphic features, internal organ anomalies	Chromosomal imbalance caused by trisomy 21	≈1:800; increased risk with advanced maternal age
Fragile X-associated mental retardation	Mental retardation, characteristic facial features, large testes	X-linked; progressive expansion of unstable DNA causes failure to express gene encoding RNA-binding protein	≈1:1500 males; can be manifest in females; multistep mechanism
Sickle cell anemia	Recurrent painful crises, increased susceptibility to infections	Autosomal recessive; caused by a single missense mutation in beta globin	≈1:400 blacks
Cystic fibrosis	Recurrent pulmonary infections, exocrine pancreatic insufficiency, infertility	Autosomal recessive; caused by multiple loss-of-function mutations in a chloride channel	≈1:2000 whites; very rare in Asians
Neurofibromatosis	Multiple café au lait spots, neurofibromas, increased tumor susceptibility	Autosomal dominant; caused by multiple loss-of-function mutations in a signaling molecule	≈1:3000; about 50% are new mutations
Duchenne's muscular dystrophy	Muscular weakness and degeneration	X-linked recessive; caused by multiple loss-of-function mutations in muscle protein	≈1:3000 males; about 33% are new mutations
Osteogenesis imperfecta	Increased susceptibility to fractures, connective tissue fragility	Phenotypically and genetically heterogeneous	≈1:10,000
Phenylketonuria	Mental and growth retardation	Autosomal recessive; caused by multiple loss-of-function mutations in phenylalanine hydroxylase	≈1:10,000

stature, is usually said to be autosomal dominant. However, rare matings between two affected individuals have a 25% probability of producing offspring with two copies of the mutant gene. This results in homozygous achondroplasia, a condition that is very severe and usually fatal in the perinatal period. Huntington's disease, a dominantly inherited neurologic disease, is the only known human condition in which the homozygous mutant phenotype is identical with the heterozygous mutant phenotype (sometimes referred to as a "true dominant").

Dominant Negative Mutations

A special kind of mutation referred to as a dominant negative occurs frequently in human diseases that involve polymeric structural proteins. In these disorders, the mutant allele gives rise to a structurally abnormal protein that interferes with the function of the normal allele. The presence of a dominant negative allele can be proved in experimental organisms by showing that one copy of the putative dominant negative allele has an effect similar to two copies of a loss-of-function allele. Such a mutation is said to be "antimorphic." Note that any molecular lesion—eg, deletion, nonsense, missense, or splicing—can produce a loss-of-function allele. However, only molecular lesions that yield a protein product—eg, splicing, missense, or nonsense mutations—can result in a dominant negative allele. Type II osteogenesis imperfecta, described below, is an example of a dominant negative mutation.

The words "dominant" and "recessive" are sometimes used imprecisely. Mutations are simply molecular alterations in a strand of DNA and therefore, strictly speaking, are not in themselves dominant or recessive. The terms are instead appropriate to the *effect of a mutation* on a particular trait. Therefore when a particular mutation is characterized as "recessive," one is referring to the effect of this mutation on the trait being studied.

GENOME SIZE & THE PREVALENCE OF GENETIC DISEASE

Estimates of the total number of genes in the human genome are on the order of 50,000–100,000. However, only 5000 or so single-gene disorders have been recognized clinically, and, of these, the molecular or biochemical basis is known for less than 10%. In considering possible explanations for this disparity, it seems likely that mutations of many single genes are lethal very early in development and thus not clinically apparent, whereas mutations in other genes do not cause an easily recognizable phenotype. Not including multifactorial conditions, the overall frequency of genetic disease in the general population is approximately 1%. However, because many genetic conditions are recessively inherited and because the rate for new deleterious mutations is relatively high—approximately 10^{-6}–10^{-5} per locus per generation—every individual in the population is estimated to carry four or five deleterious genes.

Table 2–2 lists the names, major symptoms, genetic mechanisms, and prevalence of the diseases considered in this chapter as well as of several others. The most frequent conditions, such as neurofibromatosis, cystic fibrosis, and the fragile X-related mental retardation syndrome, will be encountered at some time by most health care professionals regardless of their field of interest. Other conditions such as Huntington's disease and adenosine deaminase deficiency, while of intellectual and pathophysiologic interest, are unlikely to be clinically relevant to most practitioners.

Many common conditions such as atherosclerosis and breast cancer that do not show strictly mendelian inheritance patterns have a genetic component evident from familial aggregation or twin studies. These conditions are usually described as **multifactorial,** which means that the effects of one or more mutated genes and environmental differences all contribute to the likelihood that a given individual will manifest the phenotype. Although these conditions will not be considered in detail, the principles apparent from the study of single-gene disorders are applicable to many conditions that affect human health.

SPECIAL ISSUES IN CLINICAL GENETICS

Most patients with genetic disease present during early childhood with symptoms that ultimately give rise to a diagnosis such as fragile X-associated mental retardation or Down's syndrome. The major clinical issues at presentation are arriving at the correct diagnosis and counseling the patient and family regarding the natural history and prognosis of the condition. One of the most important questions is the likelihood that the same condition will occur again in the family and whether it can be diagnosed prenatally. These issues form the core of genetic counseling and are often dealt with by a medical geneticist and a trained genetic counselor.

Currently, only a few genetic conditions such as phenylketonuria and some forms of maple syrup urine disease can be treated effectively. Efforts are under way, however, to develop treatments for some of the more common single-gene disorders such as Duchenne's muscular dystrophy and cystic fibrosis. Some forms of therapy are directed at replacing the mutant protein, while others are directed at ameliorating its effects.

1. Define gene, locus, allele, mutation, polymorphism, and phenotype.
2. How is it possible for two individuals with the same mutated gene to have differences in penetrance and expressivity?
3. How many genes are in the human genome? How many single gene disorders have been recognized clinically? For how many is there insight into the molecular or biochemical basis?

PATHOPHYSIOLOGY OF SELECTED GENETIC DISEASES

OSTEOGENESIS IMPERFECTA

Osteogenesis imperfecta is a condition inherited in a mendelian fashion that illustrates many principles of human genetics. It is a heterogeneous and pleiotropic group of disorders characterized by a tendency toward fragility of bone. Advances in the last decade demonstrate that virtually every case is caused by a mutation of the COL1A1 or COL1A2 genes, which encode the subunits of type I collagen, α1(I) and α2(I), respectively. More than 100 different mutant alleles have been described for osteogenesis imperfecta; the relationships between different DNA sequence alterations and the type of disease (genotype-phenotype correlations) illustrate several pathophysiologic principles in human genetics.

Clinical Manifestations

The clinical and genetic characteristics of four clinical subtypes of osteogenesis imperfecta are summarized in Table 2–3. The timing and severity of fractures, the radiologic findings, the presence of additional clinical features, and the family history are used to discriminate among the different subtypes. Individuals with type I or type IV osteogenesis imperfecta present in early childhood with one or a few fractures of long bones in response to minimal or no trauma; x-rays reveal mild osteopenia, little or no bony deformity, and often evidence of earlier subclinical fractures. However, most individuals with type I or type IV osteogenesis imperfecta do not have fractures in utero. Type I and type IV osteogenesis

Table 2–3. Clinical and molecular subtypes of osteogenesis imperfecta.

Type	Phenotype	Genetics	Molecular Pathophysiology
Type I	**Mild:** Short stature, postnatal fractures, little or no deformity, blue scleras, premature hearing loss	Autosomal dominant	Loss-of-function mutation in proα1(I) chain resulting in decreased amount of mRNA; quality of collagen is normal; quantity is reduced twofold
Type II	**Perinatal lethal:** Severe prenatal fractures, abnormal bone formation, severe deformities, blue scleras, connective tissue fragility	Sporadic (autosomal dominant)	Structural mutation in proα1(I) or proα2(I) chain that slows heterotrimer assembly; quality of collagen is abnormal; quantity often reduced also
Type III	**Progressive deforming**: Prenatal fractures, deformities usually present at birth, very short stature, usually nonambulatory, blue scleras, hearing loss	Autosomal dominant (rare cases autosomal recessive)	Structural mutation in proα1(I) or proα2(I) chain that has mild or no effect on heterotrimer assembly; quality of collagen is mildly abnormal; quantity can be normal
Type IV	**Deforming with normal scleras:** Postnatal fractures, mild to moderate deformities, premature hearing loss, normal or gray scleras, dentinogenesis imperfecta	Autosomal dominant	Structural mutation in proα2(I) chain that has little or no effect on heterotrimer assembly; quality of collagen is mildly abnormal; quantity can be normal

imperfecta are distinguished by the severity (less in type I than in type IV) and by scleral hue, which indicates the thickness of this tissue and the deposition of type I collagen. Individuals with type I osteogenesis imperfecta have blue scleras, while the scleras of those with type IV are normal or slightly gray. In type I, the typical number of fractures during childhood is 10–20; fracture incidence decreases after puberty, and the main features in adult life are mild short stature, a tendency toward conductive hearing loss, and occasionally dentinogenesis imperfecta. Individuals with type IV generally experience more fractures than those with type I osteogenesis imperfecta and have significant short stature due to a combination of long bone and spinal deformities, but they often are able to walk independently. Approximately one-fourth of the cases of type I or type IV osteogenesis imperfecta will represent new mutations; in the remainder, the history and examination of other family members will reveal findings consistent with autosomal dominant inheritance.

Type II osteogenesis imperfecta presents at or before birth (diagnosed by prenatal ultrasound) with multiple fractures, bony deformities, increased fragility of nonbony connective tissue, and blue scleras and usually results in death in infancy. Two typical radiologic findings are the presence of isolated "islands" of mineralization in the skull (wormian bones), and a beaded appearance to the ribs. Nearly all cases of type II osteogenesis imperfecta represent a new dominant mutation, and there is no family history. Death usually results from respiratory difficulties.

Type III osteogenesis imperfecta presents at birth or in infancy with progressive bony deformities, multiple fractures, and blue scleras. It is intermediate in severity between types II and IV; most affected individuals will require multiple corrective surgeries and lose the ability to ambulate by early adulthood. Unlike other forms of osteogenesis imperfecta, which are nearly always due to mutations that act dominantly, type III can be inherited in either a dominant or recessive fashion. From a biochemical and molecular perspective, type III osteogenesis imperfecta is the least well understood form.

Although different subtypes of osteogenesis imperfecta can often be distinguished biochemically, the classification presented in Table 2–3 is clinical rather than molecular, and the disease phenotypes for each subtype show a spectrum of severities that overlap one another. For example, a few individuals diagnosed with type II osteogenesis imperfecta based on the presence of severe bony deformities in utero will survive for many years and thus overlap the type III subtype. Similarly, some individuals with type IV osteogenesis imperfecta may have fractures in utero and develop deformities that lead to loss of ambulation. Distinguishing this presentation from type III osteogenesis imperfecta may only be possible if other affected family members exhibit a milder course.

This discussion illustrates that clinical classifications are, by their very nature, somewhat arbitrary. Nonetheless, this approach is helpful for most affected individuals in predicting the course and inheritance pattern of the illness and can serve also as a framework within which to correlate molecular abnormalities with disease phenotypes.

Pathophysiology

Osteogenesis imperfecta is a disease of type I collagen, which constitutes the major extracellular protein in the body. It is the major collagen in the dermis, the connective tissue capsules of most organs, and the vascular and gastrointestinal adventitia and is the only collagen in bone. A mature type I collagen fibril is a rigid structure that contains multiple type I collagen molecules packed in a staggered array and stabilized by intermolecular covalent cross-links. Each mature type I collagen molecule contains two α 1 chains and one α 2 chain, encoded by the COL1A1 and COL1A2 genes, respectively (Figure 2–3). These chains are synthesized as larger precursors with amino and carboxyl terminal "propeptide" extensions, assemble with each other inside the cell, and are ultimately secreted as a heterotrimeric type I procollagen molecule. During intracellular assembly, the three chains wind around each other in a triple helix which is stabilized by interchain interactions between hydroxyproline and adjacent carbonyl residues. There is a dynamic relationship between the posttranslational action of prolyl hydroxylase and assembly of the triple helix, which begins at the carboxyl terminal end of the molecule. Increased levels of hydroxylation result in a more stable helix, but helix formation prevents further prolyl hydroxylation. The nature of the triple helix causes the side chain of every third amino acid to point inward; and steric constraints allow only a proton in this position. Thus, the amino acid sequence of virtually all collagen chains in the triple helical portion is $(Gly\text{-}X\text{-}Y)_n$, where Y is proline about one-third of the time.

The fundamental defect in nearly all individuals with type I osteogenesis imperfecta is reduced synthesis of type I collagen due to loss-of-function mutations in COL1A1. Biochemical measurements of chain synthesis show that the mutant COL1A1 allele produces little or no detectable proα1(I) mRNA, corresponding to a hypomorphic or amorphic mutation, respectively. Because the nonmutant COL1A1 allele continues to produce mRNA at a normal rate (ie, there is no dosage compensation), an amorphic mutation results in a 50% reduction in the rate of proα1(I) mRNA synthesis, while a hypomorphic mutation results in a less severe reduction. Although three proα1(I) peptide chains can assemble into a stable trimer, molecules that contain one proα1(1) and two proα2(I) chains do not assemble. Thus, a reduced concentration of proα1(I) chains limits the production of type I procollagen, and the consequences of a hypomorphic or amorphic COL1A1 mutation are (1) a reduced amount of structurally normal type I collagen and (2) an excess of unassembled proα2(I) chains, which are degraded inside the cell (Figure 2–4).

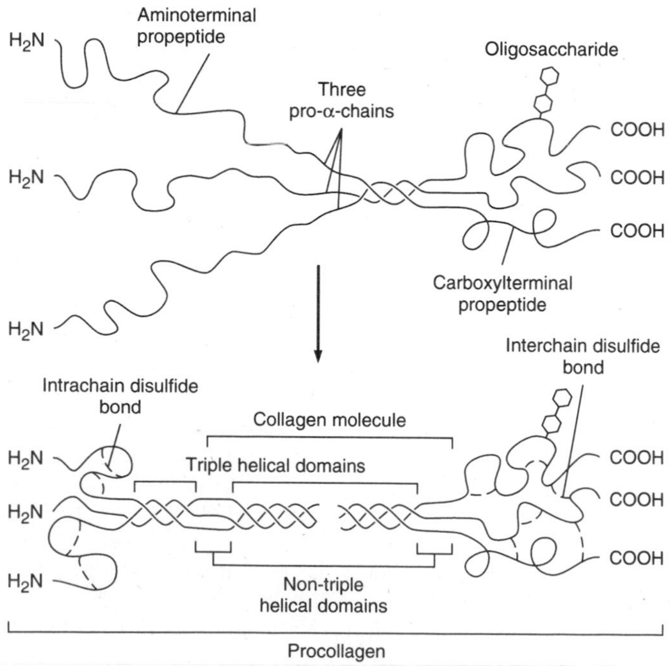

Figure 2–3. Molecular assembly of type I procollagen. Type I procollagen is assembled in the endoplasmic reticulum from three proalpha chains that associate with each other beginning at their carboxyl terminals. An important requirement for proper assembly of the triple helix is the presence of a glycine residue at every third position in each of the proalpha chains. After secretion, the amino and carboxyl terminal propeptides are proteolytically cleaved, leaving a rigid triple helical collagen molecule with very short non-triple helical domains at both ends. (Reproduced, with permission, from Alberts BA: *Molecular Biology of the Cell,* 3rd ed. Garland, 1994.)

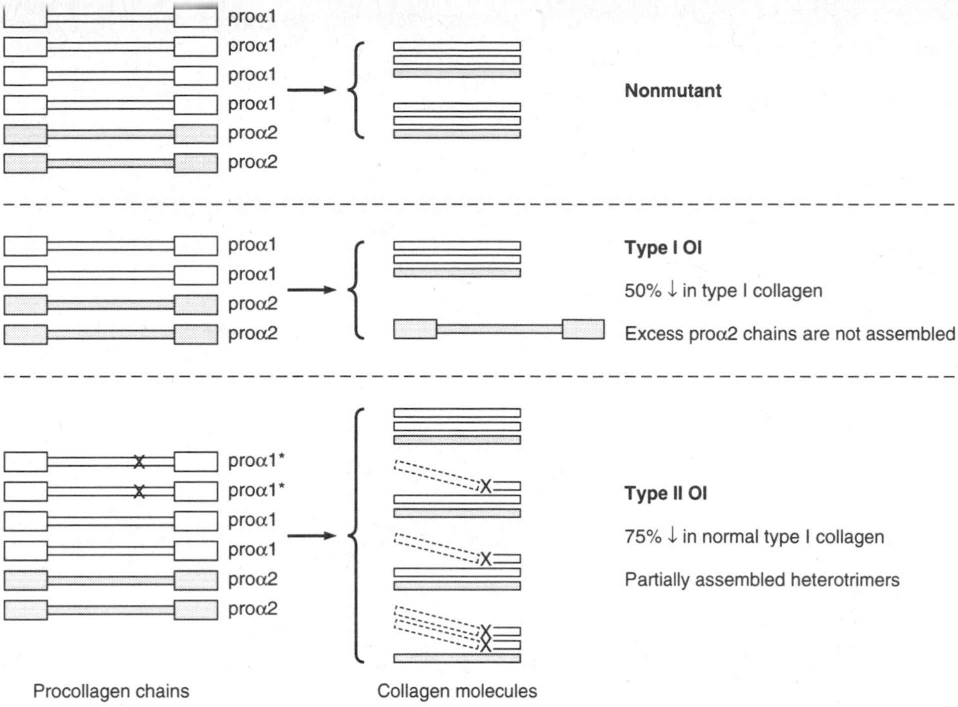

Figure 2–4. Molecular pathogenesis of type I and type II osteogenesis imperfecta (OI). The COL1A1 gene normally produces twice as many proα chains as the COL1A2 gene. Therefore, in nonmutant cells, the ratio of proα1 to proα2 chains is 2:1, which corresponds to the ratio of α1 and α2 chains in intact collagen molecules. In type I osteogenesis imperfecta, a mutation in one of the COL1A1 alleles results in failure to produce proα1 chains, leading to a 50% reduction in the total number of proα1 chains, a 50% reduction in the production of intact type I collagen molecules, and an excess of unassembled proα2 chains, which are degraded inside the cell. In type II osteogenesis imperfecta, a mutation in one of the COL1A1 alleles results in a structural alteration that blocks triple helix formation and secretion of partially assembled collagen molecules containing the mutant chain. (Adapted from Thompson MW et al: *Genetics in Medicine,* 5th ed. Saunders, 1991.)

The molecular defects responsible for COL1A1 mutations in type I osteogenesis imperfecta have not yet been identified. By analogy with other systems, possible lesions include alterations in a regulatory region leading to reduced transcription or splicing abnormalities leading to reduced steady state levels of RNA. A deletion of the entire COL1A1 gene would also cause an amorphic mutation, but this possibility has been ruled out in every case of type I osteogenesis imperfecta examined to date.

In contrast to type I osteogenesis imperfecta, type I collagen produced by patients with perinatal lethal (type II) osteogenesis imperfecta is structurally abnormal and can be caused by defects in both COL1A1 and COL1A2. Most of the actual mutations are simple DNA sequence alterations, but the effects on the peptide chain fall into two very different categories. Some type II osteogenesis imperfecta mutations affect the protein-coding sequence, in which case they usually result in an amino acid substitution at one of the conserved glycine residues within the triple helix (Figure 2–5). Other type II osteogenesis imperfecta mutations lie at intron-exon borders, in which case splicing abnormalities usually cause several internal exons to be excluded from the mature mRNA, leading to a severely shortened peptide chain.

An important principle apparent from biochemical studies of type II osteogenesis imperfecta is that in every case, the mutant peptide chain can bind to normal chains in the initial steps of trimer assembly (Figure 2–4). However, triple helix formation is ineffective, either because amino acids with large side chains are substituted for glycine or because alterations in the length of the mutant chain lead to abnormal interchain interactions. Ineffective triple helix formation leads to increased posttranslational modification by prolyl hydroxylase and a reduced rate of secretion. These appear to be critical events in the cellular pathogenesis of type II osteogenesis imperfecta, since glycine substitutions toward the carboxyl terminal end of the molecule are generally more severe than those at the amino terminus (Figure 2–4).

A second important principle apparent from these studies is that the effects of an amino acid substitution in a proα1(I) peptide chain are amplified at the

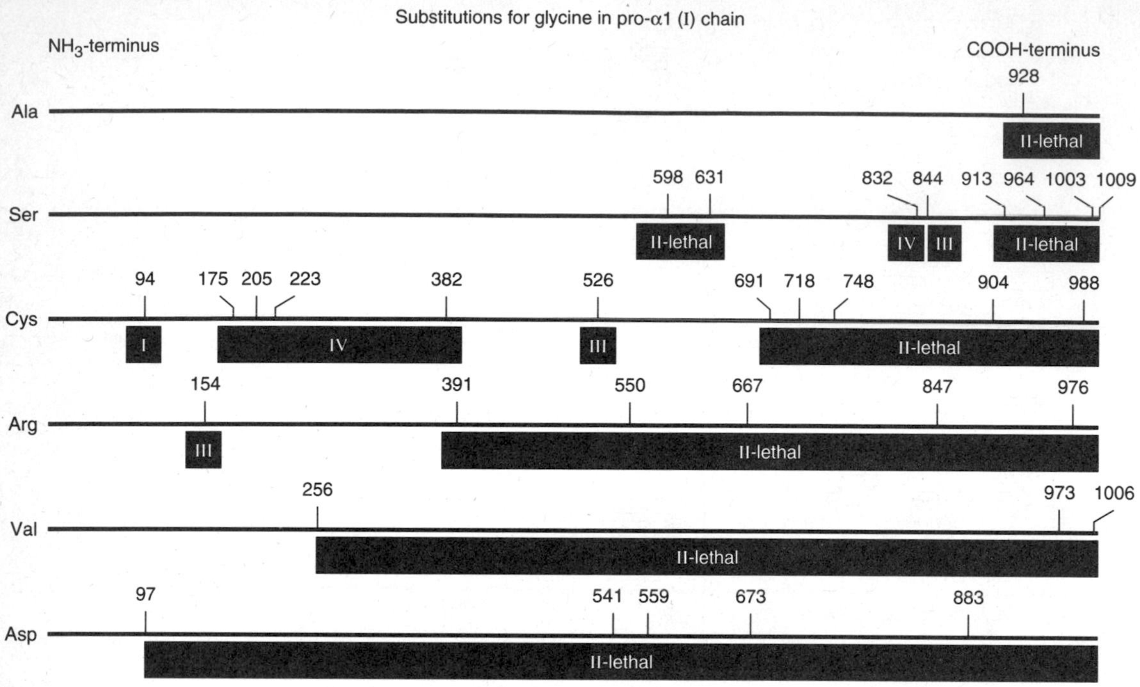

Figure 2–5. Genotype phenotype correlations for glycine substitutions in osteogenesis imperfecta. Many cases of osteogenesis imperfecta are caused by missense mutations in COL1A1 that result in substitutions of the glycine residue conserved at every third position in the triple helix. In general, substitutions of amino acids with bulky side chains like Asp and Arg are more severe than substitutions of amino acids with smaller side chains like Ser and Ala. Because assembly of the triple helix proceeds from the carboxyl terminal, the phenotypic effect of substitutions generally correlates with their distance from the amino terminal. (Reproduced, with permission, from Thompson MW et al: *Genetics in Medicine*, 5th ed. Saunders, 1991.)

levels of both triple helix assembly and fibril formation. Because every type I procollagen molecule has two proα1(I) chains, only 25% of type I procollagen molecules will contain two normal proα1(I) chains even though only one of the two COL1A1 alleles is mutated. Furthermore, because each molecule in a fibril interacts with several others, incorporation of an abnormal molecule can have disproportionate effects on fibril structure and integrity. Because this phenotype is similar to that predicted for a homozygous COL1A1 loss-of-function mutation, type II osteogenesis imperfecta provides a clinical example of "dominant negative'' gene action.

Collagen mutations that cause type III and type IV osteogenesis imperfecta are diverse and include glycine substitutions in the amino terminal portion of the collagen triple helix, a few internal deletions of COL1A1 and COL1A2 that do not significantly disturb triple helix formation, and some unusual alterations in the non-triple helical extensions at the amino and carboxyl terminals of proα chains.

Genetic Principles

Inheritance of type I and type IV osteogenesis imperfecta is autosomal dominant. However, the high frequency of new mutations (approximately 25%) and the multitude of molecular lesions that can produce a hypomorphic or an amorphic allele suggests that most families with type I osteogenesis imperfecta will have different molecular lesions in COL1A1. As a practical consequence of **allelic heterogeneity,** molecular diagnosis based on a particular DNA sequence abnormality is unfeasible, since both COL1A1 alleles would need to be sequenced in every individual at risk. Some attempts have been made to develop an efficient test for type I osteogenesis imperfecta based on measurements of COL1A1 mRNA levels. In some situations, a diagnostic approach based on linkage analysis is possible. For example, in a family in which type I osteogenesis imperfecta is known to segregate based on clinical and biochemical studies, it is usually possible to distinguish between chromosomes that carry the mutant and nonmutant alleles using closely linked DNA-based polymorphisms even though the actual COL1A1 molecular defect is not known. Once this information is established for a particular family, inheritance of the mutant allele can be predicted in future pregnancies. A similar approach is more difficult to apply for type IV osteogenesis imperfecta. In contrast to type I, in which nearly all cases are caused by defective COL1A1 alleles, mutations of both COL1A1 and COL1A2 can cause type IV osteogenesis imperfecta. As a consequence of this **genetic heterogeneity,** the type IV osteogenesis imperfecta phenotype could be linked to two different chromosomal locations.

For both type I and type IV osteogenesis imperfecta, often the most important question in the clinical setting relates to the natural history of the illness. For example, reproductive decision making in families at risk for osteogenesis imperfecta is influenced greatly by the relative likelihood of producing a child who will never ambulate and require multiple orthopedic operations versus a child whose major problems will be a few long bone fractures and an increased risk of hearing loss. As evident from the discussion above, both different mutant genes and different mutant alleles—as well as other genes that modify the osteogenesis imperfecta phenotype—can all contribute to this **phenotypic heterogeneity.** When allelic rather than genetic heterogeneity is operative, as in type I osteogenesis imperfecta, comparison of interfamilial to intrafamilial variability allows one to assess the relative contribution of different mutant alleles to phenotypic heterogeneity. For most genetic diseases, including type I osteogenesis imperfecta, intrafamilial variability is less than interfamilial variability, but in practical terms, a substantial uncertainty often remains.

In type II osteogenesis imperfecta, a single copy of the mutant allele causes the abnormal phenotype and therefore has a dominant mechanism of action. Although the type II phenotype itself is never inherited, there are rare situations in which a phenotypically normal individual will contain a COL1A1 mutant allele among their germ cells. These individuals with so-called **gonadal mosaicism** can produce multiple offspring with type II osteogenesis imperfecta (Figure 2–6), a pattern of segregation that can be confused with recessive inheritance. In fact, many other mutations, including Duchenne's muscular dystrophy, which is X-linked, and type 1 neurofibromatosis, which is autosomal dominant, also occasionally show unusual inheritance patterns explained by gonadal mosaicism.

4. When and how does type II osteogenesis imperfecta present? To what do these individuals succumb?
5. What are two typical radiologic findings in type II osteogenesis imperfecta?
6. Describe the pathophysiology of type II osteogenesis imperfecta and explain how it is an example of "dominant negative" gene action.

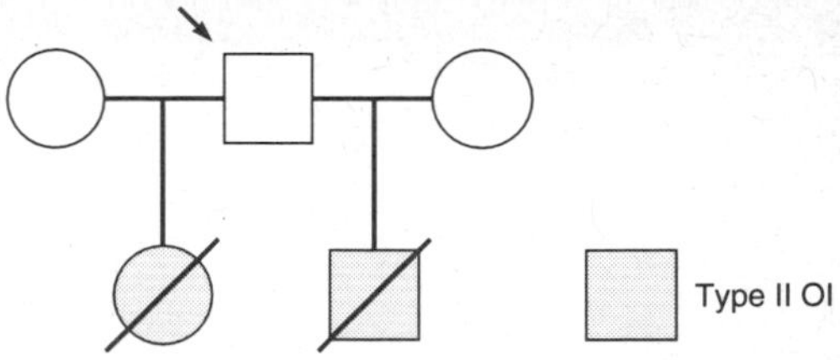

Figure 2–6. Gonadal mosaicism for type II osteogenesis imperfecta. In this idealized pedigree, the phenotypically normal father (indicated with the arrow) has had two children by different mates, each of whom is affected with autosomal dominant type II osteogenesis imperfecta. Analysis of the father showed that some of his spermatozoa carried a COL1A1 mutation, indicating that the explanation for this unusual pedigree is germline mosaicism. (Adapted from Cohn DH et al: Recurrence of lethal osteogenesis imperfecta due to parental mosaicism for a dominant mutation in a human type I collagen gene (COL1A1). Am J Hum Genet 1990; 46:591.)

FRAGILE X-ASSOCIATED MENTAL RETARDATION

Fragile X-associated mental retardation syndrome produces a unique combination of phenotypic features that affect the central nervous system, the testes, and the cranial skeleton. These features were recognized as a distinct clinical entity more than 50 years ago and have also been described as the Martin-Bell syndrome. A laboratory test for the syndrome was developed during the 1970s, when it was recognized that most affected individuals exhibit a cytogenetic abnormality of the X chromosome—failure of the region between bands Xq27 and Xq28 to condense at metaphase. Instead, this region appears in the microscope as a thin constriction that is subject to breakage during preparation, which accounts for the designation "fragile X." Advances in the past decade have helped to explain both the presence of the fragile site and the unique pattern of inheritance exhibited by the syndrome. In some respects, fragile X-associated mental retardation syndrome is similar to other genetic conditions caused by X-linked mutations—affected males are impaired more severely than affected females, and the condition is never transmitted from father to son. However, the syndrome "breaks the rules" of mendelian transmission in that at least 20% of carrier males manifest no signs of it. Daughters of these nonpenetrant but "transmitting males" are themselves nonpenetrant but produce affected offspring, male and female, with frequencies close to mendelian expectations (Figure 2–7). About a third of "carrier" females (those with one normal and one abnormal X chromosome) exhibit a significant degree of mental retardation. These unusual features of the syndrome were recently explained when the subchromosomal region spanning the fragile site was isolated and shown to contain a highly repetitive

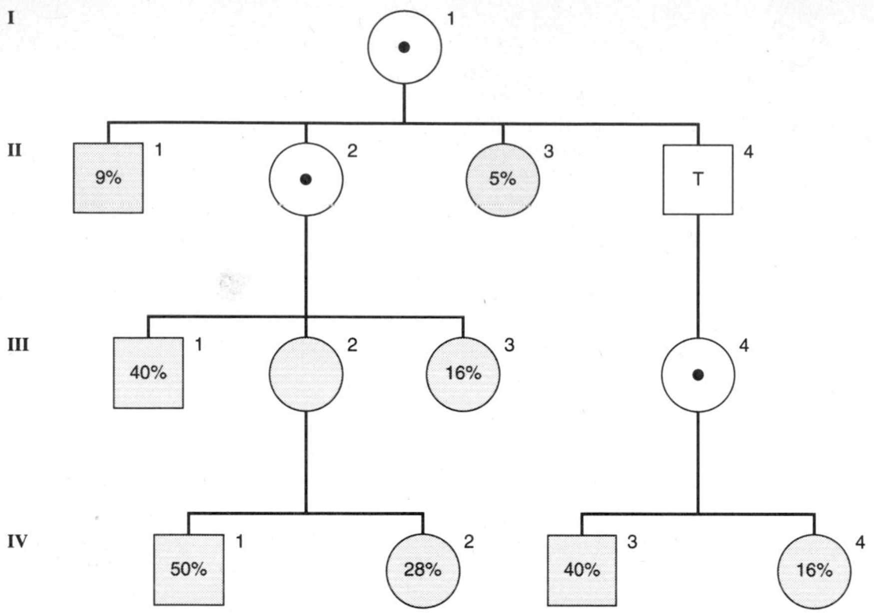

Figure 2–7. Penetrance of fragile X-associated mental retardation syndrome. This artificial pedigree of the syndrome shows the likelihood that each individual will manifest phenotypic features of the condition (penetrance). Penetrance increases with each successive generation owing to the progressive expansion of a triplet repeat element (see text). Expansion is dependent on maternal inheritance of the abnormal allele; thus, daughters of normal transmitting males (indicated with a T in II-4) are nonpenetrant. (Reproduced, with permission, from Scriver CR et al: *The Metabolic Basis of Inherited Disease,* 6th ed. McGraw-Hill, 1989.)

segment of DNA. Slight amplifications in the length of this DNA are not associated with a clinical phenotype or with the presence of a cytogenetic fragile site and therefore are described as a "premutation.'' After transmission through the female germline, this slightly lengthened segment nearly always exhibits additional amplification to a "full mutation,'' which results in the typical features of the syndrome (Figures 2–8 and 2–9).

Clinical Manifestations

Fragile X-associated mental retardation syndrome is usually recognized in affected boys because of developmental delay apparent by 1–2 years of age, small joint hyperextensibility, mild hypotonia, and a family history of mental retardation in maternally related males. Affected females generally have either mild mental retardation or only subtle impairments of visuospatial ability, and the condition may not be evident or diagnosed until it is suspected following identification of an affected male relative. In late childhood or early adolescence, affected males begin to exhibit large testes and characteristic facial features that include mild coarsening, large ears, a prominent forehead and mandible, a long face, and relative macrocephaly (considered in relation to height). The syndrome is extremely common and affects about 1:1500–1:1000 males. Virtually all affected males are born to females who are either affected or carry the premutation, and there are no well-recognized cases of new premutations in males or females.

The inheritance of fragile X-associated mental retardation syndrome is most easily described in terms of empiric risk figures for penetrance of the condition (Figure 2–9), which exhibits the following unusual features: (1) For the offspring of affected females, penetrance is 100% in sons and 56% in daughters; but for offspring of unaffected carrier females, penetrance is 80% in sons and 32% in daughters. Simply stated (and contrary to previously established genetic principles), the phenotype of an individual influences the likelihood of producing affected offspring. (2) About 20% of carrier males manifest no signs of the condition and instead are diagnosed as carriers only by retrospective pedigree analysis. Daughters of these "transmitting males'' are completely nonpenetrant, but maternal grandsons and granddaughters are 80% and 32% penetrant, respectively. This observation suggests that expression of the disease requires passage through the female germline. (3) Transmitting males tend to occur in the same sibship with each other and with nonpenetrant carrier females. This is reflected in low penetrance figures for brothers and sisters of transmitting males—18% and 10%, respectively—compared with 80% and

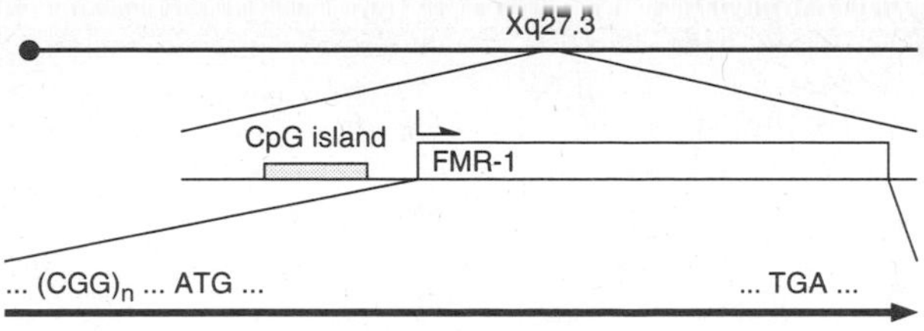

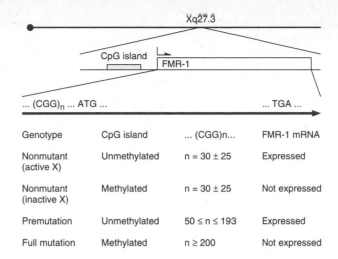

Genotype	CpG island	... (CGG)n...	FMR-1 mRNA
Nonmutant (active X)	Unmethylated	$n = 30 \pm 25$	Expressed
Nonmutant (inactive X)	Methylated	$n = 30 \pm 25$	Not expressed
Premutation	Unmethylated	$50 \le n \le 193$	Expressed
Full mutation	Methylated	$n \ge 200$	Not expressed

Figure 2–8. Molecular genetics of fragile X-associated mental retardation syndrome. The cytogenetic fragile site at Xq27.3 is located close to a small region of DNA that contains a CpG island (see text) and the *FMR-1* gene. Within the 5′ untranslated region of the *FMR-1* gene lies an unstable segment of repetitive DNA 5′-$(CGG)_n$-3′. The table shows the methylation status of the CpG island, the size of the triplet repeat, and whether the FMR-1 mRNA is expressed depending on the genotype of the X chromosome. Note that the inactive X chromosome in nonmutant females has a methylated CpG island and does not express the FMR-1 mRNA. The methylation and expression status of FMR-1 in premutation and full mutation alleles applies to males and to the active X chromosome of females; premutation and full mutation alleles on the inactive X chromosome of females will exhibit methylation of the CpG island and fail to express the FMR-1 mRNA.

32% for their maternal grandsons and granddaughters. This latter observation, which has been described as the "Sherman paradox," is sometimes referred to more generally as **genetic anticipation.**

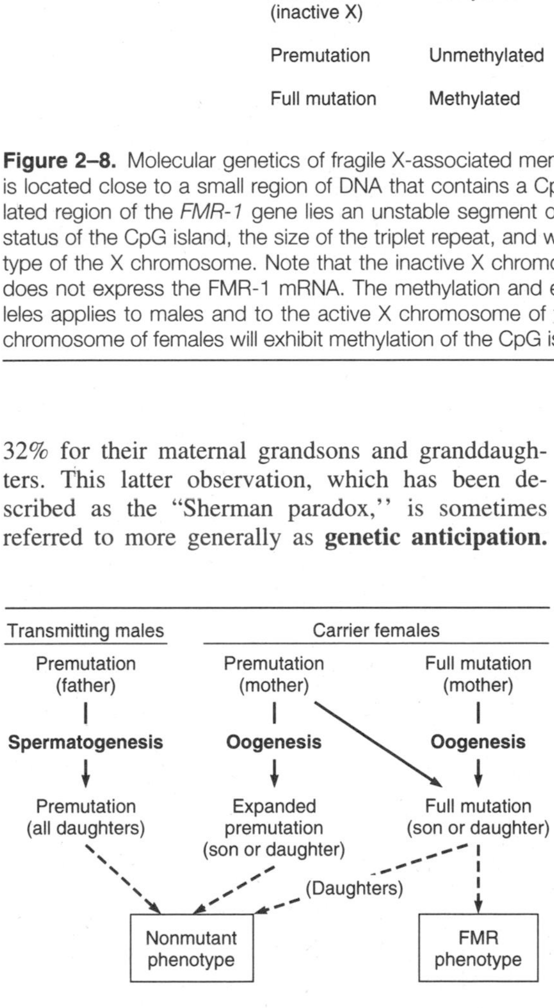

Figure 2–9. Transmission and amplification of the fragile X-associated mental retardation triplet repeat. The heavy arrows show expansion of the triplet repeat, which is thought to occur postzygotically after the premutation or full mutation is transmitted through the female germline. The dashed arrows represent potential phenotypic consequences. Daughters with the full mutation may or may not express the fragile X-associated mental retardation phenotype, depending on the proportion of cells in which the mutant allele happens to lie on the inactive X chromosome. (Adapted from Tarleton JC, Saul RA: Molecular genetic advances in fragile X syndrome. J Pediatr 1993; 122:169.)

One commonly cited explanation for genetic anticipation is **bias of ascertainment,** which occurs, for example, when a condition first diagnosed in grandchildren from a three-generation pedigree is then easily recognized in sibs or cousins of the grandchildren who are all available for examination and testing. However, recognition of the same condition in the grandparental generation is necessarily both historical and retrospective and can result in a greater *apparent* penetrance for the grandchild's than for the grandparent's generation. Although bias of ascertainment is an important feature of genetic epidemiology, it is now clear that amplification of unstable DNA accounts for genetic anticipation not only in this syndrome but also in the autosomally inherited condition myotonic dystrophy.

Pathophysiology

Amplification of the $(CGG)_n$ repeat at the fraXq27.3 site affects both methylation and expression of the *FMR-1* gene. The gene and the unstable DNA responsible for the syndrome were isolated on the basis of their physical proximity to the cytogenetic fragile site in Xq27.3. Beginning with the observation of large molecular clones that spanned the fragile site as determined by in situ hybridization and which had been closely linked to the syndrome in genetic analyses, attention was drawn to a small fragment of DNA, 5.2 kb in length, that contained a **CpG island** and exhibited several unusual features. CpG islands, which are several hundred base pairs in length and are recognized by a high frequency of 5′-CpG-3′ dinucleotides compared with the rest of the genome, are often located close to "housekeeping genes," those that code for essential intracellular functions in every cell in the body. In eukaryotes, methylation of cytosine to 5-methylcytosine occurs only when cytosine is followed by guanine, and for that reason CpG islands contain many potential sites for DNA methylation. Ironically, 5′-CpG-3′ sequences in CpG islands are usually unmethylated except when found in the context of a chromosomal region that is highly condensed and transcriptionally inactive. Such regions of so-called **heterochromatin** lie close to the centromeres on autosomes but encompass almost the entire region of the inactive X chromosome in female cells. Thus, the CpG island at Xq27.3 is normally unmethylated in male cells but methylated on one of the two X chromosomes in female cells.

A first clue to the molecular pathogenesis of fragile X-associated mental retardation syndrome came when it was discovered that the CpG island at Xq27.3 was methylated in affected males but unmethylated in nonpenetrant transmitting males. Furthermore, in affected females, the CpG island was methylated on both the active and the inactive X chromosome (Figure 2–8). Thus, for both the single X chromosome in males and for the active X chromosome in females, methylation of the CpG island correlates almost precisely with expression of the fragile X-associated mental retardation syndrome phenotype.

A second clue to the molecular basis of the syndrome was provided by the observation that the CpG island at Xq27.3 was located close to an unstable segment of DNA which contained the sequence (5′-CGG-3′)$_n$. This segment was highly variable in length; the number of repeats (n) is less than 50 in individuals who are neither affected with nor carriers for the syndrome. In transmitting males and in unaffected carrier females, the number of repeats may range from 52 to 193 and is usually between 70 and 100. Remarkably, alleles with less than 50 repeats are very stable and almost always transmitted without a change in repeat number. However, alleles with more than 52 repeats are unstable and often exhibit amplification after maternal transmission; thus, individuals with 52–193 repeats do not exhibit the fragile X-associated mental retardation syndrome phenotype but are said to carry a **premutation.** The degree of amplification is related to the number of repeats; premutation alleles with a repeat number less than 60 rarely are amplified to a full mutation, but premutation alleles with a repeat number greater than 90 are almost always amplified to a full mutation. The num-

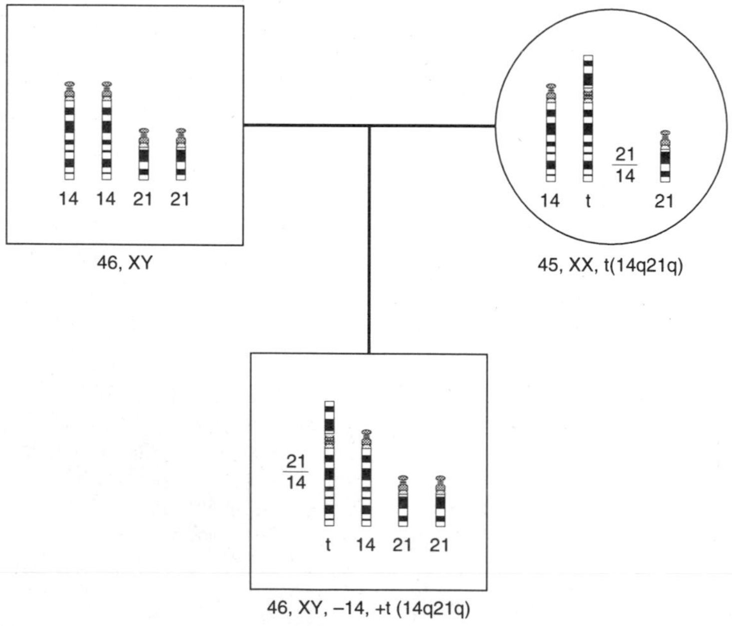

Figure 2–10. Mechanisms leading to Down's syndrome. A pedigree in which the mother is phenotypically normal yet is a balanced carrier for a 14;21 Robertsonian translocation. She transmits both the translocation chromosome and a normal chromosome 21 to her son, who also inherits a normal chromosome 21 from his father. Three copies of chromosome 21 in the son cause Down's syndrome. (Adapted from Thompson MW et al: *Genetics in Medicine*, 5th ed. Saunders, 1991.)

ber of repeats in the full mutation—observed both in affected males and in affected females—is always greater than 200 but is generally heterogeneous, suggesting that once this threshold is reached, additional amplification occurs frequently in somatic cells. For example, diagnostic testing for the cytogenetic fragile site and the number of CGG repeats is usually performed on approximately 10^7 lymphocytes taken from a small amount of peripheral blood. In individuals that carry a repeat number less than 50, each of the 10^7 cells has the same number of repeats. However, in phenotypically affected males or females, ie, those with a repeat number over 200, many of the 10^7 cells may have a different number of repeats, a circumstance described as **genetic mosaicism.** As with methylation of the CpG island, both cytogenetic expression of fraXq27.3 and the clinical fragile X-associated mental retardation syndrome phenotype correlate almost precisely with increases to a repeat number greater than 200.

The relationships of amplification and methylation to development of fragile X-associated mental retardation syndrome were integrated when it was discovered that the $(5'\text{-CGG-}3')_n$ segment of DNA lay within the 5′-untranslated region of a gene, named *FMR-1,* that encoded an RNA-binding protein, named FMR-1. The FMR-1 protein is normally expressed in brain and in testes, but amplification of the $(5'\text{-CGG-}3')_n$ segment to a repeat number greater than 200 leads to methylation of the CpG island and prevents the FMR-1 mRNA from being expressed. Amplification of the $(5'\text{-CGG-}3')_n$ segment and methylation of the CpG island at Xq23.7 may affect the expression of genes besides *FMR-1.* Recently, however, an individual affected with fragile X-associated mental retardation syndrome was discovered in which there was neither length amplification of the $(5'\text{-CGG-}3')_n$ segment, methylation, nor expression of the cytogenetic fragile site. However, in this patient, there was a de novo missense mutation in the FMR-1 protein coding sequence, which suggests that loss of FMR-1 function is sufficient to produce the fragile X-associated mental retardation syndrome phenotype.

The portion of the FMR-1 protein that binds RNA is similar to a group of proteins named hnRNPs, for *h*eterogeneous *n*uclear *RN*A-binding *p*roteins, that function in the processing or transport of nuclear mRNA precursors. It is possible that the FMR-1 protein fulfills a general role in the cellular metabolism of nuclear RNA, but only in the tissues in which it is primarily expressed, ie, the central nervous system and the testes. Although this would explain in part the unique combination of clinical features observed in fragile X-associated mental retardation syndrome, it is not yet clear whether proteins related to FMR-1 might subsume similar functions in other tissues, nor is it understood why absence of *FMR-1* expression leads to joint laxity and hyperextensibility.

Genetic Principles

In addition to the tendency of $(5'\text{-CGG-}3')_n$ premutation alleles to undergo further amplifications in length, the molecular genetics of fragile X-associated mental retardation syndrome exhibits several unusual features. As described above, each phenotypically affected individual carries a full mutation defined by a repeat number greater than 200, but the exact repeat number exhibits considerable heterogeneity in different cells and tissues. This **somatic mosaicism** in repeat number indicates that at least some of the amplification is **postzygotic,** meaning that it occurs in cells of the developing embryo after fertilization. Surprisingly, when the repeat number present in sperm DNA was examined in several affected individuals, only premutation alleles were found, even though each individual had a range of full mutation alleles present in their lymphocytes. Mature spermatozoa do not arise until after puberty, but their precursors—the **primordial germ cells**—are allocated early in development around the time of implantation and are segregated from other cells of the embryo. Thus, it is possible that expansion from a premutation to a full mutation is exclusively postzygotic and occurs only in parts of the embryo that do not give rise to primordial germ cells. In this case, the difference between individuals who carry premutation alleles and those who carry full mutation alleles would lie not in the number of repeats on the allele they inherit but in what happens to that allele after fertilization.

Analysis of pedigrees reveals that one of the most important determinants of whether a premutation allele is subject to postzygotic expansion is the sex of the parent who transmits the premutation allele (Figures 2–7 and 2–9). As discussed above, a premutation allele transmitted by a female expands to a full mutation with a likelihood proportionate to the length of the premutation; premutation alleles with a repeat number between 52 and 60 rarely expand to a full mutation, and those with a repeat number greater than 90 nearly always expand. In contrast, a premutation allele transmitted by a male rarely if ever expands to a full mutation regardless of the length of the repeat number. The concept that alleles of the same DNA sequence can behave very differently depending on the sex of the parent who transmitted them is described as **parental imprinting** and is thought to be caused by biochemical modifications (such as methylation) of the chromosome that occur during gametogenesis and do not affect the actual DNA sequence but which can be stably transmitted for a certain number of cell divisions. Parental imprinting is one example of a so-called **epigenetic** effect, which, defined broadly, is a phenotypic change not determined by the DNA sequence.

The high incidence of the fragile X-associated mental retardation syndrome—approximately 1:1000 males—is paradoxic given that affected individuals almost never reproduce. From the standpoint of population genetics, the relative probability—compared with the general population—of transmitting one's genes to the next generation is called **fitness.** For this syndrome, fitness is almost nil. Reduced fitness exhibited by many genetic conditions such as Duchenne's muscular dystrophy or type 1 neurofibromatosis is balanced by an appreciable **new mutation rate,** so that the incidence of the condition remains constant in successive generations. In fragile X-associated mental retardation syndrome, however, family studies have failed to identify any cases of a new premutation. For recessive conditions (both autosomal and X-linked), another factor that can influence disease incidence is whether heterozygous carriers experience a selective advantage or disadvantage compared with homozygous nonmutant individuals. For example, the relatively high incidence of sickle cell anemia in West Africa is thought to be due in part to **heterozygote advantage** conferring resistance to malaria, and it is possible that the high incidence of fragile X-associated mental retardation syndrome is due in part to a selective advantage of premutation carriers. A final alternative likely to contribute to the high incidence of the syndrome is the **founder effect,** ie, the high frequency of a premutation allele that occurs by chance in a population founded by a small number of ancestors. Evidence for a founder effect in the fragile X-associated mental retardation syndrome is based on the observation that rare molecular polymorphisms close to the gene are found in association with premutation alleles more frequently than expected by chance. This situation is described as **linkage disequilibrium** and is said to occur when the frequency of chromosomes that carry two distinct but genetically linked loci at the same time is significantly different from the product of their individual frequencies. Stated another way, fragile X-associated mental retardation syndrome and a closely linked locus A are in linkage disequilibrium if the frequency distribution of alleles at locus A is different in fragile X-associated mental retardation as compared to non-fragile X-associated mental retardation chromosomes.

7. How common is fragile X syndrome, and what is the phenotype of patients with fragile X syndrome?
8. What is Sherman's paradox, or genetic anticipation? What are two explanations for it?
9. What are the roles of parental imprinting and linkage disequilibrium in the molecular pathophysiology of fragile X syndrome?

DOWN'S SYNDROME

The clinical features of Down's syndrome were described over a century ago. Although the underlying cause—an extra copy of chromosome 21—has been known for more than 3 decades, the relationship of genotype to phenotype is just beginning to be understood, and many questions about the molecular pathophysiology of the condition have not yet been answered. Down's syndrome is broadly representative of **aneuploid** conditions, or those that are caused by a deviation from the normal chromosome complement **(euploidy).** Chromosome 21, which contains a little less than 2% of the total genome, is one of the **acrocentric** autosomes (the others are 13, 14, 15, and 22), which means one in which nearly all the DNA lies on one side of the centromere. In general, aneuploidy may involve part or all of an autosome or sex chromosome. Most individuals with Down's syndrome have 47 chromosomes (ie, one extra chromosome 21, or **trisomy 21**) and are born to parents with normal karyotypes. This type of aneuploidy is usually caused by **nondisjunction** during meiotic segregation, which means the failure of two homologous chromosomes to separate, or disjoin, from each other at anaphase. In contrast, aneuploid conditions that affect part of an autosome or sex chromosome must, at some point, involve DNA breakage and reunion. DNA rearrangements are an infrequent but important cause of Down's syndrome and are usually evident as a karyotype with 46 chromosomes in which one chromosome 21 is fused via its centromere to another acrocentric chromosome. This abnormal chromosome is described as a **Robertsonian translocation** and can sometimes be inherited from a carrier parent (Figure 2–10). Thus, Down's syndrome may be caused by a variety of different karyotypic abnormalities, which share in common a 50% increase in **gene dosage** for nearly all of the genes on chromosome 21.

Clinical Manifestations

Down's syndrome occurs approximately once in every 700 live births and accounts for approximately one-third of all cases of mental retardation. The likelihood of conceiving a child with Down's syndrome is related exponentially to increasing maternal age. However, screening programs detect most Down's syndrome pregnancies in pregnant women over 35 years of age (Figure 2–11). This fact, combined with the inverse relationship of maternal age to overall birth rate, means that most children with Down's syndrome are now born to women under 35 years of age. The condition is usually suspected in the perinatal period from the presence of characteristic facial and dysmorphic features such as brachycephaly, epicanthal folds, small ears, transverse palmar creases, and hypotonia (Table 2–4). Approximately 50% of

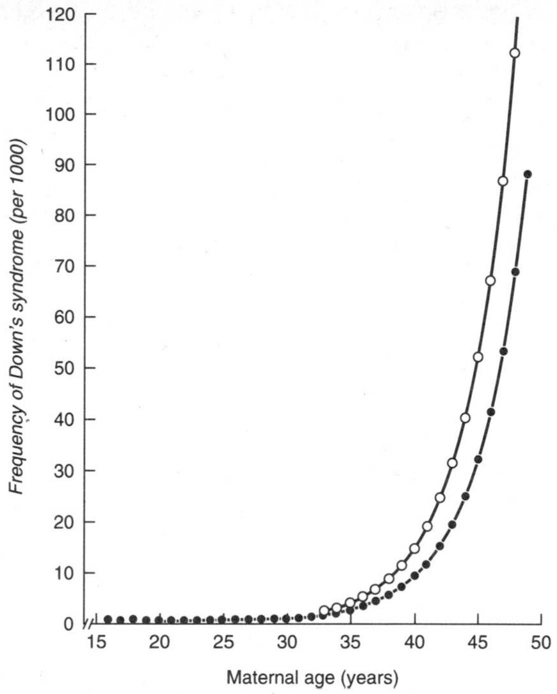

Figure 2–11. Relationship of Down's syndrome to maternal age. The frequency of Down's syndrome rises exponentially with increasing maternal age. The frequency at amniocentesis (open symbols) is slightly higher than at birth (closed symbols), because miscarriages are more likely in fetuses with Down's syndrome. Data from Scriver CR et al: *The Metabolic Basis of Inherited Disease,* 6th ed. McGraw-Hill, 1989.)

affected children have congenital heart defects that come to medical attention in the immediate perinatal period because of cardiorespiratory problems. Strong suspicion of the condition on clinical grounds is usually confirmed by karyotyping within 2–3 days.

Table 2–4. Phenotypic features of trisomy 21.

Feature	Frequency
Upslanting palpebral fissures	82%
Excess skin on back of neck	81%
Brachycephaly	75%
Hyperextensible joints	75%
Flat nasal bridge	68%
Wide gap between first and second toes	68%
Short, broad hands	64%
Epicanthal folds	59%
Short fifth finger	58%
Incurved fifth finger	57%
Brushfield spots (iris hypoplasia)	56%
Transverse palmar crease	53%
Folded or dysplastic ear	50%
Protruding tongue	47%

Data from Scriver CR et al: *The Metabolic Basis of Inherited Disease,* 6th ed. McGraw-Hill, 1989.

A great many minor and major abnormalities occur with increased frequency in Down's syndrome, yet two affected individuals rarely have the same set of abnormalities, and many single abnormalities can be seen in unaffected individuals. For example, the incidence of a transverse palmar crease in Down's syndrome is about 50%, tenfold higher than the general population, yet most individuals in which transverse palmar creases are the only unusual feature do not have Down's syndrome or any other genetic disease.

The natural history of Down's syndrome in childhood is characterized mainly by developmental delay, growth retardation, and immunodeficiency. Developmental delay is usually apparent by 3–6 months of life as a failure to attain age-appropriate developmental milestones and affects all aspects of motor and cognitive function. The mean IQ is between 30 and 70 and declines with increasing age. However, there is a considerable range in the degree of mental retardation in adults with Down's syndrome, and many affected individuals can live semi-independently. In general, cognitive skills are more limited than affective performance, and only a minority of affected individuals are severely impaired. Retardation of linear growth is moderate, and most adults with Down's syndrome have statures 2–3 SD below that of the general population. In contrast, weight growth in Down's syndrome exhibits a mild proportionate increase compared with that of the general population, and most adults with Down's syndrome are overweight for height. Although increased susceptibility to infections is a common clinical feature at all ages, the nature of the underlying abnormality is not well understood, and laboratory abnormalities can be detected in both humoral and cellular immunity.

One of the most prevalent and dramatic clinical features of Down's syndrome—premature onset of Alzheimer's disease—is not evident until adulthood. Although frank dementia is not clinically detectable in many adults with Down's syndrome, the incidence of typical neuropathologic changes—senile plaques and neurofibrillary tangles—is nearly 100% by age 35. The major causes of morbidity in Down's syndrome are congenital heart disease, infections, and leukemia. Life expectancy depends to a large extent on the presence of congenital heart disease; survival to ages 10 and 30 years is approximately 60% and 50%, respectively, for individuals with congenital heart disease and approximately 85% and 80%, respectively, for individuals without congenital heart disease.

Pathophysiology

The advent of molecular markers for different portions of chromosome 21 has provided much information about when and how the extra chromosomal material arises in Down's syndrome. In contrast, much less is known about why increased gene dosage for chromosome 21 should produce the clinical features of Down's syndrome.

For trisomy 21 (47,XX+21 or 47,XY+21), cytogenetic or molecular markers that distinguish between the maternal and paternal copies of chromosome 21 can be used to determine whether the egg or the sperm contributed the extra copy of chromosome 21. There are no obvious clinical differences between these two types of trisomy 21 individuals, which suggests that parental imprinting does not play a significant role in the pathogenesis of Down's syndrome. If both copies of chromosome 21 carried by each parent can be distinguished, it is usually possible to determine whether the nondisjunction event leading to an abnormal gamete occurred during anaphase of meiosis I or meiosis II (Figure 2–12). Studies such as these show that approximately 75% of cases of trisomy 21 are caused by an extra maternal chromosome; that approximately 75% of the nondisjunction events (both maternal and paternal) occur in meiosis I; and that both maternal and paternal nondisjunction events increase with advanced maternal age.

Several theories have been proposed to explain why the incidence of Down's syndrome increases with advanced maternal age (Figure 2–11). Most germ cell development in females is completed before birth; oocytes arrest at prophase of meiosis I (the **dictyotene** stage) during the second trimester of gestation. One proposal suggests that biochemical abnormalities that affect the ability of paired chromosomes to disjoin normally accumulate in these cells over time and that without a renewable source of fresh eggs, the proportion of eggs that undergo nondisjunction increases with maternal age. However, this hypothesis does not explain why the relationship between the incidence of trisomy 21 and advanced maternal age holds for *paternal* as well as maternal nondisjunction events.

Another hypothesis proposes that structural, hormonal, and immunologic changes that occur in the uterus with advanced age produce an environment less able to reject a developmentally abnormal embryo. Thus, an older uterus would be more likely to support a trisomy 21 conceptus to term regardless of which parent contributed the extra chromosome. This hypothesis can explain why paternal nondisjunction

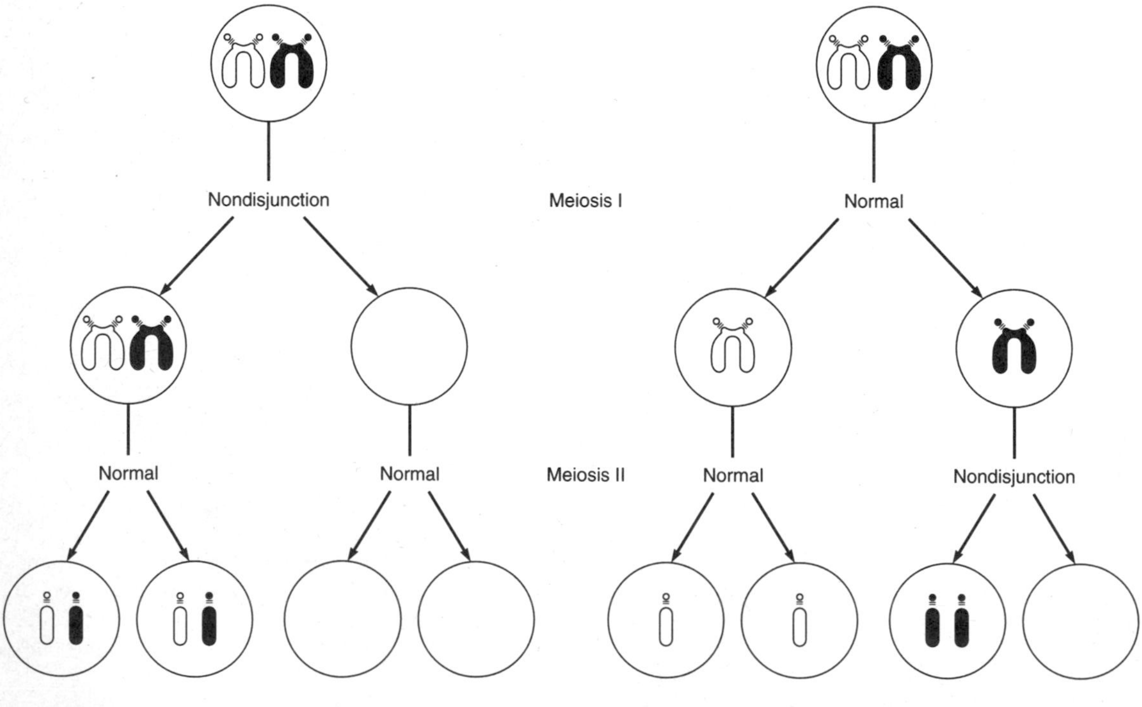

Figure 2–12. Nondisjunction has different consequences depending on whether it occurs at meiosis I or meiosis II. The abnormal gamete has two copies of a particular chromosome. When nondisjunction occurs at meiosis I, each of the copies originates from a different chromosome; but when nondisjunction occurs at meiosis II, each of the copies originates from the same chromosome. Both cytogenetic and molecular polymorphisms can be used to determine the stage and the parent in which nondisjunction occurred. (Reproduced, with permission, from Thompson MW et al: *Genetics in Medicine,* 5th ed. Saunders, 1991.)

Table 2–5. Risk for Down's syndrome depending on parental sex and karyotype.

Karyotype of Parent	Risk of Abnormal Liveborn Progeny	
	Female Carrier	Male Carrier
46,XX or 46,XY	0.5% (at age 20) to 30% (at age 30)	<0.5%
Rb(Dq;21q) (mostly 14)	10%	<2%
Rb(21q;22q)	14%	<2%
Rb(21q;21q)	100%	100%

Data from Scriver CR et al: *The Metabolic Basis of Inherited Disease,* 6th ed. McGraw-Hill, 1989.

errors increase with advanced maternal age. However, it does not explain why the incidence of Down's syndrome due to chromosomal rearrangements (see below) does not increase with maternal age.

These and other hypotheses are not mutually exclusive, and it is possible that a combination of factors is responsible for the relationship between the incidence of trisomy 21 and advanced maternal age. A number of environmental and genetic factors have been considered as possible causes for Down's syndrome, including exposure to caffeine, alcohol, tobacco, radiation, and the likelihood of carrying one or more genes that would predispose to nondisjunction. Although it is difficult to exclude all of these possibilities from consideration as minor factors, there is no evidence that any of these factors play a role in Down's syndrome.

The recurrence risk for trisomy 21 is not altered significantly by previous affected children. However, approximately 5% of Down's syndrome karyotypes are not trisomy 21 and instead are caused by Robertsonian translocations that usually involve chromosomes 14 or 22. As described above, this type of abnormality is not associated with increased maternal age; but in about 30% of such individuals, cytogenetic evaluation of the parents will reveal a so-called balanced rearrangement such as 45,XX or XY,+t(14q;21q). Because the Robertsonian translocation chromosome can pair with both of its component single acrocentric chromosomes at meiosis, the likelihood of segregation leading to unbalanced gametes is significant (Figure 2–13), and the recurrence risk to the parent with the abnormal karyotype is much higher than for trisomy 21. Approximately 1% of Down's syndrome karyotypes show mosaicism in which some cells are normal and some abnormal. Somatic mosaicism for trisomy 21 or other aneuploid conditions may initially arise either pre- or postzygotically, corresponding to nondisjunction in meiosis or mitosis, respectively. In the former case (one in which a zygote is conceived from an aneuploid gamete), the extra chromosome is then presumably lost mitotically in a clone of cells during early embryogenesis. The range of phenotypes seen in mosaic trisomy 21 is great, ranging from mild mental retardation with subtle dysmorphic features to "typical" Down's syndrome, and does not correlate with the proportion of abnormal cells detected in lymphocytes or fibroblasts. Nonetheless, on average, mental retardation in mosaic trisomy 21 is generally milder than in nonmosaic trisomy 21.

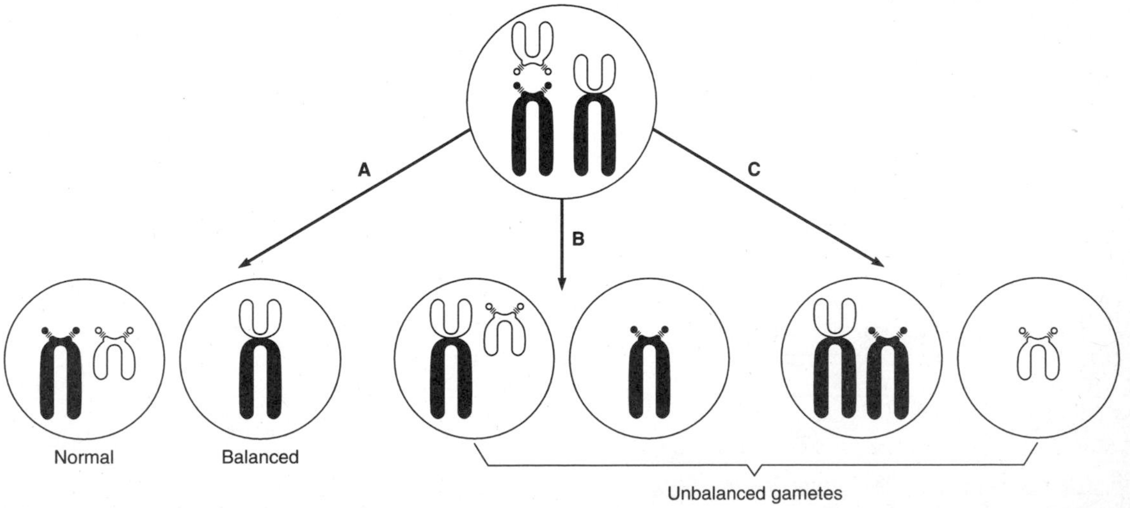

Figure 2–13. Types of gametes produced at meiosis by a carrier of a Robertsonian translocation. In a balanced carrier for a Robertsonian translocation, different types of segregation at meiosis lead to several different types of gametes, including ones that are completely normal (A), ones that would give rise to other balanced translocation carriers (B), and ones that would give rise to aneuploid progeny (C).

Genetic Principles

A fundamental question in understanding the relationship between an extra chromosome 21 and the clinical features of Down's syndrome is whether the phenotype is caused by abnormal gene expression or an abnormal chromosomal constitution. An important principle derived from studies directed at this question is that of **gene dosage,** which states that the amount of a gene product produced per cell is proportionate to the number of copies of that gene present. In other words, the amount of protein produced by all or nearly all genes that lie on chromosome 21 is 150% of normal in trisomy 21 cells and 50% of normal in monosomy 21 cells. Thus, unlike the X chromosome, there is no mechanism for dosage compensation that operates on autosomal genes.

Experimental evidence generally supports the view that the Down's syndrome phenotype is caused by increased expression of specific genes and not by a nonspecific detrimental effect of cellular aneuploidy. Rarely, karyotypic analysis of an individual with Down's syndrome reveals a chromosomal rearrangement (usually an unbalanced reciprocal translocation) in which only a very small portion of chromosome 21 is present in three copies per cell (Figure 2–14). These observations suggest that there may be a "critical region" of chromosome 21 which, when present in triplicate, is both sufficient and necessary to produce Down's syndrome. Genes that lie within or close to this critical region are candidates for contributing to the Down's syndrome phenotype and include the gene that encodes the amyloid protein found in senile plaques of Alzheimer's disease and the gene that encodes the cytoplasmic form of superoxide dismutase, which plays an important role in free radical metabolism.

The idea that altered gene dosage of a group of closely linked genes can produce a distinct clinical phenotype is also supported by the observation that several multiple congenital anomaly syndromes are due to small interstitial deletions of particular autosomes. These deletions, which often are detectable only with special cytogenetic or molecular techniques, result in monosomy for the genes located within the deleted segment. Such **contiguous gene syndromes,** described in Table 2–6, are generally rare, but they have played important roles in understanding the pathophysiology of aneuploid conditions.

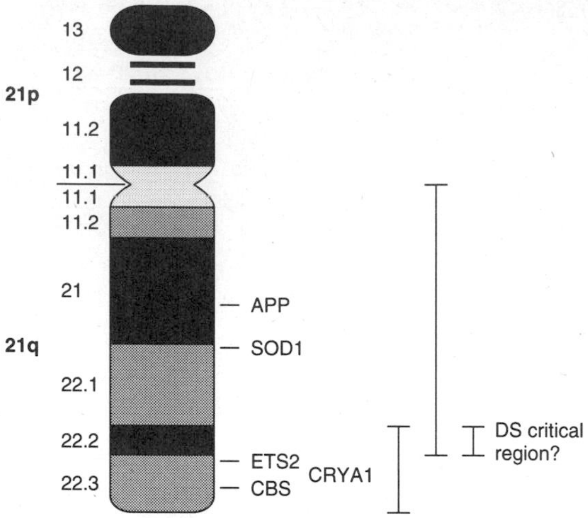

Figure 2–14. Down's syndrome critical region. Rarely, individuals with Down's syndrome will have chromosomal rearrangements that cause trisomy for just a portion of chromosome 21. Analysis of two sets of individuals (indicated by the two vertical lines) suggests that the genes responsible for Down's syndrome lie in the region of overlap. (Reproduced, with permission, from Thompson MW et al: *Genetics in Medicine*, 5th ed. Saunders, 1991.)

Carriers for Robertsonian translocations that involve chromosome 21 can produce several different types of unbalanced gametes (Figure 2–13). However, the empiric risk for such a carrier bearing an infant with Down's syndrome is higher than for other aneuploid conditions, in part because embryos with other types of aneuploidies are likely to result in miscarriages early in development. Thus, the consequences of trisomy for embryonic and fetal development are proportionate to the number of genes expressed to 150% of their normal levels. Because monosomy for chromosome 21 (and other auto-

Table 2–6. Phenotype and karyotype (deletion) of some contiguous gene syndromes.

Disorder	Phenotype	Deletion
Langer-Gideon	Mental retardation, microcephaly, bony exostoses, redundant skin	8q24.11 to q24.3
WAGR	Wilms' tumor, aniridia, gonadoblastoma, mental retardation	11p13
Prader-Willi	Mental and growth retardation, hypotonia, obesity, hypopigmentation	15q11 to q13
Angelman	Mental and growth retardation, seizures, hypertonia; paroxysmal laughter	15q11 to q13
Rubenstein-Taybi	Mental retardation, dysmorphic facial features, broad thumbs and first toes	16p13.3
Miller-Dieker	Severe mental retardation, absence of cortical gyri (lissencephaly) and corpus callosum	17p13.3
DiGeorge	Parathyroid and thymic hypoplasia, congenital heart disease	22q11

somes) is virtually never seen in liveborn infants, a similar line of reasoning suggests that a 50% reduction in gene expression is more severe than a 50% increase. Finally, female Robertsonian translocation carriers exhibit much higher empiric recurrence risks than male carriers, which suggests (1) that selective responses against aneuploidy can operate on gametic as well as somatic cells, and (2) that spermatogenesis is more sensitive to aneuploidy than oogenesis.

10. What are the common features of the variety of different karyotypic abnormalities resulting in Down's syndrome?
11. What are the major categories of abnormalities in Down's syndrome, and what is their natural history?
12. Explain why trisomy 21 is associated with such a wide range of phenotypes from mild mental retardation to that of "typical" Down's syndrome?

PHENYLKETONURIA

Phenylketonuria presents one of the most dramatic examples of how the relationship between genotype and phenotype can depend on environmental variables. Phenylketonuria was first recognized as an inherited cause of mental retardation in 1934, and systematic attempts to treat the condition were initiated in the 1950s. Treatment outcomes have been hailed, perhaps prematurely, as the pinnacle of success in applying biochemistry and molecular biology to societal problems that stem from inherited disease. The term "phenylketonuria'' denotes elevated levels of urinary phenylpyruvate and phenylacetate, which occur when circulating phenylalanine levels, normally between 0.06 and 0.1 mmol/L, rise above 1.2 mmol/L. Thus, the primary defect in phenylketonuria is **hyperphenylalaninemia,** which itself has a number of distinct genetic causes.

The pathophysiology of phenylketonuria also illustrates a number of important principles in human genetics, including the rationale for and application of population-based newborn screening programs for inherited disease. More than 10 million newborn infants per year are tested for phenylketonuria, and the focus today in treatment has shifted in several respects. First, "successful'' treatment of phenylketonuria by dietary restriction of phenylalanine is, in general, accompanied by subtle neuropsychologic defects that have been recognized only in the last decade. Thus, current investigations focus on alternative treatment strategies such as somatic gene therapy as well as on the social and psychologic factors that affect compliance with dietary management. Second, a generation of females treated for phenylketonuria are now bearing children, and the phenomenon of **maternal phenylketonuria** has been recognized, in which in utero exposure to maternal hyperphenylalaninemia results in congenital abnormalities regardless of fetal genotype. The number of pregnancies at risk has risen in proportion to the successful treatment of phenylketonuria and represents a challenge to public health officials, physicians, and geneticists in the next decade.

Clinical Manifestations

The incidence of hyperphenylalaninemia varies among different populations. In American blacks it is about 1:50,000; in Yemenite Jews, about 1:5,000; and in most Northern European populations, about 1:10,000. Postnatal growth retardation, moderate to severe mental retardation, recurrent seizures, hypopigmentation, and eczematous skin rashes constitute the major phenotypic features of untreated phenylketonuria. However, with the advent of widespread newborn screening programs for hyperphenylalaninemia, the major phenotypic manifestations of phenylketonuria today occur when treatment is partial or terminated prematurely during late childhood or adolescence. In these cases, there is usually a slight but significant decline in IQ, an array of specific performance and perceptual defects, and an increased frequency of learning and behavioral problems.

Newborn screening for phenylketonuria is performed on a small amount of dried blood obtained at 24–72 hours of age. Most screening programs are administered by state or regional governments, and the actual measurements of phenylalanine levels are performed at one or a few central laboratories. From the initial screen, there is about a 1% incidence of positive or indeterminate test results, and a more quantitative measurement of plasma phenylalanine is then performed before 2 weeks of age. In neonates who undergo a second round of testing, the diagnosis of phenylketonuria is ultimately confirmed in about 1%, providing an estimated phenylketonuria prevalence of 1:10,000, although there is great geographic and ethnic variation (see below). The false-negative rate of phenylketonuria newborn screening programs is approximately 1:70; these unfortunate individuals are usually not detected until developmental delay and seizures during infancy or early childhood prompt a systematic evaluation for an inborn error of metabolism.

Infants in whom a diagnosis of phenylketonuria is confirmed are usually placed on a dietary regimen in which a semisynthetic formula low in phenylalanine can be combined with regular breast feeding. This regimen is adjusted empirically to maintain a plasma phenylalanine concentration at or below 1 mmol/L, which is still several times greater than normal but similar to levels observed in so-called **benign hyperphenylalaninemia** (see below), a biochemical diagnosis which is not associated with phenylketonuria and has no clinical consequences. Phenylalanine is an essential amino acid, and even individuals with phenylketonuria must consume small amounts to avoid protein starvation and a catabolic state. Most children require 25–50 mg/kg/d of phenylalanine, and these requirements are met by combining natural foods with commercial products designed for phenylketonuria treatment. When dietary treatment programs were first implemented, it was hoped that the risk of neurologic damage due to the hyperphenylalaninemia of phenylketonuria would have a limited window and that treatment could be stopped after childhood. However, it now appears that even hyperphenylalaninemia greater than 1.2 mmol/L in adults is associated with neuropsychologic and cognitive deficits; therefore, dietary treatment of phenylketonuria should probably be continued indefinitely.

As an increasing number of treated phenylketonuria women reach childbearing age, a new problem—fetal hyperphenylalaninemia via intrauterine exposure—has become apparent. Newborn infants affected with maternal phenylketonuria exhibit microcephaly and growth retardation of prenatal onset, congenital heart disease, and severe developmental delay regardless of the fetal genotype. Rigorous control of maternal phenylalanine concentrations from before conception until birth reduces the incidence of fetal abnormalities in maternal phenylketonuria, but the level of plasma phenylalanine that is "safe" for a developing fetus is 0.12–0.36 mmol/L, significantly lower than what is considered acceptable for phenylketonuria-affected children or adults on phenylalanine-restricted diets.

Pathophysiology

The normal metabolic fates of free phenylalanine are incorporation into protein or hydroxylation by phenylalanine hydroxylase to form tyrosine (Figure 2–15). Because tyrosine but not phenylalanine can be metabolized to produce fumarate and acetoacetate, hydroxylation of phenylalanine can be viewed both as a means of making tyrosine a nonessential amino acid and as a mechanism for providing energy via gluconeogenesis during states of protein starvation. This may help explain why the tissue distribution of phenylalanine hydroxylase is restricted primarily to the human liver. Transamination of phenylalanine to form phenylpyruvate normally does not occur unless circulating concentrations exceed 1.2 mmol/L, but the pathogenesis of central nervous system abnormalities in phenylketonuria is related more to phenyalanine itself than to its metabolites. Besides a direct effect of elevated phenylalanine levels on energy production, protein synthesis, and neurotransmitter homeostasis in the developing brain, phenylalanine can also inhibit the transport of neutral amino acids across the blood-brain barrier, leading to a selective amino acid deficiency in the cerebrospinal fluid. Thus, the neurologic manifestations of phenylketonuria are felt to be due to a general effect on central nervous system metabolism. The pathophysiology of the eczema seen in untreated or partially treated phenylketonuria is not well understood, but eczema is a common feature of other inborn errors of metabolism in which plasma concentrations of branched-chain amino acids are elevated. Hypopigmentation in phenylketonuria is probably caused by an inhibitory effect of excess phenylalanine on the production of dopaquinone in melanocytes, which is the rate-limiting step in melanin synthesis.

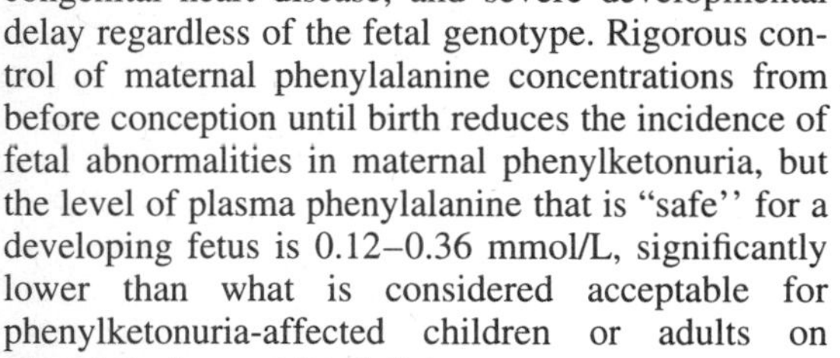

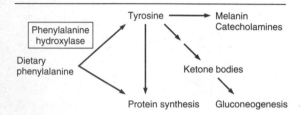

Figure 2–15. Metabolic fates of phenylalanine. Because catabolism of phenylalanine must proceed via tyrosine, the absence of phenylalanine hydroxylase leads to accumulation of phenylalanine. Tyrosine is also a biosynthetic precursor for melanin and certain neurotransmitters, and the absence of phenylalanine hydroxylase causes tyrosine to become an essential amino acid.

Approximately 90% of infants with persistent hyperphenylalaninemia detected by newborn screening have typical phenylketonuria caused by a defect in phenylalanine hydroxylase (see below). Of the remainder, most have benign hyperphenylalaninemia, in which circulating levels of phenylalanine are between 0.1 and 1 mmol/L. However, approximately 1% of infants with persistent hyperphenylalaninemia have defects in the metabolism of tetrahydrobiopterin (BH_4), which is a stoichiometric cofactor for the hydroxylation reaction (Figure 2–16). Because hydroxylation of tyrosine and tryptophan also require BH_4 as a cofactor, defects in its metabolism lead not only to phenylketonuria but also to deficiencies of catecholaminergic and serotonergic neurotransmitters that in early childhood result in a severe neurologic disorder manifested by hypotonia, inactivity, and developmental regression. Infants affected with defects in BH_4 metabolism are treated not only with dietary restriction of phenylalanine but also dietary supplementation with BH_4, dopa, and 5-hydroxytryptophan.

Shortly after the gene for phenylalanine hydroxylase was isolated in 1982, many polymorphic restriction sites at or close to the gene were identified that did not by themselves affect phenylalanine hydroxylase expression or structure. However, analysis of these RFLPs in pedigrees and in populations indicated that phenylketonuria was associated with a limited number of **haplotypes,** or certain groups of

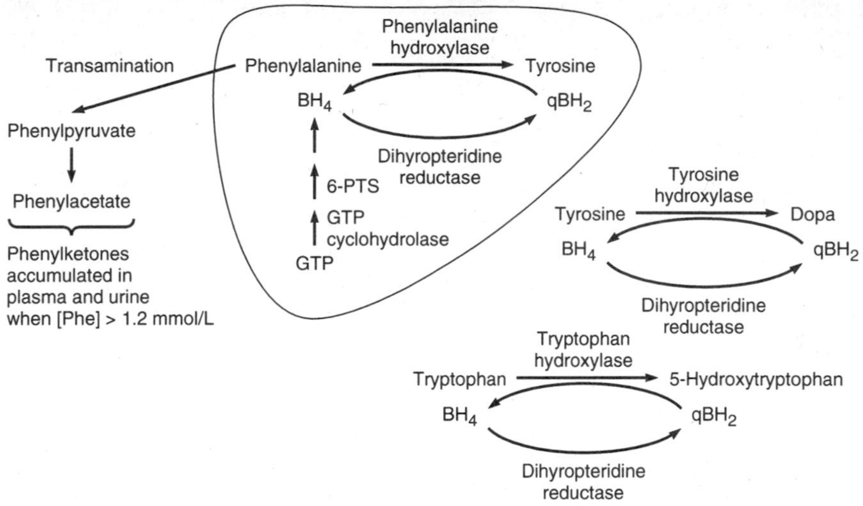

Figure 2–16. Normal and abnormal phenylalanine metabolism. Tetrahydrobiopterin (BH_4) is a cofactor for phenylalanine hydroxylase, tyrosine hydroxylase, and tryptophan hydroxylase. Consequently, defects in the biosynthesis of BH_4 or its metabolism result in a failure of all three hydroxylation reactions. The absence of phenylalanine hydroxylation has phenotypic effects due to substrate accumulation, but the absence of tyrosine or tryptophan hydroxylation has phenotypic effects due to end-product deficiency. (6-PTS, 6-Pyruvoyltetrahydrobiopterin synthetase.)

RFLPs held in linkage disequilibrium with each other. For example, the initial analysis of Danish families demonstrated 12 different RFLP haplotypes (of 1152 theoretically possible), of which four were associated with phenylalanine hydroxylase mutations (Figure 2–17; Table 2–7). The distribution of these four haplotypes among phenylalanine hydroxylase mutant chromosomes was significantly different compared with nonmutant chromosomes (Table 2–7). Comparison of haplotype data with hyperphenylalaninemia phenotypes suggested that allelic heterogeneity accounted for benign hyperphenylalaninemia as well as for phenylketonuria. For example, haplotype 1 in homozygous form or as a heterozygous compound with other haplotypes is usually associated with benign hyperphenylalaninemia or mild phenylketonuria, but haplotypes 2 or 3 in homozygous form are associated with severe phenylketonuria (Table 2–8). Measurements of phenylalanine hydroxylase activity in liver biopsy specimens correlate with these findings and demonstrate that individuals with phenylketonuria have levels of enzyme activity less than 1% of normal, while those with benign hyperphenylalaninemia generally have activity levels that are 5–30% of normal.

Most of the phenylalanine hydroxylase mutations affect the protein-coding sequence by a missense mechanism, including the one associated with benign hyperphenylalaninemia and haplotype 1, an Arg to Gln change at residue 261 (Table 2–8). A notable ex-

Haplotype	*Bgl*II	*Eco*RI	*Msp*I	*Eco*RV	Frequency
1	–	–	+	–	35
2	–	–	+	+	5
3	–	+	–	–	3
4	–	+	–	+	32
5	+	+	+	+	11
6	+	+	+	–	< 1
7	+	+	–	–	11
8	–	+	+	+	2
% – of total	**77**	**40**	**46**	**49**	
% + of total	**22**	**59**	**53**	**50**	

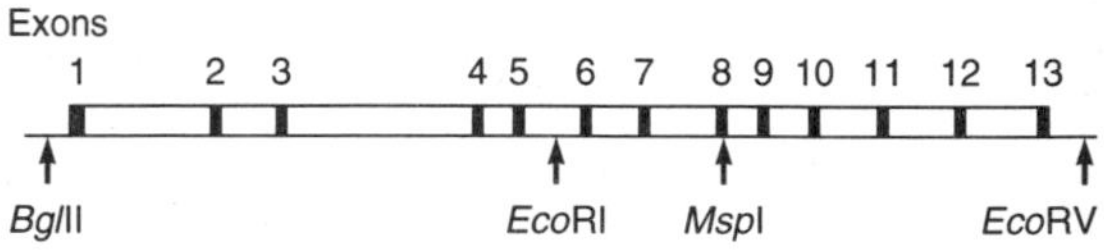

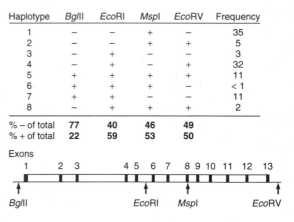

Figure 2–17. Linkage disequilibrium for phenylalanine hydroxylase haplotypes. Different haplotypes are defined by a particular combination of RFLPs whose locations are indicated relative to exons within the phenylalanine hydroxylase gene. For example, haplotype 1 is an allele that contains an *Msp*I site but not a *Bgl*II, *Eco*RI, or *Eco*RV site at the locations indicated. Shown are 8 of 12 haplotypes described initially in a large analysis of Danish families. Linkage disequilibrium is said to occur when the frequency of each haplotype differs from that predicted by the frequency of individual RFLPs. For example, 59% or 53% of all chromosomes contain *Eco*RI or *Msp*I sites, respectively. The predicted frequency of all chromosomes that contain both sites at the same time is 31% (0.59 × 0.53), which differs substantially from the observed frequency of 14%. (Adapted from Scriver et al: *The Metabolic Basis of Inherited Disease,* 6th ed. McGraw-Hill, 1989.)

Table 2–7. Linkage disequilibrium for phenylketonuria.

Haplotype	Frequency on Nonmutant Chromosomes	Frequency on Phenylketonuria Chromosomes	Molecular Basis of Phenylalanine Hydroxylase Mutation
1	35%	18%	R261Q
2	5%	20%	R408W
3	3%	38%	G→A(IVS12)
4	32%	14%	R158Q

Adapted from Thompson MW et al: *Genetics in Medicine,* 5th ed. Saunders, 1991.

Table 2–8. Phenylalanine hydroxylase (PAH) activity (%) and phenylketonuria (PKU) phenotypes for different combinations of PAH alleles.

Haplotype (Mutation)	3 (IVS12)	2 (R408W)	4 (R158Q)	1 (R261Q)
3(IVS12)	0% Classic PKU	0% Classic PKU	5% Classic PKU	15% Intermediate or mild
2(R408W)		0% Classic PKU	5% Classic PKU	15% Intermediate or mild
4(R158Q)			10% Classic PKU	20% Mild PKU
1(R261Q)				30% Benign hyperphenylalaninemia

Adapted from Okano Y et al: Molecular basis of phenotypic heterogeneity in phenylketonuria. N Engl J Med 1991; 324:1232.

ception, however, is a point mutation in the noncoding splice donor sequence immediately following exon 12 (Figure 2–18). This mutation, which was the first to be identified at a molecular level, causes exon 12 to be "skipped" from the mature mRNA and leads to production of a truncated protein associated with severe phenylketonuria.

For the 1% of infants affected with phenylketonuria in which the underlying defect is not in phenylalanine hydroxylase but in metabolism of BH_4, at least three different genetic defects have been identified. All of these are inherited in an autosomal recessive fashion and can be distinguished from each other and from phenylalanine hydroxylase deficiency by direct analysis of enzyme activity in liver biopsy samples.

Genetic Principles

Because the fitness of individuals affected with phenylketonuria has until recently been very low, the relatively high incidence of the condition could only be explained by a high mutation rate, founder effects, heterozygote advantage, or a combination of these mechanisms. New mutations of phenylketonuria are exceedingly rare, but population genetic studies provide evidence for both a founder effect and heterozygote advantage. As in the case of fragile X-associated mental retardation syndrome, linkage disequilibrium between phenylalanine hydroxylase mutations and closely linked RFLPs supports a founder effect. However, the presence of multiple phenylalanine hydroxylase mutations at relatively high frequencies and the variation in phenylketonuria prevalence between different populations suggests that reduced levels of phenylalanine hydroxylase activity in heterozygotes may have provided a selective advantage under certain environmental or geographic conditions.

The effect of dietary phenylalanine on the phenylketonuria phenotype illustrates how manipulation of an environmental variable can alter expressivity of a particular genotype. Factors that influence the expressivity of phenylalanine hydroxylase deficiency have been relevant not only to the treatment of

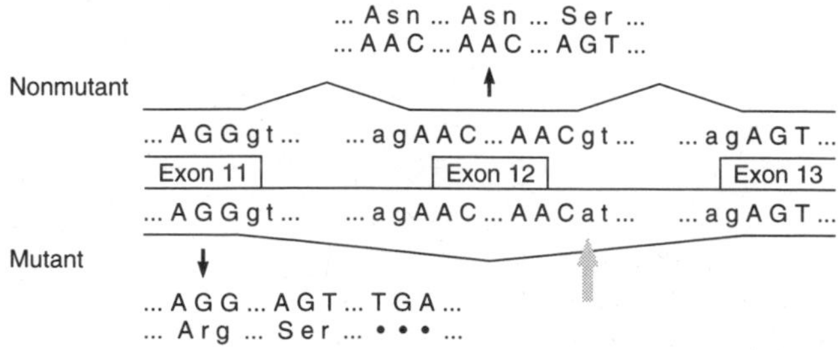

Figure 2–18. A phenylalanine hydroxylase splice donor mutation causes exon skipping in a common phenylketonuria allele. A **g** to **a** mutation in the intron sequences following exon 12 (large hatched arrow) causes the preceding exon 12 to be skipped during processing of the nuclear RNA and results in production of a truncated protein with no phenylalanine hydroxylase activity. (Adapted from Scriver CR et al: *The Metabolic Basis of Inherited Disease,* 6th ed. McGraw-Hill, 1989.)

phenylketonuria but also to public health, since aspartame, a widely used artificial sweetening agent that becomes hydrolyzed to phenylalanine and aspartic acid, can affect phenylalanine concentrations in phenylketonuria heterozygotes. Although phenylketonuria heterozygotes who consume large amounts of aspartame are not at risk of developing phenylketonuria, these considerations underscore the importance of genotypic diversity in the population when evaluating the effects of pharmaceutical, cosmetic, or dietary agents.

The different genetic forms of phenylketonuria illustrate two important pathophysiologic mechanisms by which inborn errors of metabolism can cause disease: **end-product deficiency** and **substrate accumulation.** The mental retardation in phenylalanine hydroxylase deficiency is caused not by deficiency of tyrosine or its metabolites but instead by accumulation of the substrate for phenylalanine hydroxylase. In contrast, the progressive hypotonia and developmental regression seen in disorders of BH_4 metabolism are caused by a decrease in the metabolic products of tryptophan hydroxylase and tyrosine hydroxylase.

Finally, a thorough understanding of the pathophysiology of phenylketonuria is a prerequisite for the development of gene therapy. For example, since most phenylalanine hydroxylation occurs in the liver, attempts to deliver a normal phenylalanine hydroxylase gene to affected individuals have focused on strategies to express the gene in hepatocytes. However, since individuals with benign hyperphenylalaninemia have phenylalanine hydroxylase activities that may be as low as 5% of normal, successful gene therapy of phenylketonuria might be accomplished by expressing phenylalanine hydroxylase in only a small proportion of hepatic cells.

13. What is the primary defect in phenylketonuria?
14. Why is dietary modification a less than satisfactory treatment of this condition? What might be a better therapeutic approach and why?
15. What is the false-negative rate for neonatal screening, and how do these individuals come to medical attention?
16. Explain the phenomenon of "maternal phenylketonuria."

REFERENCES

General

Caskey CT et al: Triplet repeat mutations in human disease. Science 1992;256:784.

Scriver C et al: *The Metabolic Basis of Inherited Disease,* 6th ed. McGraw-Hill, 1989.

Osteogenesis Imperfecta

Byers PH: Brittle bones—fragile molecules: Disorders of collagen gene structure and expression. Trends Genet 1990 6:293.

Byers PH, Steiner RD: Osteogenesis imperfecta. Annu Rev Med 1992:43:269.

Cohn DH et al: Recurrence of lethal osteogenesis imperfecta due to parental mosaicism for a dominant mutation in a human type I collagen gene (COL1A1). Am J Hum Genet 1990;46:591.

Wenstrup RJ et al: Distinct biochemical phenotypes predict clinical severity in nonlethal variants of osteogenesis imperfecta. Am J Hum Genet 1990;46:975.

Willing MC et al: Osteogenesis imperfecta type I is commonly due to a COL1A1 null allele of type I collagen. Am J Hum Genet 1992;51:508.

Fragile X-Associated Mental Retardation

Fu YH et al: Variation of the CGG repeat at the fragile X site results in genetic instability: Resolution of the Sherman paradox. Cell 1991;67:1047.

Kremer EJ et al: Mapping of DNA instability at the fragile X to a trinucleotide repeat sequence $p(CCG)_n$. Science 1991;252:1711.

Pieretti M et al: Absence of expression of the *FMR-1* gene in fragile X syndrome. Cell 1991;66:817.

Siomi H et al: The protein product of the fragile X gene *FMR1* has characteristics of an RNA-binding protein. Cell 1993;74:291.

Yu S et al: Fragile X genotype characterized by an unstable region of DNA. Science 1991;252:1179.

Down's Syndrome

Epstein CJ: Down syndrome. In: *The Metabolic Basis of Inherited Disease,* 6th ed. Scriver CR et al (editors). McGraw-Hill, 1989.

Phenylketonuria

Dilella AG, Woo SLC: Molecular basis of phenylketonuria and its clinical applications. Mol Biol Med 1987;4:183.

Eisensmith RC et al: Multiple origins for phenylketonuria in Europe. Am J Hum Genet 1992;51:1355.

Okano Y et al: Molecular basis of phenotypic heterogeneity in phenylketonuria. [See comments.] N Engl J Med 1991;324:1232.

Scriver CR, Kaufman S, Woo SLC: The hyperphenylalaninemias. In: *The Metabolic Basis of Inherited Disease.* Scriver CR et al (editors). McGraw-Hill, 1989.

3 Disorders of the Immune System

Richard S. Shames, MD, &
Daniel C. Adelman, MD

The function of the immune system is to protect the host from invasion of foreign organisms by distinguishing "self" from "nonself." Such a system is necessary for survival in all living animals. A well-functioning immune system not only protects the host from external factors such as microorganisms or toxins but also prevents and repels attacks by endogenous factors such as tumors or autoimmune phenomena. Dysfunction or deficiency of components of the immune system leads to a variety of clinical diseases of varying expression and severity, ranging from atopic disease to rheumatoid arthritis, severe combined immunodeficiency, or cancer. This chapter will introduce the intricate physiology of the immune system and abnormalities which lead to diseases of hypersensitivity and immunodeficiency.

NORMAL STRUCTURE & FUNCTION OF THE IMMUNE SYSTEM

ANATOMY

Cells of the Immune System

The immune system consists of both specific and nonspecific components that have distinct yet overlapping functions. The antibody-mediated and cell-mediated immune systems provide specificity and memory of previously encountered antigens. The nonspecific cellular component consists of phagocytic cells, whereas the complement proteins constitute the primary nonspecific plasma factors. Despite their lack of specificity, these components are essential because they are largely responsible for the natural immunity to a vast array of environmental microorganisms. Basic appreciation of the components and physiology of normal immunity are central to understanding the pathophysiology of diseases of the immune system.

The major cellular components of the immune system consist of monocytes and macrophages, lymphocytes, and the family of granulocytic cells, including neutrophils, eosinophils, and basophils.

Monocytes and **macrophages** play a central role in the immune response. Macrophages are derived from blood monocytes. These cells leave the circulation to become active tissue macrophages. In response to antigenic stimulation, macrophages engulf the antigen (phagocytosis), then process and present that antigen in a form recognizable to T lymphocytes. Activated macrophages secrete proteolytic enzymes, active metabolites of oxygen (including superoxide anion and other oxygen radicals), arachidonic acid metabolites, cyclic adenosine monophosphate (cAMP), and cytokines such as interleukin-1 (IL-1), IL-6, tumor necrosis factor (TNF), and IL-8, among others. Many tissue-specific cells are of macrophage lineage and function to process and present antigen (Langerhans' cells, oligodendrocytes, etc).

Lymphocytes are responsible for the initial specific recognition of antigen. They are functionally and phenotypically divided into B lymphocytes and T lymphocytes. Structurally, B and T lymphocytes cannot be distinguished visually from each other under the microscope, although about 70–80% of circulating blood lymphocytes are T lymphocytes and 10–15% B lymphocytes; the remainder are neither B nor T lymphocytes and are often referred to as "null cells."

Null cells probably include a number of different cell types, including a group called **natural killer (NK) cells.** These cells appear distinct from other lymphocytes in that they are slightly larger, with a kidney-shaped nucleus, and have a granular appearance (large granular lymphocytes, or "LGLs"). NK cells are capable of binding IgG because they have a membrane receptor for the IgG molecule (FcγR). Antibody-dependent cell-mediated cytotoxicity (ADCC) occurs when an organism or a cell is coated by antibody and undergoes NK cell-mediated destruction. Alternatively, NK cells can destroy virally infected cells or tumor cells without involvement of antibody. Other characteristics of NK cells include recognition of antigens without major histocompatibility restrictions, lack of immunologic memory, and regulation of activity by cytokines and arachidonic acid metabolites.

Polymorphonuclear leukocytes (neutrophils) (PMNs) are granulocytic cells that originate in the bone marrow and circulate in blood and tissue. Their primary function is antigen-nonspecific phagocytosis and destruction of foreign particles and organisms. The presence of Fcγ receptors on the surface of neutrophils also facilitates the clearance of opsonized microbes through the reticuloendothelial system.

Eosinophils are often found in inflammatory sites or at sites of immune reactivity and play a crucial role in the host's defense against parasites. Despite many shared functional similarities to neutrophils, eosinophils are considerably less efficient than neutrophils at phagocytosis. Eosinophils do exhibit modulatory or regulatory functions in various types of inflammation. However, in the airway inflammatory response in asthma, eosinophil-derived mediators of inflammation, including major basic protein (MBP), eosinophil-derived neurotoxin (EDN), eosinophil cationic protein (ECP), and lysophospholipase (LPL) are toxic to respiratory epithelium.

Basophils play an important role in both the immediate and late phase allergic responses. These cells release many of the potent mediators of allergic-inflammatory diseases, including histamine, leukotrienes, prostaglandins, and platelet activating factor (PAF), all of which have significant effects on the vasculature and on the inflammatory response. Basophils are present in the circulation, possess high-affinity receptors for IgE (FcϵRI), and mediate immediate hypersensitivity (allergic) responses.

Organs of the Immune System

Several tissues and organs play roles in host defenses and are functionally classified as the immune system. In mammals, the primary lymphoid organs are the thymus and the bone marrow.

All cells of the immune system are originally derived from **bone marrow.** Pluripotent stem cells differentiate into lymphocyte, granulocyte, monocyte, erythrocyte, and megakaryocyte populations. In humans, B lymphocytes, which are the antibody-producing cells, undergo early antigen-independent maturation into immunocompetent cells in the bone marrow. Deficiency or dysfunction of the pluripotent stem cell or the various cell lines developing from it can result in immune deficiency disorders of varying expression and severity.

The **thymus,** derived from the third and fourth embryonic pharyngeal pouches, functions to produce T lymphocytes and is the site of initial T lymphocyte differentiation. Its reticular structure allows a significant number of lymphocytes to migrate through it to become fully immunocompetent thymus-derived cells. A large number of cells undergo **clonal deletion** in the thymus by a mechanism in which autoreactive lymphocyte clones (ie, clones of cells that react with self antigens) are eliminated. The thymus also regulates immune function by secretion of multiple soluble hormones that promote T lymphocyte differentiation and are essential for T lymphocyte-mediated immunity.

The **lymph nodes, spleen,** and **gut-associated lymphoid tissue** are secondary lymphoid organs in mammals connected by blood and lymphatic vessels. Through these vessels, lymphocytes circulate and recirculate, respond to antigen, and spread the specific experience of this antigen exposure to all parts of the lymphoid system.

Lymph nodes are strategically dispersed throughout the vasculature and are the principal organs of the immune system that localize and prevent the spread of infection. Lymph nodes have a framework of reticular cells and fibers that are arranged into a **cortex** and **medulla.** B lymphocytes, the precursors of antibody-producing cells, or plasma cells, are found in the cortex (the follicles and germinal centers) as well as in the medulla. Areas of the lymph node rich in T lymphocytes are found chiefly in the medullary and paracortical areas of the lymph node (Figure 3–1).

The spleen is functionally and structurally divided into B lymphocyte and T lymphocyte areas similar to those of the lymph nodes. The spleen filters and processes antigens from the blood.

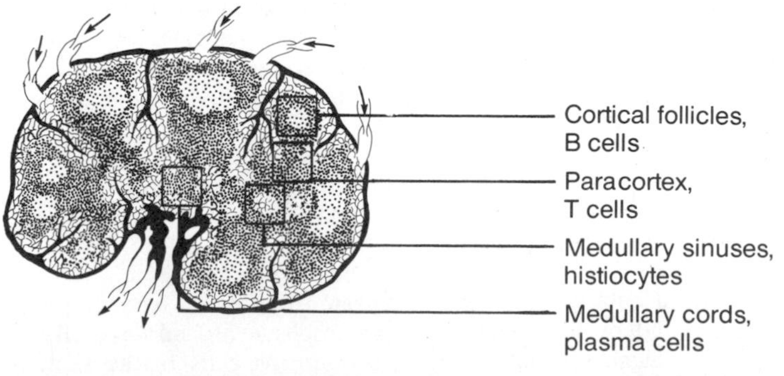

Figure 3–1. Anatomy of a normal lymph node. (Reproduced, with permission, from Chandrasoma P, Taylor CR: *Concise Pathology,* 2nd ed. Appleton & Lange, 1994.)

Gut-associated lymphoid tissue includes the tonsils, Peyer's patches of the small intestine, and the appendix. Similar to the lymph nodes and spleen, these tissues exhibit similar separation into B lymphocyte-dependent and T lymphocyte-dependent areas. Many lymphocytes are also seen within the lamina propria of the small intestinal villi and between the epithelial cells of the intestinal mucosal surface.

It is this network of dispersed immune organs that facilitates the rapid and efficient response to antigenic assaults on the host organism.

1. What are the specific and nonspecific components of the cellular and noncellular limbs of the immune system?
2. What is the role of macrophages in the immune system, and what are some of the products they secrete?
3. What are the categories of lymphocytes, and how are they distinguished?
4. What is the role of lymphocytes in the immune system, and what are some of the products they secrete?
5. What is the role of eosinophils in the immune system, and what are some of the products they secrete?
6. What is the role of basophils in the immune system, and what are some of the products they secrete?
7. What are the primary and secondary lymphoid organs, and what roles do they play in the proper functioning of the immune system?

PHYSIOLOGY

1. INNATE & ADAPTIVE IMMUNITY

Living organisms have two levels of response against external invasion: an **innate system** of natural immunity and an **adaptive system** which is acquired. Innate immunity is present from birth and is nonspecific in its activity. The skin surface serves as the first line of defense of the innate immune system, while enzymes, the alternative complement system pathway, acute phase proteins, natural killer cells, and certain cytokines provide additional layers of protection. Higher organisms have evolved the adaptive immune system, which is triggered by encounters with foreign agents that have evaded or penetrated the innate immune defenses. The adaptive immune system is characterized both by **specificity** for individual foreign agents and by **immunologic memory,** which makes possible an intensified response to subsequent encounters with the same or closely related agent. The introduction of a stimulus into the adaptive immune system triggers a complex sequence of events initiating the activation of lymphocytes, the production of antibodies and effector cells, and ultimately the elimination of the inciting organism.

2. ANTIGENS (Immunogens)

Foreign substances that can induce an immune response are called **antigens,** or **immunogens.** Antigenicity (immunogenicity) implies that the substance has the ability to react with products of the adaptive immune system (ie, antibodies). Complex foreign agents possess distinct and multiple immunogenic components. Most antigens are proteins, though pure carbohydrates may be antigenic as well. The immune response to a particular antigen may depend on the route of entry of the foreign substance. Blood-borne substances are normally removed by the spleen. Antigens entering through the skin may provoke a local inflammatory response involving afferent lymphatic channels and regional lymph nodes. Entry of agents through mucosal surfaces (respiratory or gastrointestinal systems) stimulate the production of local antibodies. Activated lymphocytes are then carried to other lymphoid organs to amplify the initial response.

3. THE IMMUNE RESPONSE (Figure 3–2)

The primary role of the immune system is to discriminate self from nonself and to eliminate the foreign substance. A complex network of specialized cells, organs, and biologic factors is necessary for the recognition and subsequent elimination of foreign antigens. The major pathways of antigen elimination include the direct killing of target cells by a subset of T lymphocytes called **cytotoxic T lymphocytes (cellular response)** and the elimination of antigen through antibody-mediated events arising from T and B lymphocyte interactions **(humoral response)**. The series of events that embody the immune response include antigen processing and presentation, lymphocyte recognition and activation, cellular or humoral immune responses, and antigenic destruction or elimination.

Antigen Processing & Presentation

Most foreign immunogens are not recognized by the immune system in their native form and require capture and processing by specialized **antigen-presenting cells.** Antigen-presenting cells include macrophages, dendritic cells in lymphoid tissue, Langerhans cells in the skin, Kupffer cells in the liver, microglial cells in the nervous system, and B lymphocytes. Following encounter with immuno-

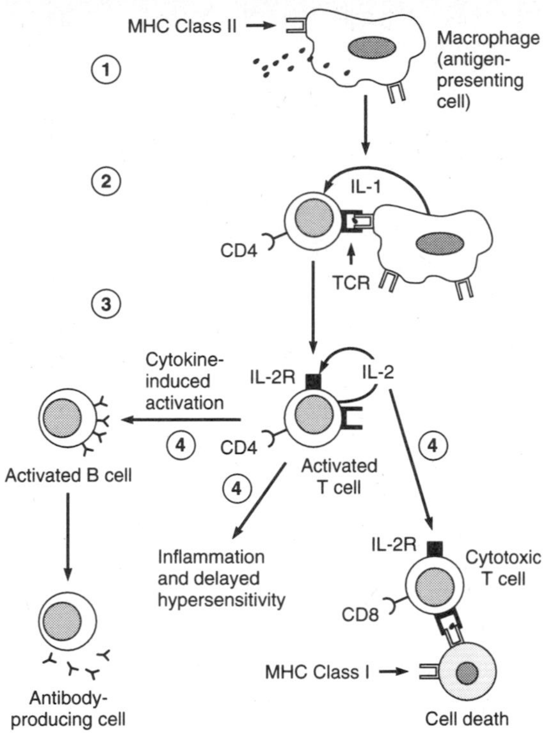

Figure 3–2. The normal immune response. ① Antigen processing and presentation by antigen-presenting cells. ② Recognition of antigen-MHC complex by CD4 T lymphocytes induces IL-1 secretion by antigen-presenting cells and subsequent cellular activation. ③ Activated T lymphocytes express IL-2 receptors and secrete IL-2, which up-regulates IL-2 receptor expression in an autocrine fashion. ④ Activated CD4 T lymphocytes can stimulate CD8 cytotoxic T lymphocytes to mediate cellular cytotoxicity, B lymphocyte activation, and differentiation into antibody-producing plasma cells, which mediate humoral immunity or mediate delayed hypersensitivity and other inflammatory reactions.

gens, the antigen-presenting cells internalize the foreign substance by phagocytosis or pinocytosis, modify its parent structure, and display antigenic fragments of the native protein on its surfaces in association with the MHC Class II Molecule.

T Lymphocyte Recognition & Activation

The recognition of processed antigen by specialized T lymphocytes known as **T helper (CD4) lymphocytes** constitutes the critical event in the immune response. The T helper lymphocytes orchestrate the many cells and biologic signals that are necessary to carry out the immune response. T helper lymphocytes recognize processed antigen displayed by antigen-presenting cells only in association with polymorphic cell surface proteins called the **major histocompatibility (MHC) complex.** The process of dual recognition is referred to as **MHC restriction.** Endogenously synthesized viral proteins are processed in association with **MHC class I** molecules, while exogenous foreign antigens that require an antibody-mediated response are expressed in association with **MHC class II** structures. All somatic cells express MHC class I, while only the specialized antigen-presenting cells can express MHC class II. Cytotoxic T lymphocytes expressing the surface protein **CD8** antigen recognize target cells bearing MHC class I complexed to antigen, while helper T lymphocytes expressing the **CD4** antigen recognize antigen in the context of MHC class II.

T helper lymphocyte recognition of the antigen-MHC class II complex thereby activates the T helper lymphocytes. Two signals are required for activation of these cells: (1) binding of the antigen-specific **T lymphocyte receptor** to the antigen-MHC complex and (2) the release of **interleukin-1 (IL-1),** a soluble protein produced by the antigen-presenting cell. These two signals induce the expression of **IL-2 receptors** on the surface of the CD4 lymphocytes as well as the production of various cell growth and differentiation factors **(cytokines)** by the activated CD4 T lymphocytes. The cytokine **IL-2,** produced and elaborated by activated CD4 T lymphocytes, stimulates the growth of more cells expressing IL-2 receptors **(autocrine effect),** thus amplifying the initial response. Activated CD4 T lymphocytes subsequently trigger the **effector cells** that mediate the cellular and humoral arms of the immune response.

Activation of Cytotoxic T Lymphocytes (Cellular Immune Response)

Cytotoxic T lymphocytes (CD8 T lymphocytes) eliminate target cells (virally infected cells, tumor, or foreign tissues), thus constituting the cellular immune response. Cytotoxic T lymphocytes differ from helper T lymphocytes in their expression of the surface antigen CD8 and by the recognition of MHC class I. Cytotoxic T lymphocytes become activated under the influence of two signals: (1) binding to the MHC class I antigen complex and (2) following stimulation by IL-2 elaborated by helper T lymphocytes. Activated cytotoxic T lymphocytes then release substances called **cytotoxins** that lead to the killing of infected target cells.

Activation of B Lymphocytes (Humoral Immune Response)

Activated T helper cells may also induce the growth and differentiation of B lymphocytes, which mediate the humoral or **antibody-mediated response.** Release of cytokines with growth and differentiation activity by CD4 T lymphocytes promotes the proliferation and terminal differentiation of B cells into high-rate antibody-producing cells called "plasma cells,'' which secrete antigen-specific antibody. B lymphocytes may also bind and internalize foreign antigen directly, process that antigen, and present it to CD4 T lymphocytes. A pool of activated B lymphocytes may differentiate to form **memory cells,** which respond more rapidly and efficiently to subsequent encounters with identical or closely related antigenic structures.

Antibody Structure & Function

The primary function of B lymphocytes is to make antibodies. Antibodies are **immunoglobulins** directed toward specific antigens. Antibodies are proteins that combine specifically with antigens to initiate the humoral (antibody-mediated) immune response. Circulating immunoglobulins have specificity that enables them to combine with one particular antigenic structure. Humoral immune responses result in the production of a diverse repertoire of antibodies that makes them able to combine with a broad range of antigens. This diversity is a function of complex DNA rearrangements and RNA processing within B lymphocytes early in ontogenic development.

All immunoglobulin molecules share a four-chain polypeptide structure consisting of two heavy and two light chains (Figure 3–3). Each chain includes an amino terminal portion, containing the **variable (V) region,** and a carboxyl terminal portion, containing four or five **constant (C) regions.** V regions are highly variable structures that form the antigen-binding site, while the C domains support effector functions of the molecules. The five classes **(isotypes)** of immunoglobulins are termed **IgG, IgA, IgM, IgD,** and **IgE** and are defined on the basis of differences in the C region of the heavy chains. Digestion of an immunoglobulin molecule by the enzyme papain produces two antigen-binding F(ab′) fragments and the Fc (crystallizable) fragment. Pepsin digestion of the immunoglobulin molecule results in single $F(ab)_2$ fragment joined by a disulfide bond. Immunoglobulins serve a variety of secondary

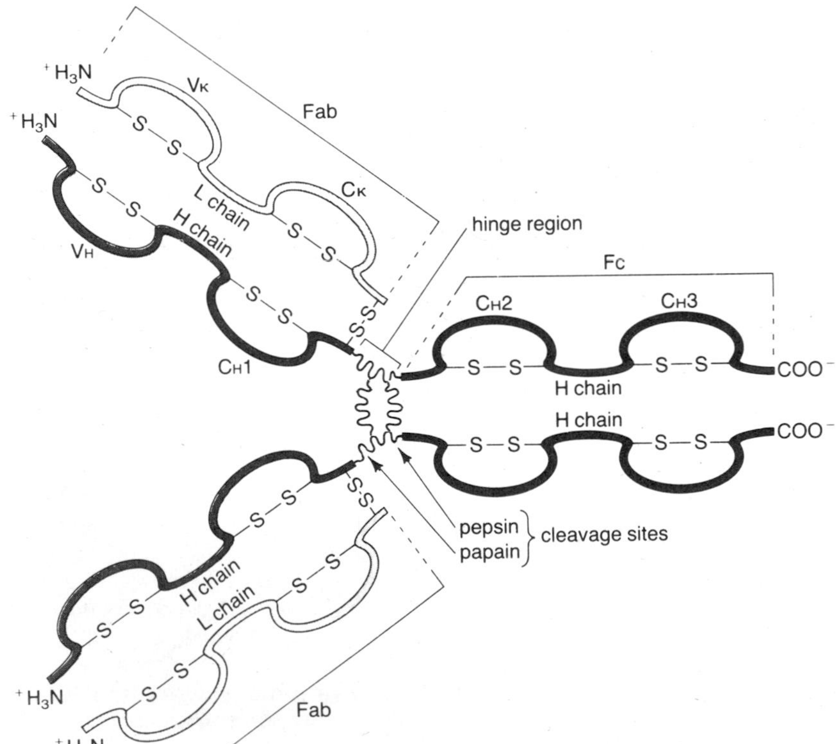

Figure 3–3. Structure of a human IgG antibody molecule. Depicted are the four chain-structure and the variable and constant domains. (V, variable region; C, constant region. The sites of pepsin and papain cleavage are shown.) (Reproduced, with permission, from Stites DP, Terr AL: *Basic & Clinical Immunology*, 7th ed. Appleton & Lange, 1991.)

biologic roles, including complement fixation, transplacental passage, and facilitation of phagocytosis **(opsonization),** all of which participate in host defenses against disease.

The IgE molecule is a monomeric structure of molecular weight 190,000. It constitutes only 0.004% of the total serum immunoglobulins and binds with very high avidity via its Fc region to the high-affinity Fcε receptor on mast cells and basophils. IgE specifically mediates the release of chemical mediators from mast cells and basophils in allergic hypersensitivity diseases as well as in the host defense against parasites.

Humoral Mechanisms of Antigen Elimination

Antibodies may induce the elimination of foreign antigen through a number of different mechanisms. Binding of antibody to bacterial toxins or foreign venoms promotes elimination of these antigen-antibody complexes through the reticuloendothelial system. Antibodies may also coat bacterial surfaces, allowing clearance by macrophages in a process known as opsonization. Some classes of antibodies may complex with antigen and activate the complement system of cascading component activation, which culminates in lysis of the target cell. Finally, the major class of antibody, IgG, can bind to natural killer cells that subsequently complex with target cells and release cytotoxins (see antibody-dependent cellular cytotoxicity, above).

Hypersensitivity Immune Responses

Gell and Coombs devised a classification scheme to define the mechanisms of immune responses to antigen into four distinct types of reactions to allow for clearer understanding of the immunopathogenesis of disease.

A. Type I: Anaphylactic or immediate hypersensitivity reactions occur following the binding of antigen to preformed IgE antibodies attached to the surface of the mast cell or basophil and result in the release of inflammatory mediators (see Mechanisms of Inflammation, below) that produce the clinical manifestations. Examples of type I-mediated reactions include anaphylactic shock, allergic rhinitis, allergic asthma, and acute drug allergic reactions.

B. Type II: Cytotoxic reactions involve the binding of either IgG or IgM antibody to antigens covalently bound to cell membrane structures. Antigen-antibody binding activates the complement cascade and results in the destruction of the cell to which the antigen is bound. Examples of tissue injury by this mechanism include immune hemolytic anemia and Rh hemolytic disease in the newborn. Another example of the type II-mediated disease process is autoimmune hyperthyroidism, a disorder in which thyroid-stimulating antibodies stimulate the thyroid tissue or TSH-binding inhibitory antibodies inhibit the binding of TSH to its receptor. Similarly, in myasthenia gravis, antibodies are directed to the acetylcholine receptor, blocking this neuromediator from interacting with its receptor. In these latter diseases, cytolysis is not a component of these reactions.

C. Type III: Immune complex-mediated reactions occur when immune complexes are formed by the binding of antigens to antibodies. Complexes are usually cleared from the circulation by the phagocytic system. However, deposition of these complexes in tissues or in vascular endothelium can produce immune complex-mediated tissue injury by leading to complement activation, anaphylatoxin generation, chemotaxis of polymorphonuclear leukocytes, phagocytosis, and tissue injury. Serum sickness, certain types of nephritis, and certain features of infective endocarditis are clinical examples of type III-mediated diseases.

D. Type IV: Delayed hypersensitivity reactions are mediated not by antibody but by T lymphocytes (cell-mediated immunity). Classic examples are the tuberculin skin test reactions and contact dermatitis.

Mechanisms of Inflammation

Elimination of foreign antigen by cellular or humoral processes is integrally linked to the inflammatory response, in which cytokines and antibodies trigger the recruitment of additional cells and the release of endogenous vasoactive and proinflammatory enzymatic substances **(inflammatory mediators).**

Inflammation may have both positive and deleterious effects. Tight control of inflammatory mechanisms promotes efficient elimination of foreign substances and prevents uncontrolled lymphocyte activation and unregulated antibody production. However, dysregulation of the system can perpetuate inflammatory processes that lead to tissue damage and organ dysfunction. Inflammation is responsible for hypersensitivity reactions and for many of the clinical effects of autoimmunity. The major type of immunologic inflammation—important in allergic diseases—involves the type I IgE-directed release of chemical mediators from mast cells and basophils (immediate-type hypersensitivity). Clinical allergy represents a hypersensitivity response arising from deleterious inflammation against normally harmless environmental antigens. Other pathways of immunologic inflammation include cell-mediated immunity and immune complex-mediated inflammation. Cell-mediated immunity is responsible for host defenses against intracellular pathogenic organisms, though dysregulation of this system may result in allergic contact dermatitis (eg, type IV delayed-type hypersensitivity responses). Similarly, immune complex-mediated (type III) inflammation is an important aspect of complement-mediated processes in normal host defenses, including opsonization and antibody-dependent cell-mediated cytotoxicity (ADCC), while hypersensitivity of immune complex-mediated immunity is responsible for the cutaneous Arthus reaction, systemic serum sickness, and some aspects of clinical autoimmunity. Imbalances in the inflammatory system may result from genetic defects, infection, neoplasms, and hormonal disturbances, though precise mechanisms which promote dysregulation and persistence of inflammatory processes are complex and poorly understood.

Synthesis of IgE in Allergic Reactivity

As IgE plays a critical role in processes of allergic hypersensitivity, attention has focused on the mechanisms underlying the synthesis and regulation of IgE. Induction of B lymphocytes to synthesize IgE requires two signals which are primarily elaborated by helper T lymphocytes: one that influences IgE isotype expression and another that serves to activate B lymphocytes. Isotype switching is regulated by mitogens and cytokines. The cytokine IL-4 is a critical factor for isotype switching to IgE and is sufficient to initiate germ line transcription of IgE. Additional B lymphocyte activation and differentiation factors are required for the expression of mature mRNA and subsequent IgE synthesis. In humans, a variety of secondary signals work in concert with IL-4 to promote IgE synthesis, including IL-5 and IL-6, which promote terminal differentiation of the B lymphocyte into an antibody-producing plasma cell. In contrast, gamma interferon-γ (IFNγ) inhibits IL-4-dependent IgE synthesis in humans. Thus, an imbalance favoring IL-4 over IFNγ may induce IgE formation.

Helper (CD4) T lymphocytes play a central role in the induction of normal immune responses. In allergic inflammatory processes, T lymphocytes represent a source of both IL-4 as well as secondary signals necessary to drive the production of IgE by B lymphocytes. Two subsets of CD4 helper T lymphocytes have been identified, differing in their phenotypic patterns of cytokine synthesis and release. **T_H1** cells elaborate IL-2, IFNγ, IL-3, and GM-CSF (granulocyte-macrophage colony-stimulating factor) and have been found to participate in type IV delayed hypersensitivity reactions. **T_H2** cells secrete IL-3, -4, -5 and GM-CSF and have been implicated in allergic and inflammatory responses. IL-3, together with other cytokines, induces mast cell differentiation and proliferation. IL-5 promotes activation and chemotaxis of eosinophils. GM-CSF drives the growth and differentiation of granulocytes, macrophages, and eosinophils. Activated T lymphocytes exhibiting T_H2-characteristic cytokines have been demonstrated at sites of inflammation in allergic airway disease and are believed to direct the immune response toward allergic inflammation. It is not known what drives undifferentiated CD4 T lymphocytes to become either T_H1 or T_H2 cells.

8. What are the components of and distinctions between the innate and adaptive forms of immunity?
9. Indicate the primary role of the immune system and the major classes of events by which this is accomplished.
10. What is the phenomenon of MHC restriction?
11. What two signals are necessary for activation of cytotoxic T lymphocytes?
12. What are the common structural features of antibodies?
13. What are some (four) different mechanisms by which antibodies can induce the elimination of foreign antigens?
14. What are the four types of immune reactions in the Gell and Coombs classification scheme, and what are some examples of disorders in which each is involved?
15. What is the critical factor in switching Ig synthesis to the IgE isotype? What are some secondary factors which contribute to, or inhibit, IgE synthesis?

PATHOPHYSIOLOGY OF SELECTED IMMUNE DISORDERS

ALLERGIC RHINITIS

Clinical Presentation

The clinical expression of allergic airways disease, manifested by allergic rhinitis and asthma, is local tissue damage and organ dysfunction arising from an abnormal hypersensitivity immune response to normally harmless and ubiquitous environmental allergens. Allergens that cause airway disease are predominantly seasonal inhalants in the form of tree, grass, and weed pollens or perennial inhalants (eg, house dust mite antigen, cockroach, mold, animal dander, and other protein antigens). Occasionally, ingested allergens, including foods and drugs, may produce allergic airway disease. Allergic disease is a common cause of pediatric and adult acute and chronic airway problems. Both allergic rhinitis and asthma account for significant morbidity, and asthma has increased in prevalence and severity (and as a cause of death) since the 1970s. The diagnosis of allergic airway disease is based on the history and physical examination confirmed by the demonstration of allergen-specific IgE in the serum or at the tissue level. As asthma is considered elsewhere in this volume (see Chapter 7), allergic rhinitis will be discussed here as a model for the pathophysiology of allergic airway disease.

Etiology

Upper airway disease may be either acute or chronic. Acute (nonallergic) rhinitis arises most commonly from infectious causes or, in children, occasionally as a result of foreign body obstruction. Chronic rhinitis occurring episodically or continuously is frequently a result of allergic hypersensitivity, though other causes may underlie this syndrome (Table 3–1).

Allergic rhinitis implies the existence of hypersensitivity to environmental allergens that impact the respiratory mucosa physically and directly. The allergic or atopic state is characterized by a tendency, generally inherited, to generate IgE antibodies to specific environmental allergens and the inflammatory response that subsequently ensues from the interaction of allergen with cell-bound IgE. The clinical presentation of stereotypical allergic rhinitis includes nasal, ocular, and palatal pruritus, paroxysmal sneezing, rhinorrhea, and nasal congestion. A personal or family history of other allergic diseases such as asthma or atopic dermatitis supports a diagnosis of allergy. Physical stigmas that support the diagnosis include bilateral infraorbital edema ("allergic shiners''), a horizontal nasal crease, pale and boggy nasal mucosa, nasal obstruction, and eczema involving the flexural surfaces of the extremities. Evidence of tissue eosinophilia or basophilia by nasal smear or scraping may support the diagnosis also. Confirmation of allergic rhinitis requires the demonstration of specific IgE antibodies to common allergens by in vitro tests such as the radioallergosorbent test (RAST) or in vivo (skin) testing.

In addition to allergic causes, chronic perennial rhinitis may result from infection, anatomic obstruction, drugs or hormones, nonallergic entities, systemic endocrine and granulomatous disease, mastocytosis, and, rarely, nasal tumors (Table 3–1). Persistent nasal congestion with discharge and cough may suggest sinusitis or otitis media. Anatomic defects such as a large septal deviation, nasal polyps, or septal spurs may cause chronic nasal obstruction. Overuse of topical nasal decongestants, resulting in an inflammatory condition called **rhinitis medicamentosa,** can induce a rebound vasodilation and cause rhinitis. Rhinitis may also be a consequence of adverse effects of certain drugs, including reserpine, aspirin, or oral contraceptives.

Vasomotor rhinitis is a nonallergic entity characterized by variable nasal obstruction and hypersecretion triggered by physical stimuli such as changes in temperature or exposure to inhaled irritants (eg, strong odors, perfumes, diesel exhaust, and other noxious substances). Systemic conditions, including pregnancy, diabetes mellitus, and hypothyroidism, may be associated with chronic rhinitis. Unusual causes of chronic rhinitis include nasal mastocytosis, granulomatous conditions such as Wegener's granulomatosis, sarcoidosis, or midline granuloma, and neoplasms. Infections, including tuberculosis, syphilis, leprosy, and mycoses (such as mucormycosis) may produce symptoms of nasal obstruction, bleeding, and eschar formation.

Table 3–1. Causes of chronic rhinitis.

A. Seasonal or perennial allergic rhinitis
B. Anatomic obstruction
  1. Anatomic defects
  2. Nasal polyps
  3. Foreign body
C. Sinusitis or otitis media
D. Vasomotor (nonallergic) rhinitis
E. Rhinitis medicamentosa
F. Rhinitis induced by drugs or hormones
  1. Antihypertensive agents
  2. Aspirin or nonsteroidal anti-inflammatory drugs
  3. Pregnancy, use of oral contraceptives, or conjugated estrogens
  4. Cocaine abuse
G. Rhinitis induced by systemic disease
  1. Endocrine
    a. Hypothyroidism
    b. Diabetes mellitus
  2. Granulomatous rhinitis
    a. Sarcoidosis
    b. Wegener's granulomatosis
    c. Relapsing polychondritis
    d. Midline granuloma
    e. Infection: tuberculosis, syphilis, leprosy, fungal disease
H. Nasal mastocytosis
I. Nasal neoplasms

Pathology & Pathogenesis

The clinical and laboratory manifestations of allergic rhinitis are due to local tissue inflammation and organ dysfunction of the upper airway arising from type I, IgE-mediated immune response. The inflammatory response mediated by the interaction of antigen with IgE bound to mast cells and basophils triggers the release of vasoactive, enzymatic, and chemotactic mediators. Activation of mast cells and basophils induces both the release of preformed mediators (histamine, chemotactic factors, and enzymes) and the synthesis and release of newly generated mediators (prostaglandins, leukotrienes, and platelet activating factor). Mast cells and basophils also have the ability to synthesize and release proinflammatory cytokines, growth and regulatory factors that interact in complex networks.

The interaction of mediators with various target organs and cells of the upper airway frequently induces a biphasic response: an early effect on blood vessels, smooth muscle, and secretory glands marked by vascular leakiness, smooth muscle constriction, and mucus hypersecretion; and a late response characterized by mucosal edema and the influx of inflammatory cells. Early phase events are mediated chiefly by histamine, while late phase events are induced by cytokines, preformed chemotactic mediators, arachidonic acid metabolites (leukotrienes), and platelet-activating factor.

The **early phase response** occurs within minutes after an antigen exposure. Atopic individuals challenged intranasally with pollen allergen or with cold, dry air release vasoactive and smooth muscle constrictive mediators, including histamine, N-α-*p*-tosyl-L-arginine methylester-esterase (TAME), leukotrienes, prostaglandin D_2 (PGD_2), and kinins and kininogens from mast cells and basophils. The **early phase response** is marked grossly by erythema, localized edema, and pruritus resulting largely from the interaction of histamine with target tissues of the upper airway. Histologically, the early response is characterized by vasodilation, edema, and a mild cellular infiltrate of mostly granulocytes.

The **late phase response** may either follow the early phase response (dual response) or occur as an isolated event. Late phase reactions begin 2–4 hours following initial antigen exposure, reach maximal activity at 6–12 hours, and usually resolve within 12–24 hours. Mediators of the early phase response—except for PGD_2—reappear during the late phase response in the absence of antigen rechallenge. Absence of PGD_2, an exclusive product of mast cell release, suggests that basophils and not mast cells are an important source of mediators in the late phase response. The late phase response is characterized grossly by erythema, induration, local heat, burning, and itching and microscopically by an influx of mainly eosinophils and mononuclear cells. There is strong circumstantial evidence that eosinophils are important proinflammatory cells in allergic airway disease (particularly asthma). Eosinophils are frequently found in secretions from the nasal mucosa of patients with allergic rhinitis and in the sputum of asthmatics. Products of activated eosinophils such as major basic protein and eosinophilic cationic protein, which are destructive to airway epithelial tissue and predispose to persistent airway reactivity, have also been localized to the airways of patients with allergic disease. Epithelial disruption is a clinical feature in patients with both atopic dermatitis and asthma. Inflammatory cells infiltrating tissues in the late response may further elaborate cytokines and histamine-releasing factors that may perpetuate the late phase response, leading to a sustained hyperresponsiveness and disruption of the target tissue (eg, bronchi, skin, or nasal mucosa). Release of proinflammatory mediators and cytokines can thus precipitate a sustained inflammatory response, resulting in localized edema, mucus secretion, epithelial disruption, and influx of eosinophils, neutrophils, and mononuclear cells. Pathophysiologic events of the late phase response characterize a persistent inflammatory state thought to most closely mimic clinical allergic disease. Indeed, late phase reactivity has been described in naturally occurring conditions, including allergic rhinitis and conjunctivitis, asthma, food-sensitive atopic dermatitis, and anaphylaxis. Inflammatory changes in the airways are recognized as critical features of both allergic rhinitis and chronic asthma. Therefore, therapeutic interventions that prevent or reverse inflammatory processes are most effective in the control of chronic and severe allergic disease.

Clinical Manifestations

The clinical manifestations of allergic airways disease arise from the interaction of mast cell and basophil mediators with target organs of the upper and lower airway (Table 3–2). The characteristic symptoms of allergic rhinitis often appear immediately following exposure to a relevant allergen (early phase response), though many patients appear to experience chronic and recurrent symptoms on the basis of the late phase response. Complications of severe or untreated allergic rhinitis may include sinusitis, eustachian tube dysfunction, dysosmia, sleep disturbances, and chronic mouth breathing.

A. Sneezing, Pruritus, Mucus Hypersecretion: Allergic rhinitis is characterized by chronic or episodic paroxysmal sneezing; nasal, ocular, or palatal pruritus; and watery rhinorrhea triggered by exposure to a specific allergen. Patients may demonstrate signs of chronic pruritus of the upper airway, including a horizontal nasal crease from frequent nose rubbing and palatal "clicking" from rubbing the itching palate with the tongue. These symptoms often occur immediately following allergen exposure, though the symptoms may occur during the late phase in patients with chronic or severe disease when early phase mediators may reappear. Sneezing is caused by stimulation of local irritant nerve endings, initiating central neural reflexes. Mucus hypersecretion results primarily from excitation of parasympathetic-cholinergic pathways. Pruritus results from the actions of histamine secreted by mast cells and basophils during the early response. Early phase symp-

Table 3–2. Clinical manifestations of allergic rhinitis.

Symptoms and signs
Sneezing paroxysms
Nasal, ocular, palatal itching
Clear rhinorrhea
Nasal congestion
Pale, bluish nasal mucosa
Transverse nasal crease
Periorbital cyanosis ("allergic shiners")
Serous otitis media
Laboratory findings
Nasal eosinophilia
Evidence of allergen-specific IgE by skin or RAST testing

toms are often effectively treated with avoidance of relevant allergens and oral antihistamines, which competitively antagonize H_1 receptor sites in target tissues. Effective treatment of late phase or chronic symptoms requires the use of topical anti-inflammatory medications (nasal cromolyn or nasal steroids) with or without allergen-specific immunotherapy (hyposensitization). Anti-inflammatory treatment appears to reduce cellular inflammation during the late phase.

B. Nasal Stuffiness: Nasal congestion results from swelling of the mucus membranes of the nose following secretion of mast cell mediators of inflammation and from the physical barrier caused by increased viscid secretions. Symptoms of nasal obstruction frequently occur during the late phase response and are characteristic of chronic perennial allergic rhinitis. Nasal mucosal membranes may appear pale blue and boggy. Children frequently show signs of obligate mouth breathing, including long facies, narrow maxillae, flattened malar eminences, marked overbite, and high-arched palates. These symptoms are not mediated by histamine and are poorly responsive to antihistamine therapy. Oral sympathomimetics that induce vasoconstriction by stimulation of alpha-adrenergic receptors are often used in conjunction with antihistamines to treat nasal congestion. Topical decongestants have limited value in patients with allergic rhinitis, as frequent use results in rebound vasodilation and the syndrome of rhinitis medicamentosa. Chronic nasal stuffiness in allergic rhinitis requires therapy with anti-inflammatory agents or allergen immunotherapy.

C. Airway Hyperresponsiveness: Late phase inflammation induces a state of nasal airway hyperresponsiveness to both irritants and allergens in patients with chronic allergic rhinitis. Airway hyperreactivity can cause heightened sensitivity to both environmental irritants such as tobacco smoke and noxious odors as well as to allergens such as pollens. The phenomenon of heightened nasal sensitivity to allergen following initial exposures to the allergen is known as "priming.'' Airway hyperresponsiveness is also a characteristic feature of allergic asthma and has been correlated with disease severity and medication requirements. There are no standardized clinical tools to accurately assess late phase hyperresponsiveness in allergic rhinitis. Bronchial provocation with antigen or pharmacologic bronchoconstrictors may be used to assess airway hyperresponsiveness in asthma. Airway hyperresponsiveness appears to result from late phase cellular infiltration and mucosal edema. Eosinophil by-products may inflict airway epithelial damage, which in turn can predispose to airway hyperreactivity in asthma. Mechanisms contributing to nasal airway hyperresponsiveness are unclear. Effective treatment of late phase airway responsiveness requires the use of anti-inflammatory medications with or without immunotherapy.

D. Nasal Eosinophilia: Infiltration of nasal mucosa with eosinophils is a characteristic finding in patients with allergic rhinitis. Release of IL-5 and GM-CSF and mast cell mediators (platelet-activating factor and leukotrienes) induces the development and accumulation of eosinophils in late phase reactions. Basophils may occasionally appear in both early and late phases. Examination of nasal secretions for eosinophils can be a useful adjunct to the evaluation of patients with suspected allergic rhinitis. Specimens from patients with atopic disease frequently show moderate to large numbers of eosinophils, while nonatopic patients demonstrate an absence of these cells. The degree of nasal eosinophilia is related to the extent of allergic exposure and symptomatology, so that findings may vary in and out of allergy season. Specimens may be collected by instructing patients to blow their nose into wax paper or by scraping the medial third of the inferior turbinate with a plastic curette. The secretions are applied to a glass slide and stained with Wright's or Hansel's stain. Both techniques have approximately 70% sensitivity and 95% specificity in the diagnosis of allergic rhinitis. Because the eosinophil is primarily a tissue-dwelling cell, quantification of peripheral blood eosinophils to diagnose allergic disease is of limited value.

E. In Vivo or in Vitro Measurement of Allergen-Specific IgE: In vivo or in vitro measurement of allergen-specific IgE is the primary tool for the confirmation of suspected allergic disease. In vivo skin testing with allergens suspected of causing hypersensitivity constitutes an indirect bioassay for the presence of allergen-specific IgE on tissue mast cells or basophils. Percutaneous or intradermal administration of dilute concentrations of specific antigens elicits an immediate wheal and flare response in a sensitized individual. This response marks a "local anaphylaxis" resulting from the controlled release of mediators from activated mast cells. Positive skin tests for inhalant allergens, combined with a history and examination suggestive of allergy, strongly implicate the allergen as a cause of the patient's symptoms. Negative skin tests with an unconvincing allergy history argue strongly against an allergic origin. Major advantages to skin testing include simplicity, rapidity of performance, and low cost.

In vitro tests provide quantitative assays of allergen-specific IgE in the serum. In these assays, patient serum is reacted initially with antigen bound to a solid phase material and then labeled with a radioactive or enzyme-linked anti-IgE antibody. These immunoallergosorbent tests show a 70–80% correlation with skin testing to pollens, dust mites, and danders and are useful in patients receiving chronic antihistamine therapy who are unable to undergo skin testing and in patients with extensive dermatitis.

F. Serous Otitis Media and Sinusitis: Serous otitis and acute and chronic sinusitis are the major morbid features in patients with allergic rhinitis. Both conditions are secondary to the obstructed nasal passages and sinus ostia observed in patients with chronic allergic or nonallergic rhinitis. Complications of chronic rhinitis should be considered in patients with protracted rhinitis unresponsive to therapy, refractory asthma, or persistent bronchitis. Serous otitis results from eustachian tube obstruction by mucosal edema and hypersecretion. Children with serous otitis media often present with conductive hearing loss, delayed speech, and recurrent otitis media associated with chronic nasal obstruction. Sinusitis may be acute, subacute, or chronic depending on the duration of symptoms. Obstruction of osteomeatal drainage in patients with chronic rhinitis predisposes to bacterial infection in the sinus cavities. Patients manifest symptoms of persistent nasal discharge, cough, sinus discomfort, and nasal obstruction. Examination may reveal chronic otitis media, infraorbital edema, inflamed nasal mucosa, and purulent nasal discharge. Radiographic diagnosis by x-ray or CT scan reveals sinus opacification, membrane thickening, or the presence of an air-fluid level. Effective treatment of infectious complications of chronic rhinitis requires antibiotics, systemic antihistamine and decongestants, and perhaps intranasal corticosteroids.

16. What are the major clinical manifestations of allergic rhinitis?
17. What are the major etiologic factors in allergic rhinitis?
18. What are the pathogenetic mechanisms in allergic rhinitis?

PRIMARY IMMUNODEFICIENCY DISEASES

Clinical Presentation

Because of the intricate complexities of the immune system, there are many potential sites where developmental aberrations in the immune system can lead to abnormalities in immunocompetence. When these defects are genetic in origin, they are referred to as the primary immunodeficiency disorders. This is in contrast to the compromised immunity secondary to extrinsic factors such as iatrogenic immunodeficiency resulting from the treatment of cancer or autoimmune disorders or due to the human immunodeficiency virus (HIV) that causes AIDS.

Traditionally, the primary immunodeficiencies are classified according to which cellular component of the immune response is principally involved. It is perhaps more useful to conceptualize these disorders according to their functional abnormalities than according to their morphologic characteristics (Table 3–3). The physiology of the normal immune response to antigen is summarized in Figure 3–2. There are distinct developmental stages that characterize the maturation and differentiation of the cellular components of the immune system. Rather than attempting to present for memorization the morphologic classifications and clinical manifestations of these disorders, the clinician should focus on understanding the predominant functional defects of a limited number of the primary immunodeficiency disorders. This can facilitate clearer insights into underlying pathogenesis and potential therapies for these disorders. The primary immunodeficiency disorders discussed below will include those characterized by (1) early developmental defects in cellular maturation, (2) specific enzyme defects, (3) abnormalities in cellular proliferation and functional differentiation, (4) abnormalities in cellular regulation, and (5) abnormal responses to cytokines.

Clinically, the primary immunodeficiency disorders typically present early in the neonatal period. In patients with severe combined immunodeficiency, there is an absence of normal thymic tissue, and the lymph nodes, spleen, and other peripheral lymphoid tissues are devoid of lymphocytes. In these patients, the complete or near-complete failure of development of both the cellular and humoral components of the immune system results in severe infections with organisms that otherwise are considered to be of low virulence, and death usually occurs within the first year.

Some of the other primary immunodeficiencies present more mildly. Children with primary immune defects in antibody production present clinically at about 6 months of age with onset of intractable infections. These infections do not become chronic until after the transplacentally transferred maternal IgG antibodies have waned, which occurs 4–6 months after birth. These children will have a more insidious onset of symptoms, including the development of progressively more severe chronic mucosal, gut, and respiratory infections, as well as slowed growth and development and sometimes failure to thrive. Patients with common variable immunodeficiency are usually born with adequate immunity and enjoy good health throughout childhood. They most commonly present with recurrent and chronic infections in late adolescence or early adulthood but can manifest these symptoms as early as birth or as late as the sixth or seventh decade. These patients will typically present with recurrent sinopulmonary infections and may manifest a variety of autoimmune-like illnesses, including, among others, thrombocytopenic purpura, hemolytic anemias, and symmetric (seronegative) arthritis.

Table 3–3. Primary immunodeficiency disorders.

Functional Abnormality	Disease Category	Primary Cellular Component	Stage of Defect
Abnormal maturation	SCID (Swiss type)	Progenitor cell	Early
	X-linked agammaglobulinemia	B lymphocyte	Early
	DiGeorge's syndrome	T lymphocyte	Early
Abnormal proliferation and differentiation	Common variable immunodeficiency	B lymphocyte[1]	Late[1]
	Selective IgA deficiency	B lymphocyte	Late
	Hyper-IgM immunodeficiency	B lymphocyte	Late
	Ataxia-telangiectasia	T lymphocyte	Early
Abnormal regulatory cell function	Common variable immunodeficiency	T lymphocyte, B lymphocyte, macrophage	Late
	Chronic mucocutaneous candidiasis	T lymphocyte, macrophage	Late
Enzyme defect	SCID-ADA deficiency	B and T lymphocytes	Late
	PNP deficiency	T lymphocyte	Late
Abnormal cytokine response	Hyper-IgE syndrome	B lymphocyte	Late

Key:
ADA = adenosine deaminase
PNP = purine nucleoside phosphorylase
SCID = severe combined immunodeficiency disease
[1] Variable defects, though the most common is in terminal differentiation of B lymphocytes.

Pathology & Pathogenesis

A. Disorders With Early Defects In Cellular Maturation:

1. Severe combined immunodeficiency disease (SCID)–This is a heterogeneous group of disorders that typically present shortly after birth and are characterized by repeated and often overwhelming infections. Without treatment, death is inevitable. Patients typically develop persistent oral candidiasis, chronic diarrhea, pulmonary infections, and sepsis caused by bacterial, viral, or fungal organisms.

Patients have reduced function of both B and T lymphocytes, hypogammaglobulinemia, and nonfunctioning circulating immature T lymphocytes. The genetic and cellular defects vary and in many cases can be traced to defective maturation of a lymphoid stem cell. Some of the B lymphocyte abnormalities are thought to result from dysfunctional T and B lymphocyte interactions. Two inheritance patterns have been identified: an autosomal recessive form (classically known as "Swiss type") and an X-linked form in which the maturation defect is mainly in the T lymphocyte lineage. The two forms are clinically indistinguishable, though the X-linked form is the most prevalent. The specific genetic defect has recently been isolated for the X-linked inherited form. The genetic defect is due to a point mutation in the gamma chain of the IL-2 receptor. This same gamma chain is shared by the receptors for IL-4 and IL-7, and defects in this chain thus result in dysfunction of all of these cytokine receptors. Identification of specific mutations allows for improved genetic counseling, prenatal diagnosis, and carrier detection. Moreover, specific gene transfer offers hope as a future therapy.

Recently, the genetic defect for a new autosomal recessive inherited form of SCID has been identified. This form is due to a deficiency of ZAP-70, a protein tyrosine kinase important in normal T lymphocyte function. Deficiency of this kinase results in a total absence of CD8 T lymphocytes as well as functionally defective CD4 T lymphocytes which do not proliferate or differentiate normally.

2. Congenital thymic aplasia (DiGeorge's syndrome)–In this syndrome, the spectrum of immunologic deficiency is wide, ranging from no clinically apparent immunologic abnormalities to severe, life-threatening infections with organisms of typically low virulence. The associated immunologic defects result from thymic abnormalities arising from defective embryonic development of the pharyngeal arches in association with structural abnormalities in the cardiovascular and endocrine (parathyroid) systems. Patients affected by the complete syndrome have a profound T lymphocytopenia due to defective thymic T lymphocyte maturation, severely depressed cell-mediated immunity, and decreased suppressor T lymphocyte activity. B lymphocyte numbers and morphology—as well as immunoglobulin production—are unaffected in most patients. Occasional patients may present with mild hypogammaglobulinemia and absent or poor antibody responses to neoantigens.

DiGeorge's syndrome is classified as complete or partial depending on the presence or absence of immunologic abnormalities. Patients typically present with neonatal tetany or seizures caused by the associated hypoparathyroidism, low serum calcium, and high serum phosphorus. In addition, it is common for patients to exhibit multiple anatomic cardiac abnormalities as well as facial abnormalities such as micrognathia, hypertelorism, low-set ears with notched pinnae, and a short philtrum. Affected children also present very early with the signs and symptoms of immunodeficiency.

3. X-linked (infantile) agammaglobulinemia (XLA)–is thought to be pathophysiologically and clinically more homogeneous than SCID. It is principally a disease of childhood, presenting clinically within the first 2 years of life with multiple and recurrent sinopulmonary infections caused by encapsulated bacteria, viruses, or parasites. The patients are panhypogammaglobulinemic and exhibit poor to absent responses to antigen challenge even though virtually all demonstrate normal functional T lymphocyte responses to in vitro as well as in vivo tests (ie, delayed hypersensitivity skin reactions).

The basic defect in this disorder appears to be arrested cellular maturation at the pre-B lymphocyte stage. Indeed, normal numbers of pre-B lymphocytes can be found in the bone marrow, though B lymphocytes in the circulation are virtually absent. Lymphoid tissues lack fully differentiated B lymphocytes (plasma cells), and lymph nodes lack developed germinal centers. The gene responsible for X-linked agammaglobulinemia has been recently isolated and is termed *bpk* and is part of the cytoplasmic tyrosine kinase family. Gene deletions and point mutations in the catalytic domain of this gene appear to be responsible for the syndrome.

B. Disorders Due to Defective Enzyme Function:

1. Adenosine deaminase (ADA) deficiency– About 40–50% of patients with the autosomal recessive form of SCID have deficiency of the enzyme ADA, which is responsible for the metabolism of adenosine. This severe immunodeficiency disorder is known as SCID-ADA. Absence of the ADA enzyme results in an accumulation of toxic metabolites of adenosine within the cells (Figure 3–4). These metabolites inhibit normal lymphocyte proliferation and lead to immunodeficiency of both B and T lymphocytes. The clinical presentation of this disorder is identical to that of the other forms of SCID.

2. Purine nucleoside phosphorylase (PNP) deficiency–In this disorder, the enzymatic activity of PNP is severely depressed, resulting in the accumulation of intracellular purine metabolites (Figure 3–4), which in turn leads to severe functional abnormalities in T lymphocytes. Despite normal levels of antibody production, patients with PNP deficiency

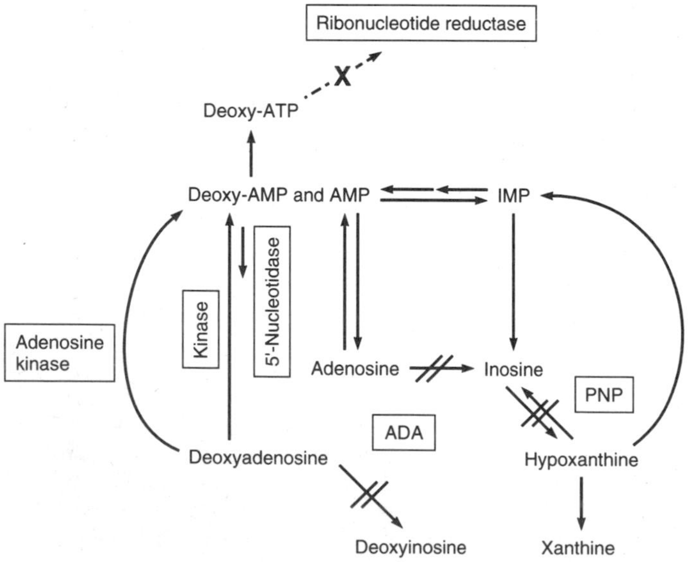

Figure 3–4. Simplified schema of the portion of the purine catabolic pathways affected by adenosine deaminase deficiency and purine nucleoside phosphorylase deficiency disorders. (ATP, adenosine triphosphate; AMP, adenosine monophosphate; IMP, inosine monophosphate; ADA, adenosine deaminase; PNP, purine nucleoside phosphorylase.) ADA catalyzes the metabolism of adenosine to inosine and deoxyadenosine to deoxyinosine. Similarly, PNP catalyzes the metabolism of inosine to hypoxanthine. In SCID-ADA, lymphocyte kinases rapidly convert deoxyadenosine to deoxy-AMP, though they are deficient in the 5′-nucleotidase that drives the reverse reaction. The result of the accumulation of deoxy-AMP and deoxy-ATP is the inhibition of ribonucleotide reductase, an enzyme critical to purine and pyrimidine biosynthesis. Inhibition of this enzyme effectively shuts down DNA synthesis in the cell.

develop severe opportunistic infections due to the cellular defects in immune function.

The clinical manifestations of this extremely rare form of SCID are similar to those of the other forms, though as many as 50% of affected individuals will develop such neurologic abnormalities as spastic diplegia, quadriparesis, and hypotonia.

C. Disorders With Defective Proliferation and Differentiation Responses:

1. Common variable immunodeficiency (CVI)–is often referred to as acquired or adult-onset hypogammaglobulinemia and is the most common serious primary immune deficiency disorder in adults, affecting an estimated 1:75,000–1:50,000 North Americans. The clinical spectrum in this disorder is broad and presents usually within the first 2 decades of life. Affected individuals commonly develop recurrent sinopulmonary infections, gastrointestinal malabsorption, autoimmune disorders, and an increased incidence of several neoplasms, including lymphomas, gastric carcinoma, and skin cancer. Treatment is primarily symptomatic, in addition to replacement of IgG with monthly infusions of intravenous gamma globulin (IGIV) in doses sufficient to maintain serum concentrations adequate to reduce the infection rate substantially.

The primary immunologic abnormality is a marked reduction in antibody production, with normal or reduced numbers of circulating B lymphocytes. The vast majority of patients will demonstrate an in vitro defect in terminal differentiation of B lymphocytes in response to T lymphocyte-dependent (antigen-activated T lymphocyte supernatants) and T lymphocyte-independent stimuli (EBV transformation), though defects in B lymphocyte development have been reported to occur at any stage of the maturation pathway. Over half of patients also have some degree of T lymphocyte dysfunction as determined by absent or diminished cutaneous responses to recall antigens. A variety of T lymphocyte abnormalities in a small minority of patients are responsible for the phenotypic expression of hypogammaglobulinemia. These rare T lymphocyte abnormalities include increased suppressor T lymphocyte activity, decreased production of IL-2 and other cytokines, and defective synthesis of B lymphocyte growth factors such as IL-4 and IL-6. In some patients, there is also evidence of defective cytokine gene expression in T cells, decreased T cell mitogenesis, and deficient lymphokine-activated killer (LAK) cell function.

2. Selective IgA deficiency–This is the most common primary immunodeficiency in adults, with a prevalence of 1:700–1:500 individuals. Most individuals with this defect have few or no clinical manifestations, though others may note an increased incidence of upper respiratory tract infections, allergy, asthma, and associated autoimmune disorders. Whereas the other immunoglobulin isotype concentration levels in serum are typically normal, serum IgA levels in these individuals are markedly depressed and are often less than 5 mg/dL.

The primary functional defect is similar to the B lymphocyte differentiation defect in common variable immunodeficiency, ie, an inability of B cells to terminally differentiate to IgA-secreting B lymphocytes. An associated deficiency of IgG subclasses (mainly IgG2 and IgG4) and low-molecular-weight monomeric IgM is not uncommon. Other cellular abnormalities have been suggested, including primary or secondary increase in suppressor T lymphocyte activity or defective T lymphocyte inducer function. Because of the role of secretory IgA in mucosal immunity, patients with this immunodeficiency are at greater risk to develop significant infections involving the mucous membranes of the gut, conjunctiva, and respiratory tract.

3. Hyper-IgM immunodeficiency–In patients with Hyper-IgM immunodeficiency, serum levels of IgG and IgA are very low or absent, associated with an elevation of serum IgM (and sometimes IgD). The inheritance of this disorder may be autosomal, though it is most often X-linked. Clinically, this syndrome is manifested by recurrent pyogenic infections and an array of autoimmune phenomena, such as Coombs-positive hemolytic anemia and immune thrombocytopenia.

T lymphocyte function is usually normal, and the principal abnormality is a defect in the gene product of a T lymphocyte surface ligand called CD40-ligand (gp39). The most common genetic defect appears to be due to point mutations in the extracellular domain of the gene product, which results in interference in the receptor binding site. Ligand-receptor interactions normally initiate B lymphocyte proliferation and isotype switch. When soluble gp39 or monoclonal antibodies directed toward the CD40 membrane receptor are incubated with B cells from these patients, the cells will undergo normal class-switching and produce IgG and IgA.

D. Disorders Due to Defective Cytokine Response:

1. Hyper-IgE immunodeficiency (HIE)–This is often referred to as "Job's syndrome" because affected individuals have diseases similar to those which tormented the biblical figure Job. The initial description of this immunodeficiency disorder was in two fair-skinned girls with chronic recurrent staphylococcal "cold" skin abscesses which were associated with furunculosis, cellulitis, recurrent otitis, sinusitis, and a coarse facial appearance. In this disorder, the predominant organism isolated from sites of infection is *Staphylococcus aureus,* though other organisms such as *Haemophilus influenzae,* pneumococci, gram-negative organisms, and *Candida albicans* are often identified also. Characteristically, patients have a chronic pruritic eczematoid dermatitis, growth retardation, and hyperkeratotic fingernails. Extremely high IgE levels

(> 3000 IU/mL) have also been observed in patients' serum.

The high IgE levels are thought to be related to nonresponsivness of terminally differentiated B lymphocytes to regulatory signals such as the interferons. The cellular basis of the immune deficiency in this disorder has not been clearly elucidated, though several mechanisms have been postulated. Humoral immunodeficiency is suggested by poor antibody responses to neoantigens, deficiency of IgA antibody against *S aureus,* and low levels of antibodies to carbohydrate antigens. T lymphocyte functional abnormalities are suggested by decreased absolute numbers of suppressor T lymphocytes, poor in vitro proliferative responses, and defects in cytokine production. Several reports have also documented abnormalities in neutrophil chemotaxis.

Clinical Manifestations

The very nature of a defect in host immune responses places the susceptible individual at high risk for the development of a variety of infectious, malignant, and autoimmune diseases and disorders. Some of the underlying mechanisms are discussed in the following paragraphs.

A. Infections: The nature of the specific functional defect will significantly influence the type of infection that affects the host. Table 3–4 lists some of the typical organisms causing infection in patients with various immunodeficiency disorders. The T lymphocyte plays a central role in inducing and coordinating immune responses; thus, any immunopathogenic mechanism that impairs T lymphocyte function predisposes the host to the development of serious chronic and potentially life-threatening infections with viruses, mycobacteria, fungi, and protozoa involving any or all organ systems. Similarly, immunopathogenic dysfunction of B lymphocytes resulting in antibody deficiency will predispose the host to pyogenic sinopulmonary and mucosal infections.

B. Malignancies: Patients with impaired immune responses are at greater risk for certain malignancies than the general population. For example, patients with common variable immunodeficiency have an increased incidence of certain non-Hodgkin lymphomas, gastric carcinoma, and various skin cancers. The occurrence of cancer may be related to an underlying impairment of **immune surveillance,** a theory that suggests that neoplastic changes occur frequently in cells but are manifested as malignant neoplasms only if they escape recognition and destruction by the immune system. Alternatively, others have speculated that chronic immune stimulation of an inadequate immune system may result in unregulated cellular proliferation and the subsequent development of malignancy (eg, B cell lymphomas).

C. Autoimmune Phenomena: Patients with antibody deficiency or complement system deficiency disorders have an increased incidence of associated autoimmune phenomena, including diseases clinically similar to rheumatoid arthritis, systemic lupus erythematosus, autoimmune hemolytic anemia, and immunologically based thrombocytopenic purpura. The underlying pathogenetic mechanisms have not been clearly elucidated.

Outlook for Management or Prevention

The greatest efforts in therapeutics are typically directed at those disorders with the highest incidence or those whose defective mechanisms are best understood. Genetic counseling for disorders with well-characterized inherited patterns is usually offered, whereas attempts at preventive care are irrelevant for the majority of the primary immunodeficiencies. The current treatment of choice for many of the primary immunodeficiency disorders developing from defective cellular components in the bone marrow is bone marrow transplantation. Because of the many problems associated with bone marrow transplantation, development of other more specifically directed therapies are constantly being sought. With advances in mapping the human genome, gene transfer may become an important form of therapy. A new era of specific functional defect directed therapies will become clinically useful and should offer exciting new challenges to physicians in the twenty-first century.

19. What are the major clinical manifestations of each of the five categories of primary immune deficiency?
20. What are the major pathogenetic mechanisms in each category of primary immune deficiency?

ACQUIRED IMMUNODEFICIENCY SYNDROME (AIDS)

Clinical Presentation

AIDS is the most common immunodeficiency disorder in the world and is among the greatest epidemics in human history. AIDS is a disease defined by the presence of any of a variety of indicator diseases and the presence of antibodies directed to the virus that causes AIDS. Table 3–5 lists the most recent criteria for defining and diagnosing AIDS.

Acute HIV infection may present as an acute, self-limited, febrile viral syndrome. A long clinically silent period follows, leading to the eventual development of signs and symptoms suggestive of chronic, slowly progressive immunosuppression. The

Table 3–4. Relationship of various pathogens to infection in primary immunodeficiency disorders.[1]

	Pyogenic Bacteria	Mycobacteria	Fungi	Viruses	Parasites			
					Pneumocystis carinii	*Giardia lamblia*	*Toxoplasma gondii*	*Cryptosporidium, Isospora*
SCID	+	+	+	+	+	–	–	–
Thymic hypoplasia	–	+	+	+	–	–	–	–
X-linked agammaglobulinemia	+	–	–	–	–	+	–	–
Common variable immunodeficiency	+	–	–	–	–	+	–	–
Complement deficiency	+	–	–	–	–	–	–	–
Phagocytic defects	+	–	–	–	–	–	–	–

Key: SCID = severe combined immunodeficiency disease; + = association; – = no association.

Table 3–5. 1993 revised classification system for HIV infection and expanded AIDS surveillance case definition for adolescents and adults.[1,2,3]

I. Clinical and lymphocyte categories:

	Clinical Categories		
CD4 T Cell Categories	**(A) Asymptomatic, Acute (Primary) HIV or PGL[4]**	**(B) Symptomatic, Not (A) or (C) Conditions**	**(C) AIDS-Indicator Conditions**
(1) ≥500/μL	A1	B1	C1
(2) 200–499/μL	A2	B2	C2
(3) <200/μL	A3	B3	C3

II. Conditions included in the 1993 AIDS surveillance case definition:

- Candidiasis of the esophagus, bronchi, trachea, or lungs
- Cervical cancer, invasive
- Coccidioidomycosis, disseminated or extrapulmonary
- Cryptococcosis, extrapulmonary
- Cryptosporidiosis, chronic intestinal (>1 month's duration)
- Cytomegalovirus disease (other than liver, spleen, or nodes); cytomegalovirus retinitis (with loss of vision)
- Encephalopathy, HIV-related
- Herpes simplex: chronic ulcers (>1 month's duration); or bronchitis, pneumonitis, or esophagitis
- Histoplasmosis, disseminated or extrapulmonary
- Isosporiasis, chronic intestinal (>1 month's duration)
- Kaposi's sarcoma
- Lymphoma, Burkitt's (or equivalent term); immunoblastic lymphoma (or equivalent term); primary brain lymphoma
- *Mycobacterium avium* complex or *Mycobacterium kansasii,* disseminated or extrapulmonary
- *Mycobacterium tuberculosis,* any site (pulmonary or extrapulmonary)
- *Mycobacterium,* other species or unidentified species, disseminated or extrapulmonary
- *Pneumocystis carinii* pneumonia
- Pneumonia, recurrent
- Progressive multifocal leukoencephalopathy
- *Salmonella* septicemia, recurrent
- Toxoplasmosis of brain
- Wasting syndrome due to HIV

III. Clinical Categories:

A. Category A consists of one or more of the conditions listed below in an adolescent or adult (>13 years) with documented HIV infection. Conditions listed in categories B and C must not have occurred.
- Asymptomatic HIV infection
- Persistent generalized lymphadenopathy
- Acute (primary) HIV infection with accompanying illness or history of acute HIV infection

B. Category B consists of symptomatic conditions in an HIV-infected adolescent or adult that are not included among conditions listed in clinical category C and that meet at least one of the following criteria: (a) the conditions are attributed to HIV infection or are indicative of a defect in cell-mediated immunity; or (b) the conditions are considered by physicians to have a clinical course or to require management that is complicated by HIV infection.

Examples of conditions in clinical category B include but are not limited to:
- Bacillary angiomatosis
- Oropharyngeal candidiasis (thrush)
- Vulvovaginal candidiasis, persistent, frequent, or poorly responsive to therapy
- Cervical dysplasia (moderate or severe) or cervical carcinoma in situ
- Constitutional symptoms, such as fever (38.5 °C) or diarrhea lasting >1 month
- Hairy leukoplakia
- Herpes zoster (shingles), involving at least two distinct dermatomes or more than one episode
- Idiopathic thrombocytopenic purpura
- Listeriosis
- Pelvic inflammatory disease, particularly if complicated by tubo-ovarian abscess
- Peripheral neuropathy

For classification purposes, category B conditions take precedence over those in category A. For example, someone previously treated for oral or persistent vaginal candidiasis (and who has not developed a category C disease) but who is now asymptomatic should be classified in clinical category B.

C. Category C includes the clinical conditions listed in the AIDS surveillance case definition (section II above). For classification purposes, once a category C condition has occurred, the person will remain in category C.

[1] Including the expanded AIDS surveillance case definition. Persons with AIDS-indicator conditions (category C) as well as those with AIDS-indicator CD4 T lymphocyte counts <200/μL (categories A3 or B3) have been reportable as AIDS cases in the United States and Territories since January 1, 1993.
[2] Modified from MMWR Morbid Mortal Wkly Rep 1992;41[RR-17].
[3] Sections II and III of this table are modified and reproduced, with permission, from Lawlor GL Jr, Fischer TJ, and Adelman DC (editors). *Manual of Allergy and Immunology.* Little, Brown, 1994.
[4] PGL = persistent generalized lymphadenopathy. Clinical category A includes acute (primary) HIV infection.

time course for progression of the disease may vary, with the majority of individuals remaining asymptomatic for as long as 5–10 years. Typically, up to 70% of individuals will develop AIDS after a decade of infection. The reasons why the other 30% fail to progress to full-blown AIDS within that time period are not known.

Etiology

AIDS is the consequence of a chronic retroviral infection that produces severe, life-threatening CD4 helper T lymphocyte dysfunction and destruction. The disease is caused by the human immunodeficiency virus (HIV). Virtually all HIV-infected individuals progress from health to AIDS over several years, though the immunologic determinants of the clinical fate of persons infected with HIV are unknown.

Pathology & Pathogenesis

With HIV infection there is an absolute reduction of CD4 T lymphocytes, an accompanying deficit in CD4 T lymphocyte function, and an associated increase in CD8 suppressor/cytotoxic T lymphocytes, most of which have a cytotoxic phenotype. In addition to the CD4 T lymphocyte functional defects, B lymphocyte function is also altered such that many infected individuals have marked hypergammaglobulinemia. HIV-infected patients with advanced disease (AIDS) will fail to respond normally to immunization with neoantigens. Autoantibodies and circulating immune complexes commonly are present.

Once an individual becomes infected with HIV, there is a progressive decline in CD4 T lymphocytes and a reversal of the normal CD4:CD8 T lymphocyte ratio. Between 1:10,000 and 1:1000 circulating CD4 lymphocytes are infected with HIV during the early stages of HIV infection. The percentage of HIV-infected T lymphocytes increases as the disease progresses and absolute CD4 T lymphocyte counts decline. The increase in the infected CD4 T lymphocytes is associated with an increase in viral burden as measured by p24 antigen by polymerase chain reaction (PCR) quantification or by direct viral culture of plasma.

The marked decline in CD4 T lymphocyte counts following infection is due to several mechanisms, including (1) autoimmune destruction of CD4 T lymphocytes, (2) direct viral infection and destruction of CD4 T lymphocytes, (3) depletion by fusion and formation of multinucleated giant cells (syncytium formation), (4) toxicity of viral proteins to CD4 T lymphocytes and marrow suppression, and (5) apoptosis (programmed cell death). Evidence that all of these mechanisms may potentially contribute to CD4 T lymphocyte decline exists. Data from several large clinical cohorts have shown that there is a direct correlation between the CD4 T lymphocyte count number and the risk of AIDS-defining opportunistic infections. The degree of CD4 T lymphocyte depletion serves as an important clinical indicator of immune status in HIV-infected individuals. Prophylaxis for opportunistic infections such as *Pneumocystis carinii* pneumonia is started when CD4 T lymphocyte counts reach the 200–250 cells/μL range. Similarly, patients with HIV infection with fewer than 50 CD4 T lymphocytes/μL have a significantly increased risk of developing cytomegalovirus (CMV) retinitis and *Mycobacterium avium* complex (MAC) infection.

Cells other than CD4 T lymphocytes contribute to the pathogenesis of HIV infection. Monocytes and macrophages are infected with HIV and facilitate transfer of virus to sites in the central nervous system. Lymph nodes from HIV-infected individuals can contain large amounts of virus that are sequestered around infected follicular dendritic cells in the germinal centers. Lymph nodes are centers for massive viral replication during "silent" or asymptomatic stages of HIV infection despite an absence of detectable virus in the peripheral blood. Infected mononuclear cells also show functional defects, including reduced chemotaxis and nonspecific killing capability. HIV-infected monocytes will also release large quantities of the acute phase reactant cytokines, including IL-1, IL-6, and TNF, the latter of which can contribute to marked wasting and cachexia, which are noted in patients with advanced disease.

Clinical Manifestations

The clinical manifestations of AIDS are the direct consequence of the progressive and severe immunologic deficiency induced by HIV. Systemic manifestations of **fever, night sweats,** and **weight loss** frequently occur in HIV-infected individuals. These patients can also manifest **rheumatic syndromes,** including Reiter's syndrome, psoriatic arthritis, sicca syndrome, and systemic lupus erythematosus. Other clinical manifestations of HIV include myopathy, gastrointestinal syndromes, endocrinologic dysfunction of the adrenal and thyroid glands; viral, bacterial, or fungal skin lesions; and gynecologic complications.

HIV-infected patients commonly develop fever, night sweats and weight loss even in the absence of opportunistic infections, though patients should be thoroughly evaluated to identify treatable causes. In HIV-infected patients, persistent fevers can be caused by a wide variety of diseases, including *Pneumocystis carinii* pneumonia, bacterial sepsis, and mycobacterial, cryptococcal, or cytomegalovirus (CMV) infections.

Weight loss and cachexia in advanced HIV infection are caused by anorexia, nausea, vomiting, and diarrhea. Anorexia can result from any systemic condition that produces nausea. In HIV-infected patients with more advanced immune dysfunction, nausea is often due to esophageal candidiasis and patients are frequently treated empirically with oral antifungal drugs. Progressive weight loss portends a poor prognosis for survival in patients with long-standing HIV infection.

As a direct consequence of HIV-induced immune dysfunction, the incidence of infection increases as the CD4 T lymphocyte declines. Lung infection with *Pneumocystis carinii* is the most common opportunistic infection, affecting three quarters of patients. Patients present clinically with fevers, cough, and shortness of breath ranging in severity from mild to life-threatening. A definitive diagnosis of pneumocystis pneumonia is made in 50–80% of cases by substantiation of the clinical history and physical findings with chest radiographs and Wright-Giemsa or silver methenamine staining (or both) of induced sputum samples. A negative sputum stain does not rule out disease in patients in whom there is a strong clinical suspicion of disease, and further diagnostic maneuvers such as bronchoalveolar lavage or fiberoptic transbronchial biopsy may be required to establish the diagnosis. Complications of pneumocystis pneumonia include pneumothoraces, progressive parenchymal disease with severe respiratory insufficiency, or, most commonly, adverse reactions to the medications used for treatment and prophylaxis of the infection. For reasons which are not clear, HIV-infected patients have an unusually high rate of adverse reactions to a wide variety of antibiotics and frequently develop severe debilitating cutaneous reactions.

As a consequence of chronic immune dysfunction, HIV-infected individuals are also at high risk for other pulmonary infections, including bacterial infections with *Haemophilus influenzae* and mycobacterial infections with *Mycobacterium tuberculosis* and *Mycobacterium avium-intracellulare*. Clinical suspicion followed by early diagnosis and aggressive treatment are required.

Chronic bacterial paranasal sinusitis is another common clinical problem in the HIV-infected patient. Symptoms commonly noted are headache, fever, nasal congestion, and purulent nasal discharge. Because the ethmoid sinuses have the highest incidence of involvement and are poorly visualized on plain radiographs, CT is often required to confirm the diagnosis. Prolonged treatment with antibiotics (3–6 weeks) is usually required, and in some patients surgical drainage of the sinuses may be needed.

The presence on physical examination of **oral candidiasis** and **hairy leukoplakia** is highly correlated with HIV infection and portends rapid progression to AIDS. Both oral infections result from the immunologic dysfunction associated with HIV infection. Abnormal outgrowth of *Candida* from normal mouth flora is the cause of persistent oral candidiasis, while Epstein-Barr virus is the cause of hairy leukoplakia. Neither widespread oral candidiasis nor hairy leukoplakia is commonly seen in immunocompetent individuals. HIV-infected individuals with oral candidiasis are at much greater risk for extension of the disease to the esophagus. Patients with **esophageal candidiasis** typically complain of substernal pain and dysphagia. This infection and its characteristic clinical presentation are so common that most practitioners will begin empiric oral antifungal therapy. Should the patient not respond rapidly, other (less common) explanations for the symptoms should be explored, including herpes simplex and CMV infections.

The protozoan *Cryptosporidium* is frequently implicated as the cause of the **biliary disease** typical of HIV. Cryptosporidial cholangitis may present clinically as cholecystitis, sclerosing cholangitis, or papillary stenosis.

Enterocolitis caused by bacteria (*Campylobacter, Salmonella, Shigella, Mycobacterium avium* complex), and protozoans (*Cryptosporidium, Entamoeba histolytica, Giardia lamblia*)—and even HIV itself—is a common problem associated with HIV infection. Persistent diarrhea, especially when accompanied by high fevers and abdominal pain, should be aggressively evaluated and treated when possible. HIV-associated **gastropathy** and **malabsorption** are commonly noted in these patients and are associated with decreased gastric acid production. Because of their reduced gastric acid concentrations, patients have an increased susceptibility to infection with *Campylobacter, Salmonella,* and *Shigella.*

Adrenal insufficiency associated with HIV infection is commonly due to *M avium* complex infections. Although complete adrenal insufficiency is uncommon, secretory mineralocorticoid defects may lead to salt wasting and hypokalemia that require treatment with fludrocortisone. Treatment of the underlying mycobacterial infection is usually unsuccessful because of the low susceptibility of these organisms to multidrug therapy.

Skin lesions commonly associated with HIV infection are typically classified as infectious (viral, bacterial, fungal), neoplastic, or nonspecific. Herpes simplex and herpes zoster are the most common skin lesions in HIV infection. The risk of disseminated disease appears to be correlated with the extent of immunoincompetence. Similarly, molluscum contagiosum is more likely to spread in severely immunocompromised patients. *Staphylococcus* is the cause of the **folliculitis, furunculosis,** and **bullous impetigo** commonly observed in HIV-infected patients. Because these patients are immunocompromised, aggressive treatment is required to prevent dissemination and sepsis.

Fungal skin infections commonly affect HIV-infected patients, particularly the dermatophytes and *Candida albicans* causing aggressive cutaneous fungal infections in the inguinal region. Seborrheic dermatitis is more common in HIV-infected patients and differs from that disorder in uninfected individuals in that skin scrapings from HIV-infected patients contain the fungus *Pityrosporum ovale,* which responds to topical antifungal medications.

Central nervous system manifestations in HIV-infected patients may be direct consequences of central nervous system infections or malignancies. **Toxoplasmosis** frequently causes a space-occupying lesion in HIV-infected patients. Clinically, toxoplasmosis may present as headache, altered mental status, seizures, or a focal neurologic deficit. **Cryptococcal meningitis** commonly manifests as headache and fever. Up to 90% of patients with cryptococcal meningitis exhibit a positive serum test for *Cryptococcus neoformans* antigen.

HIV-associated cognitive-motor complex, or the **AIDS dementia complex,** is the most frequently diagnosed cause of altered mental status in HIV-infected patients. Patients typically have difficulty with cognitive tasks, slowed motor function, and waxing and waning dementia. When evaluating altered mental status in these patients, it is critical that metabolic abnormalities such as hypoglycemia, hyponatremia, hypoxemia, and toxic encephalopathy due to drugs be considered and ruled out. Other causes of altered mental status include syphilis, cytomegalovirus and herpes simplex encephalitis, and progressive multifocal leukoencephalopathy.

Peripheral nervous system manifestations of HIV infection include sensory, motor, and inflammatory **polyneuropathies.** Almost a third of patients with advanced HIV disease will develop peripheral tingling, numbness, and pain in their extremities. These symptoms are likely to be due to loss of nerve axons. It is crucial that alcoholism, thyroid disease, syphilis, and vitamin B_{12} deficiency be considered when evaluating patients with peripheral neuropathies. HIV-infected patients can also develop an **inflammatory demyelinating polyneuropathy** similar to Guillain-Barré syndrome; but unlike the sensory neuropathies, the inflammatory demyelinating neuropathy typically presents before the onset of clinically apparent immunodeficiency. The origin of this condition is not known, though an autoimmune reaction is suspected because the disease typically responds favorably to treatment with plasmapheresis. Other causes of peripheral neuropathies include **cytomegalovirus ascending polyradiculopathy,** and **transverse myelitis** associated with CMV or herpes zoster.

Retinitis due to CMV infection is the most common cause of rapidly progressive visual loss in HIV infection. The diagnosis can be difficult to make, and prompt ophthalmologic consultation is warranted if ocular involvement is suspected, as minor visual disturbances can rapidly progress to blindness if left untreated.

Monarticular and **polyarticular arthritides** of unknown cause are frequently noted in HIV-infected patients. In patients with large effusions, particularly when the joint is warm to palpation, arthrocentesis may be warranted to rule out suppurative arthritis caused by bacteria, fungi, or mycobacteria. Several other rheumatologic disorders have been noted in HIV-infected patients, including Reiter's syndrome, psoriatic arthritis, sicca syndrome, and systemic lupus erythematosus. It is not clear whether the incidence of these diseases is substantially higher than in the uninfected population.

HIV-related malignancies commonly seen in AIDS include Kaposi's sarcoma, non-Hodgkin's lymphoma, primary central nervous system lymphoma, invasive cervical carcinoma, and anal squamous cell carcinoma. The mechanisms underlying the development of these associated malignancies may be similar to that of the neoplasms seen in the primary immunodeficiency disorders.

Kaposi's sarcoma is the most common HIV-associated cancer. In San Francisco, 15–20% percent of HIV-infected homosexual men develop Kaposi's sarcoma during the progression of their disease. Kaposi's sarcoma is uncommon in women and children for reasons which are not clear. Unlike "classic" Kaposi's sarcoma, which affects elderly men in the Mediterranean, Kaposi's sarcoma in HIV-infected patients may present with either localized cutaneous lesions or disseminated visceral involvement and is often a progressive and fatal disease. Histopathologically, the lesions of Kaposi's sarcoma consist of a mixed cell population that includes vascular endothelial cells. HIV appears to induce growth factors that stimulate tumor cell proliferation rather than causing malignant cellular transformation.

Clinically, cutaneous Kaposi's sarcoma typically presents as a purplish nodular skin lesion. The disease may also present as painless oral lesions. Sites of visceral involvement include the lung, lymph nodes, liver, and gastrointestinal tract. Kaposi's sarcoma lesions in the gastrointestinal tract can produce chronic blood loss and acute hemorrhage. Kaposi's sarcoma in the lung often presents as nodular coarse infiltrates bilaterally, frequently associated with pleural effusions. These infiltrates can be difficult to distinguish from opportunistic pulmonary pathogens.

Non-Hodgkin's lymphoma is particularly aggressive in HIV-infected patients. The majority of these tumors are of B lymphocyte origin and are most commonly extranodal in origin. In HIV infections, the central nervous system is the most common presenting site.

Anal dysplasia and squamous cell carcinoma are also more commonly found in HIV-infected homosexual men. These tumors appear to be associated with concomitant anal or rectal infection with **human papillomavirus (HPV).**

HIV infection also produces a variety of gynecologic manifestations. In HIV-infected women, **vaginal candidiasis, cervical dysplasia,** and **cervical neoplasia** are more common and more severe than in uninfected women. The incidence of cervical dysplasia is as high as 40% in HIV-infected women, and dysplasia can progress rapidly to cervical neoplasia.

Prompt diagnosis and treatment of dysplasia are needed, as cervical neoplasia is particularly aggressive and usually fatal in these patients.

Since the disease was first described in 1981, medical knowledge of the underlying pathogenesis of AIDS has increased at a rate unprecedented in medical history. This knowledge has led to the rapid development of novel and innovative therapies directed at destroying or controlling HIV infection as well as toward improved treatment for the multitude of complicating opportunistic infections and cancers.

21. What are the major clinical manifestations of AIDS?
22. What are the major steps in development of AIDS following infection with HIV?

REFERENCES

General

Adelman DC, Kesarwala H, Fischer TJ: Introduction to the immune system. In: *Manual of Allergy and Immunology,* 3rd ed. Lawlor GJ, Fischer TJ, Adelman DC (editors). Little, Brown, 1994.

Adelman DC, Saxon A: Immediate hypersensitivity: Approach to diagnosis. In: *Manual of Allergy and Immunology,* 3rd ed. Lawlor GJ, Fischer TJ, Adelman DC (editors). Little, Brown, 1994.

Adelman DC, Terr A: Allergic and immunologic disorders. In: *Current Medical Diagnosis and Treatment 1994.* Tierney LM, McPhee SJ, Papadakis M (editors). Appleton & Lange, 1994.

Goodman JW: The immune response. In: *Basic and Clinical Immunology,* 8th ed. Stites DP, Terr AI (editors). Appleton & Lange, 1994.

Allergic Rhinitis

Kaliner MA, Lemanske RF: Rhinitis and asthma. JAMA 1992;268:2807.

Naclerio RN: Allergic rhinitis. N Engl J Med 1991; 325:860.

Shames RS: Allergy: Mechanisms and disease processes. In: *Fundamentals of Pediatrics.* Rudolph AM, Kamei R (editors). Appleton & Lange, 1993.

Primary Immunodeficiency Diseases

Hassner A, Adelman DC: Biologic response modifiers in primary immunodeficiency disorders. Ann Intern Med 1991;115:294.

Waldman TA: Immunodeficiency diseases: primary and acquired. In: *Immunological Diseases.* Samter M et al (editors). Little, Brown, 1988.

AIDS

Barnes PJ: Pathophysiology of allergic inflammation. In: *Allergy: Principles and Practice,* 4th ed. Middleton E et al (editors). Mosby-Year Book, 1993.

Chernoff D: Human immunodeficiency virus disease and related opportunistic infections. In: *Manual of Allergy and Immunology,* 3rd ed. Lawlor GJ, Fischer TJ, Adelman DC (editors). Little, Brown, 1994.

Concorde Coordinating Committee: Concorde: MRC/ANRS randomised double-blind controlled trial of immediate and deferred zidovudine in symptom-free HIV infection. Lancet 1994;343:871.

Hollander H, Katz M: HIV infection. In: *Current Medical Diagnosis and Treatment 1994.* Tierney LM, McPhee SJ, Papadakis M (editors). Appleton & Lange, 1994.

Lifson AR, Rutherford GW, Jaffe HW: The natural history of HIV infection. J Infect Dis 1988;263:1497.

Masur HK et al: CD4 counts as predictors of opportunistic pneumonias in human immunodeficiency virus (HIV) infection. Ann Intern Med 1989;111:223.

Neoplasia

4

Debasish Tripathy, MD

Cell growth and maturation are normal events in organ development during embryogenesis, growth, and tissue repair and remodeling after injury. Disordered regulation of these processes can result in loss of control over cell growth, differentiation, and spatial confinement. Human neoplasia collectively represents a spectrum of diseases characterized by abnormal growth and invasion of cells. Although cancers are typically classified by their tissues of origin or anatomic location, many features are shared by all types. There is also considerable variation among patients with a given type of cancer in the nature of cellular alterations as well as the clinical presentation and course of disease. The recognition of overt malignancy by physical examination or imaging requires the presence in the body of about one billion malignant cells. A **preclinical phase** may sometimes be recognized. Preclinical signs may consist of (among others) polyps in the colon or dysplastic nevi on the skin—potential precursors of colon carcinoma and malignant melanoma, respectively. Such precursor lesions usually exhibit features of abnormal cell proliferation without the demonstration of invasiveness and may precede the development of an invasive malignancy by months to years—or may not progress to cancer within the individual's lifetime. More commonly, the preclinical phase goes undetected until invasive cancer, occasionally with regional or distant metastases, is already present. As is the case with other medical disorders, our understanding of the pathophysiology of neoplasia has been based on clinical and pathologic observations of large series of patients. More recently, cellular and molecular features of cancer cells have been described, and their relationships to certain neoplastic entities and clinical situations have extended our knowledge in this field.

1. What is the preclinical phase of cancer?
2. How many malignant cells must be present before overt signs of cancer are evident?

THE MOLECULAR & BIOCHEMICAL BASIS OF NEOPLASIA

The process of neoplasia is a result of stepwise alterations in cellular function. These phenotypic changes confer proliferative, invasive, and metastatic potential that are the hallmarks of cancer. It is generally believed—though not conclusively proved—that genetic alterations underlie all cellular and biochemical aberrations responsible for the malignant phenotype. An increasing number of genetic and cellular changes are being catalogued from the study of cancer cells—both in vivo, from the primary tumors of patients, and in vitro, from established cancer cell lines grown in tissue culture. Some of these changes tend to be specific to a tumor type or to a particular behavior, such as a high proliferative rate or metastatic potential. It can sometimes then be inferred—and subsequently proved experimentally—that a given genetic change can directly or indirectly lead to a certain phenotype. Some genetic alterations can be observed either across tumor types or can be seen at a high frequency or in combination with other aberrations such that the exact role of these changes cannot be easily ascertained.

3. What stepwise phenotypic changes are the hallmarks of cancer?

GENETIC CHANGES IN NEOPLASIA

Genetic changes in cancer can occur at random owing to the inherent genetic instability of malignant cells. Certain alterations, however, appear to produce or contribute to the malignant phenotype. These generally occur within the DNA base pair sequences that encode for a gene and can be broadly classified into two categories. Genes in which alterations result in a gain of function are referred to as **oncogenes,** whereas genes in which deletions or mutations result in loss of control function are defined as **tumor suppressor genes**. Activation of oncogenes and loss of tumor suppressor genes can be shown to cause cancer by several laboratory methods, including in vitro cell culture and in vivo transgenic mouse models. Oncogene activation can occur as a result of a **point mutation, chromosomal translocation,** or **amplification** of genetic material. In some instances, an oncogene may be a transcribed unaltered gene that is normally silent or expressed only in a regulated fashion during specific times, including embryogenesis and tissue repair. Alternatively, an oncogene can consist of a new **fusion gene** that is the result of a chromosomal translocation, and the corresponding **fusion protein** may exert a novel action that contributes to the malignant phenotype. Loss of tumor suppressor gene function can be the result of a **point mutation** or **frameshift mutation** or a **deletion,** either within the gene or over a large chromosomal segment that includes the tumor suppressor gene. In most instances, both tumor suppressor gene alleles must be inactivated, either by deletion or by mutation, to result in a loss of function. There is increasing evidence that human neoplasia is the result of serial oncogene activation and tumor suppressor gene inactivation. For some tumor types, stereotypical oncogene and tumor suppressor gene alterations and the order in which the alterations occur have been described.

Most genetic changes thus far described in human cancers are acquired somatic alterations seen only in the tumor cells of the affected individual. These changes can be produced by a variety of carcinogens or ionizing radiation. It is possible that some may arise without an inciting event, representing a net effect of DNA damage and natural repair processes. Populations of cells that normally exhibit a high growth fraction, such as hematopoietic and epithelial cells—or mesenchymal cells in growing children—may be particularly susceptible to genetic alterations introduced upon cellular division. In animals, many malignancies are the result of the activation or introduction of an oncogene by viral infection. In humans, however, few cancers are known to be directly caused by viral infection. One such virus, human T cell leukemia virus, is closely related to the human immunodeficiency virus and can cause a type of T cell leukemia due to proteins encoded by the viral genome which are able to activate latent human genes. Human papillomavirus has long been linked epidemiologically to cervical cancer, and the most often linked serotypes have recently been found to encode for proteins that can bind and inactivate host tumor suppressor gene products. In this situation, a causative gene is not necessarily introduced by the virus, but the viral genome is able to direct the inactivation of tumor suppressor gene products and thereby favor growth and proliferation as well as malignant potential. The ability of viruses to modulate the host cellular machinery—and in some cases retain altered mammalian genes that are oncogenic—is likely to have developed over the course of mammalian evolution, since an actively proliferating cell provides the optimal conditions for replication of virions and propagation of viral infections.

Inherited susceptibility to certain cancers has long been appreciated given the known increased risk of certain types of cancer if present in a family member. Certain tumors are passed on to progeny with high penetrance, suggesting that the genetic abnormality bears a strong causal relationship to the malignancy. Most of these rare familial malignancies are due to inherited allelic alterations of tumor suppressor genes, such that a somatic mutation or deletion in the remaining allele can then lead to expression of the malignant phenotype. Over recent years, tumor suppressor genes have been cloned and characterized through the study of families with malignancies such as retinoblastoma, neurofibromatosis (not itself a malignancy, but associated with a variety of tumors), and inherited colon cancer. The same tumor suppressor genes can be involved in much more common nonheritable malignancies. In these cases, tumor suppression gene changes are somatic and are only seen in the primary tumor and not other host cells. Oncogenes, on the other hand, have not generally been found to be inherited. One exception is the familial syndrome of **multiple endocrine neoplasia type II,** in which heterozygotes carrying an oncogene on chromosome 10 are at increased risk of developing two rare neural crest tumors: pheochromocytoma and medullary carcinoma of the thyroid.

ONCOGENES & TUMOR SUPPRESSOR GENES IN NORMAL PHYSIOLOGY & NEOPLASIA

The observation that cell-free tumor lysates could transform immortalized cells in tissue culture into cells with a more malignant phenotype has led to isolation of the responsible genetic elements. These proved to be genes that are homologous to normal human genes, termed **proto-oncogenes,** that encode for proteins responsible for a variety of physiologic cellular functions. In the altered form or in excessive amounts, however, proteins encoded by oncogenes possess deranged function which can confer proliferative or invasive properties on the cell. The functions of proteins encoded by known proto-oncogenes and their oncogene counterparts can be classified into surface membrane proteins, cytoplasmic proteins involved in signal transduction, and DNA-binding nuclear proteins that can modulate the expression of specific genes. By virtue of overexpression or activating mutation, surface membrane oncogene products can exhibit augmented or ligand-independent signal initiation compared with their physiologic counterparts. Cytoplasmic signaling modulator pro-

Table 4–1. Representative oncogenes identified in human neoplasia.[1]

Oncogene	Physiologic Function of Oncogene Product	Tumor Type
HER2/*neu*	Cell surface receptor	Breast, gastric, ovarian
ras	G protein	Lung, colonic, pancreatic
myc	Transcription factor	Multiple tumor types
fos	Transcription factor	Multiple tumor types
int-2	Morphogen	Esophageal, gastric, head and neck
RET	Tyrosine kinase	Pheochromocytoma, medullary carcinoma of the thyroid (MEN type 2)
myb	Transcription factor	Leukemia
fes	Tyrosine kinase	Leukemia

[1]Oncogenic fusion genes are listed in Table 4–8.

teins can be similarly activated. Examples of this functional class are the *ras* family members, which are G proteins capable of being maintained in an active signal-transducing state when containing certain stereotypic mutations. Table 4–1 sets forth a partial list of oncogenes identified in human malignancies along with the tumor types in which they are commonly observed and the cellular function encoded by their proto-oncogene counterparts. Not surprisingly, these proteins are integral parts of the cellular machinery involved in growth, differentiation, and entry into the S phase of the cell cycle. Other cellular functions such as the inhibition of programmed cell death have also been described. However, the disordered function of one or several of the individual components can be manifested as a malignant phenotype.

Tumor suppressor genes have been found to encode for proteins responsible for a variety of functions. These include regulatory proteins that regulate the cell cycle, adhesion proteins that govern cell-to-cell communication, and cytoplasmic proteins that modulate or attenuate signal transduction. Presumably, these functions are intended to keep the cell's proliferative and invasive potential in check. Since some cells need to proliferate, recruit vasculature, and invade tissue during embryogenesis, growth, and tissue repair, feedback mechanisms mediated by tumor suppressor gene products are presumably necessary physiologic controls. Table 4–2 presents a representative list of tumor suppressor genes, encoded functions, and tumor types in which somatic mutations or loss of function are common. Most of the tumor suppressor genes listed are also

Table 4–2. Representative tumor suppressor genes identified in human neoplasia.

Tumor Suppressor Gene	Chromosomal Location	Physiologic Function of Oncogene Product	Tumor Type
p53	17p13	Cell cycle regulator	Several
Retinoblastoma (Rb)	13q14	Cell cycle regulator	Retinoblastoma, small cell lung cancer, sarcoma
NF-1	17q11	GTPase activating protein	Sarcoma, glioma
NF-2	22q12	Membrane-cytoskeleton interface	Schwannoma
VHL	3p25	Surface receptor or cell adhesion	Hemangioblastoma, kidney, pheochromocytoma
WT-1	11p13	Transcription factor	Wilms' tumor
DCC	18q21	Cell adhesion	Colon
APC	5q21	Membrane/cell adhesion	Colon
MCC	5q21	Unknown, ? G protein	Colon
hMSH2	2p16	DNA repair	Colon
hMLH1	3p21	DNA repair	Colon
nm23	17q21	Nucleoside kinase	Colon, breast, others
BRCA-1	17q21	Unknown	Breast, ovarian

known to be involved in germline mutations that cause an inherited predisposition to one type or a spectrum of tumors. For example, the **p53 gene** encodes for a nuclear phosphoprotein involved in the regulation of the cell cycle. Abnormalities in this gene are seen in a variety of tumor types and are thus by far the most commonly observed genetic lesions in human malignancies. An inherited mutation in the p53 gene can cause the rare Li-Fraumeni syndrome, characterized by the early development of soft tissue, bone, breast, and brain tumors.

A paradigm for sequential genetic alterations has been proposed as a necessary set of events leading to tumorigenesis. These include both gain of oncogenic function and loss of tumor suppressor function, occurring in series or in parallel. The largest body of evidence to support this theory has been generated from the molecular study of colon cancer and identifiable preneoplastic lesions, including adenomas and colonic polyps. In this model, the progressive development of neoplasia from premalignant to malignant to invasive lesions is associated with an increasing number of genetic abnormalities, including both oncogene activation and tumor suppressor gene inactivation. This theory is further supported by the identification of inherited abnormalities of several tumor suppressor genes, all associated with a strong familial tendency to develop colon cancer at a young age. Molecular techniques have been used to study many tumor types, and most abnormalities of oncogenes and tumor suppressor genes have been found in more than one tumor type, though certain aberrations tend to be common in certain tumor types as outlined in Table 4–1. In some cases, changes at the gene, messenger RNA, or protein level have also been found to correlate with certain clinical features, including clinical aggressiveness and survival. Given the pivotal role of oncogenes and tumor suppressor genes in human cancer, their targeting for diagnostic and therapeutic modalities is an area of active research.

HORMONES, GROWTH FACTORS, & GROWTH INHIBITORS

Specialized proteins are required for the normal growth, maturation, development, and function of cells and specialized tissue. The complexity of the human organism requires that these proteins be expressed at precisely coordinated points in space and time. An essential component of this regulation is the system of hormones, growth factors, and growth inhibitors, hereinafter referred to collectively as **factors.** These proteins, upon binding to specific receptor proteins on the cell surface or in the cytoplasm, lead to a complex set of signals that can result in a variety of cellular effects, including mitogenesis, growth inhibition, differentiation, and the induction of a secondary set of genes. The actual end effects are not only dependent on the particular type of interacting factor and receptor but also on the cell type and milieu in which factor-receptor coupling occurs. This system allows for cell-to-cell interactions, whereby a factor secreted by one cell or tissue can influence another set of distant cells (endocrine action) or adjacent cells (paracrine action). An autocrine action is also possible when a cell produces a factor that can bind to a receptor on or in the same cell. Altered factor concentration as well as receptor mutations or overexpression can also change the signaling end effect, contributing to a malignant phenotype. Some growth factor receptors have actually been found to be the products of genes originally identified as transforming oncogenes. An example of this is the HER2/*neu* oncogene, which encodes for a receptor homologous to the epidermal growth factor receptor, yet its natural function remains unknown. Artificial overexpression of this receptor can reproduce a malignant phenotype in laboratory models. The HER2/*neu* oncogene has been found to be amplified and overexpressed in human breast, ovarian, and gastric cancers, and in some of these cancer cell lines, inhibition of its function by specific antibodies can partially inhibit cell proliferation.

Other factor systems known to have physiologic effects can also be expressed aberrantly in some human malignancies. Insulin, for example, exerts well-known metabolic effects upon binding to the insulin receptor. Overexpression of the receptor can also lead to insulin-dependent malignant transformation in transfected cell lines, yet the overexpression of the insulin receptor seen in some breast cancers is of unclear significance. Therefore, gene amplification or other transcriptional regulatory mechanisms that allow for the overexpression or enhanced function of growth factor receptors can provide a growth advantage to cells. It is plausible that these changes are favored in the clonal evolution of a tumor. Some growth factor-mediated actions are not necessarily mitogenic—such as the fibroblast growth factor system, which can induce angiogenesis. This is another example of a controlled physiologic activity that can help support tumor growth when it is aberrantly controlled.

Naturally occurring growth inhibitors such as **transforming growth factor β (TGFβ)** may also be physiologic mediators of growth suppression in situations such as embryonic development and tissue repair. Although not directly implicated in tumorigenesis, it is possible that cell responsiveness to these inhibitors may be altered in cancer.

Steroid hormones and their cytoplasmic receptors constitute separate signaling pathways that mediate normal growth, development, and metabolism and are also known to interact with other factor systems. The expression of **estrogen receptors** on certain breast tumors can predict a greater likelihood of response to hormonal therapies, and the determination of their presence is therefore useful in clinical management.

Other functional membrane proteins not related to growth can also be present on tumors cells. The MDR-1 gene product belongs to a class of ATP-dependent channel transporter proteins and is present on some normal epithelial cells. Its physiologic role may be to pump toxic molecules out of the cell, but in some tumor cells its overexpression causes efflux of certain chemotherapeutic agents, leading to drug resistance. In some situations, its expression can be induced by long-term exposure to chemotherapy.

STROMAL, ADHESIVE, & PROTEOLYTIC PROTEINS

Several structural proteins such as actin, which is involved in scaffolding and movement, are known to be associated with signaling surface proteins. Adhesive proteins, most notably a class known as the **integrins,** are also felt to be involved in signaling to the nucleus. It is also likely that these interactions are altered in malignancy. Stromal proteins that constitute extracellular matrix, including basement membrane, are necessary for normal cell anchorage and separation of epithelial layers. Highly regulated proteolytic enzymes normally coordinate tissue remodeling at times of development, physical stress, or damage. In neoplasia, abnormal cell growth is also accompanied by cell invasion and the establishment of metastatic colonies. The invasive phenotype is therefore due in part to abnormalities of stromal proteins and disruption of the basement membrane. There is now evidence that these alterations can be directed by malignant tumor cells through elaboration of soluble factors that cause the synthesis and release of proteolytic enzymes by surrounding stroma. Likewise, tumor cells may be able to recruit other activities, such as angiogenesis, necessary to form a metastatic focus.

CELLULAR CHANGES IN NEOPLASIA

Functional and morphologic changes accompany molecular and biochemical changes in malignancy at both the cellular and tissue levels. These abnormalities may exist in a spectrum from normal to preinvasive to frankly malignant and invasive cells. Tissue architecture is also disrupted by the abnormal growth and invasive capacity of malignant cells. This disruption results in a violation of the normal microanatomy at the site of origin of the tumor and at the site of distant metastases. At both sites, the tumor cells not only possess the capacity to proliferate abnormally but also to break tissue boundaries such as the basement membrane in the case of epithelial malignancies.

Molecular and cellular changes in tumor cells are, in a sense, a modification of normal physiology that benefits their growth and spread. The initial alterations may be "preprogrammed" in rare inherited malignancies, or they may be acquired as a consequence of mutations brought about by environmental exposure or occurring by chance during normal cell division. In a process akin to evolution, albeit in a fast time frame, additional genetic changes occur that favor further growth, invasion, and spread. Evasion of the host's immune system, enhanced proliferative and invasive potential, and resistance to therapy are examples of early, middle, and late changes in the progression of neoplasia.

4. What is an oncogene?
5. What is a tumor suppressor gene?
6. What are the genetic mechanisms by which oncogenes can be activated or tumor suppressor genes inactivated?
7. Which is the more common mechanism of oncogene activation in humans, viral infection or somatic alteration?
8. What is a potential molecular explanation for the epidemiologic correlation of human papilloma virus infection with cervical cancer?
9. What is the molecular basis for most inherited susceptibilities to certain cancers?
10. Name some factors which support or inhibit tumor growth, although not directly implicated in tumorigenesis.
11. What is the role of proteolytic enzymes in metastasis?
12. Give some examples of early, middle, and late changes in the progression of neoplasia.

PATHOPHYSIOLOGY OF NEOPLASIA

The common property of all neoplasia is uncontrolled growth and invasion. From both the clinical and the pathophysiologic standpoints, the tissue type from which the malignant cells originate is also associated with certain unique characteristics. This uniqueness is due to underlying normal architecture and machinery possessed by the cells and tissue from which the tumor originates. Three general classifications of neoplasia have been chosen in this chapter to highlight the pathophysiology of all types of neoplasia: (1) epithelial neoplasia; (2) mesenchymal, neuroendocrine, and germ cell neoplasia; and (3) hematologic neoplasia. The malignant potential of these cells is related to the proliferative rate and perhaps to exposure to environmental, dietary, and endogenous hormonal or growth factor stimuli. In the growing infant and child, mesenchymal tumors from growing muscle, cartilage, and bone are common, whereas in adults, tumors arising from epithelial elements in the colon, lung, breast, and prostate predominate.

EPITHELIAL NEOPLASIA

Epithelial cells are in constant turnover, arising from a basal layer that continually generates new cells. The mature and functional layer of cells performs specialized tissue or organ functions, and with senescence is eventually sloughed off. Proliferating epithelial cells normally observe anatomic boundaries such as the basement membrane that underlies the basal layer. The potential to divide, migrate, and differentiate is tightly controlled. The stimulus to divide may be autonomous or exogenous as a response to factors from adjacent or distant cells. The neoplastic phenotype of epithelial cells can be seen as a spectrum from **hyperplasia** to **preinvasive** to frankly **invasive and metastatic** neoplasia as illustrated in Figure 4–1. By convention, malignancies of epithelial origin are termed **carcinomas.** Hyperplasia can be a normal physiologic response in some situations, such as that which occurs in the lining of the uterus in response to estrogens prior to the ovulatory phase of the menstrual cycle. It may also be a pathologic finding and associated with a predisposition to progress to invasive carcinoma. In such instances of hyperplasia, there are usually accompanying disorders of maturation that may be recognizable by microscopic examination. These changes are termed **dysplasia, atypical hyperplasia,** or **metaplasia,** depending on the type of epithelium in which they are observed. More aggressive proliferation without the ability to invade through the basement membrane is termed **preinvasive carcinoma,** or **carcinoma in situ.** Technically, these cells do not have the capacity to metastasize, though they may progress to invasive carcinoma over time. The term **invasive carcinoma** implies that tissue boundaries, especially the basement membrane, have been breached. **Metastatic carcinoma** occurs via the lymphatic system to regional lymph nodes and via the bloodstream to distant organs and other tissues. This pattern of metastasis, however, is not unique to epithelial malignancies. Epithelial neoplasms in general have a variable propensity to spread to regional nodes and distant sites. It is assumed that the natural history of most tumors is to follow this pattern of spread over time. The specific genotypic and phenotypic changes necessary to accomplish this spread are not well understood and may in some cases be shared across tumor types and in other cases are unique to a given neoplasia. Certain molecular characteristics have been linked to clinical characteristics, though the exact mode of action is not fully understood.

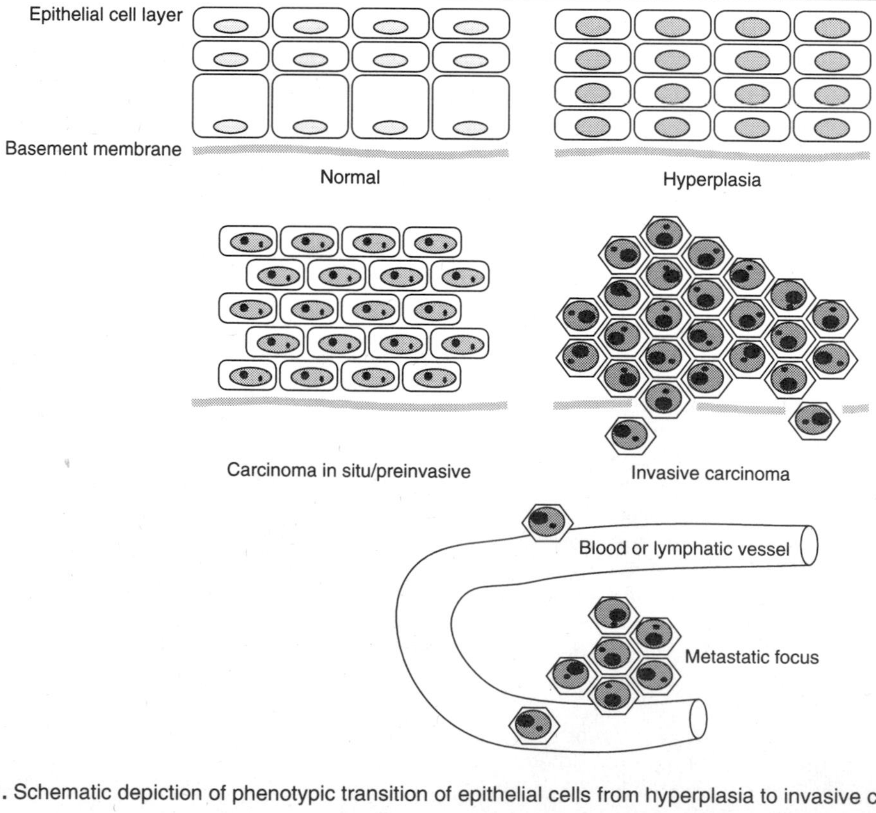

Figure 4–1. Schematic depiction of phenotypic transition of epithelial cells from hyperplasia to invasive carcinoma.

From a pathophysiologic standpoint, certain structural and functional characteristics must be acquired by malignant cells as outlined in Table 4–4. An increase in growth rate through several mechanisms has been described for different tumor types. It is known that the proliferative fraction (the percentage of cells in S phase, or actively synthesizing DNA) is elevated—and more so in histologically and clinically aggressive tumors. Changes in the tightly regulated cell cycle machinery have been observed, including abnormal levels of **cyclins** and other proteins that bind to kinases responsible for entry of the cell into S phase. Likewise, alterations of intermediate signaling proteins have been noted that couple external growth factor and hormonal stimuli to proliferation. The ability of cells to migrate and pass through cellular and extracellular matrix barriers can be enhanced in tumor cells. This can occur through the activation of proteolytic enzyme cascades from within the tumor cell or by the action of stromal cells that are directed to do so as a result of factors produced by nearby tumor cells. Through similar mechanisms, malignant cells can induce the formation of a microvasculature that is essential to support the continued growth of a tumor colony. Other functions necessary to breach the immune defenses and survive destruction by antitumor drugs can be mediated by genetic factors already possessed in latent form by tumor cells. Examples include modulation of antigens and alterations in drug metabolism or metabolic pathways that are targeted by certain drugs.

As described earlier, there is evidence that discrete phenotypic changes which arise from specific genetic alterations account for the progression from hyperplasia to metastatic neoplasia. Moreover, there is an interplay between these genetic changes and the inherent program of gene expression of a given epithelial type. This creates a specific spectrum of anatomic, pathophysiologic, and clinical entities for neoplasia of each epithelial type as listed in Table 4–3. Other highly regulated functions of epithelial cells include active or passive transport of ions or

Table 4–3. Epithelial neoplasia.

Epithelial Type	Hyperplasia or Dysplasia	Preinvasive	Invasive
Head and neck	Leukoplakia, erythroplakia (these lesions may contain dysplasia or carcinoma in situ)		Squamous cell carcinoma
Lung	Squamous metaplasia	Carcinoma in situ	Non-small cell carcinoma (squamous cell or adenocarcinoma)
Esophagus	Barrett's esophagus, chronic scarring	Carcinoma in situ	Squamous cell or adenocarcinoma
Stomach	Gastric ulcer, ?*Helicobacter pylori* infection	Carcinoma in situ	Adenocarcinoma
Colon	Adenomatous polyp	Carcinoma in situ (may be within polyp)	Adenocarcinoma
Liver and biliary tree	Hepatonodular liver regeneration, cirrhosis, biliary inflammation	Carcinoma in situ (biliary tree and gallbladder)	Adenocarcinoma
Exocrine pancreas	Chronic pancreatitis	Not seen clinically	Adenocarcinoma
Anus	Condyloma (anogenital warts)	Carcinoma in situ	Squamous cell or cuboidal (cloacogenic) carcinoma
Cervix	Dysplasia (cervical intraepithelial neoplasia grades I and II)	Carcinoma in situ (cervical intraepithelial neoplasia grade III)	Squamous carcinoma (rarely adenocarcinoma)
Uterus	Hyperplasia	Carcinoma in situ	Adenocarcinoma
Ovary	Preneoplastic ovary; epithelial lesions not seen clinically		Adenocarcinoma
Breast	Atypical hyperplasia	Ductal or lobular carcinoma in situ	Infiltrating ductal or lobular adenocarcinoma
Bladder and ureter	Hyperplasia, atypical hyperplasia and dysplasia	Carcinoma in situ	Squamous cell, transitional cell, or adenocarcinoma
Kidney	Papillary hyperplasia	Not seen clinically	Adenocarcinoma
Prostate	Prostatic hypertrophy	Not seen clinically	Adenocarcinoma
Skin	Many clinical entities, including actinic keratosis, acanthoma, cutaneous horn, and Bowen's disease	Carcinoma in situ	Basal cell and squamous cell carcinoma

Table 4–4. Serial phenotypic changes in the progression of neoplasia.

1. Enhanced proliferation
   - Autonomous growth
   - Abnormalities of cell cycle control
   - Exaggerated response to hormonal or growth factor stimuli
   - Lack of response to growth inhibitors or cell contact inhibition
2. Evasion of immune system
   - Antigen modulation and masking
   - Elaboration of immune response antagonistic molecules
3. Invasion of tissue and stroma
   - Attachment to extracellular matrix
   - Secretion of proteolytic enzymes
   - Recruitment of stromal cells to produce proteolytic enzymes
   - Loss of cell cohesion
4. Ability to gain access to and egress from lymphatics and bloodstream
   - Enhanced cell motility
   - Recognition of endothelial protein sequences
   - Cytoskeletal modifications
5. Establishment of metastatic foci
   - Cell adhesion and attachment
   - Tissue-specific tropism
6. Ability to recruit vascularization to support growth of primary or metastatic tumor
7. Drug resistance
   - Altered drug metabolism and drug inactivation
   - Increased synthesis of targeted enzymes
   - Enhanced drug efflux
   - Enhanced DNA damage repair

molecules as well as the synthesis and secretion of specific proteins. These functions may also be lost, altered, or even enhanced for specific tumor types and likewise can create specific pathophysiologic and clinical entities. Two epithelial neoplasms are discussed in further detail. Colon cancer is an example of an epithelial neoplasm for which precursor lesions have been well studied because we can seek out and biopsy such lesions by colonoscopy. Breast epithelial tissue is responsive to steroid hormones and growth factors which may play a role in the development and behavior of breast cancer.

13. What factors determine the malignant potential of epithelial vs mesenchymal tumors?
14. What is the term applied to malignancies of epithelial origin?
15. What is the spectrum of characteristics of the neoplastic phenotype in epithelial cells?

1. COLON CARCINOMA

The model of stepwise genetic alterations in cancer is best illustrated by observations made in colonic lesions representing different stages of progression to malignancy. Certain genetic alterations are found commonly in early stage adenomas, while others tend to occur with significant frequency only after the development of invasive carcinoma. These changes are in keeping with the concept that serial phenotypic changes must occur in a cell for it to exhibit full malignant properties (Table 4–4). One early alteration seen in adenomas is a point mutation in the *ras* gene that results in enhanced cytoplasmic signaling. The end result of this mutation is not known, but it appears to be associated with a more rapid cell division rate. A later genetic abnormality is the loss of part or all of the *DCC* gene, which encodes for an adhesive protein. This may contribute to the loss of cell cohesion and the tendency to metastasize, an expected phenotypic change late in the neoplastic pathway.

Two principal lines of evidence support the model of stepwise genetic alterations in colon cancer:

(1) The rare familial syndromes associated with predisposition to colon cancer at an early age are now known to result from germline mutations. **Familial adenomatous polyposis** is the result of a mutation in the *APC* gene. In the tumors that subsequently develop, the remaining allele has been lost. Similarly, **hereditary nonpolyposis colorectal cancer** is associated with germline mutations in the *hMSH2* and *hMLH1* genes, which encode for DNA repair enzymes. These genes can also be affected in sporadic cancers.

(2) The carcinogenic effects of factors known to be linked to an increased risk of developing colon cancer constitute the second line of evidence for a genetic basis for colon cancer. Substances derived from bacterial colonic flora, ingested foods, or endogenous metabolites such as fecapentaenes, 3-ketosteroids, and benzo[*a*]pyrenes are mutagenic. Levels of these substances can be reduced by low-fat and high-fiber diets, and several epidemiologic studies confirm that such diets reduce the risk of colon cancer. Furthermore, since the risk of sporadic colon cancer in older individuals is mildly elevated in the presence of a positive family history, there may be other inherited genetic abnormalities that interact with environmental factors to cause colon cancer. The sequence of genetic changes may not need to be exact to lead to the development of an invasive cancer, though there is mounting evidence that some genetic lesions tend to develop early, while others may develop late in the course of the natural disease. At present, all phenotypic changes cannot be explained by a known genetic abnormality, nor do all identified genetic alterations have a known phenotypic result.

The earliest change in the progression to colon cancer is the increase in cell number (hyperplasia) on the epithelial (luminal) surface. This produces an **adenoma,** which is characterized by gland-forming cells exhibiting increases in size and cell number but no invasion of surrounding structures (Figure 4–2).

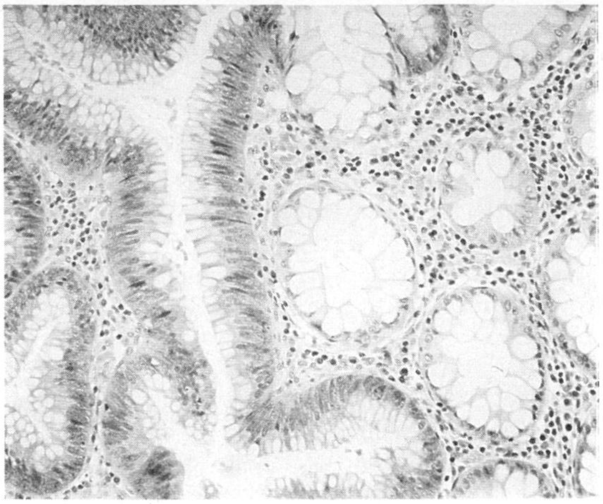

Figure 4–2. Edge of an adenomatous polyp, showing adenomatous change (left), compared with normal mucosal glands (right). Adenomatous change is characterized by increased size and stratification of nuclei and loss of cytoplasmic mucin. Note arrangement of nuclei of the adenoma perpendicular to the basement membrane (polarity). (Reproduced, with permission, from Chandrasoma P, Taylor CE: *Concise Pathology,* 2nd ed. Appleton & Lange, 1995.)

Presumably, these changes are due to enhanced proliferation and loss of cell cycle control but prior to acquisition of the capacity to invade extracellular matrix. Additional dysplastic changes such as loss of mucin production and altered cell polarity may be present to a variable degree. Some adenomas may progress to carcinoma in situ and ultimately to invasive carcinoma. An early feature associated with disrupted architecture even before invasion occurs is the development of fragile new vessels or destruction of existing vessels that can cause microscopic bleeding. This can be tested for clinically as a fecal occult blood determination used for screening and early diagnosis of preinvasive and invasive colon cancer. It is not known if all invasive colon cancers pass through a hyperplastic or preinvasive stage, nor is this information available for epithelial malignancies in general.

Further functional changes in the cell and surrounding tissue are also manifested in the preinvasive and invasive stage. Once the basement membrane is penetrated by invasive malignant cells, access can be gained to the regional lymphatics and spread to regional pericolic lymph nodes can occur. Entry of cells into the bloodstream can lead to distant spread in a pattern that reflects venous drainage. Therefore, hematogenous spread from primary colon tumors to the liver is common, whereas rectal tumors usually disseminate to liver, lung, and bone. In addition to anatomic considerations, there may exist specific tropism of malignant cells mediated by surface proteins that cause the cells to preferentially home in on certain organs or sites.

Colonic epithelium is specialized to secrete digestive enzymes and mucus proteins and to absorb specific nutrients (Chapter 9). The maintenance of a tight luminal barrier, intracellular charge differences, and the ability to exclude toxins are additional specialized functions. Some of these functions are maintained in the progression to neoplasia and may contribute to a specific phenotype of the malignant cell. One example is the expression of a transporter membrane protein, MDR-1, present on several types of epithelium including the colon. MDR-1 is known to cause the efflux of several compounds out of the cells, presumably as a protective mechanism to exclude toxins. In advanced colon cancer, this protein may contribute to the relative resistance of this and other tumor types to a variety of chemotherapeutic agents that are transported by MDR-1. In some cases, the activation of a latent gene encoding **carcinoembryonic antigen** (CEA) can result in measurable levels of the CEA protein in the serum of patients with localized or metastatic colon cancer as well as other adenocarcinomas.

16. What are the two principal lines of evidence in favor of the model of stepwise genetic alterations in colon cancer?
17. What is an explanation for the frequent appearance of occult blood in stools of patients with even early colon carcinoma?
18. What are two genes whose products contribute to the classic phenotype of colon carcinomas?

2. BREAST CARCINOMA

The breast is a specialized gland that develops after female puberty out of rudimentary ducts emanating downward from the nipples. Acinar cells and the terminal ductule they surround compose the lobular unit from which most breast carcinomas arise. Breast tissue also responds to menstrual cycling of estrogen and progesterone, but both epithelial and stromal cells are also under the control of a variety of growth factors, including insulin-like growth factor-1 (IGF-1) and TGFβ. **Hypertrophy** of breast epithelial cells in response to preovulatory estrogen surge and **hyperplasia** during pregnancy are examples of physiologic responses. Early stages of disordered growth through loss of cell cycle control or abnormalities in hormonal or growth factor response can result in benign proliferative changes such as adenosis or apocrine metaplasia. These changes by themselves are not necessarily associated with an increased risk of the subsequent development of breast cancer. Breast epithelial hyperplasia in the absence of pregnancy is associated with an increased risk of carcinoma, especially if cell atypia is present.

Factors associated with an increased risk of breast cancer development may provide clues to early driving forces. Prolonged usage of high doses of exogenous estrogen is a risk factor that implicates some excessive mitogenic stimulus. Increased risk with a positive family history of breast cancer, as with other cancers, is evidence that inherited genes may on their own—or in concert with environmental factors—represent key steps toward breast neoplasia.

The scheme depicted in Figure 4–1 applies to progressive changes toward invasive breast carcinoma, and this full spectrum may be seen in patients who undergo biopsy to evaluate breast masses or mammographic abnormalities. Carcinoma in situ of the breast represents a preinvasive lesion in which enhanced proliferation and malignant cell morphology are observed but no invasion of the basement membrane can be demonstrated. Therefore, lymph nodal or distant metastases cannot occur at this stage, presumably because the invasive phenotype has not yet been acquired. Certain molecular abnormalities can be seen at this stage, including HER2/*neu* oncogene overexpression and p53 tumor suppressor gene mutations, though the mechanisms through which these abnormalities operate are not well understood.

The pathophysiology of breast cancer is illustrative of how stromal cells can be recruited to propagate tumor growth and invasion. A dense reaction of fibroblasts and extracellular matrix by breast tumors **(desmoplastic response)** can occasionally be seen. Soluble factors suspected of mediating this response include **TGFβ** and **platelet-derived growth factor (PGDF),** which are known to be secreted by breast tumor cells or nearby stromal cells in response to tumor cells. The desmoplastic response may be a mechanism to wall off the tumor or, conversely, may actually facilitate growth and cell migration. Stromal cell production of the metalloprotease **stromolysin 3** is elicited by uncharacterized soluble factors produced by breast tumor cells. Stromolysin 3 may be pivotal in allowing tumor cells to penetrate the basement membrane or blood and lymphatic vessels. Angiogenic factors such as fibroblast growth factor can also be produced by tumor or stromal cells and promote the formation of the new microvasculature that is necessary to support a growing tumor colony in the breast or site of metastases.

The overexpression of HER2/*neu,* a growth factor receptor oncogene product, is associated with a higher growth rate and more aggressive clinical behavior. This suggests that in excessive amounts HER2/*neu* as a growth factor receptor turns on the cell division machinery in an exaggerated fashion. This may occur in response to its natural ligand or independently of any outside stimulus. Loss of expression of ***nm* 23,** which encodes for a nucleoside kinase, has been linked to an increased likelihood of lymph node metastases as well as a lower survival rate. This putative tumor suppressor gene may therefore behave as an "antimetastasis gene" such that loss of its function could lead to increased potential for invasion and metastasis, though its mode of function remains unknown. The spread of tumor cells past the basement membrane to regional lymph nodes and to distant organs is therefore the result of several discrete changes in cellular function. The tendency for breast cancer to metastasize to certain organs such as bone, lung, and liver may be a result of cell surface recognition proteins on both tumor cells and target tissue cells. The **integrins** are a class of widely expressed adhesion and recognition proteins that may be altered in malignancy and may mediate invasion and distant metastases. Furthermore, the ability of a metastatic focus to continue to grow to a clinically significant size requires additional phenotypic changes, which may explain the clinical variability in the course of advanced cancer between tumor types and from patient to patient.

MESENCHYMAL, NEUROENDOCRINE, & GERM CELL NEOPLASIA

The pathophysiology of certain types of neoplasia can be described in terms of the embryonic tissue of origin. Table 4–5 is a representative list of mesenchymal, neuroendocrine, and germ cell tumors and the embryologic cell groups from which they arise. Owing to the extensive migration and convolution of embryonic cell layers during early development, these tumor types may not evolve in specific anatomic sites. Mesenchymal, neuroendocrine, and germ cell neoplasms account for a large proportion of the tumors of childhood and young adulthood, ostensibly because these cells are actively dividing and more subject to mutational events. These tumor cells may produce specific proteins or appear morphologically similar to normal cells that derive from the same germ layer. Alternatively, they may exhibit no differentiated features at all or may maintain the ability to differentiate in an array of different directions.

1. CARCINOID TUMORS

Carcinoid tumors arise from neural crest tissue and, more specifically, from enterochromaffin cells, whose final resting place after embryonic migration is along the submucosal layer of the intestines and pulmonary bronchi. Reflecting this embryonic origin, carcinoid cells express the necessary enzymes to produce bioactive amines such as **5-hydroxytryptamine** and other vasoactive serotonin metabolites as well as a variety of small peptide hormones. Cytoplasmic granules typical of neuroendocrine cells are also

Table 4–5. Neoplasia of mesenchymal, neuroendocrine, and germ cells.

Neoplasia Type	Embryonic Derivation
Wilms' tumor	Metanephric blastema
Neuroblastoma Retinoblastoma Ganglioneuroma	Neuroblasts
Neuroendocrine tumors Small cell carcinoma Ewing's sarcoma Primitive neuroectodermal tumor Malignant melanoma Pheochromocytoma Carcinoid Gastrointestinal endocrine tumors Insulinoma Glucagonoma Somatostatinoma Gastrinoma VIPoma, GRFoma Pituitary tumors	Neural crest
Intracranial brain tumors Glioblastoma/astrocytoma Ependymoma, oligodendroglioma, medulloblastoma	Glial precursors
Germ cell tumors Teratoma (benign) Germinoma, dysgerminoma Testicular, extragonadal germ cell tumors Seminoma Choriocarcinoma Embryonal carcinoma Endodermal sinus, yolk sac tumors Ovarian germ cell tumors	Germ cell
Sarcomas	Mesenchymal cell
Rhabdomyosarcoma	Striated muscle
Leiomyosarcoma	Smooth muscle
Liposarcoma	Adipocyte
Osteosarcoma	Osteoblast
Chondrosarcoma	Chondrocyte
Malignant fibrous histiocytoma	Fibroblast
Synovial sarcoma	Synovial cell
Lymphangiosarcoma	Lymphatic endothelium
Hemangiosarcoma	Blood vessel endothelium
Kaposi's sarcoma	Endothelial cell + fibroblasts?
Hepatoblastoma	Mesenchymal cell + hepatocytes
Mesothelioma	Mesothelial cell
Schwannoma	Peripheral nerve sheath
Meningioma	Arachnoidal fibroblast

commonly seen. These features may also be shared by other tumors of neural crest origin. In contrast to epithelial neoplasms, morphologic changes observed with the light microscope do not distinguish between malignant and benign cells. The anatomic distribution of primary carcinoid tumors is consistent with embryonic development patterns as listed in Table 4–6. Carcinoid tumors and other mesenchymal neoplasms have similar patterns of tissue invasion followed by local and distant spread to regional lymph nodes and distant organs. The characteristics of increased mitotic count (an indicator of rapid proliferation), nuclear pleomorphism, lymphatic and vascular invasion, and an undifferentiated growth pattern are associated with a higher rate of metastases and a poorer clinical prognosis.

A frequent site of carcinoid metastasis is the liver. In this setting, especially with midgut carcinoid, there can be a constellation of symptoms **(carcinoid syndrome)** as a consequence of substances secreted into the blood (Table 4–7). These substances reflect the neuroendocrine origin of carcinoid and the latent machinery that can be activated inappropriately in the malignant state. Many of these peptides are vasoactive and can cause intermittent flushing as a result of vasodilation. Other symptoms often observed

Table 4–6. Carcinoid tumor location by site of embryonic origin.

Foregut	Midgut	Hindgut
Esophagus	Jejunum	Rectum
Stomach	Ileum	
Duodenum	Appendix	
Pancreas	Colon	
Gallbladder and bile duct	Liver	
Ampulla of Vater	Ovary	
Larynx	Testes	
Bronchus	Cervix	
Thymus		

include secretory diarrhea, wheezing, and excessive salivation or lacrimation. Long-term tissue damage can also occur by exposure to these substances and their metabolites. Fibrosis of the pulmonary and tricuspid heart valves, mesenteric fibrosis, and hyperkeratosis of the skin have all been reported in patients with carcinoid syndrome. A urinary marker commonly used to aid in the diagnosis or to follow patients being treated is a metabolite of serotonin, **5-hydroxyindoleacetic acid (5-HIAA),** since the production of serotonin is also characteristic of carcinoid and other neuroendocrine tumors that are able to take up and decarboxylate amine precursors.

19. What are some of the hormones and growth factors to which breast tissue responds?
20. What are some factors associated with increased risk of breast cancer?
21. How do stromal cells contribute to the propagation of breast cancer growth?
22. To what tissues do breast cancers tend to metastasize and why?
23. What products produced by carcinoid tumors reflect their embryonic origin?
24. What are some common short-term symptoms and long-term complications precipitated by release of excessive amounts of these products?

2. TESTICULAR CANCER

Testicular cancer arises chiefly from germinal elements within the testes. Germ cells are the population of cells that give rise to spermatozoa through meiotic division and can therefore theoretically retain the ability to differentiate into any cell type. Some testicular neoplasms arise from remnant tissue outside the testes owing to the midline migration of germline epithelium that occurs during early embryogenesis. This is followed by the formation of the urogenital ridge and eventually by the aggregation of germline cells in the ovary or testes. As predicted by this pattern of migration, extragonadal testicular neoplasms are found in the midline axis of the lower cranium, mediastinum, or retroperitoneum. The pluripotent ability of the germ cell—ie, the ability of one cell to give rise to an entire organism—is most evident in benign germ cell tumors such as **mature teratomas.** These tumors often contain differentiated elements from all three germ cell layers, including teeth and hair in lesions termed **dermoid cysts.** Malignant teratomas can also exist as a spectrum bridging other germ cell layer-derived neoplasms such as sarcomas and epithelium-derived carcinomas. Malignant testicular cancers may coexist with benign mature teratomas, and the benign component sometimes becomes apparent only after the malignancy has been eradicated with chemotherapy.

Proteins expressed during embryonic or trophoblastic development such as alpha-fetoprotein and human chorionic gonadotropin can be secreted and measured in the serum. Testicular carcinoma follows a lymphatic and hematogenous pattern of spread to regional retroperitoneal nodes and distant organs such as lung, liver, bone, and brain. The exquisite sensitivity of even advanced testicular cancers to radiation and chemotherapy may be a result of the foreign nature of malignant germ cells when present in a mature organism. This foreign nature may create more specific activity of cytotoxic insults and stimulate a more vigorous immune rejection of tumor.

25. From what cellular elements of the testes does testicular cancer generally arise?
26. How can the peculiar distribution of extragonadal testicular tumors be explained?
27. What are some characteristic markers that may be followed in testicular tumor progression?

Table 4–7. Peptides secreted by carcinoid cells.

Adrenocorticotropic hormone (ACTH)
Calcitonin
Gastrin
Glicentin
Glucagon
Growth hormone
Insulin
Melanocyte-stimulating hormone (β-MSH)
Motilin
Neuropeptide K
Neurotensin
Somatostatin
Pancreatic polypeptide
Pastrin
Substance K
Substance P
Vasoactive intestinal polypeptide

3. SARCOMAS

The sarcomas consist of a family of mesenchymal neoplasms whose morphologic appearance and anatomic distribution mirror the early mesenchymal elements from which they derive (Table 4–5). They arise in structures composed of the mesenchymal cell type or in locations where remnant cells eventually come to rest in the path of early tissue migration. Several of the less mature sarcomas that resemble more primitive cells are seen in children, since this compartment of cells is usually dividing more rapidly. These sarcomas include **rhabdomyosarcoma** and **osteosarcoma,** which tend to be less common in adults. The morphologic appearance of sarcomas does not involve perceptible architectural changes, since cell polarity and gland formation do not occur in normal mature mesenchymal cells such as muscle or cartilage. Nuclear pleomorphism and mitotic rate determine the grade of a tumor, with higher grade correlating with a higher propensity to invade local and distant structures and a poorer survival. Sarcomas also have a tendency to retain the cell appearance and repertoire of expressed proteins of the cell of origin. Bone matrix of calcium and phosphorus can form within osteosarcomas, and calcification of these tumors can be observed on radiography. There is less of a propensity for direct tissue invasion by sarcomas than by epithelial malignancies. However, tissue destruction can result when a sarcoma compresses but does not invade adjacent tissue, leading to the formation of a **pseudocapsule.** Sarcomas exhibit metastatic dissemination to regional lymph nodes and distant organs, especially the lungs. High-grade histologic features and anatomic location are factors influencing the likelihood and timing of metastases.

Various genetic abnormalities have been detected in sarcomas. Mutations in the **p53 tumor suppressor gene** are the most commonly detected lesion, though such changes are also seen in epithelial neoplasms. The ***NF-1* tumor suppressor gene** was originally identified through a germline mutation of this gene in patients with type I neurofibromatosis. This inherited syndrome is characterized by café au lait hyperpigmented skin spots and multiple benign **neurofibromas** (benign tumors of Schwann cells) under the skin and throughout the body. These can degenerate into malignant **neurofibrosarcomas (malignant schwannoma).** *NF-1* mutations have since been detected in sporadic sarcomas of different types. Defective or absent activity of the NF-1 protein is known to cause enhanced activation of the G protein-signaling pathways. Given the complex set of cellular activities governed by G protein-mediated pathways, the mechanisms by which NF-1 abnormalities contribute to the malignant phenotype is not known.

28. From what two kinds of locations do sarcomas arise?
29. What kinds of sarcomas are more common in children?
30. Are sarcomas more or less likely to directly invade tissues compared with epithelial malignancies?
31. To what sites do sarcomas commonly metastasize?
32. What is the most common genetic lesion in sarcomas?
33. What are the characteristics of type 1 neurofibromatosis, and what is a likely molecular basis for the development of neoplasia in this syndrome?

HEMATOLOGIC NEOPLASMS

Hematologic neoplasms are malignancies of cells derived from hematopoietic precursors. The true hematopoietic stem cell has the capacity for self-renewal and the ability to give rise to precursors **(colony-forming units)** that proliferate and terminally differentiate toward one of any lineage, as shown in Figure 4–3. Distinct hematologic neoplasms can arise from each of the mature cell types. Many of these arise in the bone marrow, circulate in the blood stream, and can infiltrate certain organs and tissues. Others may form tumors in lymphoid tissue—particularly lymphomas, which arise from lymphoblasts, as illustrated in Figure 4–4.

The cellular ultrastructure and machinery of the malignant cell can somewhat resemble that of its cell of origin. A markedly enhanced proliferative rate and arrest of differentiation are the hallmarks of these neoplasms. Examination of the interphase nucleus of cells can sometimes reveal chromosomal abnormalities such as **deletions** (monosomy), **duplications** (trisomy), or **balanced translocations.** Certain types of hematologic neoplasms tend to have stereotypical chromosomal abnormalities. Given their clonal nature, these abnormalities will be evident on all malignant cells. In some cases of chromosomal translocation, a new fusion gene is formed and can result in production of a **fusion protein** possessing abnormal function compared with the original gene products (Table 4–8). This function usually involves loss of cell cycle control, abnormal signal transduction, or reprogrammed gene expression as a result of an aberrant **transcription factor.** In contrast to hematologic malignancies, solid tumors often contain multiple chromosomal abnormalities that are not as well characterized or as reproducible. Other genetic changes described in hematologic malignancies include mutations or deletions of the p53, retinoblastoma (Rb), and Wilms (*WT1*) tumor suppressor genes and acti-

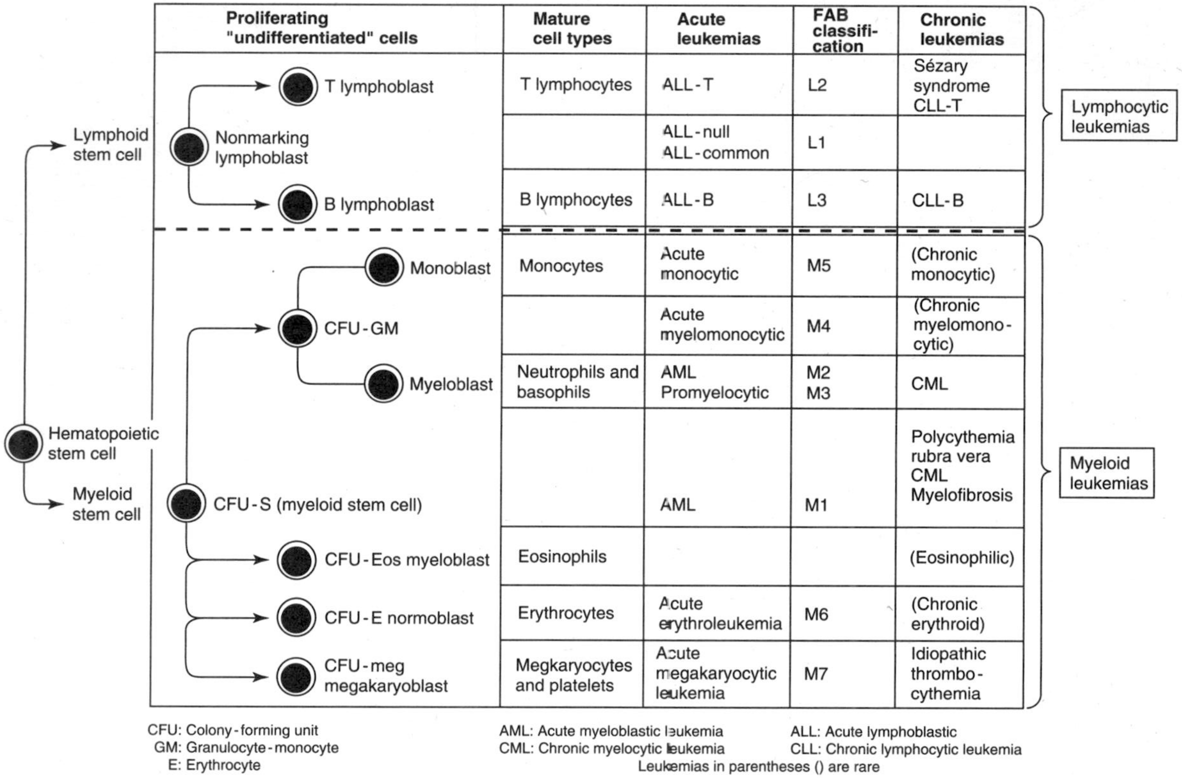

Figure 4–3. Classification of leukemias according to cell type and lineage. (Reproduced, with permission, from Chandrasoma P, Taylor CE: *Concise Pathology,* 2nd ed. Appleton & Lange, 1995.)

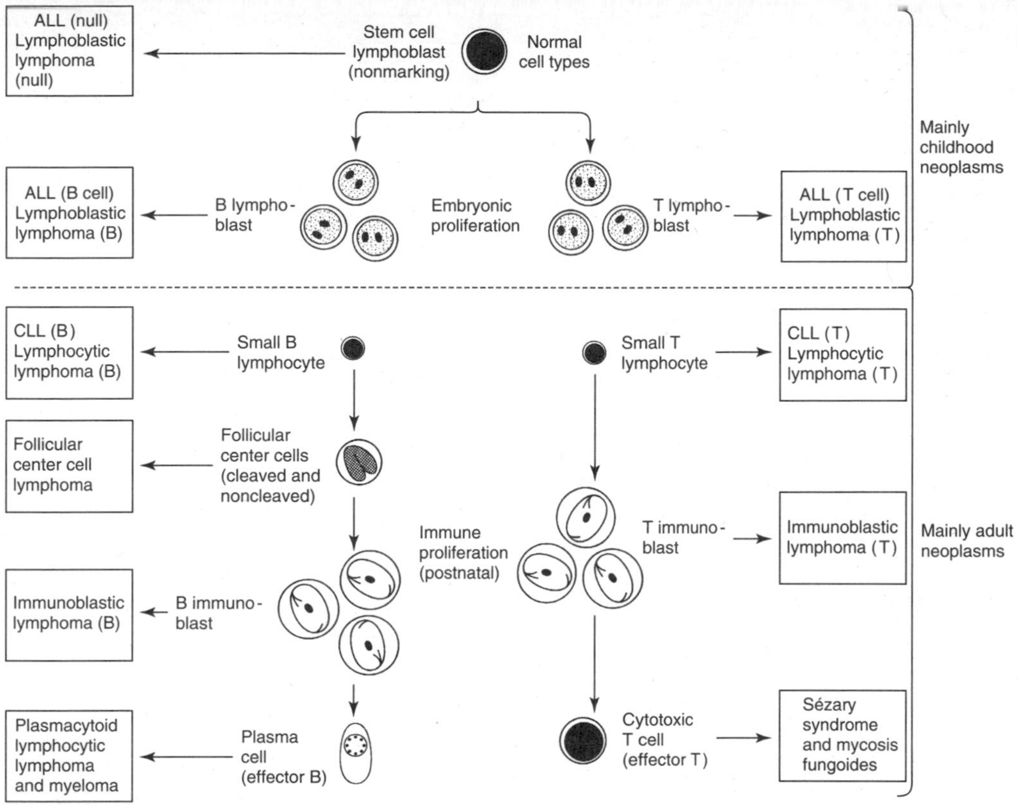

Figure 4–4. Lymphomas and leukemias derived from lymphocytes, showing relationships of the neoplastic lymphoid cells to normal lymphocyte counterparts. The cells drawn in the central area represent normal embryonic and adult lymphoid cells. Neoplasms derived from these cells are shown at top (T cell neoplasms) and bottom (B cell neoplasms). (ALL, acute lymphoblastic leukemia; CLL, chronic lymphocytic leukemia.) (Reproduced, with permission, from Chandrasoma P, Taylor CE: *Concise Pathology,* 2nd ed. Appleton & Lange, 1995.)

vating mutations in the N-*ras* oncogene. Additional genetic changes can be detected in the clonal evolution of leukemias as disease progresses to a more aggressive form in the patient's course. This finding lends further support to the theory that neoplasia is the result of stepwise genetic alterations that correspond to the sequential acquisition of additional phenotypic changes that favor abnormal growth, invasion, and resistance to normal host defenses.

1. LYMPHOMA

The lymphomas comprise a set of entities characterized by the uncontrolled proliferation and potential dissemination of lymphocytes. Normal lymphocytes are able to proliferate under conditions of antigen stimulation and migrate to specific locations such as lymph nodes or lymphoid tissue surrounding the gastrointestinal tract and other mucosal surfaces. Following this tissue tropism, lymphomas typically arise in lymph nodes, though they may also develop in other tissues or organs where lymphoid elements normally reside. Normal lymphocytes also become committed upon maturation to respond to a given antigen by rearranging genes encoding immunoglobulins in the case of B cells and surface T cell receptors in the case of T cells. Analysis of these genes can prove that a given lymphoma population is clonal, or derived from a single cell, as would be expected in a dividing neoplasm. The association of lymphoma with AIDS has raised the possibility that chronic immune stimulation or modulation may be an early step in lymphomagenesis. This is further supported by the increased risk of developing lymphoma in patients with an assortment of autoimmune diseases. Iatrogenic immunosuppression in transplant patients can also increase the risk of B cell lymphoma, often seen with evidence of infection with the Epstein-Barr virus, though a causal relationship of the virus with lymphoma remains controversial. Many classification schemes for lymphomas have been devised, addressing different characteristics such as morphology, cell of origin, and cell surface

Table 4–8. Chromosomal translocations of hematologic neoplasms.

Neoplasm	Chromosomal Translocation	Fusion Gene Resulting From Translocation	Fusion Protein Function
Follicular lymphoma	t(14;18)	IgH-*bcl*-2	Inhibitor of apoptosis
Follicular lymphoma	t(11;14)	IgH-*bcl*-1	Cyclin
Follicular lymphoma	t(14;19)	IgH-*bcl*-3	Transcription inhibitor
Burkitt's lymphoma	t(8;14)	IgH-*myc*	Transcription factor
CML	t(9;22)	*bcr-abl*	Tyrosine kinase
AML M3	t(15;17)	*PML-RAR*	Transcription factor
AML	t(8;21)	*AML*1	Unknown
T cell ALL	t(1;14)	*tal-1*-TCR	Transcription factor

Key: IgH = immunoglobulin heavy chain enhancer; TCR = T cell receptor.

antigen expression. Themost commonly used is the clinical and treatment-based Working Formulation as listed in Table 4–9. Staging is based on the extent of spread by clinical (physical examination plus radiographic studies) or surgical methods.

Lymphomas classified as well-differentiated or **low-grade** retain the morphology and patterns of gene expression of mature lymphocytes. Surface immunoglobulin in the case of B cell lymphomas and surface T cell receptor in the case of T cell lymphomas can usually be demonstrated. The appearance of individual malignant lymphocytes as well as the follicular architecture of the tumor reflect the preserved function of the cells. A slower growth rate and more favorable clinical course is also seen in low-grade lymphomas. Paradoxically, there is a tendency for patients with low-grade lymphomas to present at a more advanced stage than those with high-grade lymphoma. A common chromosomal translocation seen in low-grade follicular lymphomas juxtaposes the immunoglobulin heavy chain enhancer on chromosome 14 in front of the *bcl-2* gene on chromosome 18, leading to enhanced expression of an inner mitochondrial protein encoded by *bcl*-2. This protein has been found to inhibit the natural process of programmed cell death, morphologically recognized as **apoptosis.** Apoptosis is required to expunge certain lymphoid clones whose function is not needed, and disordered regulation of this process may be a contributing feature in low-grade lymphomas.

Table 4–9. The working formulation of non-Hodgkin's lymphomas for clinical use.[1,2]

Low-grade
- Small lymphocytic lymphoma; includes chronic lymphocytic leukemia and plasmacytoid lymphocytic lymphoma
- Follicular, small, cleaved cell lymphoma
- Follicular, mixed small cleaved and large cell lymphoma

Intermediate-grade
- Follicular, large cell lymphoma
- Diffuse, small cleaved cell lymphoma
- Diffuse, mixed small and large cell lymphoma
- Diffuse, large cell (cleaved and noncleaved) lymphoma

High-grade
- Large cell, immunoblastic lymphoma
- Lymphoblastic (convoluted and nonconvoluted cell) lymphoma
- Small noncleaved cell (Burkitt's) lymphoma

Miscellaneous
- Composite, mycosis fungoides, histiocytic lymphoma, extramedullary plasmacytoma, unclassifiable, others

[1]Reproduced, with permission, from Chandrasoma P, Taylor CR: *Concise Pathology,* 2nd ed. Appleton & Lange, 1994.
[2]Assignment to grades is based on overall pattern (follicular or diffuse) and cell type.

High-grade lymphomas, on the other hand express immature antigens and may fail to express differentiation markers such as immunoglobulin or T cell receptors. The nucleus is larger, with less organized chromatin and the presence of nucleoli, suggesting a higher growth rate and a greater loss of regulation of cell cycle. Effacement of the lymph node with an absence of follicular architecture and a tendency to exist in extranodal tissue such as the gastrointestinal tract and the central nervous system are other indications of a greater degree of genetic and cellular changes compared with low-grade lymphomas. In some cases, these changes can evolve in the clinical course of a patient with low-grade lymphoma and result in the emergence of high-grade lymphoma with a correspondingly aggressive clinical course. In these cases, additional chromosomal aberrations such as trisomy of chromosomes 7 or 3 may be seen.

Lymphomas cause a mass effect in lymph nodes or extranodal tissues and can occasionally invade and destroy adjacent tissue. Infiltration of the lungs, liver, and marrow can occur as a primary site or late in the course of the disease. Constitutional signs such as fever and weight loss, known as B symptoms, can also be seen, and these may be mediated through a variety of cytokines produced by lymphoma cells or as a reaction by normal immune cells. These cytokines include IL-1 and TNFα. In some cases of B cell lymphomas, the immunoglobulins produced by malignant cells are autoantibodies that can cause various syndromes. Among these are hemolytic anemia and thrombocytopenia, caused by autoantibodies to red cell and platelet surface proteins, respectively.

Table 4–10. Classification of acute myelogenous leukemias (AML).

M1	Myeloblasts without differentiation
M2	Myeloblasts with some degree of differentiation
M3	Acute promyelocytic leukemia
M4	Acute myelomonocytic leukemia
M5	Acute monocytic leukemia
M6	Erythroleukemia
M7	Megakaryoblastic leukemia

2. ACUTE MYELOGENOUS LEUKEMIA

Acute myelogenous leukemia (AML), also termed acute nonlymphocytic leukemia (ANLL), is a rapidly progressive neoplasm derived from hematopoietic precursors, or myeloid stem cells, that give rise to granulocytes, monocytes, erythrocytes, and platelets. There is increasing evidence that genetic events occurring early in stem cell maturation can lead to leukemia. First, there is a lag time of 5–10 years to the development of leukemia after exposure to known causative agents such as chemotherapy, radiation, and certain solvents. Second, many cases of secondary leukemia evolve out of a prolonged "preleukemic phase" manifested as either a **myeloproliferative syndrome** of hyperproduction of a cell lineage type or a **myelodysplastic syndrome** of hypoproduction with abnormal maturation without actual malignant behavior. Finally, examination of precursor cells at a stage earlier than the malignant expanded clone in a given type of leukemia can reveal genetic abnormalities such as monosomy or trisomy of different chromosomes. In keeping with the general molecular theme of neoplasia, additional genetic changes are seen in the malignant clone compared with the morphologically normal stem cell that developmentally precedes it.

Acute myelocytic leukemias are classified by morphology and cytochemical staining, as shown in Table 4–10. **Auer rods** are crystalline cytoplasmic inclusion bodies characteristic of—though not uniformly seen in—all myeloid leukemias. In contrast to mature myeloid cells, leukemic cells have large immature nuclei with open chromatin and prominent nucleoli. The appearance of the individual types of AML mirrors the cell type from which they derive. M1 leukemias originate from early myeloid precursors with no apparent maturation toward any terminal myeloid cell type. This is apparent in the lack of granules or other features that mark more mature myeloid cells. M3 leukemias are a neoplasm of promyelocytes, precursors of granulocytes, and M3 cells exhibit abundant azurophilic granules that are typical of normal promyelocytes. M4 leukemias arise from myeloid precursors that can differentiate into granulocytes or monocytes, while M5 leukemias derive from precursors already committed to the monocyte lineage. Therefore, M4 and M5 cells both contain the characteristic folded nucleus and gray cytoplasm of monocytes, while M4 cells contain also granules of a granulocytic cytochemical staining pattern. M6 and M7 leukemias cannot be readily identified on morphologic grounds, but immunostaining for erythrocytic proteins is positive in M6 cells, and staining for platelet glycoproteins is appreciated on M7 cells.

Chromosomal **deletions, duplications,** and **balanced translocations** had been noted on the leukemic cells of some patients prior to the introduction of molecular genetic techniques. Cloning of the regions where balanced translocations occur has in some cases revealed a preserved translocation site that reproducibly fuses one gene with another, resulting in the production of a new fusion protein. M3 leukemias show a very high frequency of the t(15;17) translocation that juxtaposes the *PML* gene with the *RARα* gene. *RARα* encodes for a retinoic acid steroid hormone receptor, and *PML* encodes for a transcription factor whose target genes are unknown. The fusion protein possesses novel biologic activity that presumably results in enhanced proliferation and a block of differentiation. Interestingly, retinoic acid can induce a temporary remission of M3 leukemia, supporting the importance of the RARα-PML fusion protein. Monosomy of chromosome 7 can be seen in leukemias arising out of the preleukemic syndrome of **myelodysplasia** or in de novo leukemias, and in both cases this finding is associated with a worse clinical prognosis. This monosomy as well as other serial cytogenetic changes can also be seen after relapse of treated leukemia, a situation which is characterized by a more aggressive course and resistance to therapy.

As hematopoietic neoplasms, acute leukemias involve the bone marrow and usually manifest abnormal circulating leukemic (blast) cells. Occasionally, extramedullary leukemic infiltrates known as **chloromas** can be seen in other organs and mucosal surfaces. A marked increase in the number of circulating blasts can sometimes cause vascular obstruction accompanied by hemorrhage and infarction in the cerebral and pulmonary vascular beds. This **leukostasis** results in symptoms such as strokes, retinal vein oc-

Table 4–11. Direct systemic effects of neoplasms.

Effect	Clinical Syndrome
Vessel compression	Edema, superior vena cava syndrome
Vessel invasion and erosion	Bleeding
Lymphatic invasion	Lymphedema
Nerve invasion	Pain, numbness, dysesthesia
Brain metastases	Weakness, numbness, headache, coordination and gait abnormalities, visual changes
Spinal cord compression	Pain, paralysis, incontinence
Bone invasion and destruction	Pain, fracture
Bowel obstruction and perforation	Nausea, vomiting, pain, ileus
Airway obstruction	Dyspnea, pneumonia, lung volume loss
Ureteral obstruction	Renal failure, urinary infection
Liver invasion and metastases	Hepatic insufficiency
Lung and pleural metastases	Dyspnea, chest pain
Bone marrow infiltration	Pancytopenia, infection, bleeding

34. What are the hallmarks of hematologic malignancies?
35. What observations suggest an association between chronic immune stimulation and the development of lymphoma?
36. What are some characteristics of low-grade lymphomas?
37. What are some characteristics of high-grade lymphomas?
38. What are "B symptoms," and what are they caused by?

clusion, and pulmonary infarction. In most cases of AML and other leukemias, peripheral blood counts of mature granulocytes, erythrocytes, and platelets are decreased. This is probably due to crowding of the bone marrow by blast cells as well as the elaboration of inhibitory substances by leukemic cells or alteration of the bone marrow stromal microenvironment and cytokine milieu necessary for normal hematopoiesis. Susceptibility to infections due to depressed granulocyte number and function and abnormal bleeding as a result of low platelet counts are common problems in patients initially presenting with leukemia.

SYSTEMIC EFFECTS OF NEOPLASIA

Many effects of malignancies are mediated not by the tumor cells themselves but by direct and indirect effects as outlined in Tables 4–11 and 4–12. Direct effects (Table 4–11) include compression or invasion of vital structures such as blood and lymphatic vessels, nerves, spinal cord or brain, bone, airways, gastrointestinal tract, or urinary tract. These may cause a typical pain pattern as well as dysfunction of the involved organ and obstruction of a conduit. On occasion, an inflammatory or desmoplastic host response rather than the tumor itself can eventuate in the same effect.

Indirect effects (Table 4–12) are widely heterogeneous and poorly understood. Likewise, the onset and clinical course are unpredictable. These may occur at distant targets uninvolved by tumor and are then collectively termed **paraneoplastic syndromes.** Some of these effects are stereotypical syndromes due to the elaboration of peptide hormones or cytokines with specific biologic activity, as shown in Table 4–12. The peptides secreted by a given neoplasm may reflect the tissue of origin or may be the result of activation of latent genes not normally expressed. In some malignancies such as carcinoid, several active peptides may act in concert to produce a constellation of symptoms and tissue effects. Cytokines such as the interleukins and tumor necrosis factor may be responsible for tumor-related fevers and weight loss. Some paraneoplastic syndromes are associated with the development of autoantibodies as a result of an immune response to tumor-associated antigens or an inappropriate production of antibody, as can be seen in lymphoid neoplasms. Finally, the nucleic acid, cytoplasmic, and membrane products of cell breakdown can result in electrolyte and other metabolic abnormalities as well as coagulopathic disorders, resulting in clotting or bleeding.

Table 4–12. Indirect systemic effects of neoplasms.

Tumor Type	Cause of Indirect Effect	Clinical Syndrome
EFFECTS OF HORMONE OR PEPTIDE SECRETION		
Lung	ACTH	Cushing's syndrome
Lung, breast, kidney, others	PTH or PTH-related protein	Hypercalcemia
Lung	ADH, ANP	SIADH, hyponatremia
Germ cell, trophoblastic, hepatoblastoma	Gonadotropins (FSH, LH, βhCG)	Gynecomastia, precocious puberty
Lung, gastric	Growth hormone	Acromegaly
Carcinoid, neuroendocrine	Various vasoactive peptides	Flushing, wheezing, diarrhea
Sarcoma, mesothelioma, insulinoma	Insulin, insulin-like growth factor	Hypoglycemia
CUTANEOUS EFFECTS		
Gastrointestinal	Unknown	Acanthosis nigricans (hyperkeratosis and hyperpigmentation in skin folds)
Gastrointestinal, lymphoma	Unknown	Leser-Trelat (large seborrheic) keratoses
Lymphoma, hepatoma, melanoma	Melanin deposits	Melanosis (skin darkening)
Lymphoma	Autoantibodies to subepidermal proteins	Skin bullae (blisters)
Myeloid leukemia	Neutrophilic skin infiltrates	Sweet's syndrome
NEUROLOGIC EFFECTS		
Lung, prostate, colorectal, ovarian, cervical, others	Unknown	Subacute cerebellar degeneration
Lung, testicular, Hodgkin's disease	Unknown	Limbic encephalitis
Lung	Unknown	Dementia
Lung, others	Unknown	Amyotrophic lateral sclerosis
Lung, others	Unknown	Peripheral sensory or sensorimotor neuropathy
Lymphoma	Unknown, ?autoantibodies	Ascending radiculopathy (Guillain-Barré syndrome)
Lung, gastrointestinal	Unknown, ?autoantibodies	Eaton-Lambert (myasthenia-like) syndrome
HEMATOLOGIC AND COAGULOPATHIC EFFECTS		
Several	Unknown	Anemia
Adenocarcinomas (especially gastric)	Unknown	Microangiopathic hemolytic anemia
Several	Interleukin-1, -3 and hematopoietic growth factors	Granulocytosis
Hodgkin's, others	Eosinophilic hematopoietic growth factors	Eosinophilia
Several	Unknown	Thrombocytosis
Adenocarcinoma (especially pancreatic), others	Unknown, ?exposed phospholipids from cell membranes	Thrombosis
Adenocarcinoma (especially prostate)	Urokinase, other mediators of fibrinolysis	Disseminated intravascular coagulation
METABOLIC EFFECTS		
Various	Interleukin-1, tumor necrosis factor α	Cachexia, anorexia
Lymphoma, others	Interleukins-1, -6	Fever
Hematologic neoplasms	Hypermetabolism/cell breakdown products	Hyperuricemia, hyperkalemia, hyperphosphatemia
Lymphoma, others	Tumor hypoxia	Lactic acidosis

Key: ACTH = adrenocorticotropic hormone
ADH = antidiuretic hormone (arginine vasopressin)
ANP = atrial natriuretic protein
FSH = follicle-stimulating hormone
βhCG = human chorionic gonadotropin
LH = luteinizing hormone
PTH = parathyroid hormone
SIADH = syndrome of inappropriate secretion of antidiuretic hormone

REFERENCES

General

DeVita VT, Hellman S, Rosenberg SA: *Cancer: Principles and Practice of Oncology,* 4th ed. Lippincott, 1993.

Rowley J, Aster J, Sklar J: The clinical applications of new DNA diagnostic technology on the management of cancer patients. JAMA 1993;270:2331.

Colon Cancer

Fearon ER, Vogelstein B: A genetic model for colorectal tumorigenesis. Cell 1990;61:759.

Weisburger JH: Causes, relevant mechanisms, and prevention of large bowel cancer. Semin Oncol 1991;18:316.

Breast Cancer

Harris JR et al: Breast cancer. (Three parts.) N Engl J Med 1992;327:319, 390, 473.

Tripathy D, Benz CC: Activated oncogenes and putative tumor suppressor genes involved in human breast cancers. In: *Oncogenes and Tumor Suppressor Genes in Human Malignancies.* Benz CC, Liu E (editors). Kluwer, 1993.

Carcinoid

Kvols LK, Reubi JC: Metastatic carcinoid tumors and the malignant carcinoid syndrome. Acta Oncol 1993;32:197.

Moertel CG: An odyssey in the land of small tumors. J Clin Oncol 1987;5:1502.

Testicular Cancer

Boyle P, Zaridze DG: Risk factors for prostate and testicular cancer. Eur J Cancer 1993;29:1048.

Oliver T, Mead G: Testicular cancer. Curr Opin Oncol 1993;5:559.

Sarcomas

Diller L: Rhabdomyosarcoma and other soft tissue sarcomas of childhood. Curr Opin Oncol 1992;4:689.

Shipley J, Crew J, Gusterson B: The molecular biology of soft tissue sarcomas. Eur J Cancer 1993;29:2054.

Lymphoma

Foon K et al: Genetic relatedness of lymphoid malignancies. Ann Intern Med 1993;119:63.

Paraneoplastic Syndromes

Pierce ST: Paraendocrine syndromes. Curr Opin Oncol 1993;5:639.

Posner JB: Paraneoplastic syndromes. Neurol Clin 1991;9:919.

Richardson GE, Johnson BE: Paraneoplastic syndromes in lung cancer. Curr Opin Oncol 1992;4:323.

Nervous System Disorders

5

Robert O. Messing, MD

The extent and complexity of the nervous system requires an anatomic approach to the analysis of neurologic disorders. Ignoring this precept would be like trying to diagnose the cause of chest pain without first determining whether the source is in the heart, lungs, pleura, or chest wall. The diverse expression of disease states results from abnormal excitation or inhibition of networks of neurons. Knowledge of neuroanatomy is thus very important in understanding the pathogenesis of signs and symptoms. The first part of this chapter reviews several basic aspects of neuroanatomy needed to interpret findings on a screening neurologic examination.

Understanding the causes of neurologic diseases requires knowledge of molecular and biochemical mechanisms. For several neurologic diseases, the mechanisms are not known. However, recent discoveries in neuroscience have uncovered important information about the mechanisms of some disease states. Four neurologic disorders in which some of the molecular mechanisms of pathogenesis are known are discussed later in this chapter: Parkinson's disease, myasthenia gravis, epilepsy, and stroke.

Acknowledgements

The following illustrations in this chapter are from Greenberg DA, Aminoff MJ, Simon RP: *Clinical Neurology,* 2nd ed. Appleton & Lange, 1993: Figures 5–1, 5–3, 5–7, 5–8, 5–9, 5–10, 5–18, 5–19, 5–21, 5–22, 5–23, 5–24, 5–25, 5–26, and 5–28.

The following are from deGroot J: *Clinical Neuroanatomy,* 21st ed. Appleton & Lange, 1991: Figures 5–2, 5–4, 5–5, 5–6, 5–12, 5–13, 5–14, 5–15, 5–16, 5–17, and 5–20.

FUNCTIONAL NEUROANATOMY

To understand the nervous system, it is useful to study structures as parts of functional systems.

MOTOR SYSTEM

Large motor neurons of the spinal cord ventral horns and brain stem motor nuclei (facial nucleus, trigeminal motor nucleus, nucleus ambiguus, hypoglossal nucleus) extend axons into spinal and cranial nerves to innervate skeletal muscles. Damage to these **lower motor neurons** results in loss of all voluntary and reflex movement, since they comprise the output of the motor system. Neurons in the precentral gyrus and neighboring cortical regions **(upper motor neurons)** send axons to synapse with lower motor neurons. Axons from these upper motor neurons comprise the **corticospinal and corticobulbar tracts.** The motor cortex and spinal cord are connected with other deep cerebral and brain stem motor nuclei, including the caudate nucleus, putamen, globus pallidus, red nuclei, subthalamic nuclei, substantia nigra, reticular nuclei, and neurons of the cerebellum. Neurons in these structures are distinct from cortical motor **("pyramidal")** neurons and are referred to as **"extrapyramidal"** neurons. Many parts of the cerebral cortex are connected by fiber tracts to the primary motor cortex. These connections are important for complex patterns of movement and for coordinating motor responses to sensory stimuli.

1. Where do lower motor neurons emanate from, and where do they send axons to?
2. Where do upper motor neurons emanate from, and what do they synapse with?

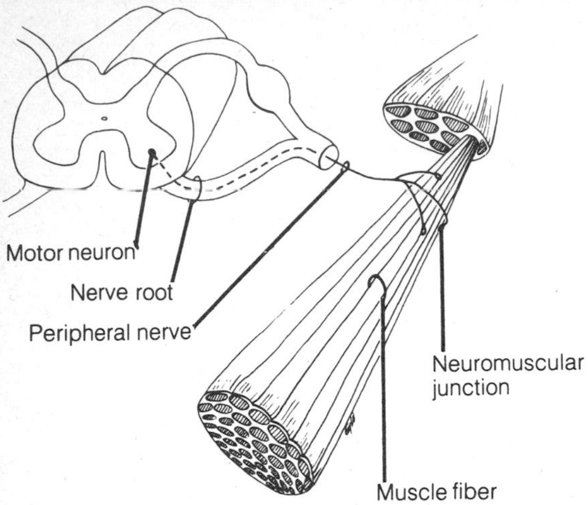

Figure 5–1. Anatomic components of the motor unit.

1. LOWER MOTOR NEURONS & SKELETAL MUSCLES

Anatomy

Each alpha motor neuron axon contacts up to about 200 muscle fibers, and together they constitute the **motor unit** (Figure 5–1). Axons of the motor neurons intermingle to form spinal ventral roots, plexuses, and peripheral nerves. Muscles are innervated from specific segments of the spinal cord, and each muscle is supplied by at least two roots. In contrast, each peripheral nerve innervates one muscle or a group of muscles, but each muscle is supplied by only one nerve. Thus, the distribution of muscle weakness differs in spinal root and peripheral nerve lesions.

Pathophysiology

The lower motor neurons are the final common pathway for all voluntary movement. Therefore, damage to lower motor neurons or their axons causes flaccid weakness of innervated muscles. In addition, muscle tone or resistance to passive movement is reduced, and deep tendon reflexes are impaired or lost. Tendon reflexes and muscle tone depend on the activity of alpha motor neurons, specialized sensory receptors known as muscle spindles, and smaller **gamma motor neurons** whose axons innervate the spindles (Figure 5–2). Some gamma motor neurons are active at rest, making the spindle fibers taut and sensitive to stretch. Tapping on the tendon stretches the spindles, which causes them to send impulses that activate alpha motor neurons. These in turn fire, producing the brief muscle contraction observed during the **myotactic stretch reflex.** Alpha motor neurons of antagonist muscles are simultaneously inhibited. Both alpha and gamma motor neurons are influenced by descending fiber systems, and their state of activity determines the level of tone and activity of the stretch reflex.

Each point of contact between nerve terminal and muscle forms a **neuromuscular junction** composed of the presynaptic motor nerve terminal and a postsynaptic muscle endplate (Figure 5–3). Presynaptic terminals store synaptic vesicles that contain the neurotransmitter acetylcholine. The amount of neurotransmitter within a vesicle constitutes a quantum of neurotransmitter. Action potentials depolarize the motor nerve terminal, opening voltage-gated calcium channels and stimulating calcium-dependent release of neurotransmitter from the terminal. Released acetylcholine traverses the synaptic cleft to the postsynaptic (endplate) membrane, where it binds to nicotinic acetylcholine receptors. These receptors are receptor-gated cation channels and, upon binding acetylcholine, they allow an entry of extracellular sodium into the muscle fiber. This depolarizes the motor endplate and stimulates contraction of the muscle fiber. Following activation, acetylcholine receptors rapidly inactivate, reducing sodium entry. They remain inactive until acetylcholine dissociates from the receptor. This is facilitated by the enzyme acetylcholinesterase, which is present in the postsynaptic zone, degrades acetylcholine, and decreases the concentration of the neurotransmitter at the synapse.

Neuromuscular transmission may be disturbed in several ways (Figure 5–3). In the **Lambert-Eaton myasthenic syndrome,** antibodies to calcium channels inhibit calcium entry into the nerve terminal and reduce neurotransmitter release. In these cases, repetitive nerve stimulation facilitates accumulation of calcium in the nerve terminal and increases acetylcholine release. Clinically, limb muscles are weak, but if contraction is maintained, power increases. Electrophysiologically, there is an increase in the amplitude of the muscle response to repetitive nerve stimulation. Aminoglycoside antibiotics also impair

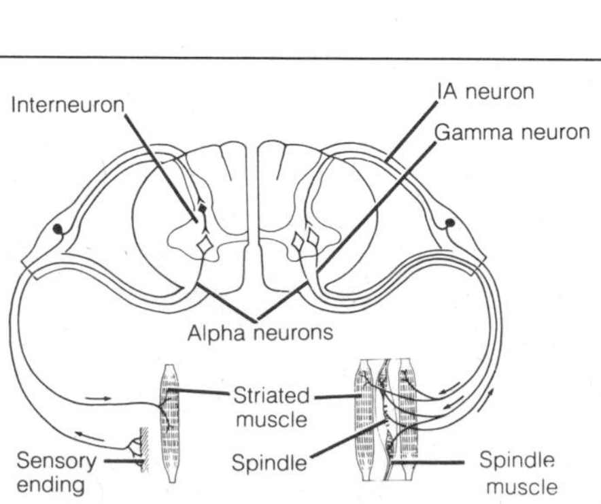

Figure 5–2. Schematic illustration of the neurons involved in the simple reflex arc (left half) and the stretch reflex (right half).

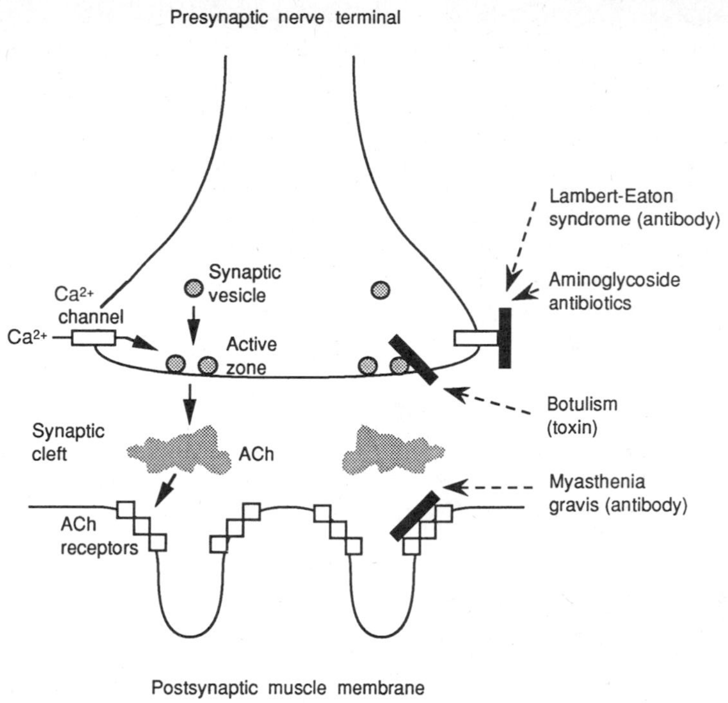

Figure 5–3. Sites of involvement in disorders of neuromuscular transmission. At left, normal transmission involves depolarization-induced influx of calcium (Ca^{2+}) through voltage-gated channels. This stimulates release of acetylcholine (ACh) from synaptic vesicles at the active zone and into the synaptic cleft. ACh binds to ACh receptors and depolarizes the postsynaptic muscle membrane. At right, disorders of neuromuscular transmission result from blockage of Ca^{2+} channels (Lambert-Eaton syndrome or aminoglycoside antibiotics), impairment of Ca^{2+}-mediated ACh release (botulinum toxin), or antibody-induced internalization and degradation of ACh receptors (myasthenia gravis).

calcium channel function and cause a similar syndrome. Proteolytic toxins produced by *Clostridium botulinum* cleave specific presynaptic proteins, preventing neurotransmitter release at both neuromuscular and parasympathetic cholinergic synapses. As a result, patients with botulism develop weakness, blurred vision, diplopia, ptosis, and large unreactive pupils. In myasthenia gravis, autoantibodies to the nicotinic acetylcholine receptor block neurotransmission by inhibiting receptor function and activating complement-mediated lysis of the postsynaptic membrane. Myasthenia gravis is discussed in greater detail later in this chapter.

Motor nerves exert trophic influences on the muscles they innervate. Denervated muscles undergo marked atrophy, losing more than half of their original bulk in 2–3 months. Nerve fibers are also required for organization of the muscle endplate and for the clustering of acetylcholine receptors to that region. Receptors in denervated fibers fail to cluster and become spread across the muscle membrane. Muscle fibers within a denervated motor unit may then discharge spontaneously, giving rise to a visible twitch **(fasciculation)** within a portion of a muscle. Individual fibers may also contract spontaneously, giving rise to **fibrillations,** which are not visible to the examiner but can be detected by electromyography. Fasciculations and fibrillations usually appear 10–14 days after damage to lower motor neurons or their axons.

3. What constitutes a motor unit?
4. Why does the distribution of weakness differ between spinal root and peripheral nerve lesions?
5. What are the features of lower motor neuron damage?
6. Describe the events in neuromuscular transmission.
7. What are some clinical syndromes in which neuromuscular transmission is disturbed?
8. What are some consequences of denervation on muscle structure and function?

Clinical Manifestations

The major manifestation of diseases affecting motor components of the peripheral nervous system is weakness. Additional characteristics are present depending on whether the weakness is due to disease affecting muscle **(myopathy),** the neuromuscular junction (eg, myasthenia gravis), peripheral nerves, nerve plexuses, spinal roots, or lower motor neurons.

The pattern of weakness is usually bilateral and symmetric in myopathies, and most myopathies affect proximal muscles more than distal muscles. In certain neuromuscular junction disorders, such as myasthenia gravis or botulism, extraocular muscles are commonly involved. **Polyneuropathies** usually cause symmetric weakness that is more marked in distal muscles. In contrast, lesions of a spinal root, a plexus or an individual peripheral nerve produce focal weakness in muscles innervated by the affected motor axons.

Deep tendon (myotactic stretch) reflexes are impaired early in diseases that affect spinal roots or peripheral nerves, especially if there is loss of myelin **(demyelination)** or damage to large myelinated nerve fibers. In contrast, reflexes are preserved in diseases of the motor neuron, neuromuscular junction, or muscle until weakness becomes severe.

Variability in weakness is characteristic of neuromuscular junction disorders. For example, easy fatigability (decreased strength upon repeated use) is typical of myasthenia gravis. **Atrophy** and **fasciculations** are characteristic of motor neuron and peripheral nerve disorders resulting in denervation of muscles. Associated **sensory deficits** are found in disorders affecting spinal roots or peripheral nerves but are absent in diseases of the motor neuron, neuromuscular junction, or muscle.

9. What is the pattern of weakness in myopathies?
10. In what kinds of diseases are deep tendon reflexes spared or impaired early in the disease process?
11. What is the character of weakness in neuromuscular junction disorders?

2. UPPER MOTOR NEURONS

Anatomy

The motor cortex is defined as the region from which movements can be elicited by electrical stimuli (Figure 5–4). This includes the primary motor area (Brodmann area 4), premotor cortex (area 6), supplementary motor cortex (medial portions of 6), and primary sensory cortex (areas 3, 1, and 2). In the motor cortex, groups of neurons are organized in vertical columns, and discrete groups control contraction of individual muscles. Planned movements and those guided by sensory, visual, or auditory stimuli are preceded by discharges from prefrontal, somatosensory, visual, or auditory cortices, which are then followed by motor cortex pyramidal cell discharges that occur several milliseconds before the onset of movement.

Cortical motor neurons contribute axons that converge in the corona radiata and descend in the posterior limb of the internal capsule, cerebral peduncles, ventral pons, and medulla. These fibers constitute the **corticospinal** and **corticobulbar tracts** and, together with fibers projecting from red nuclei, vestibular nuclei, midbrain tectal neurons, and the reticular formation, are known as upper motor neuron fibers (Figure 5–5). As they descend through the diencephalon and brain stem, fibers separate to innervate extrapyramidal and cranial nerve motor nuclei. The lower brain stem motor neurons receive input from crossed and uncrossed corticobulbar fibers, though neurons that innervate lower facial muscles receive primarily crossed fibers.

In the ventral medulla, the remaining corticospinal fibers course in a tract that on cross section is pyramidal in shape—thus the name **pyramidal tract.** At the lower end of the medulla, most fibers decussate, though the proportion of crossed and uncrossed fibers varies somewhat between individuals. The bulk of these fibers descend as the lateral corticospinal tract of the spinal cord.

Different groups of neurons in the cortex control muscle groups of the contralateral face, arm, and leg. Neurons near the ventral end of the central sulcus control muscles of the face, whereas neurons on the medial surface of the hemisphere control leg muscles (Figure 5–6). Because the movements of the face, tongue, and hand are complex in humans, a large share of motor cortex is devoted to their control. A somatotopic organization is also apparent in the lateral corticospinal tract of the cervical cord, where fibers to motor neurons that control leg muscles lie laterally and fibers to cervical motor neurons lie medially (Figure 5–12).

12. Define the motor cortex and describe its organization.
13. Fibers from which nuclei and in which tracts constitute upper motor neurons? What is their path?
14. Describe the somatotopic organization of motor neurons in the cortex.

Pathophysiology

Upper motor neuron pathways can be interrupted in the cortex, subcortical white matter, internal capsule, brain stem, or spinal cord. Unilateral upper mo-

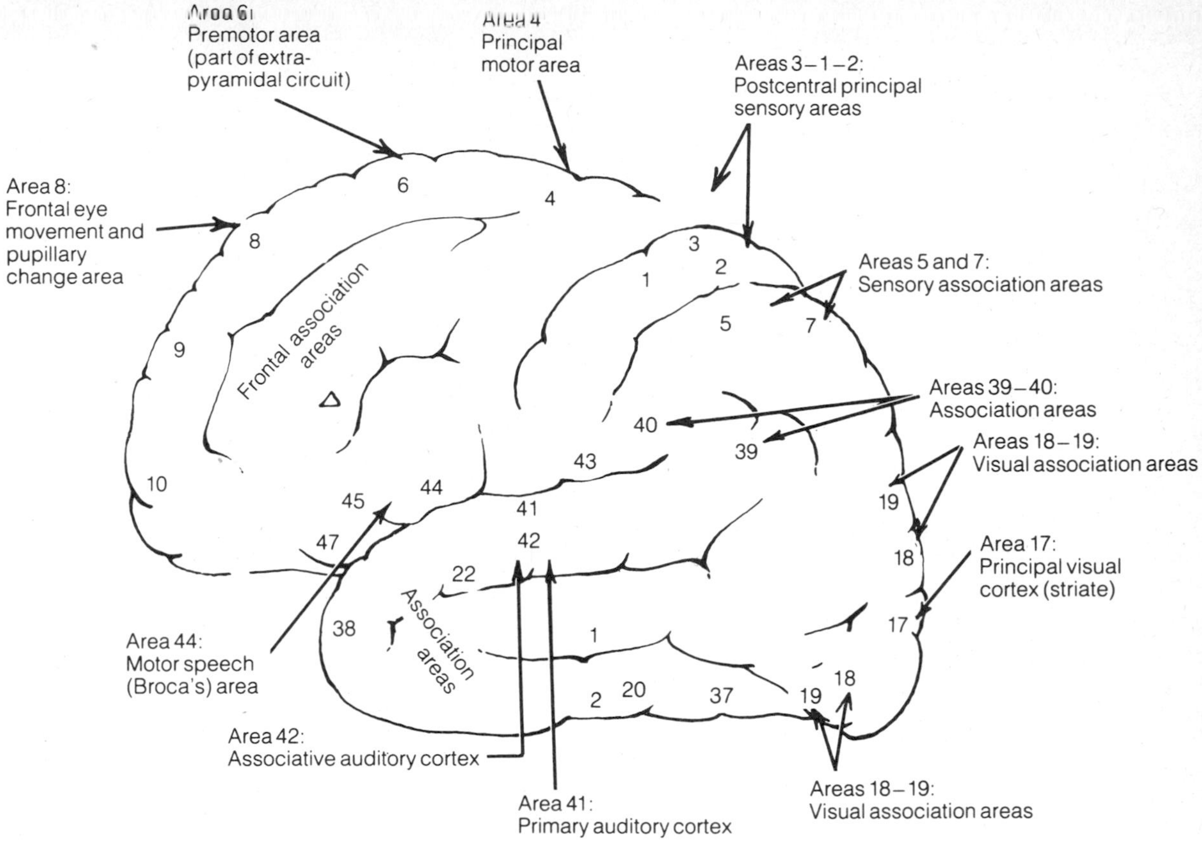

Figure 5–4. Lateral aspect of the cerebrum. The cortical areas are shown according to Brodmann, with functional localizations.

tor neuron lesions spare muscles innervated by lower motor neurons that receive bilateral cortical input, such as muscles of the eyes, jaw, pharynx, larynx, neck, thorax, and abdomen. Unlike paralysis due to lower motor neuron lesions, paralysis from upper motor neuron lesions is rarely complete for a prolonged period of time. Acute lesions, particularly of the spinal cord, often cause flaccid paralysis and absence of spinal reflexes at all segments below the lesion. With spinal cord lesions, this state is known as **spinal shock.** After a few days to weeks, a state known as **spasticity** appears, characterized by increased tone and hyperactive stretch reflexes. A similar but less striking sequence of events can occur with acute cerebral lesions.

Upper motor neuron lesions cause a characteristic pattern of limb weakness and change in tone. Antigravity muscles of the limbs become more active relative to other muscles. The arms tend to assume a flexed, pronated posture, and the legs become extended. In contrast, muscles that move the limbs out of this posture (extensors of the arms and flexors of the legs) are preferentially weakened by upper motor neuron lesions. Tone is increased in antigravity muscles (flexors of the arms and extensors of the legs), and if these muscles are stretched rapidly, they respond with an abrupt catch, followed by a rapid increase and then a decline in resistance as passive movement continues. This sequence constitutes the **"clasp knife" phenomenon. Clonus**—a series of involuntary muscle contractions in response to passive stretch—may be present, especially with spinal cord lesions.

Pure pyramidal tract lesions in animals cause temporary weakness without spasticity. In humans, lesions of the cerebral peduncles also cause mild paralysis without spasticity. It appears that spasticity is mediated by other tracts, particularly corticorubrospinal and corticoreticulospinal pathways. This may explain why the degrees of weakness and spasticity often do not correspond in patients with upper motor neuron lesions.

Clinical Manifestations

The cardinal features of upper motor neuron disease are weakness, spasticity, hyperreflexia, and impaired fine, skilled movements. There is often little

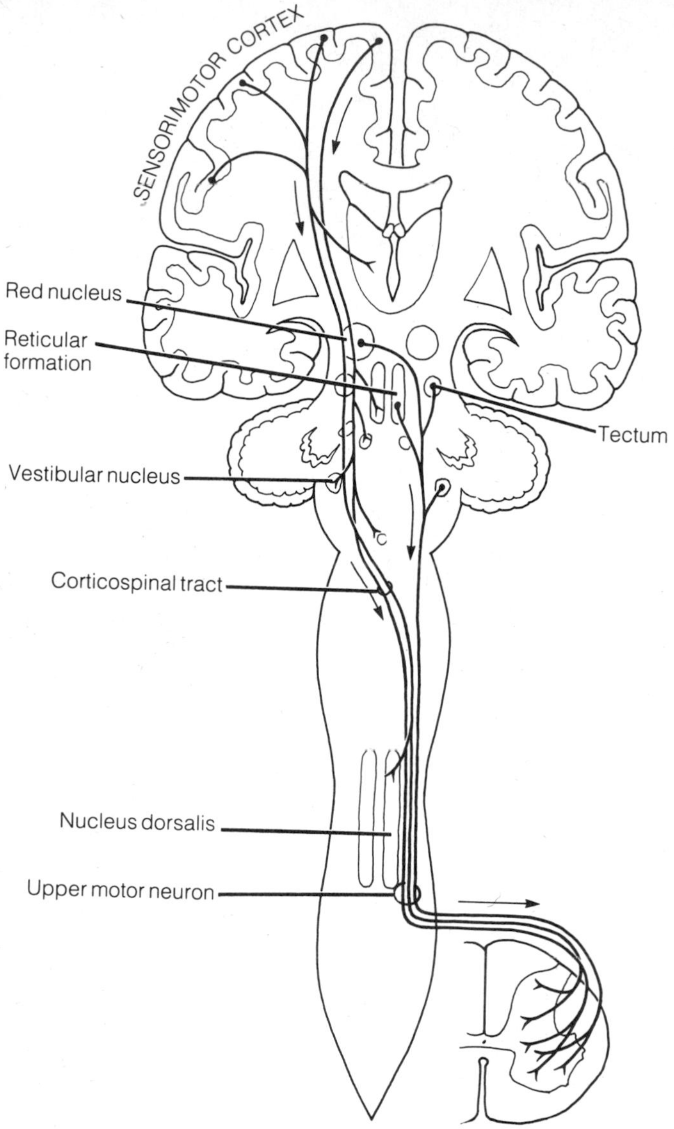

Figure 5–5. Schematic illustration of upper motor neuron pathways.

correlation between the severity of weakness, hyperreflexia, and spasticity. Thus, some patients may be extremely weak, with only a mild spastic catch, whereas others may be very spastic, with a fair degree of residual strength and movement. A **Babinski sign**—dorsiflexion of the big toe and fanning of other toes in response to stroking of the lateral plantar surface of the foot—is often present. However, this is not an essential feature of upper motor neuron dysfunction.

The distribution of paralysis due to upper motor neuron lesions varies with the location of the lesion. Lesions above the pons impair movements of the contralateral lower face, arm, and leg. Lesions below the pons spare the face. Lesions of the internal capsule often impair movements of the contralateral face, arm, and leg equally, since motor fibers are packed closely together in this region. In contrast, lesions of the cortex or subcortical white matter tend to differentially affect the limbs and face, since the motor fibers are spread over a larger area of brain. Bilateral cerebral lesions cause weakness and spasticity of cranial and trunk muscles in addition to limb muscles and lead to dysarthria, dysphonia, dyspha-

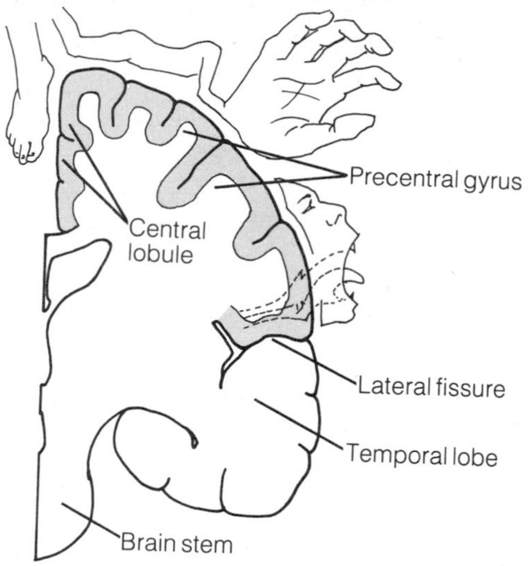

Figure 5–6. Motor homunculus, drawn on a coronal section through the precentral gyrus. The figure shows the location of cortical control of various body parts.

gia, bifacial paresis, and sometimes reflexive crying and laughing **(pseudobulbar paralysis).**

15. What is the characteristic pattern of weakness and tone in upper motor neuron lesions?
16. How is the distribution of paralysis and spasticity affected by the location of an upper motor neuron lesion?

3. CEREBELLUM

Anatomy

The cerebellar cortex can be divided into three functional regions (Figure 5–7). The **flocculonodular lobe,** composed of the flocculus and the nodulus of the vermis, has connections to vestibular nuclei and is important for the control of posture and eye movement. The **anterior lobe** lies rostrad to the primary fissure and includes the remainder of the vermis. It receives proprioceptive input (Figure 5–8) from muscles and tendons via the dorsal and ventral spinocerebellar tracts and influences posture, muscle tone, and gait. The **posterior lobe,** which comprises the remainder of the cerebellar hemispheres, receives major input from the cerebral cortex via the pontine nuclei and middle cerebellar peduncles and is important for the coordination and planning of voluntary skilled movements initiated from the cerebral cortex.

Efferent fibers from these lobes project to deep cerebellar nuclei, which in turn project to the cerebrum and brain stem through two main pathways (Figure 5–8). The fastigial nucleus receives input from the vermis and sends fibers to bilateral vestibular nuclei and reticular nuclei of the pons and medulla. Other regions of the cerebellar cortex send fibers to the **dentate, emboliform,** and **globose nuclei,** whose efferents form the superior cerebellar peduncles, enter the upper pons, decussate completely in the lower midbrain, and travel to the contralateral red nucleus. At the red nucleus, some fibers terminate, whereas others ascend to the ventrolateral nucleus of the thalamus, whence thalamic neurons send ascending efferent fibers to the motor cortex of the same side. A smaller group of fibers descend after decussation in the midbrain and terminate in reticular nuclei of the lower brain stem. Thus, the cerebellum controls movement through connections with cerebral motor cortex and brain stem nuclei.

Pathophysiology

The cerebellum is responsible for the coordination of muscle groups, control of stance and gait, and regulation of muscle tone. Rather than causing paralysis, damage to the cerebellum interferes with the performance of motor tasks. The major manifestation of cerebellar disease is **ataxia,** in which simple movements are delayed in onset and their rates of acceleration and deceleration are decreased, resulting in **intention tremor** and **dysmetria** ("overshooting"). Lesions of the cerebellar hemispheres affect the limbs, producing limb ataxia, whereas midline lesions affect axial muscles, causing truncal and gait ataxia and disorders of eye movement. Cerebellar lesions are often associated with **hypotonia** due to depression of activity of alpha and gamma motor neurons. If a lesion of the cerebellum or cerebellar peduncles is unilateral, the signs of limb ataxia appear on the same side as the lesion. However, if the lesion lies beyond the decussation of efferent cerebellar fibers in the midbrain, the clinical signs are on the side opposite the lesion.

Clinical Manifestations

Patients with cerebellar symptoms involving the limbs complain of clumsiness and tremor upon attempted movement. Movements of a limb towards a target typically overshoot and are followed by corrective movements that also overshoot. The result is a somewhat rhythmic wavering of volitional movement known as an **intention tremor.** This tends to worsen when the limbs are flexed, since the flexed posture depends heavily on the coordinate action of several muscles, whereas extension is partly stabilized by extended joints. The tremor is thus accentuated when the patient flexes the arm to touch the nose with an index finger or flexes the leg to touch the op-

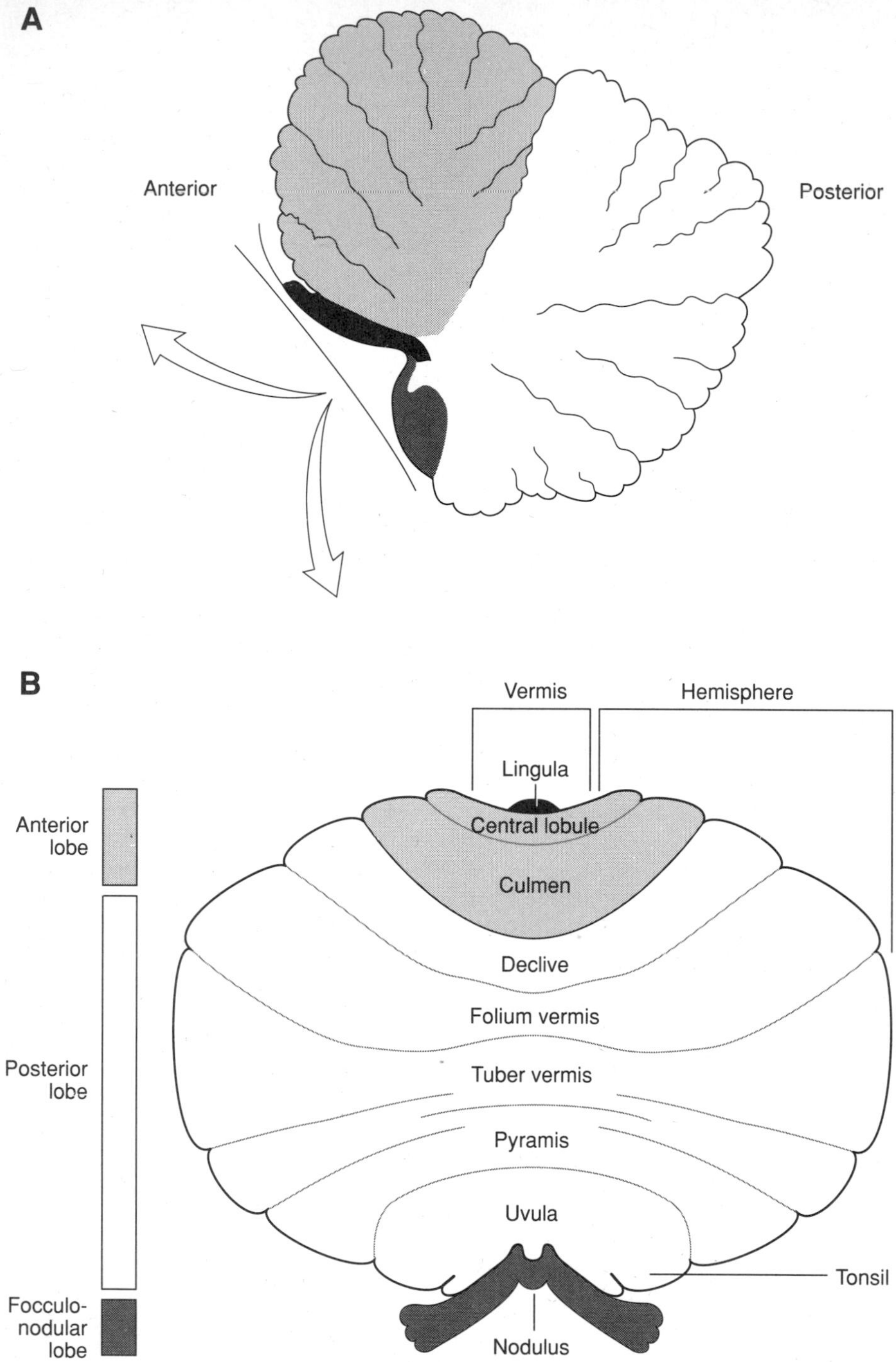

Figure 5–7. Anatomic divisions of the cerebellum in midsagittal view (***A***); unfolded (arrows) and viewed from behind (***B***).

posite knee with the heel. The tremor is most severe when lesions affect large areas of cerebellar cortex, the deep cerebellar nuclei, or efferent cerebellar fibers in the brain stem. Such lesions can cause a coarse, irregular tremor, known as a **rubral tremor,** that appears with any attempted movement.

Lesions of anterosuperior midline portions of the cerebellum cause **gait ataxia.** Patients feel unsteady

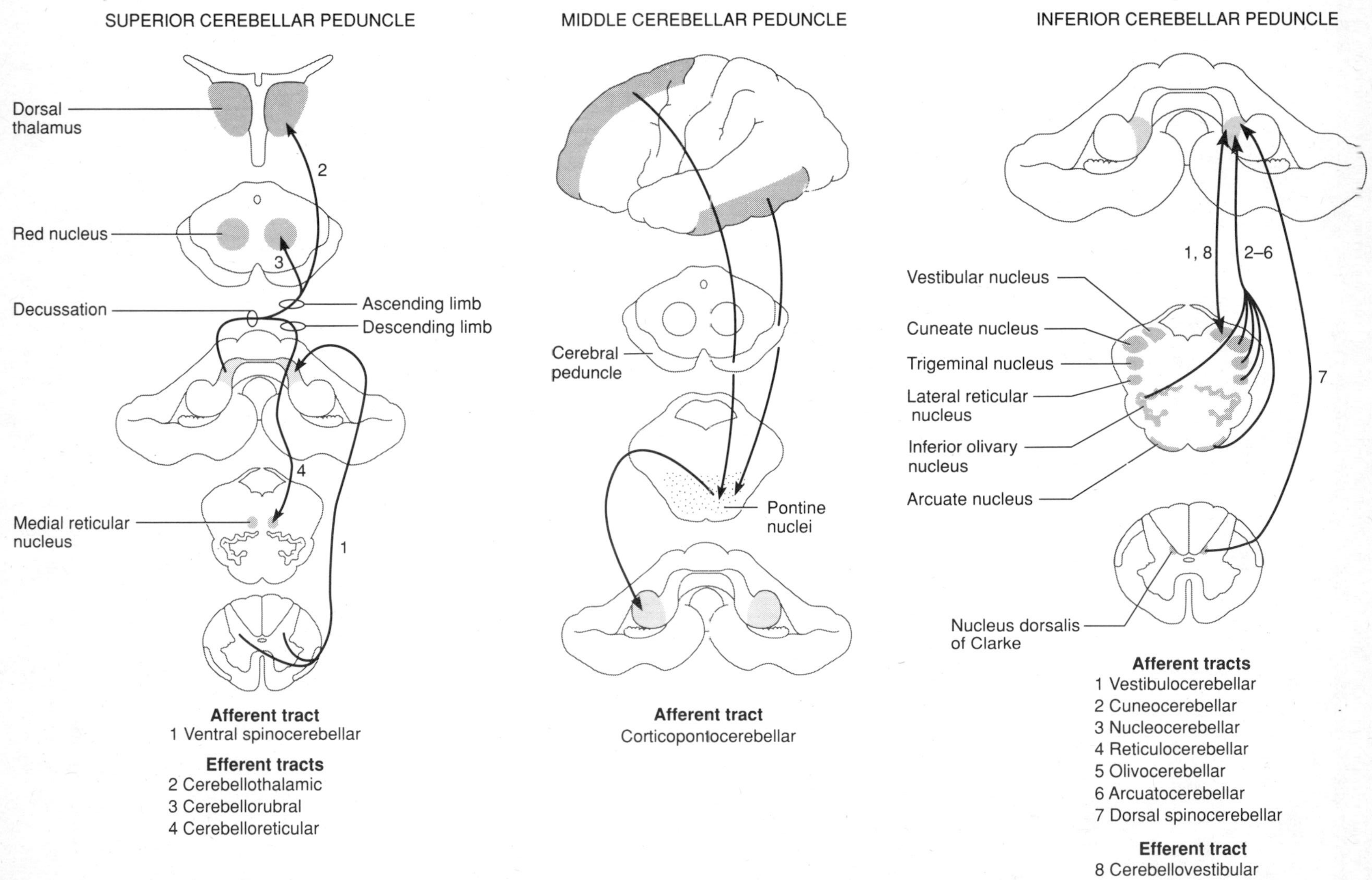

Figure 5–8. Cerebellar connections in the superior, middle, and inferior cerebellar peduncles. The peduncles are indicated by light shading and the areas to and from which they project by dark shading.

and complain of difficulty walking a straight line, walking quickly, turning, or starting or stopping walking. Bending over to pick up objects may cause a fall. Gait ataxia may occur without limb ataxia, since limb ataxia results from more lateral lesions of the cerebellar hemispheres. Patients with acute midline cerebellar dysfunction stagger as if drunk, but with chronic dysfunction they adopt a wide-based gait with short steps for greater control. Tests that impose a narrow base (eg, tandem walking) or that require sudden changes in direction bring out unsteadiness and irregular swaying of the trunk. **Titubation**—a slow oscillation or bobbing of the head or trunk—may also be present.

Hypotonia due to cerebellar lesions may be demonstrated by shaking the patient's limbs and observing greater excursion of the hands or feet of the affected limb. Sudden release of resistance against a flexed arm may cause the hand to strike the patient's face—a result of decreased tone and delayed contraction of the triceps muscle, causing impairment of the check reflex that normally prevents overflexion of the arm. The leg may swing several times after elicitation of the knee jerk reflex. This **pendular reflex** is due to decreased tone in the quadriceps and hamstring muscles.

Patients with cerebellar disease often have difficulty maintaining eccentric positions of gaze and can develop jerking movements of the eyes in the direction of gaze **(gaze-paretic nystagmus).** Cerebellar disease may also interrupt the smoothness of eye movements, causing overshoots in volitional gaze **(ocular dysmetria)**.

17. What is the overall role of the cerebellum?
18. What are the functional regions of the cerebellum, what do they control, and through which other regions of the brain do they make connections?
19. What are the consequences of damage to particular areas of the cerebellum, and how do those lesions present in patients?
20. Below what point do unilateral cerebellar lesions manifest on the opposite side?

Cerebellar lesions can cause slurring of speech. **Slurring dysarthria** due to cerebellar disease may be difficult to distinguish from slurring due to upper or lower motor neuron diseases involving the face and tongue muscles. Cerebellar lesions may also produce speech that is broken into syllables with improper emphasis and pauses that interrupt the flow of words **("scanning dysarthria").** This form of speech is especially characteristic of cerebellar disease.

4. BASAL GANGLIA

Anatomy

Several subcortical, thalamic, and brain stem nuclei are critical for regulating voluntary movement and maintaining posture. These include the caudate nucleus and putamen (corpus striatum), globus pallidus, claustrum, substantia nigra, subthalamic nuclei, red nuclei, and mesencephalic reticular nuclei. The major pathways that involve these structures form three neuronal circuits (Figure 5–9). The first is the cortical-basal ganglionic-thalamic-cortical loop. Inputs mainly from premotor, primary motor, and primary sensory cortices (areas 1, 2, 3, 4, and 6) project to the corpus striatum, which sends fibers to the medial and lateral portions of the globus pallidus. Fibers from the globus pallidus form the ansa and fasciculus lenticularis, which sweep through the internal capsule and project onto ventral and intralaminar thalamic nuclei. Axons from these nuclei project to the premotor and primary motor cortices (areas 4 and 6), completing the loop. In the second loop, the substantia nigra sends dopaminergic fibers to the corpus striatum, which has reciprocal connections with the substantia nigra. The substantia nigra also projects to the ventromedial thalamus. The third loop is

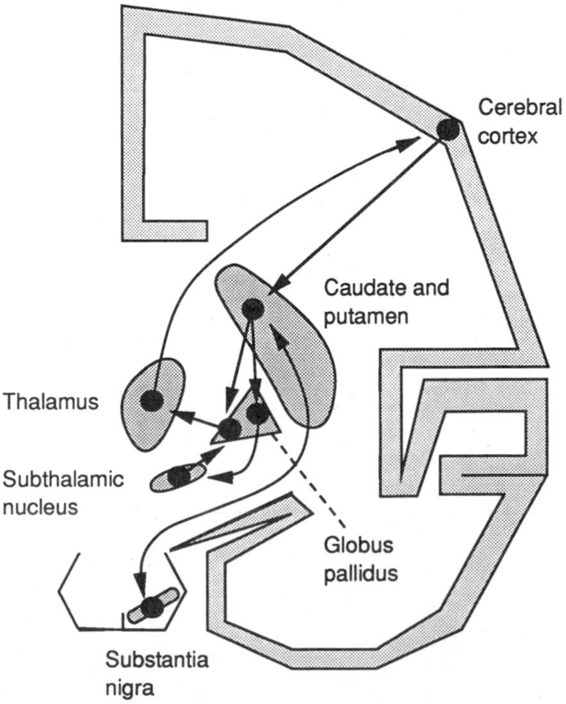

Figure 5–9. Basic neuronal circuitry of the basal ganglia.

composed of reciprocal connections between the globus pallidus and the subthalamic nucleus. The subthalamic nucleus also sends efferents to the substantia nigra and corpus striatum.

Pathophysiology

Basal ganglia circuits regulate the amplitude, speed, and initiation of movements. Diseases of the basal ganglia cause abnormalities of movement and are collectively known as **movement disorders.** They are characterized by motor deficits (bradykinesia, akinesia, loss of postural reflexes) or abnormal activation of the motor system, resulting in rigidity, tremor, and involuntary movements (chorea, athetosis, ballismus, and dystonia).

Several neurotransmitters are found within the basal ganglia, but their role in disease states is only partly understood. **Acetylcholine** is present in high concentrations within the corpus striatum, where it is synthesized and released by large Golgi type 2 neurons (Figure 5–10). Acetylcholine acts as an excitatory transmitter at medium-sized spiny striatal neurons that synthesize and release the inhibitory neurotransmitter **γ-aminobutyric acid (GABA)** and project to the globus pallidus. **Dopamine** is synthesized by neurons of the substantia nigra, whose axons form the nigrostriatal pathway that terminates in the corpus striatum. Dopamine released by these fibers inhibits striatal GABAergic neurons. In Parkinson's disease (Figure 5–11), degeneration of nigral neurons leads to loss of dopaminergic inhibition and a relative excess of cholinergic activity. This increases GABAergic output from the striatum and contributes to the paucity of movement that is a cardinal manifestation of the disease. Anticholinergics and dopamine agonists tend to restore the normal balance of striatal cholinergic and dopaminergic inputs and are effective in treatment. The pathogenesis of Parkinson's disease is discussed later in this chapter.

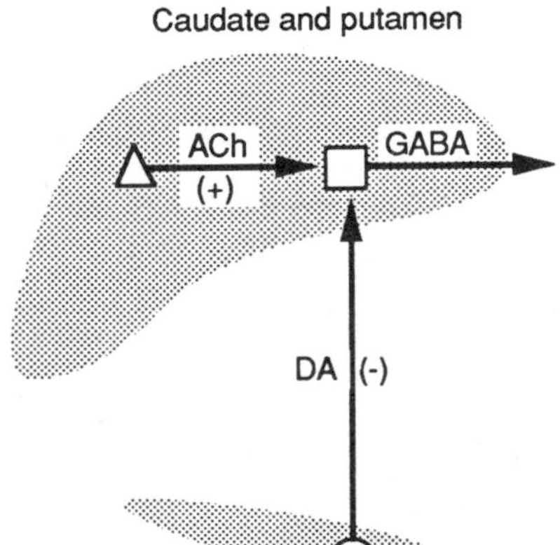

Figure 5–10. Simplified neurochemical anatomy of the basal ganglia. Dopamine (DA) neurons exert a net inhibitory effect and acetylcholine (ACh) neurons a net excitatory effect on the GABAergic output from the striatum.

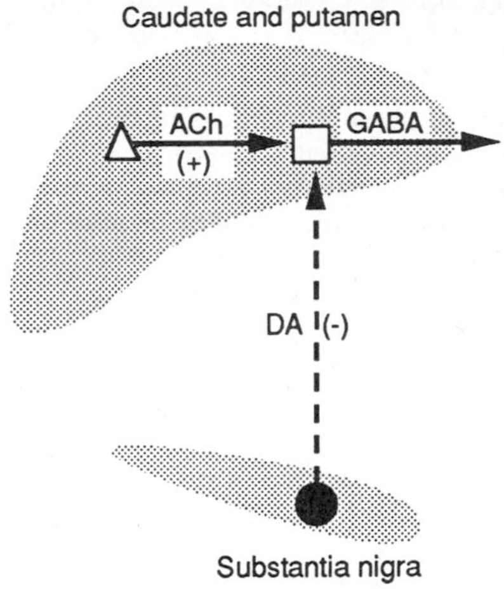

Figure 5–11. Neurochemical pathology of basal ganglia in Parkinson's disease. Dopamine (DA) neurons degenerate (black circle and dashed line), upsetting the normal balance between dopaminergic inhibition and cholinergic (ACh) excitation of striatal output (GABA) neurons. The net effect is to increase GABAergic output from the striatum.

Huntington's disease is inherited as an autosomal dominant disorder. In this disease, the spiny GABAergic neurons of the striatum preferentially degenerate, resulting in a net decrease in GABAergic output from the striatum. This contributes to the development of chorea and athetosis. Dopamine antagonists, which block inhibition of remaining striatal neurons by dopaminergic striatal fibers, reduce the involuntary movements. The gene for the disease has been recently mapped to chromosome 4 and encodes for a protein, huntingtin, of unknown function. The gene is unique in that it contains a polymorphic trinucleotide (CAG) repeat of 11–34 copies that is expanded in patients with the disease. The expanded repeat is thought to alter the structure or expression of huntingtin, but it is not known how this causes striatal neurons to degenerate.

Clinical Manifestations

Akinesia and **bradykinesia** refer to an inability to move rapidly. Voluntary and habitual movements such as blinking, smiling, touching the face, and crossing the legs are affected. The face may show a paucity of movement with infrequent blinking. Swallowing may fail to keep pace with saliva production, resulting in drooling. Speech is monotonic, soft, and dysarthric owing to limited movements of the mouth and tongue. Handwriting is often small and cramped. Immobility may predispose to pressure sores. Bradykinesia may be caused by any disorder that interrupts nigrostriatal fibers or the corticostriatal-thalamic circuit. Bradykinesia is a common feature of Parkinson's disease.

Rigidity is a form of increased tone that differs from spasticity and is commonly associated with bradykinesia. Rigidity is characterized by increased resistance to passive movement that is uniform throughout the range of movement and present in both flexors and extensors. Deep tendon reflexes are not increased. **Postural disturbances** include involuntary flexion of the trunk, limbs, and head when upright, difficulty in standing up from a reclining position, and difficulty in adjusting posture to prevent falling. Abnormalities of posture are common in Parkinson's disease. **Resting tremor** at a frequency of 4–5/s may also be present in Parkinson's disease and related disorders.

Chorea consists of involuntary, rapid, jerky random movements that may be severe enough to interrupt deliberate movements. Patients may try to incorporate chorea into voluntary movements to make them less obvious. There is often associated **hypotonia** and **pendular reflexes,** as observed with cerebellar diseases. In some patients, movements involve proximal muscles on one side of the body and are severe and flinging in character. This condition is known as **hemiballismus** and is usually due to an ischemic lesion of the opposite subthalamic nucleus. **Athetosis** is characterized by involuntary slow, writhing movements. Commonly there is eversion and inversion of the feet, pursing of the lips, twisting of the neck and trunk, alternate wrinkling and relaxing of the forehead, and opening and closing of the eyes. When associated with chorea, the condition is known as **choreoathetosis.** Voluntary movements are performed more slowly and are interrupted by the sinuous involuntary movements.

Chorea is a feature of diseases that involve the striatum, such as Huntington's disease, Sydenham's chorea, and rarely hyperthyroidism and systemic lupus erythematosus. Athetosis is common in adults with Huntington's disease and occasionally follows ischemia of the striatum, globus pallidus, or thalamus. It is also a common feature of Wilson's disease, an autosomal recessive disorder characterized by increased copper deposition in tissues and subsequent neurologic and hepatic dysfunction. The gene for this disorder has been localized to the long arm of chromosome 13, but the identity of the gene product and the exact nature of the biochemical abnormality are not known. Treatment with copper-chelating agents and restriction of dietary copper (eg, in shellfish, organ meats, legumes) reduce symptoms and neurologic damage.

Dystonia consists of persistence of a posture derived from an athetoid movement. There may be persistent hyperextension or hyperflexion of the hands or feet, lateral flexion or rotation of the head, torsion of the spine, forced closure of the eyes **(blepharospasm),** or a fixed grimace. It is seen in its most severe form in idiopathic torsion dystonias, a heterogeneous group of sporadic and inherited disorders involving the limbs, neck **(torticollis),** trunk, and muscles of the face and jaw. It also occurs in Parkinson's disease and in several disorders that cause athetosis such as Wilson's disease and Huntington's disease. Dystonia may complicate the use of certain drugs, particularly neuroleptics, and in these cases relief is usually obtained with administration of anticholinergics. Limited forms of dystonia may involve muscles of the face, neck, or hand (eg, writer's cramp).

21. Which are the component nuclei of the basal ganglia, and what is their functional role?
22. What are the clinical consequences of lesions in particular regions of the basal ganglia?
23. What are the neurotransmitters within the basal ganglia, and what is their role in disorders of basal ganglia function?

SOMATOSENSORY SYSTEM

Somatosensory pathways confer information about touch, pressure, temperature, pain, vibration, and the position and movement of body parts. This information is relayed to thalamic nuclei and integrated in the sensory cortex of the parietal lobes to provide conscious awareness of sensation. Information is also relayed to cortical motor neurons to adjust fine movements and maintain posture. Some ascending sensory fibers, particularly pain fibers, enter the midbrain and project to the amygdala and limbic cortex, where they contribute to emotional responses to pain. In the spinal cord, painful stimuli activate local pathways that induce the firing of lower motor neurons and cause withdrawal (Figure 5–2). Thus, somatosensory pathways provide tactile information, guide movement, and serve protective functions.

Anatomy

A variety of specialized end organs and free nerve endings transduce sensory stimuli into neural signals and initiate the firing of sensory nerve fibers. Fibers that mediate cutaneous sensation travel in sensory or mixed sensorimotor nerves to the spinal cord (Figure

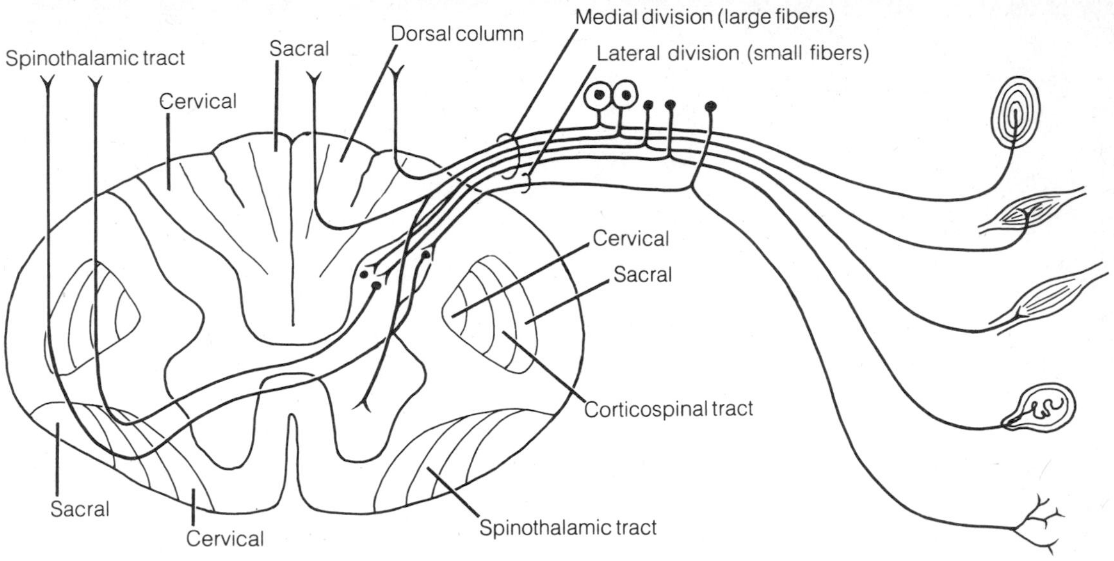

Figure 5–12. Schematic illustration of a spinal cord segment with its dorsal root, ganglion cells, and sensory organs. Sensory organs (from top to bottom) shown are the pacinian corpuscle, muscle spindle, tendon organ, encapsulated ending, and free nerve endings. The somatotopic arrangement of fibers in the dorsal columns, spinothalamic tract, and corticospinal tract is also shown.

5–12). Cutaneous sensory nerves contain small myelinated Aδ fibers that transmit information about pain and temperature, larger myelinated fibers that mediate touch and pressure sensation, and more numerous unmyelinated pain and autonomic fibers. Myelinated proprioceptive fibers and afferent and efferent muscle spindle fibers are carried in the larger sensorimotor nerves. The cell bodies of all sensory neurons are in the dorsal root ganglia, and their central projections enter the spinal cord via the dorsal spinal roots. Innervation of the skin, muscles, and surrounding connective tissue is segmental, and each root innervates a region of skin known as a **dermatome** (Figure 5–13). Cell bodies of neurons that innervate the face reside in the trigeminal ganglion and send their central projections in the trigeminal nerve to enter the brain stem (Figure 5–14). The trigeminal innervation of the face is subdivided into three regions, each innervated by one of the three divisions of the trigeminal nerve.

The dorsal roots enter the dorsal horn of the spinal cord (Figure 5–12). Large myelinated fibers divide into ascending and descending branches and either synapse with dorsal gray neurons within a few cord segments or travel in the **dorsal columns,** terminating in the gracile or cuneate nuclei of the lower medulla on the same side. Secondary neurons of the dorsal horn also send axons up the dorsal columns. Fibers in the dorsal columns are displaced medially as new fibers are added, so that in the cervical cord, leg fibers are located medially and arm fibers laterally (Figure 5–12). The gracile and cuneate nuclei send fibers that cross the midline in the medulla and ascend to the thalamus as the **medial lemniscus.** The dorsal column-lemniscal system carries information about pressure, limb position, vibration, direction of movement, recognition of texture and shape, and two-point discrimination.

Thinly myelinated and unmyelinated fibers enter the lateral portion of the dorsal horn and synapse with dorsal spinal neurons within one or two segments. The majority of secondary fibers from these cells cross in the anterior spinal commissure and ascend in the anterolateral spinal cord as the **lateral spinothalamic tracts.** Crossing fibers are added to the inner side of the tract, so that in the cervical cord the leg fibers are located superficially and arm fibers are deeper (Figure 5–12). These fibers carry information about pain, temperature, and touch sensation.

Sensation from the face is carried by trigeminal sensory fibers that enter the pons and descend to the medulla and upper cervical cord (Figure 5–14). Fibers carrying information about pain and temperature sensation terminate in the **nucleus of the spinal tract of cranial nerve V,** which is continuous with the dorsal horn of the cervical cord. Touch, pressure, and postural information are conveyed by fibers that terminate in the **main sensory and mesencephalic nuclei of the trigeminal nerve.** Axons arising from trigeminal nuclei cross the midline and ascend as the

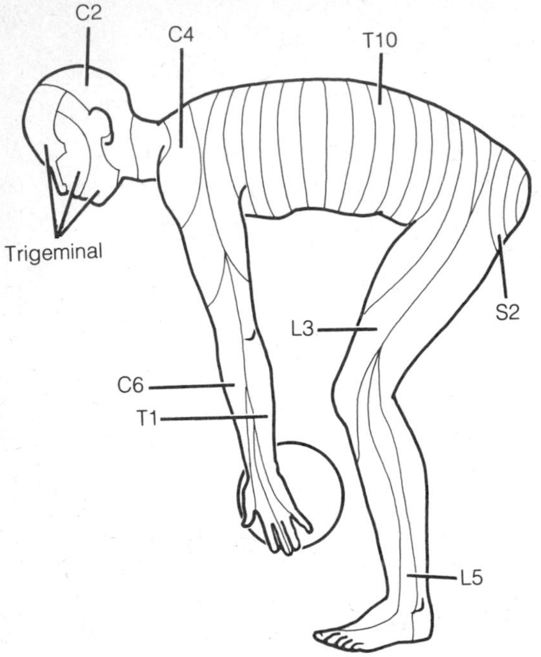

Figure 5–13. Segmental distribution of the body viewed in the approximate quadruped position.

trigeminal lemniscus just medial to the spinothalamic tract. Fibers from the spinothalamic tract, medial lemniscus, and trigeminal lemniscus merge in the midbrain and terminate along with sensory fibers ascending from the spinal cord in the posterior thalamic nuclei, mainly in the nucleus ventralis posterolateralis. These thalamic nuclei project to the primary somatosensory cortex (Brodmann areas 3, 1, and 2) and to a second somatosensory area on the upper bank of the sylvian fissure (lateral cerebral sulcus). The primary somatosensory region is organized somatotopically like the primary motor cortex (Figure 5–6).

Pathophysiology

Free nerve endings of unmyelinated C fibers and thinly myelinated Aδ fibers convey pain information in response to chemical, thermal, or mechanical stimuli. Peripheral nerve disorders that preferentially injure these fibers frequently cause unpleasant and often painful sensations **(dysesthesias)** and reduce the threshold for sensing pain and temperature. In contrast, diseases such as the demyelinating neuropathies, which injure larger myelinated fibers, can cause abnormal sensations **(paresthesias)** but usually not painful ones. Large-fiber neuropathies tend to impair deep tendon reflexes, vibration sense, and position sensation, since impulses mediating these functions are carried by the larger myelinated nerves.

In the spinal cord, the dichotomy between pain sensation and proprioception is maintained by anatomic segregation of pain fibers anterolaterally and position sense fibers posteriorly. In addition, the pain fibers cross shortly after entering the cord, which explains the appearance of "crossed" sensory deficits with unilateral spinal cord lesions that impair proprioception on the same side but impair pain and temperature sensation on the side opposite the lesion.

Since sensory fibers converge at the thalamus, lesions there tend to cause fairly equal loss of pain, temperature, and proprioceptive sensation on the contralateral half of the face and body. As fibers project to the sensory cortex, it remains difficult to distinguish fibers and neurons that respond to one type of sensory stimulus. Primary and association sensory cortices integrate sensory with visual and auditory information, which is critical to perception of space, the position of body parts in relation to the environment, and the integration of language with somatosensory information.

Several descending pathways modulate the activity of ascending pain fibers (Figure 5–15). One pathway is composed of cells in the periaqueductal gray matter of the midbrain that receive afferents from the frontal cortex and hypothalamus and project to rostroventral medullary neurons. These in turn project to the dorsolateral white matter of the spinal cord and terminate on dorsal horn neurons. Additional descending pathways arise from other brain stem nuclei

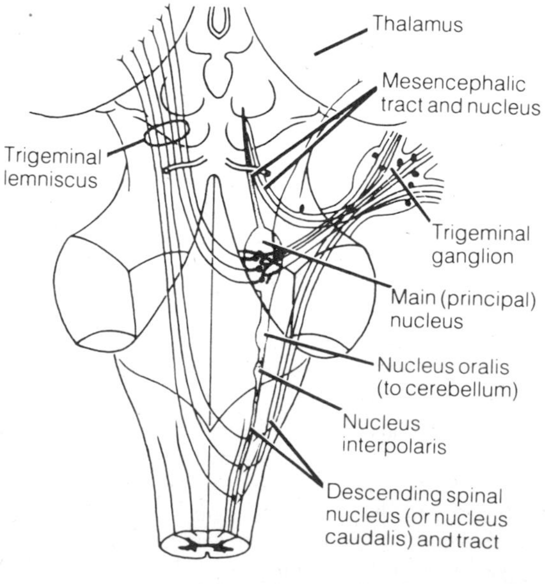

Figure 5–14. Schematic drawing of the trigeminal system.

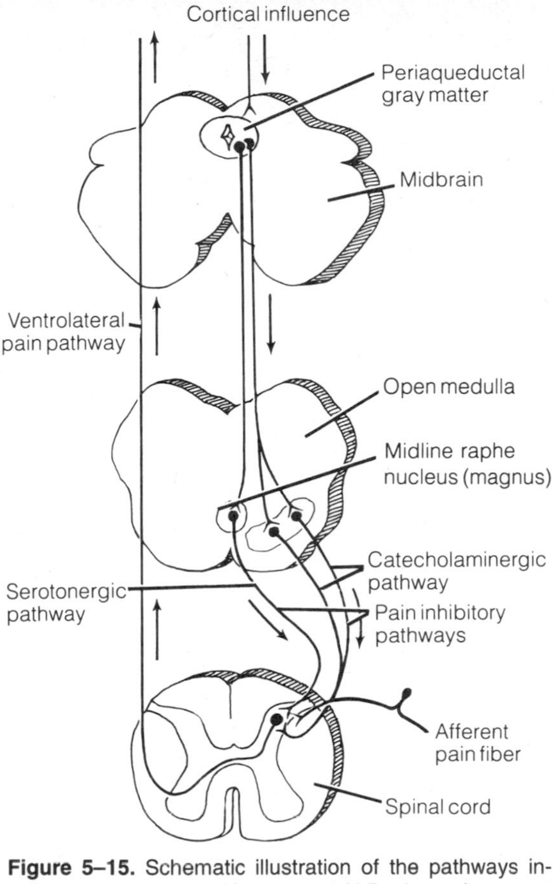

Figure 5–15. Schematic illustration of the pathways involved in pain control. (Courtesy of Al Basbaum.)

(locus ceruleus, dorsal raphe nucleus, and nucleus reticularis gigantocellularis). Major neurotransmitters utilized by these systems include endorphins, serotonin, and norepinephrine, and this provides the rationale for the use of opioids, serotonin agonists, and serotonin and norepinephrine reuptake inhibitors in the treatment of pain.

Clinical Manifestations

Somatosensory disorders not only cause loss of sensory perception but commonly cause abnormal sensations (**paresthesias** or, if unpleasant, **dysesthesias**). Often these are painful if there is disease of the unmyelinated or thinly myelinated pain fibers, spinothalamic tracts, or thalamus. Since pain and temperature sensation are carried by the same fibers, loss of both modalities confirms the presence of a deficit. Some decrease in threshold to light touch is also often detected. With peripheral nerve, plexus, spinal cord, or thalamic lesions, sensory loss can usually be detected within the dysesthetic region. However, sensory loss may be absent with lesions involving a single spinal nerve root, since there is considerable overlap in the dermatomes supplied by adjacent roots.

Disorders affecting heavily myelinated fibers or posterior columns commonly cause loss of vibratory and joint position sense. Severe loss of joint position sense in the upper extremities can lead to incoordination of fine movements and a characteristic wavering of outstretched fingers and hands when the eyes are closed, a finding known as **sensory ataxia.** Similar proprioceptive loss in the feet leads to an inability to stand quietly with the feet together and eyes closed **(Romberg's sign).** The loss of proprioception is documented by testing joint position sense in the toes and fingers. Since similar fibers and tracts carry vibratory information, vibration sense is often impaired as well, though there may be a discrepancy between the loss of vibratory and proprioceptive sensation. Loss of discriminative touch (eg, two-point discrimination) may also be impaired in the affected limb.

The patterns of sensory loss often indicate the level of nervous system involvement. Thus, symmetric distal sensory loss in the limbs, affecting the legs more than the arms, usually indicates a **polyneuropathy.** Sensory symptoms and deficits may be restricted to the distribution of a single peripheral nerve (**mononeuropathy**) or two or more peripheral nerves **(mononeuropathy multiplex).** Symptoms and signs limited to a dermatome indicate a spinal root lesion **(radiculopathy).** Pain from root lesions is often made worse by moving the limb into a position that stretches the affected root. Thus, having the patient raise an extended leg and dorsiflex the foot while lying supine can elicit a **sciatic stretch sign** if an L5 or S1 root lesion is present. Similarly, extending the hip and flexing the knee can elicit a **femoral stretch sign,** indicating an L3 or L4 root lesion.

The segregation of fiber tracts and the somatotopic arrangement of fibers in the spinal cord give rise to distinct patterns of sensory loss in spinal cord lesions. Loss of pain and temperature sensation on one side of the body and loss of proprioception on the opposite side occurs with lesions that involve one half of the cord, on the side of the proprioceptive deficit (**Brown-Séquard's syndrome;** Figure 5–16). Compression of the upper spinal cord causes loss of pain, temperature, and touch sensation first in the legs, since the leg's spinothalamic fibers are most superficial. More severe cord compression compromises fibers from the trunk, and the examiner may detect a level on the trunk above which sensation is normal. It is important to note that the spinal cord lesion is often above the level indicated by the highest dermatome involved in the deficit. This is important in deciding which level of the spinal cord to examine in radiographic studies. Intrinsic cord lesions that involve the central portions of the cord often impair pain and temperature sensation at the level of the lesion, since the fibers crossing the anterior commis-

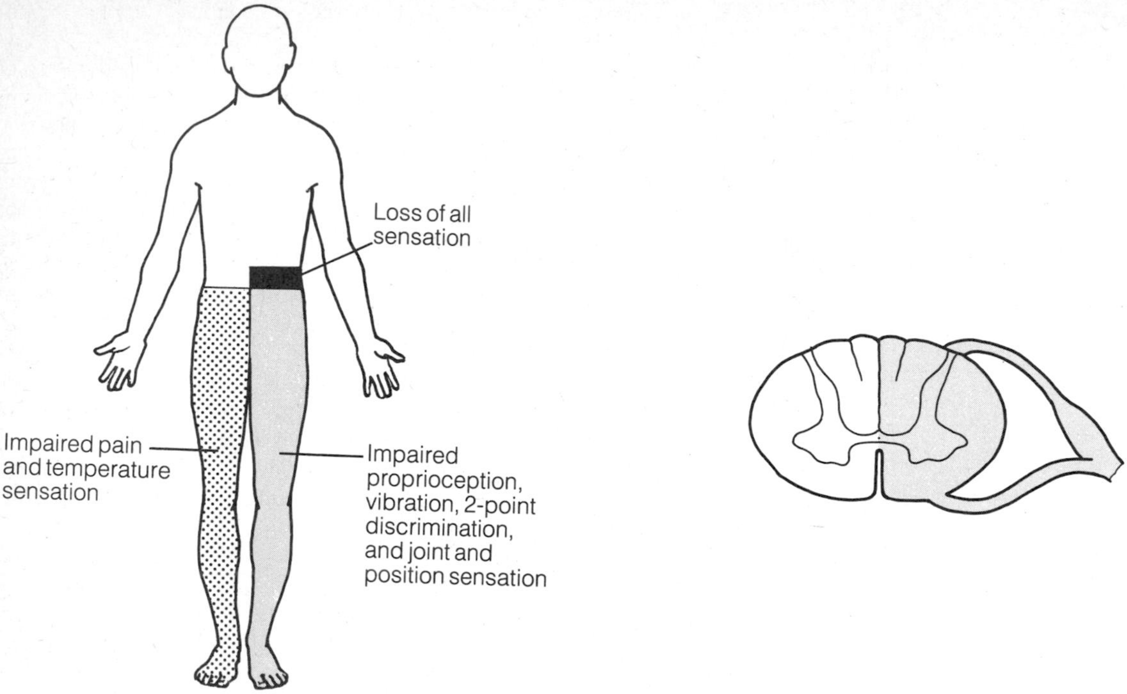

Figure 5–16. Brown-Séquard's syndrome with lesion at left tenth thoracic level (motor deficits not shown).

sure and entering the spinothalamic tracts lie most centrally. Thus, enlargement of the central cervical canal in **syringomyelia** typically causes loss of pain and temperature sensation across the shoulders and upper arms (Figure 5–17).

Brain stem lesions involving the spinothalamic tract cause loss of pain and temperature sensation on the opposite side of the body. In the medulla, such lesions can involve the neighboring spinal trigeminal nucleus, resulting in a "crossed" sensory deficit involving the ipsilateral face and contralateral limbs. Above the medulla, the spinothalamic and trigeminothalamic tracts lie close together, and lesions there cause contralateral sensory loss of the face and limbs. In the midbrain and thalamus, medial lemniscal fibers run together with pain and temperature fibers, and lesions are more likely to impair all primary sensation contralateral to the lesion.

Lesions of sensory cortex or the parietal lobe impair sensation on the opposite side of the body. In some cases, primary sensation is relatively normal, but there is impairment of discriminative sensation that requires integration of multiple stimuli. In such cases, patients may be unable to identify objects by touch or estimate their size, shape, and texture **(astereognosis),** and they may be less perceptive of sensory stimuli on the affected side when both sides of the body are stimulated simultaneously. Integration of tactile information and language may also be impaired, resulting in **agraphesthesia,** the inability to identify, with the eyes closed, a number or letter drawn on the skin. Perception of the position of body parts in space may also be abnormal, and patients may be unable to localize stimuli on the affected side.

24. What fibers carry pain, and how are they segregated from fibers that carry proprioception information in the spinal cord?
25. What are the differences in characteristics of sensory loss at different levels of the nervous system?

VISION & CONTROL OF EYE MOVEMENTS

The visual system provides our most important source of sensory information about the environment. The visual system and pathways for the control of eye movements are among the best-characterized pathways in the nervous system. Familiarity with these neuroanatomic features is often extremely valuable in localization of neurologic disease.

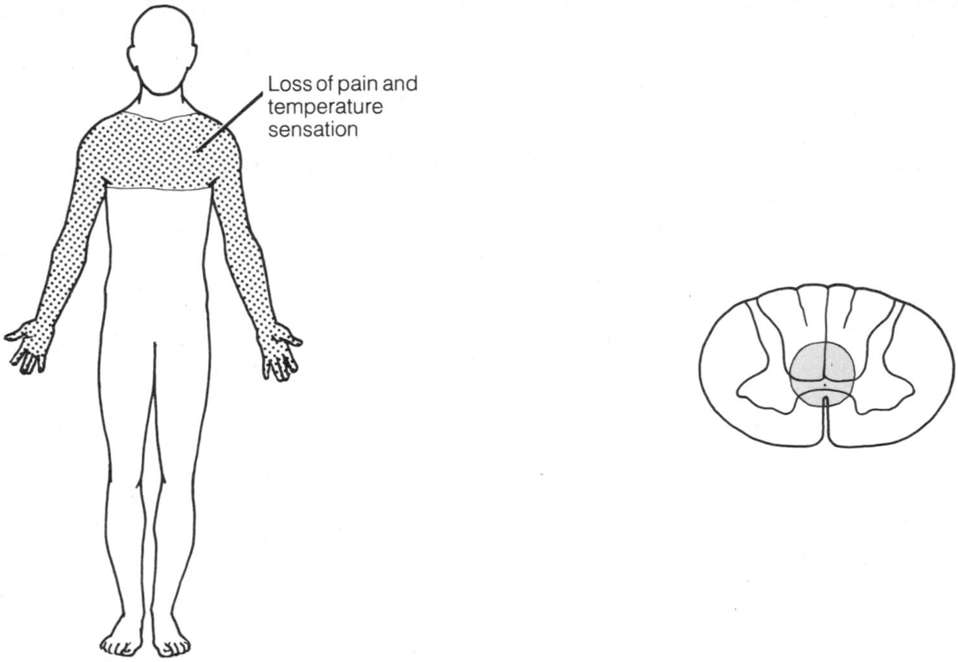

Figure 5–17. Syringomyelia involving the cervicothoracic portion of the spinal cord.

Anatomy

The cornea and lens of the eye refract and focus images on the photosensitive posterior portion of the retina. The posterior retina contains two classes of specialized photoreceptor cells, **rods** and **cones,** which transduce photons into electrical signals. At the retina, the image is reversed in the horizontal and vertical planes so that the inferior visual field falls upon the superior portions of the retina and the lateral field is detected by the nasal half of the retina.

Fibers from the nasal half of the retina traverse the medial portion of the optic nerve and cross to the other side at the **optic chiasm** (Figure 5–18). Each **optic tract** contains fibers from the same half of the visual field of both eyes. The optic tracts terminate in the **lateral geniculate nuclei** of the thalamus. Lateral geniculate neurons send fibers to the primary visual cortex in the occipital lobe (area 17, **calcarine cortex;** see Figure 5–4). These fibers form the **optic radiations,** which extend through the white matter of the temporal lobes and the inferior portion of the parietal lobes.

Eye movements are controlled by the extraocular muscles, which function in pairs to move the eyes along three axes (Figure 5–19). These muscles are innervated by the **oculomotor** (III), **trochlear** (IV), and **abducens** (VI) nerves. The oculomotor nerve innervates the ipsilateral **medial, superior,** and **inferior rectus muscles** and the **inferior oblique muscles.** It also supplies the ipsilateral levator palpebrae, which elevates the eyelid. The oculomotor nerve also carries parasympathetic fibers that mediate pupillary constriction (see below). Trochlear nerve fibers decussate before leaving the brain stem, and each trochlear nerve supplies the contralateral **superior oblique muscle.** The abducens nerve innervates the **lateral rectus muscle** of the same side.

Cortical and brain stem gaze centers innervate the extraocular motor nuclei and provide for supranuclear control of gaze (Figure 5–20). A **vertical gaze center** is located in the midbrain tegmentum, and **horizontal gaze centers** are present in the pontine paramedian reticular formation. Each lateral gaze center sends fibers to the neighboring ipsilateral abducens nucleus and, via the **medial longitudinal fasciculus,** to the contralateral oculomotor nucleus. Therefore, activation of the right lateral gaze center stimulates conjugate deviation of the eyes to the right. Rapid **saccadic eye movements** are initiated by the **frontal eye fields** in the premotor cortex that stimulate conjugate movement of the eyes to the opposite side. Slower eye movements involved in pursuit of moving objects are controlled by parieto-occipital gaze centers, which stimulate conjugate gaze to the side of the gaze center. These cortical areas control eye movements through their connections with the brain stem gaze centers.

The size of the pupils is determined by the balance between parasympathetic and sympathetic discharge to the pupillary muscles. The parasympathetic oculo-

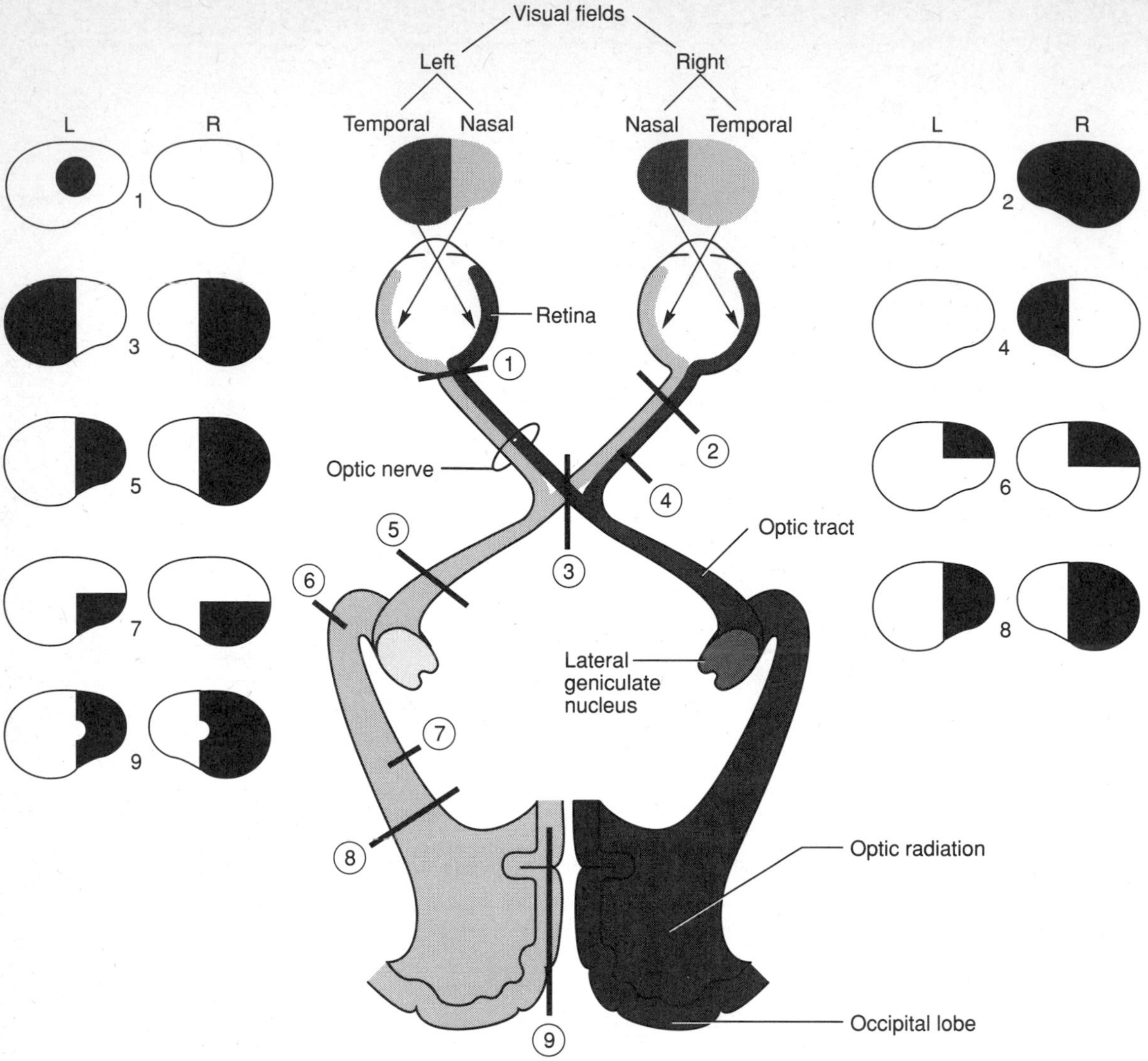

1. **Central scotoma** caused by inflammation of the optic disk (optic neuritis) or optic nerve (retrobulbar neuritis).
2. **Total blindness of the right eye** from a complete lesion of the right optic nerve.
3. **Bitemporal hemianopia** caused by pressure exerted on the optic chiasm by a pituitary tumor.
4. **Right nasal hemianopia** caused by a perichiasmal lesion (eg, calcified internal carotid artery).
5. **Right homonymous hemianopia** from a lesion of the left optic tract.
6. **Right homonymous superior quadrantanopia** caused by partial involvement of the optic radiation by a lesion in the left temporal lobe (Meyer's loop).
7. **Right homonymous inferior quadrantanopia** caused by partial involvement of the optic radiation by a lesion in the left parietal lobe.
8. **Right homonymous hemianopia** from a complete lesion of the left optic radiation. (A similar defect may also result from lesion 9.)
9. **Right homonymous hemianopia (with macular sparing)** resulting from posterior cerebral artery occlusion.

Figure 5–18. Common visual field defects and their anatomic bases.

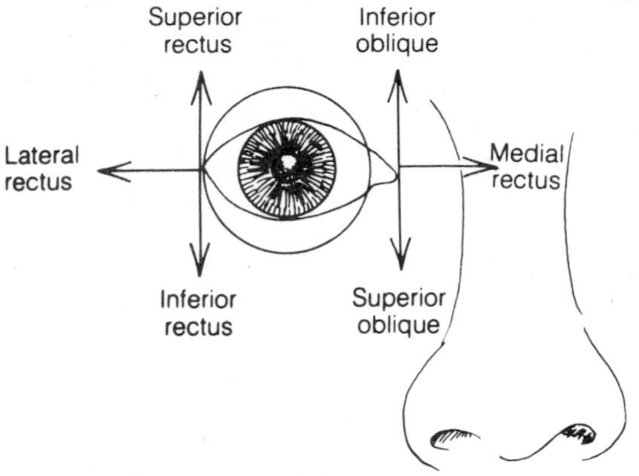

Figure 5–19. Extraocular muscles subserving the six cardinal positions of gaze. The eye is adducted by the medial rectus and abducted by the lateral rectus. The adducted eye is elevated by the inferior oblique and depressed by the superior oblique; the abducted eye is elevated by the superior rectus and depressed by the inferior rectus.

motor **nuclei of Edinger-Westphal** send fibers in the oculomotor nerves that synapse in the ciliary ganglia within the orbits and innervate the pupillary constrictor muscles.

Dilation of the pupil is controlled by a three-neuron system (Figure 5–21). It is composed of axons from neurons in the posterolateral hypothalamus that descend through the lateral brain stem tegmentum and the intermediolateral column of the cervical spinal cord to the level of T1. There they terminate on preganglionic sympathetic neurons within the lateral gray matter of the thoracic cord. These neurons send axons that synapse with postganglionic neurons in the superior cervical ganglion. Postganglionic neurons send fibers that travel with the internal carotid artery and the first division of the trigeminal nerve to innervate the iris. The fibers also innervate the tarsal muscles of the eyelids.

Pathophysiology

The rods are sensitive to low levels of light and are most numerous in the peripheral regions of the retina. In retinitis pigmentosa, there is degeneration of the retina that begins in the periphery. Poor twilight vision is thus an early symptom of this disorder. Cones are responsible for perception of stimuli in bright light and for discrimination of color. They are concentrated in the macular region, which is crucial for visual acuity. In disorders of the retina or optic nerve that impair acuity, diminished color discrimination is often an early sign.

The anatomic organization of the visual system is useful for localizing neurologic disease (Figure 5–18). Lesions of the retina or optic nerves **(prechiasma lesions)** impair vision from the ipsilateral eye. Lesions that compress the central portion of the chiasm, such as pituitary tumors, disrupt crossing fibers from the nasal halves of both retinas, causing **bitemporal hemianopia.** Lesions involving structures behind the chiasm **(retrochiasmal lesions)** cause visual loss in the contralateral field of both eyes. Lesions that completely destroy the optic tract, lateral geniculate nucleus, or optic radiations on one side produce a contralateral **homonymous hemianopia.** Selective destruction of temporal lobe optic radiations causes **superior quadrantanopia,** and lesions of the parietal optic radiations cause **inferior quadrantanopia.** The posterior portions of the optic radiations and the calcarine cortex are supplied mainly by the posterior cerebral artery, though the macular region of the visual cortex receives some collateral supply from the middle cerebral artery. Therefore, a lesion of primary visual cortex generally causes contralateral homonymous hemianopia, but if it is due to posterior cerebral artery occlusion, it may spare macular vision.

Conjugate eye movements are regulated by proprioceptive information from neck structures and information about head movement and position from the vestibular system. This information is used to maintain fixation on a stationary point when moving the head. In a comatose patient, the integrity of these oculovestibular and oculocephalic pathways can be assessed by the "doll's-eye" maneuver. This is elicited by briskly turning the head, which normally results in conjugate movement of the eyes in the opposite direction in a comatose patient. Irrigation of the ear with 10–20 mL of cold water reduces the activity of the labyrinth on that side and elicits jerk nystagmus, with the fast component away from the irrigated ear in a conscious individual. In coma, the fast saccadic component is lost, and the vestibular influence on eye movements predominates. Cold water irrigation then results in deviation of the eyes toward the irrigated ear (Figure 5–22). These caloric responses are lost with midbrain or pontine lesions, with damage to the labyrinths, or with drugs that inhibit vestibular function.

The size of the pupils is controlled by the amount of ambient light sensed by the retina (Figure 5–23). Fibers from each retina terminate within midbrain pretectal nuclei that send fibers to both Edinger-Westphal nuclei to activate pupillary constriction in bright light. In dim light, this reflex is inhibited and the influence of sympathetic fibers predominates, causing pupillary dilation.

Clinical Manifestations

A. Visual Disorders: Monocular visual loss occurs with lesions of an eye or optic nerve. Ischemic and inflammatory disorders of the optic nerve are common causes of monocular blindness. Ischemia

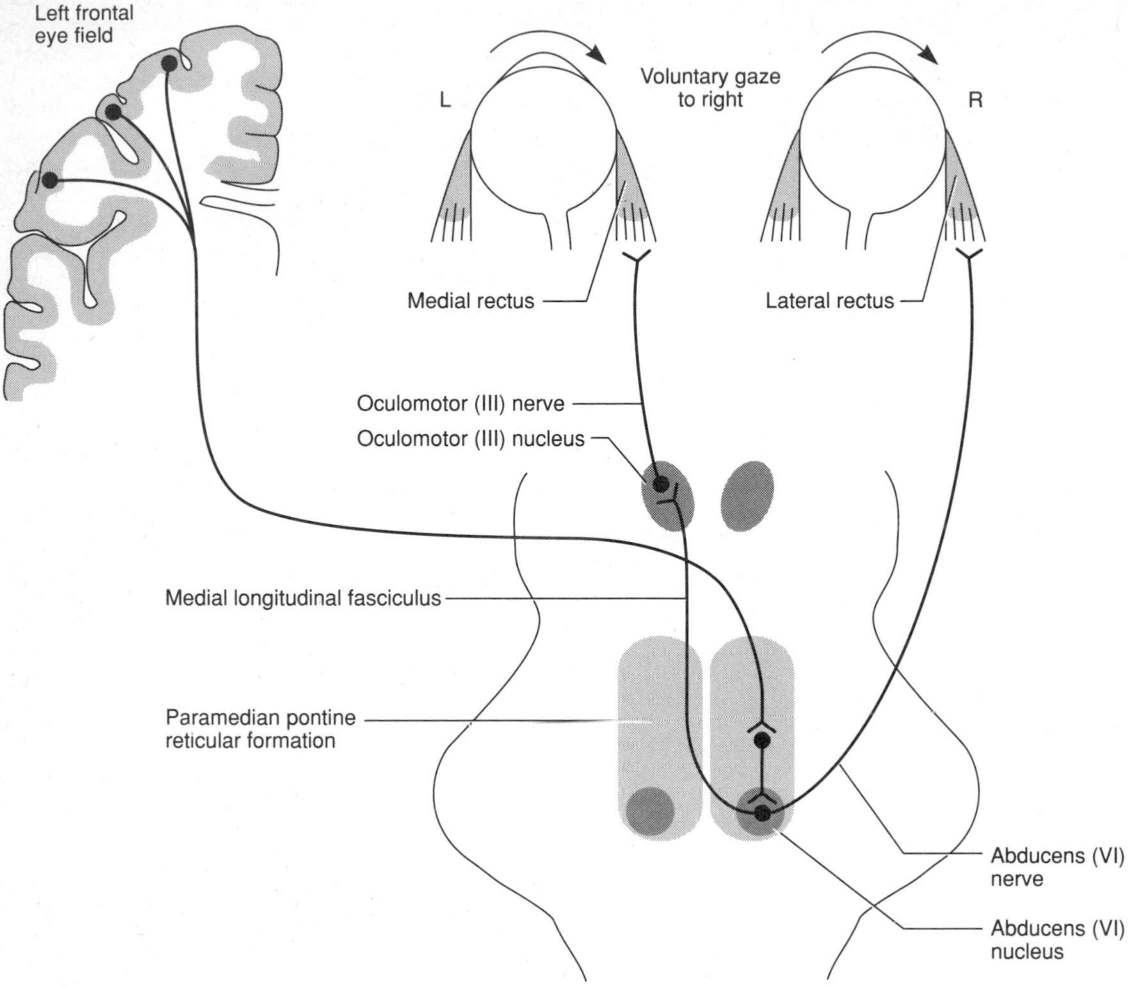

Figure 5–20. Neuronal pathways involved in horizontal gaze.

may be reversible if due to emboli from atherosclerotic lesions of the carotid arteries or from cardiac sources. Less common ischemic causes of monocular blindness include ischemic optic neuropathy and giant cell arteritis. Both conditions directly affect the ophthalmic artery or its branches. Treatment with corticosteroids usually arrests optic nerve damage due to giant cell arteritis and prevents visual loss.

Optic neuritis may produce monocular visual loss that progresses over hours to days, becoming maximal within 1 week. Often there is associated headache and eye pain. The condition may be idiopathic or may be due to demyelination or to meningeal, extraocular, or parameningeal inflammation. If inflammation involves the optic nerve head, the disk appears swollen on funduscopic examination and may resemble papilledema (see below). Visual acuity is impaired, and visual field testing often reveals a central area of visual loss (scotoma). The pupillary light response is markedly reduced upon illumination of the affected eye.

Optic neuritis may be the first manifestation of multiple sclerosis. Less common causes of optic nerve damage include methanol poisoning, syphilis, systemic lupus erythematosus, vitamin B_{12} deficiency, and tumors involving the orbit or optic nerve. Tumors generally cause unilateral visual loss, whereas the other disorders commonly affect both optic nerves.

Inflammation of the optic nerve head must be distinguished from passive edema and swelling of the optic nerves, a condition known as **papilledema.** Papilledema results from disorders that increase intracranial pressure such as brain tumor, abscess, intraparenchymal hemorrhage, meningitis, subarachnoid hemorrhage, malignant hypertension, or venous thrombosis. Unlike optic neuritis, papilledema does not impair visual acuity, cause a central scotoma, or

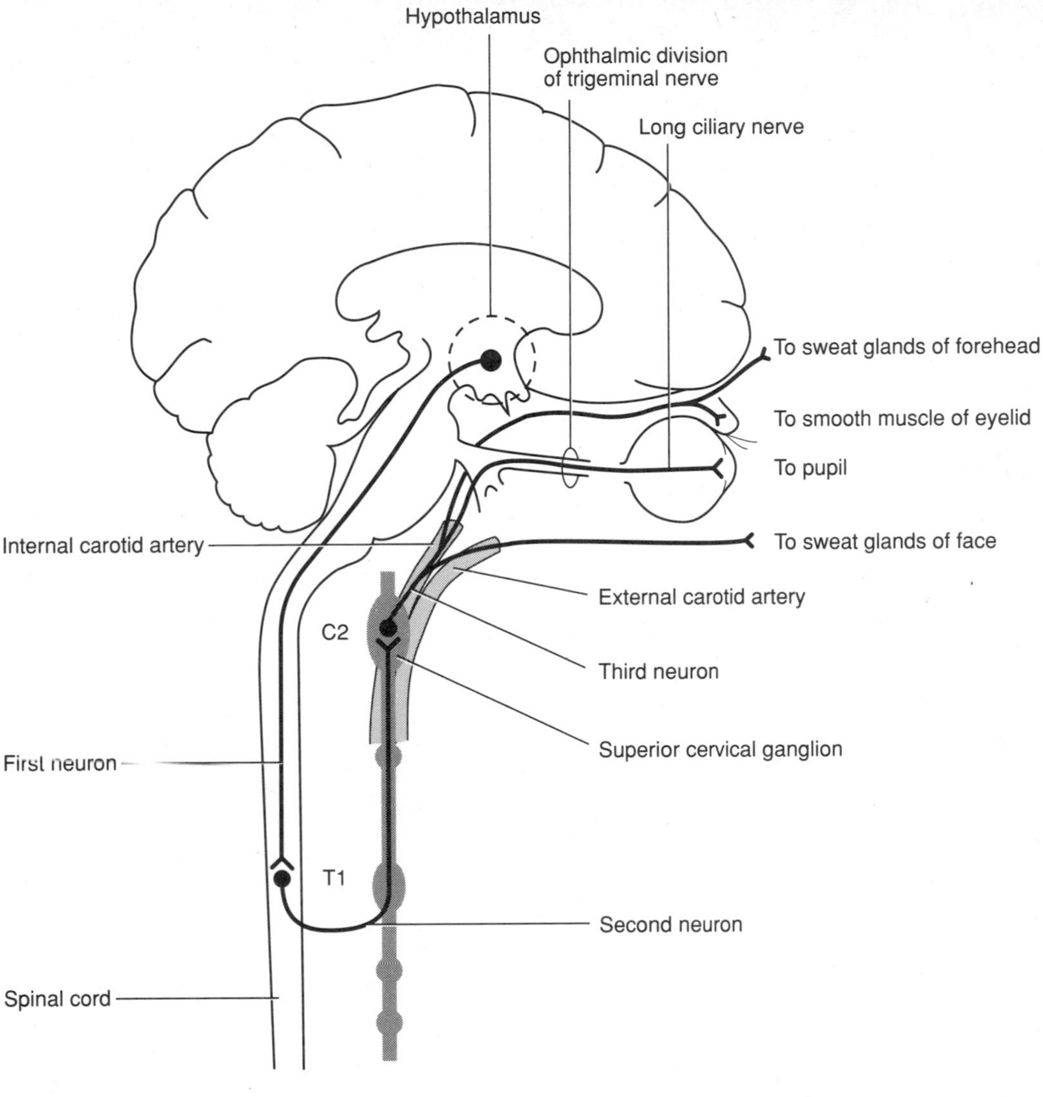

Figure 5—21. Oculosympathetic pathways. This three-neuron pathway projects from the hypothalamus to the intermediolateral column of the spinal cord, then to the superior cervical (sympathetic) ganglion, and finally to the pupil, the smooth muscle of the eyelids, and the sweat glands of the forehead and face. Interruption of these pathways results in Horner's syndrome.

impair the pupillary light response until chronic effects of prolonged disk swelling begin to damage the optic nerve. The visual fields are usually normal unless the edema has spread from the nerve head into neighboring regions of retina. In that case, the normal physiologic blind spot (due to the absence of photoreceptors at the optic nerve head) may be enlarged.

Binocular visual loss occurs with lesions involving the optic chiasm or retrochiasmal pathways. Tumors--particularly those arising from the pituitary gland--are the most common causes of chiasmal visual loss. Visual loss is usually gradual in onset and causes bitemporal hemianopia. Lesions behind the chiasm cause homonymous deficits and are usually due to ischemia or tumors. In the temporal lobe, tumors are the most common cause, producing superior quadrantanopia. Lesions of the parietal lobe are commonly ischemic and produce either complete homonymous hemianopia or inferior quadrantanopia. Occipital lesions cause homonymous hemianopia of the contralateral visual field and are most often due to infarction in the territory of the posterior cerebral artery. Tumors and vascular malformations may cause visual loss and may also induce well-formed visual hallucinations in the involved visual field.

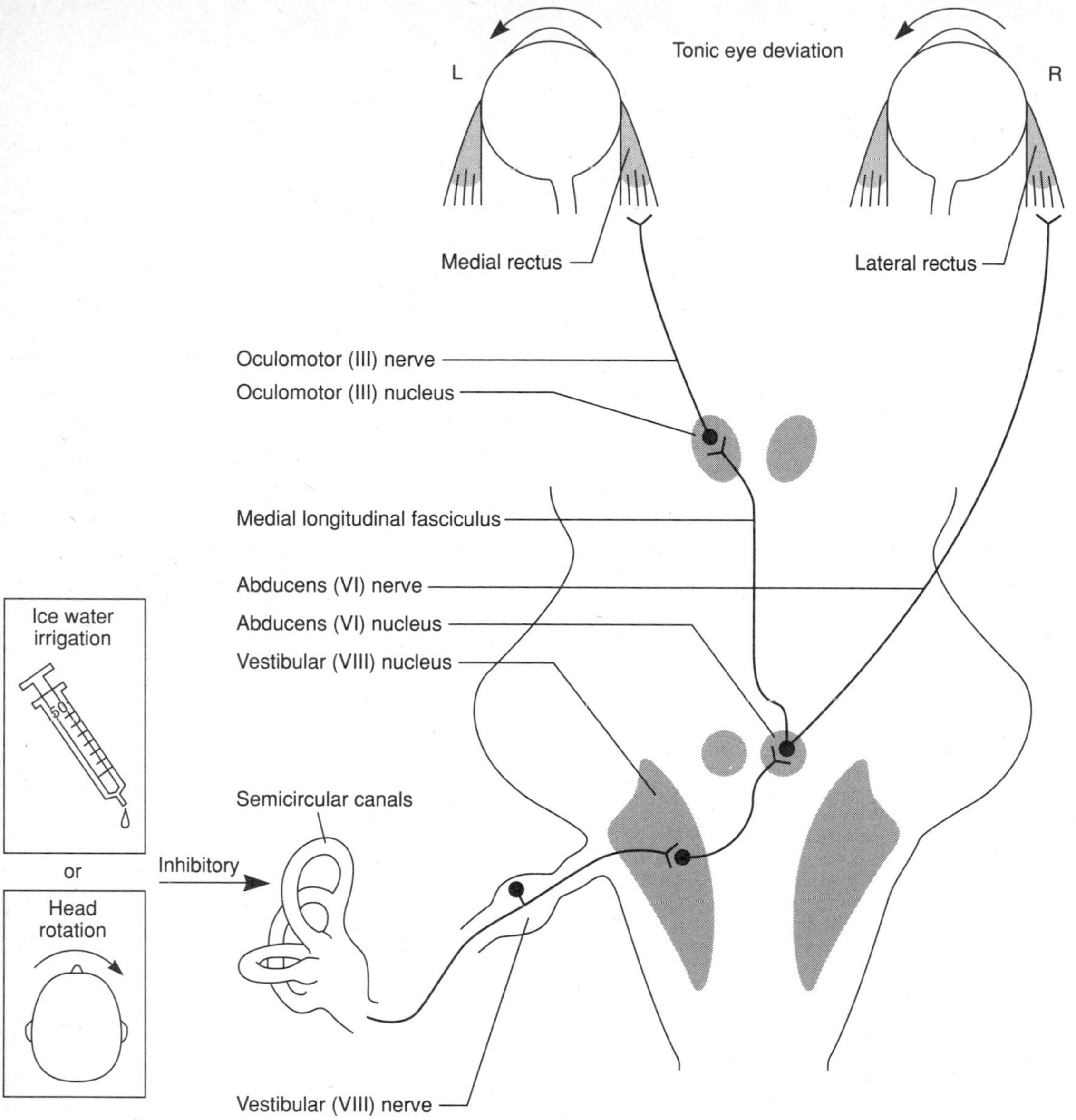

Figure 5–22. Brain stem pathways mediating conjugate horizontal eye movements. In a comatose patient with intact brain stem function, irrigation of the tympanic membrane with ice water inhibits the vestibulo-ocular pathways shown, resulting in tonic deviation of both eyes toward the irrigated side; head rotation causes eye deviation away from the direction of rotation.

Bilateral damage to occipital lobes may occur with basilar artery ischemia and produce cortical blindness. Patients with parietal or occipital lesions may be unaware of their visual defect, and with bilateral occipital lesions there may be denial of blindness **(Anton's syndrome).**

B. Oculomotor Disorders: Disorders of eye movements arise from lesions involving gaze centers (supranuclear palsies) or cranial nerves III, IV, or VI (nuclear palsies). Acute ischemic lesions involving the frontal gaze centers produce tonic deviation of the eyes toward the side of the lesion, whereas seizure discharges from a frontal gaze center cause eyes to deviate to the side opposite the epileptic focus. Midbrain lesions impinging on vertical gaze centers and pretectal nuclei can impair upward gaze and pupillary responses to light **(Parinaud's syndrome).** Abnormalities of gaze induced by cerebral

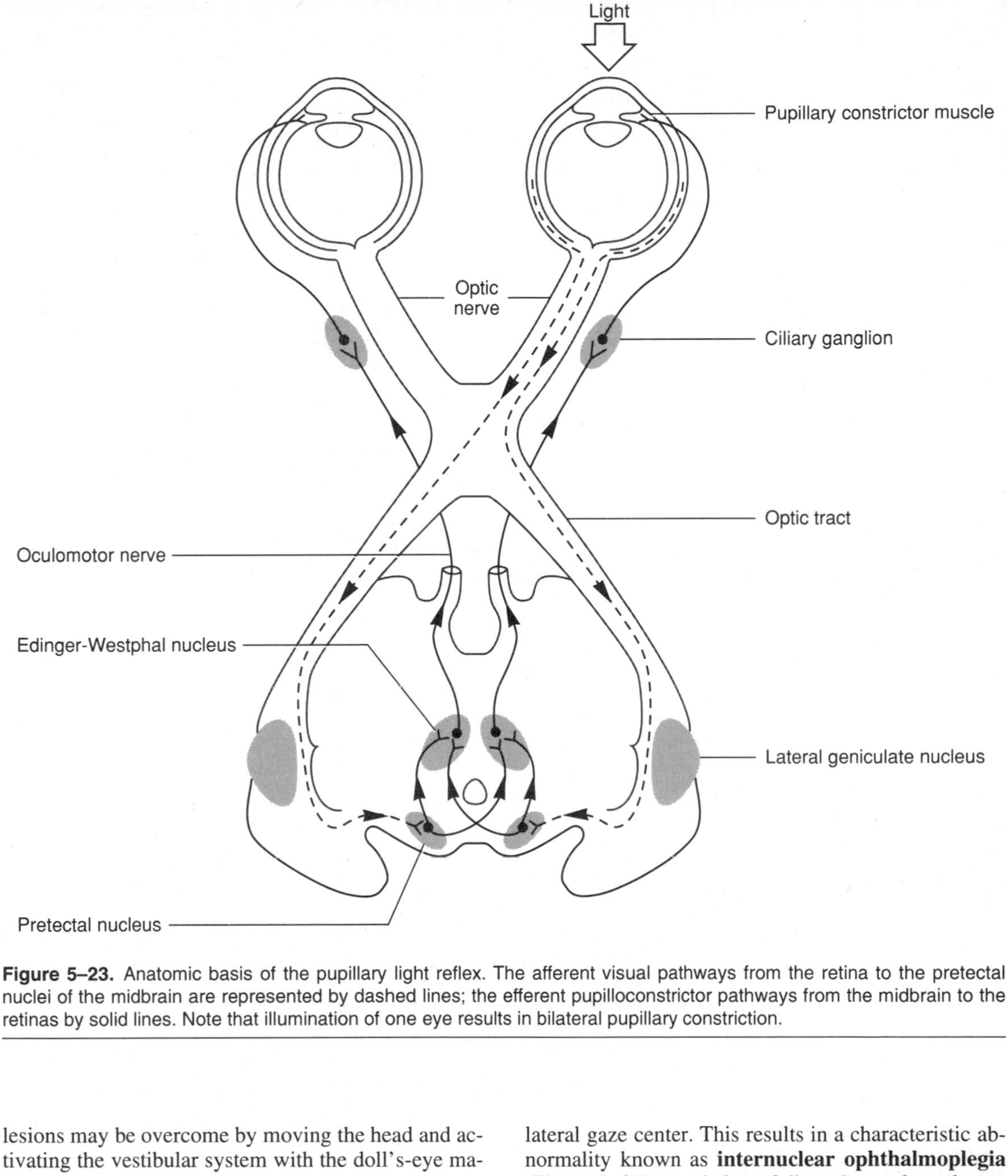

Figure 5–23. Anatomic basis of the pupillary light reflex. The afferent visual pathways from the retina to the pretectal nuclei of the midbrain are represented by dashed lines; the efferent pupilloconstrictor pathways from the midbrain to the retinas by solid lines. Note that illumination of one eye results in bilateral pupillary constriction.

lesions may be overcome by moving the head and activating the vestibular system with the doll's-eye maneuver.

Pontine lesions involving one of the lateral gaze centers cause deviation of the eyes away from the side of the lesion. Attempts to stimulate eye movements by the doll's-eye maneuver fail to overcome the gaze deviation. Such lesions commonly cause paralysis of the lateral rectus muscle on that side because of involvement of the neighboring abducens nucleus.

Lesions of the medial longitudinal fasciculus between the mid pons and the oculomotor nerve nuclei disconnect the oculomotor nuclei from the opposite lateral gaze center. This results in a characteristic abnormality known as **internuclear ophthalmoplegia** (Figure 5–24), consisting of disconjugate lateral gaze with impaired adduction of one eye and nystagmus of the abducting eye. In young adults or patients with bilateral disease, multiple sclerosis is the most common cause, whereas in the elderly, ischemic causes are more common.

Disorders that alter the function of the oculomotor, abducens, or trochlear nerves give rise to **diplopia.** The oculomotor nerve may be compressed within the subarachnoid space by expansion of an underlying posterior communicating artery aneurysm or by herniation of the ipsilateral temporal lobe. The abducens

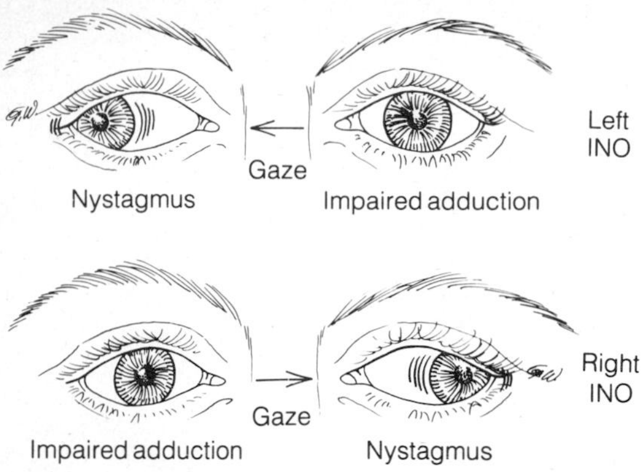

Figure 5–24. Eye movements in internuclear ophthalmoplegia (INO) resulting from a lesion of the medial longitudinal fasciculus.

nerve has a long course within the subarachnoid space and may be affected by a variety of meningeal diseases and disorders that cause increased intracranial pressure. In the cavernous sinus, diseases commonly involve the oculomotor, trochlear, and abducens nerves simultaneously along with the first and sometimes the second division of the trigeminal nerve. In contrast, lesions at the superior orbital fissure do not involve the second division of the trigeminal nerve. On the other hand, lesions within the orbit may include the optic nerve and produce protrusion of the eye **(exophthalmos).** CT or MRI is necessary to definitively localize such lesions.

Isolated oculomotor, abducens, or trochlear palsies may occur in patients with diabetes mellitus, after trauma, or without obvious cause. Diabetic oculomotor lesions characteristically do not involve parasympathetic pupillary fibers, whereas pupillary dysfunction is common in compressive oculomotor lesions. This may be due to infarction of the central fibers in diabetes, with relative sparing of the more peripherally located pupillary fibers. Pupillary dysfunction may also result from interruption of sympathetic fibers. This may occur with lesions of the sympathetic pathway in the brain stem, the cervical and upper thoracic cord, the cervical portion of the sympathetic chain, along the course of the internal carotid artery, or within the orbit. This causes **Horner's syndrome,** which consists of miosis, ptosis, and sometimes impaired sweating ipsilateral to the lesion (see Figure 5–21).

Certain myopathies and disorders of neuromuscular transmission can impair eye movements. The most common ocular myopathy is associated with hyperthyroidism. The neuromuscular junction disorders myasthenia gravis and botulism also commonly impair eye movement. Careful examination distinguishes these disorders from diseases involving gaze centers or the oculomotor, trochlear, or abducens nerves.

26. What is the pathway of fibers from the retina to the visual cortex?
27. What is the innervation of the extraocular muscles?
28. Describe the anatomic organization of the visual system and how it can be used to localize lesions.
29. What are some clinical manifestations of different visual and oculomotor system disorders, and what is their pathophysiologic explanation?

HEARING & BALANCE

Anatomy

Structures of the middle ear serve to amplify and transmit sounds to the cochlea, where specialized sensory neurons are organized to detect ranges in amplitude and frequency of sound. The semicircular canals contain specialized sensory neurons (hair cells) that detect movement of endolymphatic fluid contained within the canals. Similar hair cells in the saccule and utricle detect movement of the otolithic membrane, which is composed of calcium carbonate crystals embedded in a matrix. The semicircular canal hair cells detect angular acceleration, while the hair cells of the utricle and saccule detect linear accelaration. Axons from auditory and vestibular neurons comprise the eighth cranial nerve, which traverses the petrous bone, is joined by the facial nerve, and enters the posterior fossa through the auditory canal. Auditory fibers terminate in the cochlear nuclei of the pons, and vestibular fibers terminate in the vestibular nuclear complex.

Cochlear neurons send fibers bilaterally to a network of auditory nuclei in the midbrain, and impulses are finally relayed through the medial geniculate thalamic nuclei to the auditory cortex in the superior temporal gyri. Vestibular nuclei have connections with the cerebellum, red nuclei, brain stem gaze centers, and brain stem reticular formation. The vestibular nuclei exert considerable control over posture through descending vestibulospinal, rubrospinal, and reticulospinal pathways.

Pathophysiology

Bilateral temporal lesions can cause cortical deafness. More often, hearing loss is due to diseases of the ear or eighth cranial nerve. Secondary acoustic fibers arising from cochlear nuclei ascend bilaterally in the brain stem. Therefore, brain stem lesions rarely cause hearing loss unless severe and bilateral. Usually such extensive lesions disturb consciousness.

In contrast, vestibular function is commonly disturbed by small brain stem lesions. The vestibular nuclei occupy a large portion of the lateral brain stem, extending from medulla to midbrain. Although there are extensive bilateral connections between vestibular nuclei and other motor pathways, these connections are not redundant but are highly lateralized and act in concert to control posture, balance, and conjugate eye movement. Unilateral injury or irritation of a labyrinth results in an intense sensation of movement of the body known as **vertigo.** Diseases of the semicircular canal neurons or their fibers frequently cause rotational vertigo, whereas disease involving the utricle or saccule causes sensations of tilting or listing to one side or the other. Lesions of the vestibular nuclei or their connections within the central nervous system also cause vertigo.

Clinical Manifestations

A. Disorders of Hearing: There are three types of hearing loss: (1) **conductive deafness,** which is due to diseases of the external or middle ear that impair conduction and amplification of sound from the air to the cochlea; (2) **sensorineural deafness,** due to diseases of the cochlea or eighth cranial nerve; and (3) **central deafness,** due to diseases affecting the cochlear nuclei or auditory pathways in the central nervous system. Because of the redundancy of central pathways, almost all cases of hearing loss are due to conductive or sensorineural deafness. Besides hearing loss, auditory diseases may cause tinnitus, the subjective sensation of noise in the ear. Tinnitus due to disorders of the cochlea or eighth cranial nerve sounds like a constant nonmusical tone and may be described as ringing, whistling, hissing, humming, or roaring. Transient episodes of tinnitus occur in most individuals and are not associated with disease. When persistent, tinnitus is often associated with hearing loss.

Conductive and sensorineural deafness may be distinguished by examining hearing with a vibrating 512 Hz tuning fork. In the **Rinne test,** the tuning fork is held on the mastoid process behind the ear and then is placed at the auditory meatus. If the sound is louder at the meatus, the test is positive. Normally the test is positive, since sound transmitted through air is amplified by middle ear structures. In sensorineural deafness, although sound perception is reduced, the Rinne test is still positive since middle ear structures are intact. In conductive deafness, sounds are heard less well through air and the test is negative. In the **Weber test,** the tuning fork is applied to the forehead at the midline. In conductive deafness, the sound is heard in the abnormal ear, whereas with sensorineural deafness, the sound is heard in the normal ear. **Audiometry** can distinguish types of hearing loss. In general, sensorineural deafness causes greater loss of high-pitched sounds, whereas conductive deafness causes more loss of low-pitched sounds.

Trauma involving the middle ear, otitis media, and otosclerosis are common causes of conductive deafness. Otosclerosis is most common and is due to overgrowth of bone around the oval window with fixation of the stapes. A variety of hereditary syndromes may cause sensorineural deafness in infants and children. Acquired sensorineural deafness in children may be due to rubella, mumps, hypothyroidism (cretinism), meningitis, or infection spreading from the middle ear. Common causes of sensorineural deafness in adults include excessive exposure to loud noise; vascular disease involving the internal auditory artery; ototoxic drugs such as aminoglycoside antibiotics, quinine, and aspirin; bacterial, viral, and syphilitic infections; trauma; and hypothyroidism. In the elderly, the most common cause is **presbyacusis,** which appears to result from degenerative changes in the cochlea. Tinnitus, progressive hearing loss, and attacks of vertigo occur in **Meniere's disease.** This disorder is due to excessive accumulation of endolymph and subsequent rupture of the membranous labyrinth. Diuretics may reduce the volume of endolymph, but in severe cases, shunting of endolymph into the subarachnoid space or mastoid cavity may be necessary to prevent further hearing loss.

The auditory portion of the eighth cranial nerve may be damaged by tumors at the cerebellopontine angle. The most common tumor is an **acoustic neuroma,** which arises from the neurilemmal sheath of the vestibular portion of the eighth cranial nerve in the internal auditory canal The most common symptom is slowly progressive hearing loss. Less commonly, patients complain of mild vertigo, headache, and facial pain. Because of the proximity of the trigeminal nerve to the eighth cranial nerve, facial sensation and the corneal reflex may be diminished on the side of the affected ear.

Acoustic neuromas usually occur in isolation but may be a manifestation of **neurofibromatosis.** This disorder exists in two forms. **Neurofibromatosis 1 (NF-1)** is more common and is an autosomal dominant disorder associated with unilateral acoustic neuromas, optic nerve gliomas, cutaneous neurofibromatosis, café au lait spots, hyperpigmentation and freckling of the skin, hamartomas of the iris, and dysplastic bone lesions. Posterior fossa astrocytomas, neurofibrosarcomas, chronic myelogenous leukemia, pheochromocytomas, and carcinoid tumors are more common in patients with NF-1 than in the general population. The gene for this disorder resides on chromosome 17 and encodes for a protein, neurofibromin, which regulates the function of the proto-oncogene, *ras*. *Ras* is a key mediator of growth and differentiation. Mutations in *ras* or proteins that regulate *ras* have been found in many tumors. *Ras* is active when bound to GTP. Neurofibromin and related proteins cause the formation of inactive *ras*-GDP from *ras*-GTP by activating the intrinsic GTPase activity of *ras*. In NF-1, expression of neurofibromin is impaired, leading to increased activation of *ras* and tumor formation. **Neurofibromatosis 2 (NF-2)** is a rare autosomal dominant disorder characterized by bilateral acoustic neuromas and other neural tumors, including meningiomas, ependymomas, astrocytomas, neurofibromas, and schwannomas. The gene responsible resides on chromosome 22 but has not been identified.

B. Vestibular Disorders: Patients with diseases of the vestibular system complain of disequilibrium and dizziness. Cerebellar disease also causes disequilibrium, but this is often described as a problem with coordination rather than a feeling of dizziness in the head. Interpretation of the complaint of dizziness can often be difficult. Many patients use the term loosely to describe sensations of light-headedness, weakness, or malaise. Directed questioning is often required to establish whether there is truly an abnormal sensation of movement (vertigo).

Once the symptom of vertigo is established, the examiner must decide if it is due to disease of the labyrinth or vestibular nerve (peripheral vertigo) or to dysfunction of brain stem and central nervous system pathways (central vertigo). In general, peripheral vertigo is more severe and associated with nausea and vomiting, especially if the onset is acute. Traumatic and ischemic lesions may cause associated hearing loss. Damage to one labyrinth causes horizontal and rotatory **jerk nystagmus.** The slow phase of the nystagmus is caused by the unopposed action of the normal labyrinth, which drives the eyes to the side opposite the lesion. The fast jerk phase is due to a rapid saccade, which maintains fixation. Occasionally, the patient notes oscillation of vision **(oscillopsia).** Nystagmus due to labyrinthine damage is more prominent when the patient looks toward the side of the lesion, thereby opposing the action of the normal labyrinth. More commonly, labyrinthine diseases such as Meniere's disease cause irritation of a labyrinth and severe vertigo. In these cases, the irritated labyrinth becomes hyperactive and drives the eyes to the side of the lesion. This produces jerk nystagmus that is worse with the fast phase to the opposite side when the patient looks away from the affected ear.

In contrast, vertigo due to lesions of the central nervous system is usually less severe than peripheral vertigo and is often associated with other findings of brain stem dysfunction. In addition, nystagmus associated with central lesions may be present in vertical or multiple directions of gaze. Common causes of central vertigo include brain stem ischemia, brain stem tumors, and multiple sclerosis.

AROUSAL & DISTURBANCES OF CONSCIOUSNESS

Anatomy

The ascending reticular activating system (Figure 5–25) is composed of neurons within the central mesencephalic brain stem, the lateral hypothalamus, and the medial, intralaminar, and reticular nuclei of the thalamus. Widespread projections from these nuclei synapse on distal dendritic fields of large pyramidal neurons in the cerebral cortex and generate an arousal response.

Pathophysiology

The reticular activating system is excited by a wide variety of sensory stimuli, especially somatosensory stimuli. It is most compact in the midbrain and can be damaged by central midbrain lesions, resulting in failure of arousal, or **coma.** Higher nuclei and projections are less localized, and lesions rostrad to the midbrain must therefore be bilateral to cause coma. Certain metabolic disorders, drugs, and toxins can also disturb brain function diffusely and cause coma.

Less severe dysfunction causes **confusional states** in which consciousness is clouded and the patient is sleepy, inattentive, and disoriented. The EEG is usually abnormal, with generalized slowing of back-

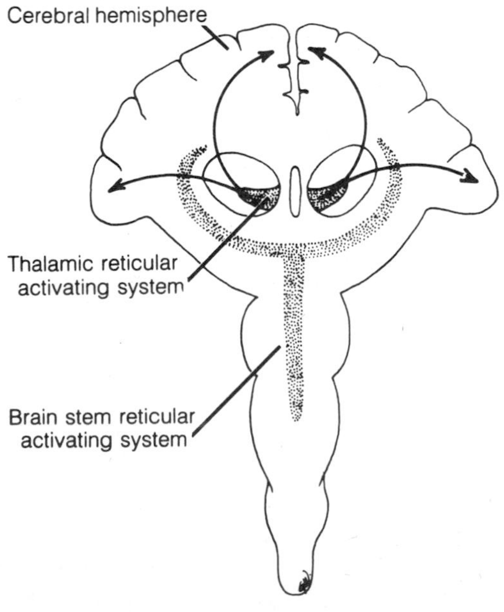

Figure 5–25. Brain stem reticular activating system and its ascending projections to the thalamus and cerebral hemispheres.

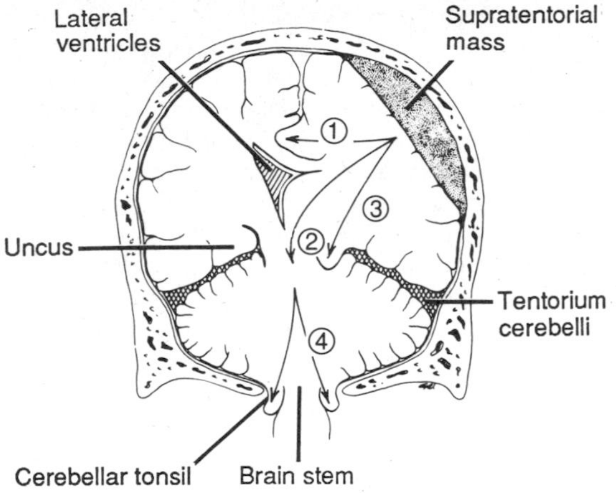

Figure 5–26. Anatomic basis of herniation syndromes. An expanding supratentorial mass lesion may cause brain tissue to be displaced into an adjacent intracranial compartment, resulting in (1) cingulate herniation under the falx, (2) downward transtentorial (central) herniation, (3) uncal herniation over the edge of the tentorium, or (4) cerebellar tonsillar herniation into the foramen magnum. Coma and ultimately death result when (2), (3) or (4) produces brain stem compression.

ground rhythms reflecting the diffuse impairment of cerebral function. In some cases, the confusional state presents as delirium, which is characterized by heightened alertness, disordered perception, agitation, delusions, hallucinations, convulsions, and autonomic hyperactivity (sweating, tachycardia, hypertension).

Neurons in the dorsal midbrain and especially nuclei within the pontine reticular formation are important for **sleep.** Thus, lesions involving the pons may preserve consciousness but disturb sleep. In contrast, diffuse lesions of the neocortex, such as those resulting from global cerebral ischemia, may preserve the reticular activating system and brain stem sleep centers; patients with these lesions have preserved sleep-wake cycles but cannot interact in any meaningful way with the environment (coma vigil or apallic state).

Clinical Manifestations

Some structural lesions of the cerebral hemispheres, such as hemorrhages, large areas of ischemic infarction, abscesses, or tumors can expand over minutes or a few hours and cause brain tissue to herniate into the posterior fossa (Figure 5–26). If lateral within the temporal lobe, the expanding mass may drive the uncus of the temporal lobe into the ambient cistern surrounding the midbrain, compressing the ipsilateral third cranial nerve **(uncal herniation).** This causes pupillary dilation and impaired function of eye muscles innervated by that nerve. Continued pressure distorts the midbrain, and the patient lapses into coma with posturing of the limbs. With continued herniation, pontine function is impaired, causing loss of oculovestibular responses. Eventually, medullary function is lost, and breathing ceases. Hemispheric lesions closer to the midline compress thalamic reticular formation structures and can cause coma before eye findings develop **(central herniation).** With continued pressure, midbrain function is affected, causing the pupils to dilate and the limbs to posture. With progressive herniation, pontine vestibular and then medullary respiratory functions are lost.

Several nonstructural disorders that diffusely disturb brain function can produce a confusional state or, if severe, coma (Table 5–1). Most of these disorders are acute, and many—particularly those due to drugs and metabolic toxins—are reversible. Clues to the etiology of these "metabolic" encephalopathies are provided by the general physical examination, drug screens, and certain blood studies. When these disorders cause coma, pupillary light responses are usually preserved despite impaired oculovestibular or respiratory function. This finding is of great help in distinguishing metabolic from structural causes of coma.

In patients who are confused but not comatose, examination of the patient's level of consciousness, perceptions, memory, and thinking uncovers a suspected confusional state. Alertness is reduced, and the patient will appear drowsy or fall asleep easily without frequent stimulation. More awake patients perceive stimuli slowly and fail to synthesize multiple stimuli correctly. They become distractible, assigning equal significance to important and trivial stimuli. Perceptions may be distorted, leading to hallucinations, and the patient may be unable to organize and interpret all elements of a complex set of

Table 5–1. Nonstructural causes of confusional states and coma.

Drugs (sedative-hypnotics, ethanol, opioids)
Global cerebral ischemia
Hepatic encephalopathy
Hypercalcemia
Hyperosmolar states
Hyperthermia
Hypoglycemia
Hyponatremia
Hypoxia
Hypothyroidism
Meningitis and encephalitis
Seizure or prolonged postictal state
Subarachnoid hemorrhage
Uremia
Wernicke's encephalopathy

stimuli. Perceptual difficulties interfere with learning and memory and with problem-solving. Thoughts become disorganized, tangential, and fragmented. In combination with distorted perceptions, patients may maintain false beliefs even in the face of compelling discrediting evidence **(delusions).**

Often a confusional state is obvious from the patient's behavior. In mild cases, careful examination of the patient's mental state is required. Observing spontaneous conversation for lack of continuity, breaks in eye contact, and interruptions because of drowsiness or distractibility can reveal subtle deficits in concentration and attention. Attention and the capacity for sustained mental activity can be further assessed by asking the patient to cross out certain letters on a printed page, count forward and backward, and repeat groups of four to six numbers in forward or reverse sequence. Serial subtraction of sevens, saying the months of the year backward, and spelling words backward are also useful tests of sustained mental activity. Attempts to engage the patient in normal conversation reveal incoherent and fragmented thinking. Having the patient recall four simple, familiar items after 5 minutes tests retentive memory and learning.

It is sometimes difficult to distinguish confusional states from other disorders that affect the speed and clarity of thinking. In dementing diseases (see below), the content of thought is reduced, and there may be delusions, incoherent conversation, and agitation. The level of consciousness may also be impaired in advanced cases. However, dementias can usually be distinguished from confusional states by their mode of onset and course. Confusional states often begin abruptly and cause fluctuating changes in the level of consciousness. In contrast, dementias have a slow onset, progress over months to years, and disturb the level of consciousness late in their course. Manic-depressive psychosis and schizophrenia can usually be separated from confusional states by the presence of a normal level of consciousness and intact memory.

COGNITIVE FUNCTION & DEMENTIA

Several disorders disturb the content rather than the level of consciousness. Affected patients have difficulty learning, remembering, calculating, drawing, using language, perceiving spatial relationships, making decisions, or performing complex motor tasks despite being alert and attentive. When several of these abilities are impaired, the patient is said to suffer from **dementia.** In other patients, focal brain lesions produce selective deficits such as **amnesia** or **aphasia.**

Anatomy

Dementia results from diseases that cause widespread disturbance in the function of cortical neurons. The major categories of disease that cause dementia are listed in Table 5–2. **Alzheimer's disease** is the most common cause and results in loss of neurons in widespread areas of the cerebral cortex, especially in cortical association areas and the basal forebrain. **Pick's disease** is a much less common degenerative disorder in which neuronal loss is more limited to frontal and temporal cortex. These disorders are distinguished by severe disturbances in memory, language, calculation, and spatial orientation; impaired performance of complex motor tasks **(apraxias);** and impaired recognition of objects, faces, colors, and sounds **(agnosias).** In contrast, several other degenerative disorders such as **Huntington's disease** or **Parkinson's disease** cause degeneration of subcortical nuclei and prominent motor abnormalities early in their course. Dementia may appear later and is characterized by forgetfulness, slowed thought, apathy, and depression rather than by aphasia, agnosia, and apraxia. The terms "cortical dementia" and "subcortical dementia" have been used to distinguish these two patterns of dementia. The terms are somewhat misleading, because the pathologic effects of these disorders are not strictly limited to cortical or subcortical structures. However, the terms help to emphasize differences in presentation and character.

Pathophysiology

A striking pathologic feature of Alzheimer's disease is the presence of argyrophilic plaques in the cerebral cortex and subcortical gray matter. These are composed of large extracellular collections of degenerated cellular processes surrounding a central mass of amyloid material (Figure 5–27). A current hypothesis proposes that deposition of β-amyloid in brain parenchyma is involved in the pathogenesis of Alzheimer's disease. β-Amyloid is processed from the β-amyloid precursor protein (APP). A role for deposition of β-amyloid in the disease is supported by

Table 5–2. Major causes of dementia.

Alzheimer's disease (>50% of cases)
Multiple cerebral infarcts
Alcoholism
Low-pressure hydrocephalus
Primary or metastatic central nervous system neoplasms
Parkinson's disease
Huntington's disease
Pick's disease
Prion diseases (eg, Creutzfeldt-Jacob disease)
Neurosyphilis
HIV infection
Hypothyroidism
Deficiency of vitamin B_{12}, B_6, B_1, or niacin
Chronic meningitis
Subdural hematoma

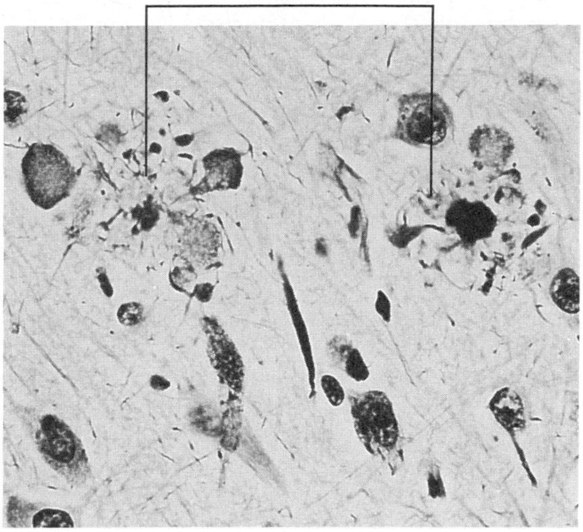

Figure 5–27. Amyloid plaques in cerebral cortex in Alzheimer's disease.

evidence that mutations or duplications in the gene for APP on chromosome 21 are found in some cases of familial Alzheimer's disease. The observation that patients with Down's syndrome (trisomy 21) show lesions of Alzheimer's disease and loss of cognitive function in adulthood also supports this hypothesis. Recently, the E4 allele of the apolipoprotein E (ApoE) gene on chromosome 19 has been strongly associated with an increased risk of developing Alzheimer's disease. ApoE binds amyloid, and the E4 isoform appears to promote the formation of aggregates of β-amyloid fibrils. Presumably this leads to neuronal damage and cell death. However, not all cases of Alzheimer's disease can be explained by the mutations in APP or the presence of ApoE4. Recently, a locus on chromosome 14 has been linked to the majority of familial cases of early-onset Alzheimer's disease. The molecular basis for this association is not yet known.

In addition to degenerative disorders, a variety of other conditions cause dementia (Table 5–2). Although most causes of meningitis or encephalitis produce acute confusional states, some, such as tertiary neurosyphilis or the AIDS-dementia complex, present slowly, with features more characteristic of dementia. Paretic neurosyphilis results from chronic meningoencephalitis and can present with behavioral disturbances and dementia before tremor, impaired gait, unsteadiness, and dysarthria appear. AIDS-dementia complex often presents like a "subcortical" dementia, with motor deficits, apathy, depression, and slowed thinking. AIDS-dementia complex may result from neurotoxic effects of cytokines (eg, TNFα), metabolites (quinolinic acid), and viral proteins (gp120) released from infected macrophages and microglia as well as from direct infection of oligodendrocytes and astrocytes with HIV.

Extensive multifocal brain lesions due to trauma or vascular disease can cause dementia. In dementia due to vascular disease, the underlying lesion is often atherosclerosis. Usually there is a history of stepwise decline and the presence of multifocal motor, sensory, or visual deficits on examination. Compression of the hemispheres by chronic subdural hematomas or compression of cerebral white matter by chronic hydrocephalus can impair mentation without obvious lateralized neurologic signs, thereby mimicking a degenerative dementia. Certain brain tumors—especially those involving the corpus callosum, frontal lobes, or temporal lobes—may impair mentation before more obvious focal signs and seizures appear. Dementia may also complicate certain endocrine and toxic disorders.

30. What are the levels at which vestibular disorders may occur, and what are characteristic clinical manifestations of each?
31. What is the pathway of neurons that maintain normal arousal and consciousness?
32. What are the signs and symptoms of cerebral herniation due to focal brain lesions?
33. How would you distinguish confusional states, dementias, and psychoses?

PATHOPHYSIOLOGY OF SELECTED NEUROLOGIC DISORDERS

The past decade has witnessed an explosion in information about nervous system function and the molecular basis of neurologic disease. The four disorders discussed below demonstrate how recent knowledge and theories about pathophysiology have influenced treatment.

PARKINSON'S DISEASE

Clinical Presentation

Parkinsonism is a clinical syndrome of rigidity, bradykinesia, tremor, and postural instability. Most cases are due to Parkinson's disease, an idiopathic disorder with a prevalence of about 1–2:1000. In the first half of this century, parkinsonism was a common sequela of von Economo's encephalitis, but since this infection no longer occurs, this type of parkinsonism is rare. Parkinsonism can also result from exposure to certain toxins such as manganese, carbon disulfide, or carbon monoxide. Several drugs, particularly butyrophenones, phenothiazines, metoclopramide, reserpine, and tetrabenazine, can cause reversible parkinsonism. Parkinsonism may also result from repeated head trauma or may be a feature of several basal ganglia diseases, including Wilson's disease, some cases of Huntington's disease, Shy-Drager syndrome, striatonigral degeneration, and progressive supranuclear palsy. In these disorders, other symptoms and signs are present along with parkinsonism.

Pathology & Pathogenesis

In Parkinson's disease there is selective degeneration of monoamine-containing cell populations in the brain stem and basal ganglia, particularly of pigmented dopaminergic neurons of the substantia nigra. In addition, scattered neurons in basal ganglia, brain stem, spinal cord, and sympathetic ganglia contain eosinophilic inclusion bodies **(Lewy bodies).**

The mechanism by which dopaminergic neurons of the substantia nigra degenerate in Parkinson's disease is not understood. However, much has been learned about the pathogenesis of Parkinson's disease through study of the potent neurotoxin MPTP (1-methyl-4-phenyl-1,2,3,6-tetrahydropyridine). MPTP is a by-product of synthesis of a synthetic opioid derivative of meperidine. Illicit use of opioid preparations heavily contaminated with MPTP led to several cases of parkinsonism in the early 1980s. MPTP selectively injures monoamine cell populations in the brain and produces a clinical syndrome very similar to Parkinson's disease.

MPTP enters the brain (Figure 5–28) and is converted by monoamine oxidase B present in glia and serotonergic nerve terminals to N-methyl-4-phenyldihydropyridine ($MPDP^+$), which diffuses across glial membranes and then undergoes nonenzymatic oxidation and reduction to the active metabolite N-methyl-4-phenylpyridinium (MPP^+). MPP^+ is taken up by plasma membrane transporters that normally act to terminate the action of monoamines by removing them from synapses. Internalized MPP^+ inhibits oxidative phosphorylation by interacting with complex I of the mitochondrial electron transport chain. This inhibits ATP production and reduces metabolism of molecular oxygen, allowing for increased formation of peroxide, hydroxyl radicals, and superoxide radicals that react with lipids, proteins, and nucleic acids to cause cell injury.

Despite clinical and pathologic similarities between MPTP toxicity and Parkinson's disease, no toxin has been identified in Parkinson's disease. However, exogenous dopamine is toxic to neurons in culture. Dopamine undergoes auto-oxidation to generate superoxide radicals or is metabolized by monoamine oxidase to generate hydrogen peroxide. The enzyme superoxide dismutase catalyzes the conversion of superoxide to H_2O_2, which is converted by glutathione peroxidase and catalase to water. However, H_2O_2 can also react with ferrous iron to form highly reactive hydroxyl radicals. In Parkinson's disease, conditions favor the formation of free radicals, since iron deposition in the substantia nigra is increased while levels of glutathione are reduced.

Treatment

Treatment is directed toward restoring the balance of dopaminergic and cholinergic activity in the striatum and preventing further neural degeneration. This

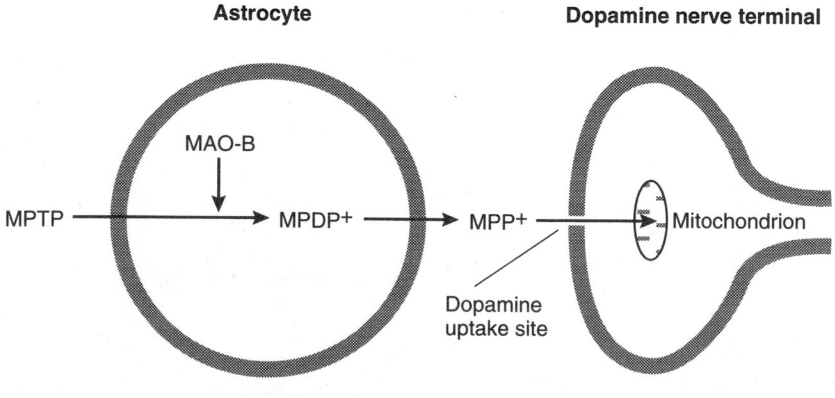

Figure 5–28. Proposed mechanism of MPTP-induced parkinsonism. MPTP enters brain astrocytes and is converted to $MDPD^+$ through the action of monoamine oxidase type B (MAO-B). $MPDP^+$ is then metabolized extracellularly to MPP^+, which is taken up through dopamine uptake sites on dopamine nerve terminals and concentrated in mitochondria. The resulting disturbance of mitochondrial function can lead to neuronal death.

is accomplished by blocking the effect of acetylcholine with anticholinergic drugs or by increasing the effect of dopamine. For reasons that are not clear, anticholinergic drugs are more helpful in reducing tremor and rigidity than relieving bradykinesia, which is often the more disabling symptom. In contrast, dopaminergic drugs are quite effective in alleviating bradykinesia and rigidity. Levodopa, which is converted to dopamine, or ergot derivatives such as bromocriptine and pergolide that are dopamine agonists, can be given orally to relieve symptoms. Amantadine, an antiviral agent, also reduces manifestations of Parkinson's disease, probably by increasing the release of dopamine. Selegiline is an inhibitor of MAO-B that prevents experimental MPTP toxicity. Selegiline also inhibits metabolism of dopamine and therefore increases the antiparkinsonian effect of levodopa. Selegiline also delays the onset of disability in early Parkinson's disease, perhaps by inhibiting dopamine metabolism, which may reduce free radical formation and oxidative stress in surviving dopaminergic neurons.

34. What are the clinical features of parkinsonism?
35. What are some of the causes of this syndrome?
36. What is the pathophysiology of Parkinson's disease?

MYASTHENIA GRAVIS

Clinical Presentation

Myasthenia gravis is an autoimmune disorder of neuromuscular transmission. The major clinical features are fluctuating fatigue and weakness that improve after a period of rest and after administration of acetylcholinesterase inhibitors. Muscles with small motor units, such as ocular muscles, are most often affected. Oropharyngeal muscles, flexors and extensors of the neck, proximal limb muscles, and the erector spinae muscle are involved less often. In severe cases, all muscles are weak, including the diaphragm and intercostal muscles, and death may result from respiratory failure.

About 5% of patients have coexistent hyperthyroidism. Rheumatoid arthritis, systemic lupus erythematosus, and polymyositis are also more common in patients with myasthenia gravis than in the general population, and up to 30% of patients have a maternal relative with an autoimmune disorder. These associations suggest that patients with myasthenia gravis share a genetic predisposition to autoimmune disease.

Pathology & Pathogenesis

The major structural abnormality in myasthenia gravis is a simplification of the postsynaptic region of the neuromuscular synapse. The muscle endplate shows sparse, shallow, and abnormally wide or absent synaptic clefts. In contrast, the number and size of the presynaptic vesicles are normal. Scattered collections of lymphocytes, some within the vicinity of motor endplates, may be present. IgG and the C3 component of complement are present at the postsynaptic membrane.

Electrophysiologic studies indicate that the postsynaptic membrane has a decreased response to applied acetylcholine. Studies with ^{125}I-labeled α-bungarotoxin, which binds with high affinity to muscle nicotinic acetylcholine receptors, show a 70–90% decrease in the number of receptors per endplate in affected muscles. Antibodies to the receptor are present in 70–90% of patients, and the disorder may be passively transferred to animals by administration of IgG from affected patients. Moreover, immunization with acetylcholine receptor protein from muscle can produce myasthenia in experimental animals. The antibodies block acetylcholine binding and receptor activation. In addition, the antibodies cross-link pairs of receptor molecules, increasing receptor internalization and degradation. Bound antibody also activates complement-mediated destruction of the postsynaptic region, resulting in simplification of the endplate.

During repetitive stimulation of a motor nerve, the number of quanta released from the nerve terminal declines with successive stimuli. Normally, this causes no clinical impairment because a sufficient number of acetylcholine receptor channels are opened by the reduced level of neurotransmitter. However, in myasthenia gravis, where there is a deficiency in the number of functional acetylcholine receptors, neuromuscular transmission fails at lower levels of quantal release. Electrophysiologically, this is measured as a decremental decline in the compound muscle action potential during repetitive stimulation of a motor nerve. Clinically, this is manifested by muscle fatigue with sustained or repeated activity.

Treatment

Treatment has reduced the mortality rate from approximately 30% to 5% in generalized myasthenia gravis. The two basic strategies for treatment are to increase the amount of acetylcholine at the neuromuscular junction and to inhibit immune-mediated destruction of acetylcholine receptors.

By preventing metabolism of acetylcholine, cholinesterase inhibitors can compensate for the normal decline in released neurotransmitter during repeated stimulation. The diagnosis of myasthenia gravis can also be confirmed by administration of the short-acting cholinesterase inhibitor edrophonium. A positive result consists of a brief improvement in strength of affected muscles.

Therapy with cholinesterase inhibitors can cause a paradoxical increase in weakness known as a **cholinergic crisis.** This is due to an excess of acetylcholine. At the microscopic level, binding of acetylcholine first opens nicotinic cation channels, but with continued exposure to the agonist, the channels desensitize and shut down again. The desensitized channels recover their sensitivity to acetylcholine only after the neurotransmitter is removed. Removal of acetylcholine is impaired when cholinesterase activity is inhibited. This can result in depolarization block of neurotransmission similar to the effect of the depolarizing paralytic agent succinylcholine or organophosphate insecticides and nerve gases that markedly inhibit acetylcholinesterase. Therefore, the dose of cholinesterase inhibitors must be carefully regulated to reduce myasthenia but avoid a cholinergic crisis.

Immunotherapy of myasthenia gravis includes thymectomy, plasmapheresis, corticosteroids, and immunosuppressant drugs such as azathioprine. With initiation of steroids, patients may first deteriorate and in some cases become ventilator-dependent. This may result from inhibitory effects of steroids on neurotransmitter release. The thymus is thought to play an important role in the pathogenesis of the disease by supplying helper T cells sensitized against thymic nicotinic receptors. In most patients with myasthenia gravis, the thymus is hyperplastic, and 10–15% have thymomas. Thymectomy is indicated if a thymoma is suspected. In patients with generalized myasthenia without thymoma, thymectomy induces remission in 35% and improves symptoms in another 45% of patients.

37. What is the clinical presentation of myasthenia gravis?
38. What causes this disorder?
39. What is the pathophysiology of symptoms in myasthenia gravis?

EPILEPSY

Clinical Presentation

Seizures are paroxysmal disturbances in cerebral function caused by an abnormal synchronous discharge of cortical neurons. The epilepsies are a group of disorders characterized by recurrent seizures. Approximately 0.6% of people in the United States suffer from recurrent seizures, and idiopathic epilepsy accounts for more than 75% of all seizure disorders. In some forms of idiopathic epilepsy, a genetic basis is apparent. Other forms of epilepsy are secondary to brain injury from stroke, trauma, a mass lesion, or infection. About two-thirds of new cases arise in children, and most of these cases are idiopathic or due to trauma. In contrast, seizures or epilepsy with onset in adult life are more often due to underlying brain lesions or metabolic causes.

Seizures are classified by behavioral and electrophysiologic data (Table 5–3). **Generalized tonic-clonic seizures** are attacks characterized by sudden loss of consciousness followed rapidly by tonic contraction of muscles, causing limb extension and arching of the back. The tonic phase lasts 10–30 seconds and is followed by a clonic phase of limb jerking. The jerking builds in frequency to a peak after 15–30 seconds and then slows gradually over another 15–30 seconds. The patient then remains unconscious for several minutes. As consciousness is regained, there is a period of postictal confusion lasting several more minutes. In patients with recurrent seizures or an underlying structural or metabolic abnormality, confusion may persist for a few hours. Focal abnormalities may be present on neurologic examination during the postictal period. Such findings suggest a focal brain lesion requiring further laboratory and radiologic study.

Typical **absence seizures** begin in childhood and usually remit by adulthood. Seizures are characterized by brief lapses in consciousness lasting several seconds without loss of posture. These spells may be associated with eyelid blinking, slight head movement, or brief jerks of limb muscles. Immediately following the seizure, the patient is fully alert. The spells may occur several times through the day and impair school performance. The EEG shows characteristic runs of spikes and waves at a rate of three per second, particularly following hyperventilation. The disorder is transmitted as an autosomal dominant trait with incomplete penetrance.

Some forms of epilepsy cause seizures with only a tonic or a clonic phase. In others, the seizure is manifested by sudden loss of muscle tone (atonic seizures). In myoclonic epilepsy, sudden, brief contractions of muscles occur. Myoclonic seizures are found in certain neurodegenerative diseases or following diffuse brain injury, as occurs during global cerebral ischemia.

Table 5–3. Simplified classification of seizures.

I. Partial (focal seizures)
   A. Simple partial seizures with motor, sensory, psychic, or autonomic symptoms
   B. Complex partial seizures
   C. Partial seizures with secondary generalization
II. Generalized seizures
   A. Absence seizures
   B. Tonic-clonic seizures
   C. Other (myoclonic, tonic, clonic, atonic)

Partial seizures are caused by focal brain disease. Therefore, in general, patients with simple or complex partial seizures should be investigated for underlying brain lesions. **Simple partial seizures** begin with motor, sensory, visual, psychic, or autonomic phenomena depending on the location of the seizure focus. Consciousness is preserved unless the seizure discharge spreads to other areas, producing a tonic-clonic seizure **(secondary generalization). Complex partial seizures** are characterized by the sudden onset of impaired consciousness with stereotyped, coordinated, involuntary movements **(automatisms).** Immediately prior to impairment of consciousness, there may be an aura consisting of unusual abdominal sensations, olfactory or sensory hallucinations, unexplained fear, or illusions of familiarity (déjà vu). Seizures usually last for 2–5 minutes and are followed by postictal confusion. Secondary generalization may occur. The seizure focus usually lies in the temporal or frontal lobe.

Pathogenesis

Normal neuronal activity occurs in a nonsynchronized manner, with groups of neurons inhibited and excited sequentially during the transfer of information between different brain areas. Seizures occur when neurons in a focal region or in the entire brain are activated synchronously. The kind of seizure depends on the location of the abnormal activity and the pattern of spread to different parts of the brain.

Interictal spike discharges are often observed on electroencephalographic recordings from epileptic patients. These are due to synchronous depolarization of a group of neurons in an abnormally excitable area of brain. Experimentally, this is known as the **paroxysmal depolarizing shift** and is followed by a hyperpolarizing afterpotential that is the cellular correlate of the slow wave that follows spike discharges on the EEG. The shift is produced by depolarizing currents generated at excitatory synapses and by subsequent influx of sodium or calcium through voltage-gated channels.

Normally, discharging excitatory neurons activate nearby inhibitory interneurons that suppress the activity of the discharging cell and its neighbors. Most inhibitory synapses utilize the neurotransmitter γ-aminobutyric acid (GABA). Voltage-sensitive and calcium-dependent potassium currents are also activated in the discharging neuron to suppress excitability. In addition, adenosine generated from ATP released during excitation further suppresses neuronal excitation by binding to adenosine receptors present on nearby neurons. Disruption of these inhibitory mechanisms by alterations in ion channels, or by injury to inhibitory neurons and synapses, may allow for the development of a seizure focus. In addition, groups of neurons may become synchronized if local excitatory circuits are enhanced by reorganization of neural networks after a brain injury.

Spread of a local discharge occurs by a combination of mechanisms. During the paroxysmal depolarizing shift, extracellular potassium accumulates, depolarizing nearby neurons. Increased frequency of discharges enhances calcium influx into nerve terminals, increasing neurotransmitter release at excitatory synapses by a process known as **posttetanic potentiation.** This involves increased calcium influx through voltage-sensitive channels and through the N-methyl-D-aspartate (NMDA) subtype of glutamate receptor-gated ion channels. NMDA receptor-gated channels preferentially pass calcium ions but are relatively quiescent during normal synaptic transmission because they are blocked by magnesium ions. Magnesium block is relieved by depolarization. In contrast, the effect of inhibitory synaptic neurotransmission appears to decrease with high-frequency stimulation. This may be partly due to rapid desensitization of GABA receptors at high concentrations of released GABA. The net effect of these changes is to recruit neighboring neurons into a synchronous discharge and cause a seizure.

In secondary epilepsy, loss of inhibitory circuits and sprouting of fibers from excitatory neurons appear to be important for the generation of a seizure focus. In the idiopathic epilepsies, the biochemical or structural defects are generally not known. Studies in the lethargic mouse (lh/lh), however, reveal a possible mechanism for absence seizures. Absence seizures arise from synchronous thalamic discharges that are mediated by activation of low-threshold calcium currents (T or "transient" currents) in thalamic neurons. The anticonvulsant ethosuximide blocks T channels and suppresses absence seizures in humans. T channels are more likely to be activated following hyperpolarization of the cell membrane. Activation of $GABA_B$ receptors hyperpolarizes thalamic neurons and facilitates T channel activation. Lethargic mice demonstrate frequent absence spells accompanied by 5–6 Hz spike-wave discharges on the EEG and respond to drugs used in human absence epilepsy. A single mutation on chromosome 2 results in this autosomal recessive disorder. There is an increase in the number of $GABA_B$ receptors in the cerebral cortex in these mice, and the $GABA_B$ agonist baclofen worsens the seizures, whereas antagonists alleviate them. This suggests that abnormal regulation of $GABA_B$ receptor function or expression may be important in the pathogenesis of absence seizures.

Treatment

The main targets for anticonvulsants are (1) voltage-gated ion channels that maintain the resting membrane potential and are involved in the generation of action potentials and neurotransmitter release, and (2) ligand-gated channels that modulate synaptic excitation and inhibition. Many agents act by more than one mechanism. Several anticonvulsants and their presumed mechanisms of action are listed in Table 5–4.

40. What is the clinical presentation of seizures?
41. What are some of the causes of seizure disorders?
42. What is the pathophysiology of seizures?

STROKE

Clinical Presentation

Stroke is a clinical syndrome characterized by the acute onset of focal neurologic deficits due to an abnormality in cerebral circulation. Symptoms may be maximal at onset or progress over a few seconds to hours. Symptoms that resolve within 24 hours constitute a **transient ischemic attack.** A variety of vascular, cardiac, or hematologic disorders can impair circulation and cause stroke (Table 5–5). These disorders produce stroke by causing focal ischemia or hemorrhage.

Pathology & Pathogenesis

A. Ischemia: Most ischemic strokes result from narrowing of arteries or arterioles and damage to the endothelial surface. This promotes platelet aggregation and thrombosis, which can occlude the vessel lumen. In addition, fragments of clotted blood can break away and travel downstream to occlude narrower distal vessels. This process is known as **thromboembolism** and is most often due to atherosclerosis of large cerebral vessels. Atherosclerosis produces fibrous plaques on the intimal surface of arteries and narrows the lumen. The plaque contains lipid material that can be released into the circulation if the plaque ruptures, occluding smaller branch arteries and arterioles. Vessels may also be damaged locally by inflammation **(arteritis).** Chronic hypertension may damage small arteries and arterioles, causing small areas of infarction known as **lacunar infarctions.** These typically occur in the corpus striatum, internal capsule, thalamus, pons, and subcortical white matter.

In several cardiac disorders, thrombi may be generated within the heart and form fragments that embolize to the brain. In addition, emboli formed within large veins may embolize to the arterial system if a patent atrial septal defect is present. Some hematologic disorders (polycythemia vera, leukemia) are associated with a marked increase in the number of circulating red or white blood cells, respectively, which increases blood viscosity and predisposes to thrombosis.

In thromboembolic stroke and strokes due to cardiac emboli, neurologic deficits result from focal ischemia to the area of brain supplied by the affected blood vessel. The history and neurologic examination help localize the damage to a particular vascular territory. Usually there is enough information to localize the deficit to the anterior or posterior cerebral circulation and—within the anterior circulation—to the right or left hemisphere. The anterior circulation comprises branches of the anterior and middle cerebral arteries (Figure 5–29), which supply most of the cerebral cortex, subcortical white matter, and striatum. The posterior circulation comprises branches of the vertebral, basilar, and posterior cerebral arteries (Figure 5–29) and supplies much of the thalamus, portions of the occipital and temporal lobes, and the

Table 5–4. Known mechanisms of action of some anticonvulsant drugs.

Drug	Main Indications	Mechanisms of Action
Phenytoin	Generalized tonic-clonic and partial seizures	Inhibition of voltage-gated sodium and calcium channels
Carbamazepine	Generalized tonic-clonic and partial seizures	Inhibition of voltage-gated sodium and calcium channels
Phenobarbital	Generalized tonic-clonic and partial seizures	Enhancement of $GABA_A$ receptor function
Valproate	Generalized tonic-clonic, absence, myoclonic, and partial seizures	Increases levels of GABA; inhibits low-threshold (T-type) voltage-gated calcium channels
Ethosuximide	Absence seizures	Inhibition of low-threshold (T-type) voltage-gated calcium channels
Felbamate	Generalized tonic-clonic and partial seizures	Antagonist of NMDA subtype of glutamate receptors; enhances action of GABA at $GABA_A$ receptors
Lamotrigine	Generalized tonic-clonic and partial seizures	Inhibition of voltage-gated sodium channels
Vigabatrin	Partial and secondarily generalized seizures	Increases GABA levels by inhibiting GABA transaminase

Table 5–5. Conditions associated with focal cerebral ischemia.[1]

Vascular disorders
Atherosclerosis
Fibromuscular dysplasia
Inflammatory disorders
Giant cell arteritis
Systemic lupus erythematosus
Polyarteritis nodosa
Granulomatous angiitis
Syphilitic arteritis
AIDS
Carotid or vertebral artery dissection
Lacunar infarction
Drug abuse
Migraine
Multiple progressive intracranial occlusions (moyamoya syndrome)
Venous or sinus thrombosis
Cardiac disorders
Mural thrombus
Rheumatic heart disease
Arrhythmias
Endocarditis
Mitral valve prolapse
Paradoxic embolus
Atrial myxoma
Prosthetic heart valves
Hematologic disorders
Thrombocytosis
Polycythemia
Sickle cell disease
Leukocytosis
Hypercoagulable states

Reproduced, with permission, from Greenberg DA, Aminoff MJ, Simon RP: *Clinical Neurology,* 2nd ed. Appleton & Lange, 1993.

entire brain stem. Anterior circulation strokes produce signs and symptoms of hemispheric dysfunction, including apraxia, aphasia, agnosia, hemisensory loss, hemianopia, and hemiparesis. Posterior circulation strokes produce signs and symptoms of brain stem, cerebellar, thalamic, and occipital dysfunction, including vertigo, crossed sensory deficits, hemiparesis or quadriparesis, ataxia, dysarthria, diplopia, hemianopia, cortical blindness, and in some cases coma.

B. Intracerebral Hemorrhage: Strokes may also result from rupture of vessels and the formation of an intracerebral hematoma. Certain disorders such as chronic hypertension cause intracerebral hemorrhage by damaging and weakening vessels. Hemorrhage is common with arteriovenous malformations that contain abnormal vessels unable to withstand arterial pressures. Certain platelet and coagulation disorders may also predispose to intracerebral hemorrhage by inhibiting coagulation. In all of these disorders, the resultant hematoma causes a neurologic deficit by compressing adjacent structures. Metabolic effects of extravasated blood on neighboring neurons may also disturb their function. In addition, nearby vessels may be compressed, causing ischemia to neighboring brain regions.

C. Excitotoxicity: Neurons deep within an ischemic focus die from energy deprivation. However, at the edge of the ischemic region, neurons appear to die because of excessive stimulation of glutamate receptors. Glutamate is the major excitatory neurotransmitter in the brain. Following its release, glutamate is normally cleared from the extracellular space by sodium-dependent uptake systems in neurons and glia. Ischemia deprives the brain of oxygen and glucose, and the resultant disruption in cellular metabolism depletes neurons and glial cells of energy reserves required to maintain normal transmembrane ion gradients. This leads to accumulation of intracellular sodium and collapse of the transmembrane sodium gradient, which, in turn, inhibits the glutamate uptake system, allowing glutamate to accumulate extracellularly within an ischemic focus. Glutamate receptors on surrounding neurons are thus stimulated, resulting in entry of calcium and sodium. Depolarization of these neurons stimulates additional calcium influx through voltage-dependent channels. The resultant overload in intracellular calcium may exceed the ability of the neuron to extrude or sequester the cation, resulting in sustained activation of a variety of calcium-sensitive enzymes, including proteases, phospholipases, endonucleases, and kinases, leading to cell death. In support of an excitotoxic mechanism of cell death in stroke are animal studies that demonstrate a reduction in the size of ischemic lesions following treatment with glutamate receptor antagonists.

Treatment

Traditional goals of therapy in stroke are to treat underlying vascular, cardiac, or hematologic causes and, in cases of ischemic stroke, prevent stroke recurrence by inhibiting coagulation. Experimental approaches include using antagonists of voltage-sensitive calcium channels and glutamate receptors to improve neuronal survival and stimulating fibrinolysis to restore circulation.

Hypertension is the most important risk factor for stroke. However, the regulation of cerebral blood flow in response to changes in systemic blood pressure is compromised in patients with chronic hypertension due to structural changes in vessel walls. In addition, many patients with acute strokes have elevated blood pressures, and attempts to reduce blood pressure may severely compromise the blood supply to ischemic but viable brain tissue. Therefore, it is best to wait 2–3 weeks after an acute stroke before carefully instituting antihypertensive therapy. **Hypercholesterolemia** is another important risk factor for atherosclerosis and should be regulated by dietary or pharmacologic measures.

Therapy with **antiplatelet agents** (aspirin, ticlopidine) reduces stroke risk in patients with atherosclerosis of cerebral vessels. In patients with a cardiac source for emboli, **anticoagulation** with heparin fol-

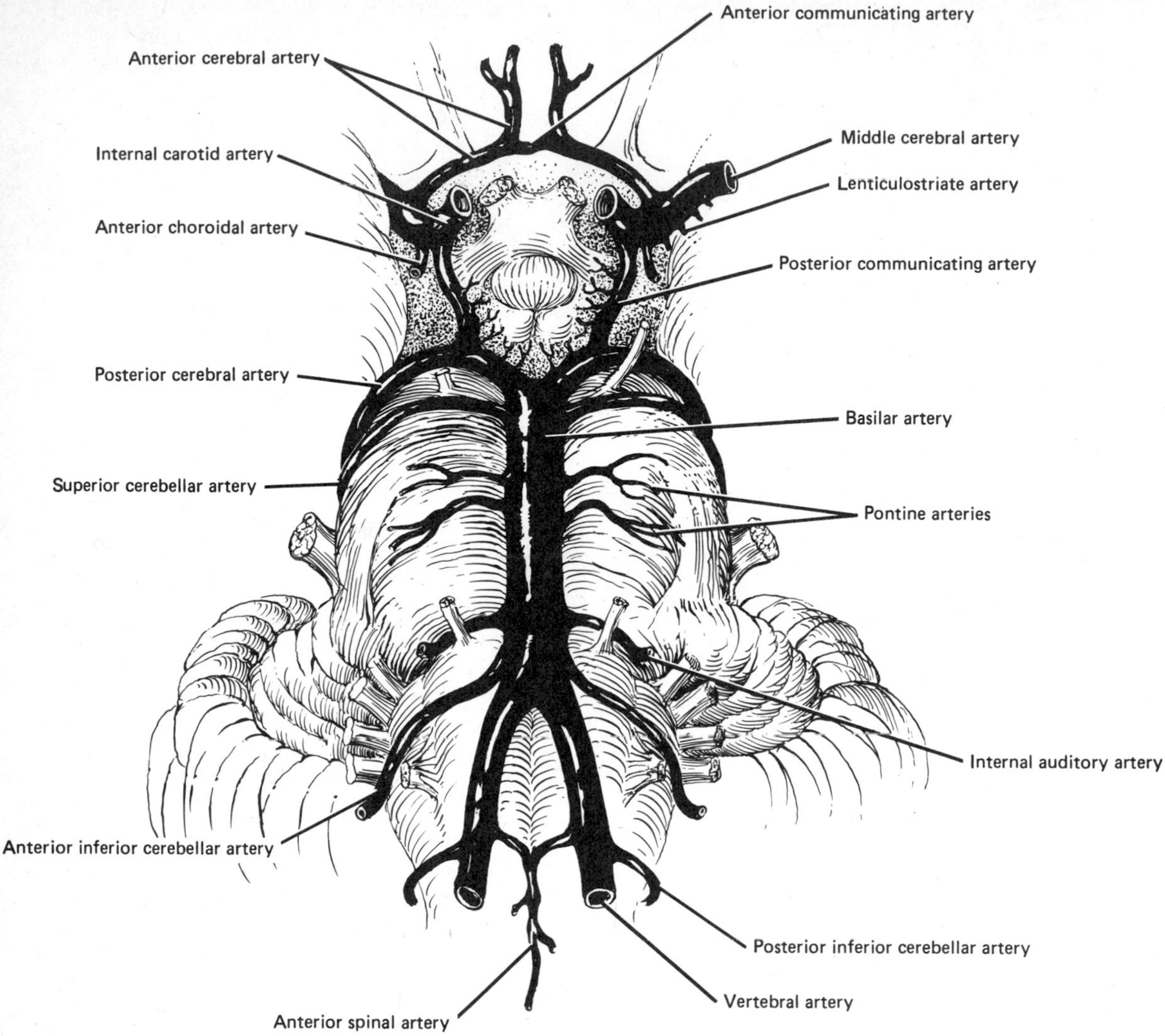

Figure 5–29. Circle of Willis and principal arteries of the brain. (Reproduced, with permission, from Chusid JG: *Correlative Neuroanatomy & Functional Neurology,* 19th ed. Lange, 1985.)

lowed by warfarin can reduce the risk of stroke. **Thrombolytic agents** such as recombinant tissue plasminogen activator (T-PA), streptokinase, and urokinase are effective in reducing cardiac ischemia. T-PA and urokinase are currently being evaluated in early ischemic stroke to restore circulation and reverse ischemic symptoms.

Several drugs are being investigated for use as neuroprotective agents that reduce brain injury by inhibiting glutamate receptors and voltage-sensitive calcium channels. The voltage-gated calcium channel antagonist nimodipine has been found to modestly reduce the mortality rate and improve outcomes in some studies of ischemic stroke. Several antagonists of glutamate receptors are currently in clinical trials.

43. What is the clinical presentation of stroke?
44. What are some of the causes of stroke?

REFERENCES

General

Kandel ER, Schwartz JH, Jessell TM (editors): *Principles of Neural Science,* 3rd ed. Appleton & Lange, 1991.

Plum F, Posner JB: The Diagnosis of Stupor and Coma. 3. Vol 19 of: *Contemporary Neurology Series.* Davis, 1980.

Sanders DB: Electrophysiologic study of disorders of neuromuscular transmission. In: *Electrodiagnosis in Clinical Neurology,* 2nd ed. Aminoff MJ (editor). Churchill Livingstone, 1986.

Functional Neuroanatomy

Albin RL, Young AB, Penney JB: The functional anatomy of basal ganglia disorders. Trends Neurol Sci 1989;12:366.

Baloh RW, Honrubia V: *Clinical Neurophysiology of the Vestibular System.* 2. Vol 32 of: *Contemporary Neurology Series.* Davis, 1990.

Gilman S, Bloedel JR, Lechtenberg R: *Disorders of the Cerebellum.* Vol 21 of: *Contemporary Neurology Series.* Davis, 1981.

Lipton SA, Rosenberg PA: Excitatory amino acids as a final common pathway for neurologic disorders. N Engl J Med 1994;330:613.

Parkinson's disease

Jenner P, Schapira AHV, Marsden CD: New insights into the cause of Parkinson's disease. Neurology 1992;42:2241.

Olanow CW: An introduction to the free radical hypothesis in Parkinson's disease. Ann Neurol 1992;32 (Suppl):S2.

Snyder SH, D'Amato RJ: MPTP: A neurotoxin relevant to the pathophysiology of Parkinson's disease. Neurology 1986;36:250.

Myasthenia Gravis

Levinson AI, Zweiman B, Lisak RP: Immuno-pathogenesis and treatment of myasthenia gravis. J Clin Immunol 1987;7:187.

Epilepsy

Dichter MA: Cellular mechanisms of epilepsy and potential new treatment strategies. Epilepsia 1989; 30(Suppl 1):S3.

Dichter MA, Buchhalter JR: The genetic epilepsies. In: *The Molecular and Genetic Basis of Neurological Disease.* Rosenberg RN et al (editors). Butterworth-Heinemann, 1993.

Hille B: *Ionic Channels of Excitable Membranes,* 2nd ed. Sinauer, 1992.

Hosford DA et al: The role of $GABA_B$ receptor activation in absence seizures of lethargic (lh/lh) mice. Science 1992;257:398.

MacDonald RL: Antiepileptic drug actions. Epilepsia 1989;30(Suppl 1):S19.

Stroke

Barnett HJM et al: *Stroke: Pathophysiology, Diagnosis and Management.* Churchill Livingstone, 1986.

Gelmers HJ et al: A controlled trial of nimodipine in acute ischemic stroke. N Engl J Med 1988;318:203.

6 Infectious Diseases

Tomás J. Aragón, MD, MPH

Infectious diseases cause significant morbidity and mortality, especially in segments of the population who are the most vulnerable to illness: the very young, the elderly, and the poor.

An understanding of the pathogenesis of infectious diseases can begin by conceptualizing the relationships between the host, the infectious agent, and the environment. Figure 6–1 portrays a host-agent-environment paradigm for the study of infectious diseases. The infectious agent can be either exogenous or endogenous. An infection results when the host, the agent, and the environment interact in a way that favors host invasion by the agent. Clearly, host susceptibility plays an important role in this process. The environment includes vectors and zoonotic hosts that transmit infectious agents.

The study of infectious diseases requires understanding of pathogenesis at the population and individual levels as well as at the cellular and molecular levels. For example, at the population level, tuberculosis results from complex interactions of infectious hosts (with different levels of infectivity) with susceptible hosts (with different levels of susceptibility) in the community over time. At the individual level, tuberculosis results from inhalation of airborne tubercle bacilli, primary infection, and progression to active tuberculosis (early progression) versus late progression ("reactivation").

In addition, because of different pathogenetic mechanisms, specific microorganisms have a tendency to cause certain types of infections: *Streptococcus pneumoniae* most commonly causes pneumonia, meningitis, bacteremia, and occasionally endocarditis; *Escherichia coli* most commonly causes gastrointestinal and urinary tract infections; *Plasmodium* species infect red blood cells and liver cells to cause malaria; *Entamoeba histolytica* causes amebic dysentery and liver abscesses, etc. Therefore, the specific approach differs for each patient. Table 6–1 presents a unifying clinical approach that incorporates knowledge of the microorganisms associated with specific clinical syndromes and the host-agent-environment paradigm in obtaining the history of the patient's illness.

NORMAL DEFENSES AGAINST INFECTION

NORMAL MICROBIAL FLORA

The human body normally harbors thousands of species of bacteria, viruses, fungi, and protozoa. The great majority of them are commensals and do not result in disease. Our bodies live in a delicate balance with these microorganisms. We can define "normal flora" as those microorganisms that are found on or in the body of a healthy human host. Some of these organisms are found in humans or animals only; others can also live freely in the environment. Few microorganisms are absolute pathogens. For example, *Neisseria meningitidis* (meningococcus) and *S pneumoniae* (pneumococcus) are well-known pathogens causing meningitis, pneumonia, and sepsis. However, these bacteria can also be found in the oropharynx in as many as 10% of healthy people and thus can be considered transient normal flora in a small percentage of the general population.

Colonization is the presence in a host—without causing disease—of a microorganism that is usually pathogenic. Colonization can be transient (normal flora) or persistent. Patients with debilitating conditions and those taking multiple medications will sometimes alter their endogenous normal flora in such a way as to become colonized with pathogenic bacteria. Not uncommonly, these patients will become infected with these organisms. For example, patients hospitalized for long periods frequently become colonized with nosocomial gram-negative organisms (eg, *Pseudomonas aeruginosa*). Depending on predisposing conditions, they can develop life-threatening infections such as pneumonia. Bacteria colonized in this way are not considered transient normal flora.

While normal flora are usually commensals, under the right conditions they can become pathogenic, invade, and cause severe disease. Consequently, many

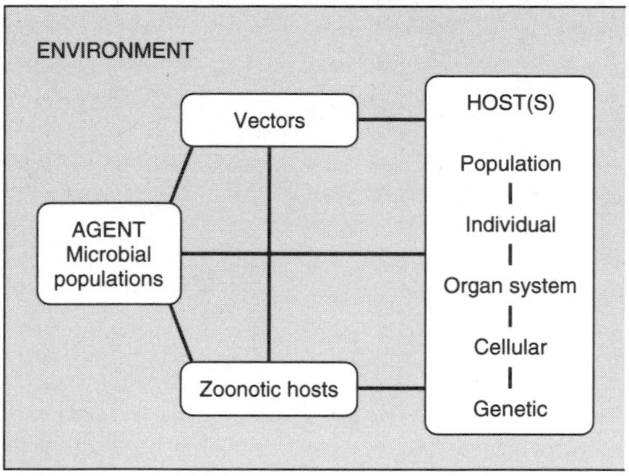

Figure 6–1. The fundamental relationships involved in the host-agent-environment paradigm. Note the role of zoonotic hosts and vectors in the environmental pathogenesis of infectious diseases. In the host, pathogenetic mechanisms extend from the level of populations (eg, person-to-person transmission) to the level of cellular and molecular processes (eg, genetic susceptibility).

common bacterial infections are caused by normal flora. Therefore, knowledge of the most common normal flora at specific body sites can help predict the cause of an infection and lead to institution of appropriate empiric antibiotic therapy while awaiting definitive isolation of the organism.

Normal bacterial flora are found on the skin, the upper respiratory tract (nasal passages and oropharynx), the gastrointestinal tract (small intestine, colon, and rectum), the anterior urethra, and the vagina. The most common members of the normal flora are listed in Table 6–2. At some of these sites (eg, the colon), bacteria proliferate, while at other sites (eg, the small intestine), their presence is only transient. Isolation of bacteria from such sites is generally not diagnostic of an infection. However, isolation of an organism that is usually considered to be pathogenic (eg, *M tuberculosis*) from such sites is diagnostic of infection. Sites of the body normally considered sterile are blood, cerebrospinal fluid, synovial fluid, and deep tissues of the body. Isolation of any microorganism from these sites is diagnostic of infection. Knowledge of the bacterial inhabitants at specific sites helps a clinician to initiate empiric antimicrobial therapy for common infections.

To colonize the host, an invading microorganism must be able first to resist host defenses, then to compete successfully with normal host flora. Before a virulent strain of pneumococcus can cause an infection, it must first colonize the oropharynx of the host. Once the oropharynx is colonized with pneumococcus, it can cause pneumonia if the respiratory tract defenses are compromised (eg, by a poor cough reflex due to a stroke or by diminished ciliary clearance in a person with a long history of smoking). Even if the oropharynx is not colonized with pathogens, significant aspiration of oropharyngeal secretions into the lung can cause disease. For example, patients with stroke or intoxication who are prone to significant aspiration frequently develop a smoldering anaerobic pneumonia, reflecting the fact that anaerobic bacteria in the oropharynx outnumber aerobic bacteria by a factor of 100:1 to 1000:1.

Similarly, in other sites heavily occupied by normal flora, colonization by a pathogenic microorganism is unlikely unless the organism is adept at resisting host and microbial defenses. The colonization of sites that are normally sterile or have very few microbes is generally easier because there is no microbial competition. However, host defenses at these sites are often vigorous. Such sites include the upper gastrointestinal tract (stomach and small intestine) and all deep body tissues. In the stomach, not many microbes can survive the alternating acidic and alkaline environment; in deep tissues, invading microbes must fight off antibodies, complement, and phagocytic cells of the host immune system.

In general, the host resists colonization by pathogenic bacteria by the following mechanisms: (1) sweeping microbes away in fluid currents, (2) killing them with phagocytes, and (3) starving them of needed nutrients. Potentially pathogenic organisms, such as gonococci, will resist being swept away by adhering to epithelial cells of the urogenital tract. Pneumococci resist phagocytosis by encapsulation within a slimy coat that impairs uptake by neutrophils. Some staphylococci resist starvation of needed nutrients by elaborating hemolysins that lyse host red blood cells, thus giving them access to host hemoglobin as a source of iron.

The normal flora plays a definite role in the balance between health and disease. Normal flora helps to prevent colonization by pathogenic bacteria by competing for nutrients and by adhering to host sites. However, normal flora can be the source of many common infections. When commensal organisms find themselves in unfamiliar body sites, under the right conditions they may cause disease. For example, the genus *Bacteroides* is abundant in the large intestine. However, when these bacteria make their way into deeper tissues (eg, by surgery or trauma) they often cause intra-abdominal abscesses. *Staphylococcus epidermidis* is the most common bacterium on the skin and can cause severe bloodborne infections if it gains access to the bloodstream through an indwelling intravenous catheter. *E coli,* the most common enteric gram-negative rod in the large intestine, is the most common cause of urinary tract infections because of common perineal contamination and because virulent strains have enhanced adherence to vaginal and uroepithelial cells. Under the right conditions, any microorganism in the normal flora can cause disease.

Table 6–1. Obtaining a history in the diagnosis of infectious diseases.

Usual History	Host-Specific History	Environment-Specific History	Agent-Specific History
Chief complaint	Chief complaint	Chief complaint	Chief complaint
History of present illness	Demographics: Age Sex Race/ethnicity Mild versus life-threatening Acute versus subacute versus chronic Endogenous versus exogenous Primary versus reactivation Relapse versus recurrent (reinfection) Pattern of symptoms (fevers, night sweats)	Person-to-person transmission Animal-to-person transmission Vector-borne transmission Water-borne transmission Food-borne transmission Airborne transmission Nosocomially acquired Community-acquired Occupational exposure Seasonal transmission	Viral versus bacterial versus parasitic Infections or infectious agents associated with host-specific or environment-specific factors (eg., measles in a child; pelvic inflammatory disease in a female; *Salmonella* infection in a black child with sickle cell disease; outbreak of food-borne hepatitis A infection; influenza epidemic in winter)
Past medical history (including medications and allergies)	Conditions predisposing to infections: HIV infection Chronic obstructive pulmonary disease Diabetes mellitus Sickle cell disease Asplenia (after spleen removal) Lack of immunizations	Previous exposures to probable exogenous infectious agents: Day-care centers Nurseries Schools Correctional facilities	Infections or infectious agents associated with host's predisposing comorbid or past medical conditions (eg, *Pneumocystis carinii* pneumonia in HIV-infected patients)
Habits	Substance use: Smoking Alcohol Injection drug use Cocaine (smoked or nasal)	Sexual contacts (exchange of body fluids) Sharing of syringes or needles	Infections or infectious agents associated with host-specific habits (eg, HIV infection or *S aureus* endocarditis in injection drug users)
Social history	Socioeconomic status (lack of access to health care): Occupation Recent immigration	Crowded housing Homelessness Congregated living facility: Shelters, prisons Nursing home, hospital Recent travel	Infections or infectious agents epidemiologically associated with host-specific or environment-specific factors (eg, outbreak of tuberculosis in homeless shelter, prison, or hospital; typhoid fever or malaria in recent traveler)
Family history	Immune deficiency syndromes	Exposure to environment in severe combined immune deficiency (SCID)	Specific infections or infectious agents associated with inherited immune deficiency (Table 3-4)
Review of systems	Review by organ system: Nonspecific constitutional symptoms (fever, chills, night sweats, weight loss) Central nervous system (photophobia) Cardiovascular system (light-headedness) Lung (productive cough) Kidney and urinary tract (dysuria) Gastrointestinal system (diarrhea) Hematologic system Reproductive organs (genital discharge) Skin and subcutaneous tissues (rash) Muscle and bone (myalgia, bone pain)	Organ-specific host-environment interaction (eg, penetrating CNS trauma; indwelling intravenous catheters; endotracheally intubated, mechanically ventilated patient; indwelling Foley catheter; contraceptive intrauterine device; postoperative wound; penetrating soft tissue injury)	Infections or infectious agents associated with organ-specific host-environment interaction (eg, epidemic of meningococcal meningitis; intravenous catheter-related *S aureus* bacteremia; nosocomial *Pseudomonas* pneumonia; pelvic inflammatory disease; postoperative wound infection; osteomyelitis in injured bone)

Table 6–2. Examples of normal flora by body location.[1]

Location	Gram-Positive		Gram-Negative		Others
	Cocci	Rods	Cocci	Rods	
Skin	*Staphylococcus*	Diphtheroids			
Oronasopharynx	*Streptococcus*		*Neisseria*	*Haemophilus* *Bacteroides*	Spirochetes
Large intestine	*Streptococcus* *Enterococcus*	*Clostridia*		Enteric bacilli *Bacteroides*	
Vagina		*Lactobacillus*			*Mycoplasma*

[1]Modified and reproduced, with permission, from Eisenstein BI, Schaechter M: Normal microbial flora. In: *Mechanisms of Microbial Disease,* 2nd ed. Schaechter M, Medoff G, Eisenstein BI (editors). Williams & Wilkins, 1993.

Second, the body's repertoire of immunoglobulins to fight infections is influenced by antigenic stimulation by normal flora. Among the antibodies produced in response to bacterial stimulation are those of the IgA class, which are secreted through the mucous membranes. These immunoglobulins probably act as the first line of humoral defense against colonization of deeper tissues by commensal organisms. In addition, antibodies elicited by the antigenic challenge of the normal flora sometimes cross-react with surface antigens from pathogenic microbes. For example, some of these antibodies will cross-react with the polysaccharide capsule of meningitis-producing strains of meningococci.

Third, by occupancy of certain sites in the host, normal flora prevent the colonization of pathogenic bacteria and thus prevent disease. Survival at these sites implies that they have developed the ability to adhere to the epithelial surfaces, to utilize the available nutrients specific to that environment, and to elaborate substances (bacteriocidins) that inhibit colonization by other bacterial strains or species. When normal flora are altered—eg, by the administration of broad-spectrum antibiotics—one bacterial species may predominate or pathogenic bacteria from the outside may colonize the site and predispose the host to infection.

CONSTITUTIVE DEFENSES OF THE BODY

Constitutive defenses of the human body are defenses against infectious diseases that do not require prior contact with the microorganism. These defenses begin when organisms first make contact with the skin or mucous membrane. They consist of simple physical and chemical barriers that prevent easy entry of microorganisms into the body. Some infectious agents utilize a vector (such as an insect) to gain direct access to the blood or soft tissues of the body. Once an agent has entered the body, the major constitutive defenses are the acute inflammatory response and the complement system. These defenses attempt neutralization of the agent, recruit phagocytic cells, and induce a more specific response through humoral and cell-mediated immunity. The constitutive defenses of the body are nonspecific but are important from an evolutionary perspective in enabling humans to encounter and adapt to a variety of new and changing environments.

Physical & Chemical Barriers to Infection

The squamous epithelium of the skin is the first line of defense against microorganisms encountered in the outside world. As keratinized epithelial surface cells desquamate, the skin maintains its protective barrier by generating new epithelial cells beneath the surface. Any break in the skin—abrasion or laceration—will eventually heal and close that avenue of microbial invasion. The skin is also bathed with oils and moisture from the sebaceous and sweat glands. These secretions contain fatty acids that inhibit bacterial growth. Poor circulation to the skin may result in skin breakdown and increased susceptibility to infection. For example, chronically debilitated patients may suffer from decubitus ulcers, predisposing to severe infections by otherwise harmless skin flora.

The mucous membranes also provide a physical barrier to microbial invasion. The mucous membranes of the mouth, pharynx, esophagus, and lower urinary tract are composed of several layers of epithelial cells, whereas those of the lower respiratory tract, the gastrointestinal tract, and the upper urinary tract are delicate single layers of epithelial cells. Mucous membranes are covered by a protective layer of mucus, which provides a mechanical and chemical barrier. The mucus traps foreign particles and prevents them from reaching the mucous membranes. Because the mucus is hydrophilic, many substances produced by the body easily diffuse to the surface, including enzymes with antimicrobial activity such as lysozyme and peroxidase.

Inflammatory Response

If a microorganism crosses the epidermis of the skin or the epithelial surface of the mucous membranes, it encounters other components of the host constitutive defenses. These responses are constitutive because they are nonspecific and do not require prior contact with the organism to be effective. Clinically, signs of inflammation (heat, erythema, pain, and swelling) are the characteristic features of localized infection and secondary tissue injury. Infected viscera become recognizable by tenderness upon palpation, by the inflammatory changes present in adjacent body fluids, or by altered organ function. Like fever, an increased peripheral blood neutrophil count gives information about the presence and severity of infection. Blood supply to the affected areas increases in response to vasodilation, and the capillaries become more permeable, allowing antibodies, complement, and white blood cells to cross the endothelium and reach the site of injury. An important consequence of inflammation is that the pH of the inflamed tissues is lowered, creating an antimicrobial environment. The increased blood flow to the area allows continued recruitment of inflammatory cells as well as the necessary components for tissue repair and recovery.

When a microorganism enters host tissue, it activates the complement system and components of the coagulation cascade (such as Hageman factor) and induces the release of chemical mediators of the inflammatory response. These mediators result in the vascular permeability and vasodilation characteristic of inflammation. For example, the anaphylatoxins C3a, C4a, and C5a, produced by the activation of complement, stimulate the release of histamine from mast cells. Histamine dilates the blood vessels and increases their permeability. Bradykinin is also released, increasing vascular permeability.

Proinflammatory cytokines include interleukin-1, interleukin-6, tumor necrosis factor, and gamma interferon. These factors, singly or in combination, promote fever, stimulate hepatic acute phase responses, produce local inflammatory signs, and trigger catabolic responses.

During severe infection, hepatic synthesis of proteins is altered, changing the profile of serum proteins. This altered profile has been termed the **acute phase reaction.** Typically, serum albumin concentration is reduced while serum amyloid A protein, C-reactive protein, and various proteinase inhibitors increase. Serum levels of zinc and iron decrease at the same time. A catabolic state is further augmented by simultaneous increases in levels of circulating cortisol, glucagon, catecholamines, and other hormones.

When mild to moderate in intensity, inflammatory responses serve important host defense functions. For example, elevated body temperature seems to accentuate lymphocyte responses and may inhibit viral replication. Inflammatory hyperemia and systemic neutrophilia optimize phagocyte delivery to sites of infection. The decreased availability of iron inhibits the growth of microbes that require this element as a nutrient. However, when the inflammatory responses become extreme, extensive tissue damage can result, as in the case of sepsis.

Complement System

The complement system is composed of a series of plasma protein and cell membrane receptors that are important mediators of host defenses and inflammation. Most of the biologically significant effects of the complement system are mediated by the third component (C3) and the terminal components (C5–9). In order to carry out their host defense and inflammatory functions, C3 and C5–9 must first be activated. Two pathways of complement activation have been recognized and have been termed the **classic** and **alternative pathways.** The classic pathway is activated by antigen-antibody complexes or antibody-coated particles, and the alternative pathway is activated by mechanisms independent of antibodies, usually by interaction with bacterial surface components. Both pathways form C3 convertase, which cleaves the C3 component of complement, a key protein common to both pathways. The two pathways then proceed in identical fashion to bind late-acting components to form a membrane attack complex (C5–9), which results in target cell lysis.

Once activated, complement functions to enhance the antimicrobial defenses in several ways: It makes invading microorganisms susceptible to phagocytosis; it lyses some of the infectious agents directly; it produces substances that are chemotactic for white blood cells; and it promotes the inflammatory response. Two of the activities of complement are specifically directed toward enhancing phagocytosis. In addition to the recruitment of white cells by chemotactic proteins, complement facilitates phagocytosis by proteins called **opsonins.** Other components of complement are responsible for the lysis of bacteria, some viruses, and foreign cells. The membrane attack complex inserts itself into the target membrane, leading to increased permeability and subsequent lysis.

Inherited disorders of complement are usually expressed as a complement deficiency state with an increased risk of bacterial infections. The kinds of infections seen in complement-deficient patients relate to the biologic functions of the missing component. Typically, patients with a deficiency of C3 or of a component in either of the two pathways necessary for the activation of C3 usually have an increased susceptibility to infections caused by bacteria for which C3b-dependent opsonization is an important defense. For example, these patients are at increased risk for infections with encapsulated bacteria such as *S pneumoniae* and *Haemophilus influenzae.* In contrast, patients with deficiencies of C5–9 have normal resistance to *S pneumoniae* and *H influenzae* since C3b-mediated opsonization is intact, but they are unusually susceptible to life-threatening infections with *N meningitidis* and *Neisseria gonorrhoeae,* since they lack C5–9-mediated serum bactericidal activity, an important host defense against *Neisseria.* Interestingly, complement deficiency diseases may be more common among patients with certain infectious diseases than was heretofore appreciated. For example, about 15% of patients with systemic meningococcal infections have a genetically determined deficiency of a terminal component.

Phagocytosis

After the natural barriers of the skin or mucous membranes have been penetrated, the phagocytes—neutrophils, monocytes, and macrophages—constitute the next line of defense. The process of internalizing particles by these cells is termed phagocytosis and involves attachment of the particle to the cell surface, which in turn triggers the extension of a pseudopod to enclose the particle in an endocytic vesicle or **phagosome.** The circulating neutrophil or polymorphonuclear leukocyte (PMN) is the best-studied and best-understood phagocyte. Before activation by chemoattractants, neutrophils circulate in a metabolically quiescent state. When chemotactic factors, arachidonic acid metabolites, or complement cleavage fragments interact with specific membrane receptors, the neutrophil rapidly becomes activated and crawls by ameboid action toward the chemoattractants. After phagocytosis, the mechanisms by which the phagolysosome kills the microorganism can be divided into oxygen-independent and oxygen-dependent processes. The former consists of those factors that contribute to phagocytic killing of microbes in an anaerobic environment. In the oxygen-dependent process, neutrophils are triggered to produce hydrogen peroxide and other microbicidal oxidants. Functional or quantitative defects of neutrophils result in infections with pyogenic bacteria.

Neutropenia—a neutrophil count < 1000 cells/μL—secondary to the myelosuppressive effects of chemotherapy is a common predisposing factor for bacterial and fungal infections. The risk of infection rises significantly with neutrophil counts < 500 cells/μL and is especially high with counts < 100 cells/μL. The longer the duration of profound neutropenia, the higher the risk of infection. At the first sign of infection (eg, fever), these patients should immediately be given broad-spectrum antibacterial agents to cover the most likely bacterial pathogens. Ironically, antibiotics are often so effective at killing a broad spectrum of bacteria that patients' mucous membranes, already colonized with fungi, become overgrown with fungi. Such patients are then at increased risk of fungal sepsis.

In addition, several inherited disorders of neutrophil function have been described, including Chédiak-Higashi syndrome, myeloperoxidase deficiency, and chronic granulomatous disease. **Chédiak-Higashi syndrome** is a rare autosomal recessive hereditary disorder in which the neutrophils have a profound defect in the formation of intracellular granules. Opsonized bacteria, such as *S aureus,* are ingested normally, but viable bacteria persist intracellularly, presumably because of the inability of normal granules to fuse with phagosomes to form phagolysosomes. Patients with Chédiak-Higashi syndrome experience recurrent bacterial infections, most frequently involving the skin and soft tissues and the upper and lower respiratory tracts. **Myeloperoxidase deficiency** is the most common neutrophil disorder, with a prevalence of 1:2000 individuals. In this disorder, phagocytosis, chemotaxis, and degranulation are normal, but microbicidal activity for bacteria is delayed. In general, these patients do not suffer from recurrent infections. In contrast, **chronic granulomatous disease** is a genetically heterogeneous group of inherited disorders with a common phenotype characterized by the failure of phagocytic cells to produce superoxides. The defect involves neutrophils, monocytes, eosinophils, and some macrophages. The normal array of microbicidal oxidants are not produced, and these patients are susceptible to recurrent, often life-threatening infections. Patients with chronic granulomatous disease also tend to form granulomas in tissues, particularly in the lungs, liver, and spleen.

INDUCED DEFENSES OF THE BODY

Constitutive host defenses to infectious agents are generally nonspecific and do not require prior exposure to the invading agent. However, induced defenses or acquired host immunity is highly specific for the invading infectious agent and is qualitatively and quantitatively altered by prior antigenic exposure. Details of the pathophysiology of the host immune system are covered in Chapter 3. Infections associated with common defects in the induced immune response are shown in Table 6–3.

ESTABLISHMENT OF INFECTIOUS DISEASES

An infectious disease occurs when a pathogenic organism causes signs or symptoms of inflammation or organ dysfunction. This may be caused directly by the infection itself, as when the etiologic agent multiplies in the host, or indirectly from the effects of toxins generated by the infecting organism. Many infections are subclinical, not producing the usual manifestations of disease. To cause disease, all microorganisms must go through the following stages (Table 6–4): The microorganism must (1) **encounter**

Table 6–3. Infections associated with common defects in humoral and cellular immune response.[1]

Host Defect in Immune Response	Examples of Diseases Associated With Defects	Common Etiologic Agents of Infections
T lymphocyte deficiency or dysfunction	Thymic aplasia/hypoplasia Hodgkin's disease Sarcoid Lepromatous leprosy	*Listeria monocytogenes, Mycobacterium, Candida, Aspergillus, Cryptococcus neoformans,* herpes simplex, herpes zoster
	AIDS	*Pneumocystis carinii,* cytomegalovirus, herpes simplex, *Mycobacterium avium* complex, *Cryptococcus neoformans, Candida*
	Mucocutaneous candidiasis	*Candida*
B cell deficiency or dysfunction	Bruton's X-linked agammaglobulinemia Agammaglobulinemia Chronic lymphocytic leukemia Multiple myeloma	*Streptococcus pneumoniae,* other streptococci, *Haemophilus influenzae, Neisseria meningitidis, Staphylococcus aureus, Klebsiella pneumoniae, Escherichia coli, Giardia lamblia, Pneumocystis carinii,* enteroviruses
	Selective IgM deficiency	*Streptococcus pneumoniae, Haemophilus influenzae, Escherichia coli*
	Selective IgA deficiency	*Giardia lamblia,* hepatitis viruses, *Streptococcus pneumoniae, Haemophilus influenzae*
Mixed T and B cell deficiency or dysfunction	Common variable hypogammaglobulinemia	*Pneumocystis carinii,* cytomegalovirus, *Streptococcus pneumoniae, Haemophilus influenzae,* various other bacteria
	Ataxia-telangiectasia	*Streptococcus pneumoniae, Haemophilus influenzae, Staphylococcus aureus,* rubella virus, *Giardia lamblia*
	Severe combined immunodeficiency	*Candida albicans, Pneumocystis carinii,* varicella virus, rubella virus, cytomegalovirus
	Wiskott-Aldrich syndrome	Infections seen in T and B cell abnormalities

[1]Modified and reproduced, with permission, from Masur H, Fauci AS: Infections in the compromised host. In: *Harrison's Principles of Internal Medicine,* 12th ed. McGraw-Hill, 1991.

the host, (2) **gain entry** into the host, (3) **multiply and spread** from the site of entry, and (4) **cause host tissue injury,** either directly (eg, cytotoxins) or indirectly (inflammatory response). The course of infection can be characterized as mild versus life-threatening and as acute, subacute, or chronic. Whether infection is clinically evident or not, the outcome is either (1) eradication of the infecting agent (resolution), (2) chronic infection, (3) prolonged excretion of the agent (carrier state), or (4) latency of the agent within host tissues (Figure 6–2).

Except for those with congenital infections caused by agents such as rubella, syphilis, and cytomegalovirus, most human beings first encounter microorganisms at birth. During parturition, the newborn comes into contact with microorganisms present in the mother's vaginal canal and on her skin. Most of the bacteria that the newborn encounters do not cause harm, and for those that might cause infection, the newborn usually has antibodies that were acquired from the mother in utero. For example, for the first 6 months of life, infants carry maternal protective antibodies against *H influenzae;* the greatest risk of *H influenzae* infection occurs after 6 months, when infants lose their maternal antibodies and are left unprotected. On the other hand, newborns whose mothers are colonized with group B streptococci at birth are at increased risk of serious infection (sepsis, meningitis). Otherwise, newborns rapidly adapt to their new microbiologic environment of normal flora and the other microbes they encounter.

Infectious diseases, therefore, arise from two sources: from **endogenous** and from **exogenous** microorganisms. Endogenous microorganisms are usually part of the normal flora that will cause infection only under the right conditions. For example, aspiration pneumonia is an anaerobic lung infection resulting from aspiration of oral flora consisting chiefly of anaerobic bacteria. Urinary tract infections are commonly caused by *E coli,* the most common enteric gram-negative bacillus in the colonic flora. Injection drug users become colonized with *S aureus* on their skin and are at risk for subsequent *S aureus* cellulitis, subcutaneous abscesses, or endocarditis.

The distinction between endogenous and exogenous microorganisms is not always clear. Exogenous microbes must first colonize the host before becoming able to cause disease. For example, the presence of *P aeruginosa* in the sputum of a hospitalized patient implies colonization unless there is evidence of disease (fever, cough, purulent sputum, leukocytosis, chest radiograph demonstrating an infiltrate). Colonization of hospitalized patients with gram-negative rods is common when the normal flora is altered because of a debilitating disease or the administration of antibiotics. Naturally, these patients are at higher risk of developing disease from these organisms.

Table 6–4. The establishment and outcome of infectious diseases.[1]

Stage of Encounter	Factors Influencing Stage of Encounter
Encounter	Time of first encounter Exogenous (colonization) Endogenous (normal flora)

Entry	Ingress
	  Inhalation
	  Ingestion
	Mucous membrane entry
	Penetration
	  Insect bites
	  Cuts and wounds
	  Iatrogenic (intravenous catheters)

Multiplication and spread	Physical factors Microbial nutrition Anatomic factors Microbial sanctuary Microbial virulence factors

Injury	Mechanical
	Cell death
	Microbial product-induced
	Host-induced
	  Inflammation
	  Immune response
	    Humoral immunity
	    Cellular immunity
	  Mediator-induced

Course of infection	Mild versus life-threatening Acute versus subacute versus chronic

Outcome of infection	Resolution (self-limited)
	Chronic
	  Carrier state (saprophytic versus parasitic)
	  Latent → Reactivation
	Death

[1]Adapted in part, with permission, from Schaechter M, Medoff G, Eisenstein BI (editors): *Mechanisms of Microbial Disease,* 2nd ed. Williams & Wilkins, 1993.

In general, exogenous infectious agents are not part of our normal flora. They represent a large variety of microbes (bacteria, viruses, fungi, parasites). After the infectious agent encounters a susceptible host, it gains entry into the host (or attaches to an appropriate epithelial surface). Direct entry into the host—ie, bypassing the usual chemical and physical barriers—occurs via direct **penetration.** These circumstances occur when (1) an insect vector directly inoculates the infectious agent into the host (mosquitoes transmitting malaria), (2) bacteria gain direct access to host tissues through cuts or wounds (trauma or surgical wounds), and (3) microbes gain access via instruments or catheters that allow communication between usually sterile sites and the outside world (eg, indwelling venous catheters). Invasion by **ingression** occurs when an infectious agent enters the host via an orifice rather than by crossing the epithelium. This primarily involves inhalation of infectious aerosolized droplets *(M tuberculosis)* or ingestion of contaminated foods (*Salmonella,* staphylococcal food poisoning).

Other infectious agents directly infect the mucous membranes or cross the epithelia to cause infection. This commonly occurs in urinary tract infections and sexually transmitted diseases. The virus that causes AIDS, the human immunodeficiency virus (HIV), is sexually transmitted across mucous membranes by the penetration of virus-laden macrophages from semen. Such a mechanism of cell-mediated entry may function at other mucous membranes as well.

Infections caused by usually nonpathogenic microorganisms that are present in very small numbers in our bodies *(Candida)* or are ubiquitous in the environment (*Mycobacterium avium* complex) are termed **opportunistic infections.** These infections occur almost exclusively in immunocompromised hosts such as HIV-infected patients or transplant recipients. These microbes are "opportunists" in the sense that they take advantage of the immune-compromised state of the host to cause infection.

Following the initial encounter with the host, the infectious agent must successfully multiply at the site of entry. When the microorganism successfully competes with normal flora and is able to multiply, this is termed colonization (eg, pneumococci colonizing the upper respiratory tract). When the microorganism multiplies at a usually sterile site, it is termed infection (eg, pneumococci multiplying in the alveoli, ie, pneumonia). Unless direct penetration occurs, agents must first successfully colonize the host to cause subsequent infection.

Factors that facilitate the multiplication and spread of the infection include inoculum size, anatomic factors (nondraining), availability of microbial nutrients, physical factors (stomach pH), microbial virulence factors, and microbial sanctuary (abscesses). An abscess is a special case where the host has contained the infection but is unable to eradicate it. The primary mode of therapy is surgical drainage, many times without the need for antibiotics. Infections that are not contained will spread. Infections can spread along the epidermis (impetigo), along the dermis (erysipelas), along subcutaneous tissue (cellulitis), along fascial planes (necrotizing fasciitis), into muscle tissue (myositis), along veins (suppurative thrombophlebitis), into the blood (bacteremia, fungemia, viremia, etc), along lymphatics (lymphangitis), and into organs (pneumonia, brain abscesses, hepatitis).

Infections cause direct injury to the host through a variety of mechanisms. An intense inflammatory response may result in significant swelling which can be life-threatening—eg, children with epiglottitis often have impending mechanical airway obstruction. Host **cell death** can occur by a variety of mechanisms. For example, Shiga toxin causes large intestinal cell death and dysentery, and poliovirus-induced

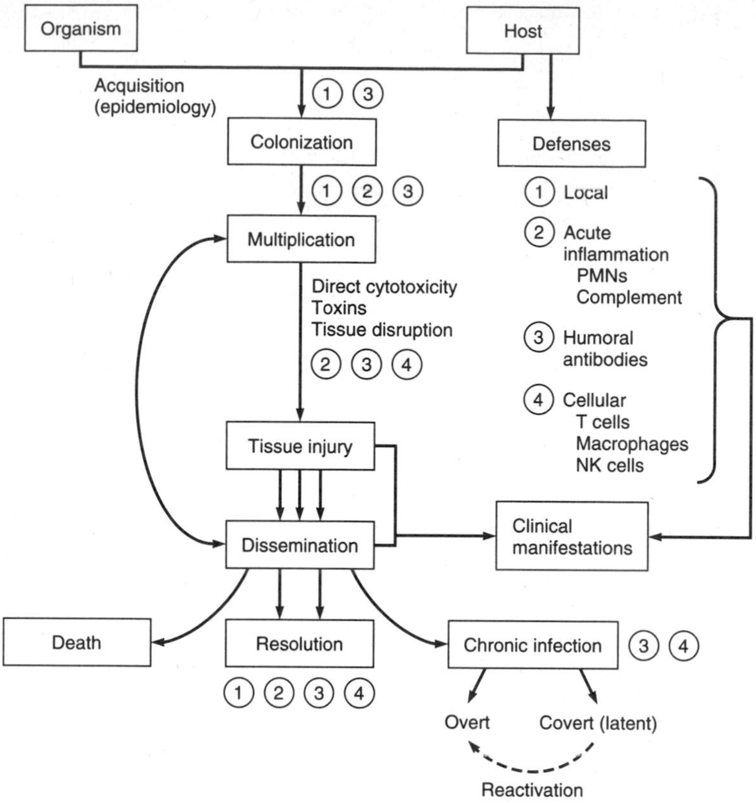

Figure 6–2. Schema of the establishment and outcome of infectious diseases. Note interplay between microorganisms and host factors that lead to infection, infectious disease, and resolution. The circled numbers indicate sites at which the designated host responses may interrupt or modify the pathogenesis of disease. (Modified and reproduced, with permission, from Heinzel FP, Root RK: Introduction to infectious diseases: Pathogenic mechanisms and host responses. In: *Harrison's Principles of Internal Medicine,* 12th ed. Wilson JD et al [editors]. McGraw-Hill, 1991.)

cell lysis of the anterior horn cells of the spinal cord causes flaccid paralysis. Gram-negative bacterial endotoxin can initiate a cascade of cytokine release, resulting in sepsis syndrome and septic shock.

The time course of an infection can be characterized as acute, subacute, or chronic, and its severity can be classified as mild or life-threatening. Many infections that start off as mild, easily curable infections can rapidly develop into life-threatening infections. Infections that are indolent for weeks, such as infective endocarditis, can be fatal unless appropriate therapy is initiated. A very small, seemingly insignificant abscess with toxic shock syndrome toxin-1 (TSST-1)-producing *S aureus* can result in fulminant toxic shock syndrome and death.

Table 6–5 summarizes some microbial strategies to overcome host immune defenses. A unifying theme is that all infectious agents, regardless of specific mechanisms, must succeed at all these levels (Tables 6–4 and 6–5). This knowledge helps the physician to plan and implement intervention strategies to prevent infections; when infection occurs, to treat and cure; and when infection cannot be cured, to prevent further transmission, recurrence, or reactivation.

1. By what three general mechanisms do hosts resist colonization by pathogenic bacteria?
2. What are three ways in which the normal flora contributes to the balance between health and disease?
3. Which host defenses against infection do not require prior contact with the would-be infecting organism?
4. What are the categories of outcomes from an infection?

Table 6–5. Selection of microbial strategies against host immune defenses.[1]

Host Defense Action	Microbial Counteraction	Example
Complement actions	Masking of complement activating substances	*Staphylococcus aureus,* surface capsule Meningococcus, coating with IgA
	Inhibition of surface complement activation	*Schistosoma mansoni,* decay accelerating factors
	Inhibition of action of membrane attack complex	*Salmonella,* long surface O antigen
	Inactivation of complement chemotaxin C5a	*Pseudomonas aeruginosa*
Phagocytic actions	Inhibition of phagocyte recruitment Microbial killing of phagocytes Escape from phagocytosis Survival of phagocytosis	*Bordetella pertussis,* toxin paralysis of chemotaxis *Pseudomonas aeruginosa,* leukocidins Staphylococci, surface protein A Trypanosomes, enter cytoplasm Rickettsiae, enter cytoplasm *Mycobacterium tuberculosis,* inhibit lysosome fusion *Chlamydia psittaci,* inhibit lysosome fusion *Legionella,* inhibit lysosome fusion
	Inhibition of phagocyte oxidative pathway	Staphylococci, catalase production against H_2O_2
Cell-mediated immunity	CD4 T cell depletion	Human immunodeficiency virus (HIV)
	Decreased B cell immunoglobulin production	Measles virus
	Inhibition of lymphokine synthesis	*Leishmania*
Humoral-mediated immunity	Changing of surface antigens	Influenza virus *Neisseria gonorrhoeae* *Trypanosoma brucei*
	Proteolysis of antibodies	*Haemophilus influenzae,* IgA proteases
Humoral- and cell-mediated immunity	DNA incorporation into host genome	Herpes simplex Herpes zoster

[1]Modified and reproduced, with permission, from Plaut A: Microbial subversion of host defenses. In: *Mechanisms of Microbial Disease,* 2nd ed. Schaechter M, Medoff G, Eisenstein BI (editors). Williams & Wilkins, 1993.

PATHOPHYSIOLOGY OF SELECTED INFECTIOUS DISEASE SYNDROMES

INFECTIVE ENDOCARDITIS

Clinical Presentation

Infective endocarditis is a bacterial or fungal infection of the heart, most commonly involving the cardiac valves and less commonly the endocardial surface. Infection of extracardiac endothelium is termed endarteritis and can cause disease which has some similarities to endocarditis. The most common predisposing factor for infective endocarditis is the presence of abnormal cardiac valves or structures. Consequently, patients with rheumatic heart disease, congenital heart disease, mitral valve prolapse with valve leaflet redundancy or an audible murmur, a prosthetic heart valve, or a history of endocarditis have an increased risk of developing infective endocarditis.

Etiology

The most common infectious agents associated with native valve infective endocarditis are bacteria and include viridans streptococci, *S aureus,* and *Enterococcus.* Infection involves the left heart (mitral and aortic valves) almost exclusively except in patients who are injection drug users or, less commonly, patients with valve injury from a pulmonary artery (Swan-Ganz) catheter, in whom infection of the right heart (tricuspid or pulmonary valves) occurs. Injection drug users most commonly develop *S aureus* tricuspid infective endocarditis with septic pulmonary emboli; not uncommonly, they also have left-sided disease. For reasons that are unclear, viridans streptococci and enterococci rarely infect the tricuspid valve. Injection drug users may also develop candidal endocarditis. Patients with prosthetic heart valves have the additional risk of developing infective endocarditis due to *S epidermidis,* gram-negative bacilli, and fungi. Prior to the availability of antibiotics, infective endocarditis was a progressively debilitating, incurable, and fatal disease. Even with antibiotics, endocarditis continues to have a significant case fatality rate, and definitive cure often requires urgent or emergent surgery to replace damaged cardiac valves.

Pathogenesis

The hemodynamic factors that predispose patients to the development of endocarditis are the following: (1) a high-velocity jet stream, (2) flow from a high- to low-pressure chamber, and (3) a comparatively narrow orifice separating the two chambers that creates a pressure gradient. The lesions of infective endocarditis tend to form just beyond the orifice through which the high-velocity stream passes—eg, they commonly form on the ventricular surface of an abnormal aortic valve and on the atrial surface of an abnormal mitral valve. Satellite lesions can also grow where the jet stream strikes the endocardium (Figure 6–3). The damaged endothelium promotes the deposition of fibrin and platelets, which form sterile vegetations **(nonbacterial thrombotic endocarditis).** Infective endocarditis occurs when microorganisms are deposited onto these sterile vegetations during the course of bacteremia. Not all bacteria adhere to these sites. For example, *E coli,* a frequent cause of bacteremia, is rarely implicated as a cause of endocarditis. Organisms that possess little inherent pathogenicity, such as viridans streptococci, usually implant only on such sites. However, more virulent organisms, such as *S aureus,* can infect apparently normal valves.

Once infected, these vegetations provide the bacteria a sanctuary from host defense mechanisms such as PMNs and complement. Consequently, once infection takes hold, the infected vegetation continues to grow in a largely unimpeded fashion. For this reason, prolonged administration of bactericidal antibiotics is required to cure this disease. Bacteriostatic antimicrobial agents are inadequate to cure the infection. Operative intervention is sometimes required for cure, particularly in infections with gram-negative bacilli or fungi or in prosthetic valve infections.

Stimulation of both the humoral and cellular immune systems by the persistent bacteremia in infective endocarditis accounts for many of the extracardiac manifestations of this disease. A variety of immunoglobulins can be expressed, resulting in immune complex deposition, circulating rheumatoid factor, and nonspecific hypergammaglobulinemia. Immune complex deposition along the glomerular basement membrane may result in the development of glomerulonephritis and renal failure.

Unless diagnosed and appropriately treated, the disease is uniformly fatal. Death is usually caused by hemodynamic collapse from rupture of the aortic or mitral valves or by septic emboli to the central nervous system, resulting in brain abscesses or mycotic aneurysms and intracerebral hemorrhage. Because of its multisystem involvement, the disease continues to have a high mortality rate, especially left-sided endocarditis.

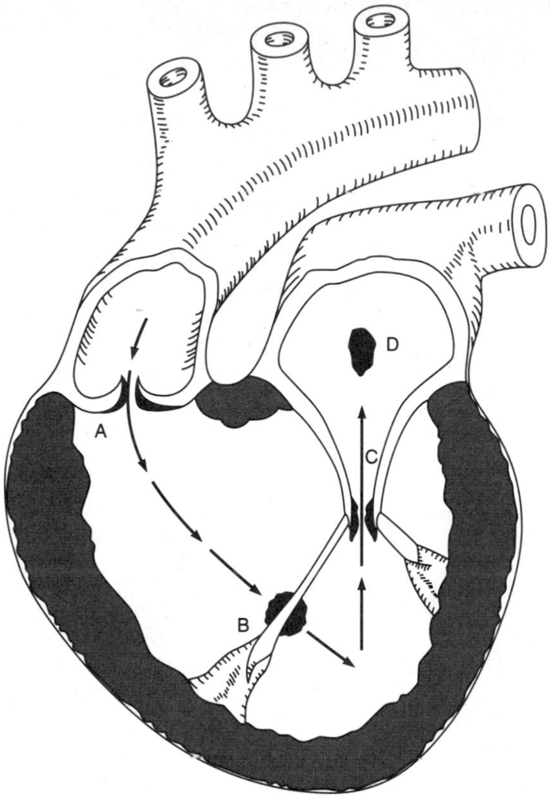

Figure 6–3. The location of endocarditic vegetations in relation to high-velocity regurgitant blood flow. The arrows indicate the high-velocity stream of blood. As a result of regurgitant flow through the orifice of the incompetent aortic valve, lesions form on the ventricular surface of the valve (***A***) or on the chordae tendineae of the anterior mitral leaflet (***B***). Regurgitant flow across the incompetent mitral valve into the low-pressure left atrium allows a vegetation to form on the atrial surface of the mitral valve (***C***) or at the site of jet stream impact on the atrial wall (***D***). (Modified and reproduced, with permission, from Karchmer AW: Intravascular infection. In: *Mechanisms of Microbial Disease,* 2nd ed. Schaechter M et al [editors]. Williams & Wilkins, 1993.)

Clinical Manifestations

Infective endocarditis is a multisystem disease with protean manifestations. For these reasons, the symptoms can be nonspecific and the diagnosis difficult to make. Table 6–6 summarizes the important features of the history, physical examination, laboratory data, and complications of infective endocarditis. The symptoms can be acute, subacute, or chronic. The clinical manifestations reflect primarily (1) hemodynamic changes from valvular damage, (2) end organ signs and symptoms from septic emboli (right-sided emboli to the lungs; left-sided emboli to the brain, spleen, kidney, gastrointestinal tract, and ex-

Table 6–6. Diagnosis of infective endocarditis and its complications.

History	Physical Examination	Laboratory Data	Complications
Fever, chills, night sweats, fatigue, malaise (nonspecific constitutional symptoms; can be acute, subacute, or chronic)	"Ill-appearing" Fever Tachycardia Hypotension	Positive blood cultures ↑ White blood cell count ↑ Erythrocyte sedimentation rate ↑ Rheumatoid factor	**Systemic** Persistent bacteremia Sepsis syndrome (?)
Headaches Back pain Focal weakness Numbness, tingling	Papilledema Focal vertebral spinal tenderness Focal neurologic exam (weakness, hyperreflexia, positive Babinski's sign, etc)	Head CT Spinal MRI (spinal CT with myelogram) Cerebral arteriogram ↑ Erythrocyte sedimentation rate	**Central nervous system** Cerebral emboli Mycotic aneurysm (with or without hemorrhage) Vertebral osteomyelitis Epidural abscess
Dyspnea Orthopnea Hepatojugular reflux Pedal edema	↑ Jugular venous pressure Pathologic cardiac murmurs Quincke's pulses Water-hammer pulses Rales	Chest radiograph Electrocardiogram Transthoracic echocardiogram Transesophageal echocardiogram Pulmonary artery (Swan-Ganz) catheter	**Cardiovascular (with left-sided endocarditis)** Mitral regurgitation Aortic regurgitation Congestive heart failure Aortic ring abscess
Pleuritic chest pain	Crackles Pleural rub	Chest radiograph	**Pulmonary (with right-sided endocarditis)** Septic pulmonary emboli
↓ Urine output Flank pain	Flank tenderness	↓ Urine output, ↑ BUN, ↑ creatinine Pyuria Renal sonogram	**Renal** Immune-complex glomerulonephritis Renal artery emboli Intrarenal abscess Perinephric abscess
Abdominal pain	Focal abdominal tenderness Hepatomegaly Splenomegaly	Abdominal radiograph Abdominal sonogram Abdominal CT	**Gastrointestinal** Liver abscesses Splenic abscesses Intestinal artery emboli (intestinal ischemia)
Rashes Focal painful lesions Visual complaints	Janeway lesions (painless macules) Osler's nodes (painful nodules) Splinter hemorrhages (nail beds) Petechiae Roth spots (funduscopic examination)	Skin biopsies (?)	**Skin, miscellaneous** Septic emboli Immune complex vasculitis

5. What is the typical presentation of infective endocarditis?
6. What is the leading etiologic agents of infectious endocarditis?
7. What features characterize infective endocarditis in intravenous drug users? In patients with prosthetic heart valves?
8. What hemodynamic features predispose to infective endocarditis?
9. What are some of the range of clinical manifestations of untreated bacterial endocarditis?
10. What is the most common cause of death in untreated infective endocarditis?

tremities), (3) end organ signs and symptoms from immune complex deposition, and (4) persistent bacteremia and distal seeding of infection (abscesses).

MENINGITIS

Clinical Presentation

In the United States, bacterial meningitis continues to be an important cause of morbidity and mortality, with an overall incidence of three cases per 100,000 persons per year. The symptoms most commonly associated with meningitis are fever, headache, neck stiffness, and confusion. Viral ("aseptic") meningitis presents as an acute illness with a self-limited clinical course. Bacterial meningitis is also acute, however, and without antibiotic therapy is associated with a significant mortality rate. Even with therapy, neurologic sequelae are common. Viral and bacterial meningitis cannot be reliably distinguished on clinical presentation, though the former more commonly has a lymphocytic pleocytosis. Chronic or subacute meningitis is caused more commonly by atypical bacteria or fungi and has a more indolent clinical course, with symptoms lasting weeks to months—sometimes with a waxing and waning course. In these cases, the etiologic diagnoses can be difficult to make in spite of extensive clinical evaluation.

Etiology

The three most frequent bacterial pathogens of community-acquired meningitis (*H influenzae, N meningitidis,* and *S pneumoniae*) account for about 80% of reported cases. Case fatality rates associated with these agents were 6%, 10%, and 26%, respectively, in the period between 1978 and 1981 (Table 6–7). These rates have not changed during the past 30 years. Approximately 10–30% of survivors of bacterial meningitis have persistent neurologic sequelae, particularly following pneumococcal meningitis.

The distribution of the causative agent varies by age (Table 6–8). In infants less than 2 months old, *E coli* (and other gram-negative bacilli) and group B streptococci are the most common causes of meningitis. For children aged 2 months to 15 years, *H influenzae* and *N meningitidis* are the most common causes. And for persons aged 16 years and older, *S pneumoniae* and *N meningitidis* are most common. Subacute or chronic meningitides are usually caused by *M tuberculosis,* fungi *(Coccidioides immitis, Cryptococcus neoformans),* and syphilis *(Treponema pallidum),* and the diagnosis can be difficult to make. In HIV-infected patients, *Cryptococcus* is the most common cause of meningitis.

Table 6–7. Pathogens causing bacterial meningitis in the United States.[1,2]

Organism	Cases		Case Fatality Rate (%)
	N	(%)	
H influenzae	6,756	(48.3)	6.0
N meningitidis	2,742	(19.6)	10.3
S pneumoniae	1,865	(13.3)	26.3
Group B streptococcus	476	(3.4)	22.5
L monocytogenes	265	(1.9)	28.5
Other	1,043	(7.5)	33.7
Unknown	827	(5.9)	16.4
Total	**13,974**	**(99.9)**	

[1]Modified and reproduced, with permission, from Swartz ML: Acute bacterial meningitis. In: *Infectious Diseases.* Gorbach SL, Bartlett JG, Blacklow NR (editors). Saunders, 1992.
[2]Reported in National Meningitis Surveillance System, 1978 through 1981.

Table 6–8. Common causes of bacterial meningitis by age group.[1]

Pathogen	Age <2 mo (%)	Age 2 mo to 15 y (%)	Age >16 y (%)
H influenzae	2	59	4
N meningitidis	0.5	24	29
S pneumoniae	2	13	46
E coli	38	0.5	4[2]
Other gram-negative bacilli	11.5	<0.2	
Group B streptococci	22	1[3]	4[3]
Other streptococci	6		
L monocytogenes	6	—	0.5
Staphylococcus	3.5	—	2.5
Miscellaneous	8	2.5	10
Total percentage	**99.5**	**100**	**100**

[1]Modified and reproduced, with permission, from Swartz M: Acute bacterial meningitis. In: *Infectious Diseases.* Gorbach SL, Bartlett JG, Blacklow NR (editors). Saunders, 1992.
[2]Combined all gram-negative bacillli.
[3]Combined all streptococci.

Pathogenesis

The pathogenesis of bacterial meningitis involves a sequence of events in which bacteria with virulence factors overcome the host's defense mechanisms (Table 6–9). Most of our knowledge of the pathogenesis of meningitis comes from studies of bacterial meningitis in animal models—inoculation of rats or rabbits with isolates of the most common bacterial pathogens associated with meningitis. The sequence of events is shown in Figure 6–4. First, bacteria colonize the host's nasopharynx, followed by local invasion of the mucosal epithelium and subsequent bacteremia. This is followed by endothelial cell injury, which increases blood-brain barrier permeability and facilitates meningeal invasion. The inflammatory response in the subarachnoid space results in cerebral edema, vasculitis, and infarction. The cascade of events leads to decreased cerebrospinal fluid outflow, hydrocephalus, worsening cerebral edema, increased intracranial pressure, and decreased cerebral blood flow.

Most cases of bacterial meningitis begin with host acquisition of a new organism by nasopharyngeal colonization. Many of the causal pathogens possess surface characteristics that enhance mucosal colonization. Different strains of *N meningitidis* have fimbriae that facilitate mucosal attachment. Bacterial

Table 6–9. Pathogenetic sequence of bacterial neurotropism.[1]

Neurotropic Stage	Host Defense	Strategy of Pathogen
1. Colonization or mucosal invasion	Secretory IgA Ciliary activity Mucosal epithelium	IgA protease secretion Ciliostasis Adhesive pili
2. Intravascular survival	Complement	Evasion of alternative pathway by polysaccharide capsule
3. Crossing of blood-brain barrier	Cerebral endothelium	Adhesive pili
4. Survival within CSF	Poor opsonic activity	Bacterial replication

[1]Reproduced, with permission, from Quagliarello V, Scheld WM: Bacterial meningitis: Pathogenesis, pathophysiology, and progress. N Engl J Med 1992; 327:864.

encapsulation may be important for nasopharyngeal colonization and systemic invasion of meningeal pathogens. Although most strains of *H influenzae* that colonize children by the age of 3 months are unencapsulated, 95% of isolates from meningitis and systemic infections are caused by encapsulated *H influenzae* type b. While all encapsulated strains of *H influenzae* have the potential for systemic invasion, type b strains are the most virulent. The polysaccharide capsule may also be an important virulence factor for invasive disease caused by *S pneumoniae.* Of the 84 strains of pneumococcal serotypes, 18 are responsible for over 80% of cases of bacteremic pneumococcal disease. Finally, in normal hosts, IgA antibodies found in mucosal secretions may inhibit the adherence of pathogenic bacteria to mucosal surfaces. However, many pathogenic *Neisseria, Haemophilus,* and *Streptococcus* species produce IgA proteases that cleave IgA and facilitate adherence of bacterial strains to the mucosal surfaces.

Once the mucosal barrier is crossed, bacteria gain access to the bloodstream, where they must overcome host defense mechanisms to survive and invade the central nervous system. The most common meningeal pathogens are all encapsulated, and the bacterial capsule is the most important virulence fac-

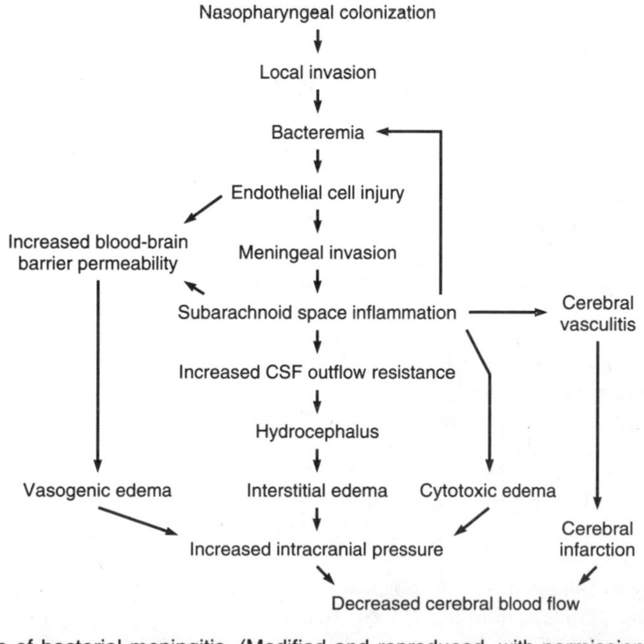

Figure 6–4. Pathogenesis of bacterial meningitis. (Modified and reproduced, with permission, from Tunkel AR, Scheld M: Pathogenesis and pathophysiology of bacterial meningitis. Clin Microbiol Rev 1993;6:118.)

tor in this regard. By inhibiting neutrophil phagocytosis and resisting classic complement-mediated bactericidal activity, the capsule enhances bacterial survival and replication in the blood. Normal host defenses counteract the antiphagocytic effects of the pneumococcal capsule by activating the alternative complement pathway, resulting in C3b activation, opsonization, phagocytosis, and intravascular clearance of the organism. This defense mechanism is impaired in patients who have undergone splenectomy. Such patients are predisposed to the development of pneumococcal bacteremia, sepsis, and meningitis. Recall that activation of the complement system is an essential host defense mechanism against invasive disease by *N meningitidis.* Patients with deficiencies in the late complement components (C5–9) are prone to invasive meningococcal disease.

The mechanisms by which bacterial pathogens gain access to the central nervous system are largely unknown. Some animal data suggest that initial bacterial entry occurs through the choroid plexus. Experimental studies have suggested that receptors for some meningeal pathogens are present on cells in the choroid plexus, which may facilitate movement of these pathogens into the subarachnoid space. Following bacterial invasion of the subarachnoid space, a secondary bacteremia may result from a local suppurative process, allowing the meningeal pathogen to continuously enter and leave the cerebrospinal fluid. Invasion of the spinal fluid by a meningeal pathogen results in increased permeability of the blood-brain barrier and is thought to occur primarily at the choroid plexus epithelium or cerebral microvascular endothelium.

Once the bacterial pathogen is in the subarachnoid space, host defense mechanisms are inadequate to control the infection. Normally, complement components are minimal or absent in the cerebrospinal fluid. Meningeal inflammation leads to increased, but low, concentrations of complement. This leads to inadequate opsonization, phagocytosis, and removal of encapsulated meningeal pathogens. Opsonic and bactericidal activities are absent or barely detectable in patients with meningitis. Immunoglobulin concentrations are also low in the cerebrospinal fluid, with an average blood:CSF IgG ratio of 800:1.

A hallmark of bacterial meningitis is the development of a neutrophilic pleocytosis in the cerebrospinal fluid. However, despite the entry of leukocytes, host defense mechanisms in spinal fluid remain suboptimal because of the relative lack of opsonic and bactericidal activity. Phagocytosis is so inefficient in the cerebrospinal fluid that there are huge numbers of bacteria in the fluid during meningitis. The ability of meningeal pathogens to induce a marked subarachnoid space inflammatory response contributes to many of the pathophysiologic consequences of bacterial meningitis.

Although the bacterial capsule is largely responsible for intravascular and cerebrospinal fluid survival of the pathogens, it does not result in the spinal fluid inflammatory response. In experimental infections, the subcapsular surface components (ie, the cell wall and lipopolysaccharide) of bacteria are more important determinants of meningeal inflammation than the bacterial surface components involved in cerebrospinal fluid invasion. The mediators of the inflammatory process are thought to be interleukin-1 and tumor necrosis factor (TNF). Within 1–3 hours after intracisternal inoculation of meningococcal lipopolysaccharide in an animal model, there is a brisk release of TNF and IL-1 into the cerebrospinal fluid; their release precedes the development of inflammation or the exudation of protein. The most direct evidence that these cytokines are involved comes from experiments in which direct inoculation of TNF and IL-1 into the cerebrospinal fluid produces the same inflammatory response.

The development of cerebral edema contributes to an increase in intracranial pressure, which may be vasogenic, cytotoxic, or interstitial in origin. This may result in life-threatening cerebral herniation. **Vasogenic cerebral edema** is principally caused by blood-brain barrier permeability. **Cytotoxic cerebral edema** results from swelling of the cellular elements of the brain due to toxic factors from bacteria or neutrophils. **Interstitial cerebral edema** reflects obstruction of flow in cerebrospinal fluid, as in hydrocephalus. Other complications of meningitis include **cerebral vasculitis** and alterations in cerebral blood flow. The vasculitis leads to narrowing or thrombosis of cerebral blood vessels, resulting in ischemia and possible brain infarction. In combination with increased intracranial pressure, cerebral vasculitis may result in altered cerebral blood flow.

Understanding the pathophysiology of bacterial meningitis has therapeutic implications. Although bactericidal therapy is necessary for the adequate treatment of bacterial meningitis, rapid bacteriolysis can release high concentrations of inflammatory bacterial fragments, thereby potentially exacerbating the inflammation and abnormalities of the cerebral microvasculature. In animal models of bacterial meningitis, antibiotic therapy has been shown to cause rapid bacteriolysis and release of bacterial endotoxin, resulting in increased cerebrospinal fluid inflammation and cerebral edema.

Clinical Manifestations

In patients who develop community-acquired bacterial meningitis, an antecedent upper respiratory tract infection is common. A smaller number of patients will have a nonspecific illness. Most patients with meningitis have a rapid onset of fever, headache, lethargy, and confusion. Other patients have prolonged respiratory tract or ear symptoms, and the meningeal symptoms develop and progress more slowly. Fewer than half of the patients complain of neck stiffness as a symptom, but nuchal rigidity is noted on physical examination in more than 75%. In young infants, manifestations of meningitis may be difficult to recognize and interpret. Other clues on physical examination include altered mental status, photophobia, stiff neck, Kernig's sign (inability of the examiner to extend the leg on the thigh with the patient supine and the thigh flexed to a right angle with the axis of the trunk and abdomen), and Brudzinki's sign (flexion of the legs occurring when the examiner passively flexes the patient's neck). About 50% of patients with meningococcal meningitis develop a petechial or purpuric rash, predominantly on the extremities. Meningococcal disease requires immediate treatment, because this infection advances rapidly.

Although a change in mental status (lethargy, confusion) is common in bacterial meningitis, up to 30% of patients present with normal consciousness. Ten to 20 percent of patients have cranial nerve dysfunction, 15–50% have seizures, and 10–20% have focal neurologic signs. Cerebral edema can occur, leading to herniation of the brain and death. Any patient suspected of having meningitis requires immediate lumbar puncture for Gram stain and culture of the cerebrospinal fluid, followed immediately by the administration of antibiotics. Alternatively, if a focal neurologic process (eg, brain abscess) is suspected, antibiotics should be initiated immediately, followed by brain imaging, either CT or MRI, followed by a lumbar puncture if it is deemed safe.

11. What is the incidence of bacterial meningitis?
12. What is the typical presentation of bacterial meningitis?
13. What are the major etiologic agents of meningitis and how do they vary with age or other characteristics of the host?
14. What is the sequence of events in development of meningitis, and what features of particular organisms predispose to meningitis?
15. What are the diverse causes of cerebral edema in patients with meningitis?
16. Why is rapid bacteriolysis theoretically dangerous in therapy of meningitis?
17. What are the associated clinical manifestations of untreated bacterial meningitis?

PNEUMONIA

Clinical Presentation

The respiratory tract is the most common site of infection by pathogenic microorganisms. Pneumonia continues to be among the leading causes of death in the United States. Over 2.5 million cases of pneumonia occur annually. Patients present with fever, cough, sputum production, and an infiltrate on chest radiograph. Diagnosis and management of pneumonia requires knowledge of host risk factors, potential infectious agents, environmental exposures, and pathogenesis. Pneumonia can be caused by viruses, bacteria, atypical bacteria (mycobacteria, chlamydiae, rickettsiae, mycoplasmas, legionellae), protozoa, parasites, or fungi.

Pneumonia is an infection of the lung parenchyma leading to inflammation (alveolitis) and the accumulation of an inflammatory exudate. With spread to the interstitium around the alveoli, consolidation and a degree of impaired gas exchange occur in the involved lung. Infection can extend to the pleural space, causing pleuritis and pain on inspiration. The exudative response of the pleura to pneumonia is termed **parapneumonic effusion,** which itself can become infected ("complicated parapneumonic effusion'') and develop into frank pus **(empyema).**

Etiology

Despite technologic advances in diagnosis, the specific agents associated with most community-acquired pneumonias often cannot be identified. Organisms most commonly associated with pneumonia in an immunocompetent adult host can be remembered by the "rule of thirds.'' In general, *one-third* of patients with a community-acquired pneumonia will have no etiologic diagnosis; *one-third* will have pneumococcal pneumonia; and *one-third* can be further categorized into thirds: *one-third* will have atypical bacterial pneumonia (including *Mycoplasma, Chlamydia,* and *Legionella*), usually diagnosed serologically; *one-third* will have viral pneumonia; and *one-third* will have *S aureus,* gram-negative bacillary, or anaerobic pneumonia. The actual distribution will vary over time and across populations, but this simple rule can assist in developing an approach to empiric antibiotic therapy.

Several other organisms require special consideration because of differences in host susceptibility, therapy, severity, or public health importance. Immunocompromised patients are at higher risk of opportunistic infections (*Pneumocystis carinii, Aspergillus, Nocardia,* cytomegalovirus). Although HIV-infected patients commonly develop pneumocystis pneumonia, *Aspergillus* and cytomegalovirus are not common causes of pneumonia in these patients. Lastly, pulmonary tuberculosis must be considered, since it has important public health and therapeutic implications.

Table 6–10 classifies by patient risk factor the most common infectious agents associated with pneumonia and the postulated primary mechanism of infection. Symptoms, though helpful, are often nonspecific. Understanding and identifying patient risk factors (smoking, HIV infection, etc), microbial pathogenetic mechanism *(M tuberculosis),* and host defense mechanisms (cough reflex, cell-mediated im-

Table 6–10. Common risk factors and causes of adult pneumonia.

Risk Factor	Etiologic Agents: Acute Symptoms	Etiologic Agents: Subacute or Chronic Symptoms	Pathogenic Mechanism and Comments
None identified	*Streptococcus pneumoniae* *Mycoplasma pneumoniae* *Chlamydia pneumoniae* *Legionella pneumophila*	*Mycobacterium tuberculosis*	Patients in the other risk categories are at higher risk for pneumonia caused by these microorganisms as well.
Immunocompromised 1. Acquired: a. HIV-infected	*Pneumocystis carinii* *Cryptococcus neoformans* (uncommon) *Toxoplasma gondii* (uncommon)	*Mycobacterium tuberculosis*	Cell-mediated immune dysfunction Granulocytopenia (These patients are at higher risk for pneumonia from all causes, especially tuberculosis.)
b. Transplant recipient	Cytomegalovirus *Aspergillus* *Pneumocystis carinii* *Nocardia*		
2. Inherited: Complement deficiency, etc	*Streptococcus pneumoniae*		
Chronic lung disease	*Streptococcus pneumoniae* *Haemophilus influenzae*		Decreased mucociliary clearance
Alcoholism		Anaerobic infection	Aspiration
Injection drug abuse	*Staphylococcus aureus*		Hematogenous
Environmental or animal exposure	*Legionella pneumophila* *Chlamydia psittaci* *Coxiella burnetti* (Q fever)	*Coccidioides immitis, Histoplasma capsulatum*	Inhalation
Institutional exposure (hospital, nursing home, etc)	Gram-negative bacilli (eg, *Pseudomonas aeruginosa, Enterobacter cloacae*) Staphylococcus epidermidis Staphylococcus aureus		Microaspirations Bypass of upper respiratory tract defense mechanisms (intubation) Hematogenous (intravenous catheters)

munity) focuses attention on the most likely etiologic agents, guides empiric therapy, and suggests possible contributing mechanisms that can be altered to decrease further risk. For example, hospital patients who have suffered a stroke are at higher risk of aspirating (or microaspirating) their oropharyngeal secretions, often colonized with nosocomial gram-negative bacteria. Likewise, a patient infected with HIV is at high risk for pneumocystis pneumonia.

Pathogenesis

Although pneumonia is a relatively common disease, it occurs infrequently in normal individuals. This can be attributed to the effectiveness of host defenses, including anatomic barriers and cleansing mechanisms in the nasopharynx and upper airways and local humoral and cellular factors in the alveoli. Normal lungs are generally sterile below the first major bronchial divisions.

Pulmonary pathogens reach the lungs by one of four routes: (1) direct inhalation, (2) aspiration of upper airway contents, (3) spread along the mucosal membrane surface, and (4) hematogenous spread. The pulmonary antimicrobial defense mechanisms are shown in Table 6–11 and Figure 6–5. The respiratory tract is exposed to potential pathogens suspended in inhaled air. Incoming air is subjected to turbulence in the nasal passages and then to abrupt changes in direction as the airstream is diverted through the pharynx and spreads along the branches of the tracheobronchial tree. Particles larger than 10 μm are trapped in the nose or pharynx; those with diameters of 2–9 μm are deposited on the mucociliary blanket; and smaller particles reach the alveoli. *M tuberculosis* and *Legionella pneumophila* are transmitted by direct inhalation. Bacteria deposited in the oropharynx can colonize the oropharynx and then be aspirated into the lungs, either by "microaspiration" or by overt aspirations (eg, in alcoholic patients who "pass out"). Likewise, chronic cigarette smokers have decreased mucociliary clearance and are often unable to clear respiratory secretions adequately. Patients who develop chronic bronchitis rely more heavily on their cough reflex to clear pathogens. The cough reflex is an important mechanism by which aspirated material, excess secretions, and foreign bodies are removed from the airway.

The respiratory epithelium has special mechanisms

Table 6–11. Pulmonary antimicrobial defense mechanisms.[1]

Aerodynamic filtration
Cough reflex
Mucociliary transport system
Phagocytic cells (alveolar macrophages and polymorphonuclear leukocytes)
Immune responses (humoral and cellular)
Pulmonary secretions (surfactant, lysozyme, iron-binding proteins)

[1]Modified and reproduced, with permission, from LaForce FM: Bacterial pneumonias. In: *Infectious Diseases.* Gorbach SL, Bartlett JG, Blacklow NR (editors). Saunders, 1992.

for fighting off infection. Epithelial cells are covered with beating cilia blanketed by a layer of mucus. Each ciliated cell has about 200 cilia that beat up to 500 times a minute and move the mucus layer upward toward the larynx. The mucus itself contains antimicrobial compounds such as lysozyme and secretory IgA antibodies. Bacteria that reach the terminal bronchioles, alveolar ducts, and alveoli are inactivated primarily by alveolar macrophages and neutrophils. Opsonization of the microorganism enhances phagocytosis. The development of humoral immunity enhances phagocytosis by macrophages and PMNs. Patients with granulocytopenia, whether acquired or congenital, are particularly susceptible to lung infections. Antigenic stimulation of T cells leads to the production of lymphokines which activate macrophages with enhanced bactericidal activity. HIV-infected patients have depleted CD4 lymphocyte counts and are predisposed to a variety of bacterial, parasitic, and fungal infections. Before the institution of prophylactic antibiotic regimens to prevent *P carinii* infection, it was the most common cause of pneumonia in HIV-infected patients and was associated with a high mortality rate.

Clinical Manifestations

Most patients with pneumonia have fever, cough, tachypnea, and tachycardia. Because upper respira-

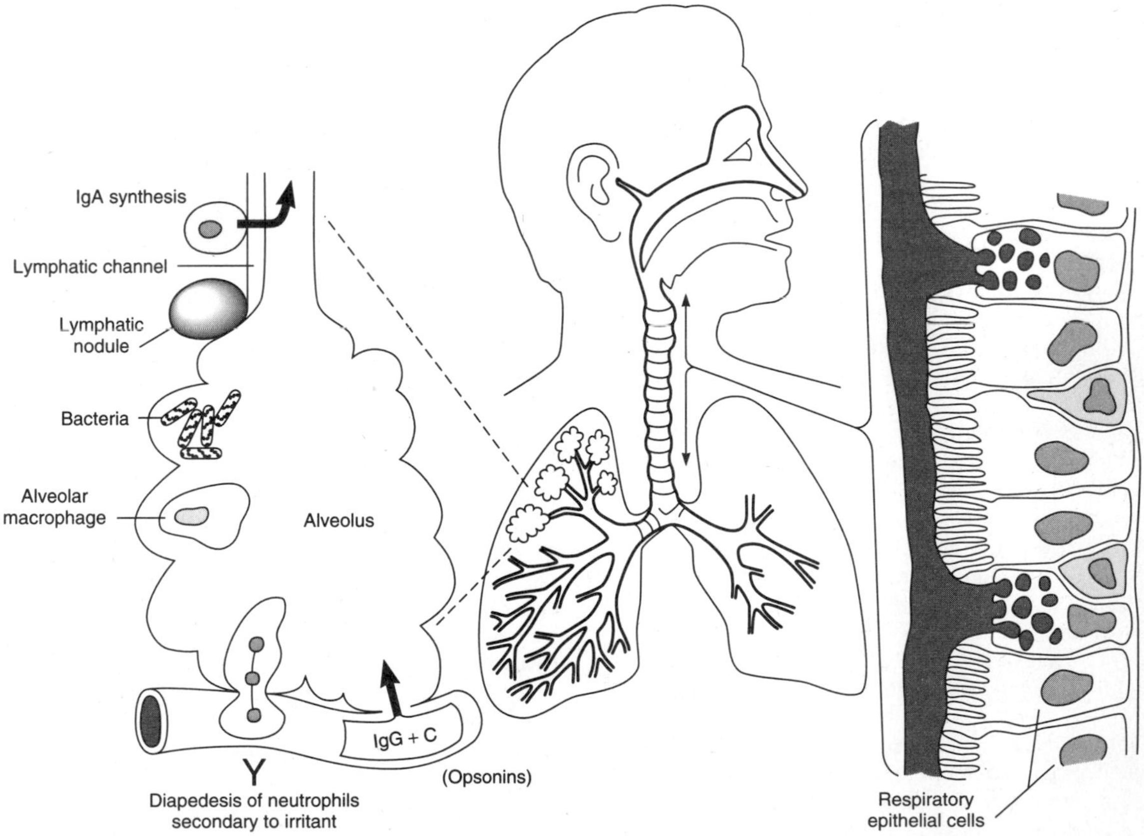

Figure 6–5. Pulmonary defense mechanisms. Abrupt changes in direction of air flow in the nasal passages can trap potential pathogens. The epiglottis and cough reflex prevent introduction of particulate matter in the lower airway. The ciliated respiratory epithelium propels the overlying mucus layer upward toward the mouth. In the alveoli, cell-mediated immunity, humoral factors, and the inflammatory response defend against lower respiratory tract infections. (Modified and reproduced, with permission, from Storch GA: Respiratory system. In: *Mechanisms of Microbial Disease,* 2nd ed. Schaechter M et al (editors). Williams & Wilkins, 1993.)

tory tract infections are common, a clinician must be prepared to recognize clues to the presence of pneumonia, such as extrapulmonary disease or systemic symptoms. Extrapulmonary manifestations occur with several important pulmonary pathogens. *S pneumoniae,* the most common identified cause of community-acquired pneumonia, is also the most common cause of meningitis in adults (Table 6–8). *S aureus* can cause a severe necrotizing pneumonia as well as endocarditis with the development of cerebritis from septic emboli. Gram-negative bacteria can cause urinary tract infections and nosocomial pneumonias in debilitated patients with chronic Foley catheters.

The following questions should be answered in every case involving a patient who presents with symptoms consistent with pneumonia:

Is this pneumonia community-acquired or institution-acquired?

Is this patient immunocompromised (HIV-infected, a transplant recipient)?

Is this patient an injection drug user?

Is this patient an alcoholic?

Has this patient had a recent loss of consciousness?

Are the symptoms acute (days) or chronic (weeks to months)?

Has this patient lived in or traveled through geographic areas associated with specific endemic infections (histoplasmosis, coccidioidomycosis)?

Has the patient had recent zoonotic exposures associated with pulmonary infections (psittacosis, Q fever)?

Could this patient have a contagious infection of public health importance (tuberculosis)?

Could this patient's pulmonary infection be associated with a common source exposure (*Legionella* outbreak)?

Is this patient hypoxemic or suffering from a potentially life-threatening complication such as pneumothorax?

18. How many cases of pneumonia occur in the U.S. annually?
19. What is the typical presentation of a patient with pneumonia?
20. What is the "rule of thirds" with regards to etiology of community-acquired pneumonias?
21. What host features influence the likelihood of particular etiologies of pneumonia?
22. What are the four mechanisms by which pathogens reach the lungs?
23. What are the defenses of the respiratory epithelium against infection?
24. How/Why does pulmonary bacterial infection result in the development of parenchymal consolidation?

INFECTIOUS DIARRHEA

Clinical Presentation

Each year throughout the world more than 5 million people—most of them children under 1 year of age—die of acute infectious diarrhea. The severity of diarrhea is due largely to the immense secretory capacity of the intestinal tract, which is greater than that of any other organ system. All segments of the intestinal tract from the proximal jejunum to the rectum secrete water and electrolytes. For example, adults with cholera, if adequately hydrated, can sometimes excrete more than 1 L of fluid per hour. Diarrheal disease can present with primarily upper gastrointestinal symptoms (nausea, vomiting, crampy epigastric pain), small intestinal symptoms (profuse watery diarrhea), or large intestinal symptoms (tenesmus, fecal urgency, less profuse diarrhea). Sources of infection include person-to-person transmission (fecal-oral spread of *Shigella*), water-borne transmission *(Cryptosporidium),* food-borne transmission (*Salmonella, S aureus* food poisoning), and overgrowth following antibiotic administration *(Clostridium difficile).*

Etiology

A wide range of microorganisms infect the gastrointestinal tract. These agents include newly identified bacterial pathogens, such as *Helicobacter pylori* and a growing number of serotypes of *E coli.* During the past 2 decades, viral causes of gastroenteritis have been identified, and viruses have joined bacteria and parasites as recognized pathogens involved in diarrheal disease. For example, rotavirus is thought to be the most common cause of severe diarrhea in infants and young children. Protozoal, algal, and fungal enteric pathogens can also produce diarrhea. In the United States, viral gastroenteritis causes 30–40% of the cases of infectious diarrhea; bacteria account for 20–30% of cases; and in 40% the cause remains unknown. HIV-infected patients with very low CD4 lymphocyte counts (usually < 100/μL) can develop a severe, often unremitting watery diarrhea caused by *Cryptosporidium* organisms for which there is no cure.

Pathogenesis

A comprehensive approach to gastrointestinal infections starts with the host-agent-environment paradigm. Host factors influencing gastrointestinal infections include age and comorbid conditions (such as HIV infection). Microbial agents responsible for gastrointestinal diarrheal illness can be categorized according to type of organism (bacterial, viral, parasitic), propensity to attach to different anatomic sites (stomach, small bowel, colon), and pathogenesis (enterotoxigenic, cytotoxigenic, or enteroinvasive). Environmental factors can be divided into four broad categories based on mode of transmission: (1) water-

Table 6–12. Approach to gastrointestinal diarrheal illness.

Paradigm	Categories	Examples	Microbes
Environment	Water-borne	Water supply	*Vibrio cholerae*
	Food-borne	Restaurants	*Staphylococcus aureus* *Bacillus cereus*
	Person-to-person	Child care centers	*Shigella* Hemorrhagic *E coli*
	Zoonotic	Farms	*Campylobacter*
Agent	Bacterial		*Salmonella* species
	Viral		Rotavirus
	Parasitic		*Entamoeba histolytica*
Host	Age	Children	Hemorrhagic *E coli*
	Comorbid conditions	HIV infection	*Cryptosporidium* Cytomegalovirus

borne diarrheal disease, (2) food-borne diarrheal disease, (3) person-to-person transmission, and (4) zoonotic transmission. Table 6–12 summarizes these relationships and provides the framework within which one can assess the pathogenesis of gastrointestinal infections.

The pathogenesis of *E coli* gastrointestinal infections is better understood than that of other types of gastrointestinal infections. *E coli,* though part of the normal human gastrointestinal microbial flora, can nonetheless cause a spectrum of diarrheal illnesses. Several different types of *E coli* can produce diarrhea by different mechanisms. One way to conceptualize the different mechanisms is to consider what bacteria must do to cause diarrheal disease (eg, elaborate a toxin). First, any pathogenic bacterium must gain entry to the gastrointestinal tract and survive gastric acidity. Next, it must adhere or attach itself to the intestinal mucosa. The adherence can be nonspecific (attaching to any part of the intestinal mucosa) or, more commonly, specific, attaching itself to specific areas of the gastrointestinal tract. Specific mechanisms of attachment differ between different strains of *E coli.* The genetic control of pathogenicity also differs; some bacterial phenotypic expression of virulence is under the control of chromosomal genes, while for others it is mediated by plasmids or bacteriophages.

Once the organism has attached itself to a specific site of intestinal mucosa, several pathogenetic mechanisms can lead to diarrhea: *First,* the bacteria may elaborate an **enterotoxin** that "poisons" intestinal cellular mechanisms. In the small bowel—the site of significant intestinal electrolyte transport—this results in profuse, sometimes explosive watery diarrhea. One common mechanism is the use of a secondary messenger system to mediate the toxin's effect (eg, cAMP in cholera). *Second,* **cytotoxins** may cause death of intestinal mucosal cells. This mechanism more often involves the large bowel intestinal mucosa, leading to a "colitis-like" clinical presentation with crampy lower abdominal pain, tenesmus, and less diarrhea. The colonic mucosa may have an inflammatory or bloody host response. An extension of this mechanism is the actual bacterial invasion of the mucosal wall, leading to a severe inflammatory, often bloody diarrhea **(dysentery).** Pathologically, microabscesses can be found in the intestinal mucosal wall. Patients are systemically ill, with severe colitis-type symptoms as well as constitutional symptoms. Shigellosis, most commonly caused by *Shigella flexneri* and *Shigella sonnei,* is noted for this clinical presentation ("bacillary dysentery"). *Third,* some bacteria can invade the host to cause systemic diseases. *Salmonella* species (most commonly *Salmonella typhi* in developing countries) can invade the bloodstream, causing bacteremia, enteric fever, and a chronic carrier state. *Shigella dysenteriae* has been associated with hemolytic-uremic syndrome.

Epidemiologic and clinical studies have since shown that *E coli* is an important diarrheal pathogen worldwide; it is probably the most common cause of diarrhea. *E coli* is the most common organism isolated in routine enteric cultures. In the 1960s, investigators isolated enterotoxin from *E coli* in animal models. Similar strains were isolated from humans in India that had a disease resembling cholera. To date, pathogenic *E coli* responsible for diarrheal diseases have been classified into the following types: enteroaggregative *E coli* (EAggEC), enteropathogenic *E coli* (EPEC), enterotoxigenic *E coli* (ETEC), enteroinvasive *E coli* (EIEC), and enterohemorrhagic *E coli* (EHEC). This classification has been based on different criteria, including known pathogenetic mechanisms, clinical syndromes, or specific reactions in cellular assay systems (Table 6–13).

Enteroaggregative *E coli* is associated with persis-

Table 6–13. *Escherichia coli* in diarrheal disease.

Class	Age at Higher Risk	Inoculum Size	Clinical Syndrome	Gastrointestinal Site	Virulence Genetic Control	Adherence	Enterotoxins or Cytotoxins	Site of Action of Toxin	Histopathologic Features
Enteroaggregative *E coli* (EAggEC)	<6 months	10^8–10^{10}	Watery diarrhea	Small bowel	Not well described	Adhesins[1]	Not well described	Not well described	Not well described
Enteropathogenic *E coli* (EPEC)	<1 year	10^8–10^{10}	Watery diarrhea	Small bowel	Chromosomal, plasmid	Adhesins[2]	Not well described	Not well described	Effacement of brush border
Enterotoxigenic *E coli* (ETEC)	>1 year	10^8–10^{10}	Watery diarrhea	Small bowel	Plasmid (toxin)	Adhesins CFA	Heat-labile toxin (LT) (cholera-like) Heat-stable toxin (ST)	Adenylyl cyclase activation Guanylyl cyclase activation	None
Enteroinvasive *E coli* (EIEC)	>2 years	10^8–10^{10}	Dysentery (bloody, inflammatory)	Small bowel, large bowel	Chromosomal, plasmid	Invasins[3]	Not well described	Not well described	Invasive and inflammatory
Enterohemorrhagic *E coli* (EHEC)	2–10 years, elderly	<10^3	Hemorrhagic colitis, hemolytic-uremic syndrome, (?thrombotic thrombocytopenic purpura)	Small bowel, large bowel	Chromosomal (adherence), phage (toxin)	Adhesins[4]	Shiga-like toxin (VT) SLT-I SLT-II SLT-IIv	Binds to 60S ribosome and inhibits protein synthesis	Effacement of brush border, not inflammatory

Key: CFA = colonization factor antigen; VT = verotoxin
[1]Autoaggregative attaching pattern.
[2]EPEC adherence factor (EAF), attaching and effacing changes, localized adherence pattern.
[3]Factors mediating cell division.
[4]Attaching and effacing changes.

tent watery diarrhea in infants. In these outbreaks, no other pathogens are isolated, including other pathogenic *E coli*. What distinguishes enteroaggregative *E coli* are the pathognomonic changes in cell assays, in which the bacteria adhere to HEp-2 cells in an autoaggregative manner—hence the descriptive name.

Enteropathogenic *E coli* has been associated with watery diarrhea in nursery outbreaks and in both endemic and sporadic disease. No toxin has been isolated from this strain of *E coli*. Infection with EPEC is associated with characteristic ultrastructural lesions in the intestine. By electron microscopy, the lesions show a dissolution of microvilli, with bacteria on the surface of the intestinal epithelial cells; these lesions are termed attaching and effacing lesions. The current model of EPEC attachment and invasion (Figure 6–6) involves three distinct processes: (1) initial adherence; (2) intimate adherence, involving formation of attaching and effacing lesions and actin polymerization; and (3) invasion.

Enterotoxigenic *E coli* strains are the most commonly isolated bacteria in acute diarrhea worldwide. In the developing world, they most frequently produce acute diarrheal disease in young children. ETEC is also the cause of up to 70% of cases of traveler's diarrhea. The common vehicle of transmission is usually fecally contaminated food. ETEC produces two **enterotoxins** that "poison" the small intestinal cells and cause watery diarrhea. The pathogenesis is very similar to that of cholera (caused by *Vibrio cholerae*) (Figure 6–7). ETEC produces a heat-labile toxin (LT) known to be closely related both structurally and antigenically to cholera enterotoxin and which produces fluid loss by the same mechanisms. Like cholera toxin, LT has A and B subunits. The B subunits attach to the intestinal cell membrane and facilitate entry of part of the A subunit, leading to activation of adenylyl cyclase, formation of cAMP, and stimulation of water and electrolyte secretion by intestinal luminal cells. ETEC also produces a heat-stable toxin (ST) that results in guanylyl cyclase activation, also causing watery diarrhea.

Enteroinvasive *E coli* (EIEC) primarily causes invasion of the colonic wall in a fashion very similar to that of *Shigella*. Some of the outer membrane proteins are identical to those of *Shigella*. EIEC is responsible for dysentery similar to that of shigellosis.

Enterohemorrhagic *E coli* (EHEC) is well known in the medical community because of recent large outbreaks in the northwestern United States that resulted in well-publicized deaths from hemolytic-uremic syndrome. It is primarily associated with serotype *E coli* O157:H7 and can cause a spectrum of illness including the following: (1) asymptomatic infection, (2) watery (nonbloody) diarrhea, (3) hemorrhagic colitis (bloody, noninflammatory diarrhea), (4) hemolytic-uremic syndrome, and (5) thrombotic thrombocytopenic purpura. In general, the gastrointestinal illness is characterized by severe crampy abdominal pain, initially watery diarrhea followed by grossly bloody diarrhea, and little or no fever. *E coli* O157:H7 produces several Shiga-like toxins (SLT) (also called verotoxins) that closely resemble *S dysenteriae* type I Shiga toxin in structure and func-

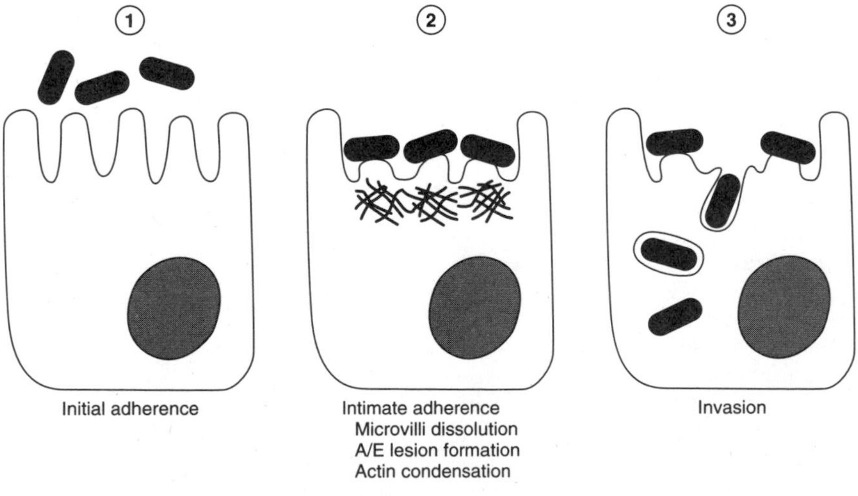

Figure 6–6. Model of enteropathogenic *E coli* (EPEC) adherence and invasion. (Modified and reproduced, with permission, from Tesh VL, O'Brien AD: Adherence and colonization mechanisms of enteropathogenic and enterohemorrhagic *Escherichia coli*. Microb Pathog 1992;12:245.)

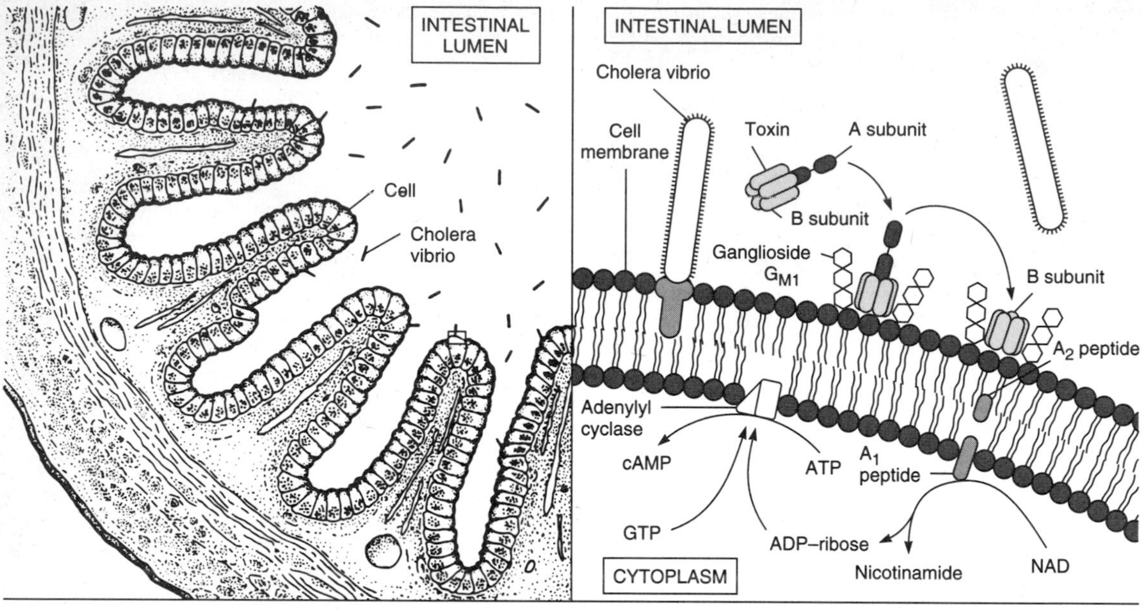

Figure 6–7. Pathogenesis of *Vibrio cholerae* and enterotoxigenic *E coli* (ETEC) in diarrheal disease. *V cholerae* and ETEC share similar pathogenetic mechanisms in causing diarrheal illness. The bacteria gain entry to the small intestinal lumen through ingestion of contaminated food (***left***). They elaborate an enterotoxin that is composed of one A subunit and five B subunits. The B subunits bind to the intestinal cell membrane and facilitate entry of part of the A subunit (***right***). Subsequently, this results in activation of adenylyl cyclase and formation of cAMP, which stimulates water and electrolyte secretion by intestinal endothelial cells. (Modified and reproduced, with permission, from Holmberg SD: Cholera and related illnesses caused by *Vibrio* species and *Aeromonas*. In: *Infectious Diseases.* Gorbach SL et al (editors). Saunders, 1992.)

tion. SLTs are proteins with one large A subunit, the active portion, and five smaller B subunits, which bind to the cell surface receptor. Following binding and internalization, the A subunit catalyzes the destructive cleavage of ribosomal RNA and halts protein synthesis, leading to cell death (Figure 6–8). The possible mechanisms whereby *E coli* O157:H7's Shiga-like toxin causes hemolytic-uremic syndrome and thrombotic thrombocytopenic purpura are shown in Figure 6–9.

Clinical Manifestations

Table 6–14 summarizes gastroenteritides and food poisoning syndromes caused by bacteria. One approach to gastrointestinal infections is to categorize the symptom complex associated with a known pathogenetic mechanism or anatomic site in the gastrointestinal tract. In staphylococcal food poisoning, symptoms develop several hours after ingestion of food contaminated with enterotoxin-producing *S aureus.* The symptoms of staphylococcal food poisoning are profuse vomiting, nausea, and abdominal cramps, followed by diarrhea. Profuse watery (noninflammatory, nonbloody) diarrhea is associated with bacteria that have infected the small intestine and elaborated an enterotoxin (eg, *V cholerae*). In contrast, colitis-like symptoms (lower abdominal pain, tenesmus, fecal urgency) and an inflammatory or bloody diarrhea occur with bacteria that more commonly infect the large intestine. In this case, the incubation period is longer (days) and colonic mucosal invasion can occur, causing fever and systemic symptoms.

25. How many individuals in the world die yearly of infectious diarrhea?
26. What are different modes of spread of infectious diarrhea? Give an example of each.
27. What are the pathogenetic mechanisms by which infectious organisms cause diarrhea?

SEPSIS, SEPSIS SYNDROME, & SEPTIC SHOCK

Clinical Presentation

Sepsis and its sequelae—sepsis syndrome and septic shock—are leading causes of death in hospital intensive care units in the United States.

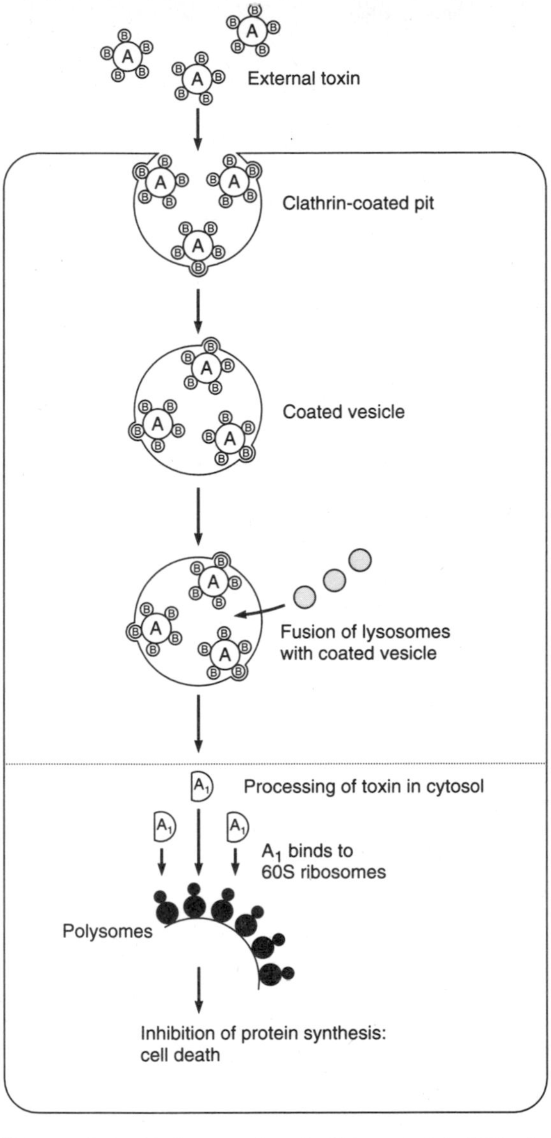

Figure 6–8. Pathogenesis of Shiga toxin (*Shigella* species) and Shiga-like toxin (enterohemorrhagic *E coli*). *Shigella* species and *E coli* O157:H7 probably cause invasive diarrheal diseases by similar pathogenetic mechanisms. The A and B subunits enter the intestinal cells through receptor-mediated endocytosis. The active A_1 fragment binds to the 60S ribosome, leading to inhibition of protein synthesis and cell death. (Modified and reproduced, with permission, from O'Brien AD, Holmes RK: Shiga and Shiga-like toxins. Microbiol Rev 1987;51:206.)

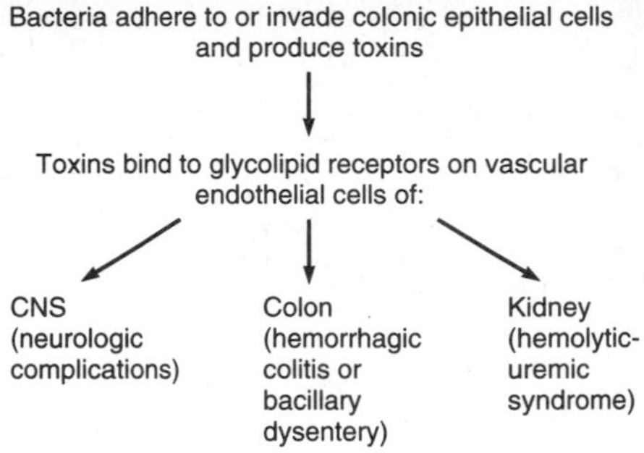

Figure 6–9. Possible mechanisms of complications of *E coli* O157:H7 and *Shigella* species. *Shigella* species and *E coli* O157:H7 may share similar pathogenetic mechanisms in diarrheal illness and extraintestinal complications. A possible mechanism is that Shiga toxin and Shiga-like toxin damage vascular endothelial cells in various target organs. (Modified and reproduced, with permission, from Tesh VL, O'Brien AD: The pathogenic mechanisms of Shiga toxin and the Shiga-like toxins. Mol Microbiol 1991;5:1817.)

Approximately 400,000 cases of sepsis and 200,000 cases of septic shock occur annually. The mortality rate from septic shock ranges from 20% to 80%. This wide range reflects differing definitions of the syndrome and the heterogeneity of the patients studied. The increasing risk of infection and subsequent sepsis is in part attributable to the increasing use of intravascular catheters and devices, implantation of prosthetic devices, and administration of immunosuppressive drugs and chemotherapeutic agents.

Sepsis is defined as a pathophysiologic process caused by an infection that can result in sepsis syndrome, septic shock, and death. The initial manifestations of sepsis are clinical signs of infection associated with a systemic response to infection such as tachycardia, tachypnea, and fever (hyperthermia) or hypothermia. Hypothermia is more common in elderly patients and in patients with severe underlying comorbidities. **Sepsis syndrome** is defined as sepsis with signs of organ hypoperfusion, including peripheral vasoconstriction, hypoxemia, elevated lactate levels, decreased urine output, and altered mental status. **Septic shock** is defined as sepsis syndrome with hypotension (systolic blood pressure < 90 mm Hg or a 40 mm Hg decrease below the baseline systolic blood pressure). **Refractory septic shock** is defined as prolonged shock that is unresponsive to administration of fluids, vasopressors, and antibiotics.

Etiology

The most common sites of infection are the genitourinary, respiratory, and gastrointestinal tracts, skin, and wounds. Any microorganism, including bacteria and fungi, can initiate sepsis. The most common causes of gram-negative sepsis are *P aeruginosa, E coli, S aureus,* and other Enterobacteriaceae. Factors that contribute to hospital-related sepsis are invasive monitoring devices and indwelling

Table 6–14. Symptom-based approach to gastroenteritis and food poisoning syndromes.[1]

Symptoms	Anatomic Site	Incubation Period	Possible Agents
Nausea, vomiting	Upper gastrointestinal tract	6 hours	*Staphylococcus aureus* *Bacillus cereus*
Watery noninflammatory diarrhea; passage of few voluminous stools	Upper small bowel	6–72 hours	*Clostridium perfringens,* type A *Bacillus cereus* Enterotoxigenic *E coli* (ETEC) Enteroaggregative *E coli* (EAggEC) Enteropathogenic *E coli* (EPEC) *V cholerae* *G lamblia*
Inflammatory ileocolitis; tenesmus, fecal urgency, dysentery; fever with invasion	Large bowel origin; colitis; with or without mucosal invasion	16–72 hours	*Salmonella* *Shigella* *Campylobacter jejuni* Enterohemorrhagic *E coli* (EHEC)[2] Enteroinvasive *E coli* (EIEC) *Yersinia enterocolitica* *Vibrio parahaemolyticus*

[1]Modified and reproduced, with permission, from Guerrant RL, Bobak DA: Bacterial and protozoal gastroenteritis. N Engl J Med 1991;325:327.
[2]EHEC gastrointestinal infections are initially watery diarrhea followed by bloody diarrhea; inflammation occurs in only a small percentage.

catheters, extensive surgical procedures, and the growing number of immunosuppressed patients. Gram-positive bacteremia, especially that due to *S aureus,* is more common because of injection drug use and the therapeutic placement of chronic venous access catheters.

Pathogenesis

Sepsis is one example of a **systemic inflammatory response** that can be triggered not only by infections but also by noninfectious disorders such as pancreatitis or trauma. The pathogenetic cascade of sepsis starts with an infection. With bacterial infections, sepsis begins with the proliferation of bacteria at the site of infection. The bacteria may then invade the bloodstream directly (leading to bacteremia and positive blood cultures) or may proliferate locally and release toxins into the bloodstream. The toxin can arise from a structural component of the bacteria (endotoxin, teichoic acid antigen, etc) or may be exotoxins, which are synthesized by the bacterial pathogen. Endotoxin derives from gram-negative bacteria. It is the lipid A component of the lipopolysaccharide-phospholipid-protein complex present in the outer cell membrane of the gram-negative bacterium (Figure 6–10). When released into the circulation of the infected host, endotoxin stimulates release of several endogenous mediators of sepsis from a variety of host cells, including plasma cells, monocytes, macrophages, and endothelial cells. When endotoxin is injected into animals, it causes a shock-like state manifested by hypotension and organ dysfunction.

A variety of host mediators have been implicated in the pathogenesis of sepsis (Figure 6–11). Gram-negative bacterial endotoxin induces activation of the coagulation cascade, the complement system, and the kinin system as well as the release of numerous endogenous mediators: cytokines (tumor necrosis factor, interleukin-1, -2, etc), platelet-activating factor, endorphins, endothelium-derived relaxing factor, arachidonic acid metabolites, myocardial depressant factors, and others. The major effects are on the myocardium and vasculature and on other organs (kidney, liver, lung, and brain). Uncontrolled sepsis leads to sepsis syndrome (evidence of organ hypoperfusion) and finally to refractory septic shock (refractory hypotension or multiple organ system failure).

A. Hemodynamic Alterations: All forms of shock result in inadequate tissue perfusion and subsequent cell dysfunction and cell death. In noninfectious forms (such as cardiogenic shock and hypovolemic shock), systemic vascular resistance is elevated as a compensatory mechanism to maintain blood pressure. In the hypoperfused tissues, there is enhanced extraction of oxygen from circulating red blood cells leading to decreased pulmonary artery oxygenation. In the early stage of septic shock, however, hypovolemia occurs as a result both of arterial and venous dilation and of leakage of plasma into the extravascular space. The hypovolemia leads to lowering of low systemic vascular resistance, increased cardiac output and tachycardia, and increased pulmonary artery oxygenation secondary to inadequate oxygen extraction in hypoperfused tissues.

A hyperdynamic circulatory state occurs that has

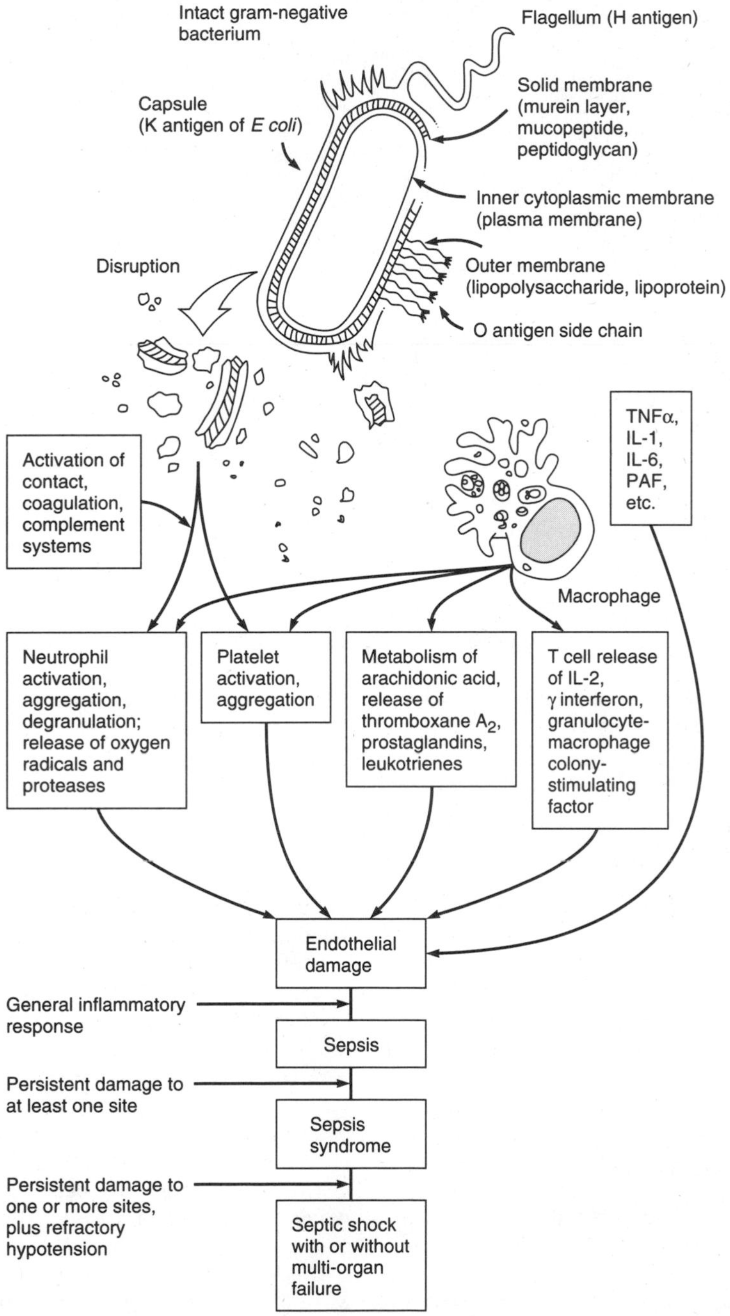

Figure 6–10. Schematic overview of sepsis. This schematic illustrates the major pathways in the pathogenesis of sepsis. See text for details. (Modified and reproduced, with permission, from Bone RC: The pathogenesis of sepsis. Ann Intern Med 1991;115:457.)

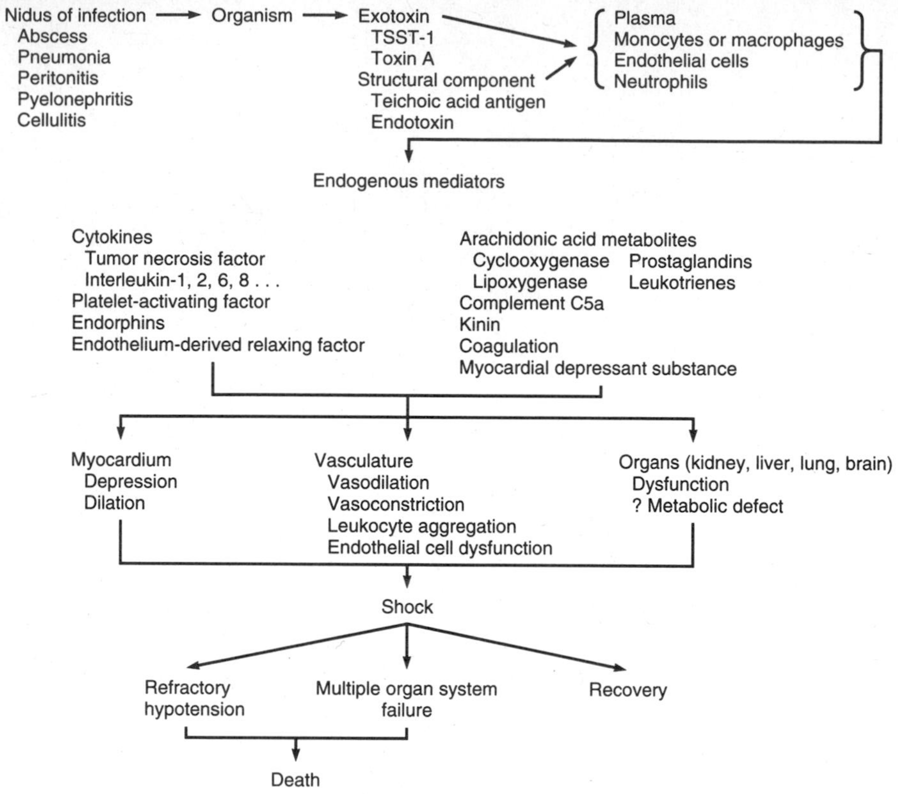

Figure 6–11. Schematic overview of sepsis. (Modified and reproduced, with permission, from Parrillo JE: Pathogenetic mechanisms of septic shock. N Engl J Med 1993;328:1471.)

been described as distributive shock to emphasize the maldistribution of blood flow to various tissues. The release of vasoactive substances results in loss of normal mechanisms of vascular autoregulation, producing regional and microcirculatory imbalances in blood flow, including regional shunting. Because the influence of vasodilatory mediators predominates, patients present with warm extremities. A mismatching of blood flow with metabolic demand causes excessive blood flow to some areas, with relative hypoperfusion of other areas, limiting optimal utilization of oxygen. Thus, these distributive changes in systemic and microcirculatory blood flow patterns are postulated to be major factors contributing to impaired oxygen utilization.

Myocardial depression is common in early septic shock. Although cardiac output is normal or increased, ventricular function is abnormal. Twenty-four to 48 hours after the onset of sepsis, left and right ventricular ejection fractions are reduced, end-diastolic and end-systolic volumes are increased, stroke volume is normal, heart rate is increased, and systemic vascular resistance is reduced. Increased end-diastolic and end-systolic volumes occur, resulting from biventricular dilation. The reduced ejection fractions and the consequent myocardial depression are reversible in patients who survive septic shock. Interestingly, patients with low ejection fractions and biventricular dilation at the onset of sepsis are more likely to survive, perhaps reflecting a greater ventricular compensation (by Frank-Starling mechanism) for sepsis-induced myocardial depression. However, patients who present with tachycardia and who fail to resolve either the tachycardia or increased cardiac index within 24 hours have decreased survival. In other words, persistence of the hyperdynamic state is associated with a higher mortality rate.

B. Vascular and Multiorgan Dysfunction: Most patients who die of septic shock have either refractory hypotension or multiple organ failure. Refractory hypotension can occur from two mechanisms. First, some patients cannot sustain a high cardiac output in response to the septic state and develop progressive cardiac failure with hypodynamic shock. Second, circulatory failure may be associated with severe vasodilation and hypotension refractory to intravenous fluid resuscitation and vasopressor therapy.

The development of multiple organ failure represents the terminal phase of a hypermetabolic process that begins during the initial stages of shock and resuscitation. Organ failure results from microvascular injury that is induced by local and systemic inflammatory responses to the infection. A large number of vascular abnormalities have been described with septic shock. Many vascular beds are dilated and others are constricted, resulting in maldistribution of blood flow. The aggregation of neutrophils and platelets may also reduce blood flow. Margination of neutrophils along vascular endothelium results in release of mediators and subsequent migration of neutrophils into tissues. Components of the complement system such as C5a are activated, attracting more neutrophils and releasing locally active substances. These inflammatory mediators (eg, arachidonic acid metabolites such as prostaglandins and leukotrienes) are released from many types of cells. They cause local vasoconstriction and vasodilation and the accumulation of still more inflammatory cells. Release of TNF results in relaxation of vascular smooth muscle and vasodilation. In the end, the release of a large number of mediators and the migration of inflammatory cells interact with endothelial and vascular smooth muscle cells to interfere with blood flow and ultimately lead to microvascular failure and subsequent organ failure.

The outcome of sepsis depends on the number of organs that fail; mortality rates of 80–100% occur in patients who sustain failure of three or more organs. A characteristic sequential pattern of pulmonary, hepatic, and renal failure is observed. Thirty to 80 percent of patients develop respiratory failure, most commonly from the adult respiratory distress syndrome (ARDS), which is characterized by severe refractory hypoxemia, decreased lung compliance, noncardiogenic pulmonary edema, and pulmonary hypertension. ARDS is often fatal. Hepatic dysfunction is frequently observed in septic shock. Its initial manifestations are hyperbilirubinemia with modest elevations in serum aminotransferase and alkaline phosphatase concentrations. Renal failure develops later in the clinical course. Its cause is multifactorial, including intrarenal shunting, renal hypoperfusion, or administration of nephrotoxic agents.

Clinical Manifestations

The clinical manifestations of sepsis include those related to the systemic response to infections (tachycardia, tachypnea, alterations in temperature, and leukocytosis) and those related to organ system dysfunction (cardiovascular, respiratory, renal, hepatic, and hematologic abnormalities). Sepsis sometimes begins with very subtle nonspecific clues that can be easily confused with more common, less serious illnesses. Awareness of these early signs of sepsis can lead to early recognition and intervention, leading to lower morbidity and mortality rates. Early signs can include isolated tachypnea (without dyspnea), isolated tachycardia (with normal blood pressure), irritability or lethargy, and unexplained fever, rigors, or myalgias. Nonspecific laboratory abnormalities can include proteinuria, leukocytosis, and mild liver function abnormalities.

A summary of the clinical manifestations of sepsis is presented in Table 6–15.

Table 6–15. Manifestations of sepsis.[1]

Common Manifestations	Less Common Manifestations, or Severe Sepsis
Fever, rigors, myalgias	Stupor, coma
Irritability, lethargy	Hypothermia
Tachycardia	Shock
Tachypnea (respiratory alkalosis)	Overt upper gastrointestinal bleeding
Hypoxemia	Cutaneous lesions
Proteinuria	Funduscopic lesions
Leukocytosis	Lactic acidosis
Eosinopenia	Acute respiratory distress syndrome
Hyperferremia	Azotemia, oliguria
Mild liver function abnormalities	Leukopenia, leukemoid reaction
Hyperglycemia in diabetics	Thrombocytopenia
	Disseminated intravascular coagulation
	Anemia
	Hypoglycemia

[1]Modified and reproduced, with permission, from Harris RL et al: Manifestations of sepsis. Arch Intern Med 1987;147:1895.

28. What is the incidence of sepsis in the U.S? Mortality?
29. What are the initial manifestations of sepsis?
30. What factors contribute to hospital-related sepsis?
31. Which organisms most commonly cause gram-negative sepsis?
32. Which host mediators have been implicated in the pathogenesis of sepsis?
33. What activates these host mediators, and on which organs do they act?
34. What are some distinctive features of septic shock vs other shock syndromes?

REFERENCES

General

Brooks GF et al: *Review of Medical Microbiology,* 20th ed. Appleton & Lange, 1994.

Committee on Emerging Threats to Health: *Emerging Infections: Microbial Threats to Health in the United States.* National Academy Press, 1992.

Finlay BB, Falkow S: Common themes in microbial pathogenicity. Microbiol Rev 1989;53:210.

Gorbach SL et al (editors): *Infectious Diseases.* Saunders, 1992.

Levinson WE, Jawetz E: *Medical Microbiology & Immunology.* Appleton & Lange, 1992.

Schaechter M et al: *Mechanisms of Microbial Disease,* 2nd ed. Williams & Wilkins, 1993.

Infective Endocarditis

Schaechter M et al: *Mechanisms of Microbial Disease,* 2nd ed. Williams & Wilkins, 1993.

Wilson JD et al (editors): *Harrison's Principles of Internal Medicine,* 12th ed. McGraw-Hill, 1991.

Meningitis

Durand ML et al: Acute bacterial meningitis in adults: A review of 493 episodes. N Engl J Med 1993;328:21.

Quagliarello V, Scheld WM: Bacterial meningitis: Pathogenesis, pathophysiology and progress. N Engl J Med 1992;327:864.

Tunkel AR, Scheld M: Pathogenesis and pathophysiology of bacterial meningitis. Clin Microbiol Rev 1993;6:118.

Tunkel AR et al: Bacterial meningitis: Recent advances in pathophysiology and treatment. Ann Intern Med 1990;112:610.

Pneumonia

Schaechter M et al: *Mechanisms of Microbial Disease,* 2nd ed. Williams & Wilkins, 1993.

Wilson JD et al (editors): *Harrison's Principles of Internal Medicine,* 12th ed. McGraw-Hill, 1991.

Infectious Diarrhea

Banwell JG: Pathophysiology of diarrheal disorders. Rev Infect Dis 1990;12(Suppl 1):S30.

Blacklow NR, Greenberg HB: Viral gastroenteritis. N Engl J Med 1991;325:252.

Cleary T: *Escherichia coli* that cause hemolytic uremic syndrome. Infect Dis Clin North Am 1992;6:163.

Cohen MB, Giannella RA: Hemorrhagic colitis associated with *Escherichia coli* O157:H7. Adv Intern Med 1991;37:173.

Field M et al: Intestinal electrolyte transport and diarrheal disease. (Two parts.) N Engl J Med 1989; 321:800, 879.

Tesh VL, O'Brien AD: The pathogenic mechanisms of Shiga toxin and the Shiga-like toxins. Mol Microbiol 1992;5:1817.

Tesh VL, O'Brien AD: Adherence and colonization mechanisms of enteropathogenic and enterohemorrhagic *Escherichia coli.* Microb Pathog 1992;12:245.

Sepsis, Sepsis Syndrome, and Septic Shock

Asitz ME, Rackow EC: Pathophysiology and treatment of shock. JAMA 1991;266:548.

Bone R: Gram-negative sepsis: A dilemma of modern medicine. Clin Microbiol Rev 1993;6:57.

Bone RC: The pathogenesis of sepsis. Ann Intern Med 1991;115:457.

Harris RL et al: Manifestations of sepsis. Arch Intern Med 1987;147:1895.

Parrillo JE: Pathogenetic mechanisms of septic shock. N Engl J Med 1993;328:1471.

Pulmonary Disease

7

Thomas J. Prendergast, MD, & Stephen J. Ruoss, MD

The principal physiologic role of the lungs is to make oxygen available to tissues for metabolism and to remove the by-product of that metabolism, carbon dioxide. The lungs perform this function by placing inspired air in close proximity to the pulmonary capillary bed to permit gas exchange by simple diffusion. This is accomplished at a minimal work load, regulated efficiently over a wide range of metabolic demand and takes place with close matching of ventilation to lung perfusion. The extensive surface area of the respiratory system must also be protected from a broad variety of infectious or noxious environmental insults.

Humans possess a complex and efficient respiratory system that satisfies these diverse requirements. When injury to components of the respiratory system occurs, the integrated function of the whole is disrupted. The consequences can be profound. Airway injury or dysfunction results in obstructive lung diseases, including bronchitis and asthma, while parenchymal lung injury can produce restrictive lung disease or pulmonary vascular disease. To understand the clinical presentations of lung disease, it is necessary first to understand the anatomic and functional organization of the lungs that determines normal function.

ABBREVIATIONS AND SYMBOLS USED IN THIS CHAPTER

V	Volume of gas
$\dot{V}$	Volume of gas per minute
$\dot{Q}$	Flow of blood per minute
$\dot{V}/\dot{Q}$ ratio	Ratio of volume of gas per minute to blood flow per minute
V_D/V_T	Ratio of wasted ventilation (dead space) to tidal volume
P_{O_2}	Partial pressure of oxygen
P_{CO_2}	Partial pressure of carbon dioxide
Pa_{O_2}	Partial pressure of oxygen in arterial blood
Pa_{CO_2}	Partial pressure of carbon dioxide in arterial blood
$F_{I}O_2$	Fractional concentration of oxygen in inspired air
A–a ΔP_{O_2}	Difference between alveolar and arterial partial pressure of oxygen
$D_{L}CO$	Diffusing capacity of the lung for carbon monoxide
cm H_2O	Pressure measured in centimeters of water
mm Hg	Pressure measured in millimeters of mercury

1. What are the two principal physiologic roles of the lungs?
2. What are the requirements for successful lung function?

NORMAL STRUCTURE & FUNCTION OF THE LUNGS

ANATOMY

The mature respiratory system consists of visceral pleura-covered lungs contained by the chest wall and diaphragm, the latter serving as the principal bellows muscle for ventilation under normal conditions. The lungs are divided into lobes, each demarcated by intervening visceral pleura. Each lung possesses an upper and lower lobe, with the middle lobe and lingula as the third lobes in the right and left lungs, respectively. At end-expiration, most of the volume of the lungs is air (Table 7–1), while almost half of the mass of the lungs is accounted for by blood volume. It is a testament to the delicate structure of the gas-exchanging region of the lungs that alveolar tissue has a total weight of only about 250 g but a total surface area of about 75 m^2.

Two anatomic elements of support serve to maintain the anatomic integrity of this organ with such a large and complex surface area: connective tissue fibers and surfactant. The connective tissue fibers are highly organized collagen and elastin structures (Figure 7–1). They radiate into the lungs, dividing

LUNG VOLUMES, CAPACITIES, AND THE NORMAL SPIROGRAM

The volume of gas in the lungs is divided into volumes and capacities as shown in the bars to the left of the figure below. Lung volumes are primary and do not overlap each other. Tidal volume (V_T) is the amount of gas inhaled and exhaled with each resting breath. A normal tidal volume in a 70-kg person is approximately 350–400 mL. Residual volume (RV) is the amount of gas remaining in the lungs at the end of a maximal exhalation. Lung capacities are composed of two or more lung volumes. The vital capacity (VC) is the total amount of gas that can be exhaled following a maximal inhalation. The vital capacity and the residual volume together constitute the total lung capacity (TLC), or the total amount of gas in the lungs at the end of a maximal inhalation. The functional residual capacity (FRC) is the amount of gas in the lungs at the end of a resting tidal breath. (IC, inspiratory capacity; IRV, inspiratory reserve volume; ERV expiratory reserve volume.)

The spirogram at right in the figure is drawn in real time. The first tidal breath shown takes 5 seconds, indicating a respiratory rate of 12 breaths per minute. The forced vital capacity (FVC) maneuver begins with an inhalation from FRC to TLC (lasting about 1 second) followed by a forceful exhalation from TLC to RV (lasting about 5 seconds). The amount of gas exhaled during the first second of this maneuver is the forced expiratory volume in 1 second (FEV_1). Normal subjects expel approximately 80% of the FVC in the first second. The ratio of the FEV_1 to the FVC (referred to as the FEV_1%) is diminished in patients with obstructive lung disease.

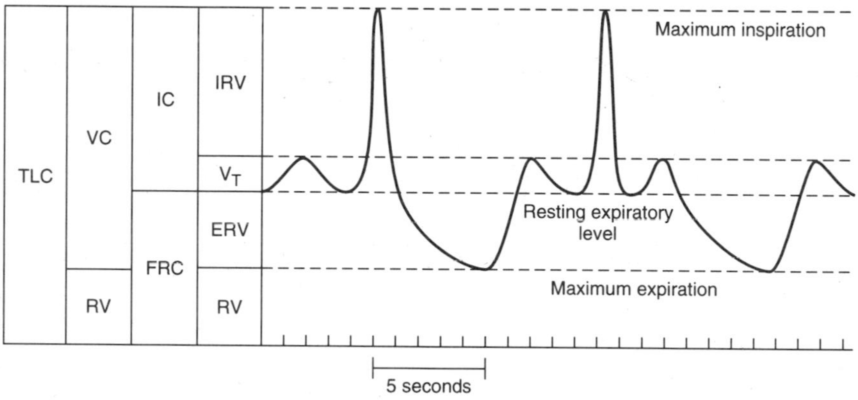

(Modified and reproduced, with permission, from Staub NC: *Basic Respiratory Physiology.* Churchill Livingstone, 1991.)

segments, investing airways and vessels, and supporting alveolar walls with a very elastic and delicate fibrous network. The multidirectional elastic support provided by this network allows the lung, from alveoli to conducting airways, to support itself and retain airway patency despite large changes in volume.

Table 7–1. Components of normal human lung.[1]

Component	Volume (mL) or Mass (g)	Thickness (μm)
Gas (functional residual capacity)	2400	
Tissue	900	
Blood	400	
Lung	500	
Support structures	250	
Alveolar walls	250–300	
Epithelium	60–80	0.18
Endothelium	50–70	0.10
Interstitium	100–185	0.22

[1]Reproduced, with permission, from Murray JF, Nadel JA: *Textbook of Respiratory Medicine,* 2nd ed. Saunders, 1994.

Surfactant provides specific anatomic assistance in reducing the surface tension of alveoli. In the absence of a surface-active layer covering the alveolar surface, increasing surface tension associated with a reduction of alveolar volume during expiration would collapse alveoli. The distending pressure required to reexpand these alveoli would be greater than normal ventilatory effort could produce. Surfactant, a complex material produced by type II alveolar cells and composed of multiple phospholipids and specific associated proteins, produces a marked reduction of surface tension, allowing expansion of alveoli with a transpulmonary distending pressure of less than 5 cm H_2O.

Airway & Epithelial Anatomy

Further anatomic division of the lungs is based primarily on the separation of the tracheobronchial tree

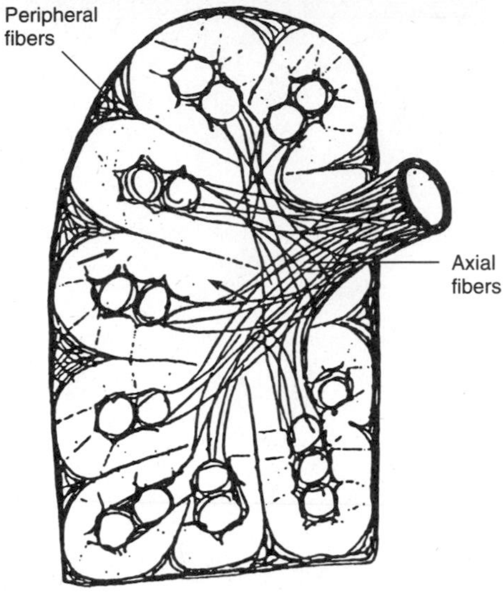

Figure 7–1. Structural fiber organization of the lung parenchyma. This schematic representation demonstrates the axial fibers, peripheral fibers, and fine septal fibers (arrows) of the alveolar walls, which provide structural integrity to the lung. (Modified and reproduced, with permission, from Weibel ER: Fleischner Lecture. Looking into the lung: What can it tell us? Am J Roentgenol 1979;133:1021.)

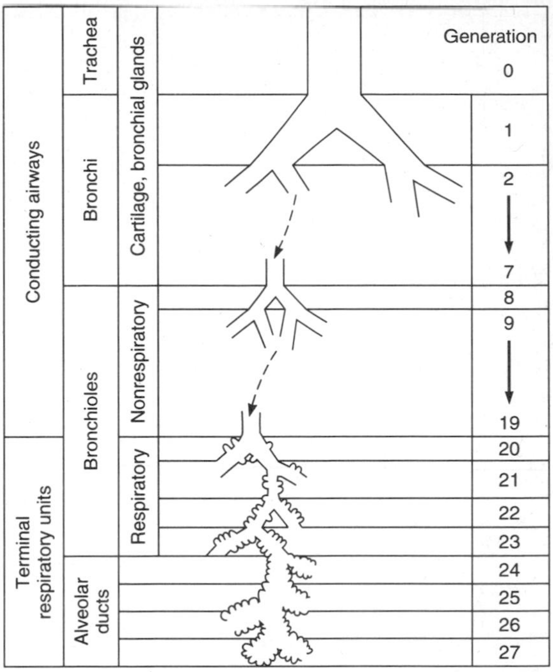

Figure 7–2. Subdivision of conducting airways and terminal respiratory units. This schematic illustration demonstrates the subdivisions of both the conducting airways and the respiratory airways. Successive branching produces increasing generations of airways, beginning with the trachea. Note that gas-exchanging segments of the lung are encountered only after extensive branching, with concomitant decrease in airway caliber and increase in total cross-sectional area (see Figures 7–3 and 7–4). (Modified and reproduced, with permission, from Weibel ER: *Morphometry of the Lung.* Springer, 1963.)

into **conducting airways,** which provide for movement of air from the external environment to areas of gas exchange, and **terminal respiratory units,** or **acini,** the airways and associated alveolar structures participating directly in gas exchange (Figure 7–2). The proximal conducting airways are lined by ciliated pseudostratified columnar epithelium, are supported by a cartilaginous skeleton in their walls, and contain secretory glands in the epithelial wall. The ciliated epithelium has a uniform orientation of cilia that beat in unison toward the pharynx. This ciliary action, together with the mucus layer produced by submucosal mucous secretory glands, provides a mechanism for the continuous transport of contaminating or excess material out of the lungs. Circumferential airway smooth muscle is also present but, as with secretory glands, is reduced and then lost as the airways branch farther into the lung and diminish in caliber. The smallest conducting airways are nonrespiratory **bronchioles.** They are characterized by a loss of smooth muscle and cartilage but retention of a cuboidal epithelium that may be ciliated and which is not a site of gas exchange. The lobes of the lung are divided into less distinct lobules, defined as collections of terminal respiratory units incompletely bounded by connective tissue septa. Terminal respiratory units are the final physiologic and anatomic unit of the lung, with walls of thin alveolar epithelial cells that provide gas exchange with the alveolar capillary bed.

The principal site of resistance to airflow in the lungs is in medium-sized bronchi (Figure 7–3). This at first seems counterintuitive, since one would expect airways of smaller caliber to be the major site of resistance. The small airways do not normally contribute significantly to airway resistance because of the profound increase in cross-sectional area in smaller airways as branching increases airway numbers (Figure 7–4). Under pathologic conditions such as asthma, where smaller bronchi and bronchioles become narrowed, airway resistance can increase dramatically.

As noted above, the pulmonary arterial system runs in close association with the branching bronchial tree throughout the lungs (Figure 7–5). By virtue of the ability to carefully regulate arterial and bronchial caliber, the anatomic arrangement provides

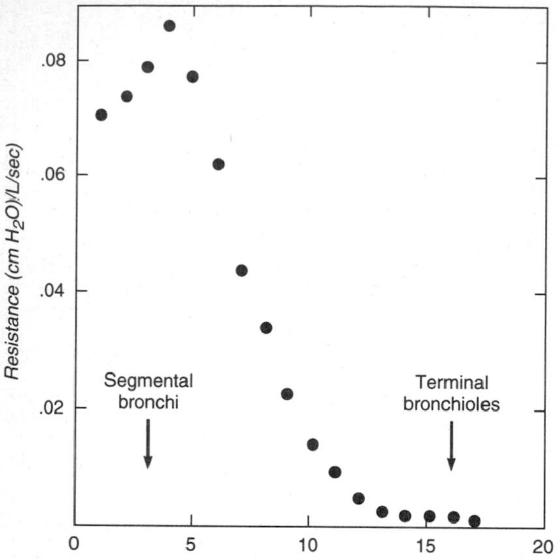

Figure 7–3. Location of the principal site of airflow resistance. The second- through fifth-generation airways include the segmental bronchi and larger bronchioles. They present the greatest resistance to airflow in normal subjects. The smaller airways contribute relatively little despite their smaller caliber because of the enormous number arranged in parallel. Compare with Figure 7–4. (Reproduced, with permission, from West JB: *Respiratory Physiology: The Essentials,* 4th ed. Williams & Wilkins, 1990.)

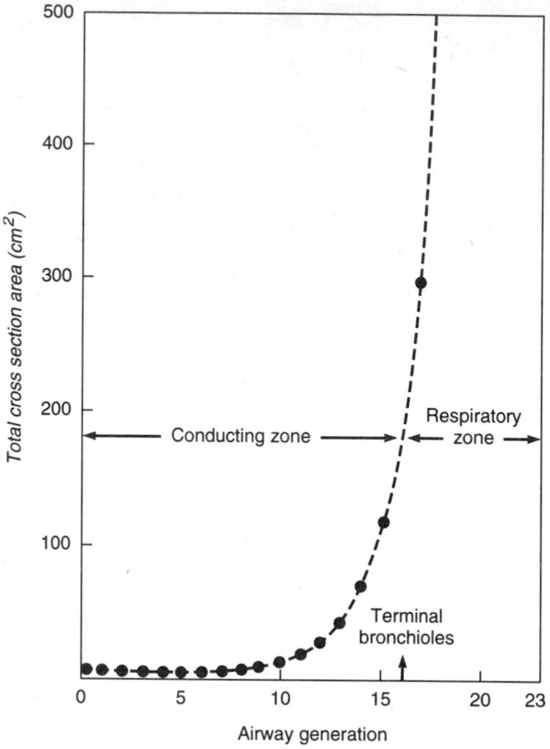

Figure 7–4. Airway generation and total airway cross-sectional area. The diagram demonstrates the relationship between airway generation and total cross-sectional area. Note the extremely rapid increase in total cross-sectional area in the respiratory zone (compare with Figure 7–2), and the fall in resistance as a consequence of the increase in cross-sectional area increase (compare with Figure 7–3). As a result, the forward velocity of gas during inspiration becomes very low at the level of the respiratory bronchioles, and gas diffusion becomes the chief mode of ventilation. (Reproduced, with permission, from West JB: *Respiratory Physiology: The Essentials,* 4th ed. Williams & Wilkins, 1990.)

the ideal setting for the continuous matching of ventilation and perfusion to lung segments.

Pulmonary Nervous System

The lungs are richly innervated with neural fibers from parasympathetic (vagal), sympathetic, and the so-called nonadrenergic, noncholinergic (NANC) systems. Efferent fibers include (1) parasympathetic fibers, with muscarinic, cholinergic efferents for bronchoconstriction, pulmonary vasodilation, and mucous gland secretion; (2) sympathetic fibers, whose stimulation produces bronchial smooth muscle relaxation, pulmonary vasoconstriction, and inhibition of secretory gland activity; and (3) the NANC system, with multiple transmitters implicated, including adenosine monophosphate (AMP), nitric oxide (NO), and peptide neurotransmitters such as substance P and vasoactive intestinal peptide (VIP). The NANC system participates in inhibitory events, including bronchodilation, and may function as the predominant reciprocal balance to the excitatory cholinergic system.

Pulmonary afferents consist principally of the vagal sensory fibers (Table 7–2). These include (1) fibers from bronchopulmonary stretch receptors, located in the trachea and proximal bronchi and responding to lung inflation with bronchodilation and heart slowing; (2) fibers from irritant receptors, which are also found in proximal airways and respond to diverse stimuli with efferent responses including cough, bronchoconstriction, and mucus secretion; and (3) C fibers, or fibers from juxtacapillary (J) receptors, which are unmyelinated fibers ending in lung parenchyma and bronchial walls and respond to mechanical and chemical stimuli. The reflex responses associated with stimulation of C fibers include a rapid shallow breathing pattern, mucus secretion, cough, and heart rate slowing with inspiration.

Vascular & Lymphatic Anatomy

The pulmonary vascular system has two main components: the pulmonary vessels and the bronchial vessels (Figure 7–5). Pulmonary arteries are smooth muscle-invested vessels running with the bronchial tree and providing perfusion to lung parenchyma. They are very sensitive to the alveolar Po_2, with a prominent hypoxic vasoconstrictor response. This provides a sensitive mechanism for maintaining matching of alveolar perfusion with ventilation. Pulmonary veins in turn drain alveolar lung parenchyma, taking a course in the intralobular septa distinct from the pulmonary bronchovascular bundle. Bronchial vessels are systemic circulation vessels that supply blood to essentially all the intrapulmonary structures except the parenchyma, including the bronchial tree, pulmonary nervous system and lymphatics, and connective tissue septa (Figure 7–6). Bronchial arteries anastomose with capillaries of the pulmonary circulation but contribute very little blood flow to the total pulmonary perfusion.

Pulmonary lymphatics develop along with the airway and vascular systems of the lung. Lymphatics are found in connective tissue spaces of the pleura, the peribronchovascular sheath, and interlobular septa. Lymphatics are found as far distally as the terminal respiratory bronchioles but do not enter the connective tissue space of the alveolar walls (Figure 7–5). Thus, fluid that finds its way into the alveolar interstitium must move the short distance to the re-

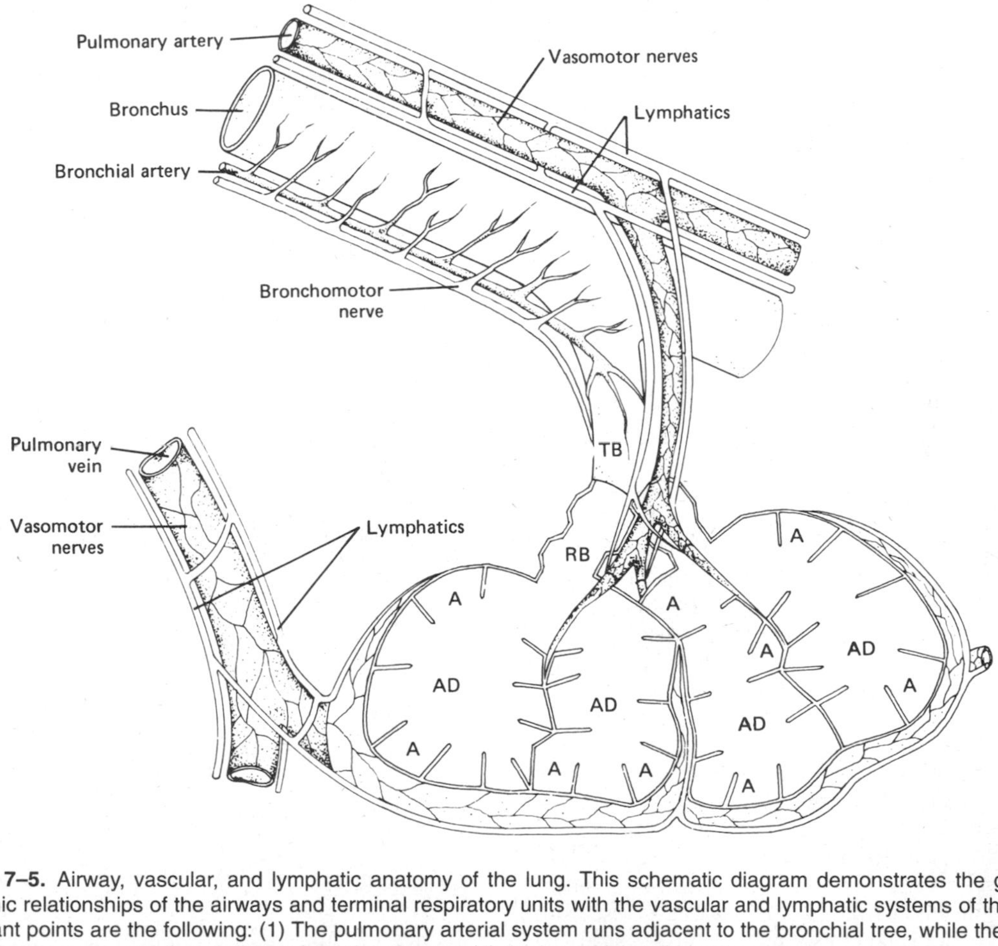

Figure 7–5. Airway, vascular, and lymphatic anatomy of the lung. This schematic diagram demonstrates the general anatomic relationships of the airways and terminal respiratory units with the vascular and lymphatic systems of the lung. Important points are the following: (1) The pulmonary arterial system runs adjacent to the bronchial tree, while the draining pulmonary veins are found distant from the airways; (2) the bronchial wall blood supply is provided by bronchial arteries, branches of systemic arterial origin; (3) lymphatics are found adjacent to both the arterial and venous systems and are very abundant in the lung; and (4) lymphatics are found as far distally as the terminal respiratory bronchioles, but they do not penetrate to the alveolar wall. (A, alveolus; AD, alveolar duct; RB, respiratory bronchiole; TB, terminal bronchiole.) (Reproduced, with permission, from Staub NC: The physiology of pulmonary edeme. Hum Pathol 1970; 1:419.)

Table 7–2. Characteristics of the three pulmonary vagal sensory reflexes.[1]

Receptor	Location	Stimulus	Response
Pulmonary stretch, slowly adapting	Associated with smooth muscle of intrapulmonary airways	1. Lung inflation 2. Increased transpulmonary pressure	1. Hering-Breuer inflation reflex 2. Bronchodilation 3. Increased heart rate 4. Decreased peripheral vascular resistance
Irritant, rapidly adapting	Epithelium of (mainly) extrapulmonary airways	1. Irritants 2. Mechanical stimulation 3. Anaphylaxis 4. Lung inflation or deflation 5. Hyperpnea 6. Pulmonary congestion	1. Bronchoconstriction 2. Hyperpnea 3. Expiratory constriction of larynx 4. Cough 5. Mucous secretion
C fibers Pulmonary type (J) Bronchial	 Alveolar wall Airway and blood vessels	 1. Increased interstitial volume (congestion) 2. Chemical injury 3. Microembolism	 1. Rapid, shallow breathing 2. Laryngeal and tracheobronchial constriction 3. Bradycardia 4. Spinal reflex inhibition 5. Mucous secretion

[1]Modified and reproduced, with permission, from Murray JF: *The Normal Lung.* Saunders, 1986.

gion of terminal bronchioles to gain access to draining lymphatics. Both visceral and parietal pleura contain associated lymphatics. These vessels—in particular the lymphatics associated with the parietal pleura—are responsible for the rapid clearance of fluid from the pleural space.

Immune Structure & Function

Of all the body's organs, the lungs are in a unique position with respect to exposure to hostile insults. Ventilatory requirements expose the lung to an enormous volume of environmental air daily—nonexertional ventilation in an adult totals about 6000 L of air per day, and the amount is increased substantially with activity. Ventilation in an open, nonsterile environment carries the continued risk of toxic or infectious insult. Furthermore, the pulmonary capillary bed is the only capillary bed in the body through which the entire circulating blood volume must flow in each cardiac cycle. As a consequence, the lung is an obligatory vascular sieve and must function as a principal site of defense against infection or other insult. Protection of the lungs from environmental and infectious injury involves a set of complex responses capable of providing a timely and successful defense against attack via the airways or the vascular bed. As outlined in Table 7–3, it is convenient for discussion to separate these responses into two major categories—nonspecific physical and chemical protections and specific immune structures and actions—all functioning in such a way as to prevent injury to or microbial invasion of the very large epithelial and vascular area of the lung (see Chapter 6).

3. What are the roles of the connective tissue and surfactant systems in lung function?
4. What is the role of ciliary action of the respiratory epithelium?
5. Why is it that medium-sized bronchi rather than small airways are the major site of resistance to airflow in the lungs?
6. What are the physiologic functions of the efferent parasympathetic, sympathetic, and NANC neural systems of the lung?
7. What are the categories of afferent vagal sensory receptors?
8. What are the different roles of the pulmonary and bronchial arteries?
9. What sensitive mechanism do the pulmonary arteries have for matching alveolar perfusion with ventilation?
10. What are the components of the nonspecific defense system of the lungs?
11. What are the humoral and cellular components of the specific immune defense system of the lungs?

PHYSIOLOGY

At rest, the lungs take 4 L/min of air and 5 L/min of blood, direct them within 0.2 μm of each other, and then return both to their respective pools. With maximal exercise, flow may increase to 100 L/min of ventilation and 25 L/min of cardiac output. The lungs thereby perform their primary physiologic function

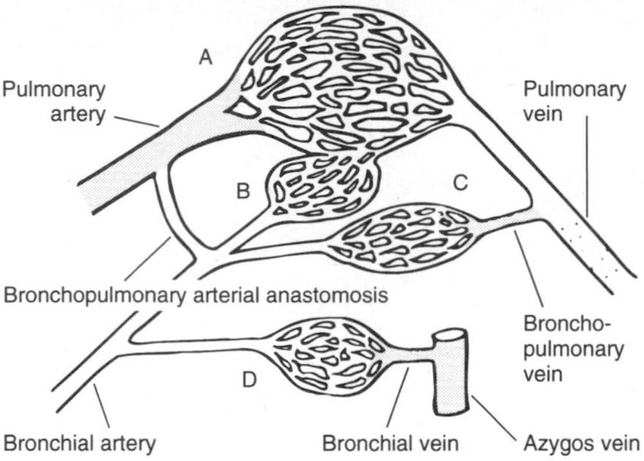

Figure 7–6. Relationship between bronchial and pulmonary circulations. The pulmonary artery supplies the pulmonary capillary network A. The bronchial artery supplies capillary networks B, C, and D. Network B represents the bronchial capillary supply to bronchioles that anastomoses with pulmonary capillaries and drains through pulmonary veins. Network C represents the bronchial capillary supply to most bronchi; these vessels form bronchopulmonary veins that empty into pulmonary veins. Network D represents the bronchial capillary supply to lobar and segmental bronchi; these vessels form true bronchial veins that drain into the azygos, hemiazygos, or intercostal veins. Shaded areas represent blood of low O_2 content. (Reproduced, with permission, from Murray JF: *The Normal Lung.* Saunders, 1986.)

Table 7–3. Lung defenses.

I. Nonspecific defenses
  1. Clearance
    a. Cough
    b. Mucociliary escalator
  2. Secretions
    a. Tracheobronchial (mucus)
    b. Alveolar (surfactant)
    c. Cellular components (lysozyme, complement, surfactant proteins, defensins)
  3. Cellular defenses
    a. Nonphagocytic
      Conducting airway epithelium
      Terminal respiratory epithelium
    b. Phagocytic
      Blood phagocytes (monocytes)
      Tissue phagocytes (alveolar macrophages)
  4. Biochemical defenses
    a. Proteinase inhibitors (α_1-protease inhibitor, secretory leukoprotease inhibitor)
    b. Antioxidants (eg, transferrin, lactoferrin, glutathione, albumin)
II. Specific immunologic defenses
  1. Antibody-mediated (B lymphocyte-dependent immunologic responses)
    a. Secretory immunoglobulin (IgA)
    b. Serum immunoglobulins
  2. Antigen presentation to lymphocytes
    a. Macrophages and monocytes
    b. Dendritic cells
    c. Epithelial cells
  3. Cell-mediated (T lymphocyte-dependent) immunologic responses
    a. Cytokine-mediated
    b. Direct cellular cytotoxicity
  4. Nonlymphocyte cellular immune responses
    a. Mast cell dependent
    b. Eosinophil-dependent

of making oxygen available to the tissues for metabolism and removing the major by-product of that metabolism, carbon dioxide. The lungs perform this task largely free of conscious control, all the while maintaining Pa_{CO_2} within 5% tolerance. It is a magnificent feat of evolutionary plumbing.

Static Properties: Compliance & Elastic Recoil

The lung maintains its extremely thin parenchyma over an enormous surface area by means of an intricate supporting architecture of collagen and elastin fibers. Anatomically as well as physiologically and functionally, the lung is an elastic organ.

The lungs inflate and deflate in response to changes in volume of the semirigid thoracic cage in which they are suspended. An analogy would be to attempt to inflate a blacksmith's bellows by pulling the handles apart, thus increasing the volume of the bellows, lowering pressure, and causing inflow of air. Air enters the lungs when the pressure in the pleural space is reduced by the expansion of the chest wall. The volume of air entering the lungs depends on the change in pleural pressure and the **compliance** of the respiratory system. Compliance is an intrinsic elastic property that relates a change in volume to a change in pressure. The compliance of the chest wall and that of the lungs both contribute to the compliance of the respiratory system (Figure 7–7). The compliance of the chest wall does not change with thoracic volume, at least within the physiologic range. The compliance of the lungs varies inversely with lung volume. At functional residual capacity (FRC), the lungs are normally very compliant, approximately 200 mL per cm H_2O. Thus, a reduction of 5 cm H_2O pressure in the pleural space will draw a breath of 1 L.

The tendency of a deformable body to return to its baseline shape is its **elastic recoil.** The elastic recoil of the chest wall is determined by the shape and structure of the thoracic cage. Two components contribute to lung elastic recoil. The first is tissue elasticity; the second is related to the forces needed to change the shape of the air-liquid interface of the alveolus (Figure 7–8). Expanding the lungs requires overcoming local surface forces that are directly proportionate to the local **surface tension.** Surface tension is a physical property that reflects the greater attraction between molecules of a liquid rather than

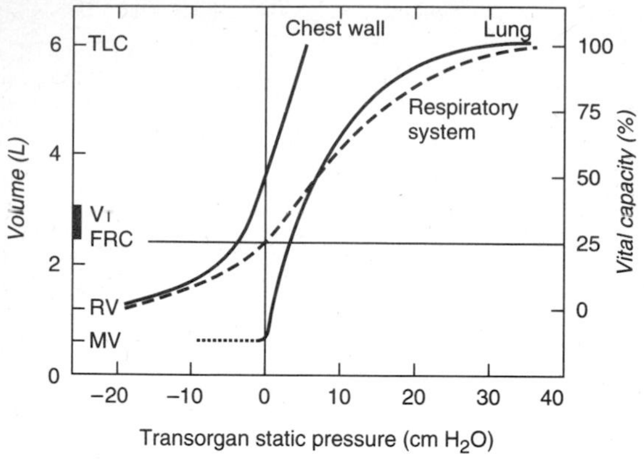

Figure 7–7. Interaction of the pressure-volume properties of the lungs and the chest wall. These curves show the pressure-volume relationships of the respiratory system, chest wall, and lungs measured at rest during deflation. Resting lung volume (functional residual capacity [FRC]) represents the equilibrium point where the elastic recoil of the lung (tendency to collapse inward) and the chest wall (tendency to spring outward) are exactly balanced. Other lung volumes can also be defined by reference to this diagram. Total lung capacity (TLC) is the point where the inspiratory muscles cannot generate sufficient force to overcome the elastic recoil of the lungs. Residual volume (RV) is the point where the expiratory muscles cannot generate sufficient force to overcome the elastic recoil of the chest wall. Compliance is calculated by taking the slope of these pressure-volume relationships at a specific volume. Note that the compliance of the lungs is greater at low lung volumes but falls considerably above two-thirds of vital capacity. (Reproduced, with permission, from Staub NC: *Basic Respiratory Physiology.* Churchill Livingstone, 1991.)

between molecules of that liquid and adjacent gas. At the air-liquid interface of the lung, molecules of water at the interface are more strongly attracted to each other than they are to the air above. This creates a net force drawing water molecules together in the plane of the interface. If the interface is stretched over a curved surface, that force acts to collapse the curve. The law of Laplace quantifies this force: The pressure needed to keep open the curve (in this case represented by a sphere) is directly proportionate to the surface tension at the interface and inversely proportionate to the radius of the sphere. (See Figure 7–9.)

Surfactant is a mixture of phospholipid (predominantly dipalmitoylphosphatidylcholine [DPPC]) and proteins. These hydrophobic molecules displace water molecules from the air-liquid interface, thereby reducing surface tension. This reduction has three physiologic implications: First, it reduces the elastic recoil pressure of the lungs, thereby reducing the pressure needed to inflate them. This results in reduced work of breathing. Second, it promotes alveolar stability and protects against atelectasis (Figure 7–9). Third, it limits the reduction of hydrostatic pressure in the pericapillary interstitium caused by surface tension. This reduces the forces promoting transudation of fluid and the tendency to accumulate interstitial edema.

Pathologic states may result from changes in lung elastic recoil related to an increase in compliance (emphysema), a decrease in compliance (pulmonary fibrosis), or a disruption of surfactant with an increase in surface forces (acute respiratory distress syndrome [ARDS]). (See Figure 7–10.)

Dynamic Properties: Flow & Resistance

Inflation of the lungs must overcome three opposing forces: elastic recoil, including surface forces; inertia of the respiratory system; and resistance to airflow. Since inertia is negligible, the work of breathing can be divided into work to overcome elastic forces and work to overcome flow resistance.

Resistance to flow depends on the nature of the flow. Under conditions of **laminar** or **streamlined flow,** resistance is described by Poiseuille's equation: Resistance is directly proportionate to the length of the airway and the viscosity of the gas and inversely

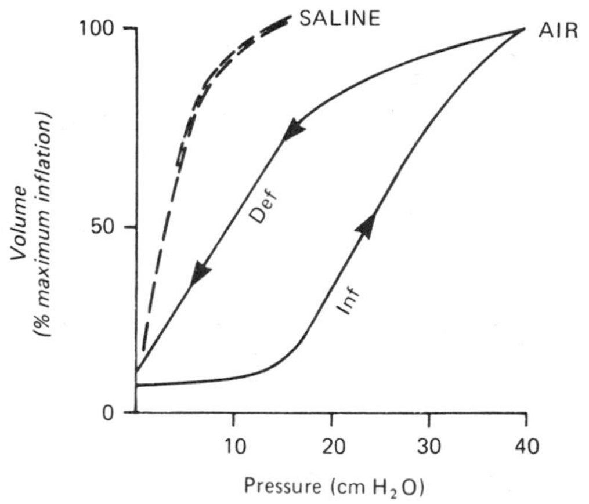

Figure 7–8. Effect of surface forces on lung compliance—a simple experiment demonstrating the effect of surface tension at the air-liquid interface of excised cat lungs. When inflated with saline, there are no surface forces to overcome and the lungs are both more compliant and show no difference (hysteresis) between the inflation and deflation curves . When inflated with air, the pressure required to distend the lung is greater at every volume. The difference between the two represents the contribution of surface forces. There is also a pronounced hysteresis that reflects surfactant recruited into the alveolar liquid during inflation (inf), where it further reduces surface forces during deflation (def). (Reproduced, with permission, from Morgan TE: Pulmonary surfactant. N Engl J Med 1971; 284:1185.)

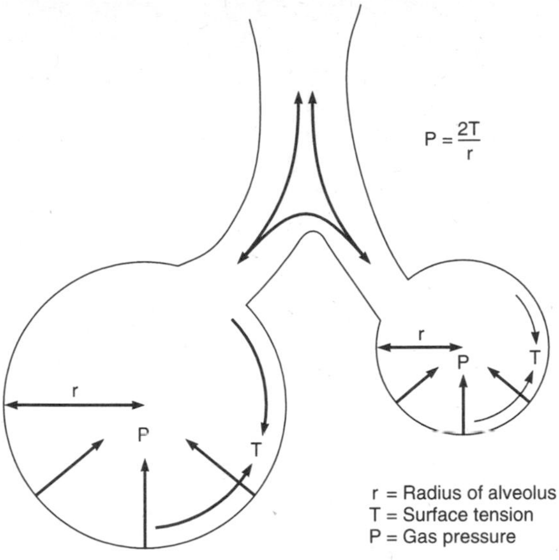

Figure 7–9. The importance of surface tension. If two connected alveoli have the same surface tension, then the smaller the radius, the greater the pressure tending to collapse the sphere. This could lead to alveolar instability, with smaller units emptying into larger ones. Alveoli typically do not have the same surface tension because surface forces are changed by the presence of surfactant. Since the relative concentration of surfactant in the surface layer of the sphere increases as the radius of the sphere falls, the effect of surfactant is increased at low lung volumes. This tends to counterbalance the increase in pressure needed to keep alveoli open at diminished lung volume and adds stability to alveoli which would otherwise tend to collapse into one another. The fact that alveoli are neither spherical nor independent (they are polyhedral and both surrounded by and connected to multiple other alveoli) is unimportant: The presence of surfactant does protect against regional collapse of lung units known as atelectasis--in addition to its other functions. (r, radius of alveolus; T, surface tension; P, gas pressure.)

proportionate to the fourth power of the radius. A reduction by one-half of airway radius leads to a 16-fold increase in airway resistance. Airway caliber is therefore the principal determinant of airway resistance under laminar flow conditions. Under conditions of **turbulent flow,** the driving pressure needed to achieve a given flow rate is proportionate to the square of the flow rate. Turbulent flow is also dependent on gas density and not on gas viscosity.

Most of the resistance to normal breathing arises in the medium-sized bronchi and not in the smaller bronchioles (Figure 7–3). There are two main reasons for this counterintuitive finding. First, airflow in the normal lung is not laminar but turbulent, at least from the mouth to the small peripheral airways. Thus, where flow is highest (in the segmental and subsegmental bronchi), resistance is dependent chiefly on flow rates. There is a transition to laminar flow approaching the terminal bronchioles as a consequence of increased cross-sectional area and decreased flow rates (Figure 7–4). In the respiratory bronchioles and alveoli, there is no bulk flow of gas, and gas movement occurs by diffusion. In small peripheral airways, airway caliber is the principal determinant of resistance. The caliber of peripheral airways is quite small, but repetitive branching creates a very large number of small airways arranged in parallel. Their resistance adds reciprocally, making their contribution to total airway resistance minor under normal conditions.

Airway resistance is determined by several factors. Many disease states affect bronchial smooth muscle tone and cause **bronchoconstriction,** an abnormal narrowing of the airways. Airways may also be narrowed by hypertrophy (chronic bronchitis) or infiltration (sarcoidosis) of the airway mucosa. Physiologically, the radial traction of the lung interstitium supports the airways and increases their caliber as lung volume increases. Conversely, as lung volume decreases, airway caliber also decreases and resistance to airflow increases. Patients with airflow obstruction often breathe at large lung volumes in an effort to minimize resistance.

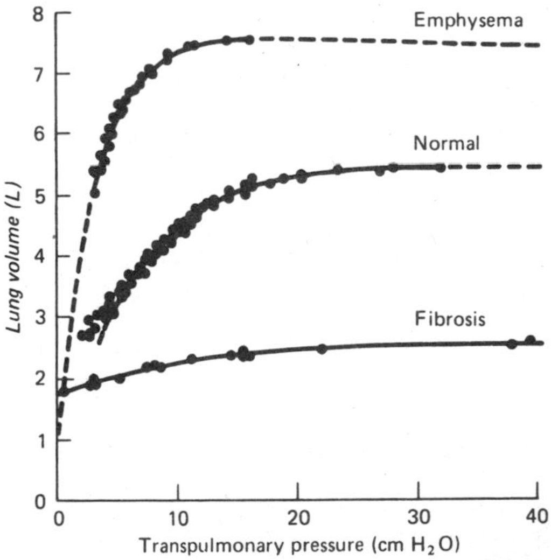

Figure 7–10. Static expiratory pressure-volume curves in normal subjects and patients with emphysema and pulmonary fibrosis. The underlying physiologic abnormality in emphysema is a dramatic increase in lung compliance. Such patients tend to breathe at very high lung volumes. Patients with pulmonary fibrosis have very noncompliant lungs and breathe at low lung volumes. (Modified and reproduced, with permission, from Pride NB, Mackem PT: Lung mechanics in disease. Pages 659–692 in Vol III, Part 2, of: *Handbook of Physiology.* Section 3. Respiratory System. Fishman AP [editor]. American Physiological Society, 1986.)

Analysis in terms of laminar and turbulent flow assumes that the airways are rigid tubes. In fact, they are highly compressible. The compressibility of the airways underlies the important phenomenon of **effort-independent flow.** It is an old clinical observation that airflow rates during expiration can be increased with effort only up to a certain point. Beyond that point, further increases in effort do not increase flow rates. The explanation for this phenomenon relies on the concept of an **equal pressure point.**

Pleural pressure is generally negative (subatmospheric) throughout quiet breathing. The peribronchiolar pressure that surrounds the conducting airways reflects pleural pressure. Hence, during quiet breathing, the airways are surrounded by negative pressure that holds them open. Pleural and peribronchiolar pressure may become positive during forced expiration. In this case, the airways are surrounded by positive pressure. The equal pressure point occurs where the airway pressure equals the surrounding peribronchiolar pressure, leading to instability and potential airway collapse (Figure 7–11).

The equal pressure point is not an anatomic site but a functional result that helps to clarify different mechanisms of airflow obstruction. Since the pressure driving expiratory airflow is lung elastic recoil pressure, a reduction in recoil pressure will cause dynamic compression of the airways. Patients with emphysema lose lung elastic recoil and may have severely impaired expiratory flow even with airways of normal caliber. Conversely, an increase in recoil pressure will oppose compression. Patients with pulmonary fibrosis may have abnormally high flow rates despite severely reduced lung volumes. The presence of airway disease augments the drop in pressure along the airways and generates an equal pressure point at high lung volumes. Patients with severe obstruction may move their equal pressure point far upstream toward the alveoli, in which case the airways will be compressed during forced expiration along their entire length. These patients breathe at larger lung volumes in order to maintain airway patency.

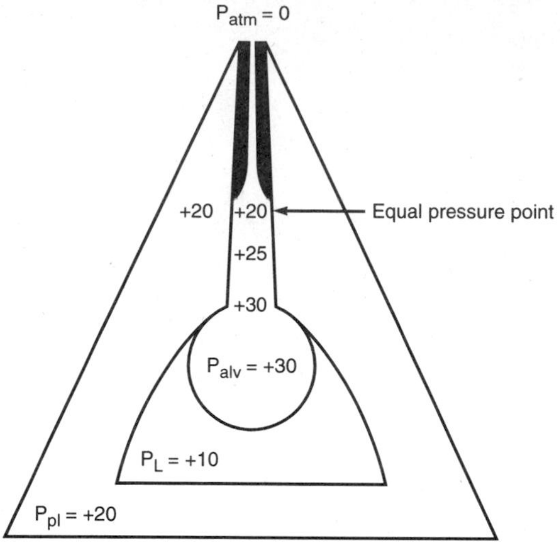

P_{pl} = Pleural pressure (cm H_2O)
P_L = Lung elastic recoil pressure (cm H_2O)
P_{alv} = Alveolar pressure (cm H_2O)
P_{atm} = Atmospheric pressure (cm H_2O)

Figure 7–11. The concept of the equal pressure point. For air to flow through a tube, there must be a pressure difference between the two ends. In the case of forced expiration with an open glottis, this driving pressure is the difference between alveolar pressure (the sum of pleural pressure and lung elastic recoil pressure) and atmospheric pressure (assumed to be zero). Frictional resistance causes a fall in this driving pressure along the length of the conducting airways. At some point, the driving pressure may equal the surrounding peribronchial pressure; in this event, the net pressure inside the airway is zero. This defines the equal pressure point. Downstream (toward the mouth) from the equal pressure point, pressure outside the airway is greater than the driving pressure inside the airway. This net negative pressure tends to collapse the airway and causes dynamic compression. At the equal pressure point, the driving pressure for flow is only lung elastic recoil pressure because the more forcefully one expires, the more the pressure surrounding the collapsible airways increases. Flow becomes effort-independent. (P_{pl}, pleural pressure; P_L, lung elastic recoil pressure; P_{alv}, alveolar pressure; P_{atm}, atmospheric pressure.)

The Work of Breathing

The amount of energy needed to maintain the respiratory muscles during quiet breathing is small, approximately 2% of basal oxygen consumption. Increasing ventilation in normal humans consumes relatively little oxygen until ventilation approaches 70 L/min. In patients with lung disease, the energy requirements are greater at rest and increase dramatically with exercise. Patients with emphysema may not be able to increase their ventilation by more than a factor of 2 because the oxygen cost of breathing exceeds the additional oxygen made available to the body.

A constant minute ventilation can be achieved through multiple combinations of respiratory rate and tidal volume. The two components of the work of breathing—elastic forces and resistance to airflow—are affected in opposite ways by changes in frequency and depth of breathing. Elastic resistance is minimized by rapid, shallow breathing; resistive forces are minimized by slow, large tidal volume breathing. Figure 7–12 shows how these two components can be summed to provide a total work of breathing for different frequencies at a constant minute ventilation. The set point for respiration is that point where the total work of breathing is minimized. In normal humans, this occurs at a frequency of approximately 15 breaths per minute. In different

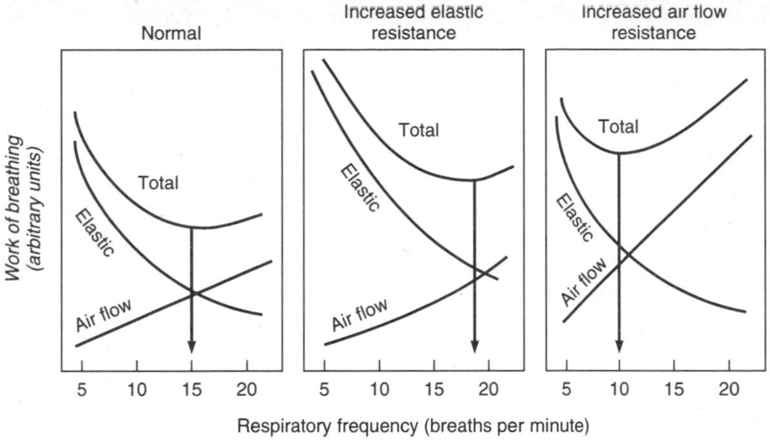

Figure 7–12. Minimizing the work of breathing. These diagrams divide the total work of breathing at the same minute ventilation into elastic and resistive components. In disease states that increase elastic forces (eg, pulmonary fibrosis), total work is minimized by rapid, shallow breathing; with increased airflow resistance (eg, chronic bronchitis), total work is minimized by slow deep breathing. (Reproduced, with permission, from Nunn JF: *Nunn's Respiratory Physiology 4th ed.* Butterworth-Heinemann, 1993.)

diseases, this pattern is altered to compensate for the underlying physiologic abnormality.

Distribution of Ventilation & Perfusion

Inhaled air is not distributed equally to all regions of the lung. In the healthy subject, this is due principally to the effects of gravity on pleural pressure. Pleural pressure varies from the top to the bottom of the lung by approximately 0.25 cm H_2O per centimeter. It is more negative at the apex and more positive at the base. The effect is shifted to an anterior-posterior distribution in the supine position and is greatly diminished (though not abolished) at zero gravity.

Regional ventilation is dependent on regional pleural pressure (Figure 7–13). More negative pleural pressure at the lung apex causes greater expansion of the apical alveoli. Given the shape of the lung's pressure-volume curve, lung compliance is greater at low lung volumes and ventilation is preferentially distributed to the lower lobes.

Pulmonary blood flow is a low-pressure system that functions in a gravitational field across 30 vertical centimeters. The distribution of blood flow to the lungs is not uniform under resting conditions. In the upright position, there is a nearly linear increase in blood flow from the top to the bottom of the lung. The details of distribution are portrayed in Figure 7–14.

Multiple factors besides gravity regulate blood flow. The most important is **hypoxic pulmonary vasoconstriction.** The smooth muscle cells of the pulmonary arterioles are sensitive to alveolar P_{O_2} (much more so than to arterial P_{O_2}). As alveolar P_{O_2} falls, there is arteriolar constriction, an increase in local resistance to flow, and redistribution of flow to regions of higher alveolar P_{O_2}. This is an extremely effective mechanism when regionalized. It can greatly diminish local blood flow without a significant increase in mean pulmonary arterial pressure when it affects less that 20% of the pulmonary circulation. Global alveolar hypoxia results in pulmonary hypertension.

Matching of Ventilation to Perfusion

The functional role of the lungs is to place ambient air in close proximity to circulating blood to permit gas exchange by simple diffusion. To accomplish this, air and blood flow must be directed to the same place at the same time. In other words, ventilation and perfusion must be matched. A failure to match ventilation to perfusion, or **$\dot{V}/\dot{Q}$ mismatch,** lies behind most abnormalities in O_2 and CO_2 exchange.

In the normal subject, a typical resting minute ventilation is 6 L/min. Approximately one-third of this amount fills the conducting airways and constitutes dead space or wasted ventilation. Resting alveolar ventilation is therefore approximately 4 L/min, while pulmonary artery blood flow is 5 L/min. This yields an overall ratio of ventilation to perfusion of 0.8. As noted above, neither ventilation nor perfusion is homogeneously distributed. Both are preferentially distributed to dependent regions at rest, though the increase in gravity-dependent flow is more marked with perfusion than with ventilation. Hence, the ratio of ventilation to perfusion is highest at the apex and lowest at the base (Figure 7–15).

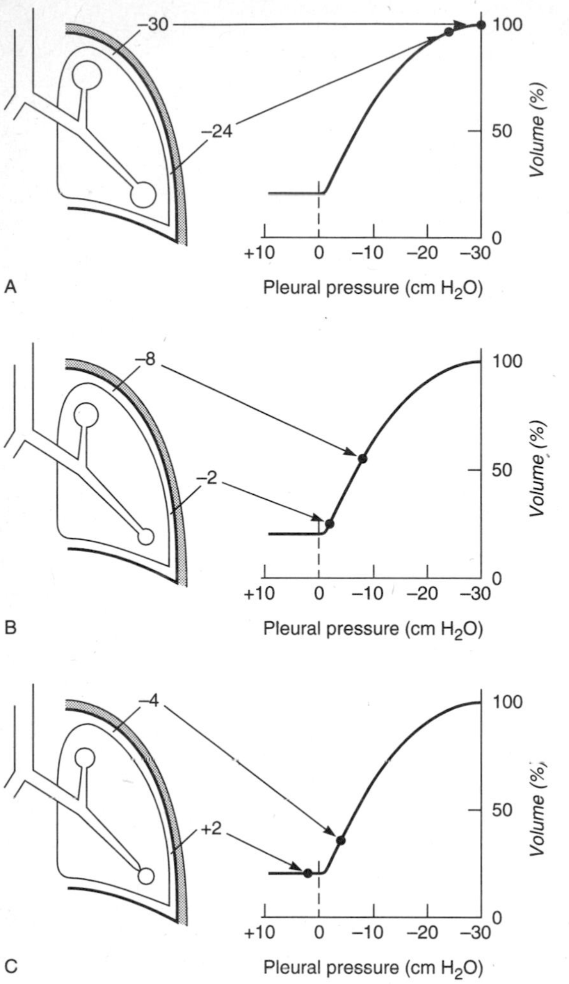

Figure 7–13. Distribution of ventilation at different lung volumes. The effect of gravity and the weight of the lung cause pleural pressure to become more negative toward the apex of the lung. The effect of this change in pressure is to increase the expansion of apical alveoli. ***A:*** Total lung capacity. At high lung volumes, the compliance curve of the lung is flat; alveoli are almost equally expanded because pressure differences cause small changes in lung volume. ***B:*** Functional residual capacity. During quiet breathing, the lower lobes are on the steep part of the pressure-volume curve. This increased compliance at lower volumes is why ventilation at FRC is preferentially distributed to the lower lobes. ***C:*** Residual volume. Below FRC, there may be dependent lung units that are exposed to positive pleural pressures. These units may collapse, leading to areas of lung that are perfused but not ventilated. (Modified and reproduced, with permission, from Murray JF: *The Normal Lung,* 2nd ed. Saunders, 1986.)

Alterations in the normal ratio of ventilation to perfusion of 0.8 are extremely important and underlie the functional impairment in many disease states. It may increase to **high $\dot{V}/\dot{Q}$ ratios,** with the limiting case being **alveolar dead space** (ventilation without perfusion, or $\dot{V}/\dot{Q} = \infty$); or toward low $\dot{V}/\dot{Q}$ ratios, with the limiting case being a **shunt** (perfusion without ventilation, or $\dot{V}/\dot{Q} = 0$). These two shifts affect respiratory function differently.

Approximately one-third of resting minute ventilation in normal subjects goes to fill the main conducting airways. This is the **anatomic dead space;** it represents ventilation to areas that do not participate in gas exchange. If gas-exchanging regions of the lung are ventilated but not perfused, as may occur in pulmonary embolism or various forms of pulmonary vascular disease, these regions also fail to function in gas exchange. They are referred to as **alveolar dead space,** or **wasted ventilation.** (See Figure 7–16 panel.) Functionally, some percentage of the work of breathing then supports ventilation that does not participate in gas exchange, thus reducing the overall efficiency of ventilation. In the absence of respiratory compensation, an increase in alveolar dead space will cause disturbances in both arterial Po_2 and arterial Pco_2: Pao_2 will fall and $Paco_2$ will rise. However, since the respiratory control center is exquisitely sensitive to small changes in $Paco_2$, the most common response to an increase in wasted ventilation is an increase in total minute ventilation that maintains $Paco_2$ nearly constant. Pao_2 is normal or may be reduced if the fraction of wasted ventilation is large. The A–a ΔPo_2 is increased (see below).

A shunt occurs when ventilation is eliminated but perfusion continues, as might happen with atelectatic lung or in areas of lung consolidation (alveoli filled with fluid or infected debris). (See Figure 7–16, panel B.) Such a right-to-left shunt permits mixed venous blood to pass to the systemic arterial circulation without coming in contact with alveolar gas. This typically causes a fall in *both* Po_2 and Pco_2. The reason can be seen in the diagram: The remaining respiratory unit is overventilated relative to its blood flow (large arrow).

The hyperventilation of some lung regions can compensate for a shunt through other regions but only for a possible rise in Pco_2 and not for the fall in Po_2. The reason is straightforward: The co_2 content of blood is linearly related and inversely proportionate to alveolar ventilation. Increased ventilation to one respiratory unit can reduce the co_2 content of blood leaving that unit. The co_2 content of the mixture is the mean of the two units. Since the Pco_2 is directly proportionate to the co_2 content, the reduced co_2 content of the hyperventilated units compensates for lack of ventilation to the dead space.

The O_2 content of blood is not linearly related to alveolar ventilation. The sigmoid shape of the hemoglobin-oxygen dissociation curve leaves blood nearly maximally saturated with oxygen at basal ventilation. Increased ventilation to one respiratory unit cannot significantly increase the O_2 content of blood

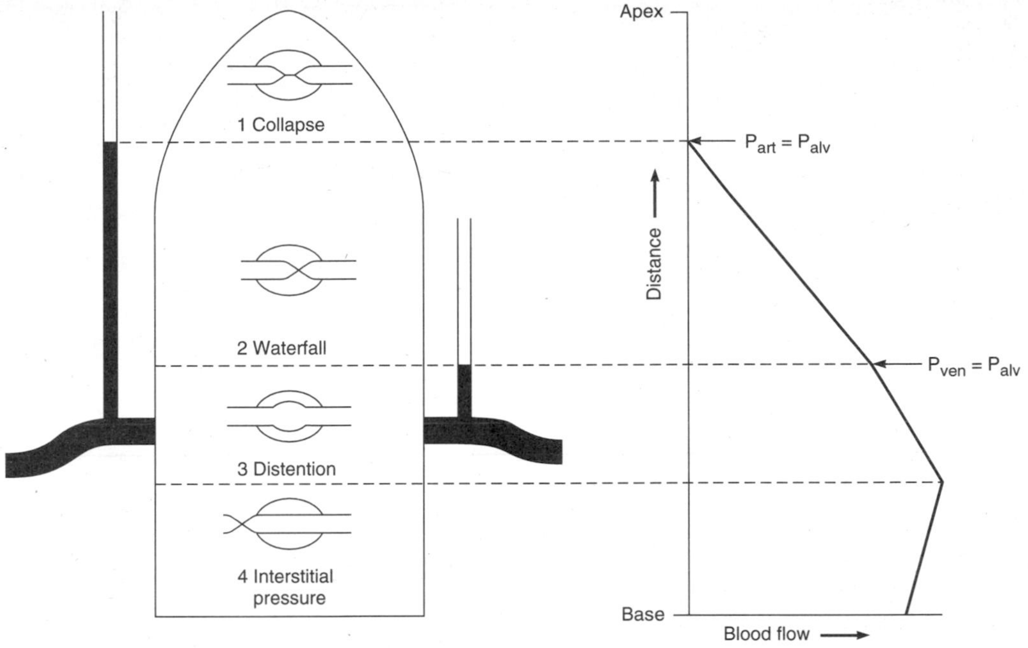

Figure 7–14. Effect of changing hydrostatic pressure on the distribution of pulmonary blood flow. Capillary blood flow in different regions of the lung is governed by three pressures: pulmonary arterial pressure, pulmonary venous pressure, and alveolar pressure. Pulmonary arterial pressure must be greater than pulmonary venous pressure to maintain forward perfusion; there are therefore three potential arrangements of these variables. ***Zone 1:*** $P_{alv} > P_{art} > P_{ven}$. There is no capillary perfusion in areas where alveolar pressure is greater than the capillary perfusion pressure. Since alveolar pressure is normally zero, this only occurs where mean pulmonary arterial pressure is less than the vertical distance from the pulmonary artery. ***Zone 2:*** $P_{art} > P_{alv} > P_{ven}$. Pulmonary arterial pressure exceeds alveolar pressure, but alveolar pressure exceeds pulmonary venous pressure. The driving pressure along the capillary is dissipated by resistance to flow until the transmural pressure is negative and compression occurs. This zone of collapse then regulates flow, which is intermittent and dependent on fluctuating pulmonary venous pressures. ***Zone 3:*** $P_{art} > P_{ven} > P_{alv}$. Flow is independent of alveolar pressure because the pulmonary venous pressure exceeds atmospheric pressure. ***Zone 4:*** Zone of extra-alveolar compression. In dependent lung regions, lung interstitial pressure may exceed pulmonary arterial pressure. In this event, capillary flow is determined by compression of extra-alveolar vessels.

The right side of the diagram shows a near-continuous distribution of blood flow from the top of the lung to the bottom, demonstrating that in the normal lung there are no discrete zones. The normal human lung at FRC spans 30 vertical centimeters, half of which distance is above the pulmonary artery and left atrium; and representative pulmonary arterial pressures are 33/11 cm H_2O with a mean of 19 cm H_2O. There is therefore no physiologic zone 1 in upright humans except perhaps in late diastole. Left atrial pressure averages 11 cm H_2O and is sufficient to create zone 3 conditions two-thirds of the distance from the heart to the apex. However, in patients undergoing positive-pressure mechanical ventilation, alveolar pressure is not atmospheric. Under conditions of positive end-expiratory pressure (PEEP), P_{alv} may be as high as 15–20 cm H_2O. This potentially shifts the entire distribution of pulmonary blood flow. (Reproduced, with permission, from Murray JF: *The Normal Lung,* 2nd ed. Saunders, 1986.)

leaving that unit. The O_2 content of the mixture is essentially the mean of normal blood oxygen content and desaturated, shunted blood. The moderately reduced oxygen content of the mixture tends to lie on the steep portion of the hemoglobin-oxygen dissociation curve. The result is that modest falls in oxygen content lead to large discrepancies in the P_{O_2}.

Ventilation/perfusion mismatching commonly falls between the extremes of shunts and wasted ventilation. In areas where the $\dot{V}/\dot{Q}$ ratio lies between 0 and 0.8 or between 0.8 and ∞, the effect on arterial blood gases can be predicted from the discussion of the limiting cases (Figure 7–17). At the top of Figure 7–17 is a respiratory unit where on one side ventilation has been reduced but perfusion maintained. This defines an area of **low $\dot{V}/\dot{Q}$ ratio.** The effect on lung function can be understood by dividing it into an area with a normal $\dot{V}/\dot{Q}$ ratio and an area of shunted blood. The physiologic effect of low $\dot{V}/\dot{Q}$ areas is similar to the effect of shunts: hypoxemia without hypercapnia. The difference between them can also be seen in this schematic. A true shunt is the

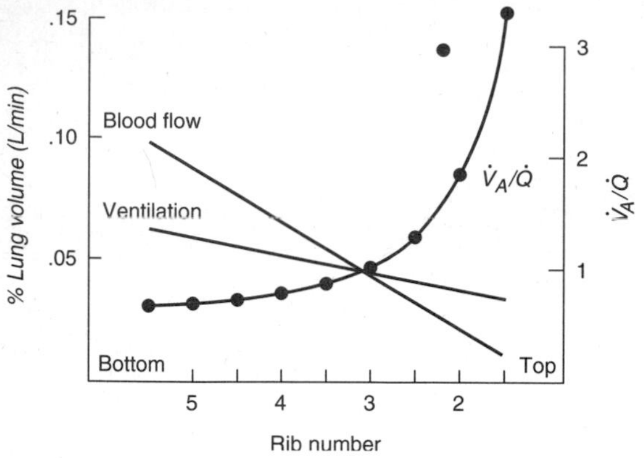

Figure 7–15. Changing distribution of ventilation and perfusion down the upright lung. The two straight lines reflect the progressive increases in ventilation and perfusion. The slope is steeper for perfusion. The ratio of ventilation to perfusion is therefore lowest at the base and highest at the apex. (Reproduced, with permission, from West JB: *Respiratory Physiology: The Essentials,* 4th ed. Williams & Wilkins, 1990.)

limiting case of a low $\dot{V}/\dot{Q}$ area where the ratio is zero. Shunted blood comes into no contact with inspired air; therefore, no amount of additional oxygen supplied to the inspired air will reverse the fall in systemic arterial Po_2. A low $\dot{V}/\dot{Q}$ area does come in contact with inspired air and can be reversed with increased inspired oxygen.

At the bottom of Figure 7–17 is a respiratory unit where on one side blood flow has been decreased but ventilation maintained. This defines an area of **high $\dot{V}/\dot{Q}$ ratio.** The effect on lung function can be understood by dividing it into an area with a normal $\dot{V}/\dot{Q}$ ratio and (this time) an area of wasted ventilation. As expected, the effect of high $\dot{V}/\dot{Q}$ ratios is to increase the amount of ventilation necessary to maintain a normal arterial Pco_2. Since the respiratory control system is very sensitive to small changes in $Paco_2$ and since the lungs have enormous excess capacity, the physiologic effect of high $\dot{V}/\dot{Q}$ areas is to increase respiration to maintain $Paco_2$. This may be done unconsciously. It becomes a clinical problem when the subject can no longer maintain an increased minute ventilation.

Arterial blood gases detect major disturbances in respiratory function. One attempt to assess more subtle abnormalities of gas exchange is to calculate the difference between the alveolar and arterial Po_2. This is referred to as the A–a ΔPo_2 or **A–a DO_2.** The alveolar-capillary membrane permits full equilibration of alveolar and arterial oxygen tension under normal $\dot{V}/\dot{Q}$ matching. There is nonetheless a small A–a ΔPo_2 in normal subjects due to right-to-left shunting through the bronchial veins and the thebe-

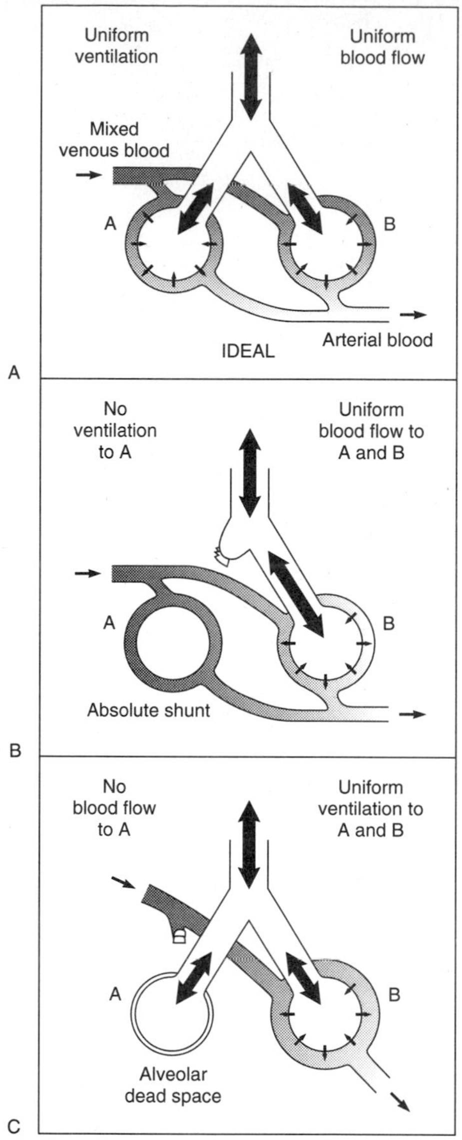

Figure 7–16. Three models of the relationship of ventilation to perfusion. In this schematic representation, the circles represent respiratory units, with tubes depicting the conducting airways. The shaded channels represent the pulmonary blood flow, which enters the capillary bed as mixed venous blood (dark) and leaves it as arterialized blood (light). Large arrows show distribution of inspired gas; small arrows show diffusion of O_2 and CO_2. In the idealized case, the Po_2 and Pco_2 leaving both units are identical. See text for details. (Reproduced, with permission, from Comroe J: *Physiology of Respiration,* 2nd ed. Year Book, 1974.)

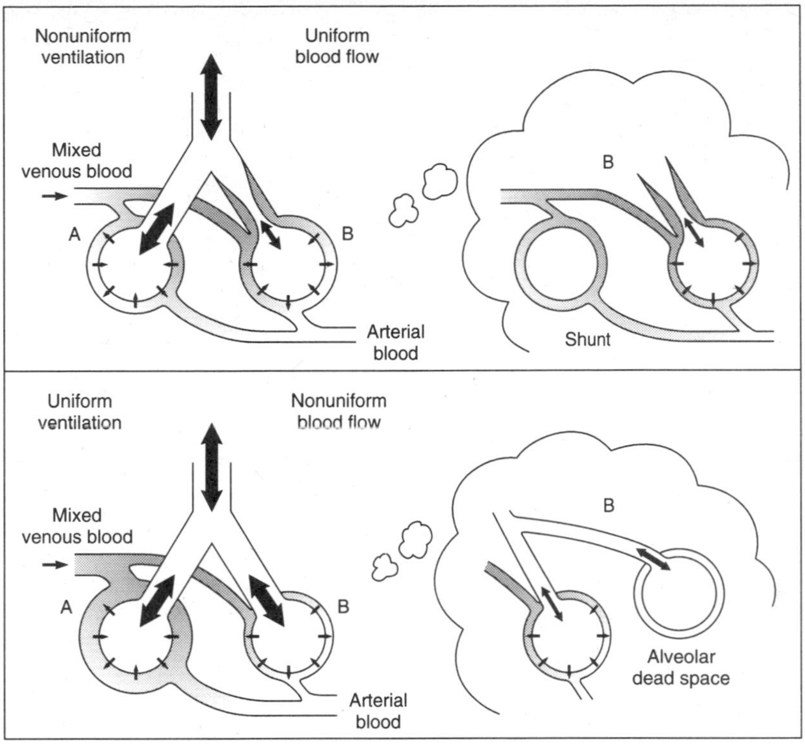

Figure 7–17. Ventilation-perfusion mismatching. See text for details. (Reproduced, with permission, from Comroe J: *Physiology of Respiration,* 2nd ed. Year Book, 1974.)

sian veins of the left heart. This accounts for approximately 2% of resting cardiac output and leads to a normal A–a ΔP_{O_2} of 5–8 mm Hg. Increasing the fractional inspired concentration of oxygen (F_{IO_2}) increases this value: A normal A–a ΔP_{O_2} breathing 100% oxygen is approximately 100 mm Hg. An increase in the A–a ΔP_{O_2} reflects areas of low $\dot{V}/\dot{Q}$ ratio, including shunting. It increases with age, presumably as a result of closure of dependent airways with an increase in regions with low $\dot{V}/\dot{Q}$ ratios.

Control of Breathing

The lungs inflate and deflate passively in response to changes in pleural pressure. Therefore, control over respiration lies in control of the striated muscles—chiefly the diaphragm but also the intercostals and abdominal wall—that change pleural pressure.

These muscles are under both automatic and voluntary control. The rhythm of spontaneous breathing originates in the brain stem, specifically in several groups of interconnected neurons in the medulla. Research into the generation of the respiratory rhythm has identified neurons with at least half a dozen distinct electrical signatures. Respiratory neurons are either inspiratory or expiratory and may fire early, late, or in an accelerating fashion during the respiratory cycle. Their integrated output is an efferent signal via the phrenic nerve (diaphragm) and spinal nerves (intercostals and abdominal wall) to generate rhythmic contraction and relaxation of the respiratory musculature. The result is spontaneous breathing without conscious input. However, by attending to breathing, the reader may hold his or her breath. Eating, speaking, singing, swimming, and defecating all depend on voluntary control over automatic breathing.

A. Sensory Input: The frequency, depth, and timing of spontaneous breathing are modified by information provided to the respiratory center from both chemical and mechanical sensors (Figure 7–18).

There are chemoreceptors in the peripheral vasculature and in the brain stem. The peripheral chemoreceptors are the **carotid bodies,** located at the bifurcation of the common carotid arteries and the aortic bodies near the arch of the aorta. The carotid bodies are particularly important in humans. They function as sensors of arterial oxygenation. There is a graded increase in firing from the carotid body in response to

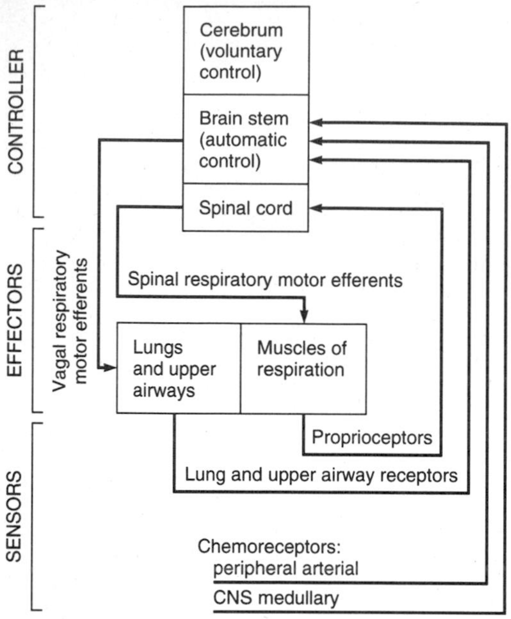

Figure 7–18. Schematic representation of the respiratory control system. The interrelationships among the central nervous system controller, effectors, and sensors are shown, as well as the connections among these components. (Reproduced, with permission, from Berger AJ et al: Regulation of respiration. [Three Parts.] N Engl J Med 1977;297:92, 138, 194.)

a fall in the Pa_{O_2}. This response is most marked below 60 mm Hg. An increase in the Pa_{CO_2} or a fall in arterial pH will potentiate the response of the carotid body to a decrease in the Pa_{O_2}.

In humans, the carotid bodies are solely responsible for the increased ventilation seen in response to hypoxia. Bilateral carotid body resection, which has been performed to treat disabling dyspnea and may happen as an unintended consequence of carotid thromboendarterectomy, results in a complete loss of this hypoxic ventilatory drive. The response to an increase in Pa_{CO_2} remains intact. The central or **medullary chemoreceptors** mediate the response to changes in Pa_{CO_2}. They lie within 200 μm of the anterolateral surfaces of the medulla and are separate from the neurons that generate the respiratory rhythm. Medullary chemoreceptors respond to changes in the hydrogen ion concentration of their extracellular fluid; this is approximated by sampling cerebrospinal fluid pH. The blood-brain barrier permits free diffusion of carbon dioxide but not hydrogen ions. Carbon dioxide is hydrated to carbonic acid, which ionizes and lowers the cerebrospinal fluid pH. The increased ventilatory response to elevations in Pa_{CO_2} are mediated through changes in cerebrospinal fluid pH. Central chemoreceptors are not stimulated by a fall in Pa_{O_2}; in fact, they are depressed by hypoxia.

There are a variety of pulmonary **stretch receptors** located in airway smooth muscle and mucosa whose afferent fibers are carried in the vagus nerve. They discharge in response to lung distention. Increasing lung volume decreases the rate of respiration by increasing expiratory time. This is known as the Hering-Breuer reflex. There are unmyelinated C fibers located near the pulmonary capillaries (hence juxtacapillary [J] receptors). These fibers are quiet during normal breathing but can be directly stimulated by intravenous administration of irritant chemicals such as capsaicin. They appear to stimulate the increased respiratory drive in interstitial edema and pulmonary fibrosis. Skeletal movement transmitted by **proprioceptors** in joints, muscles, and tendons causes an increase in respiration and may have some role in the increased ventilation of exercise. Finally, there are muscle **spindle receptors** in the diaphragm and intercostals that provide information on the work of breathing. They may be involved in the sensation of dyspnea when the work of breathing is disproportionate to ventilation.

B. Integrated Responses: Under normal conditions in healthy people, the hydrogen ion concentration in brain stem extracellular fluid determines the drive to breathe. Changes in brain stem extracellular pH occur largely via the cerebrospinal fluid pH, which itself is largely determined by the Pa_{CO_2}. The Pa_{O_2} is not an important part of the baseline respiratory drive under normal conditions.

Breathing is stimulated by a fall in the Pa_{O_2}, a rise in the Pa_{CO_2}, or an increase in the hydrogen ion concentration of arterial blood (fall in arterial pH).

Ventilation increases approximately 2–3 L/min for every 1 mm Hg rise in Pa_{CO_2}. This response occurs first through sensitization of the carotid body receptor. The carotid body will increase its firing in response to an increased Pa_{CO_2} even in the absence of changes in the Pa_{O_2}. This accounts for approximately 15% of the ventilatory response to hypercapnia. The majority of the response is mediated through changes in cerebrospinal fluid pH detected by the medullary chemoreceptors. Changes in arterial pH are additive to changes in Pa_{CO_2}. CO_2 response curves under conditions of metabolic acidosis have an identical slope but are shifted to the left (Figure 7–19). The ventilatory response to increases in Pa_{CO_2} falls with age, sleep, and aerobic conditioning and with increased work of breathing.

The individual response to hypoxemia is extremely variable. Normally, there is little increase in ventilation until the Pa_{O_2} falls below 50–60 mm Hg. At this point, there is a rapid increase in ventilation that reaches its maximum at approximately 32 mm

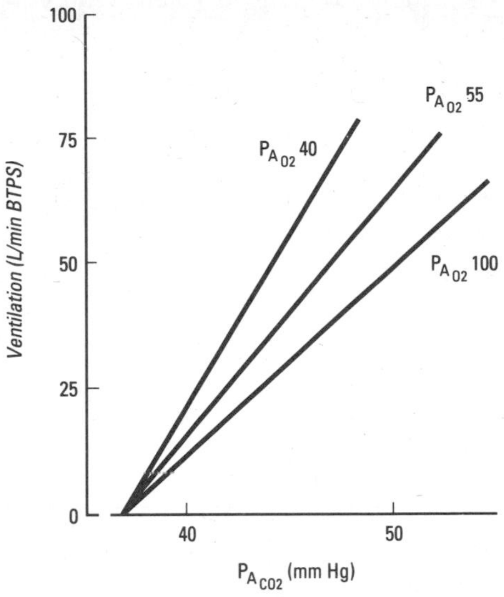

Figure 7–19. Ventilatory response to CO_2. The curves represent changes in minute ventilation plotted against changes in inspired P_{CO_2} at different values of alveolar P_{O_2}. There is a linear increase in ventilation with increasing P_{CO_2}. The rate of increase is greater at lower P_{O_2} values, but the curves begin from a common point where ventilation should cease in response to lowered P_{CO_2}. In awake humans, arousal maintains ventilation even when the P_{CO_2} falls below this level; when lightly anesthetized, apnea does occur. In the case of metabolic acidosis, this *x*-intercept is shifted to the left but the slope of the lines remains virtually unchanged. This indicates that the effects of metabolic acidosis are separate from and additive to the effects of respiratory acidosis. (Reproduced, with permission, from Ganong WF: *Review of Medical Physiology,* 16th ed. Appleton & Lange, 1993.)

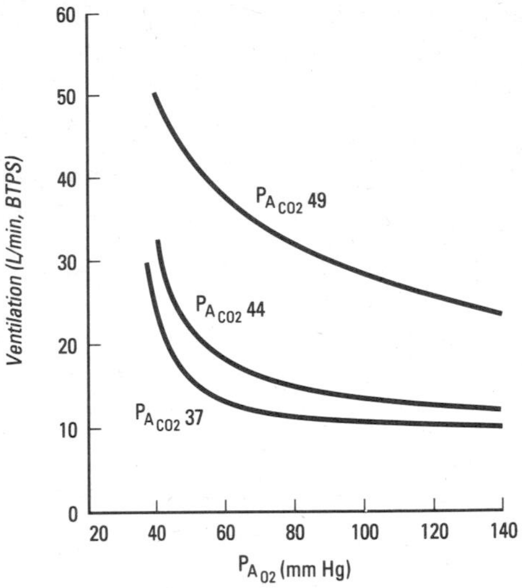

Figure 7–20. Isocapnic ventilatory response to hypoxia. These curves represent changes in minute ventilation plotted against changes in alveolar P_{O_2} when the alveolar P_{CO_2} is held constant at 37, 44, or 49 mm Hg. When the P_{CO_2} is in the normal range (37—44 mm Hg), there is little increase in ventilation until the P_{O_2} is reduced to between 50 and 60 mm Hg. This response is not linear, as is the response to an increased P_{CO_2}, but resembles a rectangular hyperbola asymptotic to infinite ventilation (at a P_{O_2} in the low 30s) and ventilation without tonic stimulation from the carotid bodies (which occurs above a P_{O_2} of 500 mm Hg). Not shown is the fall in minute ventilation that occurs with extreme hypoxia (P_{O_2} values below 30 mm Hg) due to depression of the respiratory center. (Reproduced, with permission, from Ganong WF: *Review of Medical Physiology,* 16th ed. Appleton & Lange, 1993.)

Hg. Below this level, further decreases in Pa_{O_2} lead to depression of ventilation. The response to hypoxia is affected by the Pa_{CO_2}. An increase in the Pa_{CO_2} will shift the isocapnic O_2 response curve upward and to the right (Figure 7–20).

A fall in arterial hydrogen ion concentration increases minute ventilation. This response results chiefly from stimulation of the carotid bodies and is independent of changes in Pa_{CO_2}. In acute metabolic acidosis, the cerebrospinal fluid pH is frequently *higher* than normal as a consequence of hyperventilation and the resultant fall in Pa_{CO_2}. There is a response to severe metabolic acidosis in the absence of carotid bodies. It is assumed that this response is mediated by the medullary chemoreceptors; it may represent breakdown of the blood-brain barrier.

C. Special Situations:

1. Chronic hypercapnia–In patients with chronic hypercapnia, the cerebrospinal fluid pH is returned toward normal by compensatory changes in cerebrospinal fluid bicarbonate. This makes the central chemoreceptors less sensitive to further changes in arterial Pa_{CO_2}. In this instance, a patient's minute ventilation may depend on tonic stimuli from the carotid bodies. If such a patient were given high concentrations of inspired oxygen, it could reduce carotid body output and lead to a fall in minute ventilation. In some cases, this can be extreme enough to cause a rapid rise in Pa_{CO_2} and coma.

2. Chronic hypoxia–Long-term residence at high altitude—or sleep apnea with repeated episodes of severe oxygen desaturation—may ablate the hypoxic ventilatory response. In such patients, the development of lung disease and hypercapnia may remove any endogenous stimulus to breathing. This pattern is seen in patients with obesity-hypoventilation syndrome.

3. Exercise–Exercise may increase minute ventilation up to 25 times the resting level. Strenuous but submaximal exercise in a healthy subject typically causes no change or only a slight rise in Pa_{O_2} due to increased pulmonary blood flow and better matching of ventilation and perfusion, with no change or a slight fall in Pa_{CO_2}. Changes in arterial oxygenation are therefore not a factor behind the increased ventilatory response to exercise. The reason for the increased ventilatory response is not known with certainty. Two contributing factors are the increased production of carbon dioxide and increased afferent discharge from joint and muscle proprioceptors.

12. What are the components of lung elastic recoil? What is the role of surfactant?
13. What three opposing forces must be overcome normally to inflate the lungs?
14. What are four factors affecting airway resistance?
15. What are the components of the work of breathing?
16. What factors regulate ventilation, and what factors regulate perfusion?
17. How are ventilation and perfusion normally matched?
18. What are the effects of changing CO_2 and O_2 levels on respiratory control? Which is the normal stimulus to ventilation in the resting healthy subject, O_2 or CO_2?

PATHOPHYSIOLOGY OF SELECTED LUNG DISEASES

OBSTRUCTIVE LUNG DISEASES: ASTHMA & COPD

The fundamental physiologic problem in obstructive diseases is increased resistance to airflow as a result of caliber reduction of conducting airways. This increased resistance can be caused by processes (1) within the lumen, (2) in the airway wall, or (3) in the supporting structures surrounding the airway. Examples of luminal obstruction include the increased secretions seen in asthma and chronic bronchitis. Airway wall thickening and airway narrowing can result from the inflammation seen in both asthma and chronic bronchitis or from the bronchial smooth muscle contraction in asthma. Emphysema is the classic example of obstruction due to loss of surrounding supporting structure, with expiratory airway collapse resulting from the destruction of lung elastic tissue. Though the causes and clinical presentations of these diseases are distinct, the common elements of their physiology are instructive.

1. ASTHMA

Clinical Presentation

Asthma is a disease of airway inflammation and airflow obstruction characterized by the presence of intermittent symptoms, including wheezing, chest tightness, shortness of breath (dyspnea), and cough together with demonstrable bronchial hyperresponsiveness. Exposure to defined allergens or to various nonspecific stimuli initiates a cascade of cellular activation events in the airways, resulting in both acute and chronic inflammatory processes mediated by a complex and integrated assortment of locally released cytokines and other mediators. Release of mediators can alter airway smooth muscle tone and responsiveness, produce mucus hypersecretion, and damage airway epithelium. These pathologic events result in chronically abnormal airway architecture and function.

Inherent in the definition of asthma is the possibility of considerable variation in the magnitude and manifestations of the disease within and between individuals over time. For example, while many asthmatic patients have infrequent and mild symptoms, others may have persistent or prolonged symptoms of great severity. Similarly, initiating or exacerbating stimuli may be quite different between individual patients.

Etiology & Epidemiology

Asthma is the most common chronic pulmonary disease, affecting as much as 15–17% of some populations. The highest prevalence rates are reported in Australia and New Zealand, while in the USA the prevalence is 3–5%. Asthma is more common in children and more frequent in boys than in girls. Data pertaining to deaths from asthma are incomplete and somewhat variable but suggest a trend toward an increased mortality rate in recent decades—this in spite of the greater availability of effective pharmacologic treatment. A number of explanations have been offered, including the deleterious side effects of medications and increasing exposure to industrial pollutants.

Atopy, or the production of IgE antibodies in response to exposure to allergens, is common in asthmatics and plays a role in evolution of the disease. Asthma has commonly been divided into extrinsic and intrinsic asthma depending upon the presence or absence, respectively, of accompanying atopy. There are some characteristic differences between the two groups such as, in intrinsic asthma, the later age at onset, the lack of apparent allergic sensitization by testing, and the tendency toward greater disease severity. However, the two types share the pathologic features of airway inflammation, hyperresponsiveness, and obstruction, so the distinction has not proved very useful clinically.

The fundamental abnormality in asthma is in-

Table 7–4. Asthma: Provocative factors.

- I. Physiologic and pharmacologic mediators of normal smooth muscle contraction
  - Histamine
  - Methacholine
  - Adenosine monophosphate (AMP)
- II. Physicochemical agents
  - Exercise; hyperventilation with cold, dry air
  - Air pollutants
    - Sulfur dioxide
    - Nitrogen dioxide
  - Viral respiratory infections (eg, influenza A)
  - Ingestants
    - Propranolol
    - Aspirin; NSAIDs
- III. Allergens
  - Low-molecular-weight chemicals, eg, penicillin, isocyanates, anhydrides, chromate
  - Complex organic molecules, eg, animal danders, dust mites, enzymes, wood dusts

creased reactivity of airways to stimuli. As outlined in Table 7–4, there are many known provocative agents for asthma. These can be broadly categorized as (1) physiologic or pharmacologic mediators of asthmatic airway responses, (2) allergens that can induce airway inflammation and reactivity in sensitized individuals, and (3) exogenous physicochemical agents or stimuli that produce airway hyperreactivity. Some of these provocative agents will produce responses in asthmatics only (eg, exercise, adenosine), while others produce characteristically magnified responses in asthmatics that can be used to distinguish them from normals under controlled testing conditions (eg, histamine, methacholine; see below).

Asthmatics typically have early and late responses to provocative stimuli. In the early asthmatic response, there is an onset of airway narrowing within 10–15 minutes following exposure and improvement by 60 minutes. This can variably be followed by a late asthmatic response, which appears 4–8 hours following an initial stimulus. Although the mechanisms producing these two responses are different, they are part of a common process of airway inflammation.

Pathogenesis

There is no known single mechanism that serves to explain the occurrence of asthma in all individuals. There are, however, common events that characterize the pathologic processes which produce asthma. It is important to recognize the central role of airway inflammation in the evolution of asthma.

The earliest events in asthmatic airway responses are the activation of local inflammatory cells, principally mast cells and eosinophils. This can occur by specific IgE-dependent mechanisms or indirectly via other processes, eg, osmotic stimuli or chemical irritant exposure. Acute-acting mediators, including leukotrienes, prostaglandins, and histamine, rapidly induce smooth muscle contraction, mucus hypersecretion, and vasodilation with endothelial leakage and local edema formation. Epithelial cells appear also to be involved in this process, releasing leukotrienes and prostaglandins as well as inflammatory cytokines upon activation. These preformed and rapidly acting mediators are also chemotactic agents, recruiting additional inflammatory cells such as eosinophils and neutrophils to airway mucosa.

A critical process that accompanies these acute events is the initiation of recruitment, multiplication, and activation of immune inflammatory cells through the actions of a network of locally released cytokines. These cytokines, including (among others) interleukins-2–6, -8, and -10, participate in a complex and prolonged series of events that result in perpetuation of the local airway inflammation and airway hyperresponsiveness (Table 7–5). These events include promoting growth of mast cells and eosinophils, the influx and proliferation of T lymphocytes, and the differentiation of B lymphocytes to IgE- and IgA-producing plasma cells. Thus, through their specific mediators, these cells in turn participate in the many proinflammatory processes that are active in the airways of asthmatics. Among these are injury to epithelial cells, with denuding of the airway, greater exposure of afferent sensory nerves, and consequent neurally mediated smooth muscle hyperresponsiveness; the up-regulation of IgE-mediated mast cell and eosinophil activation and mediator release, including acute and long-acting mediators; and submucosal gland hypersecretion with increased mucus volume.

Table 7–5. Asthma: Cellular inflammatory events.

- I. Epithelial cell activation or injury
  - Cytokine (IL-8) release with neutrophil chemotaxis or activation
  - Antigen presentation to lymphocytes
  - Secretory epithelial cell hyperplasia and hypersecretion
  - Epithelial death; increased magnitude of airway sensory neural reflexes
- II. Lymphocyte activation
  - Antigen exposure with lymphocyte proliferation
  - Increased cytokine expression; activation of additional effector cells (mast cells, eosinophils, macrophages)
  - Activation of B cells; increased IgE synthesis
  - Augmented lymphocyte activation by local cytokines
- III. Mast cell and eosinophil activation
  - Eosinophil release of cytotoxic and acute proinflammatory mediators
  - IgE-mediated mast cell activation, with acute mediator release (eg, histamine, leukotrienes, platelet-activating factor)
  - New expression of multiple cytokines by mast cells, with multiple effector cell activation, as with lymphocytes

Pathology

The histopathologic features of asthma reflect the cellular processes at play. Airway mucosa is thickened, edematous, and infiltrated with inflammatory cells, principally lymphocytes, eosinophils, and mast cells. Hypertrophied and contracted airway smooth muscle is seen. Bronchial and bronchiolar epithelial cells are frequently damaged, in part by eosinophil products such as major basic protein and eosinophil chemotactic protein, which are cytotoxic for epithelium. With epithelial injury and death, portions of the airway lumen are denuded, exposing autonomic and probably noncholinergic, nonadrenergic afferents that can mediate airway hyperreactivity. Secretory gland hyperplasia and mucus hypersecretion are seen, with mucus plugging of airways a prominent finding in severe asthma. Even in mildly involved asthmatic airways, inflammatory cells are found in increased numbers in the mucosa and submucosa, and subepithelial myofibroblasts are noted to proliferate and produce increased interstitial collagen; this may explain the component of relatively fixed airway obstruction seen in some asthmatics. The pathologic findings seen in severe fatal asthma parallel the pathologic events described above but reflect the greater magnitude of the insult. More severe airway epithelial injury and loss is noted, often with severe and complete obstruction of the airway lumen by mucus plugs.

Pathophysiology

Local cellular events in the airways have important effects on lung function. As a consequence of the airway inflammation, smooth muscle hyperresponsiveness, and airway narrowing, airway resistance increases significantly. As a consequence, where under normal physiologic circumstances the small-caliber peripheral airways do not contribute significantly to airflow resistance, these airways now are the site of increased resistance (Table 7–3). This will be worsened by the superimposed mucus hypersecretion and by any additional bronchoconstrictor stimuli. Bronchial neural function also appears to play a role in the evolution of asthma, though this is probably of secondary importance. Cough and reflex bronchoconstriction mediated by vagal efferents follows stimulation of bronchial irritant receptors. Peptide neurotransmitters may also play a role. The proinflammatory neuropeptide substance P can be released from unmyelinated afferent fibers in the airways and can induce smooth muscle contraction and mediator release from mast cells. Vasoactive intestinal peptide (VIP) is the peptide neurotransmitter of some airway nonadrenergic, noncholinergic neurons and functions as a bronchodilator; interruption of its action by cleavage of VIP can promote bronchoconstriction.

Airway obstruction occurs diffusely, though not homogeneously, throughout the lungs. As a result, ventilation of respiratory units becomes nonuniform and the matching of ventilation to perfusion is altered. Areas of both abnormally low and abnormally high $\dot{V}/\dot{Q}$ ratios exist, with the low $\dot{V}/\dot{Q}$ ratio regions contributing to hypoxemia. Pure shunt is unusual in asthma even though mucus plugging is a common finding, particularly in severe, fatal asthma. Arterial CO_2 tension is usually normal to low, given the increased ventilation seen with asthma exacerbations. Hypercapnia is seen as a late and ominous sign, demonstrating progressive airway obstruction, muscle fatigue, and falling alveolar ventilation.

Clinical Manifestations

The manifestations of asthma are readily explained by the presence of airway inflammation and obstruction.

A. Symptoms and Signs: The variability of symptoms and signs is an indication of the tremendous range of disease severity, from mild and intermittent disease to chronic, severe, and sometimes fatal asthma.

1. Cough–Cough results from the combination of airway narrowing, mucus hypersecretion, and the neural afferent hyperresponsiveness seen with airway inflammation. It can also be a consequence of nonspecific inflammation following superimposed infections, particularly viral, in asthmatic patients. By virtue of the compressive narrowing and high velocity of airflow in central airways, cough provides sufficient shear and propulsive force to clear collected mucus and retained particles from narrowed airways.

2. Wheezing–Smooth muscle contraction, together with mucus hypersecretion and retention, results in airway caliber reduction and prolonged turbulent airflow, producing auscultatory and audible wheezing. The intensity of wheezing does not correlate well with the severity of airway narrowing; as an example, with extreme airway obstruction, airflow may be so reduced that wheezing is barely detectable if at all.

3. Dyspnea and chest tightness–The sensations of dyspnea and chest tightness are the result of a number of concerted physiologic events. The greater muscular effort required to overcome increased airway resistance is detected by spindle stretch receptors, principally of intercostal muscles and the chest wall. Hyperinflation from airway obstruction results in thoracic distention, also detected by chest wall sensory nerves and manifested as chest tightness and dyspnea. As obstruction worsens, increased $\dot{V}/\dot{Q}$ mismatching produces hypoxemia. Rising arterial CO_2 tension and, later, evolving arterial hypoxemia (each alone, or together as synergistic stimuli) will stimulate respiratory drive through the peripheral and central chemoreceptors. This stimulus in the setting of respiratory muscle fatigue produces progressive dyspnea.

4. Tachypnea and tachycardia–Tachypnea and tachycardia may be absent in mild disease but are virtually universal in acute exacerbations.

5. Pulsus paradoxus–Pulsus paradoxus is a drop of more than 10 mm Hg in systolic arterial pressure during inspiration. It appears to occur as a consequence of lung hyperinflation, with compromise of left ventricular filling, together with augmented venous return to the right ventricle during more vigorous inspiration in severe obstruction. With increased right ventricular end-diastolic volume during inspiration, the intraventricular septum is moved to the left, compromising left ventricular filling and output. The consequence of this decreased output is a decrease in systolic pressure during inspiration, or pulsus paradoxus.

6. Hypoxemia–The presence of increasing $\dot{V}/\dot{Q}$ mismatching with airway obstruction produces areas of low $\dot{V}/\dot{Q}$ ratios, resulting in hypoxemia. Shunt is unusual in asthma.

7. Hypercapnia and respiratory acidosis–In mild to moderate asthma, normal ventilation to hyperventilation is noted, with the arterial P_{CO_2} either normal or decreased. As airway obstruction persists and increases in severe asthma attacks, respiratory muscle fatigue supervenes, with the evolution of alveolar hypoventilation and increasing hypercapnia and respiratory acidosis. It is important to note that this can occur in the face of continued tachypnea, which is not equivalent to hyperventilation.

8. Obstructive defects by pulmonary function testing–Patients with mild asthma may have entirely normal pulmonary function between exacerbations. During active asthma attacks, all indices of expiratory airflow are reduced, including FEV_1, FEV_1/FVC ratio ($FEV_1\%$) and peak expiratory flow rate. FVC is often also reduced as a result of premature airway closure before full expiration. Administration of a bronchodilator results in the improvement of airflow obstruction. As a consequence of the airflow obstruction, incomplete emptying of lung units at end-expiration results in acute and chronic hyperinflation; total lung capacity (TLC), functional residual capacity (FRC), and residual volume (RV) can be increased. Pulmonary diffusing capacity for carbon monoxide (DLCO) is often increased as a consequence of the increased lung (and lung capillary blood) volume.

9. Bronchial hyperresponsiveness–Bronchial provocation testing reveals hyperresponsiveness in all asthmatics, including those with mild disease and normal routine pulmonary function testing. Bronchial hyperresponsiveness is defined as either (1) a 20% decrease in FEV_1 in response to a provoking factor that, at the same intensity, causes less than a 5% change in a normal subject; or (2) a 20% increase in the FEV_1 in response to an inhaled bronchodilating drug. Methacholine and histamine are the agents for which standardized provocation testing has been established. Other agents have been used to establish specific exposure sensitivities; examples include sulfur dioxide and toluene diisocyanate.

19. What is the fundamental physiologic problem in obstructive lung disease? Give an example of each of its three principal sources.
20. What are the pathologic events that contribute to chronically abnormal airway architecture in asthma?
21. What are the three categories of provocative agents that can trigger asthma?
22. Which acute-acting mediators contribute to asthmatic airway responses?
23. What are some histopathologic features of asthma?
24. Name three reasons for increased airway resistance in asthma.
25. Why is arterial P_{CO_2} concentration usually low in asthma exacerbations?
26. What are some of the common signs and symptoms of acute asthma?

2. CHRONIC OBSTRUCTIVE PULMONARY DISEASE (COPD): CHRONIC BRONCHITIS & EMPHYSEMA

"Chronic obstructive pulmonary disease'' is an intentionally imprecise term used to denote a process characterized by the presence of chronic bronchitis or emphysema that may lead to the development of airway obstruction. The obstruction may be partially reversible. Although chronic bronchitis and emphysema are often regarded as independent processes, they share some common etiologic factors and are frequently encountered together in the same patient. It is for the purpose of including both under the same broad category that the definition remains imprecise--it reflects what we currently know about the evolution of these diseases.

Clinical Presentation

A. Chronic Bronchitis: Chronic bronchitis is defined by a clinical history of productive cough for 3 months out of the year for 2 consecutive years with no identifiable cause other than smoking. Dyspnea and airway obstruction, often with an element of reversibility, are intermittently to continuously present. Cigarette smoking is by far the leading cause, though other inhaled irritants may produce the same process. The predominant pathologic event is an inflammatory process in the airways, with mucosal thickening and mucus hypersecretion, resulting in diffuse obstruction.

B. Emphysema: Emphysema is properly a pathologic designation that in the lungs denotes a condition of abnormal permanent enlargement of the airspaces distal to the terminal bronchioles, accompanied by destruction of their walls without obvious fibrosis. In contrast to chronic bronchitis, the primary pathologic defect in emphysema is not in the airways but rather in the respiratory unit walls, where the loss of elastic tissue results in a loss of appropriate recoil tension to support airways during expiration. Progressive dyspnea and nonreversible obstruction accompany the airspace destruction without significant productive cough. Furthermore, the loss of alveolar surface area and the accompanying capillary bed for gas exchange contribute to the progressive hypoxia and dyspnea. Pathologic and etiologic distinctions can be made between various patterns of emphysema, but the clinical presentations of all are quite uniform.

Etiology & Epidemiology

Because of the overlap of these two diseases in individuals and the common causes encountered in both, epidemiologic data generally consider both diseases together under the rubric of COPD. COPD affects over 10 million persons in the United States, with chronic bronchitis the diagnosis in approximately 75% of cases and emphysema in the remainder. The incidence, prevalence, and mortality rates of COPD increase with age and are higher in men, whites, and persons of lower socioeconomic status. Cigarette smoking remains the principal cause of disease in up to 90% of patients with chronic bronchitis and emphysema. However, only 10–15% of smokers develop COPD. The reasons for differences in disease susceptibility are unknown but may include genetic factors. The most important identified single risk factor for the evolution of COPD—other than cigarette smoking—is deficiency of α_1-protease inhibitor. Its absence can lead to early onset of severe emphysema. **Alpha$_1$-protease inhibitor** is a circulating protein capable of inhibiting several types of proteases, including neutrophil elastase, which is implicated in the genesis of emphysema (see Pathophysiology, below). Autosomal dominant mutations, especially in northern Europeans, produce abnormally low serum and tissue levels of this inhibitor, altering the balance of connective tissue synthesis and proteolysis. A homozygous mutation (the ZZ genotype) results in inhibitor levels 10–15% of normal. The risk of emphysema, particularly in smokers who carry this mutation, is dramatically increased.

Population-based studies suggest that chronic dust (including silica and cotton) or chemical fume exposure can lead to COPD, but the contribution of these factors appears to be minor compared with tobacco use.

A. Chronic Bronchitis: A number of pathologic airway changes are seen in chronic bronchitis, though none are uniquely characteristic of this disease. The clinical features of chronic bronchitis can be attributed to chronic airway injury and narrowing. The principal pathologic features are inflammation of airways—particularly small airways—and hypertrophy of large airway mucous glands, with increased mucus secretion and accompanying mucus obstruction of airways (Figure 7–21). The airway mucosa is variably infiltrated with inflammatory cells, including polymorphonuclear leukocytes and lymphocytes. Mucosal inflammation can substantially narrow the bronchial lumen. As a consequence of the chronic inflammation, the normal ciliated pseudostratified columnar epithelium is frequently replaced by patchy squamous metaplasia. In the absence of normal ciliated bronchial epithelium, mucociliary clearance function is severely diminished or completely abolished. Hypertrophy and hyperplasia of submucosal glands is a prominent feature, with the glands often comprising over 50% of the bronchial wall thickness. Mucus hypersecretion accompanies mucous gland hyperplasia, contributing to luminal narrowing. Bronchial smooth muscle hypertrophy is common, and hyperresponsiveness to nonspecific bronchoconstrictor stimuli (including histamine and methacholine) can be seen. Bronchioles are often infiltrated with inflammatory cells and are distorted, with associated peribronchial fibrosis. Mucus impaction and

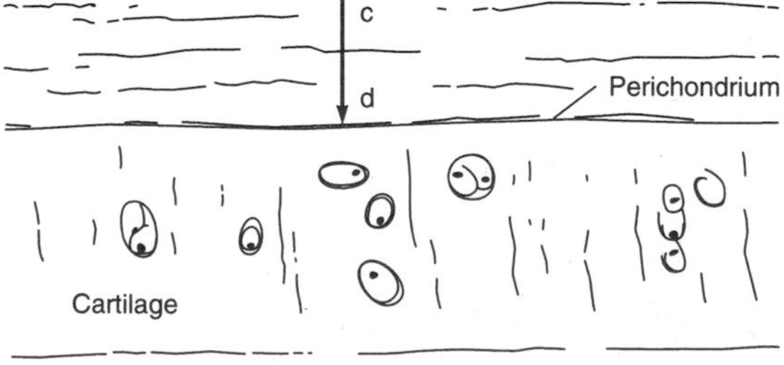

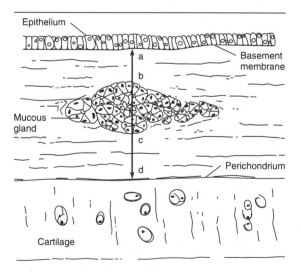

Figure 7–21. Bronchial wall anatomy. Structure of a normal bronchial wall. In chronic bronchitis, the thickness of the mucous glands increases and can be expressed as the ratio of (b–c)/(a–d); this is known as the Reid index. (Reproduced, with permission, from Thurlbeck WM: Chronic airflow obstruction in lung disease. In: *Major Problems in Pathology.* Bennington JL (editor). Saunders, 1976.)

luminal obstruction of smaller airways are often seen. In the absence of any superimposed process, such as pneumonia, the gas-exchanging lung parenchyma, composed of terminal respiratory units, is largely undamaged. The result of these combined changes is chronic airway obstruction and impaired clearance of airway secretions.

The nonuniform airway obstruction of chronic bronchitis has substantial effects on ventilation and gas exchange. Obstruction with prolonged expiratory time produces hyperinflation. Altered ventilation/perfusion relationships include areas of high and low $\dot{V}/\dot{Q}$ ratios. The latter is responsible in large part for the more significant resting hypoxemia seen in chronic bronchitis compared with emphysema. True shunt (perfusion with no ventilation) is unusual in chronic bronchitis.

B. Emphysema: The principal pathologic event in emphysema is thought to be a continuing destructive process due to an imbalance of local oxidant injury and proteolytic (particularly elastolytic) activity due to a deficiency of protease inhibitors (Figure 7–22). Oxidants, whether endogenous (superoxide anion) or exogenous (eg, cigarette smoke), can inhibit the normal protective function of protease inhibitors, allowing progressive tissue destruction.

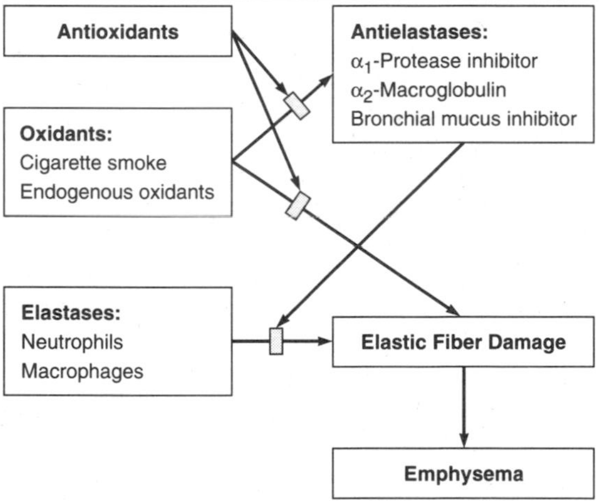

Figure 7–22. Schema of elastase-antielastase hypothesis of emphysema. The lung is protected from elastolytic damage by α_1-protease inhibitor and α_2-macroglobulin. Bronchial mucus inhibitor protects the airways. Elastase is derived primarily from neutrophils, but macrophages secrete an elastase-like metalloprotease and may ingest and later release neutrophil elastase. Oxidants derived from neutrophils and macrophages or from cigarette smoke may inactivate α_1-protease inhibitor and may interfere with lung matrix repair. Endogenous antioxidants such as superoxide dismutase, glutathione, and catalase protect the lung against oxidant injury. (Reproduced, with permission, from Snider GL: Experimental studies on emphysema and chronic bronchial injury. Eur J Respir Dis 1986;146[Suppl]:17.)

In contrast to chronic bronchitis, emphysema is a disease not primarily of the airways but of the surrounding lung parenchyma. The physiologic consequences are the result of destruction of terminal respiratory units, with loss of alveolar capillary bed and, very importantly, the supporting structures of the lung, including elastic connective tissue. The loss of elastic connective tissue produces a lung with diminished elastic recoil and increased compliance. In the absence of normal elastic recoil, the normal support of noncartilaginous airways is lost. Expiratory collapse of airways ensues, with obstructive symptoms and physiologic findings.

The pathologic picture of emphysema is one of progressive destruction of terminal respiratory units or lung parenchyma distal to terminal bronchioles. Airway inflammatory changes are minimal if present, though some mucous gland hyperplasia can be seen in large conducting airways. The interstitium of respiratory units harbors some inflammatory cells, but the chief finding is a loss of alveolar walls with enlargement of airspaces. Alveolar capillaries are also lost, which can result in decreased diffusing capacity with progressive hypoxemia, particularly with exercise.

Alveolar destruction is not uniform in all cases of emphysema. Anatomic variants have been described on the basis of the pattern of destruction of the terminal respiratory unit (or acinus, as it is also known). In **centriacinar emphysema,** destruction is focused in the center of the terminal respiratory unit, with the respiratory bronchioles and alveolar ducts relatively spared. This pattern is most frequently associated with prolonged smoking. **Panacinar emphysema** involves destruction of the terminal respiratory unit globally, with diffuse airspace distention. This pattern is typically—though not uniquely—seen in α_1-protease inhibitor deficiency. It is important to note that the distinction between these two patterns is largely pathologic—there is no significant difference in the clinical presentation. An additional emphysema pattern of clinical importance is **bullous emphysema.** Bullae are large confluent airspaces formed by greater local destruction or progressive distention of lung units. They are important because of the compressive effect they can have on surrounding lung and the large physiologic dead space associated with these structures.

Clinical Manifestations

A. Chronic Bronchitis: The clinical manifestations of chronic bronchitis are principally the result of the obstructive and inflammatory airway process.

1. Productive cough–Cough is productive of

thick, often purulent sputum owing to the ongoing local inflammation and the high likelihood of bacterial colonization and infection. Sputum viscosity is increased, largely as a result of the presence of free DNA (high-molecular-weight and highly viscous) from lysed cells. With increased inflammation and mucosal injury, hemoptysis can occur but is usually scant. The sputum usually does not have a putrid odor, as would be the case with anaerobic infection such as an abscess. Cough, which is normally very effective in clearing normal airways, is much less effective owing to the narrow airway caliber and the greater volume and viscosity of secretions.

2. Wheezing–Persistent airway narrowing and mucus obstruction can produce localized or more diffuse wheezing. This may be responsive to bronchodilators, representing a reversible component to the obstruction.

3. Inspiratory and expiratory coarse crackles–Increased mucus production, together with defective mucociliary escalator function, leaves excessive secretions in the airways, even with the increased coughing. These are heard prominently in larger airways during tidal breathing or with cough.

4. Cardiac examination–Tachycardia is common, especially with exacerbations of bronchitis or with hypoxemia. If hypoxemia is significant and chronic, pulmonary hypertension can result, with the cardiac examination revealing a prominent pulmonary valve closing sound (P_2), or elevated jugular venous pressure and peripheral edema of right heart failure.

5. Imaging–Typical chest radiographic findings include increased lung volumes with relatively depressed diaphragms consistent with hyperinflation. Prominent parallel linear densities ("tram track lines") of thickened bronchial walls are common. Cardiac size may be increased, suggesting right heart volume overload. Prominent pulmonary arteries are common and are consistent with pulmonary hypertension.

6. Pulmonary function tests–Diffuse airway obstruction is demonstrated on pulmonary function testing as a global reduction in expiratory flows and volumes. FEV_1, FVC and the ratio of FEV_1/FVC (FEV_1%), are all reduced. The expiratory flow-volume curve shows substantial limitation in flow (Figure 7–23). Some patients may respond to bronchodilators. Measurement of lung volumes reveals an increase in the RV and FRC, reflecting air trapped in the lung as a result of diffuse airway obstruction and early airway closure at higher lung volumes. DLCO is normal, reflecting a preserved alveolar capillary bed.

7. Arterial blood gases–Ventilation/perfusion mismatching is common in chronic bronchitis. The A–a ΔPo_2 is increased, with hypoxemia common, due prominently to significant areas of low $\dot{V}/\dot{Q}$ ratios (physiologic shunt); hypoxemia at rest tends to be more profound than in emphysema. With increasing obstruction, increasing Pco_2 (hypercapnia) and respiratory acidosis—with compensatory metabolic alkalosis—are seen.

8. Polycythemia–Chronic hypoxemia is associated with an erythropoietin-mediated increase in hematocrit. With more severe and prolonged hypoxia, the hematocrit may increase to well over 50%.

B. Emphysema: Emphysema presents as a noninflammatory disease manifested by dyspnea, progressive nonreversible airway obstruction, and abnormalities of gas exchange, particularly with exercise.

1. Breath sounds–Breath sounds in emphysema

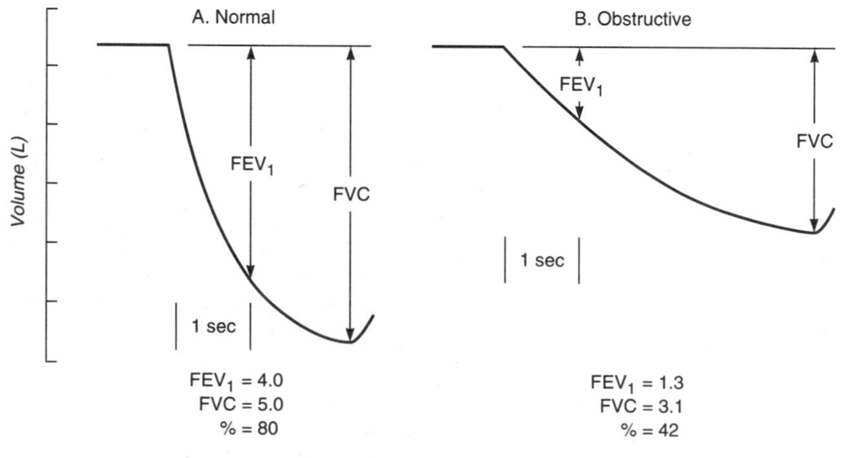

Figure 7–23. Normal and obstructive disease spirometry: FEV_1 and FVC. Demonstration of normal and obstructive patterns on forced expiratory spirometry. (Modified and reproduced, with permission, from West JB: *Pulmonary Pathophysiology: The Essentials.* Williams & Wilkins, 1992.)

are typically decreased in intensity, reflecting decreased airflow, prolonged expiratory time, and prominent lung hyperinflation. Wheezes, when present, are of diminished intensity. Airway sounds, including crackles and rhonchi, are unusual in the absence of superimposed processes such as infection.

2. Cardiac examination–Tachycardia may be present as in chronic bronchitis, especially with exacerbations or hypoxemia. Pulmonary hypertension is a common consequence of pulmonary vascular obliteration and concomitant hypoxemia; cardiac examination may reveal prominent pulmonary valve closure (increased P_2, pulmonary component of the second heart sound), or elevated jugular venous pressure and the peripheral edema of right heart failure.

3. Imaging–Hyperinflation is common, with flattened hemidiaphragms and an increased anteroposterior chest diameter. Parenchymal destruction produces attenuated lung peripheral vascular markings, often with proximal pulmonary artery dilation due to secondary pulmonary hypertension. Cystic or bullous changes may also be seen.

4. Pulmonary function tests–Lung parenchymal destruction and the loss of lung elastic recoil are the fundamental causes of the observed abnormalities of pulmonary function. The loss of elastic recoil in lung tissue supporting the airways results in increased dynamic compression of airways (Figure 7–11), especially during forced expiration; all flow rates will be reduced. With premature airway collapse, FEV_1, FVC, and the ratio of FEV_1/FVC (FEV_1%) are all reduced. As with chronic bronchitis and asthma, the expiratory flow-volume curve shows substantial limitation in flow (Figure 7–23). Expiratory time prolongation, early airway closure due to loss of elastic recoil, and consequent air trapping produce increases in the RV and FRC. TLC is increased, though often a substantial amount of this increase comes from gas trapped in poorly or noncommunicating lung units, including bullae. The DLCO is generally decreased in proportion to the extent of emphysema, reflecting the progressive loss of alveoli and their capillary beds. Incomplete hemoglobin saturation of pulmonary venous blood and arterial hypoxemia result from a combination of $\dot{V}/\dot{Q}$ mismatch, inability to increase minute ventilation with a fall in mixed venous P_{O_2}, and failure to oxygenate blood fully during capillary transit.

5. Arterial blood gases–Mild hypoxemia without hypercapnia is common in early emphysema. The A–a ΔP_{O_2} is increased; significant areas of abnormally low and high $\dot{V}/\dot{Q}$ ratios are found. With greater disease severity and greater decrease in DLCO, exercise-related (and, ultimately, even resting) arterial hemoglobin desaturation is seen. Hypercapnia, respiratory acidosis, and a compensatory metabolic alkalosis are common in severe disease.

6. Polycythemia–As in chronic bronchitis, chronic hypoxemia is frequently associated with an elevated hematocrit.

27. What is the leading cause of chronic bronchitis?
28. Describe the pathophysiologic changes in emphysema versus chronic bronchitis.
29. Mutations of which protein are strongly correlated with an increased risk of emphysema?
30. Name eight signs and symptoms of chronic bronchitis.
31. Name six signs and symptoms of emphysema.

RESTRICTIVE LUNG DISEASE: IDIOPATHIC PULMONARY FIBROSIS

The term "interstitial lung disease'' is used to denote a broad collection of pulmonary processes, some of unknown cause, whose common feature is the infiltration or inflammation and scarring of lung parenchyma (Figure 7–24). The common consequence of these diverse pathologic processes is widespread lung fibrosis, producing increased lung elastic recoil and decreased lung compliance which we know as restrictive lung disease.

The modifier "interstitial'' is an inadequate characterization of the process. Lung interstitium is considered to be the anatomic space bounded by the basement membranes of epithelium and endothelium and normally contains mesenchymal cells (eg, fibroblasts), extracellular matrix molecules (eg, collagen, elastin, and proteoglycans), and a few tissue leukocytes, including mast cells and lymphocytes. Interstitial lung diseases are not typically restricted to the anatomic interstitium but also involve inflammation of conducting airway mucosa and alveolar epithelium with an influx of recruited inflammatory cells. As a consequence, fibrosis is generally present throughout the lung parenchyma, with global effects on lung structure and function.

The pathologic events and physiologic consequences seen in idiopathic pulmonary fibrosis are shared by most of the other causes of interstitial lung disease. For that reason, idiopathic pulmonary fibrosis will be discussed as an example.

Clinical Presentation

Idiopathic pulmonary fibrosis, also known as interstitial pulmonary fibrosis or cryptogenic fibrosing alveolitis, is an uncommon disease of unknown cause marked by chronic inflammation of alveolar walls and resulting in diffuse and progressive severe fibrosis and destruction of normal lung architecture. This process produces not only a restrictive defect, with altered ventilation and increased work of breathing,

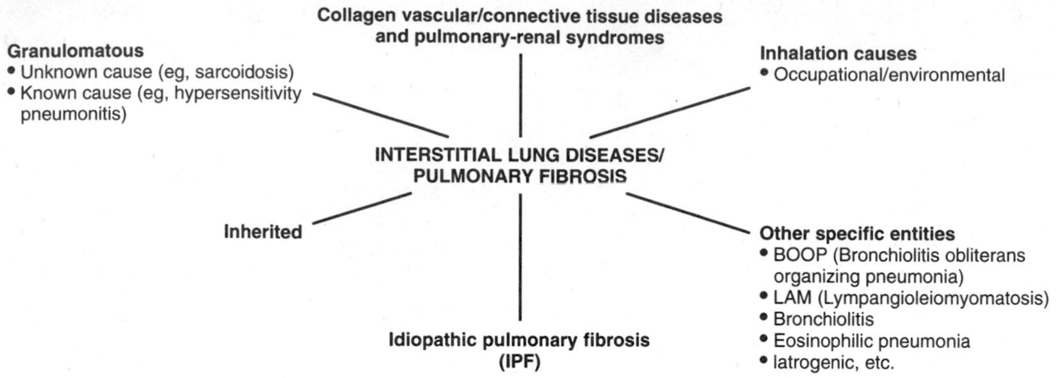

Figure 7–24. Categories of interstitial lung disease. In the absence of underlying malignancy or history of chemical or radiation therapy, interstitial lung disease can be broadly grouped into the clinical categories shown. Idiopathic pulmonary fibrosis occurs in a majority of these patients. (Reproduced, with permission, from Raghu G, Hert R: Interstitial lung diseases: Genetic predisposition and inherited interstitial lung diseases. Semin Respir Med 1993;14:323.)

but destructive and obliterative vascular injury that can severely impair normal pulmonary perfusion and gas exchange.

The usual presentation of idiopathic pulmonary fibrosis is with the insidious onset of progressive dyspnea, generally accompanied by a dry and persistent hacking cough. Fever and chest pain are generally absent. With disease progression, dyspnea often worsens and occurs even at rest. Digital cyanosis and clubbing are commonly seen. In the later stages of the disease, increasing pulmonary hypertension can lead to right heart failure and peripheral edema.

Etiology & Epidemiology

Idiopathic pulmonary fibrosis typically presents in the fifth to seventh decades of life, with a slight male predominance. There is no known causative agent. Many environmental exposures and specific systemic diseases can produce a clinical pattern similar if not identical to that seen in idiopathic pulmonary fibrosis. It is important to consider alternative causes when evaluating a patient with interstitial lung disease, as this may alter the evaluation or the treatment options. A familial form of interstitial pulmonary fibrosis has been described but is very uncommon; typical cases do not appear to have a genetic basis.

Pathophysiology

The primary insult that leads to the fibrotic response is unknown. Even in interstitial diseases of known cause, such as hypersensitivity lung disease or asbestosis, the specific events in disease initiation are not clearly established. There is, however, a common series of cellular events that mediate and regulate the inflammatory process and fibrotic response in idiopathic pulmonary fibrosis as well as in other interstitial lung diseases. This set of events, outlined in Table 7–6, includes (1) initial tissue injury; (2) vascular injury and activation, with increased permeability, exudation of plasma proteins into the extravascular space, and variable thrombosis and thrombolysis; (3) epithelial injury and activation, with loss of barrier integrity and release of proinflammatory mediators; (4) increased leukocyte adherence to activated endothelium, with transit of activated leukocytes into the interstitium; and (5) continued injury and repair processes characterized by alterations in cell populations and increased matrix production.

An extensive and complex array of effector and target cells and their specific products are thought to mediate the inflammatory and fibrotic events in idiopathic pulmonary fibrosis. A summary of the events is appropriate.

The initial pathophysiologic event in idiopathic pulmonary fibrosis is injury and activation of alveo-

Table 7–6. Cellular events involved in lung injury and fibrosis.

1. Tissue injury
2. Vascular endothelium activation and permeability changes, with thrombosis and thrombolysis
3. Epithelial injury and activation
4. Leukocyte influx, activation, and proliferation.
5. Tissue injury, remodeling and fibrosis:
   Perpetuation of tissue inflammation
   Incomplete or delayed resolution of interstitial thrombosis
   Fibroblast proliferation and matrix molecule production or deposition
   Epithelial proliferation and repopulation

lar epithelium and endothelium. Type I epithelial cells are lost and replaced by proliferating type II cells. Airway epithelial cells participate in cytokine-mediated recruitment and activation of inflammatory cells, including neutrophils and lymphocytes. Recruitment and activation of both neutrophils and lymphocytes is also mediated by the injury and activation of vascular endothelium through the coordinated action of multiple cytokines and the display of a specific repertoire of cellular adhesion molecules both on endothelial cells and on specific leukocytes. Fibroblasts are also activated by these local proinflammatory cytokines, with proliferation in the interstitium, submucosa, and alveolar lumen. Fibroblasts serve a dual role, magnifying local inflammatory events through their release of cytokines while producing the matrix molecules, including collagen, involved in tissue fibrosis. The perpetuation of this pattern of fibroblast activation and proliferation—and increased tissue matrix deposition—occurs under the influence of inflammatory cells. These include not only lymphocytes, alveolar macrophages, and neutrophils but also resident mast cells and eosinophils which are variably increased in number.

The histologic findings predict the physiologic abnormalities associated with interstitial lung disease. The process of lung injury and scarring is not uniform or synchronous. The disease is typically a nonhomogeneous process, with areas of intense injury and fibrosis often intermixed with relatively spared lung. In the early stages of disease, infiltration of alveolar structures by leukocytes accompanies patchy type II epithelial hyperplasia in alveoli. Destruction of normal alveolar epithelium also causes significant change in the production and turnover of surfactant, with an increase in the alveolar surface tension in affected lung units. This is followed by increasing tissue leukocytosis, fibroblast proliferation, and increasing scar formation. Lymphocytes—predominantly T cells—and mast cells are found in markedly increased numbers in alveolar interstitium and submucosal regions. Collagen and elastin deposition are markedly increased. Later in the course of the disease, progressive alveolar destruction is seen, with large areas of fibrosis and residual airspaces lined by cuboidal epithelium; this appears on radiographs as honeycombing. With this alveolar destruction, the accompanying vascular bed is obliterated, also in a patchy pattern.

This pattern of lung injury produces an altered physiology that includes increased elastic recoil and poor lung compliance, altered gas exchange, and pulmonary vascular abnormalities.

Clinical Manifestations

A. Symptoms and Signs:

1. Cough–With the bronchial and bronchiolar distortion that accompanies fibrotic damage to terminal respiratory units, chronic irritation of airways occurs, producing a chronic cough. Although epithelial cells may be injured, mucus hypersecretion and a productive cough are not seen.

2. Dyspnea and tachypnea–Multiple factors contribute to dyspnea in pulmonary fibrosis. With fibrosis of lung parenchyma as well as a decrease in normal surfactant effects, a greater distending pressure is required for inspiration. Increased stimuli from J receptors in fibrotic alveolar walls or stretch receptors in the chest wall may sense the increased work of inflating the less compliant lungs. In severe disease, altered gas exchange with $\dot{V}/\dot{Q}$ mismatching can produce hypoxia even at rest. The diminished capillary bed and thickened alveolar-capillary membrane contribute to limitation of diffusion and increasing hypoxia with exercise. Tachypnea is the consequence of hypoxia as well as the apparent increased drive from lung sensory receptor stimuli. A rapid and shallow breathing pattern reduces ventilatory work in the face of increased lung elastic recoil.

3. Inspiratory crackles–Diffuse fine dry inspiratory crackles are common and reflect the successive opening on inspiration of respiratory units that are collapsed owing to the fibrosis and the loss of normal surfactant.

4. Digital clubbing–Clubbing of the fingertips is a common finding, but the cause is unknown. There is no established link with any specific physiologic parameter, including hypoxemia.

5. Cardiac examination–As with hypoxemia from other causes, cardiac examination can reveal evidence of pulmonary hypertension with prominent pulmonary valve closure sound (P_2). This can be accompanied by right heart overload or decompensation, with elevated jugular venous pressure, the murmur of tricuspid regurgitation, or a right-sided third heart sound (S_3).

B. Imaging: The characteristic radiographic findings are of small lung volumes, with increased densities more prominent in the lung periphery. Fibrosis surrounding expanded small airspaces is seen as honeycombing. With pulmonary hypertension, central pulmonary arteries are enlarged, while the peripheral vascular destruction produces rapid attenuation of vessels out from the hilar regions.

C. Pulmonary Function Tests: Lung fibrosis typically produces a restrictive pattern, with reductions in TLC, FEV_1, and FVC, while maintaining a preserved or even increased ratio of FEV_1/FVC ($FEV_1\%$). The increased elastic recoil produces normal to increased expiratory flow rates when adjusted for lung volume. With increased recoil pressure on airways, the traction maintains normal to increased airway caliber, with consequent decrease in resistance. The DLCO in lung fibrosis is progressively reduced as a function of the fibrotic obliteration of lung capillaries.

D. Arterial Blood Gases: Hypoxemia is com-

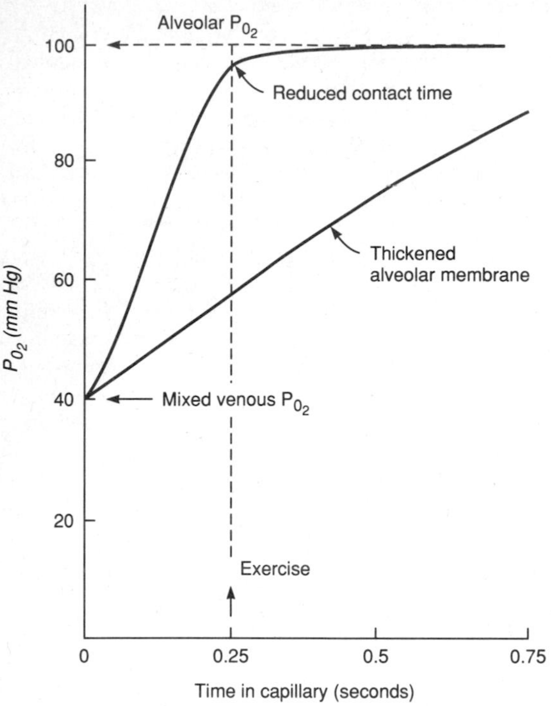

Figure 7–25. Change in Pa_{O_2} along the pulmonary capillary. The typical transit time at rest for an erythrocyte through an alveolar capillary is 0.75 s. In the normal lung, the partial pressure difference and rate of diffusion of O_2 across the alveolar-capillary barrier assure complete saturation of hemoglobin well before completion of the capillary transit. Even with exercise (and a shorter capillary transit time), the normal lung allows for essentially complete saturation of hemoglobin in the alveolar capillary. If the alveolar-capillary barrier is thickened, as is the case in lung fibrosis, diffusion rates are significantly diminished. As a consequence, alveolar-capillary blood may not be fully saturated with O_2 even at rest. Obviously, greater desaturation of arterial blood can occur with progressive exercise. (Reproduced, with permission, from West JB: *Pulmonary Pathophysiology: The Essentials.* Williams & Wilkins, 1992)

mon in pulmonary fibrosis and results from the combination of increased physiologic dead space (and therefore increased V_D/V_T) and physiologic shunt as well as an increasing component of diffusion impairment as a function of the severity of fibrosis. The contribution of diffusion impairment to hypoxemia is increased with exercise (Figure 7–25). The increased cardiac output during exercise reduces the transit time for blood through alveolar capillary beds, increasing the limitation in oxygen loading of hemoglobin. Arterial P_{CO_2} is also reduced as a consequence of increased ventilation under the stimuli of hypoxia and lung fibrosis. Only in the later stages of disease or during exercise, when the increased lung elastic recoil and work of breathing prevent appropriate ventilation, does the Pa_{CO_2} rise above normal. Hypercapnia is a grave sign, implying an inability to maintain adequate alveolar ventilation due to elevated V_D/V_T or excess work of breathing.

32. How does interstitial lung disease affect lung function?
33. Name five events in the pathophysiology of idiopathic pulmonary fibrosis.
34. Name eight signs and symptoms of idiopathic pulmonary fibrosis.

PULMONARY EDEMA

Clinical Presentation

Pulmonary edema is the accumulation of excess fluid in the extravascular space of the lungs. This accumulation may occur slowly, as in the patient with occult renal failure, or with dramatic suddenness, as in the patient with left ventricular failure following an acute myocardial infarction. Pulmonary edema most commonly presents with dyspnea. Dyspnea is breathing perceived by the patient as both uncomfortable or anxiety-provoking and disproportionate to the preceding level of activity. The patient at first notices dyspnea only with exertion but may progress to experience dyspnea at rest. In severe cases, pulmonary edema may be accompanied by edema fluid in the sputum and cause acute respiratory failure.

Etiology

Pulmonary edema is a common problem associated with a variety of medical conditions (Table 7–7). In light of these multiple causes, it is helpful to think about pulmonary edema in terms of underlying physiologic principles.

Pathophysiology

All blood vessels leak. In the adult human, leakage from the pulmonary circulation represents less than 0.01% of pulmonary blood flow, or a baseline filtration of approximately 10–20 mL/h. Two-thirds of this flow occurs across the pulmonary capillary endothelium into the pericapillary interstitial space (Figure 7–26). This is one of two extravascular spaces in the lung—the interstitial space and the airspaces—which contain the alveoli and connecting airways. These two spaces are protected by different barriers. The pulmonary capillary endothelium limits extravasation into the interstitial space while the alveolar epithelium lines the airspaces and protects them against the free movement of fluid. Edema fluid does not readily enter the alveolar space because the

Table 7–7. Causes of pulmonary edema.

Increased pulmonary capillary transmural pressure
Increased left atrial pressure
Left ventricular failure, acute or chronic
Mitral valve stenosis
Pulmonary venous hypertension
Pulmonary veno-occlusive disease
Increased capillary blood volume
Iatrogenic volume expansion
Chronic renal failure
Reduction of interstitial pressure
Rapid reexpansion of collapsed lung
Decreased plasma colloid osmotic pressure
Hypoalbuminemia: nephrotic syndrome, hepatic failure
Increased pulmonary capillary endothelial permeability
Circulating toxins: bacteremia, acute pancreatitis
Infectious pneumonia
Disseminated intravascular coagulation
Nonthoracic trauma accompanied by hypotension ("shock lung")
High-altitude pulmonary edema
Following cardiopulmonary bypass
Increased alveolar epithelial permeability
Inhaled toxins: oxygen, phosgene, chlorine, smoke
Aspiration of acidic gastric contents
Drowning and near-drowning
Depletion of surfactant through high tidal volume positive-pressure mechanical ventilation
Reduced lymphatic clearance
Lymphangitic spread of carcinoma
Following lung transplant
Mechanism uncertain
Neurogenic pulmonary edema
Narcotic overdose
Multiple transfusions

alveolar epithelium is nearly impermeable to the passage of protein. This protein barrier creates a powerful osmotic gradient that favors accumulation of fluid in the interstitium.

The amount of fluid that crosses the pulmonary capillary endothelium is determined by the surface area of the capillary bed, the permeability of the vessel wall, and the net pressure driving it across that wall (transmural or driving pressure). The transmural pressure represents the balance between the net hydrostatic forces that tend to move fluid out of the capillary and the net colloid osmotic forces that tend to keep it in. An imbalance in one or more of these four factors—capillary endothelial permeability, alveolar epithelial permeability, hydrostatic pressure, and colloid osmotic pressure—lies behind nearly all clinical presentations of pulmonary edema.

In the shorthand of clinical practice, these four factors are grouped into two types of pulmonary edema: cardiogenic, referring to edema resulting from a net increase in transmural pressure (hydrostatic or osmotic); and noncardiogenic, referring to edema resulting from increased permeability. The former is primarily a mechanical process, the latter primarily an inflammatory one. However, these two types of pulmonary edema are not exclusive but closely linked: Pulmonary edema occurs when the transmural pressure is excessive for a given capillary permeability. For instance, in the presence of damaged capillary endothelium, small increases in otherwise normal transmural pressure may cause large increases in edema formation. Similarly, if the alveolar epithelial barrier is damaged, even the baseline filtration across an intact endothelium may cause alveolar flooding.

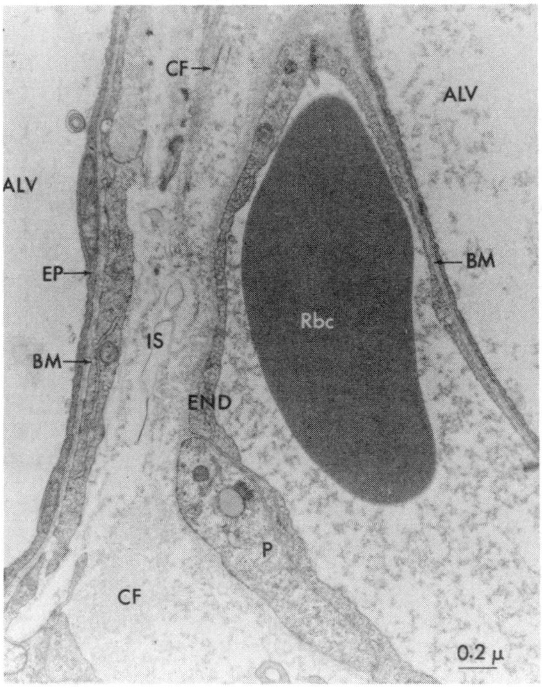

Figure 7–26. Interstitial pulmonary edema. Electron micrograph showing the alveolar septum and a pulmonary capillary in cross section. Note that the pulmonary capillary is eccentrically located. On the right, the basement membrane of the alveolar epithelium and the capillary endothelium are fused. This barrier is therefore thin (0.2 μm), which optimizes gas exchange and inhibits accumulation of edema fluid. On the other side, the basement membranes of the alveolar epithelial cell and the capillary endothelial cell are separated. This interstitial space contains connective tissue that is in continuity with the loose connective tissue of the perivascular and peribronchial interstitium. Edema fluid first accumulates in this pericapillary space. The continuity of the interstitial spaces provides a pathway for movement of edema fluid centrally away from areas of gas exchange. (Reproduced, with permission, from Fishman AP: Pulmonary edema. Circulation 1972;46:390.)

Several mechanisms aid in the clearance of ultrafiltrate and protect against its accumulation as pulmonary edema. Although there are no lymphatics in the alveolar septa, there are "juxta-alveolar" lymphatics in the pericapillary space that normally clear all the ultrafiltrate. The pericapillary interstitium is contiguous with the perivascular and peribronchial interstitium. The interstitial pressure there is negative relative to the pericapillary interstitium, so edema fluid tracks centrally, away from the airspaces. In effect, the perivascular and peribronchiolar interstitium acts as a sump for edema fluid. It can accommodate approximately 500 mL with only a small rise in interstitial hydrostatic pressure. Since this edema fluid is protein-depleted relative to blood, there is an osmotic balance that favors resorption from the interstitium into the bloodstream. This is the major source of resorption of fluid from these collection areas. The perivascular and peribronchiolar interstitium is also contiguous with the interlobular septa and the visceral pleura. In the event of pulmonary edema, there is increased interstitial flow into the pleural space where parietal pleural lymphatics are very efficient at clearance. Pleural effusions seen in patients with increased pulmonary venous pressure represent another reservoir for edema fluid, one that may compromise respiratory function less than to have the same fluid in the lung parenchyma. Finally, there is evidence that edema fluid may track along the interstitium into the mediastinum and be taken up by lymphatics there.

At some undefined critical level after the perivascular and peribronchiolar interstitium have been filled, increased interstitial hydrostatic pressure causes edema fluid to enter the alveolar space. The pathway into the alveolar space remains unknown (Figure 7–27).

In the case of cardiogenic pulmonary edema, increased transmural pressure may result from increased pulmonary venous pressure (causing increased capillary hydrostatic pressure), increased alveolar surface tension (thereby lowering interstitial hydrostatic pressure), or decreased capillary colloid osmotic pressure. When the rate of ultrafiltration rises beyond the capacity of the pericapillary lymphatics to remove it, interstitial fluid accumulates. If the rate of formation continues to exceed lymphatic clearance, alveolar flooding results. Since it is an ultrafiltrate of plasma, the edema fluid of cardiogenic pulmonary edema initially has a low protein content, generally less than 60% of the patient's plasma protein content.

Noncardiogenic (increased permeability) pulmonary edema is sometimes referred to clinically as the acute (formerly "adult") respiratory distress syndrome (ARDS). Alveolar fluid accumulates as a result of loss of integrity of the alveolar epithelium, allowing solutes and large molecules such as albumin to enter the alveolar space. These changes may result from direct injury to the alveolar epithelium by inhaled toxins or pulmonary infection, or they may occur after primary injury to the capillary endothelium by circulating toxins. This is in contrast to

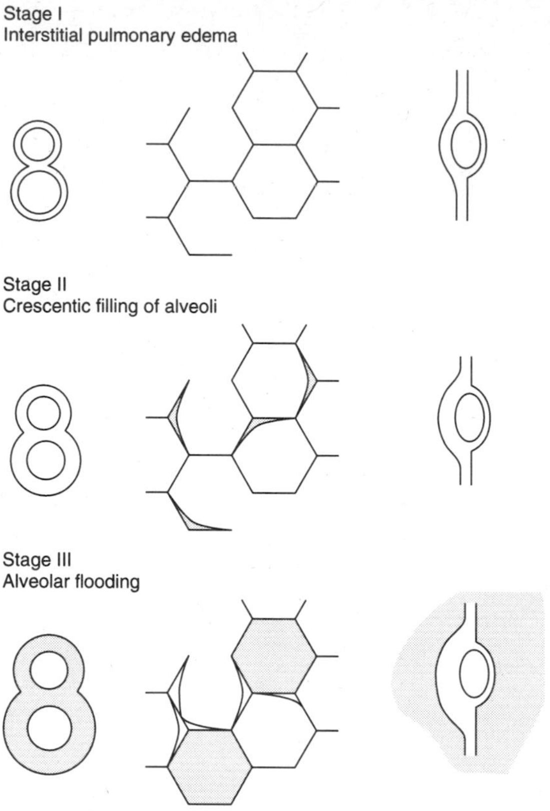

Figure 7–27. Stages in the accumulation of pulmonary edema fluid. The three columns represent three anatomic views of the progressive accumulation of pulmonary edema fluid. From left to right, the columns represent a cross section of the bronchovascular bundle showing the loose connective tissue surrounding the pulmonary artery and bronchial wall, a cross section of alveoli fixed in inflation, and the pulmonary capillary in cross section.

The first stage is eccentric accumulation of fluid in the pericapillary interstitial space. The limitation of edema fluid to one side of the pulmonary capillary maintains gas transfer better than symmetric accumulation. When formation of edema fluid exceeds lymphatic removal, it distends the peribronchovascular interstitium. At this stage, there is no alveolar flooding but there is some crescentic filling of alveoli. The third stage is alveolar flooding. Note that each individual alveolus is either totally flooded or has minimal crescentic filling. This pattern probably occurs because alveolar edema interferes with surfactant and, above some threshold, there is an increase in surface forces that greatly increases the transmural pressure and causes flooding. (Modified and reproduced, with permission, from Nunn JF: *Nunn's Applied Respiratory Physiology,* 4th ed. Butterworth-Heinemann, 1993.)

cardiogenic pulmonary edema, in which both the alveolar epithelium and the capillary endothelium are usually intact. Owing to the disrupted epithelial barrier, edema fluid in increased permeability edema has a high protein content, generally more that 70% of the plasma protein content. The list of potential causes of injury is broad and associated with a diverse group of clinical entities (Table 7–7). The reason so many different problems are grouped together in this syndrome is that they share injury to the alveolar epithelium and damage to pulmonary surfactant, which results in characteristic changes in pulmonary mechanics and function.

With inhaled injury, exemplified by the mustard gas of World War I, there is direct chemical injury to the alveolar epithelium that disrupts this normally tight cellular barrier. The presence of high-protein fluid in the alveolus—particularly the presence of fibrinogen and fibrin degradation products—inactivates pulmonary surfactant, causing large increases in surface tension. This results in a fall in pulmonary compliance and alveolar instability, leading to areas of atelectasis. Increased surface tension decreases the interstitial hydrostatic pressure and favors further fluid movement into the alveolus. A damaged surfactant monolayer may increase susceptibility to infection.

Circulating factors may act directly on the capillary endothelium or may affect it through various immunologic mediators (Table 7–8). A common instance is gram-negative bacteremia. Bacterial endotoxin does not cause endothelial damage directly; it causes neutrophils and macrophages to adhere to endothelial surfaces and release a variety of inflammatory mediators such as leukotrienes, thromboxanes, and prostaglandins as well as oxygen radicals that cause oxidant injury. Both macrophages and neutrophils may release proteolytic enzymes that cause further damage. Alveolar macrophages may also be stimulated. Vasoactive substances may cause intense pulmonary vasoconstriction, leading to capillary failure.

The pathology of increased permeability pulmonary edema reflects these changes. The lungs appear grossly edematous and heavy. The surface appears violaceous, and hemorrhagic fluid exudes from the cut pleural surface. Microscopically, there is cellular infiltration of the interalveolar septa and the interstitium by inflammatory cells and erythrocytes. Type I pneumocytes are damaged, leaving a denuded alveolar barrier. Hyaline membranes form in the absence of alveolar epithelium. These are sheets of pink proteinaceous material composed of plasma proteins, fibrin, and coagulated cell debris. Fibrosis occurs in some cases. Complete recovery with regeneration from the type II pneumocytes of the alveolar epithelium may occur.

Table 7–8. Circulating factors implicated in increased permeability pulmonary edema.

Cellular elements
Basophils
Macrophages
Platelets
Polymorphonuclear cells
Factors promoting migration and adherence of cellular elements
Complement, especially C5a
Endotoxin
Histamine
Tumor necrosis factor
Proteolytic enzymes
Kallekrein
Proteases
Substances affecting airway and vascular smooth muscle
Bradykinin
Leukotrienes
Prostaglandins
Serotonin
Thromboxane
Oxidant injury
Oxygen-derived free radicals
Others
Interleukin-1
Thrombin
Fibrin
Platelet-activating factor

Clinical Manifestations

Cardiogenic and noncardiogenic pulmonary edema both result in increased extravascular lung water, and both may result in respiratory failure. Given the differences in pathophysiology, it is not surprising that the clinical manifestations are very different in the two syndromes.

A. Increased Transmural Pressure Pulmonary Edema (Cardiogenic Pulmonary Edema): Early increases in pulmonary venous pressure may be asymptomatic. The patient may notice only mild exertional dyspnea or a nonproductive cough stimulated by irritation of the J receptors. Orthopnea and paroxysmal nocturnal dyspnea both occur when recumbency causes redistribution of blood or edema fluid, respectively, pooled in the lower extremities, thereby increasing thoracic blood volume and pulmonary venous pressures.

Clinical signs begin with the accumulation of interstitial fluid. Physical examination may reveal abnormal heart sounds, but there is a paucity of lung findings in purely interstitial edema. The earliest sign is frequently a chest radiograph showing an increase in the caliber of the upper lobe vessels ("pulmonary vascular redistribution'') and fluid accumulating in the perivascular and peribronchial spaces ("cuffing''). It may also show Kerley B lines, which represent fluid in the interlobular septa. Pulmonary compliance falls, and the patient begins to breathe more rapidly and shallowly in order to minimize the increased elastic work of breathing. As alveolar flooding begins, there are further decreases in lung volume and pulmonary compliance. With some alveoli filled with fluid, there is an increase in the fraction of the lung that is perfused but poorly ventilated. This increase in areas of low $\dot{V}/\dot{Q}$ ratios causes an increase in A–a ΔPo_2, if not frank hypoxemia. Supplemental oxygen corrects the hypoxemia. The $Paco_2$ is normal or low, reflecting the increased drive to breathe. The patient may become sweaty and cyanotic. The sputum may show edema fluid that is pink from capillary hemorrhage and frothy due to protein. Auscultation reveals inspiratory crackles—chiefly at the bases, where the hydrostatic pressure is greatest, but potentially throughout both lungs. Rhonchi and wheezing ("cardiac asthma") may occur. The radiograph shows areas of alveolar flooding.

B. Increased Permeability Pulmonary Edema (Noncardiogenic Pulmonary Edema, or ARDS): ARDS is generally a consequence of a separate serious medical condition. The range of clinical presentations includes all the diagnoses in the adult Intensive Care Unit. Nevertheless, there are clinical observations that mirror the pathophysiology.

After the initial insult—eg, an episode of high-grade bacteremia—there is generally a period of stability, reflecting the time it takes for various immunologic mediators to wreak their havoc. Surfactant is inactivated, leading to a significant increase in surface forces and markedly reduced pulmonary compliance. For the first 24–48 hours after the insult, the patient may have increased work of breathing, leading to dyspnea and tachypnea but without causing abnormalities in the chest radiograph. At this early stage, the increased A–a ΔPo_2 reflects alveolar edema and $\dot{V}/\dot{Q}$ mismatching and is corrected by increased FiO_2. Pathologically, there is alveolar edema, hemorrhage, and atelectasis. The clinical picture may improve, or there may be a further fall in compliance and disruption of pulmonary capillaries leading to areas of true shunting and refractory hypoxemia. The combination of greatly increased work of breathing and severe hypoxemia generally mandates mechanical ventilation. However, the stiffness of the lungs increases nonhomogeneous ventilation, and there is a gross increase in ventilation of poorly perfused areas. The high pressures needed to ventilate these patients may overdistend normal alveoli and reduce blood flow to areas of adequate ventilation. Hypoxemia is profound, and hypercapnia may ensue. Radiographically, there is "whiteout" of the lungs that represents diffuse confluent alveolar filling. Pathologically, there is an increase in inflammatory cells and the formation of hyaline membranes. The mortality rate averages 50–60%. Most patients die from some complication of their presenting illness. Of those who survive, many will recover essentially normal lung function, but a significant number will develop new reactive airway disease or pulmonary fibrosis.

35. What four factors determine the clinical presentation of pulmonary edema? How are they affected in cardiogenic versus noncardiogenic causes of pulmonary edema?
36. What are the common causes of noncardiogenic pulmonary edema?
37. Is lung damage from increased permeability pulmonary edema reversible? If so, how?
38. What are the two major reasons that mechanical ventilation is often required in severe pulmonary edema?

PULMONARY EMBOLISM

Clinical Presentation

The English word "embolus" derives from a Greek root meaning "plug" or "stopper." A pulmonary embolus consists of material that gains access to the venous system and then to the pulmonary circulation. Eventually, it reaches a vessel whose caliber is too small to permit free passage, and there it forms a plug, occluding the lumen and obstructing perfusion. There are many types of pulmonary embolization. The most common is pulmonary thromboembolism, which occurs when venous thrombi, chiefly from the lower extremities, migrate to the pulmonary circulation (Table 7–9).

Pulmonary thromboembolism is to some extent a normal function of the pulmonary microcirculation. The lungs possess both excess functional capacity and a redundant vascular supply, making them a superb filter for preventing small thrombi and platelet aggregates from gaining access to the systemic circulation. However, large thromboemboli—or an accumulation of smaller ones—can cause substantial

Table 7–9. Types of pulmonary emboli.

Material	Clinical Setting
Air	Cardiac surgery, neurosurgery, improper manipulation of central venous catheters
Amniotic fluid	Active labor
Fat	Long bone fracture, liposuction
Foreign body	Pieces of intravenous devices, talc
Oil	Lymphangiography
Parasite eggs	Schistosomiasis
Septic emboli	Endocarditis, thrombophlebitis
Thrombus	Deep venous thrombosis
Tumor	Renal cell carcinoma with invasion of vena cava

Table 7–10. Risk factors for venous thrombosis.

Increased venous stasis
- Bed rest
- Immobilization, especially following orthopedic surgery
- Low cardiac output states
- Pregnancy
- Obesity
- Hyperviscosity
- Local vascular damage, especially prior thrombosis with incompetent valves
- Increasing age

Increased coagulability
- Tissue injury: surgery, trauma, myocardial infarction
- Malignancy
- Presence of a lupus anticoagulant
- Nephrotic syndrome
- Oral contraceptive use, especially estrogen administration
- Genetic coagulation disorders: deficiency of antithrombin III; deficiency of protein C or its cofactor, protein S; deficiency of plasminogen; dysfunctional fibrinogen

impairment of cardiac and respiratory function, including death.

Pulmonary thromboemboli are quite common and cause significant morbidity. They are found at autopsy in 25–50% of hospitalized patients and are considered a major contributing cause of death in a third of those. However, the diagnosis is made antemortem in only 10–20% of cases.

Etiology & Epidemiology

Thromboemboli almost never originate in the pulmonary circulation. They arrive there by a venous route. Pulmonary thromboembolism is therefore a secondary consequence of another disease, ie, venous thrombosis.

More than 95% of pulmonary thromboemboli arise from thrombi in the deep veins of the lower extremity: the popliteal, femoral, and iliac veins. Venous thrombosis below the popliteal veins or occurring in the superficial veins of the leg is clinically common but not a risk factor for pulmonary thromboembolism. Thrombi in these locations rarely migrate to the pulmonary circulation without first extending above the knee. Since fewer than 20% of calf thrombi will extend into the popliteal veins, isolated calf thrombi may be observed with serial tests to exclude extension into the deep system and do not necessarily require anticoagulation. Venous thromboses occasionally occur in the upper extremities or in the right side of the heart; this happens most commonly in the presence of intravenous catheters or cardiac pacing wires.

Risk factors for pulmonary thromboembolism are therefore the risk factors for the development of venous thrombosis in the deep veins of the legs (deep venous thrombosis) (Table 7–10). The German pathologist Rudolf Virchow stated these risk factors in 1856: venous stasis, injury to the vascular wall,

Table 7–11. Risk of postoperative deep venous thrombosis or pulmonary embolus in patients who do not receive anticoagulant prophylaxis.[1]

Risk Category	Incidence of Calf Deep Venous Thrombosis	Incidence of Proximal Deep Venous Thrombosis	Incidence of Fatal Pulmonary Embolus
High risk 1. Age >40 2. Surgery > 30 minutes 3. At least one of the following: a. Orthopedic surgery b. Pelvic or abdominal cancer surgery c. History of prior deep venous thrombosis or pulmonary embolus d. Hereditary coagulopathy	40–80%	10–20%	1–5%
Moderate risk 1. Age >40 2. Surgery >30 minutes 3. At least one of the following secondary risk factors: a. Immobilization b. Obesity c. Malignancy d. Estrogen use e. Varicose veins f. Paralysis	10–40%	2–10%	0.1–0.7%
Low risk 1. Any age 2. Surgery <30 minutes 3. No secondary risk factors	<10%	<1%	<0.01%

[1]Modified and reproduced, with permission, from Merli G: Update: Deep vein thrombosis and pulmonary embolism prophylaxis in orthopedic surgery. Med Clin North Am 1993;77:397.

and increased activation of the clotting system. His observations are still valid today.

The most prevalent risk factor in hospitalized patients is stasis from immobilization, especially in those undergoing surgical procedures. The incidence of calf vein thrombosis in patients who do not receive heparin prophylaxis following total knee replacement is reported to be as high as 84%; it is more than 50% following hip surgery or prostatectomy. The risk of fatal pulmonary thromboembolism in these patients may be as high as 5%. Physicians caring for these patients must therefore be aware of the magnitude of the risk and institute appropriate prophylactic therapy (Tables 7–10 and 7–11).

Malignancy and tissue damage at surgery are the two most common causes of increased activation of the coagulation system. Genetic disorders are comparatively uncommon, representing 8% of diagnosed outpatients in one recent series. Abnormalities in the vessel wall contribute little to venous as opposed to arterial thrombosis. However, prior thrombosis can damage venous valves and lead to venous incompetence, which promotes stasis.

Pathophysiology

Venous thrombi are composed of a friable mass of fibrin, with many erythrocytes and a few leukocytes and platelets randomly enmeshed in the matrix. When a venous thrombus travels to the pulmonary circulation, it causes a broad array of pathophysiologic changes (Table 7–12).

A. Hemodynamic Changes: Every patient with a pulmonary embolus has some degree of mechanical obstruction. The effect of mechanical obstruction depends on the proportion of the pulmonary circulation obstructed and the presence or absence of preexisting cardiopulmonary disease. In patients without preexisting cardiopulmonary disease, pulmonary arterial pressure increases in proportion to the fraction of the pulmonary circulation occluded by emboli. If that fraction is greater than about one-third, pulmonary artery pressures will rise out of the normal range and cause right ventricular strain. The pulmonary circulation can adapt to increased flow, but this depends (1) on recruitment of underperfused capillaries, which may not be available because of obstruction; and (2) on relaxation of central vessels, which does not occur instantaneously. In patients with preexisting cardiopulmonary disease, increases in pulmonary artery pressures do not correlate with extent of embolization. In these studies, there were relatively few patients with both preexisting cardiopulmonary disease and extensive arterial occlusion. A correlation may be obscured by the possibility that massive emboli may either kill patients with preexisting cardiopulmonary disease or perhaps make them too unstable for angiography.

The most devastating and feared complication of acute pulmonary thromboembolism is sudden occlusion of the pulmonary outflow tract, reducing cardiac output to zero and causing immediate cardiovascular collapse and death. Large emboli that do not completely occlude vessels, particularly in patients with compromised cardiac function, may cause an acute increase in pulmonary vascular resistance. This leads to acute right ventricular strain and a fatal fall in cardiac output. Such dramatic presentations represent less than 5% of cases and are essentially untreatable. They serve to highlight the importance of primary prevention of venous thrombosis.

B. Changes in Ventilation/Perfusion Relationships: Pulmonary thromboembolism reduces or eliminates perfusion distal to the site of the occlusion. The immediate effect is to increase the proportion of lung segments with high $\dot{V}/\dot{Q}$ ratios. If there is complete obstruction to flow, then the $\dot{V}/\dot{Q}$ ratio reaches infinity. This represents alveolar dead space. An increase in dead space ventilation impairs the excretion of carbon dioxide. This tendency is generally compensated by hyperventilation. After several hours,

Table 7–12. Pathophysiologic changes in pulmonary embolism.[1]

Basic Physiology	Effect of Thromboembolism	Mechanism
Altered hemodynamics	Increased pulmonary vascular resistance	Vascular obstruction Vasoconstriction by serotonin, thromboxane A_2
Impaired gas exchange	Increase in alveolar dead space	Vascular obstruction Increased perfusion of lung units with high $\dot{V}/\dot{Q}$ ratios
	Hypoxemia	Increased perfusion of lung units with low $\dot{V}/\dot{Q}$ ratios Right-to-left shunting Fall in cardiac output with fall in mixed venous Pa_{O_2}
Ventilatory control	Hyperventilation	Reflex stimulation of irritant receptors
Work of breathing	Increased airway resistance Decreased pulmonary compliance	Reflex bronchoconstriction Loss of surfactant with lung edema and hemorrhage

[1]Modified and reproduced, with permission, from Elliot CG: Pulmonary physiology during pulmonary embolism. Chest 1992;4(Suppl):163S.

hypoperfusion interferes with production of surfactant by alveolar type II cells. Surfactant is depleted, resulting in alveolar edema, alveolar collapse, and areas of atelectasis. Edema and collapse may result in lung units with little or no ventilation. If there is perfusion to these segments, there will be an increase in lung units with low $\dot{V}/\dot{Q}$ ratios or areas of true shunting, both of which will contribute to arterial hypoxemia.

C. Hypoxemia: Mild to moderate hypoxemia with a low $Paco_2$ is the most common finding in acute pulmonary thromboembolism. This finding may be obscured by the tendency to rely on oximetry alone, since two-thirds of patients will have oxygen saturations above 90% (Figure 7–28). A more sensitive indicator is to calculate the A–a ΔPo_2 in order to compensate for the presence of hypocapnia and to account for an increased inspired FIO_2. A widened A–a ΔPo_2 is a nearly universal finding in acute pulmonary thromboembolism.

There is no one mechanism that will account for hypoxemia. Two causes have been mentioned above. An increase in lung units with low $\dot{V}/\dot{Q}$ ratios impairs oxygen delivery. In patients whose underlying disease makes them unable to increase their minute ventilation, an increase in lung units with high $\dot{V}/\dot{Q}$ ratios can also result in hypoxemia. In some patients with preexisting impaired cardiac function or with large emboli that cause acute right ventricular strain, cardiac output may fall, with a resultant fall in the mixed venous oxygen concentration. This is an important cause of hypoxemia in seriously ill patients. Finally, there may be true right-to-left shunts. Such shunts have been described in a small percentage of patients with severe hypoxemia in the setting of an acute pulmonary thromboembolism. It is presumed that these represent pulmonary artery to pulmonary venous shunting—or perhaps opening of a foramen ovale—but their exact location is unknown.

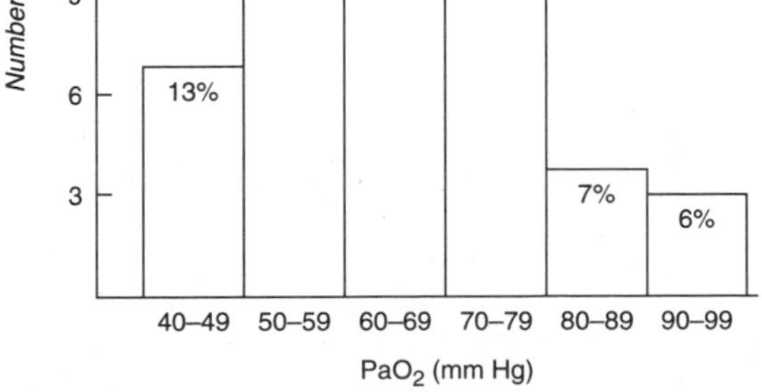

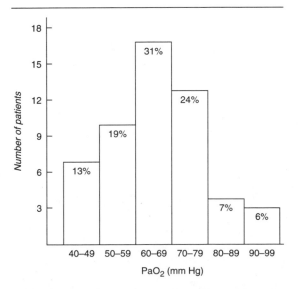

Figure 7–28. Arterial Po_2 in 54 patients with angiographically documented pulmonary embolism and no prior history of cardiopulmonary disease. (Reproduced, with permission, from Dantzker DR, Bower JS: Alterations in gas exchange following pulmonary thromboembolism. Chest 1982;81:495.)

Obstruction of small pulmonary arterial branches that act as end arteries leads to pulmonary infarction in about 10% of cases. It is generally associated with some concomitant abnormality of the bronchial circulation such as is seen in patients with left ventricular failure and chronically elevated left atrial pressures.

Clinical Manifestations

A. Symptoms and Signs: The classic triad of a sudden onset of dyspnea, pleuritic chest pain, and hemoptysis occurs in only 20% of patients. Individually, these symptoms are present in 85%, 75%, and 30% of diagnosed cases, respectively. Dyspnea probably results from reflex bronchoconstriction as well as increased pulmonary artery pressure, loss of pulmonary compliance and stimulation of J receptors. In large emboli, there may be an element of acute right heart strain. Pleuritic chest pain is much more common than pulmonary infarction; one group has suggested that the pain is caused by areas of pulmonary hemorrhage. Hemoptysis is seen with pulmonary infarction but may also result from transmission of systemic arterial pressures to the microvasculature via bronchopulmonary anastomoses, with subsequent capillary disruption. It may reflect hemorrhagic pulmonary edema from surfactant depletion or neutrophil-associated capillary injury. Syncope may signal a massive embolus.

The most compelling physical finding is not in the chest but the leg: evidence for deep venous thrombosis. The absence of such evidence does not exclude the diagnosis, since the clinical examination is insensitive, and the absence of signs may indicate that the entire thrombus has embolized. Auscultatory chest findings are common but entirely nonspecific. Atelectasis may lead to inspiratory crackles; infarction may cause a focal pleural friction rub; and the release of mediators may cause wheezing. In large embolization, one may find signs of acute right ventricular strain such as a right ventricular lift and accentuation of the pulmonary component of the second heart sound.

B. Electrocardiography: Less than 25% of cardiograms are normal in the setting of acute pulmonary thromboembolism. However, most of the findings represent sinus tachycardia or nonspecific ST and T wave changes. The classic finding of acute right ventricular strain ($S_1Q_3T_3$) was observed in 11% of patients in the Urokinase Pulmonary Embolism Trial.

C. Laboratory Findings: An increase in the A–a ΔPo_2 is nearly universal, and hypoxemia is common in the setting of acute pulmonary thromboembolism.

D. Imaging: The chest radiograph was normal in only 12% of patients with confirmed pulmonary thromboembolism in the Prospective Investigation of Pulmonary Embolism Diagnosis (PIOPED) study. The most frequent findings were atelectasis, parenchymal infiltrates, and pleural effusions. However, the prevalence of these findings was the same in hospitalized patients without suspected pulmonary thromboembolism. Local oligemia (Westermark's sign) or pleural-based areas of increased opacity that represent intraparenchymal hemorrhage (Hampton's hump) are rare. The chest radiograph is necessary to exclude other common lung diseases and to permit interpretation of the ventilation/perfusion scan, but it does not itself establish the diagnosis. Paradoxically, it may be most helpful when normal in the setting of acute severe hypoxemia.

E. Ventilation/Perfusion Scanning: A perfusion scan is obtained by injecting microaggregated albumin with a particle size of 50–100 μm into the venous system and allowing the particles to embolize to the pulmonary capillary bed (approximate diameter 10 μm). The substance is labeled with a gamma-emitting isotope of 99m Tc technetium pertechnetate that permits imaging of the distribution of pulmonary blood flow. A ventilation scan is performed by having the patient breathe radioactive xenon and doing sequential scans during inhalation and exhalation. A normal perfusion scan excludes clinically significant pulmonary thromboembolism. A segmental or larger perfusion defect in a radiographically normal area that shows normal ventilation is diagnostic. This is referred to as a "mismatched" defect and is highly specific (97%) for pulmonary thromboembolism.

A minority of ventilation/perfusion scans reveal clearly diagnostic findings. The PIOPED study demonstrated that nondiagnostic ventilation/perfusion scans can stratify a patient's risk of pulmonary thromboembolism. Furthermore, within the categories of high-, medium-, and low-probability studies, the clinician's pretest assessment of the probability of pulmonary thromboembolism can further stratify patients (Table 7–13).

F. Pulmonary Angiography: This is currently the definitive study for the diagnosis of pulmonary thromboembolism. Newer technologies such as rapid sequence computed tomography scanning (spiral CT) are being actively investigated.

G. Resolution: The variability among patients is so great that generalizations are hard to make. The largest number of patients followed serially with quantitative assessments was in the Urokinase Pulmonary Embolism Trial. In that study, serial perfusion scans showed substantial resolution in 7–14 days (Table 7–14). More modern studies, some involving quantitative angiography, have tended to support the time course of these findings.

In a small percentage of patients, pulmonary emboli do not resolve completely but become organized and incorporated into the pulmonary arterial wall as an epithelialized fibrous mass. Over time, this can

Table 7–13. Pulmonary embolism (PE) status.[1,2]

V/Q Scan Category[3]	Clinical Probability,[4] %: 80–100 PE+/No. of Pts	%	20–79 PE+/No. of Pts	%	0–19 PE+/No. of Pts	%	All Probabilities PE+/No. of Pts	%
High probability	28/29	96	70/80	88	5/9	56	103/118	87
Intermediate probability	27/41	66	66/236	28	11/68	26	104/345	30
Low probability	6/15	40	30/191	16	4/90	4	40/296	14
Near normal/normal	0/5	0	4/62	6	1/61	2	5/128	4
Total	61/90	68	170/569	30	21/228	9	252/887	28

[1]Reproduced, with permission, from The PIOPED Investigators: Value of the ventilation/perfusion scan in acute pulmonary embolism. JAMA 1990;263:2757.

[2]PE+ indicates angiogram reading that shows pulmonary embolism or determination of pulmonary embolism by the outcome classification committee on review. Pulmonary embolism status is based on angiogram interpretation for 713 patients, on angiogram interpretation and outcome classification committee reassignment for 4 patients, and on clinical information alone (without definitive angiography) for 170 patients.

[3]The division of V/Q scan into normal, high, intermediate (or indeterminate), and low probability does stratify patients at risk for pulmonary embolus.

[4]The clinical evaluation of risk adds information to this assessment. For example, in a patient with a low-probability V/Q scan, the risk of pulmonary embolus may be as high as 40% in those with a high clinical likelihood and as low as 4% in those with a low clinical likelihood. The V/Q scan functions along with clinical judgment to weight risks and benefits of pulmonary arteriography.

Table 7–14. Resolution of heparin-treated pulmonary thromboembolism assessed by serial perfusion scanning.[1]

Time After Event	Number of Patients	Resolution (% ± SD)
24 hours	70	7 ± 28
2 days	65	16 ± 30
3 days	65	21 ± 30
5 days	69	32 ± 31
7 days	67	42 ± 32
14 days	62	56 ± 30
3 months	60	75 ± 26
6 months	55	77 ± 25
12 months	50	77 ± 23

[1]From The Urokinase Pulmonary Embolism Trial: Circulation 1973;47(Suppl 2):1.

lead to **chronic pulmonary thromboembolism.** This entity presents with stenosis of the central pulmonary arteries, pulmonary hypertension, and right ventricular failure **(cor pulmonale).** Treatment is surgical.

39. Where do 95% of pulmonary thromboemboli originate?
40. What are the risk factors for pulmonary thromboemboli?
41. What hemodynamic changes are brought about by significant pulmonary thromboemboli?
42. What changes in ventilation/perfusion relationships are brought about by significant pulmonary thromboemboli?
43. Suggest some possible explanations for hypoxemia in pulmonary thromboembolism.
44. What are the clinical manifestations of pulmonary thromboembolism?

REFERENCES

General

Crystal RG et al: *The Lung: Scientific Foundations.* Raven Press, 1991.

Murray JF: *The Normal Lung,* 2nd ed. Saunders, 1986.

Murray JF, Nadel JA: *Textbook of Respiratory Medicine,* 2nd ed. Saunders, 1994.

Nunn JF: *Nunn's Applied Respiratory Physiology.* 4th ed. Butterworth-Heinemann, 1993.

Staub NC: *Basic Respiratory Physiology.* Churchill Livingstone, 1991.

West JB: *Pulmonary Pathophysiology: The Essentials,* 4th ed. Williams & Wilkins, 1992.

West JB: *Respiratory Physiology: The Essentials,* 4th ed. Williams & Wilkins, 1990.

Normal Physiology

Berger AS et al: Regulation of respiration. (Three parts.) N Engl J Med 1977;297:92, 138, 194.

Loudon R, Murphy RLH: Lung sounds. Am Rev Resp Dis 1984;130:663.

Roussos C, Macklem PT: The respiratory muscles. N Engl J Med 1982;307:786.

West JB: Ventilation-perfusion relationships. Am Rev Resp Dis 1977;116:919.

Obstructive Lung Disease

Bentley AM et al: Identification of T lymphocytes, macrophages and activated eosinophils in the bronchial mucosa in intrinsic asthma: Relationship to symptoms and bronchial hyperresponsiveness. Am Rev Respir Dis 1992;146:500.

Owens GR et al: The diffusing capacity as a predictor of arterial oxygen desaturation during exercise in patients with chronic obstructive pulmonary disease. N Engl J Med 1984;310:1218.

Robinson DS et al: Predominant TH2-like bronchoalveolar T-lymphocyte population in atopic asthma. N Engl J Med 1992;326:298.

Weinberger SE: Recent advances in pulmonary medicine. N Engl J Med 1993;328:1389.

Restrictive Lung Disease

Crystal RG et al: Interstitial lung diseases of unknown cause. (Two parts.) N Engl J Med 1984;310:154, 235.

Rochester CL, Elias JA: Cytokines and cytokine networking in the pathogenesis of interstitial and fibrotic lung disorders. Semin Respir Med 1993;14:389.

Pulmonary Edema

Matthay MA: Pathophysiology of pulmonary edema. Clin Chest Med 1985;6:301.

Staub NC: Pathophysiology of pulmonary edema. In: *Edema.* Staub NC, Taylor AE (editors). Raven Press, 1984.

Acute Respiratory Distress Syndrome

Bernard GR et al: The American-European Conference on ARDS: Definitions, mechanisms, relevant outcomes, and clinical trial coordination. Am J Resp Crit Care Med 1994;149:818.

Lewis JF, Jobe AH: Surfactant and the adult respiratory distress syndrome. Am Rev Resp Dis 1993;147:218.

Wiener-Kronish JP et al: The adult respiratory distress syndrome: Definition and prognosis, pathogenesis and treatment. Br J Anaesth 1990;65:107.

Pulmonary Embolism

Carson JL et al: The clinical course of pulmonary embolism. N Engl J Med 1992;326:1240.

Eliott CG: Pulmonary physiology during pulmonary embolism. Chest 1992;101(Suppl 4):163S.

Heijboer H et al: Deficiencies of coagulation-inhibiting

and fibrinolytic proteins in outpatients with deep-vein thrombosis. N Engl J Med 1990;323:1512.
Merli GJ: Update: Deep vein thrombosis and pulmonary embolism prophylaxis in orthopedic surgery. Med Clin North Am 1993;77:397.
The Urokinase Pulmonary Embolism Trial: A National Cooperative Study. Circulation 1973;47(Suppl 2):1.
Worsley DF et al: Chest radiographic findings in patients with acute pulmonary embolism: Observations from the PIOPED study. Radiology 1993;189:133.

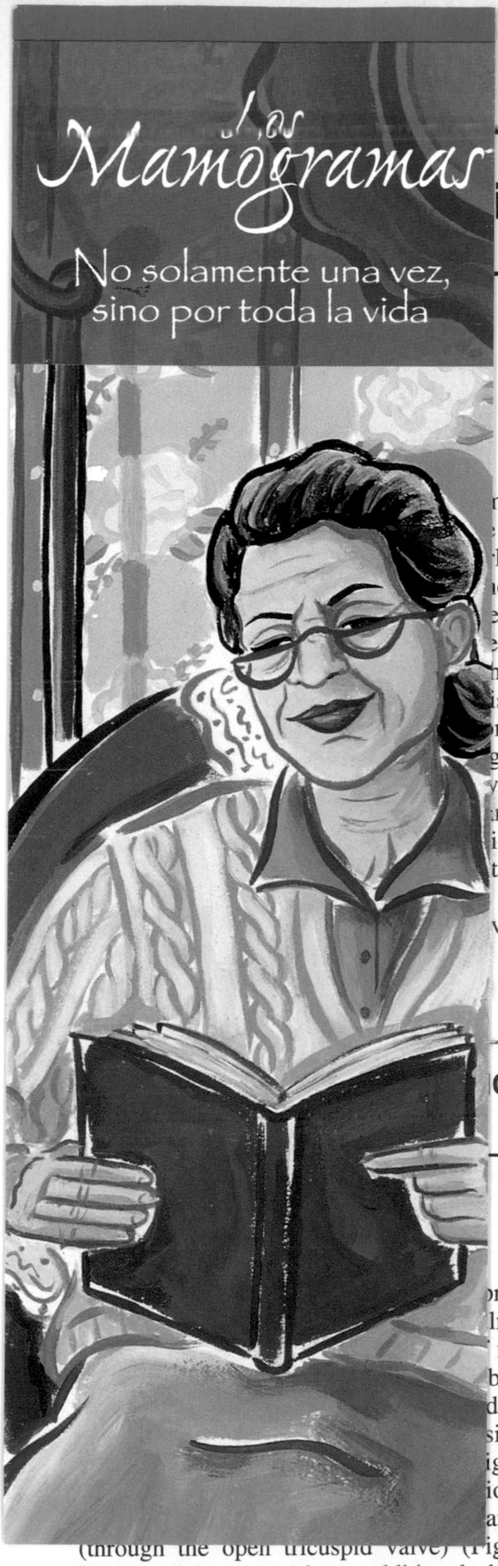
Los
Mamogramas
No solamente una vez,
sino por toda la vida

isease 8

n frequently
day-to-day
lying patho-
eart disease
ent manage-
ctions: first,
ysiology of
scussions of
mmonly en-
gestive heart
artery dis-
nd shock. A
iology of all
this chapter,
on arrhyth-
vascular dis-

CTION

rimary func-
lmonary and
four muscu-
bers, the left
d right atria
sible for the
igure 8–1A).
ior and supe-
and ventricle
(through the open tricuspid valve) (Figure 8–1B). With atrial contraction, additional blood flows through the tricuspid valve and completes the filling of the right ventricle. Unoxygenated blood is then pumped to the pulmonary artery and lung by the right ventricle through the pulmonary valve (Figure 8–1C). Oxygenated blood returns from the lung to the left atrium via four pulmonary veins (Figure 8–1D). Sequential left atrial and ventricular contraction pumps blood back to the peripheral tissues. The mitral valve separates the left atrium and ventricle, and the aortic valve separates the left ventricle from the aorta (Figures 8–1D and 8–1E).

The heart lies freely in the pericardial sac, attached to mediastinal structures only at the great vessels. During embryologic development, the heart invaginates into the pericardial sac like a fist pushing into a partially inflated balloon. The pericardial sac is composed of a serous inner layer (visceral pericardium) directly apposed to the myocardium and a fibrous outer layer called the parietal pericardium. Under normal conditions, approximately 40–50 mL of clear fluid, which probably is an ultrafiltrate of plasma, fills the space between the layers of the pericardial sac.

The left main and right coronary arteries arise from the root of the aorta and provide the principal blood supply to the heart (Figure 8–2). The large left main coronary artery usually branches into the left anterior descending artery and the circumflex coronary artery. The left anterior descending coronary artery gives off diagonal and septal branches that supply blood to the anterior wall and septum of the heart, respectively. The circumflex coronary artery continues around the heart in the left atrioventricular groove and gives off large obtuse marginal arteries that supply blood to the left ventricular free wall. The right coronary artery travels in the right atrioventricular groove and supplies blood to the right ventricle via acute marginal branches. The posterior descending artery, which supplies blood to the posterior and inferior walls of the left ventricle, arises from the right coronary artery in 80% of people (right-dominant circulation) and from the circumflex artery in the remainder (left-dominant circulation).

Contraction of the heart chambers is coordinated by several regions in the heart that are composed of myocytes with specialized automaticity (pacemaker) and conduction properties (Figure 8–3). Cells in the sinoatrial (SA) node and the atrioventricular (AV) node have fast pacemaker rates (SA node: 60–100 beats/min; AV node: 40–70 beats/min), and the His bundle and Purkinje fibers are characterized by rapid rates of conduction. Since it has the fastest intrinsic pacemaker rhythm, the SA node is usually the site of

A

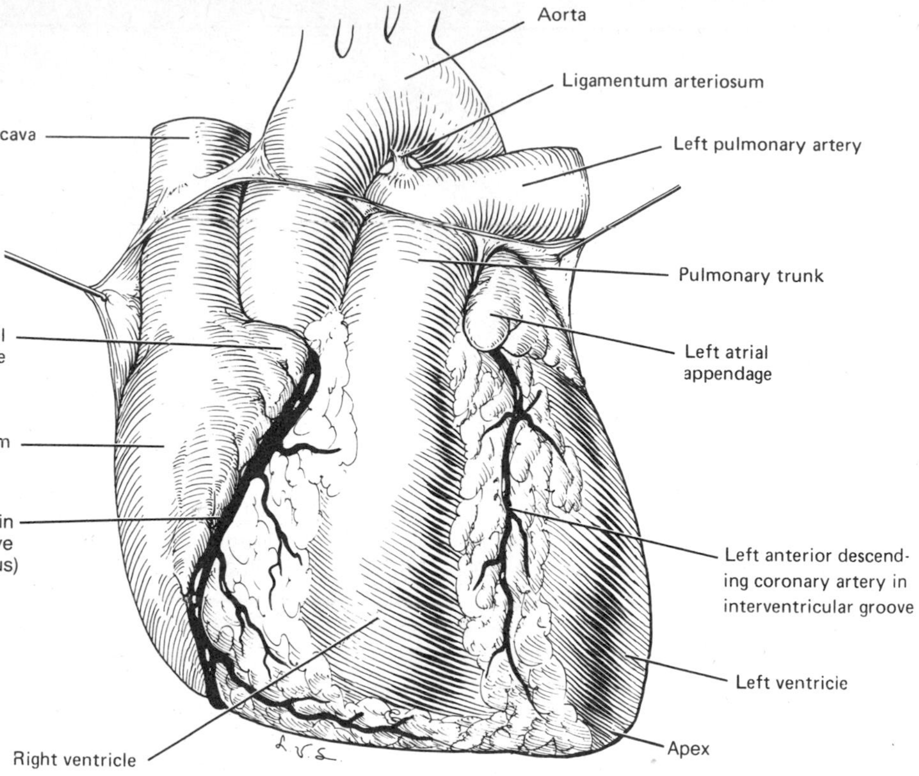

B

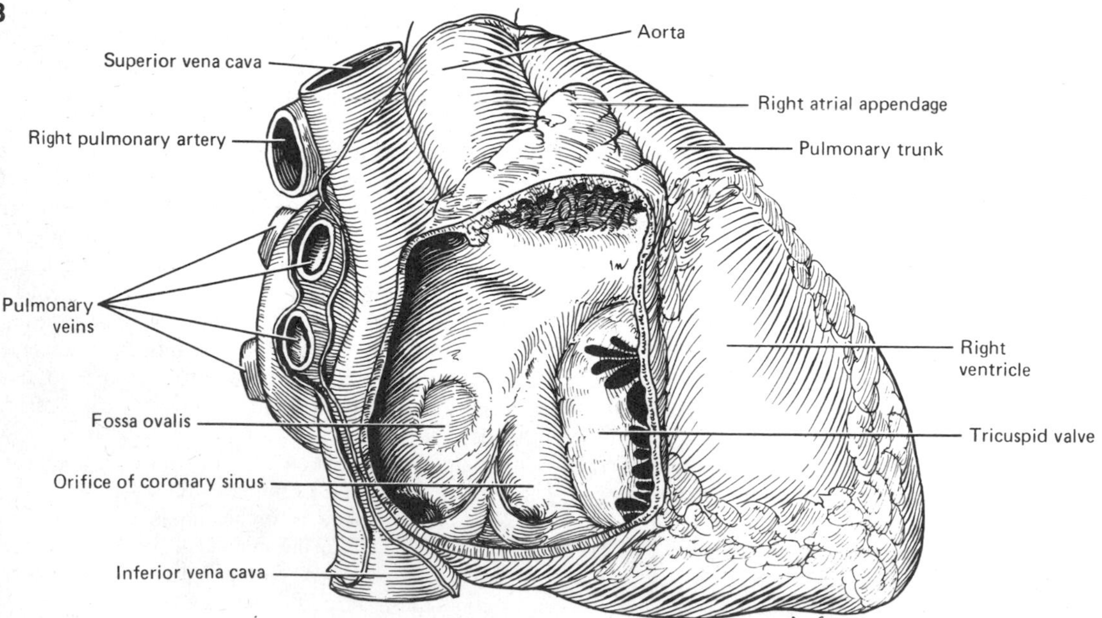

Figure 8–1. Anatomy of the heart. ***A:*** Anterior view of the heart. ***B:*** View of the right heart with the right atrial wall reflected to show the right atrium. ***C:*** Anterior view of the heart with the anterior wall removed to show the right ventricular cavity. ***D:*** View of the left heart with the left ventricular wall turned back to show the mitral valve. ***E:*** View of the left heart from the left side with the left ventricular free wall and mitral valve cut away to reveal the aortic valve. (Reproduced, with permission, from Cheitlin MD, Sokolow M, McIlroy MB: *Clinical Cardiology*, 6th ed. Appleton & Lange, 1993.)

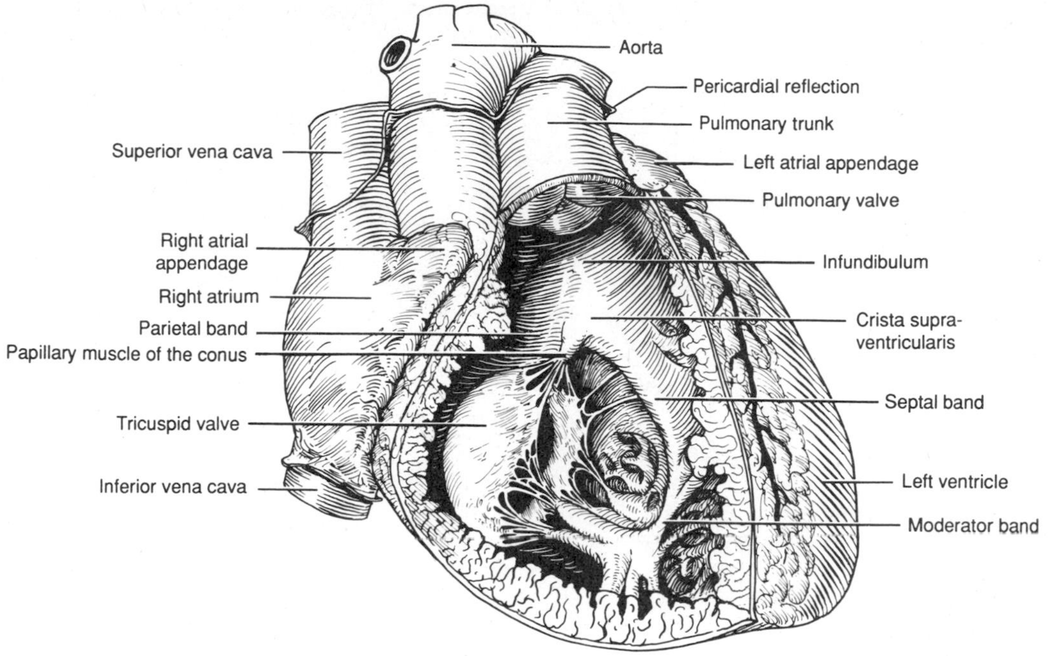

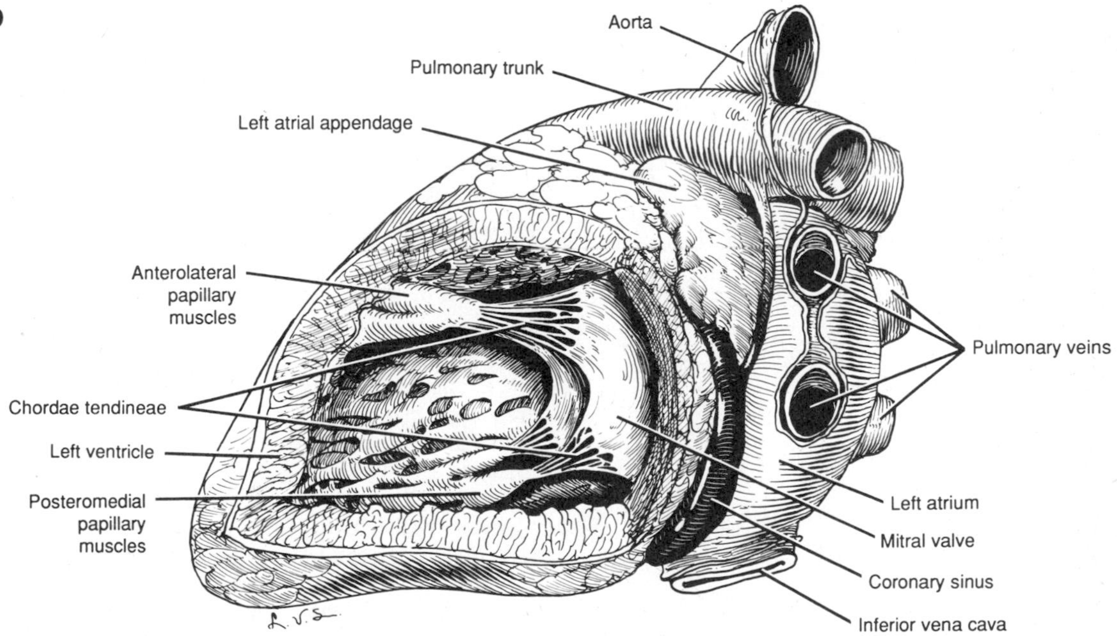

Figure 8–1 *Continued*

initiation of the cardiac electrical impulse during a normal cardiac beat. The impulse then rapidly depolarizes both the left and right atria as it travels to the AV node. Conduction velocity slows from 1 m/s in atrial tissue to 0.05 m/s in nodal tissue. After the delay in the AV node, the impulse moves rapidly down the His bundle (1 m/s) and Purkinje fibers (4 m/s) to simultaneously depolarize the right and left ventricles. The atria and ventricles are separated by a fibrous framework that is electrically inert, so that under normal conditions the AV node and the contiguous His bundle form the only electrical connection between the atria and ventricles. This arrangement allows the atria and ventricles to beat in

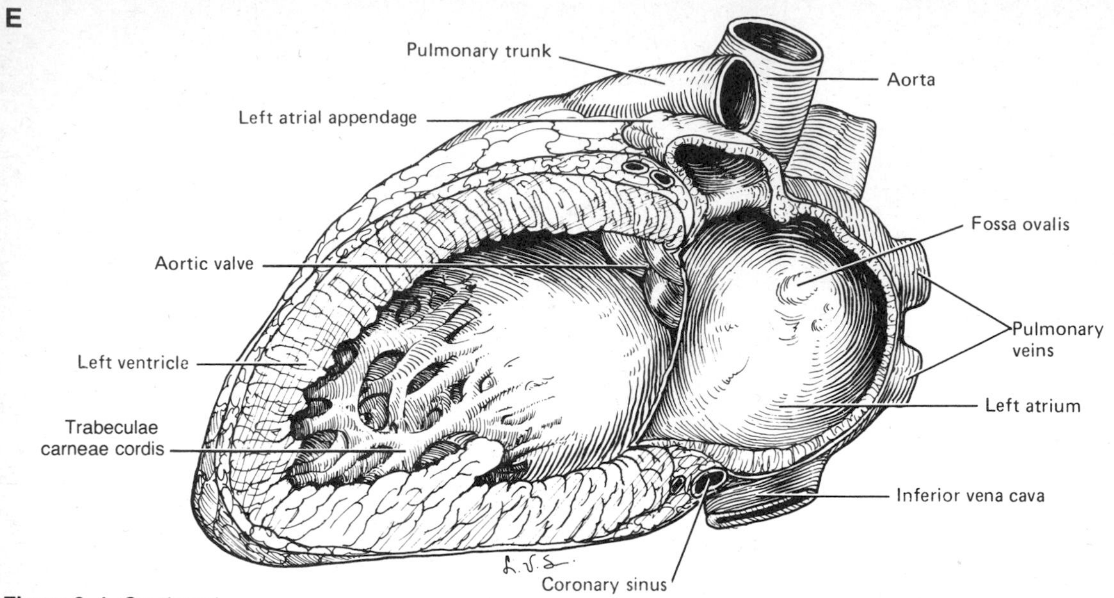

Figure 8–1 *Continued*

a synchronized fashion and minimizes the chance of electrical feedback between the chambers.

The electrical activity of the heart can be measured from the body surface at standardized positions by electrocardiography On the electrocardiogram (ECG), the P wave represents depolarization of atrial tissue; the QRS interval, ventricular depolarization; and the T wave, ventricular repolarization (Figure 8–3). Since normal ventricular depolarization occurs almost simultaneously in the right and left ventricle—usually within 60–100 ms—the QRS complex is narrow. While the electrical activity of the small specialized conduction tissues cannot be measured directly from the surface, the interval between the P wave and start of the QRS complex (PR interval) represents the conduction time of the AV node and His bundle.

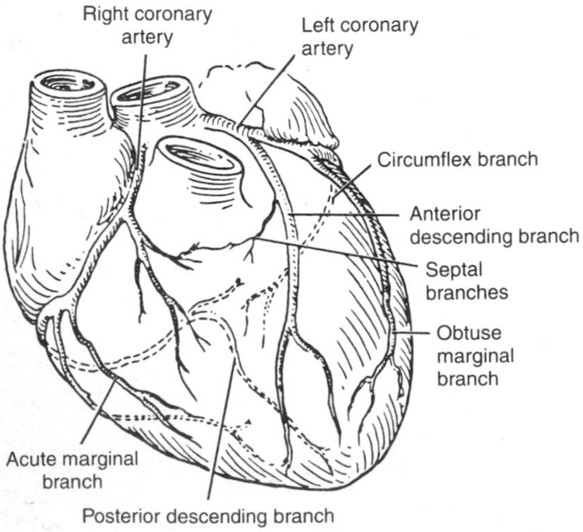

Figure 8–2. Coronary arteries and their principal branches in humans. (Modified and reproduced, with permission, from Ross G: The cardiovascular system. In: *Essentials of Human Physiology.* Ross G [editor]. Copyright © 1978 by Year Book Medical Publishers, Inc., Chicago.)

HISTOLOGY

Ventricular myocytes are normally 50–100 μm long and 10–25 μm wide. Atrial and nodal myocytes are smaller, while myocytes of the Purkinje system are larger in both dimensions. Myocytes are filled with hundreds of parallel striated bundles termed myofibrils. Myofibrils are composed of repeating units termed sarcomeres that form the major contractile unit of the myocyte (Figure 8–4). Sarcomeres are complex structures composed of interdigitating contractile proteins, myosin and actin; and a regulatory protein complex, tropomyosin. (See Cellular Physiology, below.)

PHYSIOLOGY

Physiology of the Whole Heart

Since the ventricles are the primary physiologic pumps of the heart, analysis has focused on the these chambers, particularly the left ventricle. Function of intact ventricles is traditionally studied by evaluating pressure-time and pressure-volume relationships.

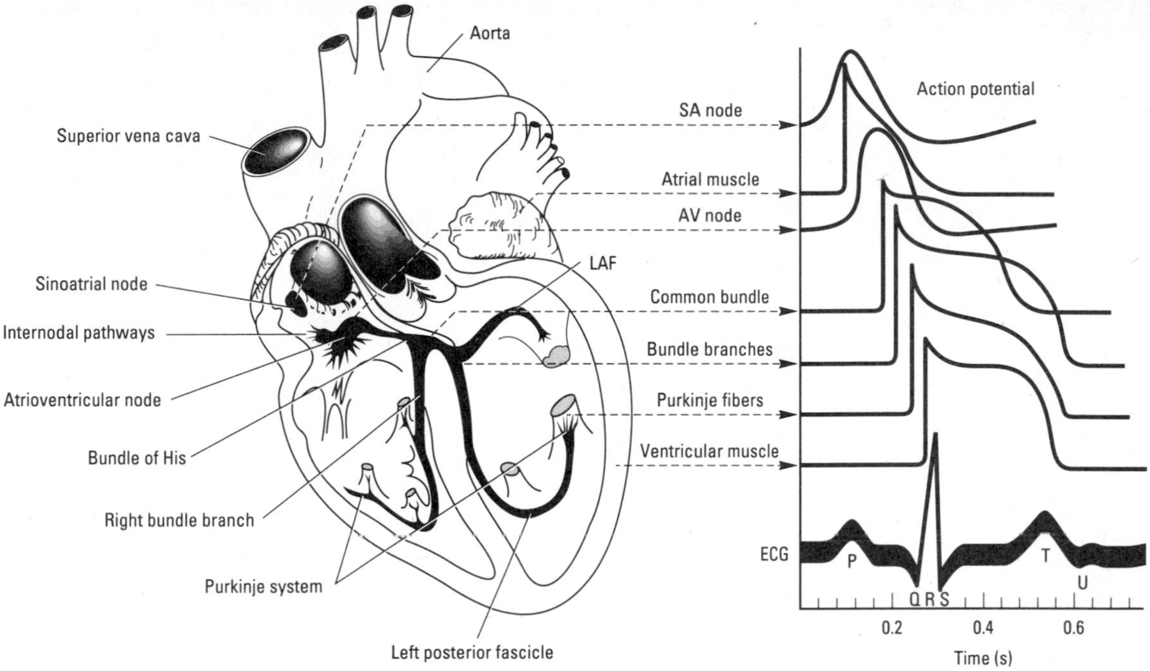

Figure 8–3. Conducting system of the heart. Typical transmembrane action potentials for the SA and AV nodes, other parts of the conduction system, and the atrial and ventricular muscles are shown along with the correlation to the extracellularly recorded electrical activity, ie, the electrocardiogram (ECG). The action potentials and ECG are plotted on the same time axis but with different zero points on the vertical scale. The PR interval is measured from the beginning of the P wave to the beginning of the QRS. (LAF, left anterior fascicle.) (Reproduced, with permission, from Ganong WF: *Review of Medical Physiology,* 16th ed. Appleton & Lange, 1993.)

In **pressure-time analysis** (Figure 8–5), pressures in the chambers of the heart and the great vessels are measured during the cardiac cycle and plotted as a function of time. At the beginning of the cardiac cycle, the left atrium contracts, forcing additional blood into the left ventricle and giving rise to an *a* wave on the left atrial pressure tracing. At end-diastole, the mitral valve closes, producing the first heart sound (S_1), and a brief period of isovolumic contraction follows during which both the aortic and the mitral valve are closed but the left ventricle is actively contracting. When intraventricular pressure rises to the level of aortic pressure, the aortic valve opens and blood flows into the aorta. After this point, the aorta and left ventricle form a contiguous chamber with equal pressures, but left ventricular volume decreases as blood is expelled. Left ventricular contraction stops and ventricular relaxation begins, and end-systole is reached when intraventricular pressure falls below aortic pressure. The aortic valve then closes, and the second heart sound (S_2) is heard. Throughout systole, blood has slowly accumulated in the left atrium (since the mitral valve is closed), giving rise to the *v* wave on the left atrial pressure tracing. During the first phase of diastole—isovolumic relaxation—no change in ventricular volume occurs, but continued relaxation of the ventricle leads to an exponential fall in left ventricular pressure. Left ventricular filling begins when left ventricular pressure falls below left atrial pressure and the mitral valve opens. Ventricular relaxation is a relatively long process that begins before the aortic valve closes and extends past mitral valve opening. The rate and extent of ventricular relaxation depends on multiple factors: heart rate, wall thickness, chamber volume and shape, aortic pressure, sympathetic tone, and the presence or absence of myocardial ischemia. Once the mitral valve opens, there is an initial period of rapid filling of the ventricle that contributes 70–80% of blood volume to the ventricle and occurs largely because of the atrioventricular pressure gradient. By middiastole, flow into the left ventricle has slowed, and the cardiac cycle begins again with the next atrial contraction. Right ventricular pressure-time analysis would be similar, but with lower pressures since the impedance to flow in the pulmonary vascular system is much lower than in the systemic circulation.

In **pressure-volume analysis** (Figure 8–6A), pressure during the cardiac cycle is plotted as a function of volume rather than time. During diastole, as ventricular volume increases during both the initial rapid filling period and atrial contraction, ventricular pressure increases (curve **da**). The shape and position of

A

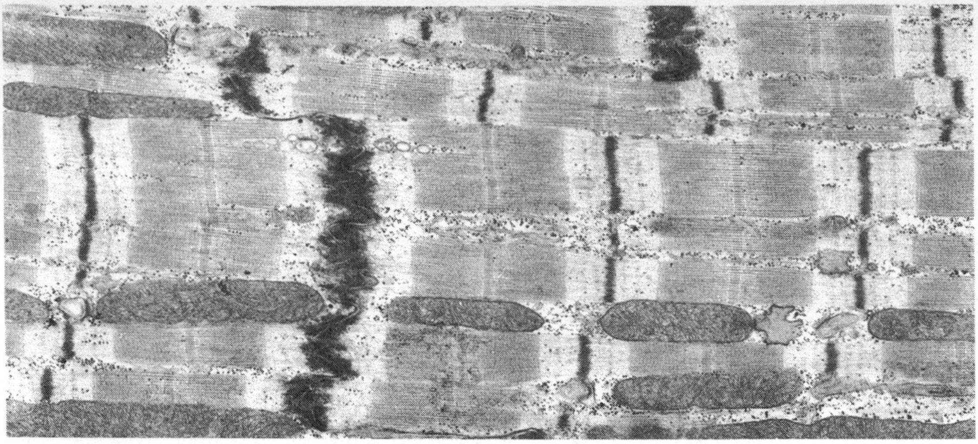

B

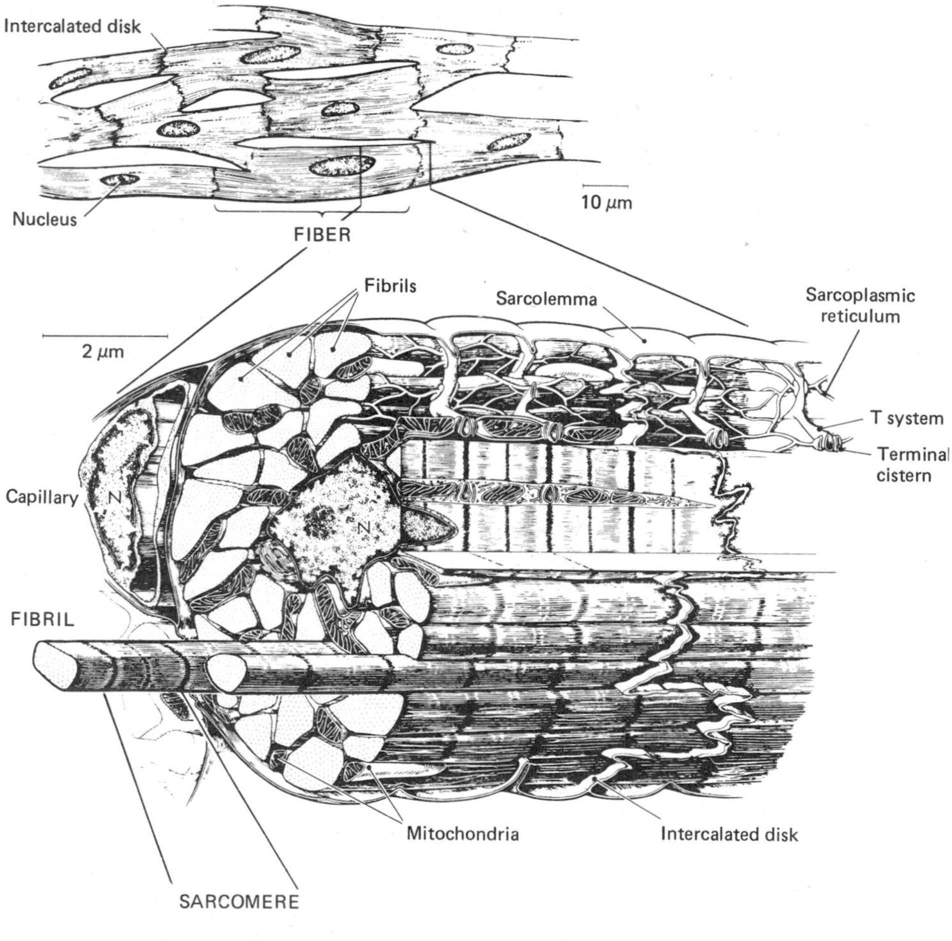
Intercalated disk
Nucleus
FIBER
10 μm
Fibrils
Sarcolemma
Sarcoplasmic reticulum
2 μm
T system
Terminal cistern
Capillary
N
N
FIBRIL
Mitochondria
Intercalated disk
SARCOMERE

C

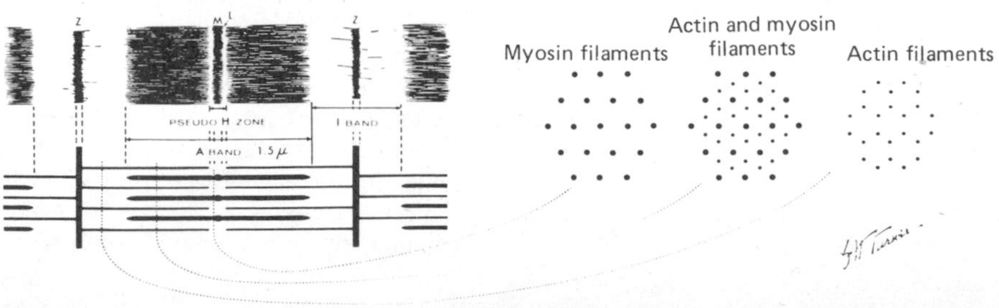
SARCOMERE
CROSS SECTIONS
Myosin filaments
Actin and myosin filaments
Actin filaments
Z
M
Z
PSEUDO H ZONE
I BAND
A BAND 1.5 μ

Figure 8–4. ***A:*** Electron photomicrograph of cardiac muscle. The fuzzy thick lines are intercalated disks (× 12,000). (Reproduced, with permission, from Bloom W. Fawcett DW: *A Textbook of Histology,* 10th ed. Saunders, 1975). ***B:*** Diagram of cardiac muscle as seen under the light microscope ***(top)*** and the electron microscope ***(bottom).*** (N, nucleus.) (Reproduced, with permission, from Braunwald E. Ross J, Sonnenblick EH: Mechanisms of contraction of the normal and failing heart. N Engl J Med 1967;277:794.) ***C:*** An individual sarcomere from a myofibril. ***At left,*** a representation of the arrangement of myofilaments that make up the sarcomere; ***at right,*** cross sections of the sarcomere, showing the specific lattice arrangement of the myofilaments. (Reproduced, with permission, from Braunwald E, Ross J Jr, Sonnenblick EH: Mechanisms of contraction of the normal and failing heart. N Engl J Med 1967;277:794.)

this curve, the **diastolic pressure-volume relationship,** is dependent on relaxation properties of the ventricle, the elastic recoil of the ventricle, and the distensibility of the ventricle. The curve will shift to the left (higher pressure for a given volume) if relaxation of the ventricle is decreased, the ventricle loses elastic recoil, or the ventricle becomes stiffer. At the beginning of systole, active ventricular contraction begins and volume remains unchanged (isovolumic contraction period) (**ab**). When left ventricular pressure reaches aortic pressure, the aortic valve opens, and ventricular volume decreases as the ventricle expels its blood (**bc**). At end-systole (**c**), the aortic valve closes and isovolumic relaxation begins (**cd**). When the mitral valve opens, the ventricle begins filling for the next cardiac cycle, repeating the entire process. The area encompassed by this loop represents the amount of work done by the ventricle during a cardiac cycle. The position of point **c** is dependent on the **isovolumic systolic pressure-volume curve.** If the ventricle is filled with variable amounts of blood (preloads) and allowed to contract but the aortic valve is prevented from opening, a relatively linear relationship exists that is termed the isovolumic systolic pressure-volume curve (Figure 8–6B). The slope and position of this line describes the inherent contractile state of the ventricle. If contractility is increased by catecholamines or other positive inotropes, the line will be shifted to the left (Figure 8–7C).

Pressure-volume relationships help illustrate the effects of different stresses on cardiac output. Cardiac output of the ventricle is the product of the **heart rate** and the volume of blood pumped with each beat (**stroke volume**). The width of the pressure-volume loop is the difference between end-diastolic volume and end-systolic volume, or the stroke volume (Figure 8–6). The stroke volume is dependent on three parameters: contractility, afterload, and preload (Figure 8–7). Changing the contractile state of the heart will change the width of the pressure-volume loop by changing the position of the isovolumic systolic pressure curve. The impedence against which the heart must work is termed **"afterload"**; increased afterload (aortic pressure for the left ventricle) will cause a decrease in stroke volume. **"Preload"** is the amount of filling of the ventricle at end-diastole. Up to a point, the more a myocyte or ventricular chamber is stretched, the more it will contract (**Frank-Starling relationship**), so that increased preload will lead to an increase in stroke volume.

Pressure-time and pressure-volume relationships are critical for understanding the pathophysiologic mechanisms of diseases that affect the entire ventricular chamber function, such as heart failure and valvular abnormalities.

Cellular Physiology

A. Ventricular and Atrial Myocytes: The cellular mechanism of myocyte contraction after electrical stimulation is too complex to be fully addressed in this section, but excellent discussions of electromechanical coupling can be found. Briefly, when the myocyte is stimulated, sodium channels on the cell surface membrane (sarcolemma) open, and sodium flows down its electrochemical gradient into the cell. This sudden inward surge of ions is responsible for the sharp upstoke of the myocyte action potential (phase 0) (Figure 8–8). A plateau phase follows during which the cell membrane potential remains relatively unchanged owing to the inward flow of calcium (Ca^{2+}–L) and outward flow of potassium through specialized potassium (IK current) channels. Repolarization occurs because of continued outward flow of potassium after inward flux of calcium has stopped.

Within the cell, the change in membrane potential from the sudden influx of sodium and the subsequent increase in intracellular calcium causes the sarcoplasmic recticulum to release large numbers of calcium ions. The exact signaling mechanism is not known. Once in the cytoplasm, however, calcium released from the sarcoplasmic reticulum binds with the regulatory proteins troponin and tropomyosin. Myosin and actin are then allowed to interact and form cross-bridges, which gives rise to contraction (Figure 8–9). The process of relaxation is poorly understood also but appears to involve return of calcium to the sarcoplasmic recticulum via a transmembrane SR-embedded protein, phospholamban. Reuptake of calcium is an active process that requires ATP.

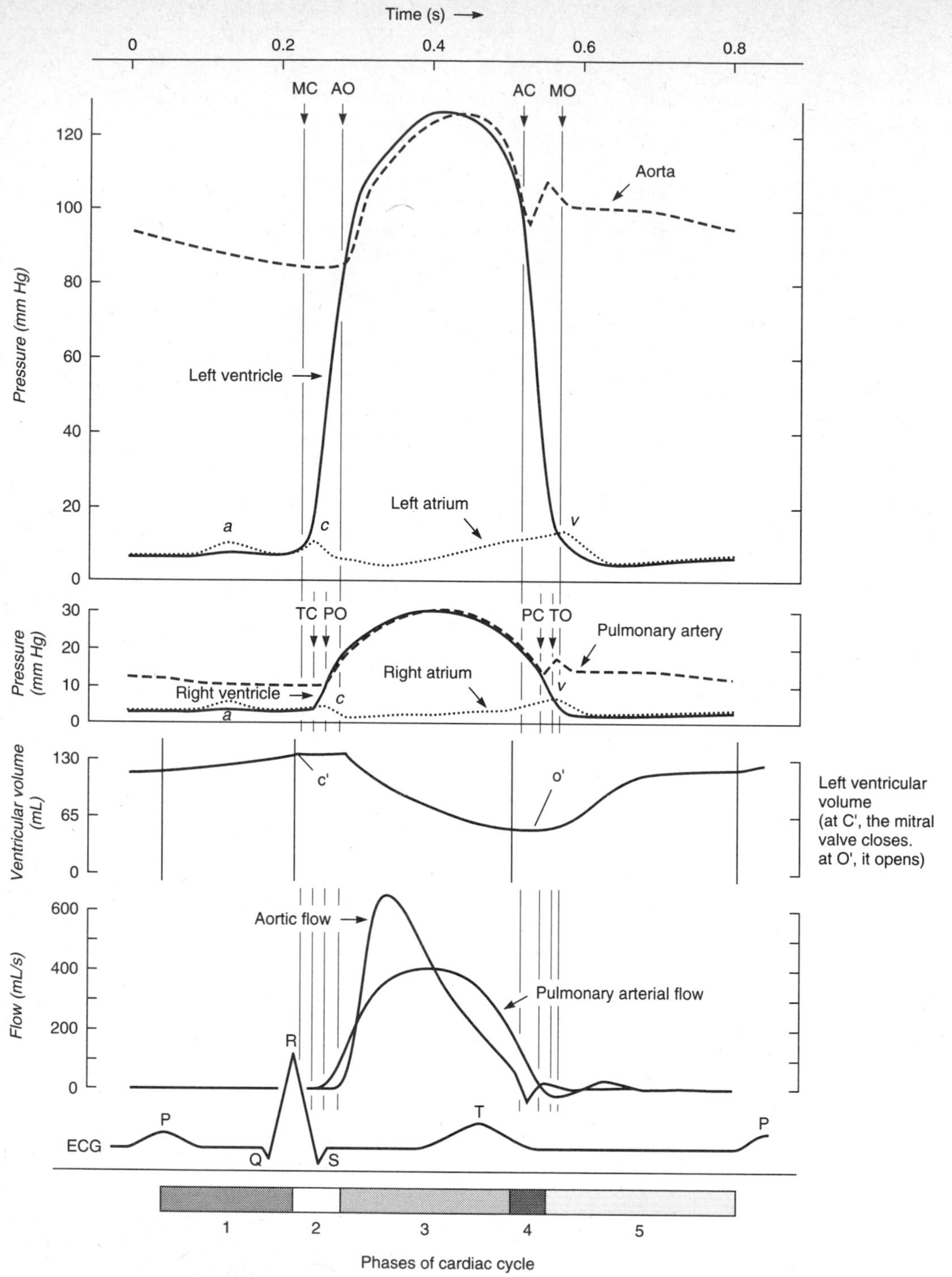

Figure 8–5. Diagram of events in the cardiac cycle (top downward). Pressure (mm Hg) in aorta, left ventricle, left atrium, pulmonary artery, right ventricle, right atrium; blood flow (mL/s) in ascending aorta and pulmonary artery; ECG. Abscissa, time (seconds). (Valvular opening and closing are indicated by AO and AC, respectively, for the aortic valve; MO and MC for the mitral valve; PO and PC for the pulmonary valve; TO and TC for the tricuspid valve.) Events of the cardiac cycle at a heart rate of 75 beats/min. The phases of the cardiac cycle identified by the numbers at the bottom are as follows: 1, atrial systole; 2, isovolumetric ventricular contraction; 3, ventricular ejection; 4, isovolumetric ventricular relaxation; 5, ventricular filling. Note that late in systole, aortic pressure actually exceeds left ventricular pressure, However, the momentum of the blood keeps it flowing out of the ventricle for a short peroid. The pressure relationships in the right ventricle and pulmonary artery are similar. (Atr. syst., atrial systole; Ventric. syst., ventricular systole.) (Modified and reproduced, with permission, from Milnor WR: The circulation. In: *Medical Physiology.* 2 vols. Mountcastle VB [editor]. Mosby, 1980.) and Ganong WF: *Review of Medical Physiology,* 16th ed. Appleton & Lange, 1993.)

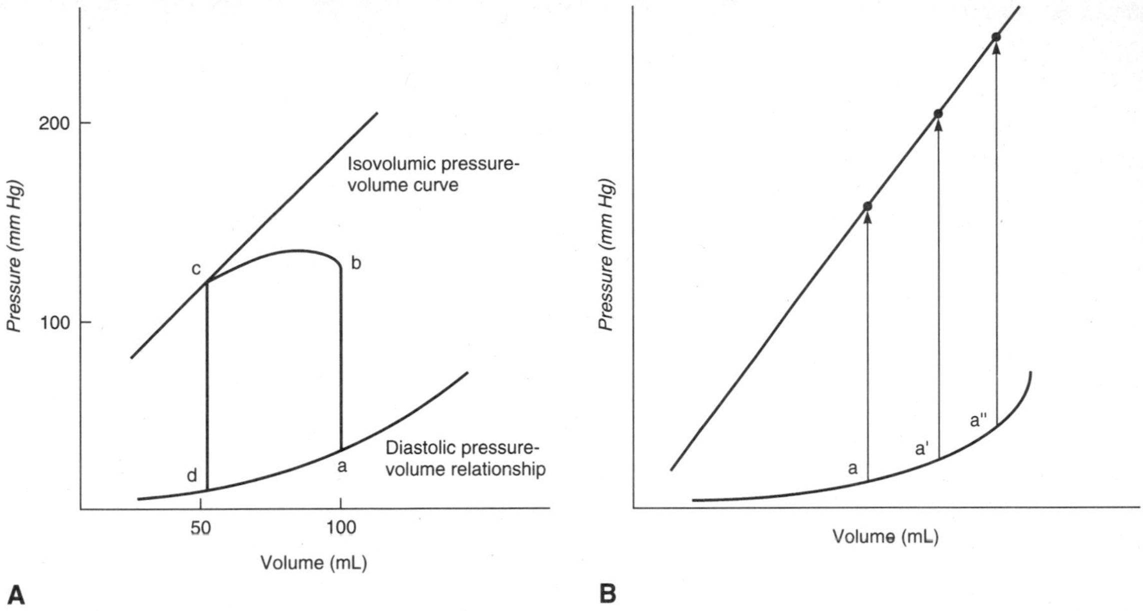

Figure 8–6. ***A:*** Pressure-volume loop for the left ventricle. During diastole the left ventricle fills and pressure increases along the diastolic pressure-volume curve from **d** to **a.** Line **ab** represents isometric contraction, and bc the ejection phase of systole. The aortic valve closes at point **c,** and pressure drops along **cd** (isovolumic relaxation), until the mitral valve opens at point **d** and the cycle repeats. The distance from **b** to **c** represents the stroke volume ejected by that beat. Point **a** represents end-diastole and point **c,** end-systole. ***B:*** If the left ventricle is filled by varying amounts **a, a′, a″,** and allowed to undergo isovolumic contraction, a relatively linear relationship, the isovolumic pressure-volume relation, can be defined.

B. Pacemaker Cells: The action potential of pacemaker cells is different from that described for ventricular and atrial myocytes (Figure 8–8). Fast sodium channels are absent, so that rapid phase 0 depolarization is not observed in SA nodal and AV nodal cells. In addition, these cells are characterized by increased automaticity from a relatively rapid spontaneous phase 4 depolarization. A specialized sodium (Na^+I_f) current and calcium (Ca^{2+}-T) channel may in part be responsible for this dynamic change in membrane potential. Myofibrils are sparse, though present, in the specialized pacemaker cells.

1. What are the differences in pacemaker and conduction properties in different regions of the heart, and why do these differences explain the observation that cardiac electrical impulses normally arise in the SA node?
2. Describe pressure-time analysis through the cardiac cycle.
3. Describe pressure-volume analysis through the cardiac cycle.
4. What are preload and afterload?
5. Briefly describe the molecular mechanism of electro mechanical coupling in cardiac myocyte contraction.

PATHOPHYSIOLOGY OF SELECTED CARDIOVASCULAR DISORDERS

CONGESTIVE HEART FAILURE

Inadequate pump function of the heart, which leads to congestion resulting from fluid in the lungs and peripheral tissues, is a common end result of many disease processes. Congestive heart failure is present in approximately 3 million people in the United States, with more than 400,000 new cases reported annually. The clinical presentation is highly variable; for an individual patient, symptoms and signs depend on how quickly heart failure develops and whether it involves the left, right, or both ventricles.

1. LEFT VENTRICULAR FAILURE

Clinical Presentation

Patients with left ventricular failure most commonly present with a sensation of breathlessness and difficulty breathing (dyspnea), particularly when ly-

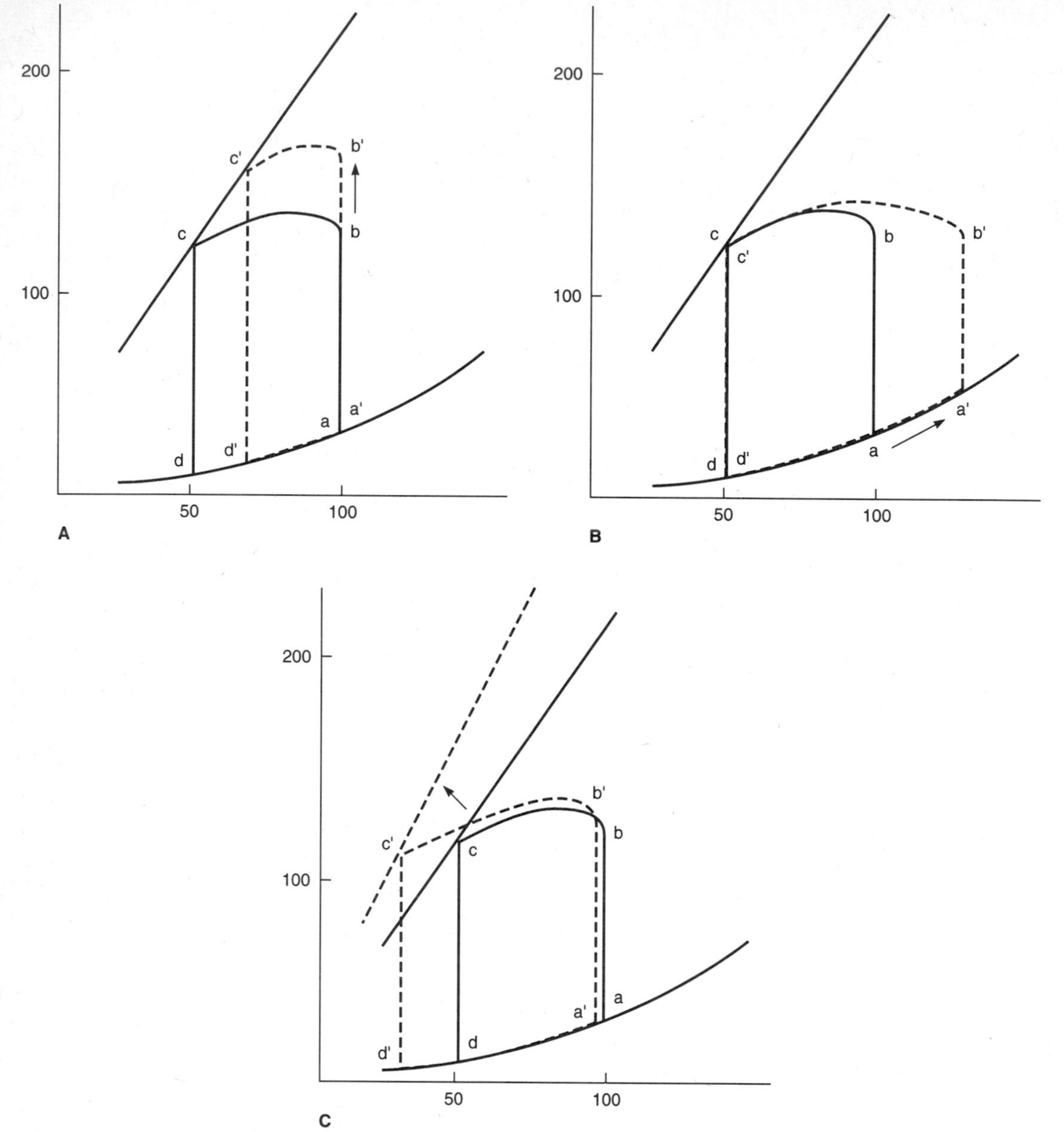

Figure 8–7. ***A:*** Increasing afterload from **b** to **b´** decreases stroke volume from **bc** to **b´c´**. ***B:*** Increasing preload from **a** to **a´** increases stroke volume from **bc** to **b´c´**, but at the expense of increased end-diastolic pressure. ***C:*** Increasing contractile state shifts the isovolumic pressure-volume relationship leftward, increasing stroke volume from **bc** to **b´c´**.

ing down (orthopnea) or at night (paroxysmal nocturnal dyspnea). In addition, the patient may complain of blood-tinged sputum (hemoptysis) and occasionally chest pain. Fatigue, nocturia, and confusion can also be caused by heart failure.

On physical examination, the patient usually has elevated respiratory and heart rates. The skin may be pale, cold, and sweaty. In severe heart failure, palpation of the peripheral pulse may reveal alternating strong and weak beats (pulsus alternans). Auscultation of the lungs reveals abnormal sounds that have been described as "crackling leaves," called rales. In addition, the bases of the lung fields may be dull to percussion. On cardiac examination, the apical impulse is often displaced laterally and sustained. Third and fourth heart sounds can be heard on auscultation of the heart. Since many patients with left ventricular failure also have accompanying fail-

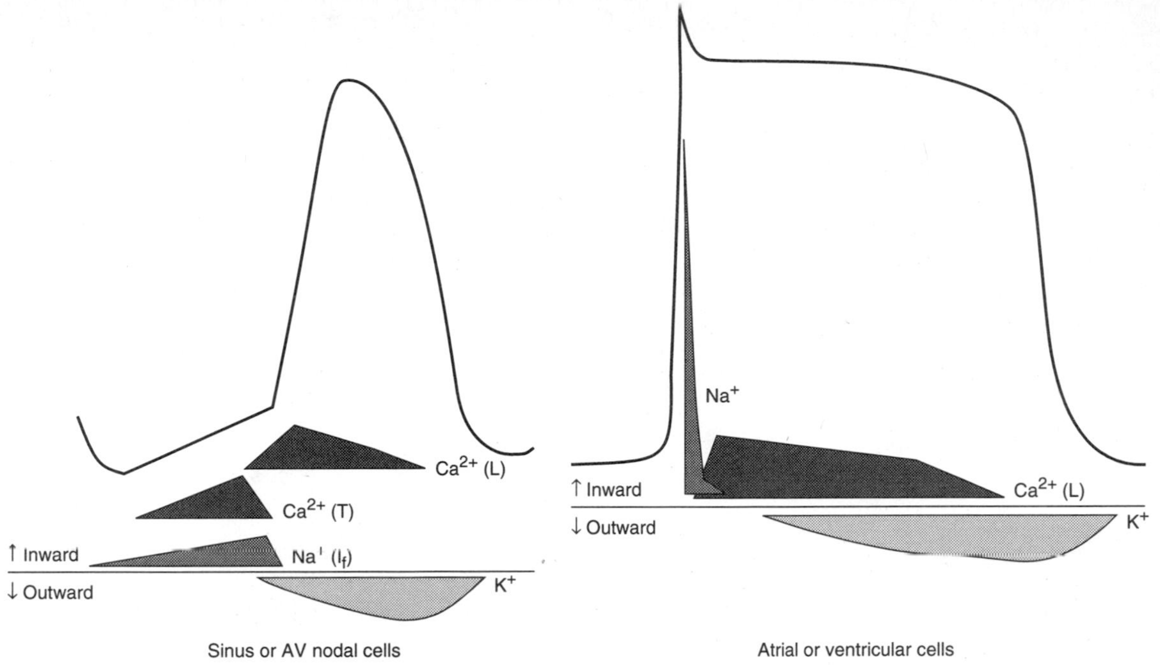

Figure 8–8. Changes in ionic conductances responsible for generating action potentials for ventricular or atrial tissue (right) and a sinus or AV node cell (left). In nodal cells rapid sodium channels are absent, so that the action potential upstroke is much slower. Diastolic depolarization observed in nodal cells is thought to be due to Ca-T channels and or a specialized pacemaker current produced by sodium flow (I_f).

ure of the right ventricle, signs of right ventricular failure may also be present (see next section).

Etiology

Heart failure is a pathophysiologic complex associated with dysfunction of the heart and is a common end point for many diseases of the cardiovascular system. As such, there are many possible causes of heart failure (Table 8–1), and the specific reason for heart failure in a given patient must always be sought. In general, heart failure can be caused by (1) inappropriate workloads placed on the heart, such as volume overload or pressure overload, (2) restricted filling of the heart, (3) myocyte loss, or (4) decreased myocyte contractility.

Pathophysiology

Pathophysiologically, heart failure can arise from worsening systolic or diastolic function or, more frequently, a combination of both. In **systolic dysfunction** the isovolumic systolic pressure curve of the pressure-volume relationship is shifted downward (Figure 8–10A). This reduces the stroke volume of the heart with a concomitant decrease in cardiac output. In order to maintain cardiac output, the heart can respond with three compensatory mechanisms: First, increased return of blood to the heart (preload) can lead to increased contraction of sarcomeres (Frank-Starling relationship). In the pressure-volume relationship, the heart operates at ***a′*** instead of ***a,*** and stroke volume increases—but at the cost of increased end-diastolic pressure (Figure 8–10D). Second, increased release of catecholamines can increase cardiac output both by increasing the heart rate and by shifting the systolic isovolumetric curve leftward (Figure 8–10C). Finally, cardiac muscle can hypertrophy and ventricular volume can increase, which shifts the diastolic curve rightward (Figure 8–10B). While each of these compensatory mechanisms can temporarily maintain cardiac output, each is of limited potential, and if the underlying reason for systolic dysfunction remains untreated, the heart ultimately fails.

In **diastolic dysfunction,** the position of the systolic isovolumic curve remains unchanged (contractility of the myocytes is preserved). However, the diastolic pressure-volume curve is shifted to the left, with an accompanying increase in left ventricular end-diastolic pressure and symptoms of congestive heart failure (Figure 8–11). Diastolic dysfunction can be present in any disease that causes decreased relaxation, decreased elastic recoil, or increased stiffness of the ventricle. Hypertension, which often leads to increases in left ventricular wall thickness, can cause diastolic dysfunction by changing all three parame-

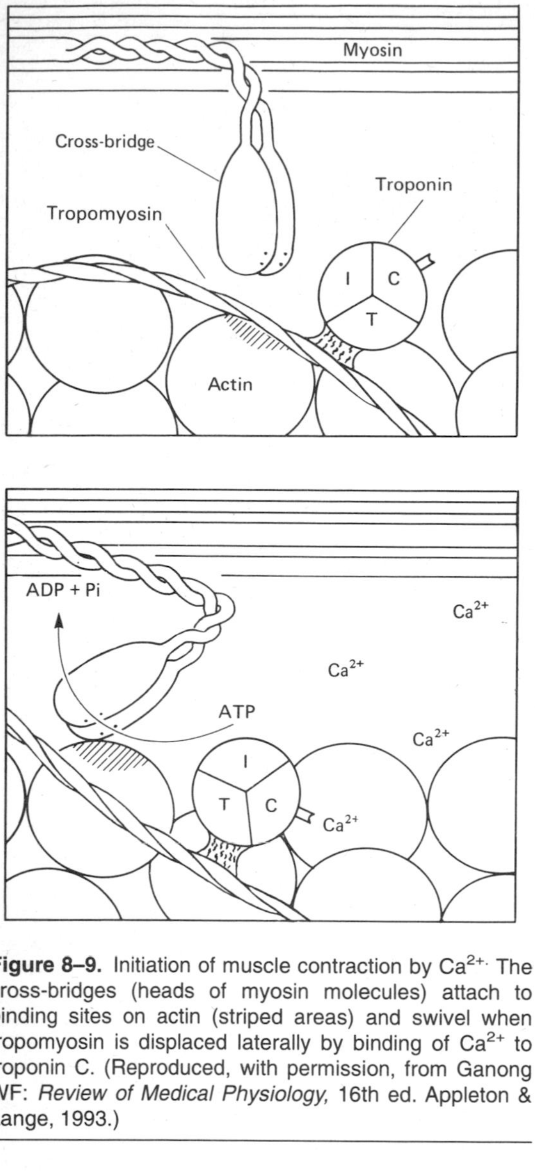

Figure 8–9. Initiation of muscle contraction by Ca^{2+}. The cross-bridges (heads of myosin molecules) attach to binding sites on actin (striped areas) and swivel when tropomyosin is displaced laterally by binding of Ca^{2+} to troponin C. (Reproduced, with permission, from Ganong WF: *Review of Medical Physiology,* 16th ed. Appleton & Lange, 1993.)

ters. Lack of sufficient blood to myocytes (ischemia) can also cause diastolic dysfunction by decreasing relaxation. If ischemia is severe, as in myocardial infarction, irreversible damage to the myocytes can occur, with replacement of contractile cells by fibrosis, which will lead to systolic dysfunction. In most patients, a combination of systolic and diastolic dysfunction is responsible for the symptoms of heart failure.

Table 8–1. Causes of left ventricular failure.

Volume overload	
	Regurgitant valves (mitral or aortic)
	High-output states: Anemia, hyperthyroidism
Pressure overload	
	Systemic hypertension
	Outflow obstruction: Aortic stenosis, asymmetric septal hypertrophy
Loss of muscle	
	Myocardial infarction from coronary artery disease
	Connective tissue disease: systemic lupus erythematosus
Loss of contractility	
	Poisons: Alcohol, cobalt, doxorubicin
	Infections: Viral, bacterial
Restricted filling	
	Mitral stenosis
	Pericardial disease: Constrictive pericarditis and pericardial tamponade
	Infiltrative diseases: Amyloidosis

Clinical Manifestations

A. Symptoms:

1. Shortness of breath, orthopnea, paroxysmal nocturnal dyspnea–Although many details of the physiologic mechanisms for the sensation of breathlessness are unclear, the inciting event probably is a rise in pulmonary capillary pressures as a consequence of elevated left ventricular and atrial pressures. The rise in pulmonary capillary pressure relative to plasma oncotic pressure causes fluid to move into the interstitial spaces of the lung (pulmonary edema), which can be seen on chest x-ray (Figure 8–12). Interstitial edema probably stimulates juxtacapillary J receptors, which in turn causes reflex shallow and rapid breathing. Replacement of air in the lungs by blood or interstitial fluid can cause a reduction of vital capacity, restrictive physiology, and air trapping due to closure of small airways. The work of breathing increases as the patient tries to distend stiff lungs, which can lead to respiratory muscle fatigue and the sensation of dyspnea. Alterations in the distribution of ventilation and perfusion result in relative ventilation/perfusion ($\dot{V}/\dot{Q}$) mismatch, with the consequent widening of the alveolar-arterial O_2 gradient, hypoxemia, and increased dead space. Edema of the bronchial walls can lead to small airway obstruction and produce wheezing ("cardiac asthma"). Shortness of breath occurs in the recumbent position (orthopnea) because of reduced blood pooling in the extremities and abdomen–and, since the patient is operating on the steep portion of the diastolic pressure-volume curve, any increase in blood return leads to marked elevations in ventricular pressures. Patients usually learn to minimize orthopnea by sleeping with the upper body propped up by two or more pillows. Sudden onset of severe respiratory distress at night—"paroxysmal nocturnal dyspnea"—probably occurs because of the reduced adrenergic support of ventricular function that occurs with sleep, the increase in blood return as described above, and normal nocturnal depression of the respiratory center.

2. Fatigue, confusion–Fatigue probably arises because of inability of the heart to supply appropriate amounts of blood to skeletal muscles. Confusion may arise in advanced heart failure because of underperfusion of the cerebrum.

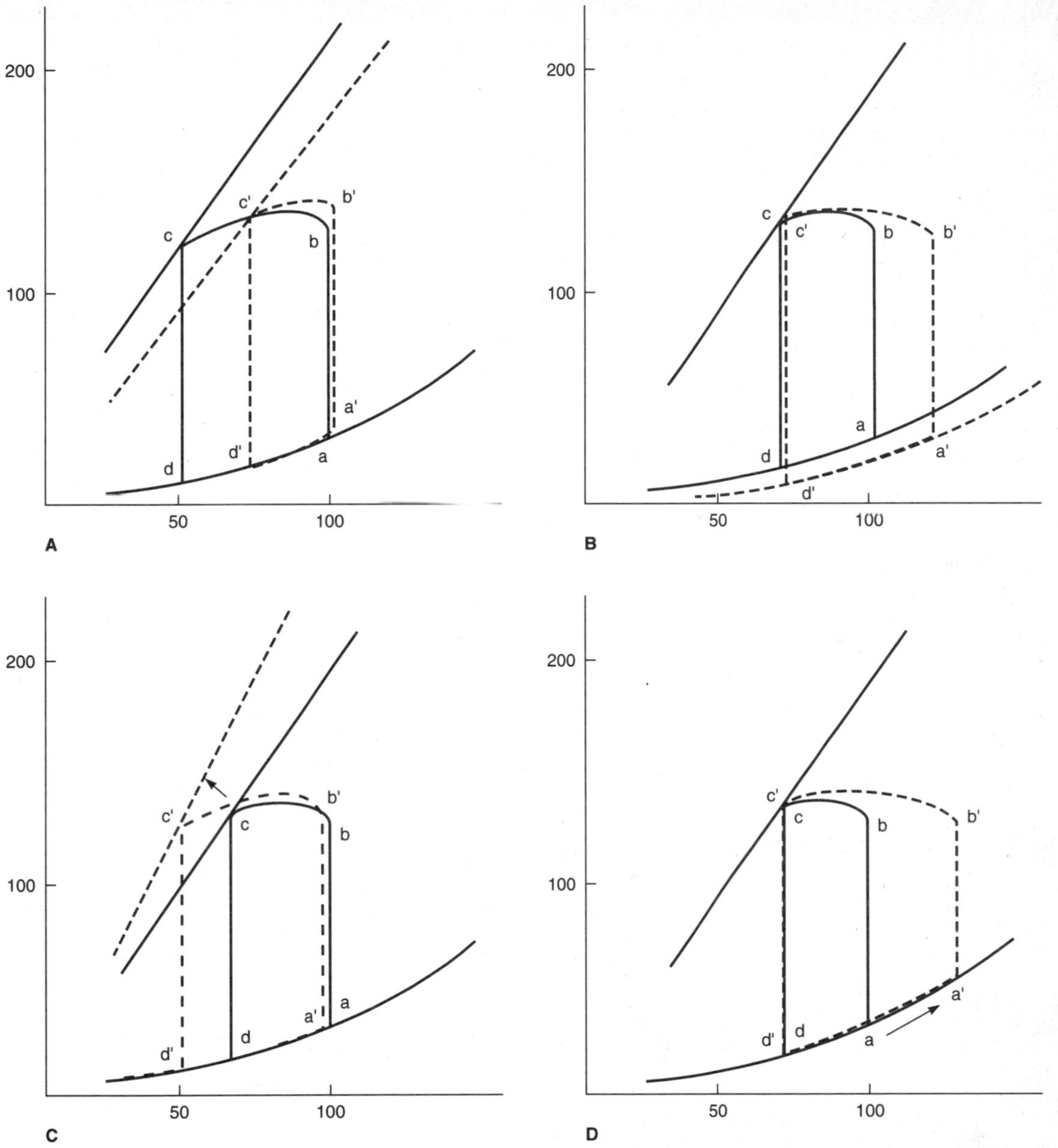

Figure 8–10. ***A:*** Systolic dysfunction is represented by shifting of the isovolumic pressure-volume curve to the right (dashed line), thus decreasing stroke volume. The ventricle can compensate by ***(B)*** shifting the diastolic pressure-volume relationship rightward (dashed line) by increasing left ventricular volume or elasticity, ***(C)*** increasing contractile state (dashed line) by activation of circulating catecholamines, and ***(D)*** by increasing filling or preload (**a** to **a´**).

3. Nocturia–Heart failure can lead to reduced renal perfusion during the day while the patient is upright, which normalizes only at night while the patient is supine, with consequent diuresis.

4. Chest Pain–If the cause of failure is coronary artery disease, patients may have chest pain secondary to ischemia (angina pectoris). In addition, even without ischemia, acute heart failure can cause chest pain from unknown mechanisms.

B. Physical Examination:

1. Rales, pleural effusion–Increased fluid in the alveolar spaces from the mechanisms described above can be heard as rales. Increased capillary pressures can also cause fluid accumulation in the pleural spaces.

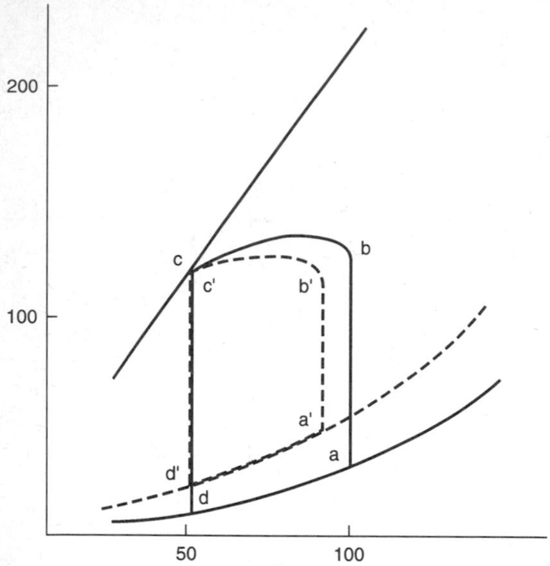

Figure 8–11. In diastolic dysfunction, the diastolic pressure-volume relation is shifted upward and to the left, which leads to an elevated left ventricular end-diastolic pressure **a´** and reduced stroke volume.

2. Displaced and sustained apical impulse– In most people, contraction of the heart can be appreciated by careful palpation of the chest wall (apical impulse). The normal apical impulse is felt in the midclavicular line in the fourth or fifth intercostal space and is palpable only during the first part of systole. When the apical impulse can be felt during the latter part of systole, it is sustained. Sustained impulses suggest that increases in left ventricular volume or mass are present. In addition, when left ventricular volume is increased as a compensatory mechanism of heart failure, the apical impulse will be displaced laterally.

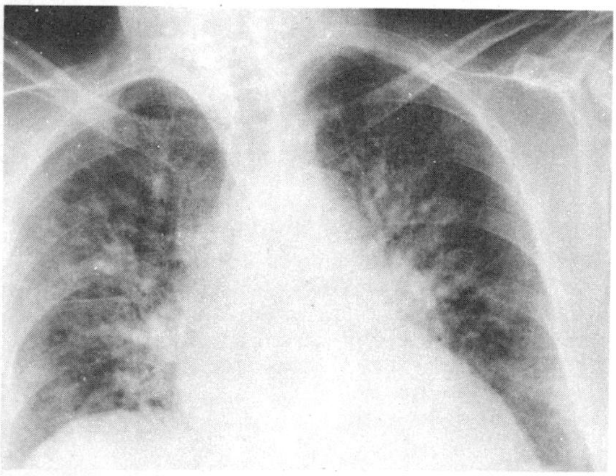

Figure 8–12. Posteroanterior chest x-ray in a man with acute pulmonary edema due to left ventricular failure. Note the bat's wing density, cardiac enlargement, increased flow to upper lobes, and pulmonary venous congestion. (Reproduced, with permission, from Cheitlin MD, Sokolow M, McIlroy MB: *Clinical Cardiology,* 6th ed. Appleton & Lange, 1993.)

3. Third heart sound (S_3)–The third heart sound is a low-pitched sound that is heard during rapid filling of the ventricle in early diastole (Figure 8–13A). The exact mechanism for the genesis of the third heart sound is not known, but the sound appears to result either from the sudden deceleration of blood as the elastic limits of the ventricular chamber are reached or from the actual impact of the ventricular wall against the chest wall. Although a third heart sound is normal in children and young adults, it is rarely heard in healthy adults over 40 years of age. The presence of a third heart sound is almost pathognomonic for ventricular failure in such adults. The increased end-systolic volumes and pressures characteristic of the failing heart are probably responsible for the prominent third heart sound. When it arises because of left ventricular failure, the third heart sound is usually heard best at the apex. It can be present in patients with either diastolic or systolic dysfunction.

4. Fourth heart sound (S_4)–Normally, sounds arising from atrial contraction are not heard. However, if there is increased stiffness of the ventricle, a low-pitched sound at end-diastole that occurs concomitantly with atrial contraction can sometimes be heard (Figure 8–13B). Like the third heart sound, the exact mechanism for the genesis of the fourth heart sound is not known. However, it probably arises from the sudden deceleration of blood in a noncompliant ventricle or from sudden impact of a stiff ventricle against the chest wall. It is best heard laterally at the apical impulse, particularly when the patient is rolled over onto the left side (left lateral decubitus position). The fourth heart sound is commonly heard in any patient with heart failure due to diastolic dysfunction.

5. Pale, cold, and sweaty skin–Patients with severe heart failure often have peripheral vasoconstriction, which maintains blood flow to the central organs and head. In some cases, the skin appears dusky because of reduced oxygen content in venous blood as a result of increased oxygen extraction from peripheral tissues that are receiving low blood flow. Sweating occurs because body heat cannot be dissipated through the constricted vascular bed of the skin.

2. RIGHT VENTRICULAR FAILURE

Clinical Presentation

Symptoms of right ventricular failure include shortness of breath, pedal edema, and abdominal pain.

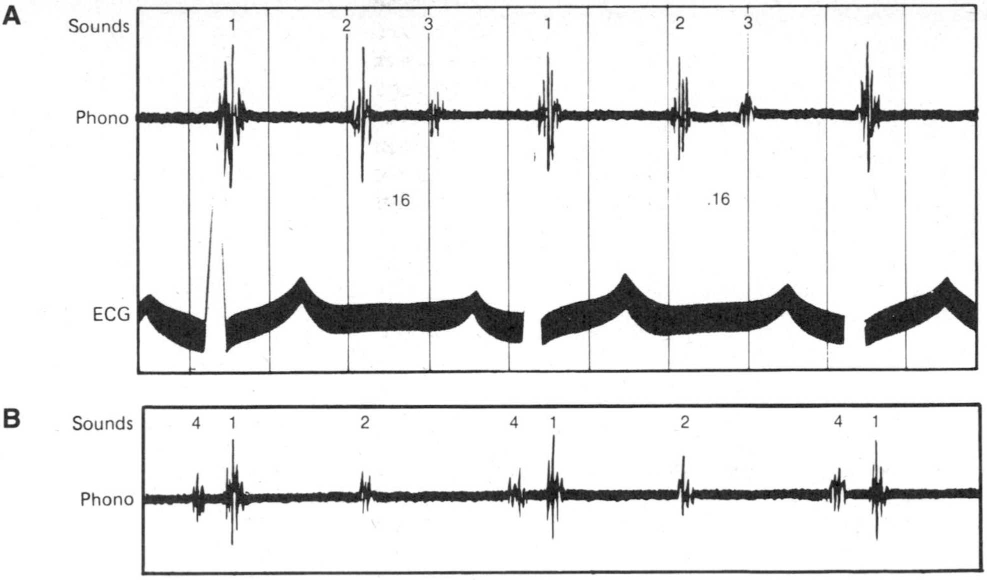

Figure 8–13. ***A:*** Phonocardiogram showing typical third heart sound (S_3). It follows the second sound (S_2) by 0.16 s. (Courtesy of Roche Laboratories Division of Hoffman-La Roche, Inc.) ***B:*** Phonocardiogram showing a fourth heart sound (S_4) and its relation to first sound (S_1).

The findings on physical examination are similar to those of left ventricular failure but in different positions, since the right ventricle is anatomically anterior and to the right of the left ventricle (Figure 8–1). Patients with right ventricular failure may have a third heart sound heard best at the sternal border or a sustained systolic heave of the sternum. Inspection of the neck reveals elevated jugular venous pressures. Since the most common cause of right ventricular failure is left ventricular failure, signs of left ventricular failure are often also present.

Etiology

Right ventricular failure can be due to several causes. As just mentioned, left ventricular failure can cause right ventricular failure because of the increased afterload placed on the right ventricle. Increased afterload can also be present from abnormalities of the pulmonary arteries or capillaries. For example, increased flow from a congenital shunt can cause reactive pulmonary artery constriction, increased right ventricular afterload, and, ultimately, right ventricular failure. Right ventricular failure can occur as a sequela to pulmonary disease (cor pulmonale) because of destruction of the pulmonary capillary bed or hypoxia-induced vasoconstriction of the pulmonary arterioles. Right ventricular failure can also be caused by right ventricular ischemia, usually in the setting of an inferior wall myocardial infarction (Table 8–2).

Table 8–2. Causes of right ventricular failure.

Type	Comments
Left-sided failure	Most common cause
Precapillary obstruction	
Congenital (shunts, obstruction)	Vasoconstriction of the pulmonary arteries occurs in response to increased flow
Idiopathic pulmonary hypertension	Also known as primary pulmonary hypertension
Primary right ventricular failure	
Right ventricular infarction	Can occur with obstruction of the right coronary artery. Often associated with inferior wall myocardial infarction.
Cor pulmonale	
Hypoxia-induced vasoconstriction	
Pulmonary embolism	
Chronic obstructive lung disease	

Pathophysiology

The pathophysiology of right ventricular failure is similar to that described for the left ventricle. Both systolic and diastolic abnormalities of the right ventricle can be present and usually occur because of inappropriate loads placed on the ventricle, or primary loss of myocyte contractility.

Patients with isolated right ventricular failure (pulmonary hypertension, cor pulmonale) can have a mechanical reason for left ventricular failure. The interventricular septum is usually bowed toward the thinner-walled and lower-pressure right ventricle. When right ventricular pressure increases relative to the left, the interventricular septum can bow to the left and prevent efficient filling of the left ventricle, which may lead to pulmonary congestion. Rarely, the bowing can be so severe that left ventricular outflow can be partially obstructed. This phenomenon is termed a "reversed Bernheim effect."

Clinical Manifestations

A. Shortness of Breath: If there is left ventricular failure, patients may be short of breath because of pulmonary edema as discussed above. In patients with right-sided failure due to pulmonary disease, shortness of breath may be a manifestation of the underlying disease (eg, pulmonary embolus, chronic obstructive pulmonary disease). In some patients with right ventricular failure, congestion of the hepatic veins with formation of ascites can impinge on normal diaphragmatic function and contribute to the sensation of dyspnea. In addition, reduced right-sided cardiac output alone can cause acidosis, hypoxia, and air hunger. If the cause of right-sided failure is a left-sided defect such as mitral stenosis, the onset of right heart failure can sometimes lessen the symptoms of pulmonary edema because of the decreased load placed on the left ventricle.

B. Elevated Jugular Venous Pressure: The position of venous pulsations of the internal jugular vein can be observed during examination of the neck (Figure 8–14A). The distance above the heart at which venous pulsations are observed is an estimate of the right atrial or central venous pressure. Since the position of the right atrium cannot be precisely determined, the height of the jugular venous pulsation is measured relative to the angle of Louis on the sternum. Right atrial pressure can then be approximated by adding 5 cm to the height of the venous column (since the right atrium is approximately 5 cm inferior to the angle). Jugular venous pulsations are usually observed less than 7 cm above the right atrium. Elevated atrial pressures are present any time this distance is greater than 10 cm. Elevated atrial pressures indicate that the preload of the ventricle is adequate but ventricular function is decreased and fluid is accumulating in the venous system. Other causes of elevated jugular pressures besides heart failure include pericardial tamponade, constrictive pericarditis, and massive pulmonary embolus.

In addition to relative position, individual waveforms of the jugular venous pulse can be assessed. Three positive waves (*a*, *c*, and *v*) and two negative waves (*x* and *y*) can be recognized (Figure 8–14B).

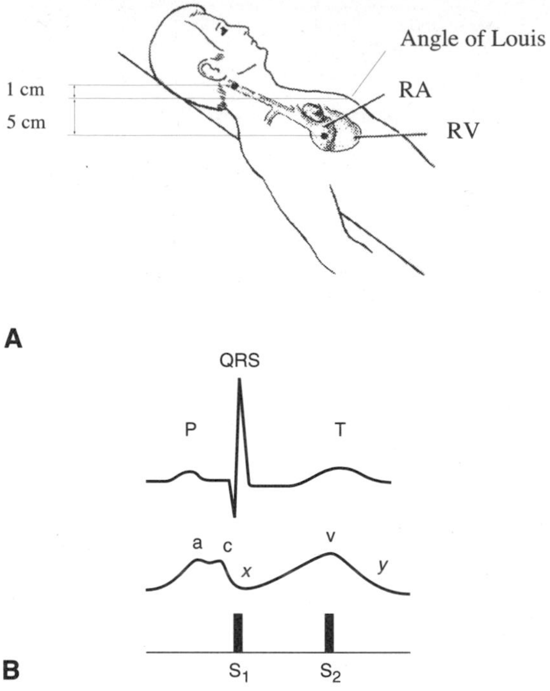

Figure 8–14. ***A:*** Examination of jugular venous pulse and estimation of venous pressure. (RA, right atrium; RV, right ventricle.) ***B:*** Jugular venous pressure waveforms in relation to the electrocardiogram (P wave, QRS, and T wave) and the first and second heart sounds (S_1 and S_2). The bottom of the *x* descent occurs coincident with the first heart sound (S_1). The *v* wave occurs just after the apical impulse is felt at the same time the second heart sound (S_2) is heard. See text for further explanation of jugular venous wave forms.

The *a* wave is caused by transmitted right atrial pressure from atrial contraction. The *c* wave is usually not present on bedside examination; it is thought to arise from bulging of the tricuspid valve during isovolumic contraction of the right ventricle. The *x* descent is thought to be due to atrial relaxation and downward displacement of the tricuspid annulus during systole. The *v* wave arises from continued filling of the right atrium during the latter part of systole. Once the tricuspid valve opens, blood flows into the right ventricle and the *y* descent begins. Evaluation of the individual wave forms will become particularly important when pericardial disease is discussed.

C. Anasarca, Ascites, Pedal Edema, Hepatojugular Reflux, Abdominal Pain: Elevated right-sided pressures leads to accumulation of fluid in the systemic venous circulation. Venous congestion can be manifested by generalized edema (anasarca), ascites (collection of fluid in the peritoneal space), and dependent edema (swelling of the feet and legs). Pressing on the liver for approximately 5 seconds can lead to displacement of blood into the vena cava; when the right ventricle cannot accommodate this additional volume, an increase in jugular venous pressure ("hepatojugular reflux") can be observed. Expansion of the liver from fluid accumulation can cause distention of the liver capsule with accompanying right upper quadrant abdominal pain.

6. What are the clinical presentations of CHF? Of right ventricular failure?
7. What are the four general categories which account for almost all causes of CHF?
8. Explain the differences between the pathophysiology of CHF due to systolic vs diastolic dysfunction.
9. What are the major clinical manifestations and complications of left- vs right-sided heart failure?

VALVULAR HEART DISEASE

Dysfunctional cardiac valves can be classified as either narrow (stenosis) or leaky (regurgitation). While the tricuspid and pulmonary valves can become dysfunctional in patients with endocarditis, congenital lesions, or carcinoid syndrome, primary right-sided valvular abnormalities are relatively rare and will not be discussed further. In this section, the pathophysiologic mechanisms of stenotic and regurgitant aortic and mitral valves will be addressed.

A general classification of heart murmurs is presented in Figure 8–15. Any disease process that creates turbulent flow in the heart or great vessels can cause a murmur. For instance, ventricular septal defect is associated with a systolic murmur because of the abnormal interventricular connection and the pressure difference between the left and right ventricle; patent ductus arteriosus is associated with a continuous murmur because of a persistent connection between the pulmonary artery and the aorta. However, valvular lesions are the principal cause of heart murmurs. Thus, an understanding of heart murmurs gives insight into the underlying pathophysiologic processes of specific valvular lesions.

Heart murmurs can be either systolic or diastolic. During systole, while the left ventricle is contracting, the aortic valve is open and the mitral valve is closed. Turbulent flow can occur either because of an incompetent mitral valve, leading to regurgitation of blood back into the atrium, or from a narrowed aortic valve. In diastole, the situation is reversed, with filling of the left ventricle through an open mitral valve while the aortic valve is closed. Turbulent flow occurs when there is narrowing of the mitral valve or incompetence of the aortic valve. Stenosis of valves usually develops slowly over time; lesions that cause valvular regurgitation can be either chronic or acute.

1. AORTIC STENOSIS

Clinical Presentation

For all causes of aortic stenosis, there is usually a long latent period of slowly increasing obstruction before symptoms appear. In descending order of frequency, the three characteristic symptoms of aortic stenosis are chest pain (angina pectoris), syncope, and congestive heart failure (see above). Once symptoms occur, the prognosis is poor if the obstruction is untreated, with life expectancies of 5, 3, and 2 years for angina pectoris, syncope, and heart failure, respectively.

On physical examination, palpation of the carotid upstroke reveals a pulsation (pulsus) that is both decreased (parvus) and late (tardus) relative to the apical impulse. Palpation of the chest reveals an apical impulse that is laterally displaced and sustained. On auscultation, a midsystolic murmur is heard, loudest at the base of the heart, and often with radiation to the sternal notch and the neck. Depending on the cause of the aortic stenosis, a crisp, relatively high-pitched aortic ejection sound can be heard just after the first heart sound. Finally, a fourth heart sound (S_4) is often present.

Etiology

Various causes of aortic stenosis are listed and described in Table 8–3 and Figure 8–16.

Pathophysiology

The normal aortic valve area is approximately 3.5–4 cm^2. As the narrowing slowly increases, critical aortic stenosis is usually defined when the area is less than 0.8 cm^2. At this point, the systolic gradient between the left ventricle and the aorta can exceed 150 mm Hg, and most patients are symptomatic (Figure 8–17A). The fixed outflow obstruction places a large afterload on the ventricle. The compensatory mechanisms of the heart can be understood by examining Laplace's law for a sphere, where wall stress (σ) is proportionate to the product of systolic pressure (P) and cavitary radius (r) and inversely proportionate to wall thickness (h):

$$\sigma \propto P \times \frac{r}{h}$$

In response to the pressure overload (increased P), left ventricular wall thickness markedly increases, while cavitary radius remains relatively unchanged, by parallel replication of sarcomeres. These compensatory changes, termed "concentric hypertrophy," are an attempt to minimize the increase in wall tension observed in aortic stenosis (see Aortic Regurgitation). Analysis of pressure-volume loops

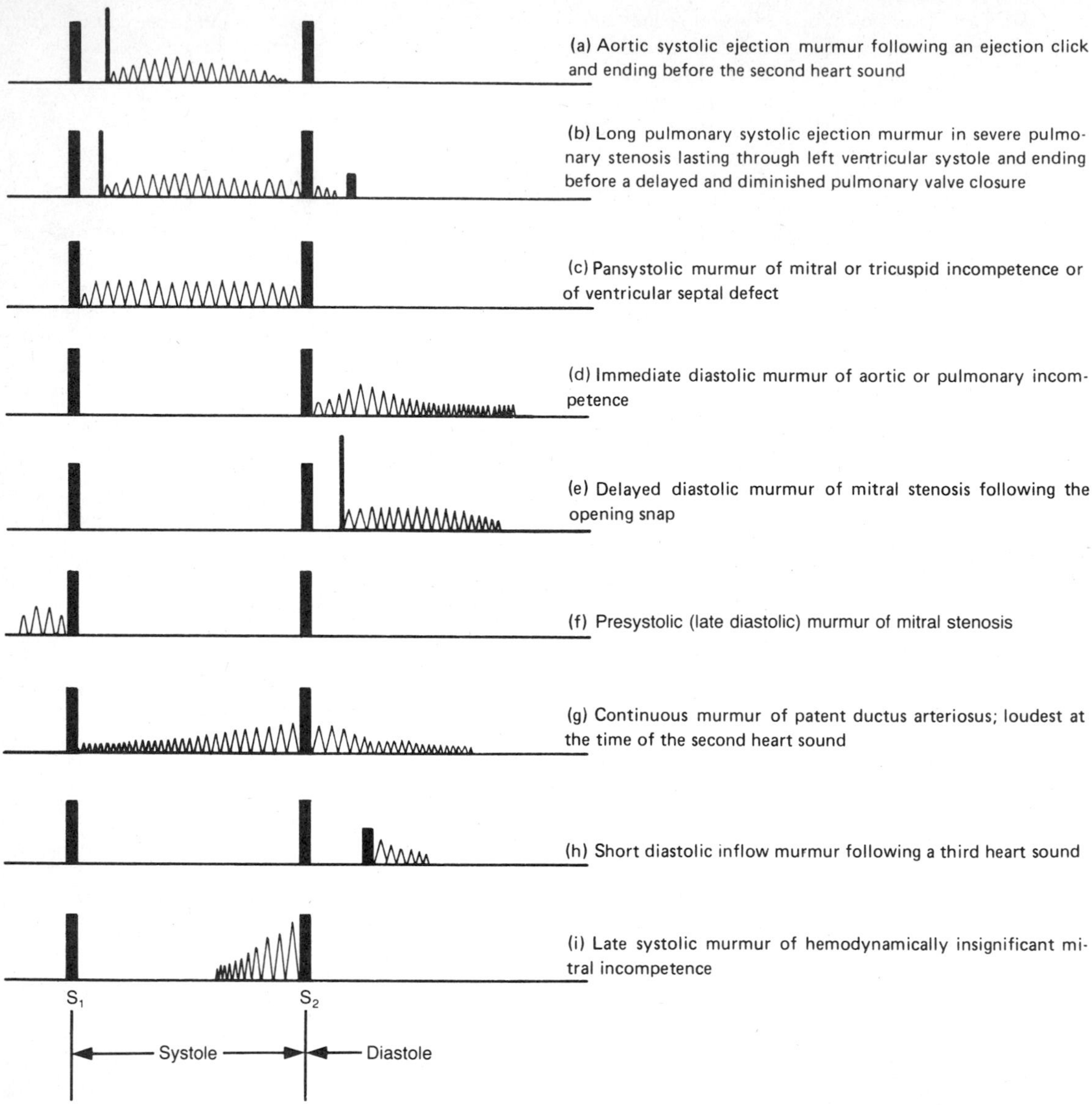
(a) Aortic systolic ejection murmur following an ejection click and ending before the second heart sound
(b) Long pulmonary systolic ejection murmur in severe pulmonary stenosis lasting through left ventricular systole and ending before a delayed and diminished pulmonary valve closure
(c) Pansystolic murmur of mitral or tricuspid incompetence or of ventricular septal defect
(d) Immediate diastolic murmur of aortic or pulmonary incompetence
(e) Delayed diastolic murmur of mitral stenosis following the opening snap
(f) Presystolic (late diastolic) murmur of mitral stenosis
(g) Continuous murmur of patent ductus arteriosus; loudest at the time of the second heart sound
(h) Short diastolic inflow murmur following a third heart sound
(i) Late systolic murmur of hemodynamically insignificant mitral incompetence
S1
S2
Systole
Diastole

Figure 8–15. The timing of the principal cardiac murmurs. (Modified and reproduced, with permission, from Wood P: *Diseases of the Heart and Circulation,* 3rd ed. Lippincott, 1968.)

reveals that in order to maintain stroke volume and because of decreases in ventricular compliance, left ventricular end-diastolic pressure increases significantly (Figure 8–17C). The thick ventricle leads to a prominent *a* wave on left atrial pressure tracings as the ventricle becomes more dependent on atrial contraction to fill the ventricle.

Clinical Manifestations

A. Symptoms:

1. Angina pectoris–Angina can occur because of several mechanisms. First, approximately half of all patients with aortic stenosis have significant concomitant coronary artery disease. Even without significant coronary artery disease, the combination of increased oxygen demands because of ventricular hypertrophy and decreased supply due to excessive compression of the vessels can lead to relative ischemia of the myocytes. Finally, coronary artery obstruction from calcium emboli arising from a calcified stenotic aortic valve has been reported, though it is an uncommon cause of angina.

2. Syncope–Syncope in aortic stenosis is usually due to decreased cerebral perfusion from the fixed obstruction, but it may also occur because of transient atrial arrhythmias with loss of effective atrial

Table 8–3. Causes of aortic stenosis.

Type	Pathology	Clinical Presentation
Congenital	The valve can be unicuspid, bicuspid, or tricuspid with partially fused leaflets. Abnormal flow can lead to fibrosis and calcification of the leaflets.	Patient usually develops symptoms before age 30.
Rheumatic	Tissue inflammation results in adhesion and fusing of the commissures. Fibrosis and calcification of the leaflet tips can occur because of continued turbulent flow.	Patient usually develops symptoms between ages 30 and 70. Often the valve will also be regurgitant. Accompanying mitral valve disease is frequently present.
Degenerative	Leaflets become inflexible because of calcium deposition at the bases. The leaflet tips remain relatively normal.	The most likely cause of aortic stenosis in patients over age 70. Particularly prevalent in patients with diabetes or hypercholesterolemia.

contribution to ventricular filling. In addition, arrhythmias arising from ventricular tissues are more common in patients with aortic stenosis and can cause syncope.

3. Congestive heart failure–(See Heart Failure.) The progressive increase in left ventricular end-diastolic pressure can cause elevated pulmonary venous pressure and pulmonary edema.

B. Physical Examination: Since there is a fixed obstruction to flow, the carotid upstroke is decreased and late. Left ventricular hypertrophy causes the apical impulse to be displaced laterally and become sustained. The increased dependence on atrial contraction is responsible for the prominent S_4. Flow through the restricted orifice gives rise to a midsystolic murmur. The murmur is usually heard best at the base of the heart but often radiates to the neck and apex. The murmur is usually crescendo-decrescendo, and, in contrast to mitral regurgitation, the first and second heart sounds are usually easily heard. As aortic valve narrowing worsens, the murmur peaks later in systole. When calcified leaflets are present, the murmur tends to have a harsher quality. An aortic ejection sound, which is caused by the sudden checking of the leaflets as they open, is heard only when the leaflets remain fairly mobile, as in congenitally malformed valves.

While obstruction of blood flow from the left ventricle is usually due to valvular disease, obstruction can also occur above or below the valve and can present in somewhat the same way as valvular aortic stenosis. A membranous shelf that partially obstructs flow just above the valve in the aorta can sometimes be present from birth. In this condition, the systolic murmur is usually heard best at the first intercostal space at the right sternal border. Subvalvular stenosis can occur in some patients who develop severe hypertrophy of the heart (Figure 8–18). This well-recognized clinical entity—hypertrophic cardiomyopathy--can also be manifested by a crescendo-decrescendo systolic murmur noted on physical examination. However, obstruction of the outflow tract in hypertrophic cardiomyopathy is dynamic, with greater obstruction when preload is decreased from decreased intraventricular volume. For this reason, having the patient stand or perform Valsalva's maneuver (forced expiration against a closed glottis), both of which cause a decrease in venous return, will cause the murmur to increase. In contrast, both of these maneuvers will cause a decrease in the murmur owing to valvular stenosis, since less absolute blood volume will flow across the stenotic aortic valve.

2. AORTIC REGURGITATION

Clinical Presentation

Aortic regurgitation can be either chronic or acute. In chronic aortic regurgitation, there is a long latent period during which the patient remains asymptomatic as the heart responds to the volume load. When the compensatory mechanisms fail, symptoms of left-sided failure become manifest. In acute aortic regurgitation, there are no compensatory mechanisms, so shortness of breath, pulmonary edema, and hypotension, often with cardiovascular collapse, occur suddenly.

Physical examination of patients with chronic aortic regurgitation reveals hyperdynamic (pounding) pulses. The apical impulse is hyperdynamic and displaced laterally. On auscultation, three murmurs may be heard: a high-pitched early diastolic murmur, a diastolic rumble called the Austin Flint murmur, and a systolic murmur. A third heart sound is often present. However, in acute aortic regurgitation, the peripheral signs are often absent, and the left ventricular impulse is in many cases normal. On auscultation, the diastolic murmur will be much softer, and the Austin Flint murmur, if present, will be short. The first heart sound will be soft and sometimes absent.

Etiology

Acute and chronic aortic regurgitation can be due to either valvular or aortic root abnormalities (Table 8–4).

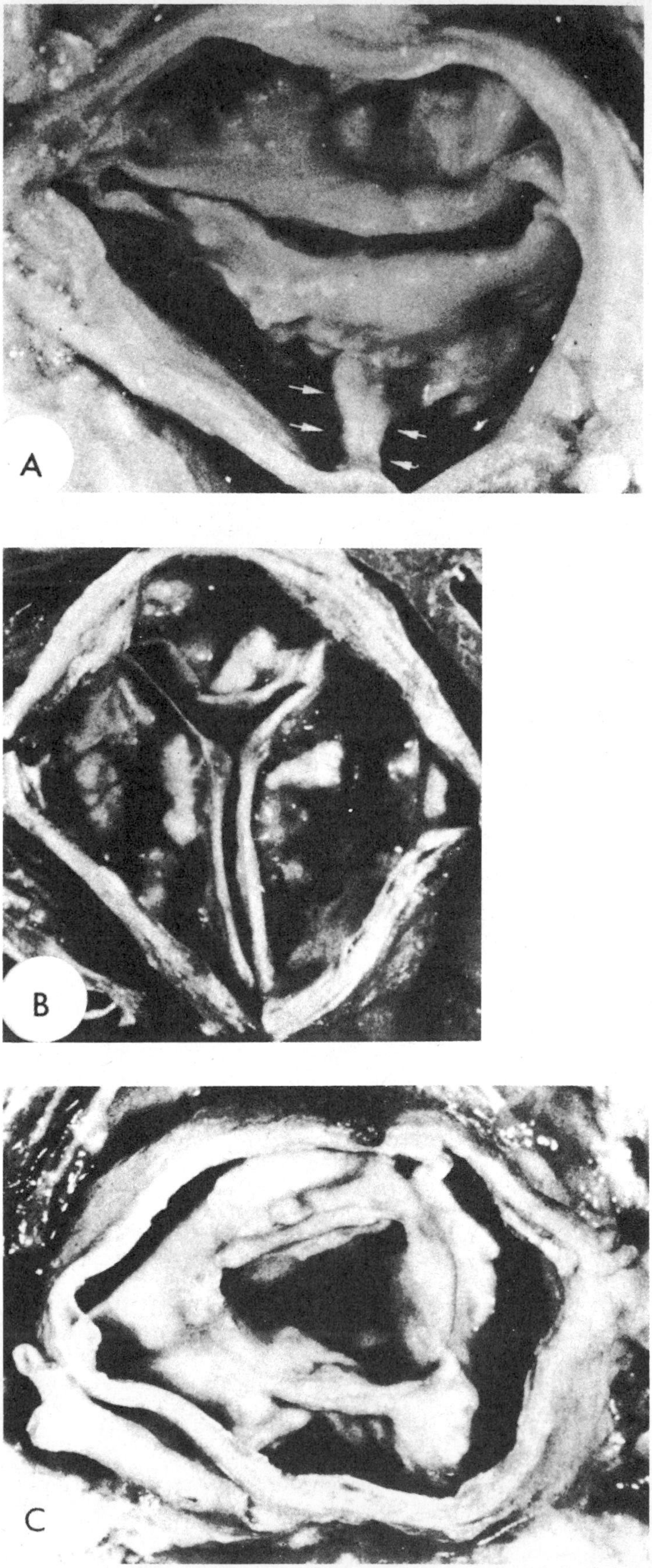

Figure 8–16. ***A:*** Calcified, stenotic, congenitally bicuspid aortic valve of a 59-year-old man. The cusps are situated anteriorly and posteriorly, with the commissures on the right and left, respectively. The valve has a raphe (white arrows) in the anterior cusp. Peak systolic gradient across the valve was 45 mm Hg, and the patient had complete heart block secondary to destruction of the atrioventricular bundle by calcium, which presumably had extended down from the aortic valvular cusps. ***B:*** Stenotic tricuspic aortic valve in an 81-year-old man. Aortic stenosis in the elderly is characterized by calcific deposits on the aortic surfaces of the cusps and typically no or little commissural fusion. ***C:*** Stenotic tricuspid aortic valve in a 55-year-old man with rheumatic heart disease. Each of the three commissures is fused, producing a triangular fixed central orifice that is both stenotic and incompetent. (Reproduced, with permission from Roberts WC: Valvular, subvalvular and supravalvular aortic stenosis: Morphologic features. In: *Clinical-Pathologic Correlations No. 2.* Edwards JE [editor]. Davis, 1973.)

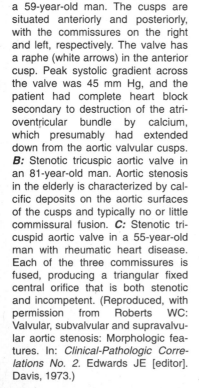

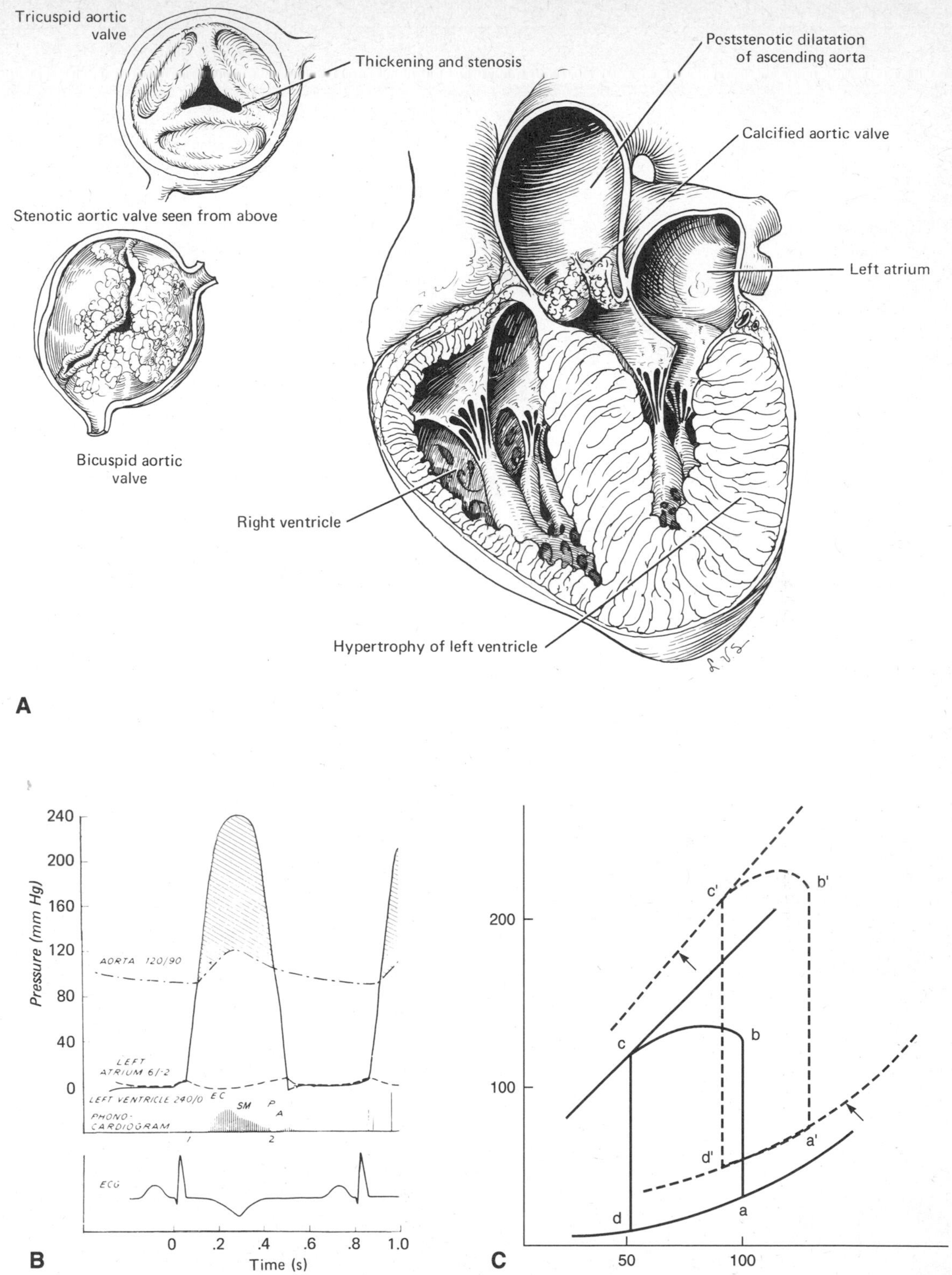

Figure 8–17. Aortic stenosis. ***A:*** Drawing of the left heart in left anterior oblique view showing anatomic features of aortic stenosis. Note structures enlarged: left ventricle (thickened); poststenotic dilation of the aorta. ***B:*** Drawing showing auscultatory and hemodynamic features of predominant aortic stenosis. Cardinal features include left ventricular hypertrophy; systolic ejection murmur. (EC, ejection click; SM, systolic murmur; P, pulmonary valve; A, aortic valve.) (Reproduced, with permission, from Cheitlin MD, Sokolow M, McIlroy MB: *Clinical Cardiology,* 6th ed. Appleton & Lange, 1993.) ***C:*** Pressure-volume loop in aortic stenosis. The left ventricle becomes thickened and less compliant, forcing the diastolic pressure-volume curve upward and to the left, which results in elevated left ventricular end-diastolic pressure (**a´**). Since the left ventricle must pump against a fixed gradient (increased afterload), **b** increases to **b´**. Finally, the hypertrophy of the ventricle results in increased inotropic force, which shifts the isovolumic pressure curve leftward.

Cardinal features: *Left ventricular (especially septal) hypertrophy; diastolic dysfunction; systolic outflow obstruction; systolic anterior motion of mitral valve; excessive left ventricular emptying.*

Variable factors: *Severity; level of peripheral resistance; low resistance and low blood volume lead to obstruction.*

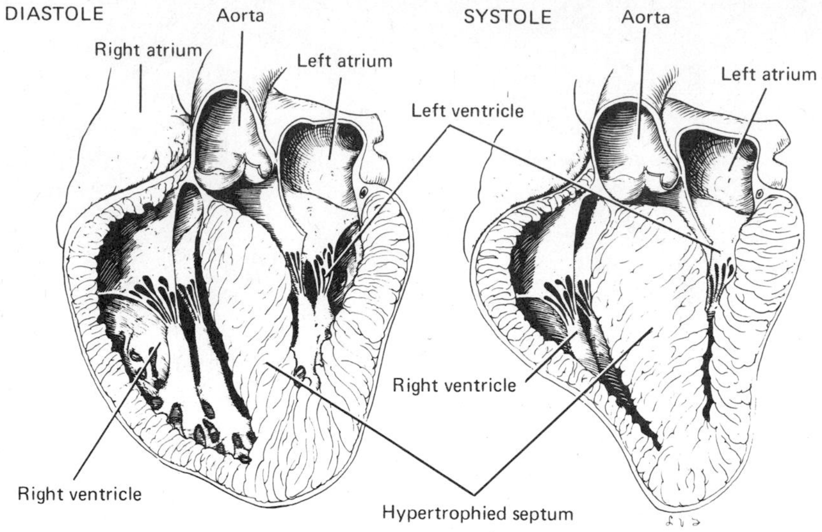

Figure 8–18. Hypertrophic cardiomyopathy (left lateral view). The cardinal features are displayed. (Reproduced, with permission, from Cheitlin MD, Sokolow M, McIlroy MB: *Clinical Cardiology*, 6th ed. Appleton & Lange, 1993.)

Pathophysiology

Aortic regurgitation places a volume load on the left ventricle, since during diastole blood enters the ventricle both from the left atrium and from the aorta. If the regurgitation develops slowly, the heart responds to the increased diastolic pressure by fiber elongation and replication of sarcomeres in series, which leads to increased ventricular volumes. Since systolic pressure remains relatively unchanged, increased wall stress—by Laplace's law—can be compensated for by an additional increase in wall thickness. This response, "eccentric hypertrophy" (so named because the ventricular cavity enlarges laterally in the chest and becomes eccentric to its normal position), explains the different ventricular geometry observed in patients with aortic regurgitation when compared with patients who have aortic stenosis (concentric hypertrophy due to the systolic pressure overload). Ultimately, chronic aortic regurgitation leads to huge ventricular volumes as demonstrated in the

Table 8–4. Causes of aortic regurgitation.

Site	Pathology	Causes	Time Course
Valvular	Cusp abnormalities	Endocarditis	Acute or chronic
		Rheumatic disease	Acute or chronic
		Ankylosing spondylitis	Usually chronic
		Congenital	Chronic
Aortic	Dilation	Aortic aneurysms	Acute or chronic
		Heritable disorders of connective tissue	Usually chronic
		Marfan's syndrome	
		Ehlers-Danlos syndrome	
		Osteogenesis imperfecta	
	Inflammation	Aortitis (Takayasu)	Usually chronic
		Syphilis	Usually chronic
		Arthritic diseases	Usually chronic
		Ankylosing spondylitis	
		Reiter's syndrome	
		Rheumatoid arthritis	
		Systemic lupus erythematosus	
		Cystic medial necrosis	Acute or chronic
	Tears with loss of commissural support	Trauma	Usually acute
		Dissection, often from hypertension	Usually acute

pressure-volume loops (Figure 8–19A). The left ventricle operates as a low-compliance pump, handling large end-diastolic and stroke volumes, often with little increase in end-diastolic pressure. In addition, no truly isovolumic period of relaxation or contraction exists because of the persistent flow into the ventricle from the systemic circulation. Aortic pulse pressure is widened. Diastolic pressure decreases because of regurgitant flow back into the left ventricle and increased compliance of the large central vessels (in response to increased stroke volume); elevated stroke volume leads to increased systolic pressures (Figure 8–19C).

Clinical Manifestations

A. Shortness of Breath: Pulmonary edema can develop, particularly if the aortic regurgitation is acute and the ventricle does not have time to compensate for the sudden increase in volume. In chronic aortic regurgitation, compensatory mechanisms eventually fail and the heart begins to operate on the steeper portion of the diastolic pressure-volume relationship.

B. Physical Examination:

1. Hyperdynamic pulses–In chronic aortic regurgitation, a widened pulse pressure is responsible for several characteristic peripheral signs. Palpation of the peripheral pulse reveals a sudden rise and then drop in pressure (water-hammer or Corrigan's pulse). Head bobbing (DeMusset's sign), rhythmic pulsation of the uvula (Müller's sign), and arterial pulsation observed in the nail bed (Quincke's pulse) have been described in patients with chronic aortic regurgitation.

2. Murmurs–Three heart murmurs can be heard in patients with aortic regurgitation: First, flow from the regurgitant volume back into the left ventricle can be heard as a high-pitched, blowing, early diastolic murmur usually heard best along the left sternal border. Second, the rumbling murmur described by Austin Flint can be heard at the apex during any part of diastole. The Austin Flint murmur is thought to result from regurgitant flow from the aortic valve impinging on the anterior leaflet of the mitral valve, producing functional mitral stenosis. Finally, a crescendo-decrescendo systolic murmur, which is thought to arise from the increased stroke volume flowing across the aortic valve, can be heard at the left sternal border.

In acute, severe aortic regurgitation, the early diastolic murmur may be softer owing to rapid diastolic equalization of ventricular and aortic pressures. The first heart sound is soft because of early mitral valve closure from aortic regurgitation and elevated ventricular pressures.

3. Third heart sound–A third heart sound can be heard because of concomitant heart failure or because of the exaggerated early diastolic filling of the left ventricle.

4. Apical impulse–The apical impulse is displaced laterally because of the increased volume of the left ventricle.

3. MITRAL STENOSIS

Clinical Presentation

The symptoms of mitral stenosis include dyspnea, fatigue, and hemoptysis. Occasionally, the patient complains of palpitations or a rapid heart beat. Finally, the patient with mitral stenosis may present with neurologic symptoms such as transient numbness or weakness of the extremities, sudden loss of vision, or difficulty with coordination.

The characteristic murmur of mitral stenosis is a late low-pitched diastolic rumble. In addition, an opening snap may be heard in the first portion of diastole (Figure 8–20). Auscultation of the lungs may reveal rales.

Etiology

Mitral stenosis is most commonly a sequela of rheumatic heart disease (Table 8–5). Infrequently, it may be caused by congenital lesions or calcium deposition. Atrial masses (myxoma) can cause intermittent obstruction of the mitral valve.

Pathophysiology

The mitral valve is normally bicuspid, with the anterior cusp approximately twice the area of the posterior cusp. The mitral valve area is usually 5–6 cm^2; clinically relevant mitral stenosis usually occurs when the valve area decreases to less than 1 cm^2. Since obstruction of flow protects the ventricle from pressure and volume loads, the left ventricular pressure-volume relationship shows relatively little abnormality other than decreased volumes. However, analysis of hemodynamic tracings shows the characteristic elevation in left atrial pressures (Figure 8–20). For this reason, the main pathophysiologic abnormality in mitral stenosis is elevated pulmonary venous and right-sided (pulmonary artery, right ventricle, and right atrium) pressures. Dilation and reduced systolic function of the right ventricle are commonly observed in patients with advanced mitral stenosis.

Clinical Manifestations

A. Symptoms:

1. Shortness of breath, hemoptysis, and orthopnea–All of these symptoms occur because of elevated left atrial, pulmonary venous, and pulmonary capillary pressures (the actual mechanisms are described in the section on congestive heart failure).

2. Palpitations–Increased left atrial size predisposes patients with mitral stenosis to atrial arrhythmias. Chaotic atrial activity, or atrial fibrillation, is commonly observed. Since ventricular filling is par-

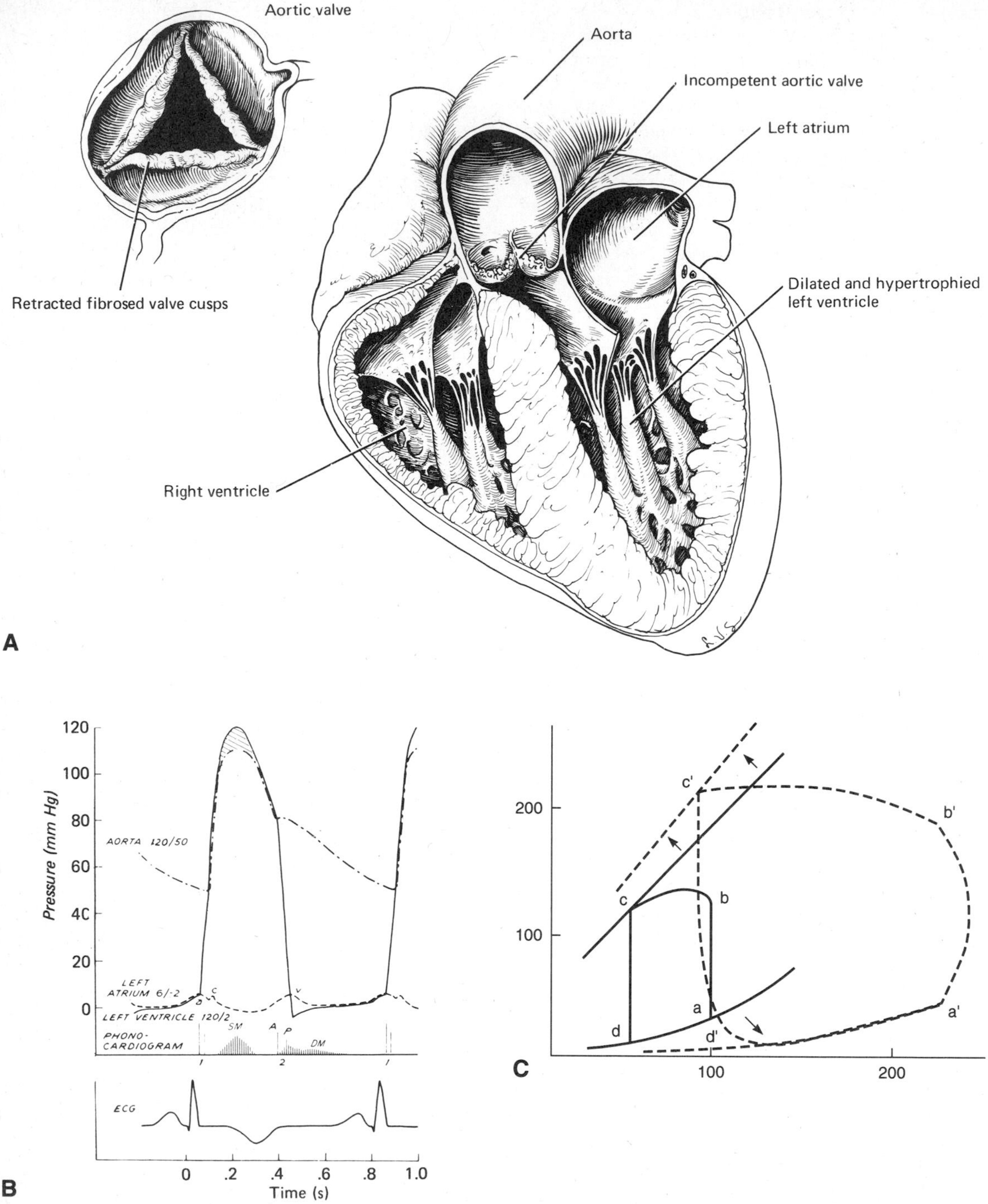

Figure 8–19. Aortic insufficiency (regurgitation). ***A:*** Drawing of the left heart in left anterior oblique view showing anatomic features of aortic insufficiency. Note structures enlarged: left ventricle, aorta. ***B:*** Drawing showing auscultatory and hemodynamic features of predominant aortic insufficiency. Cardinal features include large hypertrophied left ventricle; large aorta; increased stroke volume; wide pulse pressure; diastolic murmur. (SM, systolic murmur; A, aortic valve; P, pulmonary valve; DM, diastolic murmur.) (Reproduced, with permission, from Cheitlin MD, Sokolow M, McIlroy MB: *Clinical Cardiology,* 6th ed. Appleton & Lange, 1993.) ***C:*** Pressure-volume loop in chronic aortic insufficiency. Marked enlargement in left ventricular volume shifts the diastolic pressure-volume curve rightward. Hypertrophy of the ventricle shifts the isovolumic pressure-volume curve leftward. Stroke volume is enormous, although effective stroke volume may be minimally changed since much of the increase in stroke volume leaks back into the ventricle. Since the ventricle is constantly being filled from the mitral valve or the incompetent aortic valve, no isovolumic periods exist.

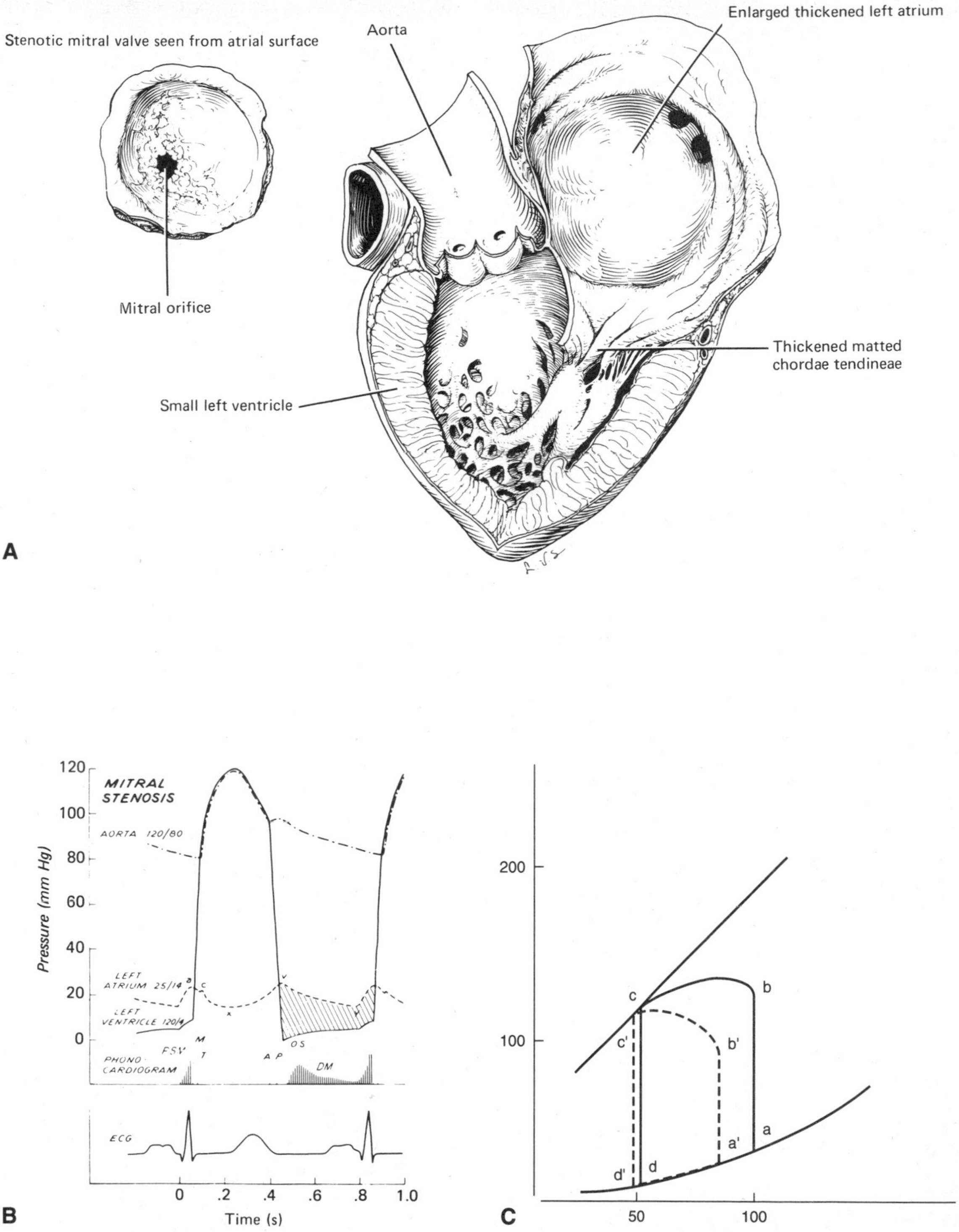

Figure 8–20. Mitral stenosis. ***A:*** Drawing of the left heart in left anterior oblique view showing anatomic features of mitral stenosis. Note enlarged left atrium, small left ventricle. ***B:*** Drawing showing auscultatory and hemodynamic features of mitral stenosis. Cardinal features include thickening and fusion of mitral valve cusps, elevated left atrial pressure, left atrial enlargement, opening snap, diastolic murmur. (PSM, presystolic murmur; OS, opening snap; M, mitral; T, tricuspid; A, aortic; P, pulmonary; DM, diastolic murmur). (Reproduced, with permission, from Cheitlin MD, Sokolow M, McIlroy MB: *Clinical Cardiology,* 6th ed. Appleton & Lange, 1993.) ***C:*** Pressure-volume loop in mitral stenosis. Filling of the left ventricle is restricted from **a** to **a´**, decreasing stroke volume to **b´c´**.

Table 8–5. Causes of mitral stenosis.

Type	Comments
Rheumatic	Most common. Narrowing results from fusion and thickening of the commissures, cusps, and chordae. Symptoms usually develop 20 years after acute rheumatic fever.
Calcific	Usually causes mitral regurgitation but can cause mitral stenosis in some cases.
Congenital	Usually presents during infancy or childhood.
Collagen vascular disease	Systemic lupus erythematosus and rheumatoid arthritis (rare).

ticularly dependent on atrial contraction in patients with mitral stenosis, acute hemodynamic decompensation may occur when organized contraction of the atrium is lost.

3. Neurologic symptoms–Reduced outflow leads to dilation of the left atrium and stasis of blood flow. Thrombus in the left atrium is observed in approximately 20% of patients with mitral stenosis, and the prevalence increases with age, the presence of atrial fibrillation, the severity of stenosis, and any reduction in cardiac output. Embolic events that lead to neurologic symptoms occur in 8% of patients in sinus rhythm and 32% of patients with chronic or paroxysmal atrial fibrillation. In addition, left atrial enlargement can sometimes impinge on the recurrent laryngeal nerve and lead to hoarseness (Ortner's syndrome).

B. Physical Examination: On auscultation of the heart, the diastolic rumble occurs because of turbulent flow across the narrowed mitral valve orifice. An opening snap, analagous to the ejection click described for aortic stenosis, may be heard in early diastole. The opening snap is heard only when the patient has relatively mobile leaflets.

Rales occur because elevated pulmonary capillary pressures lead to accumulation of intra-alveolar fluid.

4. MITRAL REGURGITATION

Clinical Presentation

The presentation of mitral regurgitation depends on how quickly valvular incompetence develops. Patients with chronic mitral regurgitation develop symptoms gradually over time. Common complaints include dyspnea, easy fatigablity, and palpitations. Patients with acute mitral regurgitation present with symptoms of left heart failure: shortness of breath, orthopnea, and shock. Chest pain may be present in patients whose mitral regurgitation is due to coronary artery disease.

On physical examination, patients have a pansystolic regurgitant murmur that is heard best at the apex and often radiates to the axilla. This murmur often obscures the first and second heart sounds. When mitral valve incompetence is severe, a third heart sound is often present. In chronic mitral regurgitation, the apical impulse is often hyperdynamic and displaced laterally.

Etiology

In the past, rheumatic heart disease accounted for most cases of mitral regurgitation. Mitral valve prolapse is now probably the most common cause, followed by coronary artery disease. The tips of the anterior and posterior mitral valve leaflets are held in place during ventricular contraction by the anterolateral and posteromedial papillary muscles. The valves are connected to the papillary muscles via thin fibrous structures called chordae tendineae. In patients with mitral valve prolapse, extra tissue present on the valvular apparatus can undergo myxomatous degeneration by the fifth or sixth decades. Mitral regurgitation follows, either from poor coaptation of the valve leaflets or from sudden rupture of the chordae tendineae. In coronary artery disease, obstruction of the circumflex coronary artery can lead to ischemia or rupture of the papillary muscles (Table 8–6).

Pathophysiology

When the mitral valve fails to close properly, regurgitation of blood into the left atrium from the ventricle occurs during systole. In chronic mitral regurgitation, the compensatory mechanism to this volume load is similar to the changes seen in aortic regurgitation. The left ventricle and atrium dilate, and to normalize wall stress in the ventricle there is also concomitant hypertrophy of the ventricular wall (see discussion of Laplace's law). Diastolic filling of the ventricle increases since it is now the sum of right ventricular output and the regurgitant volume from the previous beat. In acute mitral regurgitation, the sudden volume load on the atrium and ventricle is not compensated for by chamber enlargement and hypertrophy. The sudden increase in atrial volume leads to prominent atrial *v* waves with transmission of this elevated pressure to the pulmonary capillaries and the development of pulmonary edema (Figure 8–21).

Clinical Manifestations

A. Symptoms:

1. Pulmonary edema–Rapid elevation of pulmonary capillary pressure in acute mitral regurgitation leads to the sudden onset of pulmonary edema, manifested by shortness of breath, orthopnea, and paroxys-

Table 8–6. Causes of mitral regurgitation.

Type	Causes
Acute	
Ruptured chordae	Infective endocarditis Trauma Acute rheumatic fever "Spontaneous"
Ruptured or dysfunctional papillary muscles	Ischemia Myocardial infarction Trauma Myocardial abscess
Perforated leaflet	Infective endocarditis Trauma
Chronic	
Inflammatory	Rheumatic heart disease Connective tissue disease
Infection	Infective endocarditis
Degenerative	Myxomatous degeneration of the valve leaflets Calcification of the mitral annulus
Rupture or dysfunction of the chordae tendineae or papillary muscles	Infective endocarditis Trauma Acute rheumatic fever "Spontaneous" Ischemia Myocardial infarction Myocardial abscess
Congenital	

mal nocturnal dyspnea. In chronic mitral regurgitation, the symptoms develop gradually, but at some point the compensatory mechanisms fail and pulmonary edema develops, particularly with exercise.

2. Fatigue–Fatigue can develop because of decreased forward blood flow to the peripheral tissues.

3. Palpitations–Left atrial enlargment may lead to the development of atrial fibrillation and accompanying palpitations. Patients with atrial fibrillation and mitral regurgitation have a 20% incidence of cardioembolic events.

B. Physical Examination

1. Holosystolic murmur–Regurgitant flow into the atrium produces a high-pitched murmur that is heard throughout systole. The murmur begins with the first heart sound and continues to the second heart sound and is of constant intensity throughout systole. It finally ends when left ventricular pressure drops to equal left atrial pressure during isovolumic relaxation. Unlike the murmur of aortic stenosis, there is little variation in the intensity of the murmur as the heart rate changes. In addition, the murmur does not change in intensity with respiration. It is usually heard best at the apex and often radiates to the axilla. If rupture of the anterior leaflet has occurred, the mitral regurgitation murmur will sometimes radiate to the back.

2. Third heart sound–A third heart sound will be heard if heart failure is present. Because of increased and rapid filling of the ventricle during diastole, it may also be heard in the absence of overt failure in patients with severe mitral regurgitation.

3. Displaced and hyperdynamic apical impulse–The compensatory increase in left ventricular volume and wall thickness in patients with chronic mitral regurgitation will be manifest by a laterally displaced apical impulse. Since the ventricle now has a low pressure chamber (the left atrium) in which to eject blood, the apical impulse is often hyperdynamic. When mitral regurgitation develops suddenly, the apical impulse will not be displaced or hyperdynamic, since the left ventricle has not had enough time for compensatory volume increases.

10. What are the clinical presentations of each of the four major categorics of valvular heart disease?
11. What are the most common courses of each category of valvular heart disease?
12. What is the pathogenesis of each category of valvular heart disease?
13. What are the major clinical manifestations and complications of each category of valvular heart disease?

CORONARY ARTERY DISEASE

Clinical Presentation

Chest pain is the most common symptom associated with coronary artery disease. It is usually described as dull, and it can often radiate down the arm or to the jaw. It does not worsen with a deep breath and can be associated with shortness of breath, diaphoresis, nausea, or vomiting. This entire symptom complex has been termed **angina pectoris**, or "pain in the breast"; this phrase was first used by Heberden in 1772 to convey the sense of "strangling" that occurs with this symptom complex.

Clinically, angina is classified by the duration of symptoms and precipitating causes. If the pain occurs only with exertion and has been stable over a long period of time, it is termed **stable angina.** If the pain occurs with rest, it is termed **unstable angina.** Finally, regardless of the precipitating cause, if the chest pain persists without interruption for prolonged periods and irreversible myocyte damage has occurred, it is termed **myocardial infarction.**

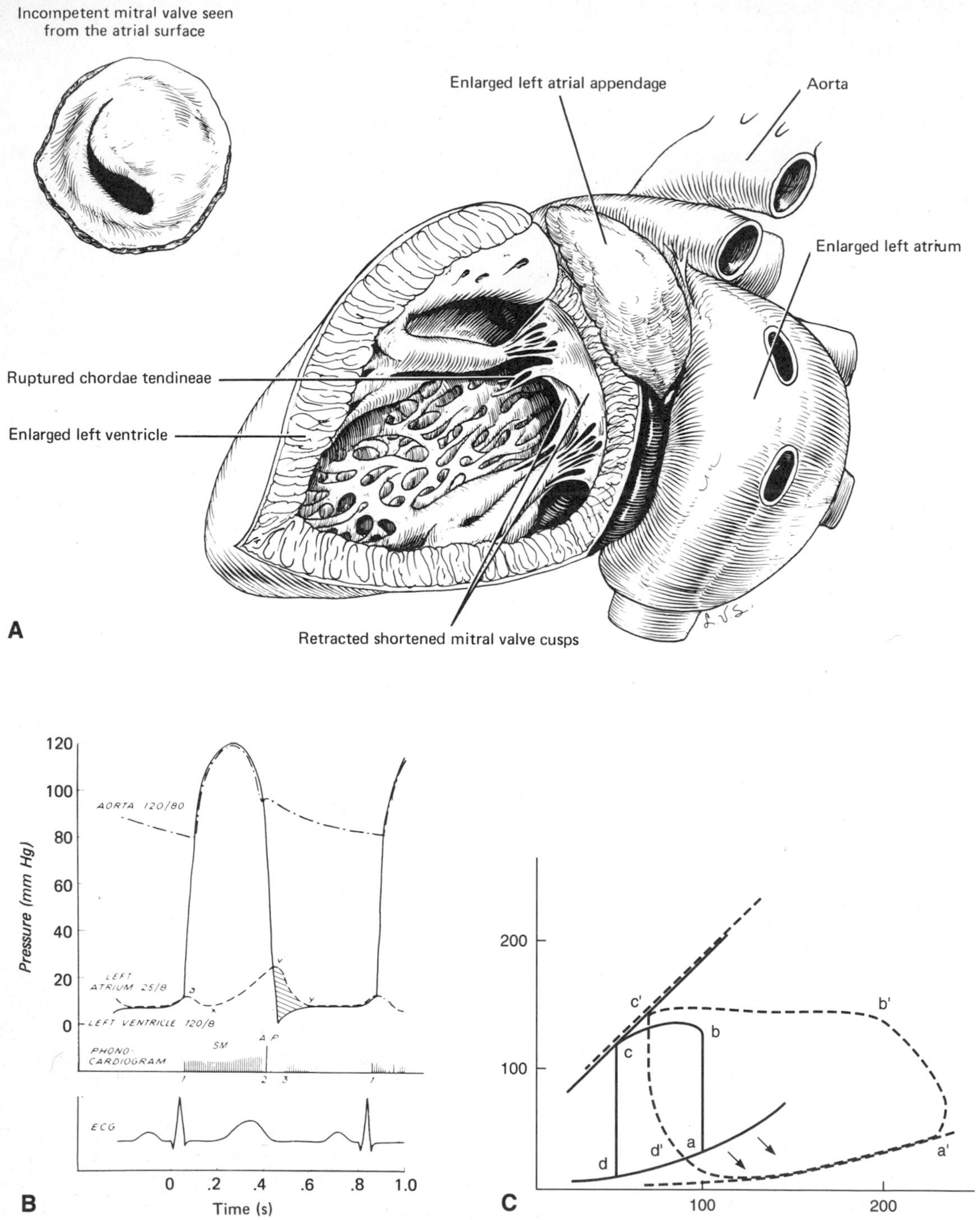

Figure 8–21. Mitral insufficiency (regurgitation). ***A:*** Drawing of the left heart in left lateral view showing anatomic features of mitral insufficiency. Note structures enlarged: left atrium, left ventricle. ***B:*** Drawing showing auscultatory and hemodynamic features of mitral insufficiency. Cardinal features include systolic backflow into left atrium, left atrial enlargement, left ventricular enlargement (hypertrophy in acute lesions), prominent v wave due to filling from both the pulmonary veins and the regurgitant jet, holosystolic murmur. (3, third heart sound; SM, systolic murmur; A, aortic; P, pulmonary.) (Reproduced, with permission, from Cheitlin MD, Sokolow M, McIlroy MB: *Clinical Cardiology,* 6th ed. Appleton & Lange, 1993.) ***C:*** Pressure-volume loop in mitral insufficiency. Increased ventricular volumes shift the diastolic pressure-volume curve rightward. Stroke volume is increased since the ventricle can now eject blood into the low-pressure left atrium.

On physical examination, the patient with coronary artery disease may have a fourth heart sound or signs of congestive heart failure and shock. However, more than any other cardiovascular problem, the initial diagnosis relies on patient history.

Etiology

Atherosclerotic obstruction of the large epicardial vessels is by far the most common cause of coronary artery disease. Spasm of the coronary arteries from various mediators such as serotonin and histamine has been well described and is more common in Japanese. Rarely, congenital abnormalities can cause coronary artery diseases (Table 8–7).

Pathophysiology

Coronary blood flow brings oxygen to myocytes and removes waste products such as carbon dioxide, lactic acid, and hydrogen ions. The heart has a tremendously high metabolic requirement; although it accounts for only 0.3% of body weight, it is responsible for 7% of the body's resting oxygen consumption. Cellular ischemia occurs when there is either increased demand for oxygen relative to maximal arterial supply or when there is an absolute reduction in oxygen supply. While situations of increased demand, such as thyrotoxicosis and aortic stenosis, can cause myocardial ischemia, most clinical cases are due to decreased oxygen supply. Reduced oxygen supply can rarely arise from decreased oxygen content in blood, such as in carbon monoxide poisoning or anemia, but more commonly stems from coronary artery abnormalities (Table 8–7), particularly atherosclerotic disease. Myocardial ischemia may arise from a combination of increased demand and decreased supply; cocaine abuse increases oxygen demand (by inhibiting reuptake of norepinephrine at adrenergic nerve endings in the heart) and can reduce oxygen supply by causing vasospasm.

Table 8–7. Causes of coronary artery disease.

Type	Comments
Atherosclerosis	Most common cause. Risk factors include hypertension, Cholesterolemia, diabetes mellitus, smoking, and a family history of atherosclerosis.
Spasm	Coronary artery vasospasm can occur in any population but is most prevalent in Japanese. Vasoconstriction appears to be mediated by histamine, serotonin, catecholamines, and endothelium-derived factors. Since spasm can occur at any time, the chest pain is often not exertion-related.
Emboli	Rare cause of coronary artery disease. Can occur from vegetations in patients with endocarditis.
Congenital	Congenital coronary artery abnormalities are present in 1–2% of the population. However, only a small fraction of these abnormalities cause symptomatic ischemia.

Atherosclerosis of large coronary arteries remains the predominant cause of coronary artery disease. Raised fatty streaks, which appear as yellow spots or streaks in the vessel walls, are seen in coronary arteries in almost all members of any population by 20 years of age. They are found mainly in areas exposed to increased shear stresses such as bending points and bifurcations and are thought to arise from isolated macrophage foam cell migration into areas of minimal chronic intimal injury. In many people this process progresses, with additional migration of foam cells, smooth muscle cell proliferation, and extracellular fat and collagen deposition (Figure 8–22). The extent and incidence of these advanced lesions varies among different geographic and ethnic groups.

The underlying pathophysiologic processes differ for each clinical presentation of coronary artery disease. In patients with **stable angina,** fixed narrowing of one or several coronary arteries is usually present. Since the large coronary arteries usually function as conduits and do not offer resistance to flow, the arterial lumen must be decreased by 90% to produce cellular ischemia when the patient is at rest. However, with exercise, a 50% reduction in lumen size can lead to symptoms. In patients with **unstable angina,** fissuring of the atherosclerotic plaque can lead to platelet accumulation and transient episodes of thrombotic occlusion, usually lasting 10–20 minutes. In addition, platelet release of vasoconstrictive factors such as thromboxane A_2 or serotonin and endothelial dysfunction may cause vasoconstriction and contribute to decreased flow. In **myocardial infarction,** deep arterial injury from plaque rupture may cause formation of a relatively fixed and persistent thrombus.

The heart receives its energy primarily from ATP generated by oxidative phosphorylation of free fatty acids, though glucose and other carbohydrates can be utilized. Within 60 seconds after coronary artery occlusion, myocardial oxygen tension in the affected cells falls essentially to zero. Cardiac stores of high-energy phosphates are rapidly depleted and the cells shift rapidly to anaerobic metabolism with consequent lactic acid production. Macroscopically, myocardial dysfunction of relaxation and contraction occurs within seconds, even before depletion of high-energy phosphates occurs. The biochemical basis for this abnormality is not known. If perfusion is not restored within 40–60 minutes, an irreversible stage of injury characterized by diffuse mitochondrial

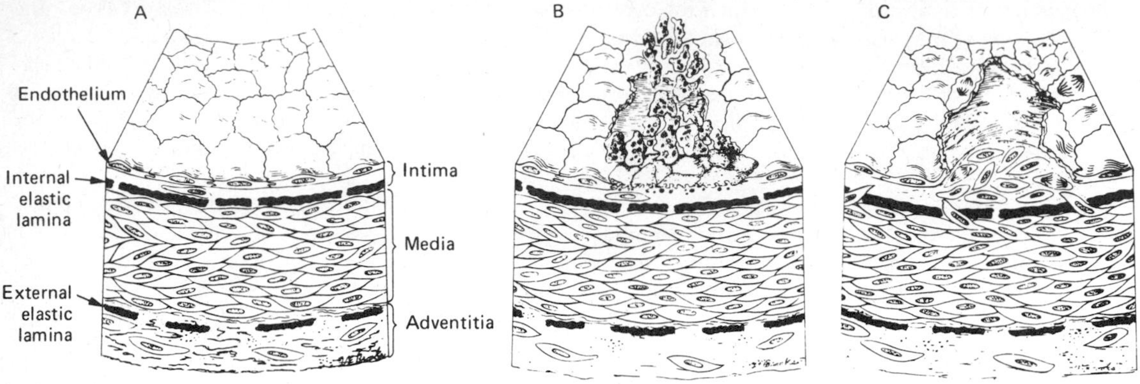

Figure 8–22. Mechanisms of production of atheroma. ***A:*** Structure of normal muscular artery. The adventitia, or outermost layer of the artery, consists principally of recognizable fibroblasts intermixed with smooth muscle cells loosely arranged between bundles of collagen and surrounded by proteoglycans. It is usually separated from the media by a discontinuous sheet of elastic tissue, the external elastic lamina. ***B:*** Platelet aggregates, or microthrombi, which may form as a result of adherence of the platelets to the exposed subendothelial connective tissue. Platelets that adhere to the connective tissue release granules whose constituents may gain entry into the arterial wall. Platelet factors thus interact with plasma constituents in the artery wall and may stimulate events shown in the next illustration. ***C:*** Smooth muscle cells migrating from the media into the intima through fenestrae in the internal elastic lamina and actively multiplying within the intima. Endothelial cells regenerate in an attempt to re-cover the exposed intima, which thickens rapidly owing to smooth muscle proliferation and formation of new connective tissue. (Reproduced, with permission, from Ross R, Glomset JA: The pathogenesis of atherosclerosis. [Part 1.] N Engl J Med 1976;295:369.)

swelling, damage to the cell membrane, and marked depletion of glycogen begins. The exact mechanism by which irreversible damage occurs is not clear, but severe ATP depletion, increased extracellular calcium concentrations, lactic acidosis, and free radicals have all been postulated as possible causes.

In experimental preparations, if ischemic myocardium is perfused within 5 minutes, systolic function returns promptly whereas diastolic abnormalities may take up to 40 minutes to normalize. With prolonged episodes of ischemia--up to 1 hour--it may take up to a month to restore ventricular function. When the heart demonstrates this prolonged period of decreased function despite normal perfusion, the myocardium is said to be "stunned." The biochemical basis for stunning is poorly understood. If reperfusion occurs later or not at all, systolic function often will not return to the affected area.

Clinical Manifestations

A. Chest Pain: Chest pain in the past has traditionally been ascribed to ischemia. However, recent evidence suggests that in patients with coronary artery disease, 70–80% of episodes of ischemia are actually asymptomatic. When present, the chest pain is thought to be mediated by sympathetic afferent fibers that richly innervate the atrium and ventricle. From the heart, the fibers connect with the upper thoracic sympathetic ganglia and the five upper thoracic dorsal roots of the spinal cord. In the spinal cord, the impulses probably converge with impulses from other thoracic structures. This convergence is probably the mechanism for chest wall, back, and arm pain that can sometimes accompany angina pectoris. The importance of these fibers can be demonstrated in patients who have had a heart transplant. When these patients develop atherosclerosis, they remain completely asymptomatic, without development of angina.

Recent evidence suggests that the actual trigger for nerve stimulation is adenosine. Adenosine infusion into the coronary arteries can produce the characteristic symptoms of angina without evidence of ischemia. In addition, blocking the adenosine receptor (P_1) with aminophylline leads to reduced anginal symptoms despite similar degrees of ischemia.

The large proportion of asymptomatic episodes of ischemia probably has three causes: (1) Dysfunction of afferent nerves may cause silent ischemia. Patients with transplanted hearts do not sense cardiac pain despite significant atherosclerosis. Peripheral neuropathy in patients with diabetes may explain the increased episodes of silent ischemia described in this patient population. (2) Insufficient ischemia may also be an important mechanism for silent ischemia. Within a few seconds after cessation of perfusion, systolic and diastolic abnormalities can be observed. Angina is a relatively late event, occurring after at least 30 seconds of ischemia. (3) Finally, differing pain threshholds between patients may explain the high prevalence of silent ischemia. The presence of angina is moderately correlated with a decreased pain tolerance. The mechanism for different pain threshholds is unknown but may be due to differences in plasma endorphins.

B. Fourth Heart Sound and Shortness of Breath: Both of these findings may occur because of diastolic and systolic dysfunction of the ischemic myocardium. (See the section on congestive heart failure.)

C. Shock: The site of coronary artery occlusion determines the clinical presentation of myocardial ischemia or infarction. As a general rule, the more myocardium that is supplied by the occluded vessel, the more significant and severe the symptoms. For example, obstruction of the left main coronary artery or the proximal left anterior descending coronary artery will usually present as severe cardiac failure, often with associated hypotension (shock). In addition, shock may be associated with coronary artery disease in several special situations. If necrosis of the septum occurs from left anterior descending artery occlusion, myocardial rupture with the formation of an interventricular septal defect can occur. Rupture of the anterior or lateral free walls from occlusion of the left anterior descending or circumflex coronary arteries, respectively, can lead to the formation of pericardial effusion and tamponade. Rupture of myocardial tissue usually occurs 4–7 days after the acute ischemic event, when the myocardial wall has thinned and is in the process of healing. Sudden hemodynamic decompensation during this period should arouse suspicion of these complications. Finally, circumflex artery occlusion may result in ischemia and dysfunction or overt rupture of the papillary muscles, which can produce severe mitral regurgitation and shock.

D. Bradycardia: Inferior wall myocardial infarctions usually arise from occlusion of the right coronary artery. Since the area of left ventricular tissue supplied by this artery is small, patients usually do not present with heart failure. However, the artery that provides blood supply to the AV node branches off the posterior descending artery, so that inferior wall myocardial infarctions are sometimes associated with slowed or absent conduction in the AV node. Besides ischemia, AV nodal conduction abnormalities can occur because of reflex activation of the vagus nerve, which richly innervates the AV node.

Dysfunction of the sinus node is rarely seen in coronary artery disease, since this area receives blood supply from both the right and the left coronary artery circulations.

E. Nausea and Vomiting: Nausea and vomiting may arise from activation of the vagus nerve in the setting of an inferior wall myocardial infarction.

F. Tachycardia: To maintain stroke volume, levels of catecholamines are usually raised in patients with a myocardial infarction which leads to increased heart rate.

14. What is the clinical presentation of CAD along the continuum from stable angina to unstable angina to myocardial infarction?
15. What are the most common causes of CAD?
16. How are the pathophysiology of stable angina, unstable angina, and myocardial infarction different?
17. What are the major clinical manifestations and complications of CAD?

PERICARDIAL DISEASE

Pericardial disease can be due to inflammation of the pericardium (pericarditis) or abnormal amounts of fluid in the space between the visceral and parietal pericardium.

PERICARDITIS

Clinical Presentation

The patient presents with severe chest pain. Descriptions of the pain are variable, but the usual picture is of a sharp retrosternal pain with radiation to the back and worse with deep breathing or coughing. The pain is often position-dependent—worse when lying flat and improved while sitting up and leaning forward.

On physical examination, the pericardial rub is pathognomonic for pericarditis. It is a high-pitched squeaking sound, often with two or more components.

Occasionally, continual inflammation of the pericardium leads to fibrosis and the development of constrictive pericarditis (Figure 8–23). Examination of the jugular venous pulsation is critical in the patient who may have constrictive pericarditis. The jugular venous pressure is elevated, and the individual waveforms are often quite prominent. In addition, there can be an inappropriate increase in the jugular venous pulsation level with inspiration (Kussmaul's sign). Hepatomegaly and ascites may be noted on

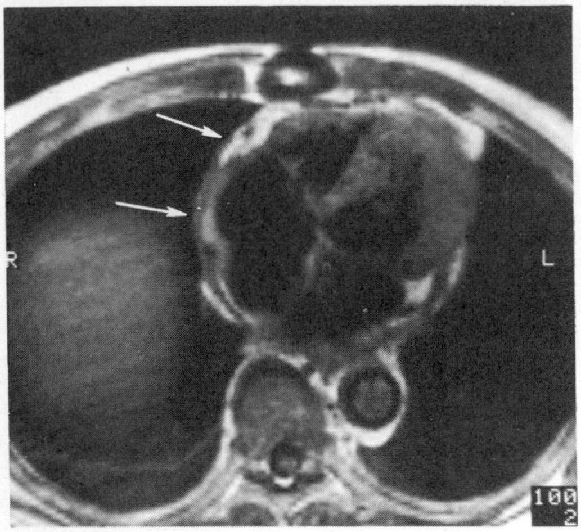

Figure 8–23. Magnetic resonance image of cross-section of thorax showing pericardial thickening (arrows) in a patient with constrictive pericarditis. (Courtesy of C Higgins. Reproduced, with permission, from Cheitlin MD, Sokolow M, McIlroy MB: *Clinical Cardiology*, 6th ed. Appleton & Lange, 1993.)

physical examination. On auscultation of the heart, a high-pitched sound called a pericardial knock can be heard just after the second heart sound, often mimicking a third heart sound.

Etiology

Table 8–8 lists the causes of acute pericarditis. Viruses, particularly the coxsackieviruses, are the most common cause of acute pericarditis. Viruses are also probably responsible for "idiopathic" pericarditis.

Pathophysiology

In pericarditis, microscopic examination of the pericardium shows signs of acute inflammation, with increased numbers of polymorphonuclear leukocytes, increased vascularity, and deposition of fibrin. If the inflammation is long-lived, the pericardium can become fibrotic and scarred, with deposition of calcium.

The heavily fibrotic pericardium can inhibit the filling of the ventricles. At this point, signs of constrictive physiology appear (see below).

Clinical Manifestations

A. Chest Pain: Chest pain is probably due to the inflammation of the pericardium. Inflammation of adjacent pleura may account for the characteristic worsening of pain with deep breathing and coughing.

B. Physical Examination:

1. Friction rub–The pericardial friction rub is thought to arise from friction between the visceral and parietal pericardial surfaces. The rub is traditionally described as having three components, each associated with rapid movement of a cardiac chamber: The systolic component, which is probably related to ventricular contraction, is most common and most easily heard. During diastole, there are two components—one during early diastole, due to rapid filling of the ventricle; and another, quieter component that occurs in late diastole, thought to be due to atrial contraction. Clinically, the diastolic components often merge so that a two-component or "to-and-fro" rub is most commonly heard.

2. Signs of constriction–In the patient with constrictive pericarditis, early diastolic filling of the ventricle occurs normally but the filling is suddenly stopped once the nonelastic thickened pericardium is reached. This leads to sudden cessation of filling that can be observed on the pressure-time curve of the ventricle. This sudden "checking" of flow is probably responsible for the diastolic knock (Figure 8–24). In addition, the rapid emptying of the atrium leads to a prominent *y* descent that makes the *v* wave more noticeable on the atrial pressure tracing (Figure 8–25). Systemic venous pressure is elevated, since flow entering the heart is limited. Usually with inspiration, the decrease in intrathoracic pressure is transmitted to the heart, and filling of the right side of the heart increases with an accompanying fall in systemic venous pressure. In patients with constrictive pericarditis, this normal response is prevented and the patient develops Kussmaul's sign (Figure 8–26). Elevated systemic venous pressure can lead to accu-

Table 8–8. Causes of pericarditis.

Infections
Viral: Coxsackievirus
Bacterial
Tuberculosis
Purulent: Staphylococcal, pneumococcal
Protozoal: Amebiasis
Mycotic: Actinomycosis, coccidioidomycosis
Connective tissue disease
Systemic lupus erytheumatosis
Scleroderma
Rheumatoid arthritis
Neoplasm
Metabolic
Renal failure
Injury
Myocardial infarction
Postinfarction
Postthoracotomy
Trauma
Radiation
Idiopathic

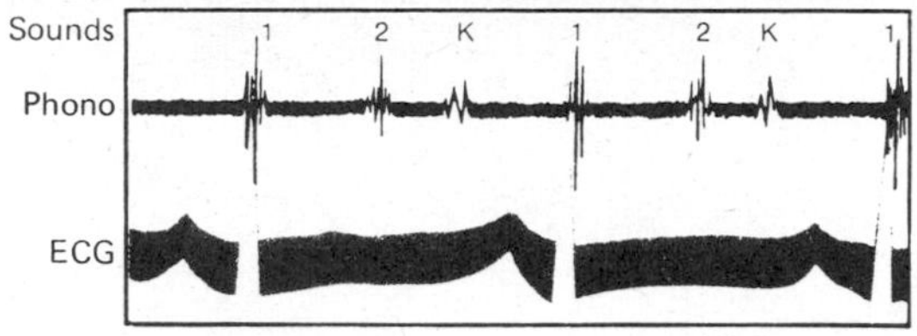

Figure 8–24. Phonocardiogram of typical sharp, early diastolic pericardial knock (K). (Courtesy of Roche Laboratories Division of Hoffman-La Roche, Inc.)

mulation of fluid in the liver and intraperitoneal space, leading to hepatomegaly and ascites.

PERICARDIAL EFFUSION & TAMPONADE

Clinical Presentation

Pericardial effusion may occur in response to any cause of pericarditis, so the patient may develop chest pain or pericardial rub as described above. In addition, pericardial effusion may develop slowly and may be asymptomatic. However, sudden filling of the pericardial space with fluid can have catastrophic consequences by limiting ventricular filling (pericardial tamponade). Patients with pericardial tamponade often complain of shortness of breath, but the diagnosis is most commonly made by noting the characteristic physical examination findings associated with pericardial tamponade.

Pericardial tamponade is accompanied by characteristic physical signs that arise from the limited filling of the ventricle. The three classic signs of pericardial tamponade are called Beck's triad after the surgeon who described them in 1935: (1) hypotension, (2) elevated jugular venous pressure, and (3) muffled heart sounds. In addition, the patient may have a decrease in systemic pressure with inspiration ("paradoxic pulse").

Etiology

Almost any cause of pericarditis can cause pericardial effusion.

Pathophysiology

The pericardium is normally filled with a small amount of fluid (30–50 mL) with an intrapericardial pressure that is usually similar to the intrapleural pressure. With the sudden addition of fluid, the pericardial pressure can increase, at times to the level of the right atrial and right ventricular pressures. The transmural distending pressure of the ventricle decreases and the chamber collapses, preventing appropriate filling of the heart from systemic venous return. The four chambers of the heart occupy a relatively fixed volume in the pericardial sac, and evaluation of hemodynamics reveals equilibration of

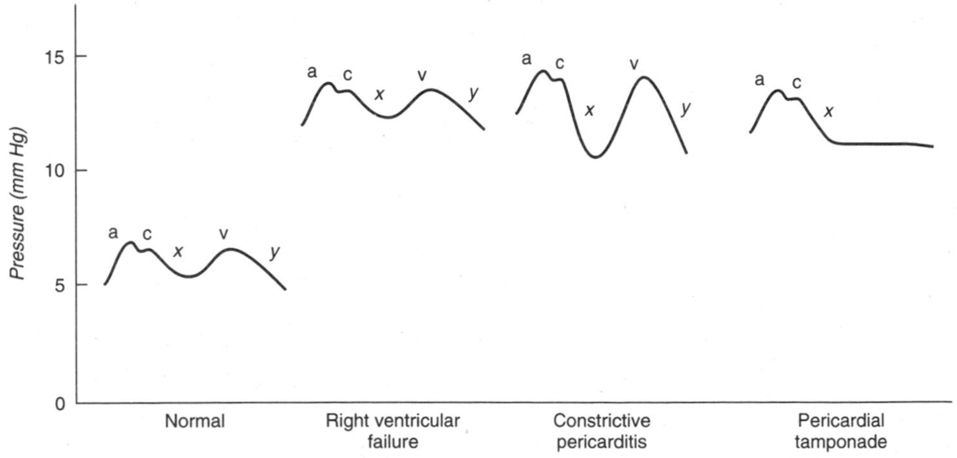

Figure 8–25. Jugular venous pressure waveforms in various kinds of heart disease. In right ventricular failure, mean jugular venous pressure is elevated, but the waveforms remain relatively unchanged. If right ventricular failure is accompanied by tricuspid regurgitation, the *v* wave may become more prominent (since the right atrium is receiving blood both from systemic venous return and the right ventricle. In constrictive pericarditis the *y* descent becomes prominent since the right ventricle rapidly fills in early diastole. In contrast, in pericardial tamponade, the right ventricle only fills during early systole, so that only an *x* descent is observed. In both constrictive pericarditis and pericardial tamponade, mean jugular venous pressure is elevated.

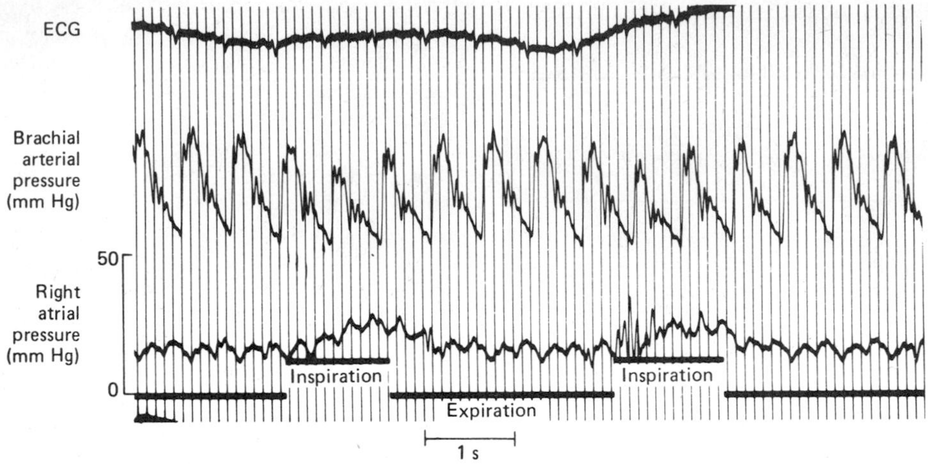

Figure 8–26. Brachial arterial and right atrial pressures showing pulsus paradoxus in a patient with constrictive pericarditis and an increase in right atrial pressure on inspiration (Kussmaul's sign). Both the systolic and diastolic atrial pressures rise with inspiration. (Reproduced, with permission, from Cheitlin MD, Sokolow M, McIlroy MB: *Clinical Cardiology,* 6th ed. Appleton & Lange, 1993.)

ventricular and pulmonary artery diastolic pressures with right atrial and left atrial pressures, all at approximately intrapericardial pressure.

Clinical Manifestations

Since the clinical manifestations of pericardial effusion without tamponade are similar to those of pericarditis, they will not be described here. Instead, the pathophysiologic mechanisms for the signs and symptoms of pericardial tamponade will be described.

A. Shortness of Breath: Dyspnea is the most common symptom of pericardial tamponade. The pathogenesis probably relates to a reduction in cardiac output and, in some patients, the presence of pulmonary edema.

B. Elevated Jugular Venous Pressure: Jugular venous pressure is elevated (Figure 8–25). In addition, cardiac tamponade alters the dynamics of atrial filling. Normally, atrial filling occurs first during ventricular ejection (*x* descent) and then later when the tricuspid valve opens (*y* descent). In cardiac tamponade, during ventricular contraction, the atrium can fill so that the *x* descent can still be seen. However, when the tricuspid valve opens, further filling of the right atrium is prevented because chamber size is limited by the surrounding pericardial fluid. For this reason, the *y* descent is not seen in the patient with pericardial tamponade. Loss of the *y* descent in the setting of elevated jugular venous pressures should always arouse suspicion of pericardial tamponade.

C. Hypotension: Hypotension occurs because of reduced cardiac output.

D. Paradoxic Pulse: Arterial systolic blood pressure normally drops 8–12 mm Hg with inspiration. Marked inspiratory drop in systolic blood pressure (> 20 mm Hg) is an important physical finding in the diagnosis of cardiac tamponade but can also be seen in severe pulmonary disease or, less commonly, in constrictive pericarditis (Figure 8–26). Marked inspiratory decline in left ventricular stroke volume occurs because of decreased left ventricular end-diastolic volume. With inspiration, increased blood return augments filling of the right ventricle which causes the interventricular septum to bow to the left and reduce left ventricular end-diastolic volume (reverse Bernheim effect). Also during inspiration, flow into the left atrium from the pulmonary veins is reduced, further reducing left ventricular preload.

E. Muffled Heart Sounds: Pericardial fluid can cause the heart sounds to become muffled or indistinct.

18. What are the clinical presentations of each form of pericardial disease discussed above?
19. What are the most common causes of pericarditis and pericardial effusion?
20. What is the pathogenesis of pericarditis and of pericardial effusion?
21. What are the major clinical manifestations and complications of pericarditis and pericardial effusion with tamponade?

HYPERTENSION

Clinical Presentation

Uncomplicated hypertension is usually asymptomatic. Symptoms ascribed to hypertension such as headache, nausea, visual changes, tinnitus, and dizziness are just as prevalent in normotensive individuals. Hypertension can be responsible for sudden weakness or numbness of the extremities or pain in the calves, thighs, or buttocks with walking (claudication).

The diagnosis of hypertension is made by measuring serial blood pressures on three separate occasions. However, even single elevated measurements should not be dismissed, since single episodes of elevated systolic blood pressure have been correlated with a higher likelihood of subsequent cardiovascular disease. Blood pressure measurements used to define hypertension under usual conditions are diastolic pressures greater than 90 mm Hg and systolic pressures greater than 160 mm Hg. Normal blood pressures for adolescents and children are much lower.

Additional physical examination findings that may be observed in the patient with hypertension include the presence of a fourth heart sound, narrowing of the arteries or frank hemorrhages on funduscopic examination, pedal edema or anasarca, and decreased peripheral pulses.

Etiology

Hypertension can be classified as primary (95% of cases) or secondary (5% of cases). A patient is said to have primary hypertension when the known causes of hypertension have been excluded and the origin of the elevated blood pressure remains unknown (Table 8–9).

Table 8–9. Causes of hypertension.

Type	Comments
Primary 1. Increased cardiac output Increases in contractility or heart rate	Elevated cardiac output is almost uniformly observed in patients with primary hypertension. Primary increases in contractility and heart rate have been suggested as possible causes of primary hypertension.
Abnormal regulation of fluid volume	Altered mineralocorticoid function or primary alteration of renal sodium transport.
2. Increased vascular resistance Sympathetic nervous defects	Abnormalities in both α- and β-adrenergic responses in patients with primary hypertension have been reported.
Abnormal humoral responses	Altered prostaglandin, kinin, and angiotensin metabolism have been suggested as possible causes of primary hypertension.
Alterations in local regulation of vascular tone	Abnormalities in autoregulation of arteriolar tone have been reported in patients with primary hypertension.
Secondary Drug	A number of drugs can cause hypertension, including oral contraceptives, alcohol, amphetamines, cocaine, sympathomimetics, and nonsteroidal anti-inflammatory agents.
Renal disease	Loss of nephrons or glomerulitis from almost any cause of renal failure can lead to hypertension.
Adrenal disease	Adrenal cortex diseases such Cushing's syndrome can cause hypertension. Adrenal medullary diseases such as pheochromocytoma can cause hypertension from catecholamine secretion.
Hyperparathyroidism	Usually associated with thiazide use and hypercalcemia. Calcium-mediated cardiac and smooth muscle contraction is thought to be the mechanism of hypertension.
Renal artery stenosis	Narrowing of the renal artery can occur because of fibrous dysplasia or atherosclerosis.

Pathophysiology

Multiple pathophysiologic mechanisms for **primary hypertension** have been postulated, and detailed descriptions of each are beyond the scope of this chapter. Briefly, blood pressure is proportionate to cardiac output and peripheral vascular resistance. Increased cardiac output may be due to (1) a primary change in heart rate or contractility, or (2) abnormal renal regulation of fluid volume such as abnormalities in renal sodium transport or altered mineralocorticoid function. Abnormalities in peripheral vascular resistance can occur because of (1) sympathetic nervous defects (abnormal alpha- or beta-adrenergic responses), (2) abnormal humoral responses (prostaglandins, kinins, angiotensin), or (3) abnormalities in local arteriolar tone. In a given patient, any one or a combination of these factors may be responsible for hypertension.

The pathophysiologic mechanisms responsible for **secondary hypertension** are also complex. **Drugs** such as alchohol, cocaine, amphetamines, and sympathomimetics can cause hypertension. About 5% of patients who use estrogen-containing oral contraceptives develop hypertension with blood pressures greater than 140/90 mm Hg. The mechanism probably involves renin-and aldosterone-mediated volume expansion from estrogen-induced increased synthesis of renin substrate. **Renal disease** can also cause elevated hypertension by relative or absolute volume excess. **Adrenal disease** can also cause hypertension by three possible mechanisms: (1) Excess secretion of aldosterone from adrenal adenomas or bilateral adrenal hyperplasia can cause elevated blood pressures. (2) Increased production of cortisol can be associated with hypertension. Cortisol stimulates the synthesis of renin substrate, which allows more angiotensin to be produced. (3) Catecholamine production from adrenal medullary tumors (pheochromocytoma) can cause wild fluctuations of blood pressures. **Hyperparathyroidism** can cause hypertension from elevated calcium. **Narrowing or blockage of large vascular arteries** such as the aorta or the renal artery can cause hypertension by generalized activation of the renin-angiotensin system.

Clinical Manifestations

A. Fourth Heart Sound: Hypertension causes an increased afterload to be placed on the heart. This leads to ventricular hypertrophy, often with associated abnormalities in relaxation. In addition, hypertension is a risk factor for the presence of coronary artery disease, and a fourth heart sound may arise from ischemia (as described earlier).

B. Funduscopic Changes: Hypertension can produce narrowing and wall thickening in the retinal arterioles (Figure 8–27). Progressive hypertension can lead to rupture of the vessels and, if unchecked, swelling of the optic nerve (papilledema).

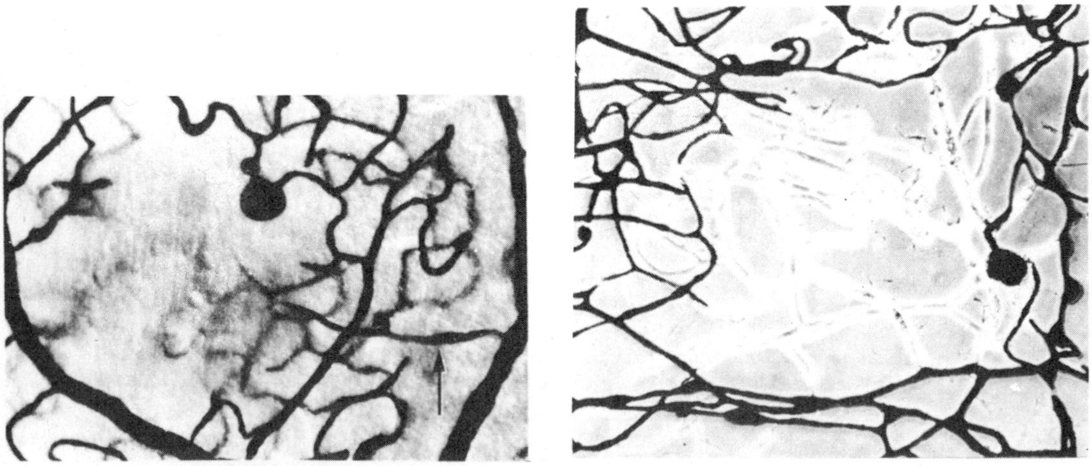

Figure 8–27. ***Left:*** Retina of a patient with malignant hypertensive retinopathy, showing a cotton-wool spot. The capillaries within the affected area have failed to become injected, whereas the capillaries at the margin are dilated and show aneurysm formation. Swollen nerve fibers may be seen in the avascular area. The terminal arteriole (arrow) showed hyalin lipid occlusion. (Injected with India ink; stain: oil red 0; × 90.) ***Right:*** Retina of a patient with malignant hypertensive retinopathy, showing a cotton-wool spot. The retina has been digested, revealing that capillaries are present within the uninjected zone; they appear patent and consist of simple basement membrane tubes without endothelial cells or pericytes. (Injected with India ink; × 130.) (Reproduced, with permission, from Ashton N: Pathophysiology of retinal cotton-wool spots. Br Med Bull 1970;26:143.)

C. Stroke: Hypertension is a major risk factor for cerebral insufficiency or stroke (see Chapter 5).

D. Peripheral Vascular Disease: Long-standing hypertension can lead to narrowing of arteries supplying blood to the lower extremities: iliac, common femoral, and superficial femoral arteries. Ischemic pain or claudication is described as a cramp or sense of fatigue that is usually reproducible at a fixed amount of exertion such as walking one block and resolves after a brief rest. Location of pain is determined by the artery where critical stenosis occurs. Pain occurs in the buttocks for aortoiliac artery occlusion, the thighs for iliofemoral disease, and in the calves for femoral artery disease. Patients with peripheral vascular disease have weak or absent distal pulses, absent foot hair, and pale and cold extremities.

E. Pedal Edema, Anasarca: Hypertension can cause a modest and symmetric decrease in kidney size. In severe cases, renal failure with accompanying fluid retention, leading to pedal edema and anasarca, can occur.

22. What are the clinical presentations of hypertension?
23. What are the most common primary vs secondary causes of hypertension?
24. What is the pathogenesis of primary vs secondary hypertension?
25. What are the major clinical manifestations and complications of hypertension?

SHOCK

Shock can be defined as a clinical syndrome characterized by systemic underperfusion of organs and cells. With such a broad definition, symptoms and signs of shock are likewise diverse and include confusion, loss of consciousness, shortness of breath, cold and clammy skin, and oliguria, all in the setting of reduced blood pressure. Shock is one of the most complex diagnostic and therapeutic challenges facing the physician involved in patient care. However, a clear understanding of the pathophysiologic mechanisms involved can make management of the patient in shock less difficult (Figure 8–28). Shock can arise from one of three causes: cardiac dysfunction, volume loss, and volume maldistribution.

SHOCK DUE TO CARDIAC DYSFUNCTION

Cardiac dysfunction can be further classified as electrical or mechanical. The first decision that must be made by a clinician confronted by a hypotensive patient is whether the cardiac rhythm is hemodynamically stable.

1. SHOCK DUE TO ELECTRICAL DYSFUNCTION

Electrical dysfunction of the heart can be defined as cardiac rhythms that are either too rapid (tachyarrhythmia) or too slow (bradyarrhythmia) to allow for efficient perfusion of end-organs.

Tachyarrhythmias

Tachyarrhythmias can arise from three basic mechanisms (Figure 8–29): (1) Increased automaticity from more rapid phase 4 depolarization can cause a more rapid heart rate. (2) Spontaneous depolarizations can sometimes occur in phase 3 or phase 4 of an action potential. If these depolarizations reach threshold, sustained tachycardia can ensue which is called "triggered activity," since it is dependent on the existence of a preceding action potential. (2) Most commonly, tachyarrhythmias arise from a reentrant circuit in abnormal cardiac tissue. Any condition that gives rise to adjacent regions with different conduction velocities (such as the border zone of a myocardial infarction) can serve as the substrate for a reentrant circuit.

Regardless of the mechanism, clinical management of tachyarrhythmias depends on whether the QRS complex is narrow or wide. If the QRS complex is narrow, depolarization of the ventricles must be occurring normally over the specialized conduction tissues of the heart and the arrhythmia must be originating at or above the AV node (supraventricular) (Figure 8–30). Initial treatment of narrow complex tachyarrhythmias should be a bolus of 6–12 mg of adenosine. Adenosine causes rapid but short-lived slowing of atrial and AV nodal conduction. Since the reentrant circuits of AV nodal reentrant tachycardia and atrioventricular reentry critically involve the AV node, these tachycardias will usually be terminated by this maneuver. Atrial tachycardia due to reentry or triggered activity will also usually terminate by slowing of atrial conduction and breaking the reentrant circuit or by shortening the action potential and abolishing the phase 3 or 4 depolarizations. In atrial tachycardia due to automaticity, atrial fibrillation, and atrial flutter, adenosine will slow the arrhythmia but usually will not terminate it. However, transient slowing will allow the appropriate diagnosis to be

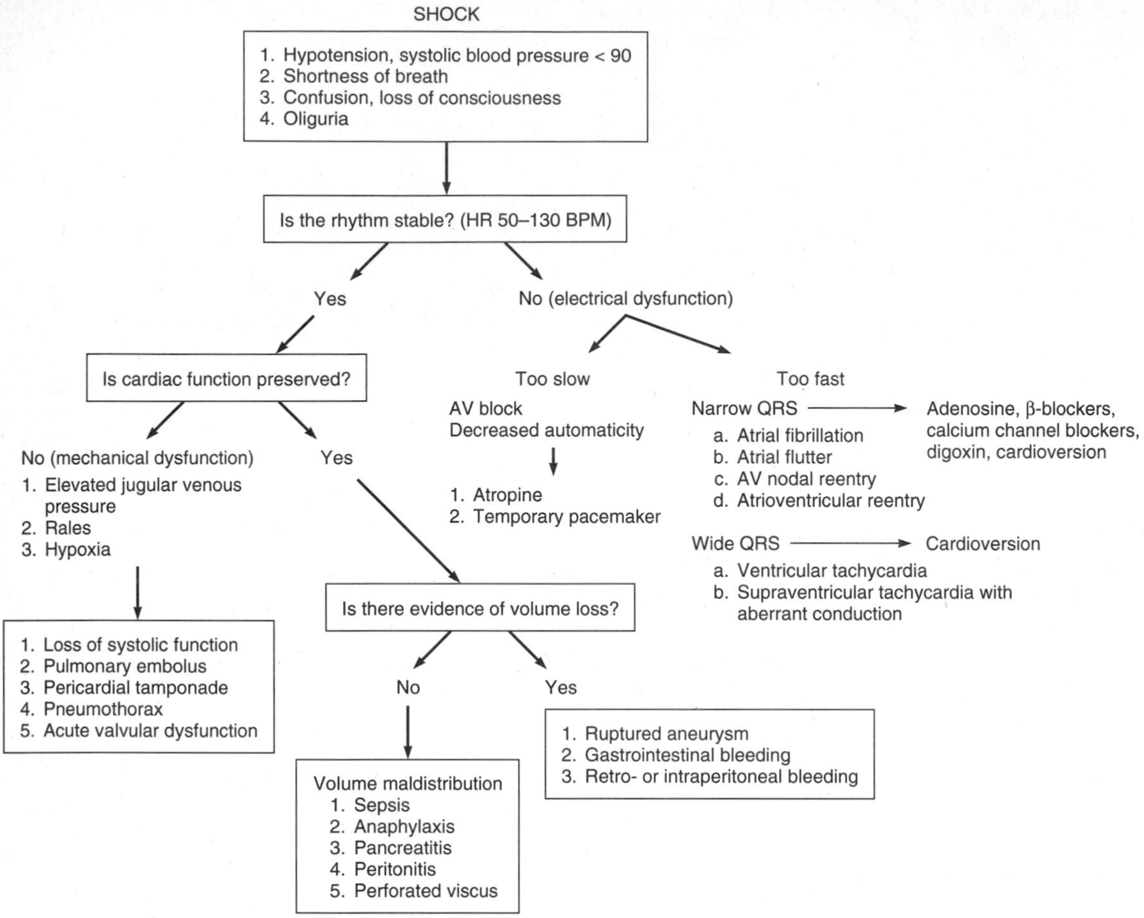

Figure 8–28. Flow sheet for management of the patient in shock.

made and often restores hemodynamic stability. Since adenosine has a short half-life, treatment of atrial flutter and fibrillation should be supplemented by drugs that slow conduction through the AV node, such as digoxin, beta-blockers, or calcium channel blockers. If adenosine is ineffective and the patient remains hypotensive and critically ill in any of the narrow complex QRS tachyarrhythmias, synchronized cardioversion should be performed.

A wide QRS complex suggests that ventricular activation is not occurring normally over the specialized conduction tissues of the heart. The tachycardia is either arising from ventricular tissue or is a supraventricular tachycardia aberrantly conducted down the Purkinje fibers. While many criteria have been developed for distinguishing between these two possibilities, regardless of cause, any wide complex tachycardia that is associated with hypotension should be immediately treated with electrical cardioversion.

Bradyarrhythmias

Bradyarrhythmias arise from loss of normal pacemaker activity in the SA and AV nodes or block of the impulse at some point in the conduction system, usually at the AV node. Treatment includes reducing parasympathetic tone by administering 0.5–2 mg of intravenous atropine and, if the bradyarrhythmias persists, placement of a temporary pacemaker.

2. SHOCK DUE TO MECHANICAL DYSFUNCTION

Mechanical dysfunction is most often due to **primary loss of systolic function** in a patient with a my-

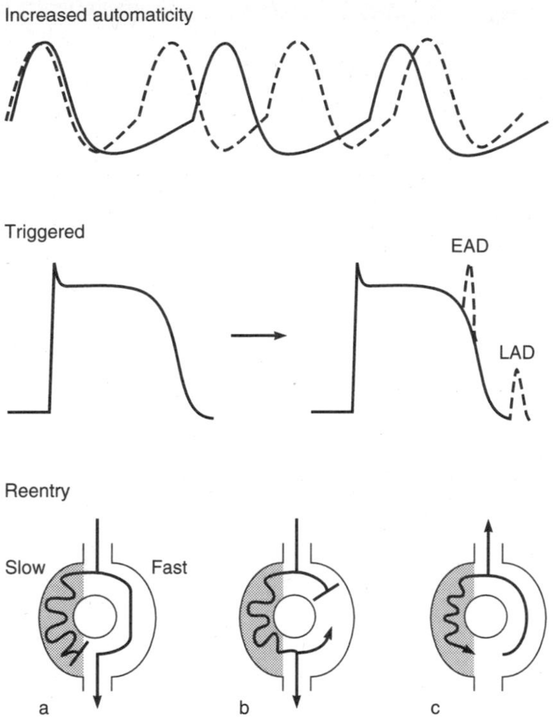

Figure 8–29. Tachyarrhythmias can arise from three different mechanisms. First, increased automaticity from more rapid phase 4 depolarization can cause arrhythmias. Second, in certain conditions, spontaneous depolarizations during phase 3 (early afterdepolarizations) or phase 4 (late afterdepolarizations) can repetitively reach threshhold and cause tachycardia. This appears to be the mechanism of the polymorphic ventricular tachycardia (torsade de pointes) observed in some patients taking procainamide or quinidine and the arrhythmias associated with digoxin toxicity. The most common mechanism for tachyarrhythmia is reentry. Third, in reentry two parallel pathways with different conduction properties exist (perhaps at the border zone of a myocardial infarction or a region of myocardial ischemia). The electrical impulse normally travels down the fast pathway and the slow pathway (shaded region), but at the point where the two pathways converge the impulse traveling down the slow pathway is blocked since the tissue is refractory from the recent depolarization via the fast pathway (a). However, when a premature beat reaches the circuit, block can occur in the fast pathway, and the impulse will travel down the slow pathway (shaded region) (b). After traveling through the slow pathway the impulse can then retrogradely enter the fast pathway (which because of the delay has recovered excitability), and then reenter the slow pathway to start a continuous loop of activation, or reentrant circuit (c).

ocardial infarction or decompensated congestive heart failure. However, several other syndromes can cause mechanical dysfunction of the heart. The pericardial space can fill with fluid in patients with trauma, neoplasm, pericarditis, or uremia. **Pericardial tamponade** occurs when the accumulation of fluid interferes with normal filling of the left and right ventricles. This syndrome is characterized by elevated venous pressure, hypotension, and a quiet precordium. Treatment consists of immediate drainage of the pericardial fluid. **Massive pulmonary embolus** can result in mechanical obstruction of the pulmonary artery and present with shock. **Tension pneumothorax** can occur in patients with traumatic injury to the chest, those with chronic obstructive lung disease, or those being maintained by mechanical ventilation. Accumulation of air in the pleural space can cause a shift in mediastinal structures that interferes with cardiac filling and ejection. Treatment of these syndromes is addressed in the chapter on respiratory pathophysiology. Finally, acute **mitral or aortic valve regurgitation** can present as shock. Prompt repair or replacement of the defective valve is required in both of these conditions.

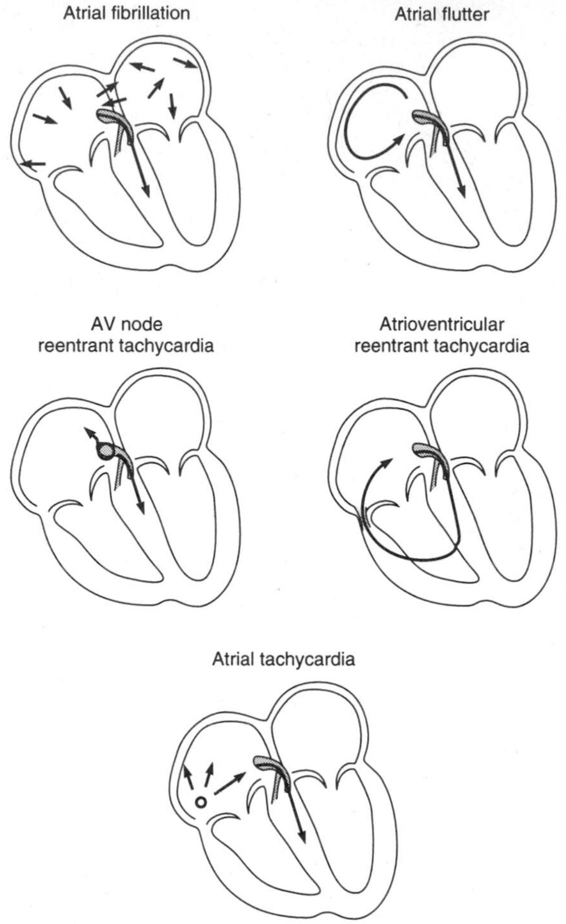

Figure 8–30. In supraventricular tachycardia, the QRS is narrow since the ventricles are depolarized over the normal specialized conduction tissues (hatched region). There are five possible arrhythmias commonly encountered. First, in atrial fibrillation, multiple microreentrant circuits can lead to chaotic activation of the atrium. Since impulses are reaching the AV node at irregular intervals, ventricular depolarization is irregular. Second, in atrial flutter, a macroreentrant circuit, traveling up the interatrial septum and down the lateral walls can activate the atria in a regular fashion at approximately 300 beats/min. The AV node can conduct only every other or every third beat, so that the ventricles are depolarized at 150 or 100 beats/min. In AV node reentrant tachycardia, slow and fast pathways exist in the region of the AV node and a microreentrant circuit can be formed. Fourth, in atrial tachycardia an abnormal focus of atrial activity due to either reentry, triggered activity, or abnormal automaticity can activate the atria in a regular fashion. Finally, in atrioventricular reentry, an abnormal connection between the atrium and ventricle exists so that a reentrant circuit can be formed with the AV node forming the slow pathway, and the abnormal atrioventricular connection, the fast pathway.

SHOCK DUE TO VOLUME LOSS

If both electrical and mechanical function of the heart appear to be normal, sources of fluid or blood loss must be searched for. Excessive **fluid loss** can occur from vomiting, diarrhea, polyuria, burns, or trauma with extensive muscle injury. **Blood loss** can occur from the gastrointestinal tract, a ruptured aortic aneurysm, retro- or intraperitoneal bleeding, and bleeding into the respiratory tract (hemoptysis) or into the pleural space (hemothorax). Treatment includes rapid resuscitation with fluid (isotonic fluids such as normal saline and lactated Ringer's solution are preferred) and blood if appropriate. After aggressive fluid resuscitation has begun, treatment of the underlying problem must be quickly addressed.

SHOCK DUE TO VOLUME MALDISTRIBUTION

Hypotension and shock may also occur because of volume maldistribution. **Sepsis,** usually from gram-negative bacteremia, can cause massive capillary leakage that results in hypotension. Patients should receive aggressive fluid resuscitation; vasopressor agents such as dopamine can also be used to reverse the hypotension. Exposure to allergens or venoms can result in **anaphylaxis,** a disorder in which chemical mediators such as serotonin and histamines cause a widespread increase in vascular permeability. Epinephrine, 0.5–1 mL of 1:1000 solution, should be administered subcutaneously or intramuscularly along with aggressive fluid replacement. **Pancreatitis, peritonitis,** or a **perforated viscus** can cause shock by increased "third-spacing'' of fluid into the interstitial spaces. Patients should first receive aggressive fluid resuscitation, and the underlying problem should then be treated.

26. What is the clinical presentation of shock?
27. What are the three basic mechanisms of tachyarrhythmias?
28. What are the most common mechanical causes of cardiac dysfunction?
29. Changes in what two features of volume status can precipitate shock? By what mechanisms?

REFERENCES

General

Hoffman BF et al: Electrophysiology and pharmacology of cardiac arrhythmias. Am Heart J 1975;89:115.

Wit AL: Cellular electrophysiologic mechanisms of cardiac arrhythmias. Cardiol Clin 1990;8:393.

Gilmour RF, Zipes DP: Basic electrophysiologic mechanisms for development of arrhythmias. Med Clin North Am 1984;68:795.

Crawford ES et al: Aortic dissection and dissecting aortic aneurysm. Ann Surg 1988;208:254.

Dobrin PB: Pathophysiology and pathogenesis of aortic aneurysm. Surg Clin North Am 1989;69:687.

Breslin DJ: Peripheral vascular disease in the elderly. Cardiol Clin 1991;9:193.

Congestive Heart Failure

Ruggie N: Congestive heart failure. Med Clin North Am 1986;70:829.

Strobeck JE, Sonnenblick EH: Pathophysiology of heart failure: Deficiency in cardiac contraction. In: *Drug Treatment of Heart Failure.* Cohn J (editor). Advanced Therapeutics Communications, 1988.

Shah PM: Diastolic heart failure. Curr Prob Cardiol 1992;7:411.

Valvular Abnormalities

Carabello B: Valvular heart disease. Cardiol Clin 1991;9:193.

Coronary Artery Disease

Opie LH: Pathophysiology and biochemistry of ischemia, necrosis, and reperfusion. In: *Acute Myocardial Infarction.* Gersh BJ, Rahimtoola SH (editors). Elsevier, 1991.

Raines EW, Ross R: Smooth muscle cells and the pathogenesis of the lesions of atherosclerosis. Br Heart J 1993;69(1 Suppl):S30.

Fisher M: Atherosclerosis: Cellular aspects and potential interventions. Cerebrovasc Brain Metab Rev 1991; 3:114.

Ip JH et al: Syndromes of accelerated atherosclerosis: Role of vascular injury and smooth muscle cell proliferation. J Am Coll Cardiol 1990;15:1667.

Pericardial Disease

Shabetai R: Diseases of the pericardium. Cardiol Clin 1990;8:579.

Hypertension

Cheitlin MD, Sokolow M, McIlroy MB: *Clinical Cardiology,* 6th ed. Appleton & Lange, 1993.

Haddy FJ: Roles of sodium, potassium, calcium, and natriuretic factors in hypertension. Hypertension 1991;18(5 Suppl):III179.

Bohr DF, Dominiczak AF, Webb RC: Pathophysiology of the vasculature in hypertension. Hypertension 1991;18(5 Suppl):III69.

Kaplan NM: Hormonal and local factors in hypertension. Am J Med Sci 1991;301:412.

Luke RG: Essential hypertension: A renal disease? A review and update of the evidence. Hypertension 1993;21:380.

Vicaut E: Hypertension and the microcirculation: A brief overview of experimental studies. J Hypertens 1992;10(5 Suppl):S59.

Shock

Ahktar M et al: Wide QRS complex tachycardia: Reappraisal of a common clinical problem. Ann Intern Med 1988;109:905.

Billhardt RA, Rosenbush SW: Cardiogenic and hypovolemic shock. Med Clin North Am 1986;70:853.

Haynes DE, DiMarco JP: Current therapy for supraventricular tachycardia. Curr Probl Cardiol 1992;7:411.

Walsh KA, Ezrii MD, Denes P: Emergency treatment of tachyarrhythmias. Med Clin North Am 1986;70:791.

Gastrointestinal Disease

9

Vishwanath R. Lingappa, MD, PhD

Gastrointestinal diseases most often present with one or more of four common classes of signs and symptoms: (1) abdominal or chest pain; (2) altered ingestion of food, eg, due to nausea, vomiting, **dysphagia** (difficulty swallowing), **odynophagia** (painful swallowing), or **anorexia** (lack of appetite); (3) altered bowel movements, ie, diarrhea or constipation; and (4) gastrointestinal bleeding, occurring either without warning or preceded by one or more of the foregoing (Table 9–1). However, not all cases of a particular gastrointestinal disease present in the same way. For example, peptic ulcer disease, while typically accompanied by abdominal pain, may be painless.

Gastrointestinal disease may be limited to the gastrointestinal tract (eg, reflux esophagitis, peptic ulcer, diverticular disease); may be a manifestation of a systemic disorder (eg, inflammatory bowel disease); or may be manifested as a systemic disease resulting from a primary gastrointestinal pathologic process (eg, vitamin deficiencies due to malabsorption). Since different parts of the gastrointestinal tract are specialized for certain functions, the most prominent causes, consequences, and manifestations of disease differ from region to region (see Table 9–2).

Acutely, gastrointestinal disease can be complicated by dehydration, sepsis, or bleeding or by their consequences, such as shock. **Dehydration** can occur as a consequence of even subtle alterations in fluid input or outflow because the volume of fluid traversing the gastrointestinal tract daily is enormous (see below). **Sepsis** can result from disruption of the barrier function against pathogens in the environment, including bacteria resident in the colon. The tendency to **bleeding** is a reflection of the tremendous vascularity of the gastrointestinal tract and the inability to apply pressure at the site of bleeding.

Chronically, gastrointestinal disease can be complicated by malnutrition and deficiency states. These occur because many primary gastrointestinal diseases result in **malabsorption** (failure to absorb one or more necessary nutrients in ingested food).

Gastrointestinal tract disease can present as partial or complete **obstruction** (blockage of movement of contents down the gastrointestinal tract) due to **adhesions** and **stenosis** resulting from proliferation of connective tissue in response to inflammation. The signs and symptoms of obstruction can range from mild nausea, abdominal pain, and anorexia to projectile vomiting, rebound tenderness with progression to perforation, infarction and bleeding, hypotension, shock, and death. The severity of symptoms depends on the extent of obstruction and the degree to which the obstruction compromises blood flow to the affected region.

1. What are the cardinal signs and symptoms of gastrointestinal disease?
2. What are some acute systemic complications of primary gastrointestinal disease?
3. What additional systemic manifestations can occur as a result of chronic gastrointestinal disease?

I. STRUCTURE & FUNCTION OF THE GASTROINTESTINAL TRACT

The gastrointestinal tract includes the continuous lumen from mouth to anus which is involved in separating ingested food into nutrients to be assimilated and wastes to be eliminated (Figure 9–1). The activities necessary to achieve these goals can be broadly categorized as motility, secretion, digestion, and absorption. **Motility** is achieved by muscular contractions of different segments of the gastrointestinal tract. **Secretion** depends upon the transport of substances derived from the epithelial cells lining the tract into the gut lumen or from gastrointestinal endocrine cells into the interstitial spaces between cells and into the bloodstream. **Digestion** consists of the breakdown of substances within the gut lumen. **Absorption** refers to transport of the modified nutrients from the gut lumen into and across the lining epithelial cells. Different regions of the gastrointestinal tract are specialized for support of these processes, which are under neural and hormonal control.

Table 9–1. Common presentations of gastrointestinal disease.

Cardinal Gastrointestinal Symptom or Sign	Esophagus	Stomach	Intestines
Pain	Achalasia, reflux	Gastric ulcer Gastric cancer	Perforation/Infarction Duodenal ulcer Irritable bowel syndrome Diverticular disease
Altered ingestion			
Dysphagia	Achalasia, reflux		
Nausea, vomiting	Achalasia, reflux Esophageal cancer	Gastroparesis	Acute gastroenteritis Obstruction
Altered bowel movements			
Constipation			Diverticular disease Diabetic autonomic neuropathy
Diarrhea		Gastric surgery, dumping syndrome	Gastroenteritis Irritable bowel syndrome Inflammatory bowel disease Diabetic autonomic neuropathy
Bleeding			
Hematemesis	Varices due to portal hypertension	Gastric ulcer Mucosal laceration (eg, after violent retching)	Duodenal ulcer
Bloody stools (including melena, frank blood and occult blood)	Varices	Gastric ulcer	Inflammatory bowel disease Duodenal ulcer Diverticular disease Colon cancer Gastroenteritis Infarction

Histologically, the wall of the gastrointestinal tract is composed of four major layers. From the lumen outward, these are the mucosa, submucosa, muscularis externa, and serosa (Figure 9–2). Each of these layers can be further subdivided into components with different structure and function. Thus, the mucosa consists not only of the epithelial cells that line the lumen of the gastrointestinal tract but also the immediately adjacent **lamina propria,** a layer of loose connective tissue rich in blood and lymph vessels and immune system cells, including both macrophages and lymphocytes active in secretion of IgA and IgM. In some regions of the gastrointestinal tract, glands and organized lymphoid tissue are also found in the lamina propria. Finally, the innermost aspect of the mucosa is demarcated by a thin layer of smooth muscle called the **muscularis mucosae.** It has both inner (circular) and outer (longitudinal) fibers. The muscularis mucosae is an important boundary in determining whether cancer of the gastrointestinal tract is still localized to its site of origin or is likely to have metastasized, ie, spread to distant regions of the body. In certain parts of the gastrointestinal tract, the mucosa is further organized into folds termed **villi** and **microvilli,** which serve to greatly increase the luminal surface area and which have important functional implications.

Table 9–2. Alteration of normal physiologic processes in common gastrointestinal disorders by site.

Physiologic Process	Esophagus	Stomach	Small Bowel	Colon
Motility	Achalasia	Diabetic gastroparesis Postsurgery (vagotomy, pyloroplasty)	Irritable bowel syndrome Obstruction Adhesions	Irritable bowel syndrome Diverticular disease Cancer
Digestion	. . .	Acid hypersecretion	Diarrhea	. . .
Absorption	. . .	Acid hypersecretion	Malabsorption	Malabsorption
Secretion	Reflux esophagitis	Gastric ulcer	Duodenal ulcer Secretory diarrhea	Diarrhea
Blood flow	Variceal bleeding	Mucosal laceration (Mallory-Weiss tear)	Ischemia, infarction Vascular telangiectasia	Cancer Inflammatory bowel disease Diverticular disease

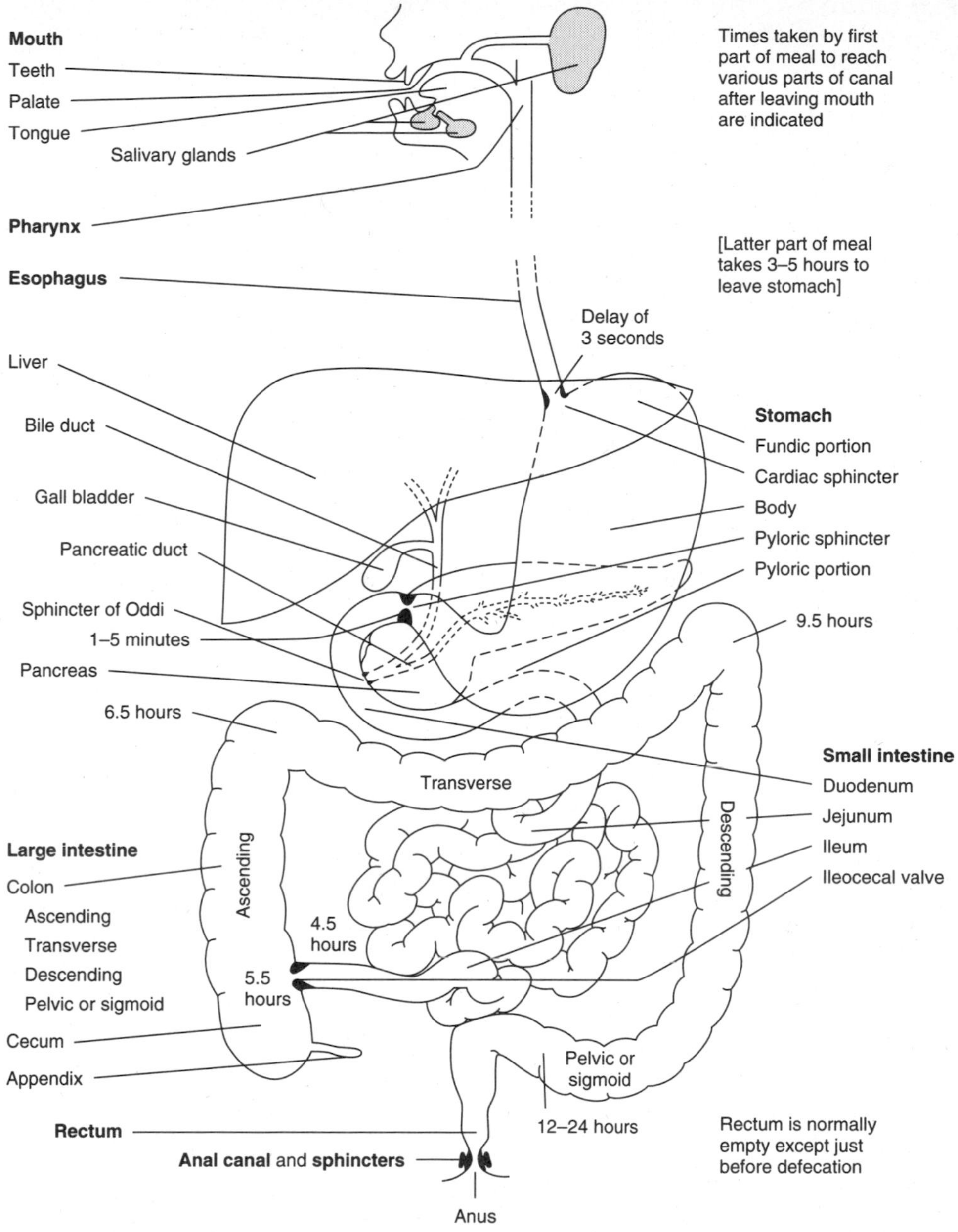

Figure 9–1. Progress of food along the alimentary canal. Food undergoes mechanical as well as chemical changes to render it suitable for absorption and assimilation. (Modified and reproduced, with permission, from Mackenna BR, Callander R: *Illustrated Physiology,* 5th ed. Churchill Livingstone, 1990.)

The **submucosa** is a layer of loose connective tissue directly beneath the mucosa containing not only larger blood and lymphatic vessels but also a nerve plexus of the intrinsic enteric nervous system termed the **submucosal nerve plexus (Meissner).** This nerve plexus is particularly important for control of secretion in the gastrointestinal tract. In some areas, the submucosa also contains glands and organized lymphoid tissue. The **muscularis externa** contains gut smooth muscle and is responsible for gastrointestinal tract motility. There are two layers of muscle fibers: an innermost circular layer, whose contraction decreases the diameter of the intestinal lumen; and an outer longitudinal layer, whose contraction shortens the tube. Between these muscle layers lies the **myenteric nerve plexus (Auerbach)** of the enteric ner-

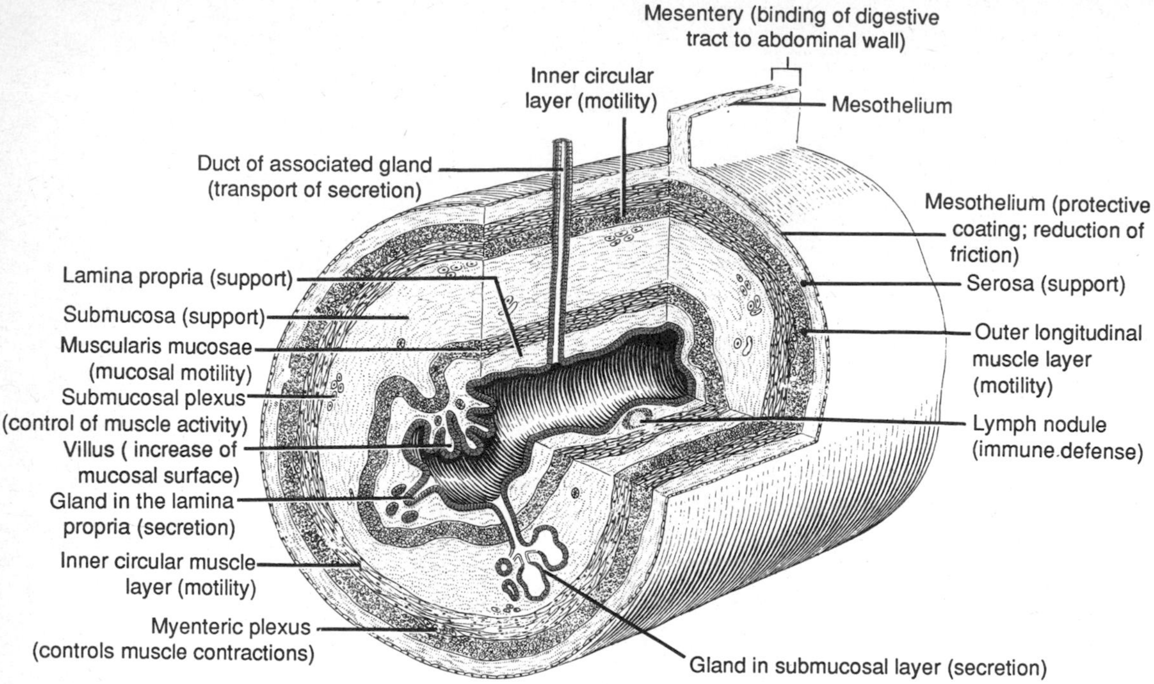

Figure 9–2. Schematic structure of a portion of the digestive tract with various possible components. (Redrawn and reproduced, with permission, from Bevelander G: *Outline of Histology,* 7th ed. Mosby, 1971.)

vous system, involved primarily in control of motility. The **serosa** is the outermost layer, where larger nerves and blood vessels travel in a bed of connective and adipose tissue.

4. What are the broad classes of gastrointestinal tract functions?
5. Describe the key microscopic anatomic features of a cross-section of the gastrointestinal tract.
6. What features of gastrointestinal tract anatomy predispose to severe bleeding?

Functions of the Gastrointestinal Tract

A. Motility: The motility of the gastrointestinal tract is due to the contraction of smooth muscle. Smooth muscle cells have a small excess of negative charge in their interior as a result of the activity of pumps in the plasma membrane. When a cell is depolarized, this potential difference is transiently abolished, generating a signal that (1) triggers events within that cell, leading to sliding of actin and myosin filaments; and (2) is propagated to neighboring cells, resulting in the coordinated response of muscle contraction. Depolarization of a cell can occur spontaneously or in response to a neural or hormonal stimulus depending on the specific characteristics of different cells. Gastrointestinal smooth muscle displays differences in contractile properties in different regions of the tract. "Slow wave" oscillating depolarizations occur in some areas and rapid "spike" depolarizations in other areas. Each type occurs with a characteristic frequency, but each can also be triggered by specific stimuli such as stretch, neuronal input, or hormones. Short bursts of spikes cause phasic motor activity; longer bursts cause tonic muscle contraction. Tonic contraction occurs at **sphincters** (locations that serve as "gates" which allow further movement down the gastrointestinal tract only during relaxation). Phasic electrical activity occurs at the intervening regions of the gastrointestinal tract (between sphincters).

The degree of central nervous system control over gut motility varies from region to region: Striated muscle of the mouth, pharynx, and proximal esophagus is under direct central nervous system control; the small intestine is almost totally independent of the central nervous system, being controlled instead by a system of neurons localized entirely to the gastrointestinal tract and termed the **enteric nervous system;** the stomach, colon, and distal esophagus are under partial central nervous system control. Generally speaking, parasympathetic nerve stimulation causes muscle contraction and secretion while sympathetic nerve stimulation inhibits blood flow and motility. These effects of the autonomic nervous system occur both directly and by interfacing with neurons of the enteric nervous system.

The myenteric plexus has two programmed responses, **segmental** and **peristaltic,** which characterize the motility of the gastrointestinal tract. The segmental program predominates in the postprandial period, the peristaltic pattern during fasting. Program selection is determined by hormonal, neural, and other factors and is manifested in different ways in different parts of the gastrointestinal tract.

B. Secretion: Certain epithelial cells lining the intestinal lumen (or glands that connect to the lumen) are specialized to secrete large volumes of fluid containing acid, digestive enzymes, or other products. The daily fluid load in the gastrointestinal tract is approximately 2 L of oral intake and 7 L of secretions (1.5 L saliva, 2.5 L gastric juice, 0.5 L bile, 1.5 L pancreatic juice, and 1 L intestinal secretions). From this total of 9 L, approximately 100 mL ends up in stool daily, with the balance recycled (Figure 9–3).

Several mechanisms can be used to transport substances in the gastrointestinal tract. Ions as well as small charged molecules such as amino acids, small peptides, and sugars are transported directly across the epithelial plasma membrane via the processes of diffusion, facilitated diffusion, and active transport. Only active transport requires metabolic energy. Active transport can be of two sorts, either primary (where energy from ATP hydrolysis is used to transport a specific molecule directly across the membrane) or secondary (where transport of one substance is coupled to that of another). An example of primary active transport is the H^+-K^+ ATPase in the stomach. An example of secondary active transport is the coupling of monosaccharide and amino acid uptake to the Na^+ gradient established by Na^+-K^+ ATPase. For large molecules such as proteins, transport occurs by pinching-off from and fusion of membrane vesicles with the plasma membrane. These processes are termed **endocytosis** (uptake into) and **exocytosis** (export out of) epithelial cells.

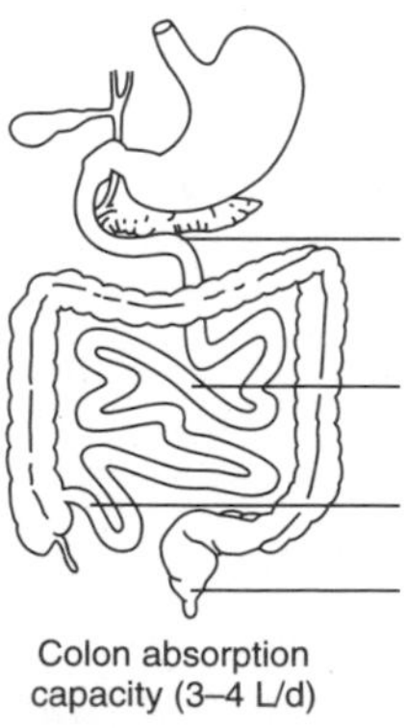

Flow rate mL/d	Ion concentrations meq/L Na^+	K^+	Cl^-	HCO_3^-	Osmolality mosm/kg
9000	60	15	60	15	Variable
3000	140	6	100	30	Isotonic
1000	140	8	60	70	Isotonic
100	40	90	15	30	Isotonic

Figure 9–3. Approximate flow rates per day and ionic constituents of fluid passing through different levels of the intestine. (Reproduced, with permission, from Fine KD, Krejs GJ, Fordtran JS: Diarrhea. In: *Gastrointestinal Disease,* 4th ed. Sleisenger MH, Fordtran JS [editors]. Saunders, 1990.)

Structures in the proximal part of the gastrointestinal tract are more directly involved in secretion. For example, saliva is secreted from the mouth, acid is secreted from the stomach, and mucus, bicarbonate, and digestive enzymes from the pancreas. Conversely, structures in the distal part of the gastrointestinal tract (ie, intestine) are more involved in absorption. For example, the products of digestion are absorbed in small intestine, while water is absorbed from the colon. Likewise, in the small intestine, epithelial cells of the villus tip are prominently involved in absorption while epithelial cells of the crypts are involved in secretion.

C. Digestion: The complex process of digestion actually starts in the mouth through the action of salivary amylase, lingual lipase, and the act of chewing. In the small intestine, the process has four phases: (1) hydrolysis in the intestinal lumen, (2) hydrolysis at the enterocyte brush border, (3) transport of nutrients into the enterocyte, and (4) processing of nutrients within and export from the enterocyte into the portal or lymphatic circulation.

7. What kind of electrical activity occurs at sphincters, and what are its consequences?
8. Describe the range in extent of central nervous system control over gut motility in different parts of the gastrointestinal tract.
9. What are the programmed responses of the myenteric plexus of the enteric nervous system, and when do they occur?
10. What are the sources and approximate daily volumes of fluids entering the gastrointestinal tract?
11. By what mechanisms can substances be transported into or out of enterocytes?
12. What is the role of the villus tip versus crypts in absorption versus secretion?
13. List the key steps in carbohydrate, fat, and protein digestion.

Mechanisms of Control of Gastrointestinal Tract Functions

Neural and hormonal factors regulate the processes of motility, secretion, digestion, and absorption in the gastrointestinal tract (Figure 9–4).

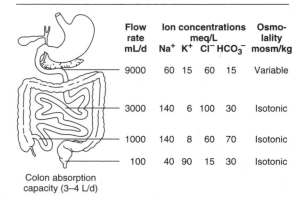

A. Neural Control: Gastrointestinal tract functions are controlled by both the central nervous system, working through autonomic components of the peripheral nervous system, and by the enteric nervous system. The size and complexity of the enteric

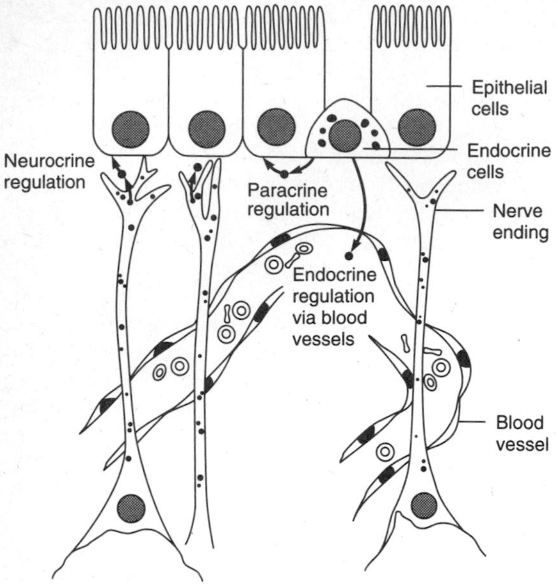

Figure 9–4. Neural and hormonal control of the intestine. (Reproduced, with permission, from Dharmsathaphorn K: Intestinal water and electrolyte transport. In: *Textbook of Internal Medicine.* Kelley WN [editor]. Lippincott, 1989.)

nervous system is remarkable: It contains more neurons than the spinal cord and receives sensory input from neurons specialized to detect chemical, osmotic, or thermal changes in the lumen or mechanical activity involving the gut wall. This information is integrated with and modified by input from the central nervous system via the sympathetic and parasympathetic neurons, which synapse with intramural neurons and provide the program for motor neurons. In this way, otherwise random and uncontrolled phasic motor and secretory activity of the gut becomes purposeful and coordinated, as manifested by characteristic gut programs such as peristalsis and sphincter control.

The enteric nervous system consists of two major networks of neurons and their processes—the myenteric plexus and the submucosal plexus—as well as several minor ones. The myenteric plexus is largely involved with muscular contraction while the submucosal plexus tonically suppresses fluid and electrolyte transport and limits the absorptive capacity of the intestine. These secretory effects are mediated by neurotransmitters released by the motor neurons that interact with receptors on intestinal epithelial cells to influence the function of ion channels.

The dependence of the enteric nervous system on central nervous system control varies with the embryologic origin of gut structures. The characteristic functions of structures derived from the embryonic foregut (proximal to the ampulla of Vater) are more dependent on central nervous system control (eg, esophageal peristalsis, relaxation of the lower esophageal sphincter, gastric accommodation and peristalsis, pyloric sphincter function). However, midgut- and hindgut-derived structures (ie, small and large intestine) function relatively well when their connections with the central nervous system are disrupted.

The clinical importance of the enteric nervous system itself is emphasized when its function is lost, which can occur at several levels. In esophageal achalasia, for example, the body of the esophagus is quiet and the lower sphincter is tonically contracted, making ingestion of food difficult or impossible. Similarly, loss of enteric nervous system function in syndromes of pseudo-obstruction of the small bowel or Hirschsprung's disease in the colon have severe clinical consequences, including abdominal pain, distention, and a risk of catastrophic intestinal perforation.

B. Hormonal Control: Unlike the other endocrine glands, the gastrointestinal endocrine system is a diffuse aggregate of individual cells distributed throughout the mucosa of the tract. Armed with apical microvilli and crammed with basal secretory granules, they are ideally situated to respond to a change in the luminal environment by releasing their secretory products into the bloodstream.

Many peptides produced in the gastrointestinal tract are neurotransmitters of the enteric nervous system rather than true hormones. Others may be involved in **paracrine** actions (affecting neighboring cells rather than distant cells via the bloodstream). Some peptides play multiple roles in the gastrointestinal tract, and some do serve as hormones and play a role in the pathophysiology of gastrointestinal disease (Table 9–3).

Mechanisms of Defense of the Gastrointestinal Tract

The gastrointestinal tract is an interface between the external and internal environments where external products are broken down into nutrients and imported into the bloodstream. The gastrointestinal tract must be defended from pathogens that would use this route to enter the body as well as from corrosive products capable of digesting the gastrointestinal tract itself. Multiple lines of defense have evolved to deal with these diverse threats to gastrointestinal integrity and systemic homeostasis (Table 9–4; Figure 9–5).

14. What are the roles of the myenteric and submucosal plexuses in control of the gastrointestinal tract?
15. What are some functions of each of the major families of gastrointestinal tract hormones?
16. Describe the defense mechanisms that serve to protect the gastrointestinal tract from acid and infection.

Table 9–3. Secretory products of the gastrointestinal tract.[1]

Products	Physiologic Actions	Site of Release	Stimulus for Release	Disease Association
True hormones				
Gastrin	Stimulates acid secretion and growth of gastric oxyntic gland mucosa	Gastric antrum (and duodenum)	Peptides, amino acids, distention, vagal stimulation	Zollinger-Ellison syndrome, peptic ulcer disease
CCK	Stimulates gallbladder contraction, pancreatic enzyme and bicarbonate secretion, and growth of exocrine pancreas	Duodenum and jejunum	Peptides, amino acids, long chain fatty acids, (acid)	
Secretin	Stimulates pancreatic bicarbonate secretion, biliary bicarbonate secretion, growth of exocrine pancreas, pepsin secretion; inhibits gastric acid secretion, trophic effects of gastrin	Duodenum	Acid, (fat)	
GIP	Stimulates insulin release; (inhibits gastric acid secretion)	Duodenum, jejunum	Glucose, amino acids, fatty acids	
Candidate hormones				
Motilin	Stimulates gastric and duodenal motility	Duodenum and jejunum	Unknown	Irritable bowel syndrome; diabetic gastroparesis
Pancreatic polypeptide	Inhibits pancreatic bicarbonate and enzyme secretion	Pancreatic islets of Langerhans	Protein, (fat and glucose)	
Enteroglucagon	Elevates blood glucose?	Ileum	Glucose and fat	
Paracrines				
Somatostatin	Inhibits release of most other peptide hormones	Gastrointestinal tract mucosa, pancreatic islets of Langerhans	Acid stimulates, vagus inhibits release	Gallstones
Histamine	Stimulates gastric acid secretion	Oxyntic gland mucosa	Unknown	
Neurocrines				
VIP	Relaxes sphincters and gut circular muscle; stimulates intestinal and pancreatic secretion	Mucosa and smooth muscle of gastrointestinal tract	Enteric nervous system	Secretory diarrhea
Bombesin	Stimulates gastrin release	Gastric mucosa	Enteric nervous system	
Enkephalins	Stimulate smooth muscle contraction; inhibit intestinal secretion	Mucosa and smooth muscle of gastrointestinal tract	Enteric nervous system	
Other products				
Intrinsic factor	Binds vitamin B_{12} to facilitate its absorption	Parietal cells of the stomach	Constitutive secretion	Autoimmune destruction resulting in pernicious anemia
Mucin	Lubrication and protection	Goblet cells along entire gastrointestinal tract mucosa	Gastrointestinal tract irritation	Viscid mucus in cystic fibrosis Attenuation in some cases of peptic ulcer.
Acid	Initiates digestion of food; prevents infection	Parietal cells of the stomach	Gastrin, histamine, acetylcholine, NSAIDs (indirectly)	Acid-peptic disease

[1]Parentheses indicate minor components and effects.

Table 9–4. Mechanisms of defense of the gastrointestinal tract (and features of structure and function involved).

Forms of Defense	Structural Adaptations	Functional Adaptations	Mechanism of Defense
Defense from acid			
Mucus production	Large numbers of mucus-secreting goblet cells.	Mucin gene expression	Prevents direct contact of acid with epithelium
Bicarbonate production (alkaline tide)	Capillary blood flow to surface		Neutralizes any acid that breaches epithelium
Prostaglandin production			Attenuates acid production
Tight junctions	Tight junction formation		Prevents breach of epithelium
Bicarbonate from pancreas	Pancreatic duct opening into duodenum	Response of secretin to gastric acid	Neutralizes acid leaving stomach
Defense from infection			
Secretory immune system		Machinery for transcytosis	Extends to gastrointestinal tract lumen the protective umbrella of blood-borne immunity
Rapid turnover of enterocytes	Villi with cell proliferation in crypts and cell release at tips.		Limits the consequences of enterocyte infection.
Normal colonic microflora			Impedes invasion or colonization by pathogenic organisms.
Stomach acid	Gastric glands containing parietal cells	Multiple humoral controls on acid secretion (histamine, acetylcholine, and gastrin)	Kills pathogenic organisms upon ingestion.

ESOPHAGUS

Anatomy & Histology

The esophagus is a hollow muscular tube, bounded by sphincters, that serves as a conduit from the pharynx to the stomach. Lined with stratified squamous epithelium, its muscular wall is notable for a transition from striated muscle (top third of its length, starting from the pharynx) to smooth muscle (bottom two-thirds). A key functional feature is the lower esophageal sphincter at the transition from low pressure (intrathoracic) to high pressure (intra-abdominal) sections of the gastrointestinal tract. The lower esophageal sphincter remains closed as a result of tonic contractions, thereby keeping acidic stomach contents out of the esophagus. A specialized neural control mechanism governs relaxation of the lower esophageal sphincter to allow passage of food into the stomach during swallowing.

17. What is the histologic difference between the proximal two-thirds and the distal one-third of the esophagus?
18. What foods affect lower esophageal sphincter pressure, and what are the potential pathologic consequences of these changes?

Physiology of Esophageal Motility & Sphincter Tone

The key features of esophageal motility are primary and secondary peristalsis and lower esophageal sphincter tone. Various foods can increase (eg, protein) or decrease (eg, fat, ethanol, chocolate) lower esophageal sphincter pressure (Table 9–5). Loss of lower esophageal sphincter tone is a major cause of esophageal reflux, presenting as "heartburn."

STOMACH

Anatomy & Histology

In the stomach, ingested food is subjected to thorough mixing and attack by hydrochloric acid and the proteolytic enzyme pepsin. The mucosal surface of the stomach is a simple columnar epithelium of mucus-secreting cells interrupted occasionally by various types of glands in the form of surface invaginations (Figure 9–6). Within these glands, the surface epithelial cells are replaced by specialized exocrine or endocrine secretory cells. The exocrine cells secrete various substances from their apical surface (eg, acid from **parietal cells** and pepsin from **chief cells** of the oxyntic glands in the fundus and

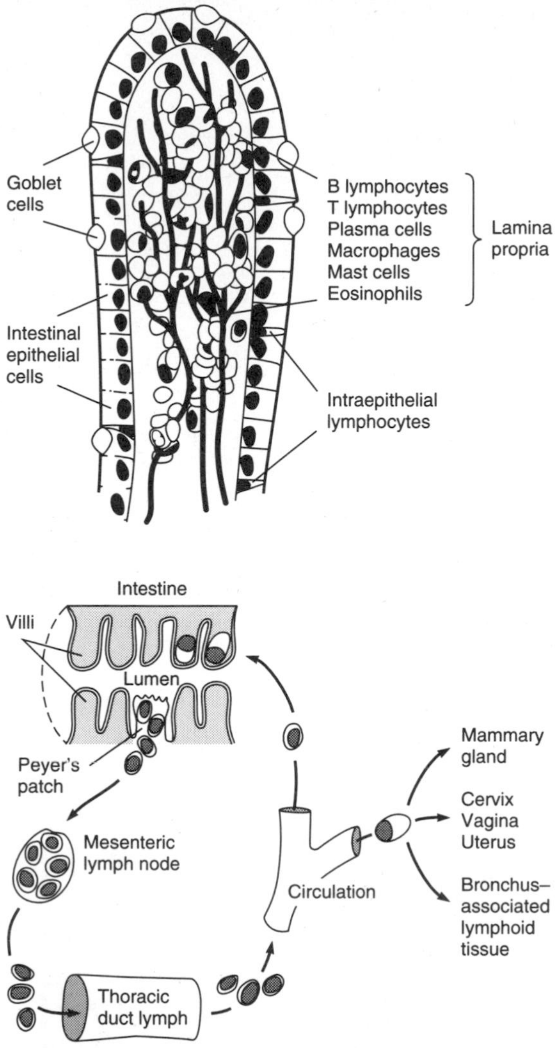

Figure 9–5. Systemic and local features of gut immunology. (Reproduced, with permission, from Kagnoff M: Immunology and disease of the gastrointestinal tract. In: *Gastrointestinal Disease,* 4th ed. Sleisenger MH, Fordtran JS [editors]. Saunders, 1989.)

Table 9–5. Factors influencing lower esophageal sphincter pressure.[1]

	Increase	Decrease
Hormones	Gastrin Motilin Substance P	Secretin Cholecystokinin Glucagon Somatostatin Gastric inhibitory polypeptide (GIP) Vasoactive intestinal polypeptide (VIP) Progesterone
Neural agents	Alpha-adrenergic agonists Beta-adrenergic antagonists Cholinergic agonists	Beta-adrenergic agonists Alpha-adrenergic antagonists Anticholinergic agents
Foods	Protein meals	Fat Chocolate Ethanol Peppermint
Other	Histamine Antacids Metoclopramide Domperidone Prostaglandin $F_{2\alpha}$ Migrating motor complex Raised intra-abdominal pressure	Theophylline Caffeine Gastric acidification Smoking Pregnancy Prostaglandins E_2, I_2 Serotonin Meperidine, morphine Dopamine Calcium channel-blocking agents Diazepam Barbiturates

[1]Reproduced, with permission, from Diamant NE: Physiology of the esophagus. In: *Gastrointestinal Disease,* 4th ed. Sleisenger MH, Fordtran JS (editors). Saunders, 1989.

body of the stomach) into the gastrointestinal tract lumen. The endocrine cells secrete hormones from their basolateral surface (eg, gastrin from so-called **G cells** of the antral glands in the antral mucosa) into the adjacent capillary bloodstream.

Physiology of Stomach Motility

The proximal and distal stomach are functionally distinct. Both parts are involved in mixing ingested materials. Tonic contraction of the proximal stomach normally prevents reflux back into the esophagus, while the distal stomach promotes transit to the duodenum. Both of these functions involve **receptive relaxation,** which is the tendency of stretch of one part of the tract (eg, by food) to induce relaxation of muscle in the part of the tract immediately beyond it. This is followed by muscle contraction when the stretch is relieved, ie, when the food has passed beyond. As a result, material can be propagated from the esophagus through the stomach and into the intestine in an efficient, coordinated fashion. Furthermore, because the pyloric sphincter is triggered to start contracting at the same time as the distal stomach, most of the contents of the stomach are churned rather than sent forward into the duodenum. As a result of this churning action, large chunks of food are converted into fine suspensions of particles—in effect, put through a "strainer"—before leaving the stomach for the duodenum. Both the small particle size and the controlled release of small spurts of nutrient suspension from stomach to duodenum are critical for subsequent absorption. This process is under the control of fibers of the vagus nerve, but it responds also to a variety of luminal receptors. Thus, neutral, isotonic, noncaloric liquids leave the stomach most rapidly. The rate of gastric emptying slows with increasing acidity, fat, and amino acid content or caloric content of ingested food.

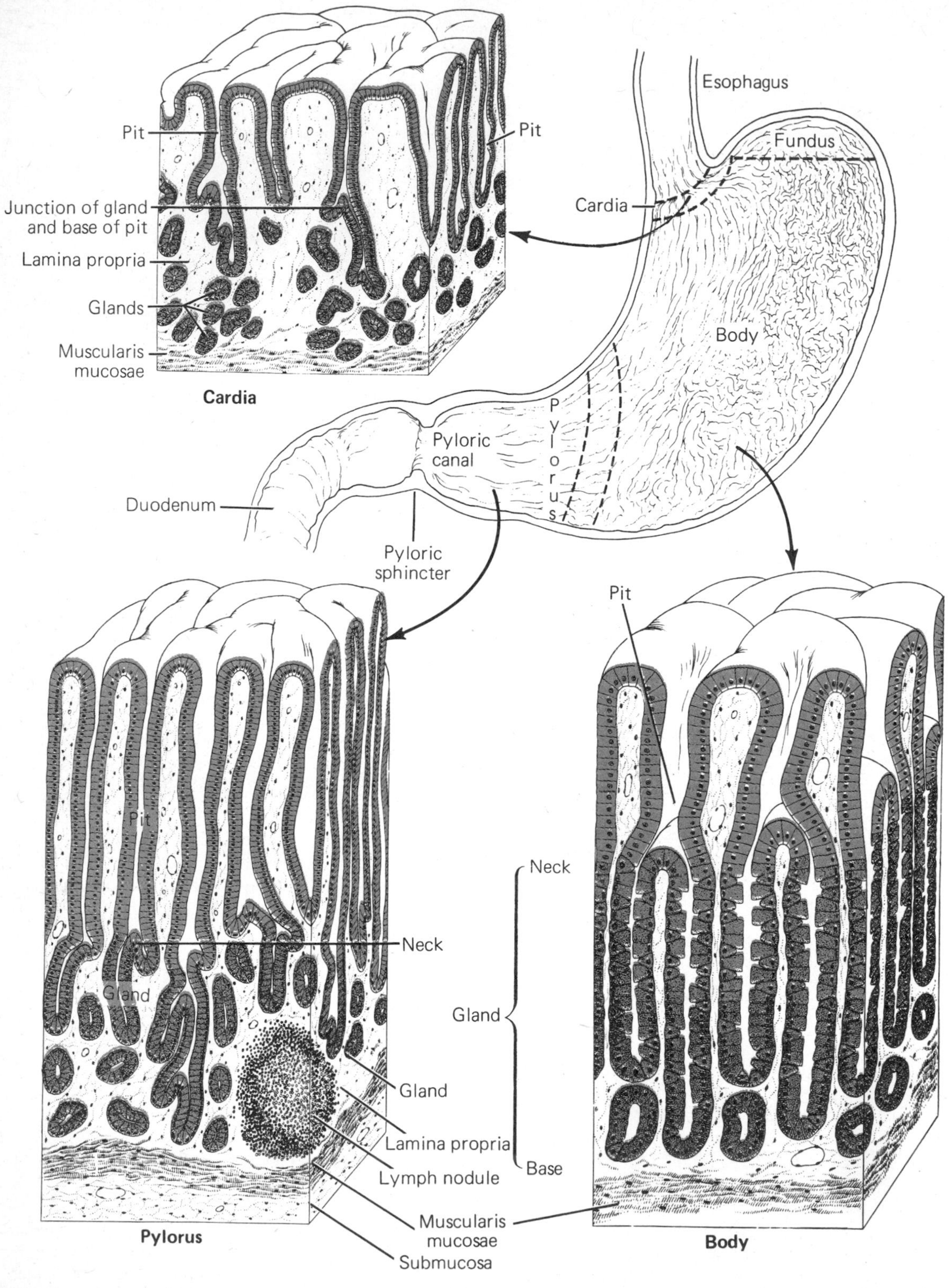

Figure 9–6. Regions of the stomach and their histologic structure. (Reproduced, with permission, from Junqueira LC, Carneiro J, Kelley RO: *Basic Histology,* 7th ed. Appleton & Lange, 1992.)

The importance of nervous system control over gastric motility is reflected in the high incidence of the so-called **dumping syndrome** (nausea, bloating, flushing, and explosive diarrhea) that occurs as a consequence of stomach dysmotility in some patients who have undergone partial gastrectomy or vagotomy.

Physiology of Stomach Secretion

A number of products are secreted from the stomach (Table 9–3). Of these, acid is perhaps the most important from a pathophysiologic standpoint. Secretion of acid occurs in a basal diurnal pattern but can be stimulated by such diverse factors as the thought of food, distention of the stomach, and protein ingestion. Hydrochloric acid is secreted by parietal cells of the gastric mucosa. Acid secretion generates an approximately millionfold concentration gradient at particular times, and myriad levels of defense and control are required to prevent crossing of the line between acid attack on ingested food and attack on the mucosal lining of the gastrointestinal tract (see Table 9–4).

At the subcellular level, acid secretion is controlled by a special mechanism that serves to deliver H^+-K^+ ATPase to the plasma membrane. Vesicle fusion causes H^+-K^+ ATPase to be localized to the plasma membrane, so that hydrogen ions pumped against a tremendous concentration gradient end up in the gastrointestinal lumen (Figure 9–7). A concentration of up to 100 mmol/L HCl (pH = 1.0) can be achieved by this mechanism. Tight junctions keep H^+ in the lumen, with electroneutrality being maintained by export of K^+ and Cl^- through appropriate apical channels. Carbonic anhydrase generates bicarbonate, which is exported into the bloodstream in exchange for Cl^- via pumps on the basolateral side. Together with other pumps to export Na^+ in exchange for K^+ and H^+ in exchange for Na^+, electroneutrality and the ionic composition of the cytosol are maintained in the mucosal cells. Thus, HCl is secreted across the apical surface of the parietal cell while at the same time an "alkaline tide" is generated by sodium bicarbonate export across the basal surface of the parietal cell into the blood flowing through the surface capillaries. This serves as another line of defense against damage from acid reflux (Table 9–4).

At the cellular level, regulation of movement of the H^+-K^+ ATPase to the cell surface is a receptor-mediated process stimulated by histamine, gastrin, and acetylcholine working via both the cAMP and inositol phosphate pathways and inhibited by prostaglandins. The role of acetylcholine as a stimulant of acid secretion reflects yet another level of control of acid secretion. This allows higher centers in the central nervous system (eg, for satiety) to control acid production in anticipation of a meal via the autonomic nervous system.

The clinical importance of regulation of acid secretion is seen in the pathogenesis and therapy of

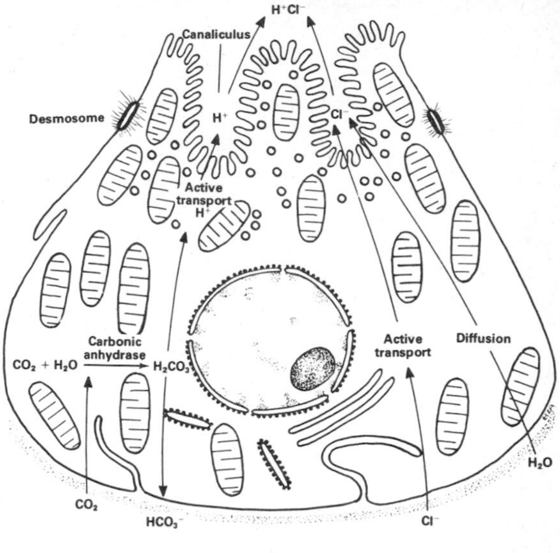

Figure 9–7. Diagram of parietal cell, showing the main steps in the synthesis of hydrochloric acid. Blood CO_2 under the action of carbonic anhydrase produces carbonic acid. This dissociates into a bicarbonate ion and a proton, H^+, which reacts with the chloride ion to produce hydrochloric acid. The tubulovesicles of the cell apex seem to be related to hydrochloric acid secretion, since they decrease in number after parietal cell stimulation. The bicarbonate ion returns to the blood and is responsible for a measurable increase in blood pH during digestion. (Reproduced, with permission, from Junqueira LC, Carneiro J, Kelley RO: *Basic Histology,* 7th ed. Appleton & Lange, 1992.)

peptic ulcer: Exacerbations are often traced to the use of drugs that inhibit prostaglandin synthesis (eg, aspirin, ibuprofen), thereby stimulating acid secretion, and to behavioral and personality features that may affect autonomic or hormonal controls in complex and poorly understood ways (Figure 9–8). Clinical management of peptic ulcer includes therapy with histamine H_2 receptor blocking agents (eg, cimetidine); avoiding stimulants of gastrin secretion (eg, protein-rich meals); and selective surgical disruption of the parasympathetic innervation to the stomach. Omeprazole, a direct inhibitor of H^+-K^+ ATPase, is another potent weapon in the arsenal of antacid therapies. The role of chronic infection by the bacterium *Helicobacter pylori* in breaching the defenses against acid-mediated attack on the gastric and duodenal mucosa has recently been recognized.

Other Stomach Products Secreted Into the Gut Lumen

Intrinsic factor is a vitamin B_{12}-binding protein required for the vitamin's uptake in the terminal ileum. It is secreted by a constitutive pathway from the same parietal cells that generate gastric acid. Thus, autoimmune destruction of parietal cells produces

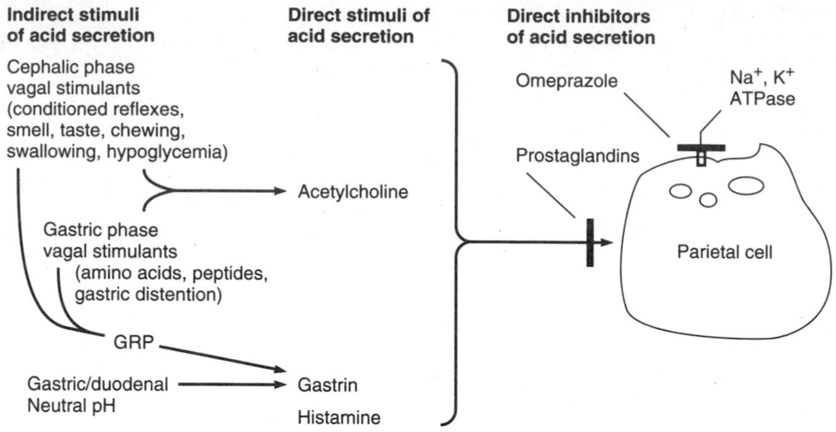

Figure 9–8. Regulation of gastric acid secretion (GRP, gastric-releasing peptide.)

not only **achlorhydria** due to lack of acid secretion but also **pernicious anemia** from vitamin B_{12} deficiency.

> 19. What are the cell types that are found in the lining of the stomach?
> 20. What are the roles of the proximal and distal stomach?
> 21. Name two products secreted by the stomach into (1) the gut lumen and (2) the bloodstream, and describe their functions.

SMALL INTESTINE

Anatomy & Histology

Three regions can be distinguished along the approximately 5-meter length of the small intestine. The pyloric sphincter marks the beginning of the **duodenum,** which is largely retroperitoneal and fixed in its location. Thanks to this sphincter, stomach contents normally enter the duodenum in small spurts containing tiny suspended particles. In the duodenum, gastric contents are mixed with the secretions of the common bile duct and pancreatic ducts.

Beyond the duodenum, the small intestine is mobile and suspended in the peritoneal cavity by a mesentery. The proximal two-fifths is called the **jejunum.** The distal three-fifths is termed the **ileum,** which ends at the ileocecal valve at the start of the large intestine.

The most striking gross structural features of the small intestine are the numerous **villi** (projections of the mucosa approximately 1 mm in height) that confer the apt name of "brush border" to its luminal surface (Figure 9–9A). Each villus contains a single terminal branch of the arterial, venous, and lymphatic trees. These allow efficient transfer to the circulatory system of substances absorbed from the gut lumen by **enterocytes** (surface epithelial cells). At electron microscopy, each enterocyte displays numerous microvilli—plasma membrane evaginations that further increase the absorptive surface area (Figure 9–9B).

The crypts between villi are the site of cell proliferation. The cells differentiate as they ascend the villus to be rapidly shed from the tip (average life span 4–6 days). In addition to serving as the reservoir for cell renewal, the crypts contain other important cell types, including goblet cells, which secrete mucus into the gastrointestinal lumen; endocrine cells, which secrete hormones into the bloodstream; and cells with the capacity for electrolyte transport and hence for fluid absorption or secretion.

Physiology of Intestinal Motility

Two patterns of motility occur in the intestine: **fasting** and **feeding.** During fasting, the pattern is called the **migrating motor complex (MMC)** and consists of a repetitive (every 80–100 minutes) three-phase cycle of activity that keeps the gastrointestinal tract clear of debris (bacteria, undigested material, desquamated cells, secretions) as one of the body's "housekeeping" duties. Phase I is quiescent, phase II is spontaneous irregular activity, and phase III is a burst of rhythmic propagated contraction. The migrating motor complex appears to be under the control of the gut hormone **motilin.** This pattern is interrupted upon feeding, with a new pattern of activity involving both segmental (to and fro) as well as propulsive contractions, and acts to promote optimal mixing and absorption.

Some common gastrointestinal tract disorders involve aberrant small intestine motility. Individuals with complaints of alternating constipation, diarrhea, and abdominal pain in whom no structural problem

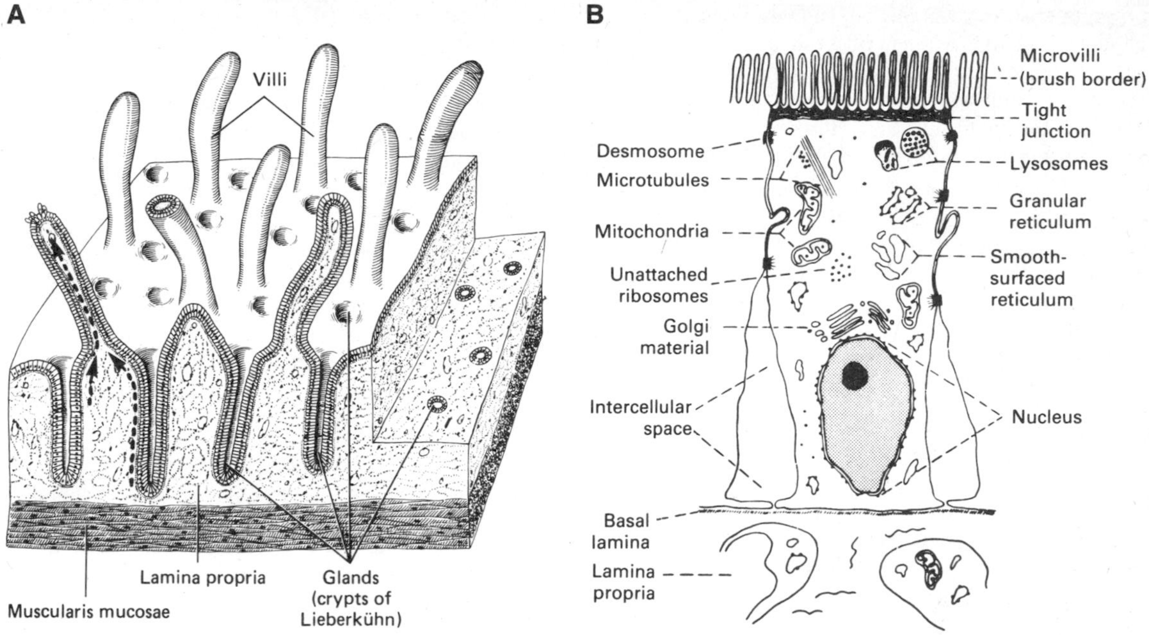

Figure 9–9. Structure of the small intestine. ***A:*** Schematic diagram illustrating the structure of the small intestine and the relationship of villi, epithelial cells, and the underlying lamina propria. (Redrawn and reproduced, with permission, from Ham AW: *Histology,* 6th ed. Lippincott, 1969.) ***B:*** Schematic diagram of an individual small intestine epithelial cell with microvilli. (Reproduced, with permission, from Sleisenger MH, Fordtran JS [editors]: *Gastrointestinal Disease,* 3rd ed. Saunders, 1986.)

or underlying disease can be identified are said to have "irritable bowel syndrome." They probably have disordered small intestine motility. Similarly, disorders in which the migrating motor complex is disrupted or lacking can be a complication of diseases such as diabetes mellitus, familial pseudo-obstruction, and scleroderma. Complications can include bezoar formation, intestinal bacterial overgrowth, excessively rapid small bowel transit time (diarrhea), nausea and vomiting, abdominal distention, and constipation.

Secretion in the Small Intestine

The intestinal mucosa is armed with an array of transporters that allow it to absorb a tremendous volume of fluids and electrolytes in the course of a normal day. Of the 9 L of fluid input, the small intestine typically absorbs 7–8 L, leaving 1–2 L to be dealt with by the colon. Much of fluid and electrolyte transport in the intestine can be compared with the same processes in the renal tubule. Absorption in the small intestine shares common features with absorption by the proximal renal tubule. Absorption in the colon resembles that in the distal renal tubule in that both the colon and the distal renal tubule have aldosterone-sensitive sodium transporters.

However, absorption in the small intestine has some distinctive features. Particularly in the crypts, chloride exits to the gastrointestinal lumen through a channel whose conductance is regulated by cAMP, with water following passively. The small intestine's capacity to reabsorb sodium (against a concentration gradient) is limited. However, because glucose and sodium uptake from the lumen are coupled, high concentrations of luminal glucose greatly stimulate small intestinal uptake of sodium and hence of water. This coupling phenomenon does not occur in the colon for lack of the cotransporter. The maximum absorptive capacity of the small intestine is probably about 12 L/d, whereas that of the colon is only 5 L/d.

Secretagogues (substances that stimulate secretion) can act from either the **apical** (gut lumen) or **basal** (blood) sides of the enterocyte. Examples of **luminal secretagogues** are bacterial enterotoxins, bile salts, fatty acids, and some laxatives. **Humoral** (blood-borne) **secretagogues** include vasoactive intestinal peptide, calcitonin, prostaglandins, and serotonin.

Digestion & Absorption in the Small Intestine

The small intestine is the most important site of both digestion and absorption. The histologic specialization of villi and microvilli greatly expands the surface area on and across which digestion and absorption can take place. Similarly, the segmental motility program ensures even mixing and efficient extraction of substances in the lumen of the small intestine.

Most nutrients (eg, lipids, proteins, and carbohydrates) are digested and absorbed along the entire length of the small intestine. However, some specialized substances are absorbed only in particular regions of the small intestine. Thus, conjugated bile acids and vitamin B_{12} are absorbed in the terminal ileum, while absorption of iron occurs in the duodenum and in the stomach.

22. What are the programs of activity in the small intestine during fasting and feeding?
23. What are some consequences of disordered small intestinal motility?
24. What substances are absorbed in specialized regions of the small intestine?
25. Give an example of a luminal and of a humoral gastrointestinal tract secretagogue.

COLON

Anatomy & Histology

The adult human colon is 1–2 meters in length. Its various segments (cecum; ascending, transverse, descending, and sigmoid colon; rectum and anal canal) are involved in absorption of water and electrolytes, secretion of mucus, and formation, propulsion, and storage of unabsorbed material (feces). The colon is also the home of the intestinal microbial flora.

The surface of the colon consists of a columnar epithelium with no villi and few folds except in the distal rectum. The epithelium has a few short, irregular microvilli. Numerous deep glands contain goblet cells, endocrine cells, and absorptive cells.

Physiology of Colonic Motility

Unlike the stomach and small intestine, the colon is rarely inactive, though its activity is less easily characterized than that of the stomach (which has the pattern known as receptive relaxation) or than that of the small intestine (which displays the pattern known as the migrating motor complex). Some patterns are discernible, however, such as the **gastrocolic reflex** (colonic mass peristalsis following a meal). Disorders of colonic motility are common complications of autonomic neuropathy in patients with diabetes mellitus and can cause severe gastrointestinal complaints.

Secretion in the Colon

The major secretory product of the colon is mucin, a complex glycoprotein conjugate that is exported via the intracellular secretory pathway. It serves lubricating and perhaps protective functions.

Digestion & Absorption in the Colon

Digestion in the colon occurs as a consequence of the action of the colonic microflora; its physiologic significance is not well understood. Absorption of fluid and electrolytes, however, has been well studied and is a major function of the colon. Up to 5 L of water can be absorbed per day across the colonic epithelium. Furthermore, the colonic epithelium can also take up sodium against a considerable concentration gradient. Aldosterone, a hormone involved in fluid and electrolyte homeostasis, increases the colonic sodium conductance in response to volume depletion, thus playing an important role in maintaining fluid and electrolyte balance.

26. How does colonic motility differ from that in the small intestine?
27. What is the major secretory product of the colon?
28. What volume of water is the colon capable of absorbing per day?

II. OVERVIEW OF GASTROINTESTINAL DISORDERS

DISORDERS OF MOTILITY

Disorders of motility affect all major regions of the gastrointestinal tract (Table 9–2). Because gastrointestinal tract motility is a complex result of smooth muscle contraction under neural and hormonal control, abnormal motility of the gastrointestinal tract can occur either through damage to gastrointestinal smooth muscle or to the neural and hormonal mechanisms by which it is controlled. An example of muscle damage leading to abnormal motility is seen in esophageal stricture as a result of caustic ingestions or acid reflux. Abnormal neural control of motility is seen in esophageal achalasia. All esophageal motility disorders are characterized by dysphagia and odynophagia.

Motility disorders of the stomach include gastroparesis, a complication of diabetes mellitus; and dysmotility as a consequence of stomach surgery, either due to resection of part of the stomach or to **vagotomy.** Vagotomy entails surgical transection of the vagus nerve trunks, which prevents vagus-stimulated acid secretion and also cuts vagal fibers, influencing motility via the enteric nervous system. Vagotomy is usually performed as treatment for Zollinger-

Ellison syndrome and for severe peptic ulcer disease or for acid hypersecretion due to a gastrin-secreting tumor.

The signs and symptoms of motility disorders in the stomach depend upon their cause. Because vagotomy cuts fibers influencing the enteric nervous system as well as the intended fibers that influence acid secretion, a classic complication of vagotomy is disordered gastric motility. More commonly, this presents clinically as too rapid movement of gastric contents into the duodenum, with resulting fluid shifts and vasomotor symptoms **("dumping syndrome").** Sometimes, however, patients may develop symptoms of stomach distention, nausea, early satiety, and vomiting suggestive of partial gastric outlet obstruction. To ameliorate the latter symptoms, **pyloroplasty** (severing the fibers of the pyloric sphincter) is done to render the sphincter less competent, so that food can pass more easily into the duodenum. Intrinsic neuropathy (eg, in diabetes mellitus) results in delayed gastric emptying, nausea, vomiting, and constipation rather than the classic dumping syndrome. The pathophysiologic basis for these differences is not known.

In the small intestine and colon, disordered motility is believed to be responsible for **irritable bowel syndrome,** characterized by recurrent episodes of abdominal pain, bloating, and diarrhea alternating with constipation. While the pathophysiology of this disorder is poorly understood, altered levels of gastrointestinal tract hormones such as motilin have been suggested as a cause, perhaps influenced by emotional and psychologic factors. Thus, a wide range of causes can result in abnormal motility as a consequence of interference with mechanisms of control of the gastrointestinal tract.

DISORDERS OF SECRETION

Disorders of secretion involve the production of acid or intrinsic factor by the stomach, digestive enzymes and bicarbonate by the pancreas, bile by the liver, and water and electrolytes by the small intestine in response to secretagogues.

Either elevated gastric acid secretion or diminished mucosal defense can predispose to development of **peptic ulcers.** These are discrete regions of erosion through the mucosa which are surrounded by apparently normal tissue. Acid-induced damage may occur in the form of an ulcer either in the stomach **(gastric ulcer)** or in the first part of the small intestine **(duodenal ulcer).** Acid-induced injury may also occur in the form of more diffuse and less clearly demarcated inflammation anywhere along the gastrointestinal tract from the lower esophagus through the duodenum. It appears that elevated acid secretion is relatively more important in the development of duodenal ulcer, while diminished mucosal defense (perhaps due to diminished mucus secretion in some cases) is the crucial factor in development of gastric ulcer. Disorders of secretion involving the pancreas and liver are discussed in Chapters 15 and 10. Diarrhea, the major secretory disorder of the small intestine, is discussed below.

DISORDERS OF DIGESTION & ABSORPTION

Physiologically significant digestion and absorption can occur throughout the gastrointestinal tract. Thus, amylase in salivary secretions initiates carbohydrate digestion. Indeed, the effectiveness of sublingual nitroglycerin therapy for patients with angina is a testimonial to the efficacy of lingual absorption. Nevertheless, the clinically prominent disorders of digestion and absorption focus on the small intestine and colon and the accessory organs (pancreas and liver) whose secretions (digestive enzymes and bicarbonate versus bile, respectively) are necessary for digestion and absorption in the small intestine.

GASTROINTESTINAL MANIFESTATIONS OF SYSTEMIC DISEASE

A wide range of systemic conditions and diseases may produce signs and symptoms in the gastrointestinal tract. These include endocrine disorders that alter control of gastrointestinal tract functions or which predispose to pancreatitis or peptic ulcer disease; complications of diabetes mellitus, including autonomic neuropathy and ketoacidosis; pregnancy; deficiency disorders, including deficiency of zinc, niacin, and iron; and neoplastic, rheumatologic, and other syndromes (Table 9–6).

29. What are some common symptoms of esophageal dysmotility?
30. Why does vagotomy often create motor disorders in the stomach?
31. What are some suggested factors in the pathogenesis of the irritable bowel syndrome?

Table 9–6. Gastrointestinal manifestations of systemic diseases and their pathophysiologic mechanisms.[1]

Disease or Condition	Commonly Associated Gastrointestinal Manifestations	Mechanism
Thyroid disease		
Autoimmune thyroiditis	Achlorhydria and pernicious anemia	Autoimmune destruction of parietal cells
Hypothyroidism	Esophageal reflux	Lower esophageal sphincter dysfunction
	Bezoars	Gastric dysmotility
	Constipation	Intestinal dysmotility
	Malabsorption	Villous atrophy and pancreatic insufficiency
Hyperthyroidism	Diarrhea and weight loss	Intestinal hypermotility with rapid transit and malabsorption
Adrenal disease		
Adrenal insufficiency	Abdominal pain	Unknown
	Diarrhea	Malabsorption due to loss of trophic effect of corticosteroids on enterocyte brush border
Parathyroid disease		
Primary hyperparathyroidism	Nausea and vomiting	Hypercalcemia-induced alteration in signal transduction resulting in gastric atony and dysmotility
	Pancreatitis	Hypercalcemia-induced premature activation of pancreatic enzymes
	Acid-peptic disease	Hypercalcemia-induced increased acid secretion
Diabetes mellitus	Esophageal, gastric, small and large intestinal and rectal dysfunction	Autonomic neuropathy
	Nausea, vomiting, abdominal pain	Ketoacidosis with gastric atony
Pregnancy	Esophageal reflux; nausea and vomiting; hematemesis; constipation and hemorrhoids	Pressure effects of gravid uterus on lower esophageal sphincter, gastric emptying, intestinal transit time, and venous return
Deficiency states		
Zinc	Malabsorption syndrome	Altered enterocyte brush border
Niacin	Malabsorption syndrome	Altered enterocyte brush border
Cancer	Pain, fever, bleeding, ascites, obstruction, perforation	Metastases (most commonly breast cancer, melanoma, bronchogenic carcinoma of lung)
	Paraneoplastic syndromes and hypercalcemia	Tumor-produced peptides
Hematologic conditions		
Bleeding disorders	Intramural hematoma	Hemorrhage
Hypercoagulable states	Bowel infarction	Intestinal ischemia
Dysproteinemias	Hemorrhage, obstruction, amyloidosis	Infiltration
Rheumatologic disorders		
Scleroderma	Dysphagia, esophageal reflux, obstruction, bleeding, perforation, pseudo-obstruction, pancreatitis, malabsorption	Inflammation, vasculitis, vascular obliteration, villous atrophy
Systemic lupus erythematosus	Nausea, vomiting, mucosal ulceration	Inflammation, vasculitis, vascular obstruction, villous atrophy
Rheumatoid arthritis	Gastric ulcers	Aspirin use
Metabolic and infiltrative disorders (dyslipidemias; sarcoidosis, amyloidosis)	Malabsorption	Infiltration, muscle atrophy, dysmotility
	Infarction	Infiltration, mucosal ischemia, infarction
Renal disorders (including chronic renal failure and transplantation)	Abdominal pain, gastrointestinal bleeding, intestinal perforation	Gastritis, duodenitis, pancreatitis
Neurologic disorders (including spinal cord injury, myotonic dystrophy, CNS disease)	Impaired gut motility with nausea, vomiting, chronic constipation	Disordered central and enteric nervous system communication
Pulmonary disorders		
Asthma	Esophageal reflux	Nocturnal aspiration
Cystic fibrosis	Diarrhea, malabsorption and weight loss	Pancreatic exocrine insufficiency

[1]Reproduced, with permission, from Hunter TB, Bjeilard JC: Gastrointestinal complications of leukemia and its treatment. AJR Am J Roentgenol 1984;143:513; from Riley SA, Tumberg LA: Maldigestion and malabsorption. In: *Gastrointestinal Disease,* 4th ed. Sleisenger MH, Fordtran JS (editors). Saunders, 1989; and from Sack TL, Sleisenger MH: Effects of systemic and extraintestinal disease on the gut. In: *Gastrointestinal Disease,* 4th ed. Sleisenger MH, Fordtran JS (editors). Saunders, 1989.

III. PATHOPHYSIOLOGY OF SELECTED GASTROINTESTINAL DISEASES

DISORDERS OF THE ESOPHAGUS

The major disorders of the esophagus are related to motor functions: Disordered peristalsis and hypertensive lower esophageal sphincter tone are seen in **esophageal achalasia,** while diminished tone results in **reflux esophagitis.**

ESOPHAGEAL ACHALASIA

Clinical Presentation

Esophageal achalasia is a motor disorder in which the lower esophageal sphincter fails to relax properly. As a result, a **functional obstruction** (ie, obstruction due to abnormal function in the absence of a visible mass or lesion) is created that is manifested as dysphagia, regurgitation, and chest pain. It is a progressive disease in which severe radiographic distortion of the esophagus develops.

Etiology

The cause of esophageal achalasia, which occurs with an incidence of 0.5–1:100,000 population per year, is unknown. It has been suggested that degenerative disease (due to any cause) of the myenteric plexus of the enteric nervous system of the lower two-thirds of the esophagus results in the clinical features of achalasia. Esophageal involvement in Chagas' disease, due to damage of the neural plexuses of the esophagus by the parasite *Trypanosoma cruzi,* bears a striking resemblance to esophageal achalasia. A number of other disorders, including malignancies, may present with manometric pressure characteristics or radiographic features similar to those observed in idiopathic esophageal achalasia (Table 9–7).

Table 9–7. Disorders with manometric and radiologic features that mimic idiopathic achalasia.[1]

Malignancy
Gastric adenocarcinoma
Esophageal squamous cell carcinoma
Lymphoma
Lung carcinoma
Pancreatic cancer
Prostate cancer
Hepatocellular cancer
Anaplastic cancer
Chronic idiopathic intestinal pseudo-obstruction
Amyloidosis
Chagas' disease
Postvagotomy disturbance
Familial glucocorticoid deficiency syndrome
Multiple endocrine neoplasia type IIb
Juvenile Sjögren's syndrome with achalasia and gastric hypersecretion

[1]Reproduced, with permission, from Clouse RE: Motor disorders. In: *Gastrointestinal Disease,* 4th ed. Sleisenger MH, Fordtran JS (editors). Saunders, 1989.

Pathology & Pathogenesis

While achalasia is manifested as a motor disorder of esophageal smooth muscle, it is actually caused by defective innervation of smooth muscle in the esophageal body and lower esophageal sphincter. Lower esophageal sphincter tone is normally characterized by tonic contraction with intermittent relaxation due to a neural reflex arc (see above). In achalasia, it is even more tightly contracted and does not relax properly in response to swallowing, due to partial loss of neurons in the wall of the esophagus.

In addition to dysfunction of the lower esophageal sphincter, loss of normal peristalsis in the esophageal body is also often seen in achalasia—consistent with the hypothesis of myenteric plexus degeneration. Variations of achalasia also exist in which normal peristalsis is replaced by simultaneous contractions of large or small amplitude.

Clinical Manifestations

Over months and years, lower esophageal sphincter dysfunction results in tremendous enlargement of the esophagus. Normally intended as a direct conduit to the stomach, the esophagus in advanced cases of achalasia can hold as much as 1 L of putrid, infected material, imposing a high risk of aspiration pneumonia. Without treatment, patients display progressive severe weight loss with worsening chest pain, mucosal ulceration, infection, and occasional esophageal rupture, culminating in death.

REFLUX ESOPHAGITIS

Clinical Presentation

The predominant presenting symptom of reflux is burning chest pain ("heartburn") due to recurrent mucosal injury, often worse at night, when lying supine, or after consumption of foods or drugs that diminish lower esophageal sphincter tone.

Etiology

Common causes of reflux esophagitis are those conditions that result in persistent or repetitive acid exposure to the esophageal mucosa, including any disorder that diminishes lower esophageal sphincter pressure (Table 9–5); conditions that increase gastric volume or pressure (eg, partial or complete gastric outlet obstruction; and conditions that increase acid production (Figure 9–8).

Pathology & Pathogenesis

Normally, the tonically contracted state of the lower esophageal sphincter provides an effective barrier to reflux of acid from the stomach back into the esophagus. Effectiveness of that barrier can be altered by loss of lower esophageal sphincter tone (ie, the opposite of achalasia), increased stomach volume or pressure, or increased production of acid, all of which make reflux of acidic stomach contents more likely. Recurrent reflux can damage the mucosa, resulting in inflammation—hence the term reflux esophagitis. Recurrent reflux itself predisposes to further reflux because the scarring that occurs with healing of the inflamed epithelium renders the lower esophageal sphincter progressively less competent as a barrier.

Although typically a consequence of acid reflux, esophagitis can also result from reflux of pepsin or bile. In most cases of esophageal reflux disease, a common pathophysiologic thread can be identified (Figure 9–10). Recurrent mucosal damage results in infiltration of granulocytes and eosinophils, hyperplasia of basal cells, and eventually the development of friable, bleeding ulcers and exudates over the mucosal surface. These pathologic changes set the stage for scar formation and sphincter incompetence, predisposing to recurrent cycles of inflammation.

Clinical Manifestations

Heartburn is the usual symptom of reflux esophagitis, typically worsening at night or upon lying flat in bed. With recurrent reflux, a range of complications may develop. The most common complication is the development of stricture in the distal esophagus. Progressive obstruction, initially to solid food and later to liquid, presents as dysphagia. Other complications of recurrent reflux include hemorrhage or perforation; hoarseness, coughing, wheezing, or pneumonia as a result of aspiration of gastric contents into the lungs, particularly during sleep; and finally, epidemiologic studies suggest that cigarette and alcohol abuse associated with recurrent reflux results in a change in the esophageal epithelium from squamous to columnar histology, termed **Barrett's esophagus.** In 2–5% of cases, Barrett's esophagus leads to the development of adenocarcinoma.

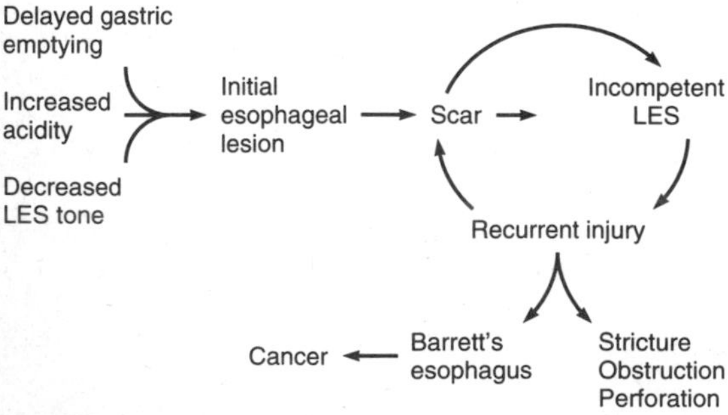

Figure 9–10. Pathophysiology of esophageal reflux disease. (LES, lower esophageal sphincter.)

> 32. What are the roles of the lower esophageal sphincter structure in achalasia and in reflux esophagitis?

DISORDERS OF THE STOMACH

Common disorders involving the stomach reflect the importance of its role as a secretory organ, in particular of acid and intrinsic factor. Disorders of acid secretion result in acid-peptic disease, while loss of intrinsic factor secretion results in inability to absorb vitamin B_{12}, manifesting as **pernicious anemia.** The major motility disorder of the stomach is gastroparesis.

> 33. How does pernicious anemia result from a secretory disorder of the stomach?
> 34. What is the typical acid secretion status of patients with pernicious anemia?
> 35. What is the relationship of esophageal reflux to Barrett's esophagus and cancer?

ACID-PEPTIC DISEASE

Clinical Presentation

Patients with acid-peptic disease typically present with chronic, mild, gnawing or burning abdominal or chest pain due to superficial or deep erosion of the gastrointestinal mucosa; with sudden complications such as gastrointestinal bleeding, resulting in hematemesis or melena; or with perforation and infection, resulting in severe abdominal pain and signs of an acute abdomen (absence of bowel sounds, guarding, rebound tenderness). The latter presentation reflects the fact that in some cases, acid-peptic disease can be painless in the early stages, to be detected only when acid-peptic disease leads to an intra-abdominal catastrophe.

Classically, duodenal ulcer presents as gnawing or burning epigastric pain occurring 1–3 hours after meals, often waking the patient at night, with antacids or food producing relief. However, many patients later documented to have duodenal ulcer do not fit this symptom profile. Elderly patients in particular often present with a complication of duodenal ulcer but no history of pain.

Etiology

Various causes of increased acid production (Figure 9–8) or decreased mucosal defenses (Table 9–4) predispose to acid-peptic disease.

Pathology & Pathogenesis

Corrosive agents (acid and pepsin) secreted by the stomach play a key role in gastric ulcer, duodenal ulcer, and acute erosive gastritis. Each of these diseases has a distinctive but overlapping pathogenesis with the common themes of either excessive acid secretion or diminished mucosal defense. Exactly why one but not another form of acid-peptic disease should develop in a given individual remains unclear. A specific infectious agent, the bacterium *Helicobacter pylori,* has been implicated in predisposition to a number of forms of acid-peptic disease, presumably by diminishing mucosal defenses through inflammation. The role of *H pylori* is particularly important to remember since conventional therapies for acid-peptic disease without eradication of *H pylori* infection are associated with much higher rates of recurrence.

1. GASTRIC ULCER

Gastric ulcer is distinguished from gastritis by the depth of the lesion, with gastric ulcers penetrating through the mucosa. The actual ulcer crater is often surrounded by an area of intact but inflamed mucosa, suggesting that gastritis is a predisposing lesion to development of gastric ulcer. Most gastric ulcers occur on the lesser curvature of the stomach. It is likely that gastric ulcer represents the outcome of a number of different abnormalities summarized below.

Some gastric ulcers are believed to be related to impaired mucosal defenses, since the acid and pepsin secretory capacity of some affected patients is normal or even below normal.

Motility defects have been proposed to contribute to development of gastric ulcer in at least three ways: (1) By a tendency of duodenal contents to reflux back through an incompetent pyloric sphincter. Bile acids in the duodenal reflux material act as an irritant and may be an important contributor to a diminished mucosal barrier against acid and pepsin. (2) By delayed emptying of gastric contents, including reflux material, into the duodenum. (3) By delayed gastric emptying and hence food retention, resulting in increased gastrin secretion and gastric acid production. It is not known whether these motility defects are a cause or a consequence of gastric ulcer formation.

Mucosal ischemia may play a role in the development of a gastric ulcer. Prostaglandins are known to increase mucosal blood flow as well as bicarbonate and mucus secretion and to stimulate mucosal cell repair and renewal. Thus, their deficiency—resulting from NSAID ingestion or other insults—may predispose to gastritis and gastric ulcer, as might diminished bicarbonate or mucus secretion due to other causes. Subsets of gastric ulcer patients with each of these defects have been identified. Thus, the risk factors (NSAID ingestion, smoking, psychologic stress, *H pylori* infection) that have been associated with gastric ulcer probably act by diminishing one or more mucosal defense mechanisms.

Gastritis (inflammation of the gastric mucosa) as a result of aspirin and other NSAIDs, bile salts, alcohol, or other insults, may predispose to ulcer formation (1) by attenuating the barrier created by the epithelial cells or the mucus and bicarbonate they secrete or (2) by reducing the quantity of prostaglandins the epithelial cells produce that might otherwise diminish acid secretion.

2. ACUTE EROSIVE GASTRITIS

Acute erosive gastritis includes inflammation due to superficial mucosal injury, mucosal erosion, or shallow ulcers due to a wide variety of insults, most notably alcohol, drugs, and stress. Ethanol ingestion predisposes to gastritis but not to development of gastric ulcer. Unlike gastric or duodenal ulcers, in erosive gastritis the submucosa and muscularis mucosae are not penetrated. Acid hypersecretion, gastric anoxia, altered natural defenses (especially diminished mucus secretion), epithelial renewal, tissue mediators (eg, prostaglandins), reduced intramucosal pH, and intramucosal energy deficits have been suggested as factors in the development of superficial gastric mucosal injury.

3. CHRONIC ATROPHIC GASTRITIS

This heterogeneous group of syndromes is characterized by inflammatory cell infiltration with gastric mucosal atrophy and loss of glands. In chronic disease—unlike acute erosive gastritis—endoscopic abnormalities may not be grossly apparent. The capacity to secrete gastric acid is progressively reduced, and the serum levels of gastrin are elevated.

Autoantibodies to parietal cells, intrinsic factor, and gastrin are common findings. Chronic atrophic gastritis is associated with *H pylori* infection, development of pernicious anemia, gastric adenocarcinoma, and gastrointestinal endocrine hyperplasia with carcinoids (neuroendocrine tumors of the gastrointestinal tract producing serotonin metabolites and associated with dramatic symptoms of flushing and diarrhea).

4. DUODENAL ULCER

Like gastric ulcer, duodenal ulcer is believed to be a consequence of excessive acid and pepsin secretion plus diminished mucosal defenses. Excessive secretion is believed to play the more important role, however, since duodenal ulcer rarely occurs in individuals who secrete less than 10 meq of acid per hour.

Since duodenal ulcer is an intermittent and recurrent disease, all of the predisposing factors may not be present in every patient at any given time (Figure 9–11). Patients found to have a duodenal ulcer are more likely to have (1) increased acid and peptic secretory capacity; (2) increased basal acid secretion; (3) increased postprandial acid secretory response; (4) increased sensitivity of gastrin secretory cells to secretagogues and impaired acid inhibition of gastrin release; (5) impairment of other feedback mechanisms of gastric acid secretion; and (6) rapid gastric emptying. However, considerable overlap exists between patients who develop duodenal ulcer and those who do not, which may mean that important variables in pathogenesis are still unrecognized.

Various risk factors, including diet, smoking, *H pylori* infection, and excessive alcohol consumption, may influence the development of duodenal ulcers, though specific associations (eg, between coffee or spicy foods and the development of ulcers, or between bland diets and the healing of ulcers) have not been demonstrated. Genetic factors also play a role, with studies supporting the existence of a heritable component in duodenal ulcers distinct from that involved in gastric ulcer. Likewise, psychologic stress has been implicated in duodenal ulcer disease, perhaps by the autonomic-mediated influence of acid secretion (Figure 9–11).

Clinical Manifestations

Those forms of acid-peptic disease characterized by exclusively superficial mucosal lesions (eg, acute erosive gastritis) can result in either acute or chronic gastrointestinal bleeding, accompanied by a significant drop in hematocrit and related complications (eg, precipitating angina in a patient with coronary artery disease). Patients with acute massive bleeding will present with hematemesis (vomiting blood), rectal bleeding, or melena (tarry stools from the effect of acid on blood) depending on the site of origin, the rate of transit of blood through the gastrointestinal tract, and the extent of hemorrhage. Acute massive hemorrhage (> 10% of blood volume over minutes to hours) is manifested by hypotension, tachycardia, and orthostatic blood pressure and heart rate changes on standing, often with dizziness.

In addition to hemorrhage, complications of duodenal ulcer and gastric ulcer include life-threatening perforation and obstruction.

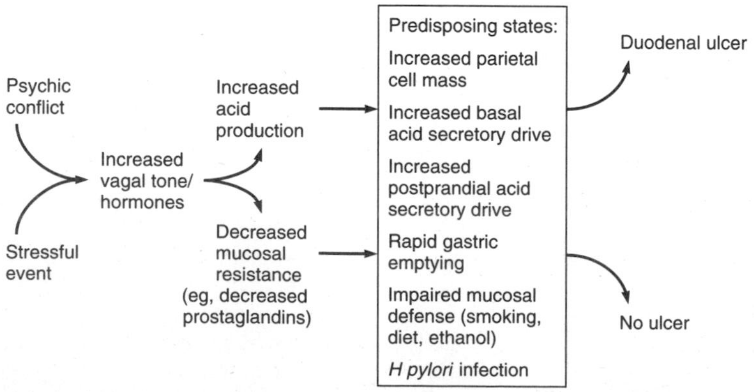

Figure 9–11. Pathophysiology of duodenal ulcer disease.

Table 9–8. Conditions producing symptomatic gastric motor dysfunction.[1]

Acute Conditions	Chronic Conditions
Abdominal pain, trauma, inflammation	Mechanical
Postoperative state	Gastric ulcer
Acute infections, gastroenteritis	Duodenal ulcer
Acute metabolic disorders:	Idiopathic hypertrophic pyloric stenosis
Acidosis, hypokalemia, hypercalcemia or hypocalcemia, hepatic coma, myxedema	Superior mesenteric artery syndrome
Immobilization	Acid-peptic disease
Hyperglycemia (glucose >200 mg/dL)	Gastroesophageal reflux
Pharmaceutical agents and hormones	Gastric ulcer disease, nonulcer dyspepsia
Opioids, including endorphins and narcotics (eg, morphine)	Gastritis
Anticholinergics	Atrophic gastritis with or without pernicious anemia
Tricyclic antidepressants	Viral gastroenteritis (acute, ?chronic gastritis)
Beta-adrenergic agonists	Metabolic and endocrine
Levodopa	Diabetic ketoacidosis (acute)
Aluminum hydroxide antacids	Diabetic gastroparesis (chronic)
Gastrin	Addison's disease
Cholecystokinin	Hypothyroidism
Somatostatin	Pregnancy?
	Uremia?
	Collagen vascular diseases
	Scleroderma
	Dermatomyositis
	Polymyositis
	Lupus?
	Pseudo-obstruction
	Idiopathic, hollow visceral myopathy
	Secondary (eg, amyloidosis, Chagas' disease, muscular dystrophies, cancer-associated syndrome)
	Postgastric surgery
	Postvagotomy or postgastric resections
	Medications
	Anticholinergic, narcotic analgesics, levodopa, tricyclic antidepressants
	Hormones (pharmacologic studies)
	Gastrin, cholecystokinin, somatostatin
	Anorexia nervosa: bulimia
	Idiopathic
	Gastric dysrhythmias: tachygastria
	Gastroduodenal dyssynchrony
	Central nervous system: tabes dorsalis, depression

[1]Reproduced, with permission, from McCallum RW: Motor function of the stomach in health and disease. In: *Gastrointestinal Disease,* 4th ed. Sleisenger MH, Fordtran JS (editors). Saunders, 1989.

36. In which acid-peptic disorder is diminished mucosal defenses more important than acid hypersecretion?
37. How might motility defects contribute to gastric ulcer?
38. What factors may predispose a patient to duodenal ulcer disease?
39. How do nonsteroidal anti-inflammatory agents contribute to acid-peptic disease?

GASTROPARESIS

Clinical Presentation

A common complication of stomach disorders is delayed gastric emptying (Table 9–8), known as gastroparesis and manifested by nausea, bloating, vomiting, and either constipation or diarrhea.

Etiology

Gastroparesis is a common complication of poorly controlled diabetes mellitus, with consequent autonomic neuropathy.

Pathology & Pathogenesis

Insight into disorders of gastric motility is provided by the discovery that the antibiotic erythromycin is an analogue of the gastrointestinal hormone motilin. Thus, loose stools occurring as a side effect of erythromycin appear to be due to a motilin-like effect. Some patients with diabetic gastroparesis—especially those in whom the symptoms of constipation and bloating are prominent—have had significant improvement in their symptoms when treated with erythromycin (or its nonantibiotic analogues).

Disorders of motilin secretion include not only excessive or insufficient secretion but also disordered secretion, where the characteristic sensing, timing, rate, and amplitude of secretion are altered even though the amount of hormone secreted may be normal. This may explain why some patients with diabetic gastroparesis do not present with the same symptoms or respond in the same way to erythromycin or other drugs.

Clinical Manifestations

Complications of gastroparesis include the development of bezoars from retained gastric contents, bacterial overgrowth, erratic blood glucose control, and, when nausea and vomiting are profound, weight loss. Elevated blood glucose can be either a cause or a consequence of delayed gastric emptying. Bacterial overgrowth itself can result in both malabsorption and diarrhea. For unknown reasons, the symptoms of gastroparesis are variable from patient to patient as well as over time in a given patient.

40. What are the symptoms of delayed versus rapid gastric emptying?
41. What are the complications of gastroparesis?
42. Why might erythromycin improve diabetic gastroparesis?

DISORDERS OF THE SMALL INTESTINE & COLON

Discussed below are diarrhea, inflammatory bowel disease, and diverticular disease. **Diarrhea** has many causes and diverse pathogenetic mechanisms, including altered motility, secretion, digestion, and absorption. While intestinal disorders are particularly prominent causes, disease of the stomach, pancreas, and biliary tract can also cause diarrhea. **Inflammatory bowel diseases** are poorly understood chronic autoimmune processes in the small intestine, colon, or both, with malabsorption as a prominent feature, and with important systemic manifestations. **Diverticular disease** occurs most prominently in the colon, in part as a direct or indirect consequence of altered motor function.

DIARRHEA

Clinical Presentation

Diarrhea is defined as bowel movements which are excessive in volume, frequency, or liquidity. Any process that increases the frequency of defecation or volume of stool makes it more loose, since time-dependent absorption of water is responsible for the normal soft but formed consistency of stool.

Patients' subjective assessments of bowel movements are influenced by their baseline bowel habits. An individual with chronic constipation, with bowel movements once every 3 days or so, may regard three soft stools in a day as "diarrhea.'' In contrast, an individual taking a high-fiber diet may normally have bowel movements twice or even three times a day.

Diarrhea may be characterized as secretory, osmotic, or malabsorptive, depending on the physiologic basis for altered gut fluid homeostasis. **Osmotic diarrhea** is due to malabsorbed nutrients or poorly absorbed electrolytes that retain water in the lumen. **Secretory diarrhea** results when secretagogues maintain elevated rates of fluid transport out of epithelial cells. **Malabsorptive diarrhea** occurs when the ability to digest or absorb a particular nutrient is defective. These physiologic distinctions are useful in both diagnosis and therapy of diarrheal disorders. In transport capacity, the small intestine far exceeds the colon (owing to the enormous surface area of the brush border). Thus, infectious, toxic, or other causes of heightened secretion in the small intestine can overwhelm absorptive mechanisms in the colon, resulting in diarrhea.

Etiology

Flow in the gastrointestinal tract is a steady state involving massive fluid secretion into and absorption from the gastrointestinal lumen. Each process is controlled by both extrinsic and intrinsic factors. Subtle aberrations in input or output at any of several levels can result in diarrhea with or without nutrient malabsorption. Thus, an excessive osmotic load, increased secretion, or diminished fluid resorption may result in diarrhea (Table 9–9).

An excessive osmotic load in the gastrointestinal tract may come about in three different ways: By direct oral ingestion of excessive osmoles; by ingestion of a substrate that may be converted into excessive osmoles (eg, when bacterial action on the nondigestible carbohydrate lactulose generates a diarrhea-causing osmotic load in the colon); and as a manifestation of a genetic disease such as an enzyme deficiency in the setting of a particular diet (eg, milk consumption by a lactase-deficient individual).

Secretion is increased by either blood-borne or intraluminal secretagogues. These include endogenous endocrine products (eg, overproduced by a tumor), exotoxins due to direct ingestion (eg, acute food poisoning) or infection (eg, cholera), or gastrointestinal luminal substances (eg, bile acids) that stimulate secretion.

Absorption of fluid, electrolytes, and nutrients can be diminished by many factors, including the toxic effects of alcohol; mucosal damage from infectious agents (Table 9–9); prokinetic agents that speed up gastrointestinal motility, thereby diminishing the time available for absorption of any given nutrient,

Table 9–9. Mechanisms of diarrhea and major specific causes.[1]

Mechanisms of Diarrhea	Specific Causes
Osmotic	Disaccharidase deficiencies (eg, lactase deficiency) Glucose-galactose or fructose malabsorption Mannitol, sorbitol ingestion Lactulose therapy Some salts (eg, magnesium sulfate) Some antacids (eg, Maalox) Generalized malabsorption
Secretory	Enterotoxins Tumor products (eg, VIP, serotonin) Laxatives Bile acids Fatty acids Congenital defects
Malabsorption	Pancreatic enzyme deficiency Pancreatic enzyme inactivation (eg, by excess acid) Defective fat solubilization (disrupted enterohepatic circulation or defective bile formation) Ingestion of nutrient binding substances Bacterial overgrowth Loss of enterocytes (eg, radiation, infection, ischemia) Lymphatic obstruction (eg, lymphoma, tuberculosis)
Motility disorder	Diabetes mellitus Postsurgical
Inflammatory exudation	Inflammatory bowel disease Infection (eg, shigellosis)

[1]Reproduced, with permission, from Fine KD, Krejs GJ, Fordtran JS: Diarrhea. In: *Gastrointestinal Disease,* 4th ed. Sleisenger MH, Fordtran JS (editors). Saunders, 1989.

fluid, or electrolyte load. Finally, inflammatory and other disorders resulting in loss of mucus, blood, or protein from the gastrointestinal tract may be manifested as diarrhea. Symptoms and signs suggesting specific causes of diarrhea are listed in Table 9–10.

Pathology & Pathogenesis

Recognition of pathophysiologic subtypes of secretory, malabsorptive (Table 9–11 and 9–12) and osmotic diarrheas provides a means of approaching diagnosis and therapy of diarrheal disorders. For example, nonbloody diarrhea that continues in the absence of oral intake must be due to a secretory mechanism, whereas diarrhea that diminishes as oral intake is curtailed (eg, in a patient receiving intravenous hydration) suggests an osmotic or malabsorptive cause. Likewise, the presence of white blood cells in the stool suggests an infectious or inflammatory origin of diarrhea, though their absence does not rule out such causes.

Of the many causes of diarrhea (Table 9–13), infectious agents are among the most important because they cause acute, sometimes life-threatening diseases whose pathogenesis is relatively well understood and because they are usually treatable. The symptoms of diarrhea due to infectious agents are due either to toxins that alter small bowel secretion and absorption or to direct mucosal invasion. The noninvasive toxin-producing bacteria are generally small bowel pathogens, while the invasive organisms are localized typically to the colon. Diarrheas due to infectious agents can be classified into five groups.

A. Cholera: Infectious diarrhea can be due to toxin elaborated by pathogenic bacteria within the gut lumen or adherent to the mucosa. The classic example is *Vibrio cholerae* infection. Cholera is characterized by an abrupt onset of massive watery diarrhea that is isotonic with plasma. Volumes of diarrhea as high as 1 L/h or up to 15 L/d can result. If fluid replacement is inadequate, profound dehydration leading to renal failure can rapidly occur. Without treatment, the mortality rate can approach 50%. The cholera toxin acts by covalently modifying a heterotrimeric G protein in the cytosol of the enterocyte—as a result of which adenylyl cyclase is activated, thereby driving chloride secretion and with it sodium and water loss. The disease is largely due to dysfunction of the small intestine, with the resulting large volumes of fluid overwhelming the colon's capacity for absorption. Since the organisms do not penetrate the mucosa, supportive therapy alone, with or without antibiotics, is lifesaving. The organism is cleared spontaneously if the patient does not succumb to dehydration. Oral rehydration with glucose-containing salt solutions has been developed for use in developing nations where cholera remains endemic. This therapy takes advantage of the fact that sodium uptake is coupled to that of glucose in enterocytes of the villus. Ingestion of large volumes of glucose-containing electrolyte solutions provides glucose that is absorbed along with sodium. Water moves with the sodium osmotically and counters the toxin-mediated chloride secretion occurring in the crypts.

B. Enteroinvasive Bacterial Gastroenteritis: Bacterial pathogens may directly invade the mucosa and proliferate within the enterocytes (see Chapter 6). These organisms may elaborate a variety of toxins, some of which are cytotoxic and may kill enterocytes, whereas others serve as secretagogues directing fluid secretion. A characteristic of these gastroenteritides is an intense submucosal inflammatory reaction with necrosis of areas of overlying mucosa. Together, the necrosis and inflammation result in the typical findings of blood, pus, and mucus in the stool. *Salmonella, Shigella, Campylobacter,* and certain strains of *E coli* are classic examples of enteroinvasive pathogens. Antibiotic therapy may limit the course of these illnesses, though typically they resolve spontaneously in an immunocompetent host. Therapy to slow or stop the diarrhea can actually pro-

Table 9–10. Clues to diagnosis of diarrhea from other symptoms and signs.[1]

Symptoms or Signs Associated With Diarrhea	Diagnoses to Be Considered
Arthritis	Ulcerative colitis, Crohn's disease, Whipple's disease, enteritis due to *Yersinia enterocolitica,* gonococcal proctitis
Liver disease	Ulcerative colitis, Crohn's disease, colon cancer with metastases to liver
Fever	Ulcerative colitis, Crohn's disease, amebiasis, lymphoma, tuberculosis, Whipple's disease, other enteric infections
Marked weight loss	Malabsorption, inflammatory bowel disease, colon cancer, thyrotoxicosis
Eosinophilia	Eosinophilic gastroenteritis, parasitic disease (particularly *Strongyloides*)
Lymphadenopathy	Lymphoma, Whipple's disease, AIDS
Neuropathy	Diabetic diarrhea, amyloidosis
Postural hypotension	Gastrointestinal bleeding, diabetic diarrhea, Addison's disease, idiopathic orthostatic hypotension
Flushing	Malignant carcinoid syndrome, pancreatic cholera syndrome
Erythema	Systemic mastocytosis, glucagonoma syndrome
Proteinuria	Amyloidosis
Collagen vascular disease	Mesenteric vasculitis
Peptic ulcers	Zollinger-Ellison syndrome
Chronic lung disease	Cystic fibrosis
Systemic arteriosclerosis	Ischemic injury to gut
Frequent infections	Immunoglobulin deficiency
Hyperpigmentation	Whipple's disease, celiac disease, Addison's disease
Good response to corticosteroids	Ulcerative colitis, Crohn's disease, Whipple's disease, Addison's disease, eosinophilic gastroenteritis, celiac disease
Good response to antibiotics	Blind loop syndrome, tropical sprue, Whipple's disease

[1]Reproduced, with permission, from Fine KD, Krejs GJ, Fordtran JS: Diarrhea. In: *Gastrointestinal Disease,* 4th ed. Sleisenger

Table 9–11. Histologic features of small intestinal diseases causing malabsorption.

Disease	Pathologic Features	Pattern of Distribution
Celiac (nontropical) sprue	Villus flattening, crypt hyperplasia, increased lymphocytes and plasma cells in lamina propria	Diffuse in proximal jejunum
Tropical sprue	Shortened villi, increased lymphocytes and plasma cells in lamina propria	Diffuse in proximal jejunum
Crohn's disease	Noncaseating granulomas with or without giant cells	Patchy lesions particularly affecting terminal ileum
Collagenous sprue	Subepithelial collagen deposits	Diffuse
Primary lymphoma	Malignant lymphocytes or histiocytes in lamina propria, variable villus flattening	Patchy
Whipple's disease	Lamina propria laden with PAS-staining foamy macrophages, bacilli in macrophages	Diffuse
Amyloidosis	Amyloid deposition in blood vessels, muscle layers	Diffuse in muscularis mucosae, mucosal sparing
Abetalipoproteinemia	Lipid-laden, vacuolated epithelial cells, normal villi	Diffuse
Radiation enteritis	Flattened villi, mucosal inflammation, fibrosis, ulceration	Patchy
Lymphangiectasia	Dilated lymphatics in lamina propria	Patchy
Eosinophilic gastroenteritis	Eosinophilic infiltrate in the intestinal wall	Patchy
Hypogammaglobulinemina	Villus flattening, *Giardia* trophozoites often present, few plasma cells	Patchy
Giardiasis	Trophozoites may be present, variable villus flattening	Patchy
Opportunistic infections	Organisms may be seen (*Isospora belli,* cryptosporidia, Microsporida), PAS-staining macrophages (*Mycobacterium avium* complex)	Patchy

Table 9–12. Symptoms and signs of malabsorption.[1]

Clinical Features	Pathophysiology	Laboratory Findings
Diarrhea	Increased secretion and decreased absorption of water and electrolytes; unabsorbed fatty acids and bile salts	Increased fat excretion, decreased serum carotene, "osmotic gap" in stool electrolytes
Weight loss with hyperphagia	Decreased absorption of fat, protein, and carbohydrate	Increased fat excretion
Bulky, foul-smelling stools	Decreased fat absorption	Increased fat excretion
Muscle wasting, edema	Decreased protein absorption	Decreased serum albumin
Flatulence, borborygmi, abdominal distention	Fermentation of carbohydrates by intestinal bacteria	Increased fat excretion Decreased D-xylose absorption
Abdominal pain	Small intestinal stricture, infiltration of the pancreas, intestinal ischemia	Increased fat excretion
Paresthesias, tetany	Decreased vitamin D and calcium absorption	Hypocalcemia, hypomagnesemia
Bone pain	Decreased calcium absorption	Hypocalcemia, increased alkaline phosphatase
Muscle cramps, weakness	Excess potassium loss	Hypokalemia, abnormal ECG
Easy bruisability, petechiae, hematuria	Decreased vitamin K absorption	Prolonged prothrombin time, increased fat excretion
Hyperkeratosis, night blindness	Decreased vitamin A absorption	Decreased serum carotene, increased fat excretion
Pallor	Decreased vitamin B_{12}, folate, or iron absorption	Macrocytic anemia, microcytic anemia
Glossitis, stomatitis, cheilosis	Decreased vitamin B_{12}, folate, or iron absorption	Decreased serum vitamin B_{12}, RBC folate, or serum iron
Acrodermatitis	Zinc deficiency	Decreased serum zinc

[1]Tables 9–11 and 9–12 reproduced, with permission, from Wright TL, Heyworth MF: Maldigestion and malabsorption. In: *Gastrointestinal Disease,* 4th ed. Sleisenger MH, Fordtran JS (editors). Saunders, 1989.

long the course of the illness by preventing elimination of toxins and organisms in diarrheal stools.

C. Toxin Ingestion: Common "food poisoning" is a constellation of self-limited syndromes resulting from ingestion of preformed bacterial toxins in contaminated food with or without live bacteria. The toxin produces nausea, vomiting, and diarrhea within hours after ingestion. These illnesses can be mild to severe but are typically self-limited and require only supportive therapy to prevent dehydration. *Clostridium perfringens, Staphylococcus aureus,* and *Bacillus cereus* elaborate these heat-stable toxins.

D. Viral Gastroenteritis: A number of viruses, including rotaviruses and Norwalk virus, when ingested, can bind to receptors on enterocytes, causing invasion and infection. In some cases, the enterocytes are killed in the process of viral replication; in others, the enterocytes are not killed but their normal protein synthetic functions are disrupted. In either case, the net effect is loss of absorptive capacity by the small intestine, resulting in diarrhea. Since the host's immune mechanisms normally respond rapidly to such viral infections with the development of humoral immunity and since the lifetime of mature enterocytes is short (3–5 days), these disorders are generally self-limited, as the infected cells are sloughed and replaced by new cells that are protected by specific antibodies.

E. Parasitic Diseases: A number of parasites, including protozoa, roundworms, and tapeworms, can colonize the small intestine and colon, producing either acute self-limited or chronic intermittent diarrheal syndromes. The most important diarrhea-producing parasites are *Giardia lamblia,* a small intestinal pathogen, and *Entamoeba histolytica,* a colon pathogen.

43. By what mechanisms do infectious agents cause diarrhea?
44. Name three ways in which an excessive osmotic load can occur in the gastrointestinal tract.

Clinical Manifestations

Dehydration, malnutrition, weight loss, and specific vitamin deficiency syndromes (eg, glossitis, cheilosis, and stomatitis) are common signs in diarrhea depending on its cause, severity, and chronicity (Tables 9–10 and 9–12).

Table 9–13. Most likely causes of diarrhea in seven different clinical categories.[1]

1. **Acute diarrhea (<2–3 weeks' duration)**
   - Viral, bacterial, parasitic, and fungal infections
   - Food poisoning
   - Drugs[2] and food additives
   - Fecal impaction
   - Pelvic inflammation
   - Heavy metal poisoning (acute or chronic)
2. **Traveler's diarrhea**
   - Bacterial infections
   - Mediated by enterotoxins produced by *E coli*
   - Mediated mainly by invasion of mucosa and inflammation, eg, invasive *E coli, Shigella*
   - Mediated by combination of invasion and enterotoxins, eg, *Salmonella*
   - Viral and parasitic infections
3. **Diarrhea in homosexual men without AIDS**
   - Amebiasis
   - Giardiasis
   - Shigellosis
   - *Campylobacter*
   - Rectal syphilis
   - Rectal spirochetosis other than syphilis
   - Rectal gonorrhea
   - *Chlamydia trachomatis* infection (lymphogranuloma venereum and non-LGV serotypes D-K)
   - Herpes simplex
4. **Diarrhea in patients with AIDS**
   - *Cryptosporidium*
   - Amebiasis
   - Giardiasis
   - *Isospora belli*
   - Herpes simplex, cytomegalovirus
   - *Mycobacterium avium intracellulare*
   - *Salmonella typhimurium*
   - *Cryptococcus*
   - *Candida*
   - AIDS enteropathy
5. **Chronic and recurrent diarrhea**
   - Irritable bowel syndrome
   - Inflammatory bowel disease
   - Parasitic and fungal infections
   - Malabsorption syndromes
   - Drugs,[2] food additives, sorbitol
   - Colon cancer
   - Diverticulitis
   - Fecal impaction
   - Heavy metal poisoning (acute or chronic)
   - Raw milk-related diarrhea
6. **Chronic diarrhea of unknown origin (previous workup failed to reveal diagnosis)**
   - Surreptitious laxative abuse
   - Defective anal sphincter competence masquerading as diarrhea
   - Microscopic colitis syndrome
   - Previously unrecognized malabsorption
   - Pseudopancreatic cholera syndrome
   - Idiopathic fluid malabsorption
   - Hypermotility-induced diarrhea
   - Neuroendocrine tumor
7. **Incontinence**
   - Causes of sphincter dysfunction:
     - Anal surgery for fissures, fistulas, or hemorrhoids
     - Episiotomy or tear during childbirth
     - Anal Crohn's disease
     - Diabetic neuropathy
   - Causes of diarrhea: same as under 5 and 6, above.

[1]Reproduced, with permission, from Fine KD, Krejs GJ, Fordtran JS: Diarrhea. In: *Gastrointestinal Disease,* 4th ed. Sleisenger MH, Fordtran JS (editors). Saunders, 1989.
[2]Digitalis, propranolol, quinidine, diuretics, colchicine, antibiotics, lactulose, antacids, laxatives, chemotherapeutic agents, bile acids, meclomen, and many others. (See drug compendiums for adverse effects of drugs the patient has been taking.)

In certain circumstances (eg, in young children), viral gastroenteritis is associated with a high mortality rate from dehydration when supportive measures (ie, oral or intravenous rehydration) are not promptly provided.

Some individuals with diarrhea due to parasitic infections remain relatively asymptomatic, while others may develop more severe symptoms and complications, including intestinal perforation.

INFLAMMATORY BOWEL DISEASE

Clinical Presentation

Inflammatory bowel disease is distinguished from infectious entities by exclusion: recurrent episodes of mucopurulent (ie, containing mucus and white cells) bloody diarrhea characterized by lack of positive cultures for infectious organisms and failure to respond to antibiotics alone. Because inflammatory bowel disease is characterized by exacerbations and remissions, favorable responses to therapy are difficult to distinguish from spontaneous remissions occurring as part of the natural history of the disease.

Etiology

The cause of inflammatory bowel disease is unknown despite recent progress in understanding its pathogenesis.

Pathology & Pathogenesis

There are two forms of chronic noninfectious gastrointestinal inflammation, one that is superficial and limited to the colonic mucosa **(ulcerative colitis)** and the other transmural and granulomatous in character and occurring anywhere along the gastrointestinal tract (**Crohn's disease,** also called **regional enteritis**). Both have been proposed to result from aberrant host immune responses to normal gastrointestinal tract antigens. In mice, targeted disruption of the genes for the T cell receptor and the cytokine IL-2 results in gastrointestinal tract disease resembling ulcerative colitis, while similar disruption of the gene for the cytokine IL-10 results in a panenteritis resem-

Table 9–14. Similarities and differences between ulcerative colitis and Crohn's disease[1].

	Ulcerative Colitis	Crohn's Disease
Clinical features		
Rectal bleeding	>90%	<50%
Diarrhea	10–30%	>70%
Abdominal mass	<1%	30%
Perianal abscesses, sinuses, and fistulas	2%	30%
Bowel perforation (free)	2–3%	<1%
Toxic megacolon	5–10%	<5%
Cancer of colon	Definite increase (5%)	Questionable increase
Pyoderma gangrenosum	<5%	1%
Erythema nodosum	5%	15%
Renal stones	<5% (uric acid stones, postcolectomy)	10% (oxalate stones)
Stomatitis	10%	10%
Aphthous ulceration	4%	4%
Uveitis	45%	5–10%
Spondylitis	<5%	15–20%
Peripheral arthritis	10%	20%
Thromboembolism with increased platelets and increased coagulant activity	Occurs	Occurs
Radiologic, endoscopic, and pathologic findings		
Rectal involvement	Almost 100%	<50%
Ulcers	Superficial, multiple Irregular	Solitary ulcers in the rectum Linear, serpiginous, and aphthoid ulcers Collar-button ulcers
Crypt abscesses, pseudopolyps, diminished goblet cells	>70%	<40%
Lymphoid aggregates and noncaseating granuloma	<10%	60–70%
Extent of disease	Mucosal and continuous	Transmural and discontinuous with "skip lesions"
Ileal involvement	Nonspecific with mild inflammation and dilation (backwash ileitis)	Ulcers, fissures, and stenosis
Fatty liver	39–40%	30–40%
Pericholangitis	30%	20%
Sclerosing cholangitis	30%	20–30%
Cirrhosis	Rare	<1%
Gallstones	Rare	10–15%
Treatment		
General	Supportive and symptomatic	Supportive and symptomatic
Definitive (drugs)	Sulfasalazine and corticosteroids	Sulfasalazine, corticosteroids, metronidazole

[1]Modified and reproduced, with permission, from Gopalswamy N: Inflammatory bowel disease. In: *Clinical Medicine Selected Problems With Pathophysiologic Correlations.* Barnes HV et al (editors). Year Book, 1988.

bling Crohn's disease. These and other studies support the hypothesis that a delicate balance between helper and suppressor T cell effects on B cell function is disrupted in these diseases. The two forms of inflammatory bowel disease have characteristic differences and in many cases considerable overlap in manner of presentation (Table 9–14). The feature common to all forms of inflammatory bowel disease is mucosal ulceration and inflammation of the gastrointestinal tract—indistinguishable, in fact, from that which can occur acutely during invasive infectious diarrhea. Other factors besides the presence of key gene products, including infectious agents, altered host immune responses, immune-mediated intestinal damage, psychologic factors, and dietary and environmental factors, may contribute to a final common pathway of disordered immune response.

Clinical Manifestations

A. Crohn's Disease: Crohn's disease typically occurs in the distal ileum or the colon, though any region of the gastrointestinal tract from mouth to anus can be involved, generally in a discontinuous fashion. It is characterized by ulceration and inflammation involving the entire thickness of the bowel wall, with recurrence of disease in previously uninvolved regions of the intestine, and can even involve adjacent mesentery and lymph nodes. The combination of deep mucosal ulceration and submucosal thickening gives the involved mucosa a characteristic "cobblestone'' appearance.

Perforation, fistula formation, abscess formation, and small intestinal obstruction are frequent complications of Crohn's disease, though an indolent course occurs in most patients. The full-thickness involvement of the bowel wall may predispose to these complications. Frank bleeding from the mucosal ulcerations can be either insidious or massive, as can **protein-losing enteropathy**. Another important complication is an increased incidence of intestinal cancer.

Patients with Crohn's disease often manifest symptoms outside of the gastrointestinal tract, including migratory arthritis. Inflammatory disorders of the skin, eye, and mucous membranes—particularly aphthous ulcers of the buccal mucosa, are also seen. Renal disorders, especially nephrolithiasis, are observed in a third of patients with Crohn's disease, probably related to increased oxalate absorption associated with steatorrhea. Amyloidosis is a serious complication of Crohn's disease, as is thromboembolic disease. Both of these complications are probably reflections of the systemic character of the inflammatory process. Patients are often malnourished and show evidence of deficiency states.

B. Ulcerative Colitis: In contrast to Crohn's disease, inflammation in ulcerative colitis is restricted to the mucosa of the colon and rectum. At one time it was believed that ulcerative colitis and Crohn's disease were distinct entities. This view was based on the observation of characteristic necrotic lesions of the colonic crypts of Lieberkühn, termed crypt abscesses in patients with ulcerative colitis. However, it is now recognized that in 10% of patients, regions characteristic of both Crohn's disease and ulcerative colitis are present. The diseases are similar in presentation (eg, bloody diarrhea and malabsorption) and in at least some of the complications (eg, protein-losing enteropathy and malnutrition), reflecting widespread involvement of the mucosa in both entities. However, since ulcerative colitis generally is limited to the mucosa, obstruction, perforation, and fistula formation are not typical complications. Most patients have mild disease, and—as with Crohn's disease—some patients will have only one or two episodes during their lifetimes. For unknown reasons, the risk of development of carcinoma appears even higher in ulcerative colitis than in Crohn's disease. Toxic megacolon is the one complication of ulcerative colitis that carries a high risk of perforation. Its cause is unknown.

Both ulcerative colitis and Crohn's disease can go into remission after treatment with anti-inflammatory agents such as sulfasalazine and glucocorticoids. The natural history of both diseases is one of periods of remission interrupted by active disease, with medical therapy during exacerbations directed toward supportive measures and attempts at inducing remission. Because these diseases can recur after resection of involved regions of the gastrointestinal tract, operative management is generally limited to relief of life-threatening intestinal obstruction or bleeding. Because of the variable response rate and the high risk of side effects, therapy with immunosuppressive agents such as mercaptopurine and azathioprine are limited to cases that have failed to respond to sulfasalazine and glucocorticoids.

45. How is inflammatory bowel disease distinguished from infectious diarrhea?
46. What are the differences between ulcerative colitis and Crohn's disease?
47. What are the complications of inflammatory bowel disease?

DIVERTICULAR DISEASE

Clinical Presentation

Nearly 80% of patients with diverticular disease are asymptomatic except for chronic constipation. Of those that develop other symptoms, the most common presentation is an intermittent and unpredictable griping lower abdominal pain. Additional features of the presentation depend on which of the two major complications of diverticular disease the patient develops.

A patient who develops diverticulitis (see below) may present with fever and signs and symptoms of peritoneal irritation (guarding, rebound tenderness, absence of bowel sounds). A patient who develops diverticular bleeding may present with either frankly bloody stools or stools that are positive for occult blood.

Etiology

Diverticular disease (diverticulosis) results from an acquired deformity of the colon in which the mucosa and submucosa herniate through the underlying muscularis (Figure 9–12). This is a disease of modern affluent life. A rarity at the turn of the century, today it afflicts 10% of the United States population. Its incidence increases with age, starting from about 40 years. Epidemiologic studies suggest that the consumption of highly refined foods and less fiber with resulting increased prevalence of chronic constipation, are responsible for the increased prevalence of diverticular disease.

Pathology & Pathogenesis

A. Diverticulosis: Most acquired diverticula occur in the colon, with the sigmoid being involved in 95% of cases. Both structural and functional factors are believed to contribute to the development of diverticulosis. Abnormalities in colonic wall connective tissue are believed to be the structural basis of diminished resistance to mucosal and submucosal herniation (Figures 9–12). Thus, individuals with genetic diseases involving connective tissue, such as Ehlers-Danlos and Marfan's syndromes, are characterized by the appearance of diverticular disease at a much earlier age. The functional abnormality is believed to be related to the development of a transmural pressure gradient from colonic lumen to peritoneal space as a result of vigorous muscle contraction of the colonic wall. This functional abnormality is probably due to the change in dietary habits, with decreased dietary fiber making forward propulsion of feces at normal transmural pressures more difficult.

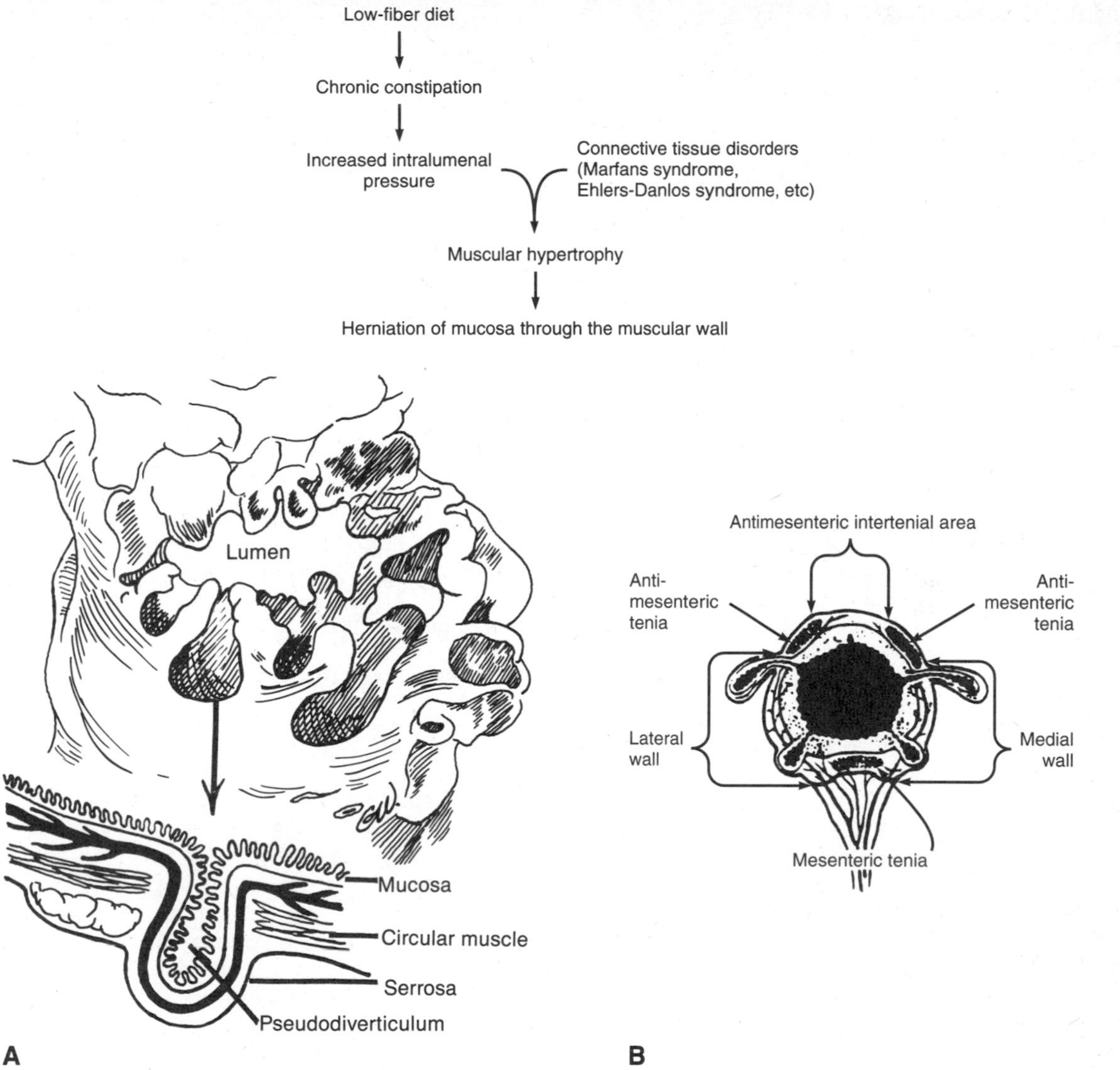

Figure 9–12. ***Top:*** Pathophysiology of diverticular disease. **A:** Herniation of mucosa of sigmoid colon between thickened folds of circular muscle, forming pseudodiverticula. (Reproduced, with permission, from Fleischner FG: Diverticular disease of the colon. New observations and revised concepts. Gastroenterology 1971;60:316. © 1971 by Williams & Wilkins.) **B:** Cross-sectional drawing of the colon, showing principal points of diverticula formation between mesenteric and antimesenteric teniae. (Reproduced, with permission, from Goligher JC: *Surgery of the Anus, Rectum and Colon,* 4th ed. Baillière Tyndall, 1980.)

This increased muscle contraction, which contributes to the development of diverticular disease, is also believed to cause the abdominal pain that is the cardinal symptom of uncomplicated diverticular disease. The pain may last hours to days, with sudden relief upon passing flatus or feces. Constipation or diarrhea and flatulence are common findings during such episodes, leading to the suggestion that there is a relationship between irritable bowel syndrome and the development of diverticulosis. Treatment of the pain of diverticular disease with opioids is contraindicated because they directly raise intraluminal pressure and hence may increase the risk of perforation.

B. Diverticular Bleeding: Branches of the colonic intramural arteries are closely associated with the diverticular sac, presumably leading to occasional rupture and bleeding. This is the most common cause of massive lower gastrointestinal bleeding in the elderly. Diverticular bleeding is typically painless and not believed to be associated with a focus of inflammation.

C. Diverticulitis: This most common complication of diverticulosis develops when a focal area of inflammation occurs in the wall of a diverticulum in response to irritation by fecal material. The patient develops symptoms of abdominal pain and fever with a risk of progression to abscess with or without perforation. The perforations usually are self-contained, but the potential for subsequent fistula formation and intestinal obstruction is high.

Clinical Manifestations

About one-fifth of all individuals with diverticular disease develop one of the two major complications—diverticular bleeding or diverticulitis—which must be distinguished from carcinoma, inflammatory bowel disease, and ischemic injury due to diffuse atherosclerosis.

48. Where in the gastrointestinal tract do most diverticula occur?
49. What predisposing factors contribute to the development of diverticular disease?
50. What are the major complications of diverticular disease?

REFERENCES

General

Wilson JD et al (editors): *Harrison's Principles of Internal Medicine,* 12th ed. McGraw-Hill, 1991.

Sleisenger MH, Fordtran JS (editors): *Gastrointestinal Disease,* 4th ed. Saunders, 1989.

Chandrasoma P, Taylor CR: *Concise Pathology,* 2nd ed. Appleton & Lange, 1995.

West JB (editor): *Best and Taylor's Physiological Basis of Medical Practice,* 12th ed. Williams & Wilkins, 1991.

Junqueira LC, Carneiro J, Kelley RO: *Basic Histology,* 7th ed. Appleton & Lange, 1992.

Achalasia and Esophageal Reflux

Aggestrup S et al: Lack of vasoactive intestinal peptide nerves in esophageal achalasia. Gastroenterology 1983;84:924.

Klauser AG, Schindlebeck NE, Mull-Lissner SA: Symptoms in gastro-esophageal reflux disease. Lancet 1990;335:205.

Acid-Peptic Disease

Feldman M, Peterson WL: *Helicobacter pylori* and peptic ulcer disease. West J Med 1993;159:555.

Gastroparesis

Rothstein RD: Gastrointestinal motility disorders in diabetes mellitus. Am J Gastroenterol 1990;85:782.

Diarrhea

Lynn RB, Friedman LS: Irritable bowel syndrome. N Engl J Med 1993;329:1940.

Perrson J: Alcohol and the small intestine. Scand J Gastroenterol 1991;26:3.

Inflammatory Bowel Disease

Strober W, Ehrhardt RO: Chronic intestinal inflammation: An unexpected outcome in cytokine or T cell receptor mutant mice. Cell 1993;75:203.

Diverticular Disease

Meyers MA et al: Pathogenesis of bleeding diverticulosis. Gastroenterology 1976;71:577.

Liver Disease

10

Vishwanath R. Lingappa, MD, PhD

Although many different pathogenic agents and processes can affect the liver (Table 10–1), they are generally manifested in individual patients in a limited number of ways that can be assessed by evaluation of some key parameters. Liver disease can be acute or chronic; focal or diffuse; mild or severe; and reversible or irreversible. Most cases of **acute liver disease** (eg, due to viral hepatitis) are so mild that they never come to medical attention. Transient symptoms of fatigue, loss of appetite, and nausea are often ascribed to other causes (eg, "flu"), and minor biochemical abnormalities referable to the liver that would be identified in blood studies are not discovered. The patient recovers without any lasting medical consequences apart from immunity in the case of hepatitis A or B infection. In other cases of acute liver injury, signs and symptoms are severe enough to call for medical attention. The entire range of liver functions may be affected or only a few, as is the case with liver injury due to certain drugs manifested as isolated impairment of the liver's role in bile formation **(cholestasis).** Occasionally, viral and other causes of acute liver injury occur in an overwhelming manner with massive liver cell death. This syndrome of **fulminant hepatitis** carries a high mortality rate, but if the patient survives, liver function returns to normal and there is no residual evidence of liver disease.

Liver injury may continue beyond the initial acute episode or may be recurrent **(chronic hepatitis).** In some cases of chronic hepatitis, liver function remains stable or the disease process ultimately resolves altogether. In other cases, there is progressive and irreversible deterioration of liver function.

Cirrhosis is an end-stage syndrome that is the consequence of progressive liver injury. Cirrhosis occurs in the subset of cases of chronic hepatitis that manifest a deteriorating course. Cirrhosis also occurs after repeated episodes of acute liver injury, as in the case of chronic alcoholism. In cirrhosis, the liver becomes hard, shrunken, and nodular and displays impaired function and diminished reserve due to a decreased amount of functioning liver tissue. More importantly, however, the physics of blood flow is altered in that blood in the hepatic portal vein is *diverted around* rather than *passing through* the liver. This phenomenon, termed **portal-to-systemic shunting,** has profound effects on the function of various organ systems and sets the stage for some of the most devastating complications of liver disease, as will be described below.

While liver disease due to many different causes may present in common ways, the reverse is also true—ie, liver diseases due to specific causes may have distinctly different presentations in different patients. For example, consider two patients with acute viral hepatitis: One may present with yellow eyes and skin—a manifestation of impaired liver function—complaining of nothing more than itching and loss of appetite, while the other may be brought to the emergency room moribund, with massive gastrointestinal bleeding and altered mental status. Such variations are probably due to genetic, immunologic, and environmental (including nutritional) factors that are at present poorly understood.

The consequences of liver disease can be either reversible or irreversible. In the first group are those arising directly from acute damage to the functional cells of the liver, most notably **hepatocytes,** without destruction of the liver's capacity for regeneration. Like many organs of the body, the liver normally has both a huge reserve capacity for the various biochemical reactions it carries out and the ability to regenerate fully differentiated cells and thereby recover completely from injury. Thus, only in the most fulminant cases or in end-stage disease are there insufficient residual hepatocytes to maintain minimal essential liver functions. More commonly, patients display transient signs of liver cell necrosis and disordered function. The signs and symptoms of this sort of acute liver injury can be best understood as an impairment of normal biochemical functions of the liver.

Other consequences of liver disease are typically seen in the patient with cirrhosis and are best understood as a result of portal-to-systemic shunting of blood flow. These include a heightened sensitivity to noxious substances absorbed from the gastrointestinal tract (encephalopathy), an increased risk of massive gastrointestinal bleeding (development of varices and coagulopathy), and malabsorption of fat

Table 10–1. Categories of liver disease by presentation.[1]

Cholestasis Familial causes (Gilbert's, Crigler-Najjar, Dubin-Johnson, and Rotor syndromes) Reactions to certain classes of drugs (including anabolic steroids, oral contraceptives, phenothiazines, erythromycins, oral hypoglycemic and antithyroid drugs) Developmental (neonatal) Secondary causes (postoperative, endotoxins, total parenteral nutrition, sickle cell crisis, hypophysectomy, some porphyrias) Direct causes (intrahepatic biliary atresia, cholangiocarcinoma, viral hepatitis, alcoholic hepatitis, primary biliary cirrhosis, pericholangitis) **Acute hepatitis** Viral (including hepatitis viruses A, B, C, D, and E and cytomegalovirus), Epstein-Barr virus, yellow fever virus) Reactions to certain classes of drugs (anesthetics such as halothane, anticonvulsants such as phenytoin, antihypertensives such as methyldopa, chemotherapeutic agents such as isoniazid, and thiazide diuretics such as hydrochlorothiazide) Poisons and toxins (such as ethanol) **Fulminant hepatitis** Infections (hepatitis A, B, C, and D, yellow fever, and cytomegalovirus; *Coxiella burnetii* infection) Poisons and toxins, chemicals, and drugs (*Amanita phalloides* toxin, phosphorus, ethanol; solvents, including carbon tetrachloride and dimethylformamide; anesthetics, including halothane; analgesics, including acetaminophen; antimicrobials, including tetracycline and isoniazid; and other drugs, including methyldopa, monoamine oxidase inhibitors, and valproate) Ischemia and hypoxia (vascular occlusion, circulatory failure, heat stroke, gram-negative sepsis with shock, congestive heart failure, pericardial tamponade) Miscellaneous metabolic anomalies (acute fatty liver of pregnancy, Reye's syndrome, jejunoileal bypass, Wilson's disease, galactosemia)	**Chronic hepatitis** Viral hepatitis (types B, C, and D) Primary autoimmune disorders (idiopathic autoimmune chronic active hepatitis, primary biliary cirrhosis, sclerosing cholangitis, and inflammatory bowel disease) Therapeutic drug-induced (methyldopa, nitrofurantoin, oxyphenisatin-containing laxatives) Genetic diseases (Wilson's disease, α_1-antiprotease deficiency) Infiltrative disorders (sarcoidosis, amyloidosis, hemochromatosis) **Cirrhosis** Infectious (viral: hepatitis B, C, and D and cytomegalovirus; toxoplasmosis, schistosomiasis, echinococcosis, brucellosis) Genetic diseases (Wilson's disease, hemochromatosis, α_1-antiprotease deficiency, glycogen storage diseases, Fanconi's syndrome, cystic fibrosis) Drugs and toxins Miscellaneous (sarcoidosis, graft-versus-host disease, inflammatory bowel disease, cystic fibrosis, jejunoileal bypass, diabetes mellitus) **Focal or extrinsic diseases with variable manifestations in the liver** Vascular (hepatic vein thrombosis, occlusion by parasites such as *Echinococcus* or *Schistosoma*) Biliary (duct obstruction due to stones or tumor or bacterial infection) Infectious (systemic sepsis; bacterial, fungal, or parasitic abscesses) Granulomatous diseases (sarcoidosis, tuberculosis) Infiltrative diseases (hemochromatosis, amyloidosis, Gaucher's disease and other lysosomal storage diseases, lymphoma)

[1]Modified from Isslebacher KJ, Podolsky DK: Biological and clinical approach to liver disease. In: *Harrison's Principles of Internal Medicine,* 12th ed. Wilson JD et al (editors). McGraw-Hill, 1991.

in the stool. In contrast to the consequences of acute hepatitis, those of cirrhosis are generally irreversible. Nevertheless, patients with cirrhosis will often present with superimposed acute liver injury (eg, due to an alcoholic binge or other drug exposure). Since they have a decreased hepatocyte mass and functional reserve, they are much more sensitive to acute liver injury than is the patient with a normal liver.

1. What parameters must you consider in assessing a patient with liver disease?
2. What factors determine the difference in severity of liver disease between two patients with acute hepatitis due to the same cause?
3. In what ways is the patient with underlying cirrhosis who presents with acute hepatitis likely to be different from the patient with a previously normal liver and acute hepatitis?

STRUCTURE & FUNCTION OF THE LIVER

ANATOMY, HISTOLOGY, & CELL BIOLOGY

The liver is located in the right upper quadrant of the abdomen in the peritoneal space just below the right diaphragm and under the rib cage (Figure 10–1). It weighs approximately 1400 g in the adult and is covered by a fibrous capsule. It receives nearly 25% of the cardiac output, approximately 1500 mL of blood flow per minute, via two sources: venous flow from the **hepatic portal vein,** which is crucial to performance of the liver's roles in bodily func-

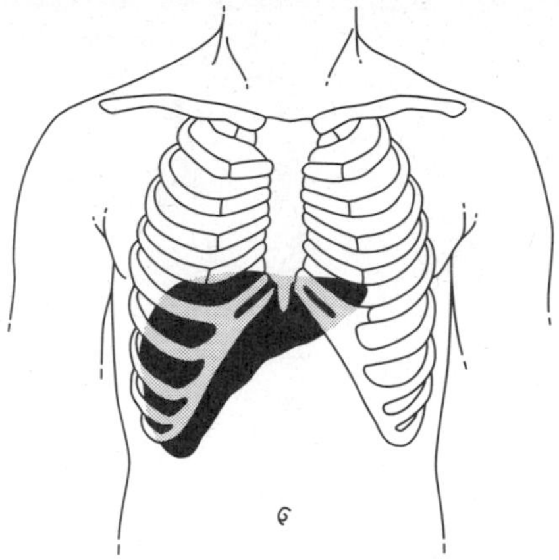

Figure 10–1. Location of the liver. (Reproduced, with permission, from Wolf DC: Evaluation of the size, shape and consistency of the liver. In: *Clinical Methods,* 3rd ed. Walker HK, Hall WD, Hurst JW [editors]. Butterworth, 1990.)

tions; and arterial flow from the **hepatic artery,** which is important for liver oxygenation. These vessels converge within the liver, and the combined blood flow exits via the so-called **central veins** (also called terminal veins) that drain into the hepatic vein and ultimately the inferior vena cava.

The portal vein carries venous blood from the small intestine, rich in freshly absorbed nutrients—as well as drugs and poisons—directly to the liver. Also flowing into the portal vein prior to its entry into the liver is the pancreatic venous drainage, rich in pancreatic hormones (insulin, glucagon, somatostatin, and pancreatic polypeptide). The portal vein forms a capillary bed that allows individual hepatocytes to be bathed directly in portal blood. In part because of this system of blood supply, the liver is a prime site for metastatic spread of neoplasms, especially from the gastrointestinal tract, breast, and lung.

Concepts of Liver Organization

The substance **(parenchyma)** of the liver is organized into plates of hepatocytes lying in a cage of supporting cells termed **reticuloendothelial cells** (Figure 10–2A). The plates of hepatocytes are generally only one cell thick, and individual plates are separated from each other by vascular spaces called **sinusoids.** It is in these sinusoids that blood from the hepatic artery is mixed with blood from the portal vein on the way to the central vein. The reticuloendothelial cell meshwork in which the hepatocytes reside includes diverse cell types, most importantly the **endothelial cells** that make up the walls of the sinusoids; specialized macrophages termed **Kupffer cells** are anchored in the sinusoidal space; and **lipocytes,** fat-storing cells involved in vitamin A metabolism, which lie between the hepatocytes and the endothelial cells. Approximately 30% of all cells in the liver are reticuloendothelial cells, and about one-third of these are Kupffer cells. Yet, because reticuloendothelial cells are smaller than hepatocytes, the reticuloendothelial system accounts for only 2–10% of the total protein in the liver. The reticuloendothelial cells are much more than just a cage for hepatocytes. They perform specific functions and communicate with each other as well as with hepatocytes. Their dysfunction has been implicated in the molecular basis for certain aspects of liver disease and its complications.

A. Lobules: Under the microscope at low-power magnification, liver architecture has been traditionally described in terms of the **lobule** (Figure 10–2B). Neat arrays of hepatocyte plates are organized around individual central veins to form hexagons with **portal triads** or **spaces** (sheath-like structures containing a portal venule, hepatic arteriole, and bile canaliculus) at their corners. The hepatocytes adjacent to the portal triad are termed the **limiting plate.** Disruption of the limiting plate is a significant diagnostic marker of some forms of immune-mediated liver disease, as may be seen, for example, at liver biopsy in a patient with liver disease of unknown cause.

B. Functional Zonation: In reality, it is physiologically more sensible to think of liver architecture in terms of the portal-to-central direction of blood flow: Blood entering the sinusoids from a terminal portal venule or hepatic arteriole flows past hepatocytes closest to those vessels first (termed zone 1 hepatocytes) and then percolates past zone 2 hepatocytes (so called because they are *not* the first hepatocytes reached by blood entering the hepatic parenchyma). The last hepatocytes reached by the blood before it enters the central vein are the zone 3 hepatocytes. Thus, the microscopic organization of the liver can be viewed in terms of functional zones. Thus, a liver **acinus** is defined as the unit of liver tissue centered around the portal venule and hepatic arteriole whose hepatocytes can be imagined to form concentric rings of cells in the order in which they come into contact with portal blood, first to last (Figure 10–2C). Hepatocytes at either extreme of the acinus (zones 1 and 3) appear to differ in both enzymatic activity and physiologic functions. Zone 1 hepatocytes, exposed to the highest oxygen concentrations, are particularly active in gluconeogenesis and oxidative energy metabolism. They are also the major site of urea synthesis (since freely diffusible substances such as ammonia absorbed from protein breakdown in the gut will be largely extracted in zone 1). Conversely, zone 3 hepatocytes are more active in glycolysis and lipogenesis (processes requiring less oxygen). Zone 2 hepatocytes display attributes of both zone 1 and zone 3 cells.

C. Receptor-Mediated Uptake: Functional zonation applies only to processes driven by the

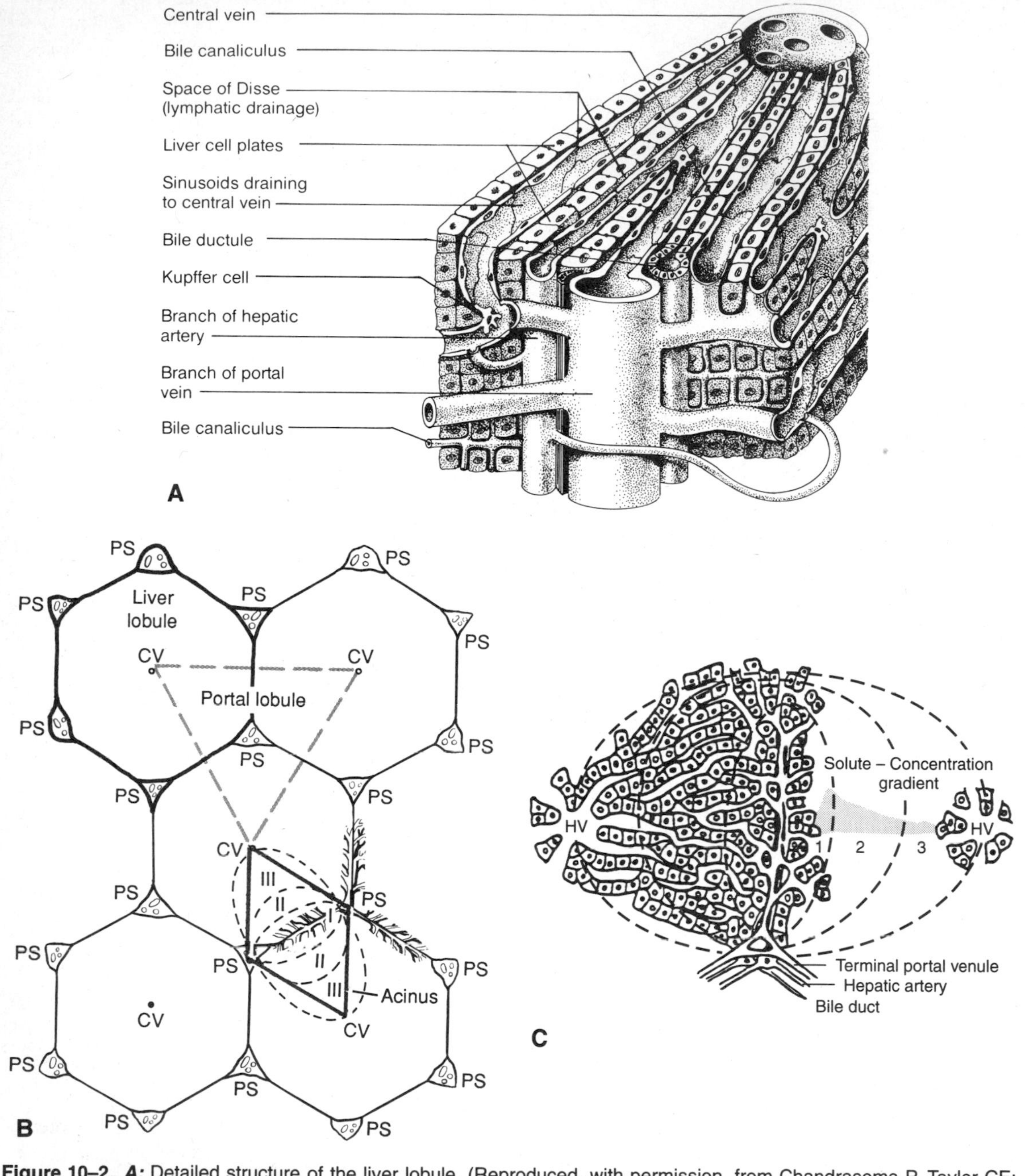

Figure 10–2. ***A:*** Detailed structure of the liver lobule. (Reproduced, with permission, from Chandrasoma P, Taylor CE: *Concise Pathology,* 2nd ed. Appleton & Lange, 1994.) ***B:*** Relationship of lobule to acinus. (Reproduced, with permission, from Junqueira LC, Carneiro J, Kelley RO: *Basic Histology,* 7th ed. Appleton & Lange, 1992.) ***C:*** Hepatic acinus. (CV, central vein; PS, portal space or triad; HV, hepatic venule; TPV, terminal portal venule.) (Reproduced, with permission, from Gumucio JJ: Hepatic transport. In: *Textbook of Medicine.* Kelley WN [editor]. Lippincott, 1989.)

presence of diffusible substances. The liver, however, is involved in many pathways participating in receptor-mediated uptake and active transport of substances unable to diffuse freely into cells. These substances will enter whichever hepatocytes have the appropriate transporters, regardless of their zone. Similarly, substances that are tightly bound to carrier proteins for which the liver does not have receptors will be cleared equally poorly by hepatocytes in all three zones.

Hepatocytes: Polarized Cells With Segregation of Functions

All surfaces of a hepatocyte are not the same. One side, the **apical surface,** forms the bile canaliculus, while the **basolateral surface** is in contact with the bloodstream via the sinusoids. Very different activities go forward at these regions of the hepatocyte plasma membrane, with **tight junctions** between hepatocytes serving to maintain segregation of apical and basolateral plasma membrane domains. Processes related to bile transport and excretion act at the apical plasma membrane (Figure 10–3A). Uptake from and secretion into the bloodstream are activities that occur across the basolateral membrane (Figure 10–3B).

Effects of Hepatocyte Dysfunction

In view of this organization, it is perhaps not surprising that hepatocyte dysfunction can sometimes involve disruption of bile flow (cholestasis) with relative preservation of other functions. There is, however, no clear line between the consequences of disturbed apical and basolateral functions: Cholestasis, while initially a disorder of apical bile flow, is ultimately manifested at the basolateral surface. This is because it is at the basolateral surface that bilirubin and other substances to be excreted across the apical plasma membrane into the bile must first be taken up from the bloodstream. Similarly, disruption of energy metabolism or protein synthesis, while initially impinging on the secretory and metabolic processes of the hepatocyte, will ultimately affect the bile transport machinery in the apical plasma membrane as well.

Capacity for Regeneration

While the normal liver harbors very few cells in mitosis, when hepatocytes are lost, poorly understood mechanisms stimulate proliferation of the remaining hepatocytes. This is why in most cases of fulminant hepatitis with massive hepatocellular death, if the pa-

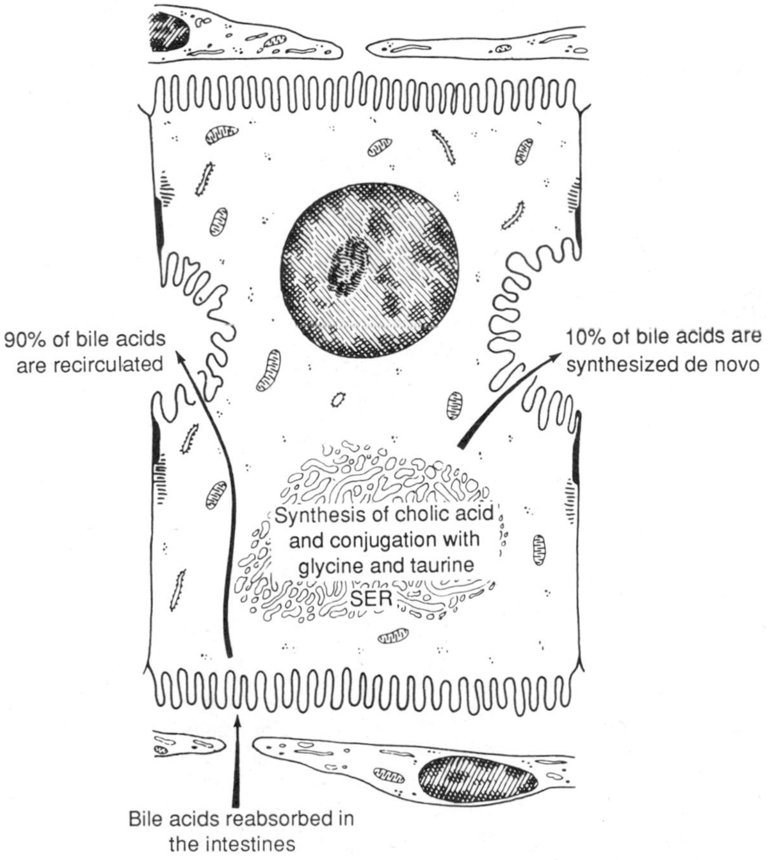

A

Figure 10–3. ***A:*** Mechanism of secretion of bile acids. About 90% of these compounds derive from bile acids absorbed in the intestinal epithelium and recirculated to the liver. The remainder are synthesized in the liver by conjugating cholic acid with the amino acids glycine and taurine. This process occurs in the smooth endoplasmic reticulum (SER). (Continued)

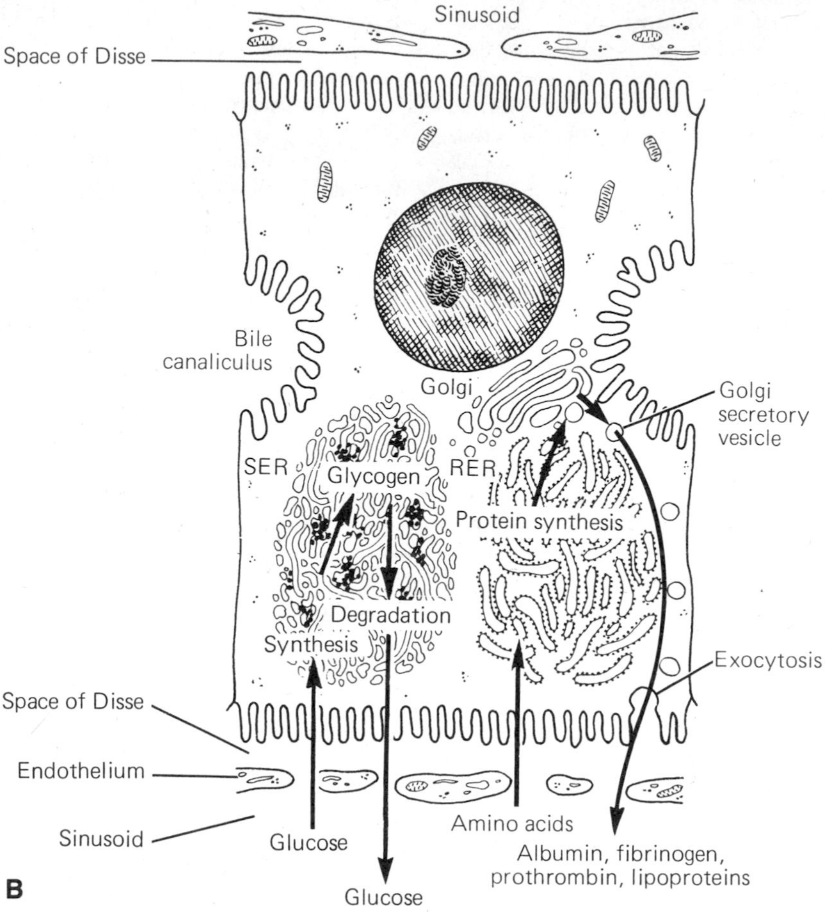

Figure 10-3. *B:* Protein synthesis and carbohydrate storage in the liver. Protein synthesis occurs in the rough endoplasmic reticulum, which explains why liver cell lesions or starvation lead to a decrease in the amounts of albumin, fibrinogen, and prothrombin in a patient's blood. In several diseases, glycogen degradation is depressed, with abnormal intracellular accumulation of this compound. (SER, smooth endoplastic reticulum; RER, rough endoplastic reticulum.) (Reproduced, with permission, from Junqueira LC, Carneiro J, Kelley RO: *Basic Histology,* 7th ed. Appleton & Lange, 1992.)

tient survives the acute period of hepatic dysfunction, recovery will be complete. Similarly, surgical resection of liver tissue is followed by proliferation of the remaining hepatocytes **(hyperplasia).** Hepatocyte regeneration, however, may be a two-edged sword. Under certain circumstances, the consequence of regeneration is not restoration of the normal liver but rather augmentation of hepatocyte mass with loss of normal liver architecture. This aberrant regenerative process, together with fibrosis, sets the stage for chronic changes that occur in cirrhosis.

LIVER BLOOD FLOW & ITS CELLULAR BASIS

The portal blood flow, being venous in nature, is normally under low hydrostatic pressure (about 10 mm Hg). Accordingly, there must be little resis-

4. From which vascular beds do the hepatic central veins derive their blood flow?
5. Why is the liver a major site for metastasis of malignant neoplasms from other parts of the body?
6. What cell types make up the liver, and what are their distinguishing characteristics?
7. What is the difference between the lobule concept and the acinus concept of liver subarchitecture?
8. What are some physiologic consequences of functional zonation in the liver?
9. What activities are found in zone 1 hepatocytes? In zone 3 hepatocytes?
10. What structures normally maintain the separation of apical and basolateral plasma membrane domains of the hepatocyte?
11. What happens to the remaining hepatocytes when part of the liver is surgically resected?

tance to its flow within the liver, allowing the blood to percolate through the sinusoids and achieve maximal contact, for exchange of substances, with hepatocytes. Two histologic specializations make these features of hepatic flow possible—namely, that the hepatic portal capillary endothelium is fenestrated and that it lacks a typical basement membrane. These features are lost in cirrhosis, resulting in profound changes in liver blood flow with devastating clinical consequences.

The spaces **(fenestrations)** between the endothelial cells that make up the walls of the portal capillary system allow plasma and its proteins—but not red blood cells—free and direct access to the surface of the hepatocytes. This feature is crucial to the liver's function of uptake from and secretion into the bloodstream. This feature also contributes to the efficiency of the liver as a filter of portal blood. (Most of the capillary beds in the body lack such fenestrations.)

Unlike most other organs, the liver has very little basement membrane between the capillary endothelial cell and the functional cells of the organ (ie, the hepatocytes). This feature further enhances the exchange of dissolved substances between liver and portal blood.

12. What are the roles of the liver in carbohydrate, protein, and lipid metabolism?
13. What are two physiologic mechanisms by which the body transports cholesterol?
14. Explain phase I and phase II reactions in drug detoxification.
15. Name and explain four clearance or protective functions of the liver.
16. What specializations allow the liver normally to be a low-pressure conduit for blood flow?

Table 10–2. Functions of the normal liver.

Energy metabolism and substrate interconversion
Glucose production through gluconeogenesis and glycogenolysis
Glucose consumption by pathways of glycogen synthesis, fatty acid synthesis, glycolysis, and the tricarboxylic acid cycle
Cholesterol synthesis from acetate, triglyceride synthesis from fatty acids, and secretion of both in VLDL particles
Cholesterol and triglyceride uptake by endocytosis of HDL and LDL particles with excretion of cholesterol in bile, beta-oxidation of fatty acids, and conversion of excess acetyl-CoA to ketones
Deamination of amino acids and conversion of ammonia to urea via the urea cycle
Transamination and de novo synthesis of nonessential amino acids
Protein synthetic functions
Synthesis of various plasma proteins, including albumin, clotting factors, binding proteins, apoliproproteins, angiotensinogen, and insulin-like growth factor I
Solubilization, transport, and storage functions
Drug and poison detoxification through phase I and phase II biotransformation reactions and excretion in bile
Solubilization of fats and fat-soluble vitamins in bile for uptake by enterocytes
Synthesis and secretion of VLDL and pre-HDL lipoprotein particles and clearance of HDL, LDL, and chylomicron remnants
Synthesis and secretion of various binding proteins, including transferrin, steroid hormone-binding globulin, thyroid hormone-binding globulin, ceruloplasmin, and metallothionein
Uptake and storage of vitamins A, D, B_{12}, and folate
Protective and clearance functions
Detoxification of ammonia through the urea cycle
Detoxification of drugs through microsomal oxidases and conjugation systems
Synthesis and export of glutathione
Clearance of damaged cells and proteins, hormones, drugs, and activated clotting factors from the portal circulation
Clearance of bacteria and antigens from the portal circulation

PHYSIOLOGY

The diverse functions of the liver are listed as four broad categories in Table 10–2. While there is considerable overlap between them, systematic consideration of each category is a useful way of approaching the patient with liver disease.

Energy Generation & Substrate Interconversion

Much of the body's carbohydrate, lipid, and protein is synthesized, metabolized, and interconverted in the liver, with products removed from or released into the bloodstream in response to the energy and substrate needs of the body.

A. Carbohydrate Metabolism: After a meal, the liver carries out net glucose consumption (eg, for glycogen synthesis and generation of metabolic intermediates via glycolysis and the tricarboxylic acid cycle). This occurs as a result of changes in the levels of substrates (eg, increase in glucose) in the portal vein and in the levels of hormones (eg, elevation of insulin with a relative decrease in glucagon) that increase the amount and activity of enzymes which control these pathways of glucose utilization in the hepatocyte. In times of fasting (low blood glucose) or stress (when higher blood glucose is needed), hormone and substrate levels in the bloodstream drive metabolic pathways of the liver responsible for net glucose production (eg, the pathways of glycogenolysis and gluconeogenesis). As a result, blood glucose levels are raised to—or maintained in—the normal range in spite of wide and sudden changes in the rate of glucose input (eg, ingestion and absorption) and output (eg, utilization by tissues) from the bloodstream (Figure 10–4).

B. Protein Metabolism: Related to its role in protein metabolism, the liver is a major site for processes of oxidative deamination and transamination (Figure 10–5). These reactions allow amino groups to be shuffled among molecules in order to generate substrates for both carbohydrate metabolism and amino acid synthesis. Likewise, the urea cycle allows nitrogen to be excreted in the form of urea, which is much less toxic than free amino groups in the form of ammonium ions. More will be said later about impairment of this function in liver disease.

C. Lipid Metabolism: Finally, the liver is the center of lipid metabolism. It manufactures nearly 80% of the cholesterol synthesized in the body from acetyl-CoA via a pathway that connects metabolism of carbohydrates with that of lipids (Figure 10–4). Moreover, the liver can synthesize, store, and export triglycerides (Figure 10–4). The liver is also the site of keto acid production via the pathway of fatty acid oxidation that connects lipid catabolism with activity of the tricarboxylic acid cycle.

In order to control the body's level of cholesterol and triglycerides, the liver assembles, secretes, and takes up various lipoprotein particles (Figure 10–6). Some of these particles **(very low density lipoproteins [VLDL])** serve to distribute lipid to adipose tissue for storage as fat or to other tissues for immediate use. In the course of these functions, the structure of VLDL particles is modified by loss of lipid and protein components. The resulting **low-density lipoprotein (LDL)** particles are then returned to the liver by virtue of their affinity for a specific receptor, the **LDL receptor,** found on the surface of various cells of the body, including hepatocytes. Other lipoprotein particles **(high-density lipoproteins [HDL])** are synthesized and secreted from the liver (in order to scavenge excess cholesterol and triglycerides from other tissues) and from the bloodstream, returning them to the liver for excretion. Thus, secretion of HDL and removal of LDL are both mechanisms by which cholesterol in excess of that needed by various tissues is removed from the circulation (Figures 10–6B and 10–6C).

Synthesis & Secretion of Plasma Proteins

The liver manufactures and secretes many of the proteins found in plasma, including albumin, several of the clotting factors, a number of binding proteins, and even certain hormones and hormone precursors. By virtue of the actions of these proteins, the liver has important roles in maintaining plasma oncotic pressure (serum albumin), coagulation (clotting

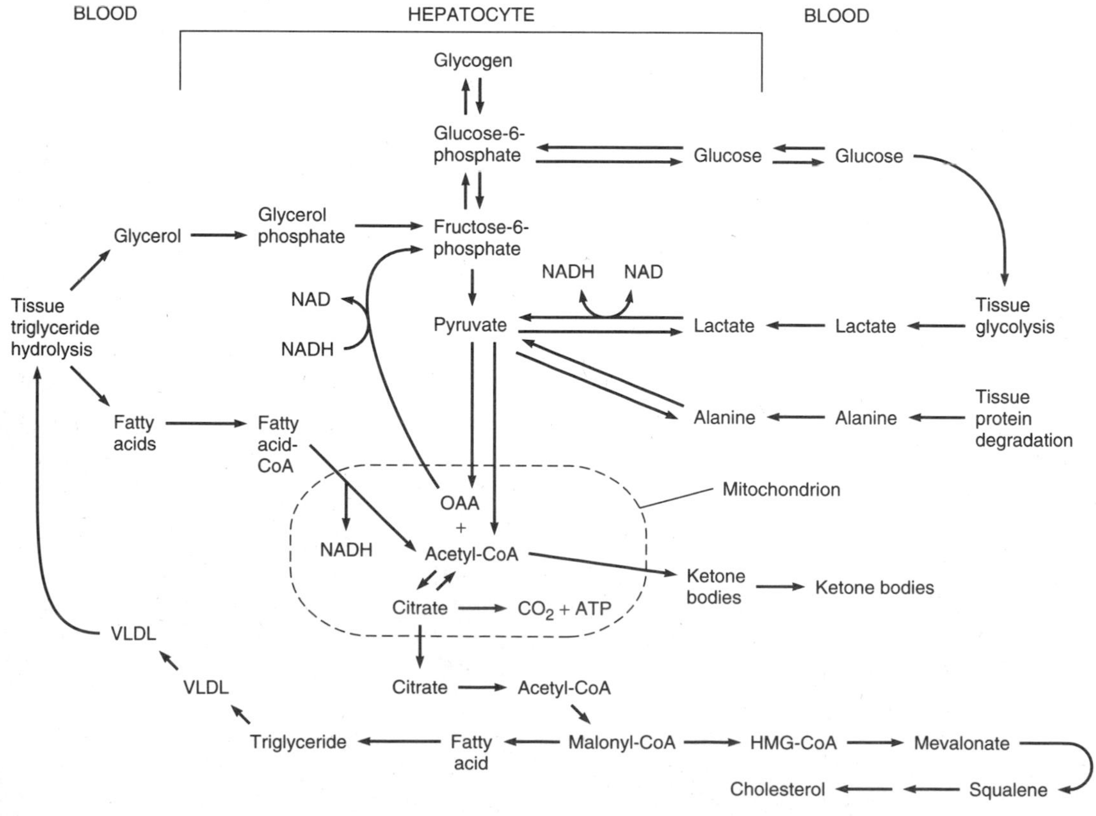

Figure 10–4. Pathways of hepatic carbohydrate and lipid metabolism. (Modified from Schwartz CC: Hepatic metabolism. In: *Textbook of Medicine.* Kelley WN [editor]. Lippincott, 1989.)

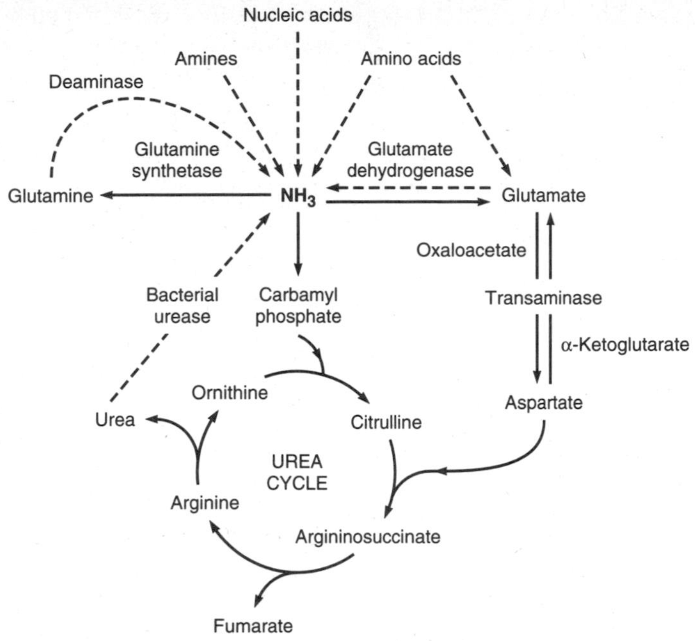

Figure 10–5. Urea cycle. (Reproduced, with permission, from Powers-Lee SG, Meister A: Urea synthesis and Ammonia Metabolism. In: *The Liver: Biology and Pathology,* 2nd ed. Arias IM et al [editors]. Raven Press, 1988.)

factor synthesis and modification), blood pressure (angiotensinogen), growth (insulin-like growth factor-1), and metabolism (steroid- and thyroid-hormone-binding proteins). Table 10–3 lists some of the proteins synthesized by the liver and their physiologic functions.

Solubilizing, Transport, & Storage Functions

The liver plays an important role in solubilizing, transporting, and storing a variety of very different substances that would otherwise be difficult for the tissues to obtain or to move in and out of cells. Specific cells in the liver perform these functions by making specialized proteins.

A. Enterohepatic Circulation of Bile: Bile is a detergent-like substance synthesized by the liver that permits a variety of otherwise insoluble substances to be dissolved in an aqueous environment for transport into or out of the body. Bile is recycled in the so-called **enterohepatic circulation** between the liver and the intestines. After synthesis and transport into the bile canaliculus (at the apical plasma membrane of the hepatocyte), bile is collected in the biliary tract (and sometimes stored in the gallbladder) and excreted via the common bile duct into the duodenum. While still in the cytoplasm of the hepatocyte, many bile acids are conjugated to sugars to increase their solubility. Once in the duodenum, bile acids serve to solubilize lipids, facilitating digestion and absorption of fats. In the terminal ileum, deconjugated bile salts are taken up and transported from enterocytes to portal blood flow, which brings them back to the liver, where specialized bile acid transporters return them to the hepatocyte cytosol for reconjugation and another cycle of enterohepatic transport.

B. Drug Metabolism and Excretion: Most of the enzymes that carry out metabolic processes necessary for the detoxification and excretion of drugs and other substances are located in the endoplasmic reticulum of hepatocytes. These pathways are used not only for metabolism of exogenous drugs but also for many endogenous substances that would otherwise be difficult for cells to excrete (eg, bilirubin and cholesterol). In most cases, this metabolism involves the conversion of **lipophilic** (hydrophobic) substances (which are difficult to excrete from cells because they tend to partition into cellular membranes) into more **hydrophilic** substances. This process involves catalysis of covalent modifications to make the substance more charged, so that it will partition more readily into an aqueous medium or at least be solubilized sufficiently in bile. As a result of these processes, collectively termed biotransformations, some substances so modified can be excreted directly in the urine while others are transported into the bile for excretion in feces.

C. Phases of Biotransformation: Biotransformation generally occurs in two phases. **Phase I reactions** involve oxidation-reductions in which an oxygen-containing functional group is added to the

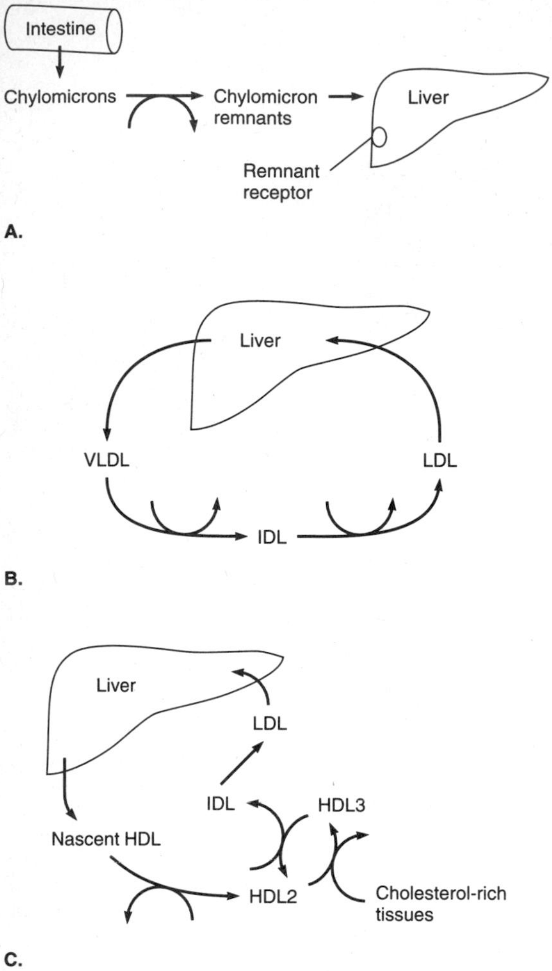

Figure 10–6. Lipoprotein metabolism in the liver. ***A:*** Exogenous fat transport pathway. ***B:*** Endogenous fat transport pathway. ***C:*** Pathway of reverse cholesterol transport. (Modified from Breslow JL: Genetic basis of lipoprotein disorders. J Clin Invest 1989;84:373.)

substance to be excreted. While oxidation itself does not necessarily have a major effect on water solubility, it usually introduces into the drug a reactive "handle" that makes possible other reactions which do render the modified substance water-soluble. These **phase II reactions** usually involve covalent attachment of the drug to a water-soluble carrier molecule such as the sugar glucuronic acid or the peptide glutathione. Unfortunately, phase I oxidation reactions often convert mildly toxic drugs into more toxic reactive intermediates, which facilitates their conjugation by phase II enzymes. This feature of drug detoxification has important clinical implications.

D. Role of Apolipoprotein in Solubilization and Transport of Lipids: The detoxification and bile transport pathways allow hepatocytes to convert a wide range of hydrophobic low-molecular-weight substances (eg, drugs and bilirubin) into a more hydrophilic and hence water-soluble form in which they can be excreted (eg, in bile or by the kidney). However, these are not the only solubilization challenges facing the body. The body also needs a mechanism that makes lipids available to various tissues (eg, to synthesize membranes) and one that removes any excess lipid the tissues do not use. To carry out these roles, lipid must be solubilized in a dispersed form that can be carried through the bloodstream. Hepatocytes synthesize for this purpose a class of specialized **apolipoproteins.** Apolipoproteins assemble into a variety of lipoprotein particles that transport lipids to and from various tissues by receptor-mediated endocytosis (see Lipid Metabolism, above).

E. Role in Production of Binding Proteins: Various cells in the liver synthesize proteins that bind certain substances very tightly (eg, some vitamins, minerals, and hormones). In some cases, this allows their transport in the bloodstream, where they would otherwise not be soluble (eg, steroids bound to steroid-binding globulin, which is synthesized and secreted by hepatocytes). In other cases, binding proteins made by the liver (eg, thyroid hormone-binding globulin) allow transport of specific substances (eg, thyroxine) in a form not fully accessible to tissues. In this way, the effective concentration of the substance is limited to its free concentration at equilibrium.

In some cases, binding proteins made by the liver allow accumulation there of specific substances in high concentrations. **Transferrin,** for example, is an iron-binding protein synthesized and secreted into the bloodstream by the liver. Upon binding of free iron at normal blood pH, transferrin develops affinity for a specific membrane receptor of the hepatocyte **(transferrin receptor).** Upon receptor binding, the transferrin–transferrin receptor complex is internalized into the endocytic pathway, a progressively more acidic environment. There, at low pH, iron no longer remains bound to transferrin. However, conformational changes at low pH allow transferrin to maintain high-affinity binding to its receptor even in the absence of bound iron. Thus, when the receptor recycles back to the surface, it brings the "empty" transferrin with it. Upon presentation to the neutral pH environment of the bloodstream, transferrin lacking bound iron is released from the receptor, and the cycle can start over again. Meanwhile, the free iron released from transferrin in the acidic environment of the endosome is transported into the cytoplasm of the hepatocyte, where it binds to **ferritin,** a cytoplasmic iron storage protein. This provides a reservoir that can be mobilized in response to the body's needs. Similar dynamics of plasma binding proteins, receptors, and cytosolic storage proteins occur for many other substances.

Whereas most solubilization functions are performed in hepatocytes, some of the binding and storage functions are properties of accessory cells. Thus, vitamin A storage occurs in fat droplets seen in the

Table 10–3. Proteins synthesized by the liver: Physiologic functions and properties.[1]

Name	Principal Function	Binding Characteristics	Serum or Plasma Concentration
Albumin	Binding and carrier protein; osmotic regulator	Hormones, amino acids, steroids, vitamins, fatty acids	4500–5000 mg/dL
Orosomucoid	Uncertain; may have a role in inflammation		Trace; rises in inflammation
α_1-Antiprotease	Trypsin and general protease inhibitor	Proteases in serum and tissue secretions	1.3–1.4 mg/dL
α-Fetoprotein	Osmotic regulation; binding and carrier protein[2]	Hormones, amino acids	Found normally in fetal blood
α_2-Macroglobulin	Inhibitor of serum endoproteases	Proteases	150–420 mg/dL
Antithrombin-III	Protease inhibitor of intrinsic coagulation system	1 : 1 binding to proteases	17–30 mg/dL
Ceruloplasmin	Transport of copper	Six atoms copper/mol	15–60 mg/dL
C-reactive protein	Uncertain; has role in tissue inflammation	Complement C1q	<1 mg/dL; rises in inflammation
Fibrinogen	Precursor to fibrin in hemostasis		200–450 mg/dL
Haptoglobin	Binding, transport of cell-free hemoglobin	Hemoglobin 1 : 1 binding	40–180 mg/dL
Hemopexin	Binds to porphyrins, particularly heme for heme recycling	1 : 1 with heme	50–100 mg/dL
Transferrin	Transport of iron	Two atoms iron/mol	3.0–6.5 mg/dL
Apolipoprotein B	Assembly of lipoprotein particles	Lipid carrier	
Angiotensinogen	Precursor to pressor peptide angiotensin II		
Proteins, coagulation factors II, VII, IX, X	Blood clotting		20 mg/dL
Antithrombin III, protein C	Inhibition of blood clotting		
Insulin-like growth factor I	Mediator of anabolic effects of growth hormone	IGF-I receptor	
Steroid hormone-binding globulin	Carrier protein for steroids in bloodstream	Steroid hormones	3.3 mg/dL
Thyroxine-binding globulin	Carrier protein for thyroid hormone in bloodstream	Thyroid hormones	1.5 mg/dL
Transthyretin (thyroid-binding prealbumin)	Carrier protein for thyroid hormone in bloodstream	Thyroid hormones	25 mg/dL

[1]Adapted from Donohue TM et al: Synthesis and secretion of plasma proteins by the liver. In: *Hepatology: A Textbook of Liver Disease.* Zakim D, Boyer TD (editors). Saunders, 1990.
[2]The function of alpha-fetoprotein is uncertain, but because of its structural homology to albumin it is often assigned these functions.

lipocytes of the reticuloendothelial system. Recently, lipocytes have been implicated in the pathogenesis of chronic liver injury and cirrhosis. These observations suggest that lipocytes have poorly understood roles other than vitamin A storage.

Protective & Clearance Functions

Many of the liver functions already discussed, such as drug detoxification and excretion of excess cholesterol by conversion to and solubilization in bile, can also be considered protective. Nevertheless, it is useful to conceptualize the protective function as a separate category because of its clinical importance in ameliorating the consequences of liver disease.

Some additional indirect liver functions, such as its role in maintaining normal sodium and water balance, are inferred from the derangements observed in patients with liver disease, as will be discussed later.

A. Phagocytic and Endocytic Functions of Kupffer Cells: The liver helps remove bacteria and antigens that breach the defenses of the gut to enter the portal blood and participates also in clearing the circulation of endogenously generated cellular debris. It appears that specialized receptors on the Kupffer cell surface bind to glycoproteins (via carbohydrate receptors), or to material coated with immunoglobulin (via the Fc receptor), or to complement (via the C3 receptor), thus allowing damaged plasma proteins, activated clotting factors, immune complexes, senescent blood cells, etc, to be recognized and removed.

B. Endocytic Functions of Hepatocytes: Hepatocytes have a number of specific receptors for damaged plasma proteins distinct from the receptors present on Kupffer cells (eg, the asialoglycoprotein receptor that specifically binds glycoproteins whose terminal sialic acid sugar residues have been removed). The precise physiologic significance of this metabolic action remains unclear.

C. Ammonia Metabolism: Ammonia generated from deamination of amino acids is metabolized within hepatocytes into the much less toxic substance urea. Loss of this function results in altered mental status, a common manifestation of severe or end-stage liver disease.

D. Hepatocyte Synthesis of Glutathione: Glutathione is the major intracellular (cytoplasmic) reducing reagent and thus is crucial for preventing oxidative damage to cellular proteins. This molecule is a nonribosomally synthesized tripeptide (γ-glutamyl-cistinyl-glycine) which is also a substrate for many phase II drug detoxification conjugation reactions. The liver may also export glutathione for use by other tissues.

OVERVIEW OF LIVER DISEASE

TYPES OF LIVER DYSFUNCTION

Most of the clinical consequences of liver disease can be understood either as a failure of one of the liver's four broad functions (summarized in Table 10–2) or as a consequence of portal hypertension, the altered hepatic blood flow of cirrhosis.

Hepatocyte Dysfunction

One mechanism of liver disease—particularly in acute liver injury—is dysfunction of the individual hepatocytes that make up the liver parenchyma. The pathway and extent of hepatocellular dysfunction determine the specific manifestations of liver disease. The outcomes to be anticipated when normal hepatic functions fail are described below.

Portal Hypertension

Some consequences of liver disease—particularly of cirrhosis—are best understood in terms of what we know about hepatic blood flow. Of greatest clinical importance are the existence under normal circumstances of a low-pressure portal venous capillary bed throughout the liver parenchyma and the functional zonation of portal blood flow.

When pathologic processes (eg, fibrosis) result in elevation of the normally low intrahepatic venous pressure, blood "backs up" and finds alternative venous routes back to the systemic circulation. Thus, blood from the gastrointestinal tract is no long er filtered—or is filtered less efficiently—by the liver prior to entering the systemic circulation. Thus, the consequences of this portal-to-systemic shunting are loss of protective and clearance functions of the liver; functional abnormalities in renal salt and water homeostasis; and a greatly increased risk of gastrointestinal hemorrhage from the development of engorged blood vessels carrying venous blood bypassing the liver (eg, **esophageal varices**).

Even in the absence of any intrinsic parenchymal liver disease, portal-to-systemic shunting of blood can produce or contribute to **encephalopathy** (altered mental status due to failure to clear poisons absorbed from the gastrointestinal tract); gastrointestinal bleeding (due to esophageal varices); and malabsorption of fats and fat-soluble vitamins (due to loss of enterohepatic recirculation of bile), with associated coagulopathy. In Table 10–4, the sydromes of aberrant liver function are categorized as a consequence of hepatocyte dysfunction, portal-to-systemic shunting, or of both.

The fact that hepatocytes in the different zones of the acinus "see" blood in a particular sequence has great pathophysiologic significance. Since zone 1 hepatocytes see blood that has just left the portal venule or hepatic arteriole, they have access to the highest concentrations of various substances—both good (eg, oxygen and nutrients) and bad (eg, drugs and toxins absorbed from the gastrointestinal tract). Zone 2 hepatocytes receive blood containing less of these substances, and zone 3 hepatocytes are bathed in blood largely depleted of them. However, zone 3 hepatocytes see the highest concentrations of products (eg, drug metabolites) released into the bloodstream by hepatocytes of zones 1 and 2. Thus, direct poisons have their most severe impact on zone 1 hepatocytes, while poisons that are generated as a result of hepatic metabolism will cause more damage to those of zone 3. Similarly, since sinusoidal blood around zone 3 has the lowest oxygen concentration, hepatocytes of this zone are at greatest risk of injury under conditions of hypoxia.

MANIFESTATIONS OF LIVER DYSFUNCTION

Whether due to hepatocyte dysfunction or portal-to-systemic shunting, prominent features of liver disease are manifestations of failure of normal functions. An understanding of these mechanisms offers insight into the probable causes of illness in a patient with acute or chronic liver disease.

Table 10–4. Pathophysiology of syndromes of aberrant function in liver disease.

Syndromes of Abberrant Function in Liver Disease	Hepatocellular Dysfunction	Portal-to-Systemic Shunting
Energy metabolism and substitute conversion		
Alcoholic hypoglycemia	✓	
Alcoholic ketoacidosis	✓	
Hyperglycemia		✓
Familial hypercholesterolemia	✓	
Hepatic encephalopathy	✓	✓
Fatty liver	✓	
Solubilization, transport, and storage function		
Drug sensitivity	✓	
Steatorrhea	✓	✓
Fat-soluble vitamin deficiency	✓	✓
Hemochromatosis	✓	✓
Coagulopathy	✓	✓
Protein synthetic function		
Edema due to hypoalbuminemia	✓	
Protective and clearance functions		
Hypergammaglobulinemia		✓
Hypogonadism and hyperestrogenism	✓	✓
Renal dysfunction		
Sodium retention		✓
Impaired water excretion		✓
Impaired renal concentrating ability		✓
Deranged potassium metabolism		✓
Prerenal azotemia		✓
Acute renal failure		✓
Glomerulopathies		✓
Impaired renal acidification		✓
Hepatorenal syndrome		✓

Diminished Energy Generation & Substrate Interconversion

A first category of altered liver function involves the intermediary metabolism of carbohydrates, fats, and proteins.

A. Carbohydrate Metabolism: Severe liver disease can result in either hypo- or hyperglycemia. Hypoglycemia results largely from decrease in functional hepatocyte mass, while hyperglycemia is a result of portal-to-systemic shunting, which decreases the efficiency of postprandial extraction of glucose from portal blood by hepatocytes, thus elevating systemic blood glucose concentration.

B. Lipid Metabolism: Disturbance of lipid metabolism in the liver can result in syndromes of fat accumulation early in the course of liver injury. Perhaps this is because the complex steps in assembly of lipoprotein particles for export of cholesterol and triglycerides from the liver are more sensitive to disruption than the pathways of lipid synthesis, resulting in a buildup of fat within the liver. In certain chronic liver diseases such as primary biliary cirrhosis, bile flow decreases as a result of destruction of bile ducts. The decrease in bile flow results in decreased lipid clearance via bile with consequent hyperlipidemia. These patients often develop subcutaneous accumulations of cholesterol termed **xanthomas.**

C. Protein Metabolism: Finally, any disturbance of protein metabolism in the liver can result in a syndrome of altered mental status and confusion known as **hepatic encephalopathy.** As with carbohydrate metabolism, altered protein metabolism can result from either hepatocyte failure or portal-to-systemic shunting, with the net effect of elevation of blood concentrations of centrally acting toxins.

Loss of Solubilization & Storage Functions

A. Disordered Bile Secretion: The clinical significance of bile synthesis can be seen in the prominence of cholestasis—failure to secrete bile—in many forms of liver disease. Cholestasis can occur as a result of extrahepatic obstruction (eg, from a gallstone in the common bile duct) or of selective dysfunction of the bile synthetic and transport machinery within the hepatocytes themselves (eg, from a reaction to certain drugs). The mechanisms responsible for cholestatic drug reactions are not well understood. Regardless of the mechanism, however, the clinical consequences of severe cholestasis may be profound: A failure to secrete bile results in a failure to solubilize substances such as dietary lipids and fat-soluble vitamins, resulting in **malabsorption** and deficiency states.

The solubilization function of bile works both to excrete and to absorb substances. Thus, in cholestasis, endogenous substances that are normally excreted via the biliary tract can accumulate to high levels. One such substance is bilirubin, a product of heme degradation (Figure 10–7). The buildup of bilirubin results in **jaundice** or **icterus** (yellow discoloration of the scleras and skin). In the adult, the most significant feature of jaundice is that it serves as a readily monitored index of cholestasis, which may occur alone or with other abnormalities in hepatocyte function (ie, as part of the presentation of acute hepatitis). In the neonate, however, elevated bilirubin concentrations can be toxic to the developing nervous system, producing a syndrome termed **kernicterus.**

Similarly, cholesterol is normally excreted either by conversion into bile salts or by forming complexes, termed micelles, with preexisting (recycled) bile salts. In cholestasis, the resultant buildup of bile salts can lead to their deposition in the skin, manifested as intense itching, or **pruritus.** Disorders of bile production are a basis for the formation of cholesterol gallstones. Nevertheless, as mentioned earlier, other hepatocyte functions are often relatively well preserved in the face of significant cholestasis. The syndromes that produce jaundice are summarized in Table 10–5.

B. Impaired Drug Detoxification: Two features of the mechanisms of drug detoxification are of particular clinical importance. One is the phenomenon of **enzyme induction.** It is observed that the presence in the bloodstream of any of the large class of drugs inactivated by phase I enzymes increases the amount and activity of these enzymes in the liver. This property of enzyme induction makes physiologic sense (as a response to the body's need for increased biotransformation) but can have undesired effects as well. A patient who chronically consumes large amounts of a substance that is metabolized by phase I enzymes (eg, ethanol) will induce high levels of these enzymes and thus speed up the metabolism of other substances metabolized by the same detoxifying enzymes (eg, antiseizure or anticoagulant medications, resulting in subtherapeutic blood levels of the drugs).

A second clinically important phenomenon in drug metabolism has already been mentioned, namely, that phase I reactions often convert relatively benign compounds into more reactive and hence more toxic ones. Normally, this heightened reactivity of phase I reaction products serves to facilitate phase II reactions, making detoxification more efficient. However, under certain conditions when phase II reactions are impaired (eg, glutathione deficiency from inadequate nutrition), enhanced phase I enzyme activity can cause increased liver injury. This is because the products of phase I reactions, in the absence of glutathione, may react with and damage cellular components. Such damage can rapidly kill a hepatocyte.

Thus, the combined effects of certain common conditions can make the individual abnormally sensitive to the toxic effects of drugs. For example, the combination of induced phase I activity (eg, due to alcoholism) with low phase II activity (eg, due to low glutathione levels from nutritional deprivation) can result in heightened generation of reactive intermediates with an inadequate capacity to conjugate and detoxify them. A classic example of this phenomenon is acetaminophen toxicity. As little as 2 g of acetaminophen can produce significant liver damage in such susceptible individuals.

C. Lipoprotein Dynamics and Dyslipidemias: The liver's role in lipid metabolism is illustrated by the genetic defect causing familial hypercholesterolemia. Lack of a functional LDL receptor in such cases renders the liver unable to clear LDL cholesterol from the bloodstream, resulting in markedly elevated serum cholesterol and accelerated atherosclerosis and coronary artery disease. Heterozygotes with one normal LDL receptor allele can be treated with drugs (eg, HMG-CoA reductase inhibitors) that inhibit endogenous cholesterol synthesis and thus upregulate LDL receptor levels. However, there is no effective drug therapy for homozygotes, since they have no normal LDL receptors. Hepatic transplantation is effective therapy for homozygous familial hypercholesterolemia because it provides a genetically unrelated liver with normal LDL receptors.

In acquired liver diseases, the serum cholesterol is elevated in biliary tract obstruction, which blocks cholesterol excretion in bile; and diminished in severe alcoholic cirrhosis, in which fat malabsorption prevents cholesterol intake.

D. Altered Hepatic Binding and Storage Functions: Liver disease influences the liver's ability to store various substances. As a result, patients with liver disease have a high risk of developing certain deficiency states such as folic acid and vitamin B_{12} deficiency. Since these vitamins are needed for DNA synthesis, their deficiency results in **macrocytic anemia** (low red blood cell count with

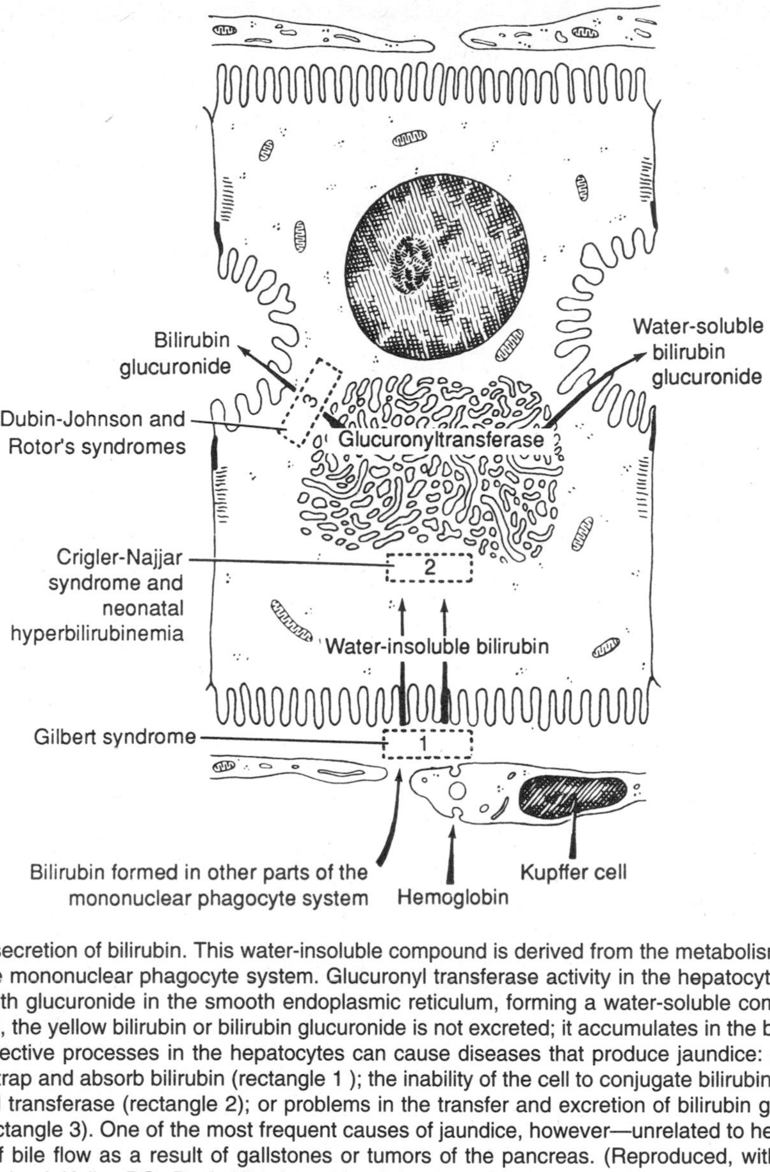

Figure 10–7. The secretion of bilirubin. This water-insoluble compound is derived from the metabolism of hemoglobin in macrophages of the mononuclear phagocyte system. Glucuronyl transferase activity in the hepatocytes causes bilirubin to be conjugated with glucuronide in the smooth endoplasmic reticulum, forming a water-soluble compound. When bile secretion is blocked, the yellow bilirubin or bilirubin glucuronide is not excreted; it accumulates in the blood, and jaundice results. Several defective processes in the hepatocytes can cause diseases that produce jaundice: a defect in the capacity of the cell to trap and absorb bilirubin (rectangle 1); the inability of the cell to conjugate bilirubin because of a deficiency in glucuronyl transferase (rectangle 2); or problems in the transfer and excretion of bilirubin glucuronide into the biliary canaliculi (rectangle 3). One of the most frequent causes of jaundice, however—unrelated to hepatocyte activity—is the obstruction of bile flow as a result of gallstones or tumors of the pancreas. (Reproduced, with permission, from Junqueira LC, Carneiro J, Kelley RO: *Basic Histology,* 7th ed. Appleton & Lange, 1992.)

large red cells), a common finding in patients with liver disease.

Diminished Synthesis & Secretion of Plasma Proteins

The clinical significance of liver protein synthesis and secretion derives from the wide range of functions carried out by these proteins. For example, since albumin is the major contributor to plasma oncotic pressure, hypoalbuminemia as a consequence of liver disease or nutritional deficiency presents with marked edema formation. Other important proteins synthesized and secreted by the liver include clotting factors and hormone binding proteins.

Loss of Protective & Clearance Functions

A crucial protective function of the liver is its role as a filter of blood from the gastrointestinal tract, by which various substances are removed from portal blood before it reenters the systemic circulation.

A. Clearance of Bacteria and Endotoxin: Clearance of bacteria by Kupffer cells of the liver is the final line of defense in keeping gut-derived bacteria out of the systemic circulation. Loss of this capacity in liver disease due to portal-to-systemic shunting may help to explain why, in patients with severe liver disease, infections can rapidly decompensate into sepsis.

Table 10–5. Laboratory findings in the differential diagnosis of jaundice.[1]

Type of Jaundice	Blood						Stool	Urine	
	Hct	Unconjugated Bilirubin (Indirect)	Conjugated Bilirubin (Direct)	Alkaline Phosphatase	Aminotransferases	Cholesterol	Color	Bilirubin	Urobilinogen
Hemolytic	↓	↑ ↑	N	N	N	N	N	0	↑
Hepatocellular Gilbert's syndrome	N	↑	N	N	N	N	N	0	N or ↓
Abnormal conjugation	N	↑	N	N	N	N	N	0	N or ↓
Hepatocellular damage	N	↑	↑	↑ ↑	↑ ↑	N	N	↑	↑
Obstructive Defective excretion	N	N	N	N	N	N	N	↑	N
Intrahepatic cholestasis	N	N	↑	N	N	N or ↑	Pale	↑	↓
Extrahepatic biliary obstruction	N	N	↑ ↑	N or ↑	N or ↑	↑	Pale	↑	↓

[1]Reproduced, with permission, from Chandrasoma P, Taylor CR: *Concise Pathology,* 2nd ed. Appleton & Lange, 1994.

B. Altered Ammonia Metabolism: Impairment of the liver's ability to detoxify ammonia to urea leads to hepatic encephalopathy, manifested as an altered mental status. This may be an early manifestation of acute fulminant hepatitis with massive hepatocellular dysfunction even before the development of maximal hepatocellular necrosis. It can be a final step in progressive chronic liver disease with diminished hepatocyte functional capacity. Most often it is a consequence of an increased ammonia load in a patient with marginal liver function or significant portal-to-systemic shunting. Hepatic encephalopathy may occur as a first sign of renewed gastrointestinal bleeding (as a result of increased production of ammonia and other products due to breakdown of blood protein and urea by gastrointestinal tract microbes) or may simply be due to increased protein intake (eg, a cheeseburger eaten by a patient with cirrhosis). Finally, the development of sepsis in these predisposed patients results in increased endogenous protein catabolism and therefore elevated ammonia production. Thus, the development of encephalopathy in a patient with chronic liver disease calls for investigation of possible acute gastrointestinal bleeding as well as potentially catastrophic infection. Pending the outcome of diagnostic studies (eg, serial hematocrit measurements and cultures of blood, urine, and ascitic fluid), therapy is designed to improve mental status by diminishing the absorption of ammonia and other noxious substances from the gastrointestinal tract. When the patient is given the nonabsorbable carbohydrate **lactulose,** whose metabolism by microbes creates an acidic environment, ammonia is trapped as the charged NH_4^+ species in the gut lumen and excreted by the resulting osmotic diarrhea. Thus, this toxin is prevented from ever entering the portal circulation, and the patient's mental status gradually improves.

C. Altered Hormone Clearance in Liver Disease: Normally, the liver removes from the bloodstream the fraction of steroid hormones not bound to steroid hormone-binding globulin. Upon uptake by hepatocytes, the hormones are oxidized, conjugated, and excreted into bile, where a fraction undergoes enterohepatic circulation. In liver disease accompanied by significant portal-to-systemic shunting, steroid hormone clearance is diminished; extraction of the enterohepatic circulated fraction is impaired; and peripheral aromatization of androgens to estrogens is increased. The net effect is an elevation of blood estrogens, which in turn alters hepatocyte protein synthesis and secretion and microsomal P450 content. Synthesis of some hepatic proteins increases, while synthesis of others is diminished. P450 content increases as the liver attempts to metabolize the higher blood estrogen. Thus, male patients with liver disease display both gonadal and pituitary suppression as well as feminization.

Sodium & Water Balance

Patients with liver disease often display renal abnormalities and complications, most commonly sodium retention and difficulty in excreting water. An intrinsic renal lesion is apparently not involved, since the kidneys of patients with liver disease typically function normally when transplanted into patients with normal livers. Instead, renal abnormalities associated with liver disease are functional, occurring because liver disease induces altered intravascular pressures. As a result, homeostatic mechanisms perceive intravascular volume as being inadequate when it is really only maldistributed. Renal mechanisms of salt and water retention are then stimulated to correct what has been sensed as volume depletion. Some of the factors influencing renal sodium retention in liver disease are summarized in Table 10–6. In addition, patients with severe liver disease are at risk of developing renal failure.

17. Under what circumstances is hypoglycemia seen in liver disease?
18. Name three clinical consequences of cholestasis.
19. Development of hepatic encephalopathy in a patient with chronic liver disease should lead you to investigate what possible precipitating factors?
20. By what mechanisms can coagulation defects be a consequence of liver disease?
21. What is an explanation for hypogonadism in male patients with liver disease?

PATHOPHYSIOLOGY OF SELECTED LIVER DISEASES

ACUTE HEPATITIS

Acute hepatitis is an inflammatory process causing liver cell necrosis. A wide range of clinical entities can cause global hepatocyte injury of sudden onset.

Table 10–6. Factors influencing renal sodium retention in liver disease.[1]

Hormonal
Elevated renal endothelin production
Hyperaldosteronism due to diminished clearance by the liver
Diminished angiotensinogen synthesis by the liver
Diminished renin and angiotensin II clearance by the liver
Altered kallikrein-kinin system
Loss of hepatic humoral natriuretic factors
Atrial natriuretic factor
Elevated blood estrogens
Prolactin
Vasoactive intestinal peptide
Elevated peripheral nitric acid production
Neural
Increased sympathetic nervous system activity
Hemodynamic
Alterations in intrarenal blood flow
Portal-to-systemic shunting
Hypoalbuminemia

[1]Modified and reproduced, with permission, from Epstein M: Functional renal abnormalities in cirrhosis: Pathophysiology and management. In: *Hepatology: A Textbook of Liver Disease,* 2nd ed. Zakim D, Boyer JD (editors). Saunders, 1990.

Acute hepatitis is usually caused by infection with one of several types of viruses. Although these viral agents can be distinguished by serologic laboratory tests based on their antigenic properties, all produce clinically similar illnesses. Other less common infectious agents can result in liver injury (Table 10–1). Hepatitis is also sometimes caused by exposure to drugs or noxious insults (eg, isoniazid, ethanol).

Clinical Presentation

The severity of illness in acute hepatitis ranges from asymptomatic and clinically inapparent to fulminant and fatal acute infections and from subclinical and persistent to rapidly progressive chronic liver disease culminating in cirrhosis and even hepatocellular carcinoma (see Figure 10–8).

The presentation of acute hepatitis can be quite variable. Some patients are relatively asymptomatic, with abnormalities noted only by laboratory studies. Others may have a range of symptoms and signs, including anorexia, weight loss, nausea, vomiting, right upper quadrant abdominal pain, jaundice, fever, splenomegaly, and ascites. The extent of hepatic dysfunction can also vary tremendously, correlating roughly with the severity of liver injury. The relative extent of cholestasis versus hepatocyte necrosis is also highly variable.

Etiology

A. Viral Hepatitis: Acute hepatitis is commonly caused by one of five major viruses (Table 10–7): hepatitis A virus (HAV) (formerly: infectious or short-incubation hepatitis); hepatitis B virus (HBV) (formerly: serum or long-incubation hepatitis); hepatitis C virus (HCV) (one form of the illness formerly called non-A, non-B hepatitis, or posttransfusion hepatitis); hepatitis D virus (HDV) (also called HBV-associated delta agent); and hepatitis E virus (HEV) (another form of non-A, non-B hepatitis causing epidemic hepatitis in Third World countries).

Table 10–7 summarizes important characteristics of these viral agents. Other viral agents that can cause acute hepatitis, though less commonly, include the Epstein-Barr virus (cause of infectious mononucleosis), cytomegalovirus (CMV), herpes simplex virus (HSV), rubella virus, and yellow fever virus.

Hepatitis A virus—a small RNA virus—causes liver disease both by direct killing of hepatocytes and by the host's immune response to infected hepatocytes. It is spread by the fecal-oral route from infected individuals. While most cases are mild, hepatitis A can occasionally present with fulminant liver failure and massive hepatocellular necrosis resulting in death. Regardless of the severity, patients who recover do so completely, show no evidence of residual liver disease, and have antibodies that protect them from reinfection.

Hepatitis B virus is a DNA virus that is transmitted by sexual and other intimate contact or by contact with infected blood. This virus does not kill the cells it infects. Rather, the infected hepatocytes die almost

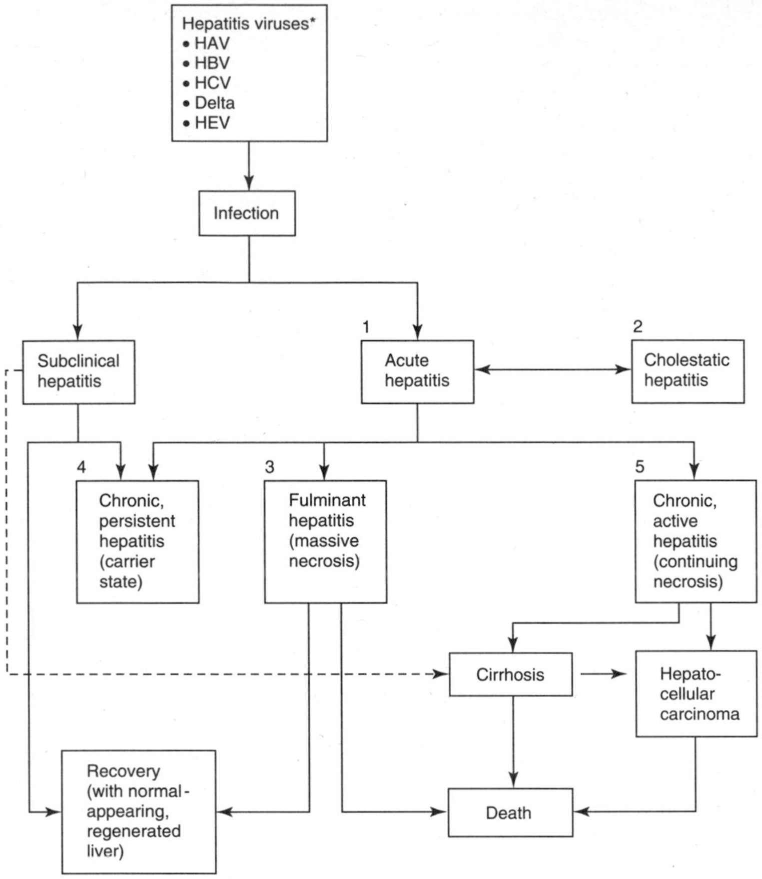

Figure 10–8. Clinical syndromes associated with viral hepatitis. The commonest clinical syndrome is acute hepatitis **(1)**, which is sometimes associated with intrahepatic cholestasis **(2)**. Fulminant hepatitis **(3)** is associated with massive necrosis and is associated with a high mortality rate. Chronic viral hepatitis may be persistent **(4)** or active **(5)**. Chronic active hepatitis commonly progresses to cirrhosis of the liver. (Reproduced, with permission, from Chandrasoma P, Taylor CE: *Concise Pathology,* 2nd ed. Appleton & Lange, 1994.)

exclusively as a consequence of attack by the immune system after recognition of viral antigens on the hepatocyte surface. While most cases of hepatitis B infection are asymptomatic or produce only mild disease before clearance of the virus, an excessive immune response may produce fulminant hepatic failure. In even fewer patients—typically those with mild acute disease—the immune response is inadequate to clear the virus completely, and chronic hepatitis develops.

Hepatitis C virus, once known as non-A, non-B hepatitis virus, causes a form of hepatitis similar to HBV infection but with a greater proportion of cases progressing to chronic active hepatitis.

Hepatitis D virus, also known as delta agent, is a defective RNA virus that requires helper functions of HBV to cause infection. Thus, individuals who are chronically infected with HBV are at high risk for HDV infection, while individuals who have been vaccinated against HBV are at no risk. HDV infection causes a much more severe form of hepatitis, both in terms of the proportion of fulminant cases and in the percentage of cases that progress to chronic hepatitis.

B. Toxic Hepatitis: Some of the various drugs, poisons, and toxins known to cause acute hepatitis and fulminant hepatitis are listed in Table 10–8. Toxic acute hepatitis can be further subdivided into those for which hepatic toxicity is predictable and dose-dependent for most individuals and those which cause unpredictable (idiosyncratic) reactions without relationship to dose. Table 10–9 summarizes speculation on the mechanisms of dose-related drug-induced hepatic disease. In contrast, idiosyncratic reactions to drugs may be due to genetic predisposition in susceptible individuals to certain pathways of drug metabolism that generate toxic intermediates.

The time course of acute hepatitis is highly variable. In hepatitis A, jaundice is typically seen 4–8 weeks after exposure, while in hepatitis B, jaundice occurs usually from weeks 8 to 20 after exposure (see Figure 10–9). Drug- and toxin-induced hepatitis

Table 10–7. Characteristics of various types of viral hepatitis.

	Hepatitis A	Hepatitis B	Hepatitis C	Hepatitis D	Hepatitis E
Clinical presentation					
Age group	Primarily young	All ages	All ages	All ages	Mostly adults
Onset	Abrupt	Insidious	Insidious	Insidious	Abrupt
Incubation period					
Range (days)	15–20	28–160	14–160		
Mean (days)	30	8	50		40
Symptoms					
Arthralgia, rash	Uncommon	Common	Uncommon	Uncommon	Common
Fever	Common	Uncommon	Uncommon	Common	Common
Nausea, vomiting	Common	Common	Common	Common	Common
Jaundice	Uncommon in children	More common in hepatitis A	Uncommon	Common	Common
Laboratory data					
Duration of liver enzyme elevation	Short	Prolonged	Like hepatitis B	Like hepatitis B	
Virus	RNA	DNA	?	RNA	?
Location of virus					
Blood	Transient	Prolonged	Prolonged	Prolonged	?Transient
Stool	Yes	No	No	No	Yes
Elsewhere	?	Yes	?	?	?
Outcome					
Severity of acute disease	Mild	Moderate	Mild	Moderate to severe	Severe
Mortality rate	Low (1%)	Low (1–3%)	Low (2%)	High (5%)	Moderate (+3%)
Chronic hepatitis	No	Yes	Yes	Yes	No
Chronic carrier	No	Yes	Yes	Yes	No
Liver carrier	No	Yes	Possible	?	No
Relapse	Yes	Yes	?	?	?
Transmission					
Oral	+	±	?No	?No	+
Percutaneous	Rare	+	+	+	−
Sexual	+	+	−	+	?
Perinatal	−	+	±	−	?

[1]Modified and reproduced, with permission, from Seeff LB: Diagnosis, therapy, and prognosis of viral hepatitis. In: *Hepatology: A Textbook of Liver Disease,* 2nd ed. Zakim D, Boyer JD (editors). Saunders, 1990.

typically occurs at any time during or shortly after exposure and resolves with discontinuance of the offending agent. This is usually the case for both idiosyncratic and dose-dependent reactions.

Acute hepatitis typically resolves in 3–6 months. Hepatic injury continuing for more than 6 months is arbitrarily defined as chronic hepatitis and suggests, in the absence of continued exposure to a noxious agent, that immune or other mechanisms are at work.

Pathogenesis

A. Viral Hepatitis: The viral agents responsible for acute hepatitis first infect the hepatocyte. During the incubation period, intense viral replication in the liver cell leads to the appearance of viral components (first antigens, later antibodies) in urine, stool, and body fluids. Liver cell necrosis and an associated inflammatory response then ensue, followed by changes in laboratory tests of liver function and the appearance of various symptoms and signs of liver disease.

1. Liver damage–The host's immunologic response plays an important though incompletely understood role in the pathogenesis of liver damage. In hepatitis B, for example, the virus is probably not directly cytopathic. (There are asymptomatic HBV carriers with normal liver function and histologic features.) Instead, the host's cellular immune response

Table 10–8. Drugs implicated in idiosyncratic liver injury leading to acute liver failure.[1]

Infrequent Causes	Rare Causes	Synergistic Causes[2]
Isoniazid	Carbamazepine	Alcohol and acetaminophen
Valproate	Ofloxacin	Trimethoprim and sulfamethoxazole
Halothane	Ketoconazole	Rifampin and isoniazid
Phenytoin	Lisinopril	Acetaminophen and isoniazid
Sulfonamides	Niacin	Amoxicillin and clavulanic acid
Propylthiouracil	Labetalol	
Amiodarone	Etoposide (VP-16)	
Disulfiram	Imipramine	
Dapsone	Interferon alfa	
	Flutamide	

[1]Reproduced, with permission, from Lee WM: Acute renal failure. N Engl J Med 1993;327:1862.
[2]These are commonly used combinations of drugs with apparent systemic toxicity.

has an important role in causing liver cell injury. Patients with defects in cell-mediated immunity are more likely to remain chronically infected with HBV than to clear the infection. Histologic specimens from patients with HBV-related liver injury demonstrate lymphocytes next to necrotic liver cells. It is thought that cytolytic T lymphocytes become sensitized to recognize hepatitis B viral antigens (eg, small quantities of HBsAg) and host antigens on the surfaces of HBV-infected liver cells.

2. Extrahepatic manifestations–Immune factors may also be important in the pathogenesis of the extrahepatic manifestations of acute viral hepatitis.

Table 10–9. Postulated mechanisms of drug-induced liver disease.[1]

Effect	Example
Alteration of the physical properties of membranes	Estrogens
Inhibition of membrane enzymes (eg, Na^+-K^+ ATPase)	Chlorpromazine metabolites
Interference with hepatic uptake processes	Rifampin
Impairment of cytoskeletal function	Chlorpromazine metabolites
Formation of insoluble complexes in bile	Chlorpromazine
Conversion to reactive intermediates Electrophils producing covalent modifications of tissue macromolecules	Acetaminophen
Free radicals producing lipid peroxidation	Carbon tetrachloride
Redox cycling with production of oxygen radicals	Nitrofurantoin

[1]Reproduced, with permission, from Bass NM, Ockner RK: Drug-induced liver disease. In: *Hepatology: A Textbook of Liver Disease,* 2nd ed. Zakim D, Boyer JD (editors). Saunders, 1990.

For example, in hepatitis B, a serum sickness-like prodrome characterized by fever, urticarial rash and angioedema, and arthralgias and arthritis appears to be related to immune complex-mediated tissue damage. During the early prodrome, circulating immune complexes are composed of HBsAg in high titer in association with small quantities of anti-HBs. These circulating immune complexes are deposited in blood vessel walls, leading to activation of the complement cascade. In patients with arthritis, serum complement levels are depressed, and complement can be detected in circulating immune complexes containing HbsAg, anti-HBs, IgG, IgM, IgA, and fibrin.

Finally, immune factors are thought to be important in the pathogenesis of some clinical manifestations in patients who become chronic HBsAg carriers following acute hepatitis. For example, in patients developing glomerulonephritis with nephrotic syndrome, histopathologic investigation demonstrates deposition of HBsAg, immunoglobulin, and complement in the glomerular basement membrane. In patients developing polyarteritis nodosa, similar deposits have been demonstrated in affected small- and medium-sized arteries.

B. Alcoholic Hepatitis: Ethanol has both direct and indirect toxic effects on the liver. Its direct effects relate to increasing the fluidity of membranes and thereby disrupting cellular functions. Its indirect effects on the liver are consequences of its metabolism. Ethanol is sequentially oxidized to acetaldehyde and then to acetate, with the generation of NADH and ATP. As a result of the high ratio of reduced to oxidized NAD that is generated, the pathways of fatty acid oxidation and gluconeogenesis are inhibited, while fatty acid synthesis is promoted. This and other biochemical mechanisms may explain the common observation of fat accumulation in the liver of alcoholics and the tendency to develop hypoglycemia in alcoholics whose liver glycogen has been depleted by fasting. Ethanol metabolism also affects the liver by generation of acetaldehyde, which

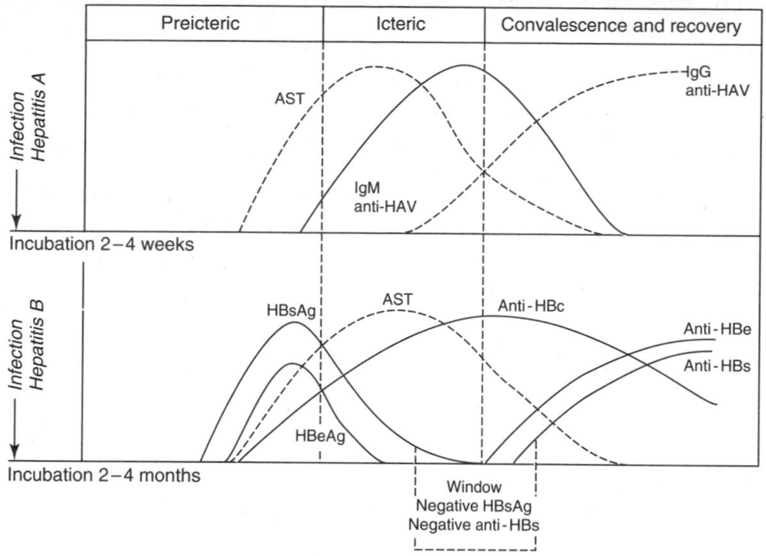

Figure 10–9. Serum antibody and antigen levels in hepatitis A and hepatitis B. (Reproduced, with permission, from Chandrasoma P, Taylor CE: *Concise Pathology,* 2nd ed. Appleton & Lange, 1994.)

reacts with primary amino groups to inactivate enzymes, resulting in direct toxicity to the hepatocyte in which it is generated.

There is considerable variation among individuals in the amount of ethanol required to cause acute liver injury. Whether nutritional, genetic, or other factors are responsible for these differences has not been determined. The mechanisms thought to be responsible for ethanol-induced liver injury are listed in Table 10–10.

Pathology

In uncomplicated acute hepatitis, the typical histologic findings consist of (1) focal liver cell degeneration and necrosis, with cell drop-out, ballooning, and acidophilic degeneration (shrunken cells with eosinophilic cytoplasm and pyknotic nuclei); (2) inflammation of portal areas, with infiltration by mononuclear cells (small lymphocytes, plasma cells, eosinophils); (3) prominence of Kupffer cells and bile ducts; and (4) cholestasis (arrested bile flow) with bile plugs. Characteristically, although the regular pattern of the cords of hepatocytes is disrupted, the reticulin framework is preserved.

Recovery from acute hepatitis is characterized histologically by regeneration of hepatocytes, with numerous mitotic figures and multinucleated cells, and by a largely complete restoration of normal lobular architecture.

Less commonly in acute hepatitis (1–5% of patients), there will be a more severe histologic lesion called **bridging hepatic necrosis** (also called subacute, submassive, or confluent necrosis). "Bridging" is said to occur between lobules because necrosis involves contiguous groups of hepatocytes, resulting in large areas of hepatic cell drop-out and collapse of the reticulin framework. Necrotic zones ("bridges") consisting of condensed reticulin, in-

Table 10–10. Mechanisms of hepatocyte injury by ethanol.[1]

I. Disorganizes the lipid portion of cell membranes, leading to adaptive changes in their composition:
- Increased fluidity and permeability of membranes
- Impaired assembly of glycoproteins into membranes
- Impaired secretion of glycoproteins
- Impaired binding and internalization of large ligands
- Formation of abnormal mitochondria
- Impairment of transport of small ligands
- Impairment of membrane-bound enzymes
- Adaptive changes in lipid composition, leading to increased lipid peroxidation
- Abnormal display of antigens on the plasma membrane

II. Alters the capacity of liver cells to cope with environmental toxins:
- Induces xenobiotic metabolizing enzymes
- Directly inhibits xenobiotic metabolizing enzymes
- Induces deficiency in mechanisms protecting against injury due to reactive metabolites
- Enhances the toxicity of O_2

III. Oxidation of ethanol produces acetaldehyde, a toxic and reactive intermediate:
- Inhibits export of proteins from the liver
- Modifies hepatic protein synthesis in fasted animals
- Alters the metabolism of cofactors essential for enzymatic activity—pyridoxine, folate, choline, zinc, vitamin E
- Alters the oxidation-reduction potential of the liver cells
- Induces malnutrition

[1]Reproduced, with permission, from Zakim D, Boyer TD, Montgomery C: Alcoholic liver disease. In: *Hepatology: A Textbook of Liver Disease,* 2nd ed. Zakim D, Boyer JD (editors). Saunders, 1990.

flammatory debris, and degenerating liver cells link adjacent portal or central areas, or they may involve entire lobules.

Rarely, in massive hepatic necrosis or fulminant hepatitis (< 1% of patients), the liver becomes small, shrunken, and soft (acute yellow atrophy). Histologic examination reveals massive hepatocyte necrosis and drop-out in most of the lobules, leading to extensive collapse and condensation of the reticulin framework and portal structures (bile ducts and vessels).

Clinical Manifestations

A. Viral Hepatitis: Acute viral hepatitis usually is manifested in three phases: the prodrome, the icteric phase, and the convalescent phase.

1. Prodrome–The prodrome is characterized by three sets of symptoms and signs: (1) nonspecific constitutional symptoms and signs: malaise, fatigue, and mild fever; (2) gastrointestinal symptoms and signs: anorexia, nausea, vomiting, altered senses of olfaction and taste (loss of taste for coffee or cigarettes), and right upper quadrant abdominal discomfort (reflecting the enlarged liver); and (3) extrahepatic symptoms and signs: headache, photophobia, cough, coryza, myalgias, urticarial skin rash, arthralgias or arthritis (10–15% of patients with HBV), and, rarely, hematuria and proteinuria.

2. Icteric phase–The constitutional symptoms usually improve, though mild weight loss may occur. Pruritus occurs if cholestasis is severe. Right upper quadrant abdominal pain as a result of the enlarged and tender liver, which was present in the prodromal phase, continues. Splenomegaly is noted in 10–20% of patients.

Jaundice may be observed as a yellowing of the scleras, skin, or mucous membranes. Jaundice is generally not appreciated on physical examination before the serum bilirubin rises above 2.5 mg/dL (41.75 μmol/L). **Direct hyperbilirubinemia** is elevation of the level of conjugated bilirubin in the bloodstream. Its occurrence indicates unimpaired ability of hepatocytes to conjugate bilirubin but a defect in the excretion of bilirubin into the bile as a result of intrahepatic cholestasis or posthepatic obstructive biliary tract disease, with overflow of conjugated bilirubin out of hepatocytes and into the bloodstream.

Changes in stool color (lightening) and urine color (darkening) often precede clinically evident jaundice. This reflects loss of bilirubin metabolites from the stool as a consequence of disrupted bile flow. Water-soluble (conjugated) bilirubin metabolites are excreted in the urine, while water-insoluble metabolites accumulate in tissues, giving rise to jaundice.

Ecchymoses suggest coagulopathy, which may be due to loss of vitamin K absorptive capacity (caused by cholestasis) or coagulation factor synthesis—or, rarely, loss of clearance of activated clotting factors, triggering the syndrome of disseminated intravascular coagulation. Coagulopathy in which the prothrombin time can be corrected by vitamin K injections but not by oral vitamin K suggests cholestatic disease, since vitamin K uptake from the gut is dependent on bile flow and enterohepatic circulation. If the prothrombin time cannot be corrected with either oral or parenteral vitamin K, inability to synthesize clotting factor polypeptides (eg, due to massive hepatocellular dysfunction) should be suspected. Correction of prothrombin time with oral vitamin K alone suggests a nutritional deficiency rather than liver disease as the basis for the coagulopathy.

Tests for serum levels of various enzymes normally localized primarily within hepatocytes provide an indication of the extent of liver cell necrosis. Misnamed "liver function tests," these enzyme assays include aspartate aminotransferase (AST), alanine aminotransferase (ALT), and alkaline phosphatase. For unclear reasons, perhaps somehow related to liver cell polarity, certain forms of liver disease typically result in disproportionate elevations in some parameters. Thus, in alcoholic hepatitis but not in viral hepatitis, AST is often disproportionately elevated relative to ALT (AST:ALT ratio > 2.0). Likewise, in cholestasis, alkaline phosphatase is disproportionately elevated relative to AST or ALT.

Measurement of antigen and antibody titers is a convenient way to assess whether an episode of acute hepatitis is due to viral infection. Moreover, since IgM antibodies are produced early after exposure to antigens (ie, soon after onset of illness), the presence of IgM antibodies to either HAV or to core antigen of HBV (HBcAg) is strong evidence that an episode of acute hepatitis is due to the corresponding viral infection. Several months after onset of illness, IgM antibody titers wane and are replaced by antibodies of the IgG class, indicating immunity to recurrence of infection by the same virus. Moreover, since the presence of surface antigen of hepatitis B virus (HBsAg) correlates well with infectivity and infectivity correlates inversely with the titer of antibody to surface antigen, such serologic studies help determine whether a patient with acute hepatitis is infectious to others (Table 10–11).

Subtle or profound mental status changes are seen in fulminant hepatic necrosis. Encephalopathy is believed to be related to failure of detoxification of ammonia (which normally occurs through the urea cycle). Other products such as γ-aminobutyric acid (GABA) may not be metabolized. Although ammonia is a demonstrable neurotoxin, it remains unclear whether it is the major agent of central nervous system dysfunction and whether elevated blood levels of other compounds such as GABA may act synergistically to alter mental status because of its role as a major inhibitory neurotransmitter.

In addition to encephalopathic changes due to accumulation of toxins, acute hepatic failure is associated with encephalopathy due to cerebral edema

Table 10–11. Commonly encountered serologic patterns in hepatitis B infection.

HBsAg	Anti-HBs	Anti-HBc	HBeAg	Anti-HBe	Interpretation
+	–	IgM	+	–	Acute HBV infection, high infectivity
+	–	IgG	+	–	Chronic HBV infection, high infectivity
+	–	IgG	–	+	Late acute or chronic HBV infection, low infectivity
+	+	+	+/–	+/–	1. HBsAg of one subtype and heterotypic anti-HBs (common) 2. Process of seroconversion from HBsAg to anti-HBs (rare)
–	–	IgM	+/–	+/–	1. Acute HBV infection 2. Anti-HBc window
–	–	IgG	–	+/–	1. Low-level HBsAg carrier 2. Remote past infection
–	+	IgG	–	+/–	Recovery from HBV infection
–	+	–	–	–	1. Immunization with HBsAg (after vaccination) 2. Remote past infection (?) 3. False-positive

[1]Reproduced, with permission, from Dienstag DL, Wards JR, Isselbacher KJ: Acute hepatitis. In: *Harrison's Principles of Internal Medicine.* Wilson JD et al (editors). McGraw-Hill, 1991.

caused by increased intracranial pressure, perhaps related to alterations in the blood-brain barrier.

Renal dysfunction may complicate fulminant hepatitis. Affected patients may develop prerenal azotemia when the glomerular filtration rate falls secondary to intravascular volume depletion. A state of intravascular volume depletion can be induced by the combination of decreased oral intake, vomiting, and formation of ascites. If uncorrected, this process can lead to acute tubular necrosis and acute renal failure.

3. Convalescent phase–The convalescent phase is characterized by complete disappearance of constitutional symptoms but persistent abnormalities in liver function tests. Symptoms and signs gradually improve.

22. Describe the range of clinical presentations of acute hepatitis.
23. Which viruses can cause hepatitis?
24. What are some extrahepatic manifestations of viral hepatitis?
25. What is the basis for the extrahepatic manifestations of viral hepatitis?

CHRONIC HEPATITIS

Chronic hepatitis is a category of disorders characterized by the combination of liver cell necrosis and inflammation of varying severity persisting for more than 6 months. It may be due to viral infection, drugs and toxins, genetic and metabolic factors, or unknown causes. The severity ranges from an asymptomatic stable illness characterized only by laboratory test abnormalities to a severe, gradually progressive illness culminating in cirrhosis, liver failure, and death. Based on clinical, laboratory, and biopsy findings, chronic hepatitis is often divided into two classes: chronic persistent and chronic active hepatitis. **Chronic persistent hepatitis** is seldom progressive despite persistent biochemical abnormalities reflecting ongoing liver cell necrosis. The clinical course is relatively benign, often characterized by spontaneous resolution (eg, clearance of persistent viral infection). **Chronic active (aggressive) hepatitis** is typically progressive, often resulting ultimately in cirrhosis and its complications or liver failure and death. The characteristics of the two types are summarized in Table 10–12.

Clinical Presentation

Patients may present with fatigue, malaise, low-grade fever, anorexia, weight loss, mild intermittent jaundice, and mild hepatosplenomegaly. Others are initially asymptomatic and present late in the course of the disease with complications of cirrhosis, including variceal bleeding, coagulopathy, encephalopathy, jaundice, and ascites. In contrast to chronic persistent hepatitis, some patients with chronic active hepatitis—particularly those without serologic evidence of antecedent HBV infection—present with extrahepatic symptoms such as skin rash, diarrhea, or arthritis (Table 10–13).

Etiology

Either type of chronic hepatitis can be caused by infection with several hepatitis viruses (eg, hepatitis B with or without hepatitis D superinfection and hepatitis C); a variety of drugs and poisons (eg, ethanol, isoniazid, acetaminophen), often in amounts insufficient to cause symptomatic acute hepatitis; genetic and metabolic disorders (eg, α_1-antiprotease (α_1-antitrypsin) deficiency, Wilson's disease, and hemochromatosis); or immune-mediated injury of

Table 10–12. Chronic persistent and chronic active hepatitis.[1]

	Chronic Persistent Hepatitis	Chronic Active Hepatitis
Clinical features		
Onset like that of acute hepatitis	≈70%	≈30%
Recurrent acute episodes	Infrequent	Common
Extrahepatic involvement	Rare	Common
Prognosis	Good	Variable; typically poor
Liver histology		
Piecemeal necrosis	Inconstant	Typical
Site of inflammation	Portal	Portal, extending into lobule
Lobular architecture	Preserved	Distorted
Fibrosis	Slight	Common
Progression to cirrhosis	Rare	Common

[1]Reproduced, with permission, from Ward JR, Isselbacher KJ: Chronic hepatitis. In: *Harrison's Principles of Internal Medicine,* 12th ed. Wilson JD et al (editors). McGraw-Hill, 1991.

unknown origin. Table 10–1 summarizes known causes of chronic hepatitis. A specific cause can be determined for only 10–20% of patients. Up to 10% of otherwise healthy individuals with acute hepatitis B remain chronically infected with HBV; of these patients, about two-thirds develop chronic persistent disease and one-third develop chronic active disease. Superinfection with HDV of a patient with chronic HBV infection is associated with a much higher rate of development of chronic active hepatitis than is seen with isolated hepatitis B infection. Hepatitis D superinfection of patients with hepatitis B is also associated with a high incidence of fulminant hepatic failure. Finally, about 50% of individuals with acute posttransfusional or community-acquired hepatitis C develop chronic hepatitis.

Pathogenesis

Many cases of chronic hepatitis are thought to represent an immune-mediated attack on the liver occurring as a result of persistence of certain hepatitis viruses or after prolonged exposure to certain drugs or noxious substances (Table 10–14); in some, no mechanism has been recognized. Evidence that the disorder is immune-mediated is that liver biopsies reveal inflammation (infiltration of lymphocytes) in characteristic regions of the liver architecture (eg, portal versus lobular) (Table 10–12). Furthermore, a variety of autoimmune disorders occur with high frequency in patients with chronic hepatitis (Table 10–13).

A. Postviral Chronic Hepatitis: In approximately 2–10% of cases of HBV infection, the im-

Table 10–13. Autoimmune disorders and extrahepatic manifestations associated with chronic active hepatitis.[1]

Thyroiditis
Thyrotoxicosis (rare)
Hypothyroidism
Autoimmune hemolytic anemia
Polyarthritis
Capillaritis
Glomerulonephritis
Pulmonary disorders
  Fibrosing alveolitis
  Primary pulmonary hypertension
Amenorrhea and other menstrual abnormalities
Ulcerative colitis
Monoclonal gammopathy
Hyperviscosity syndrome
Lichen planus
Polymyositis
Uveitis

[1]Reproduced, with permission, from Maddrey WC: Chronic hepatitis. In: *Hepatology: A Textbook of Liver Disease,* 2nd ed. Zakim D, Boyer JD (editors). Saunders, 1990.

Table 10–14. Drugs implicated in the etiology of chronic hepatitis.[1]

Drug	Use
Acetaminophen	Analgesic
Amiodarone	Antiarrhythmic
Aspirin	Analgesic
Ethanol	Abuse
Isoniazid	Antituberculous therapy
Methyldopa	Antihypertensive
Nitrofurantoin	Antibiotic
Propylthiouracil	Antithyroid therapy
Sulfonamides	Antibiotic

[1]Modified and reproduced, with permission, from Bass NM, Ockner RK: Drug-induced liver disease. In: *Hepatology: A Textbook of Liver Disease,* 2nd ed. Zakim D, Boyer JD (editors). Saunders, 1990.

mune response is inadequate to clear the liver of virus, resulting in persistent infection. The individual becomes a chronic carrier, intermittently producing the virus and hence remaining infectious to others. Biochemically, these patients are often found to have viral DNA integrated into their genomes in a manner that results in abnormal expression of certain viral proteins with or without production of intact virus. Viral antigens expressed on the hepatocyte cell surface are associated with class I HLA determinants, thus eliciting lymphocyte cytotoxicity and resulting in hepatitis. The severity of chronic active hepatitis is largely dependent on the activity of viral replication and the response by the host's immune system.

Independently of the risk of progression to cirrhosis, chronic hepatitis B infection predisposes the patient to the development of hepatocellular carcinoma. It remains unclear whether hepatitis B infection is the initiator or simply a promoter in the process of tumorigenesis.

B. Alcoholic Chronic Hepatitis: Chronic liver disease in response to some poisons or toxins may represent triggering of an underlying genetic predisposition to immune attack on the liver. In alcoholic hepatitis, however, repeated episodes of acute injury ultimately cause necrosis, fibrosis, and regeneration, leading eventually to cirrhosis (Figure 10–10). As in other forms of liver disease, there is considerable variation in the extent of symptoms prior to development of cirrhosis.

C. Idiopathic Chronic Hepatitis: Some patients develop chronic active hepatitis in the absence of evidence of preceding viral hepatitis or exposure to noxious agents (Figure 10–11). These patients typically have serologic evidence of disordered immunoregulation, manifested as hyperglobulinemia and circulating autoantibodies. Nearly 75% of these patients are women, and many have other autoimmune disorders. A genetic predisposition is strongly suggested. Patients with idiopathic autoimmune chronic active hepatitis show histologic improvement in liver biopsies after treatment with systemic corticosteroids. The clinical response, however, can be variable.

Pathology

Both forms of chronic hepatitis share the common histopathologic features of (1) inflammatory infiltra-

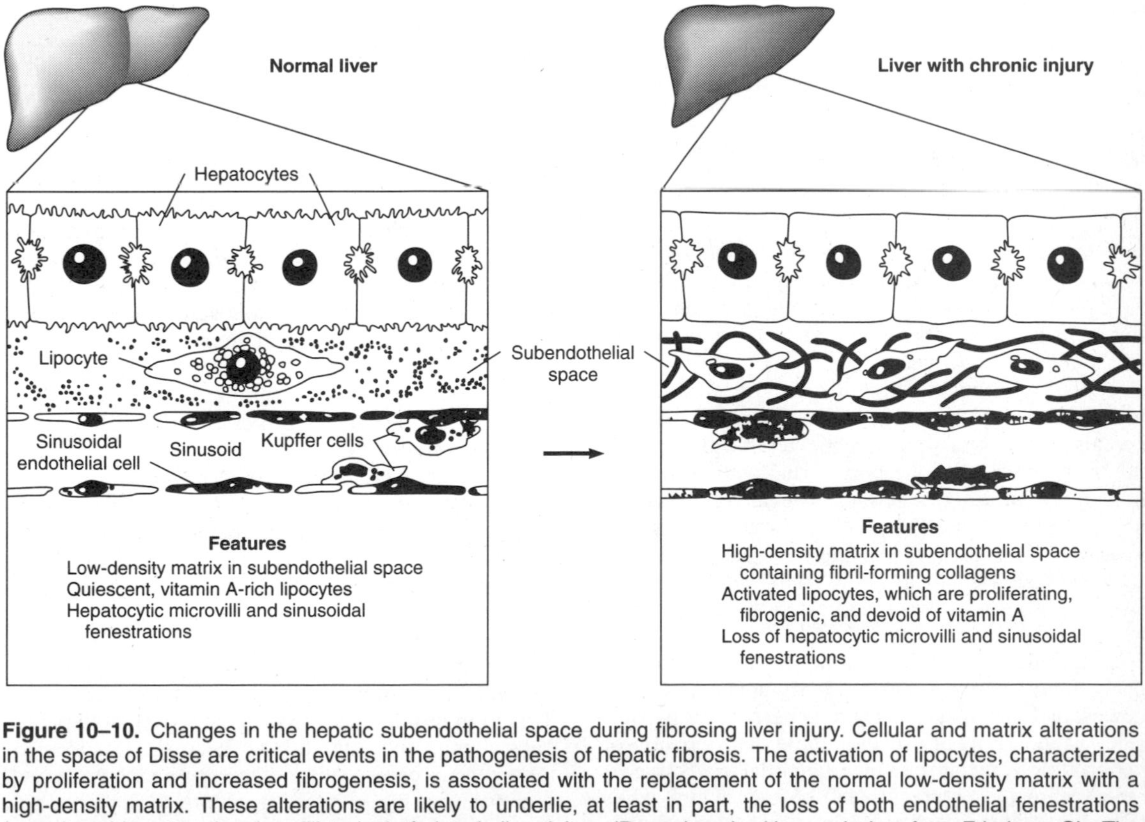

Figure 10–10. Changes in the hepatic subendothelial space during fibrosing liver injury. Cellular and matrix alterations in the space of Disse are critical events in the pathogenesis of hepatic fibrosis. The activation of lipocytes, characterized by proliferation and increased fibrogenesis, is associated with the replacement of the normal low-density matrix with a high-density matrix. These alterations are likely to underlie, at least in part, the loss of both endothelial fenestrations (pores) and hepatocytic microvilli typical of chronic liver injury. (Reproduced, with permission, from Friedman SL: The cellular basis of hepatic fibrosis. N Engl J Med 1993;328:1828.)

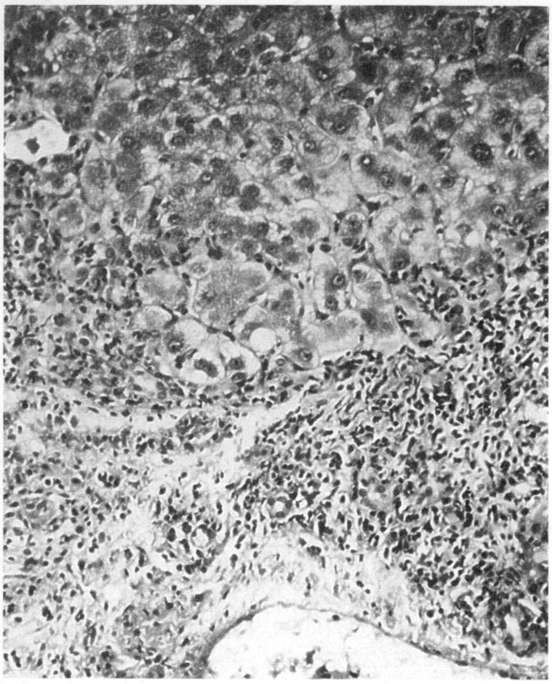

Figure 10–11. Chronic active hepatitis, showing marked lymphocytic infiltration and fibrosis of the portal areas. The lymphocytes extend into the peripheral part of the lobule through the limiting plate. There is ongoing necrosis of hepatocytes in the peripheral part of the lobule (piecemeal necrosis). (Reproduced, with permission, from Chandrasoma P, Taylor CE: *Concise Pathology*, 2nd ed. Appleton & Lange, 1994.)

tion of hepatic portal areas with mononuclear cells, especially lymphocytes and plasma cells; and (2) necrosis of hepatocytes within the parenchyma or immediately adjacent to portal areas (periportal hepatitis, or "piecemeal necrosis").

In chronic persistent hepatitis, the overall architecture of the liver is preserved. Histologically, the liver reveals a characteristic lymphocyte and plasma cell infiltrate confined to the portal triad without disruption of the limiting plate and no evidence of active hepatocyte necrosis. There is little or no fibrosis, and what there is is generally restricted to the portal area; there is no sign of cirrhosis. A "cobblestone" appearance of liver cells is seen, indicating regeneration of hepatocytes.

In chronic active hepatitis, the portal areas are expanded and densely infiltrated by lymphocytes, histiocytes, and plasma cells. There is necrosis of hepatocytes at the periphery of the lobule, with erosion of the limiting plate surrounding the portal triads (piecemeal necrosis; Figure 10–11). More severe cases also show evidence of necrosis and fibrosis between portal triads. There is disruption of normal liver architecture by bands of scar tissue and inflammatory cells that link portal areas to one another and to central areas (bridging necrosis). These connective tissue bridges are evidence of remodeling of hepatic architecture, a crucial step in the development of cirrhosis. Fibrosis may extend from the portal areas into the lobules, isolating hepatocytes into clusters and enveloping bile ducts. Regeneration of hepatocytes is seen with mitotic figures, multinucleated cells, rosette formation, and regenerative pseudolobules. Progression to cirrhosis is signaled by extensive fibrosis and regenerating nodules.

Clinical Manifestations

Some patients with chronic persistent hepatitis are entirely asymptomatic and identified only in the course of routine blood testing; others have an insidious onset of nonspecific symptoms such as anorexia, malaise, and fatigue or hepatic symptoms such as right upper quadrant abdominal discomfort or pain. Jaundice, if present, is usually mild. There may be mild tender hepatomegaly and occasional splenomegaly. Palmar erythema and spider telangiectases are seen in severe cases. Other extrahepatic manifestations are unusual. By definition, signs of cirrhosis and portal hypertension (such as ascites, collateral circulation, and encephalopathy) are absent. Laboratory studies show mild to moderate increases in serum aminotransferase, bilirubin, and globulin levels. Serum albumin and the prothrombin time are normal until late in the progression of liver disease.

The clinical manifestations of chronic hepatitis probably reflect the role of a systemic genetically controlled immune disorder in the pathogenesis of chronic active hepatitis. Acne, hirsutism, and amenorrhea may occur as a reflection of the hormonal effects of chronic liver disease. Laboratory studies in patients with chronic active hepatitis are invariably abnormal to various degrees. Moreover, these abnormalities do not correlate with clinical severity. Thus, the serum bilirubin, alkaline phosphatase, and globulin levels may be normal and aminotransferase levels only mildly elevated at the same time that a liver biopsy reveals severe chronic active hepatitis. However, an elevated prothrombin time usually reflects a severe liver disease.

The complications of chronic active hepatitis are those of progression to cirrhosis—variceal bleeding, encephalopathy, coagulopathy, hypersplenism, and ascites—and thus are largely due to portal-to-systemic shunting rather than diminished hepatocyte reserve (see below).

Patients with chronic liver disease can develop a poorly understood form of renal disease called **hepatorenal syndrome,** which has a dismal prognosis. This form of renal disease is distinct from both prerenal azotemia and acute tubular necrosis. It is characterized by progressively rising serum creatinine and diminished urine volume. It occurs typically in patients with massive tense ascites and is often precipitated by overly aggressive attempts at diuresis in hospital. The urine produced is notable for an extremely low sodium content and an absence of casts, resembling the findings in prerenal azotemia. Yet when central venous pressures are measured the patient does not show intravascular volume depletion, and the disorder does not respond to hydration with normal saline. The renal abnormalities of the hepatorenal syndrome appear to be functional, since no pathologic changes are identifiable in the kidney, and when this organ is transplanted from a patient dying of hepatorenal syndrome, it functions well in a recipient without liver disease. It remains to be determined whether this form of renal failure represents loss of an as yet unrecognized hormone produced by the liver that affects the kidneys or is the consequence of some combination of local hemodynamic effects resulting in diminished renal perfusion.

In recent years, the role of nitric oxide as an intracellular second messenger with vasodilatory effects on vascular beds and the role of endothelins, peptides synthesized by vascular endothelium which have vasoconstrictive properties, have been identified. A speculated role for nitric oxide-mediated peripheral arterial vasodilation combined with sympathetic nervous system and endothelin-mediated renal vasoconstriction has been proposed to explain the salt and water retention of cirrhosis. Those same mechanisms, in the extreme case, may give rise to the hepatorenal syndrome.

26. What are the categories of chronic hepatitis based on histologic findings on liver biopsy?
27. What are the causes of chronic hepatitis?
28. What are the consequences of chronic hepatitis?

CIRRHOSIS

Clinical Presentation

Cirrhosis is an irreversible distortion of normal liver architecture characterized by hepatic injury, fibrosis, and nodular regeneration. The clinical pre-

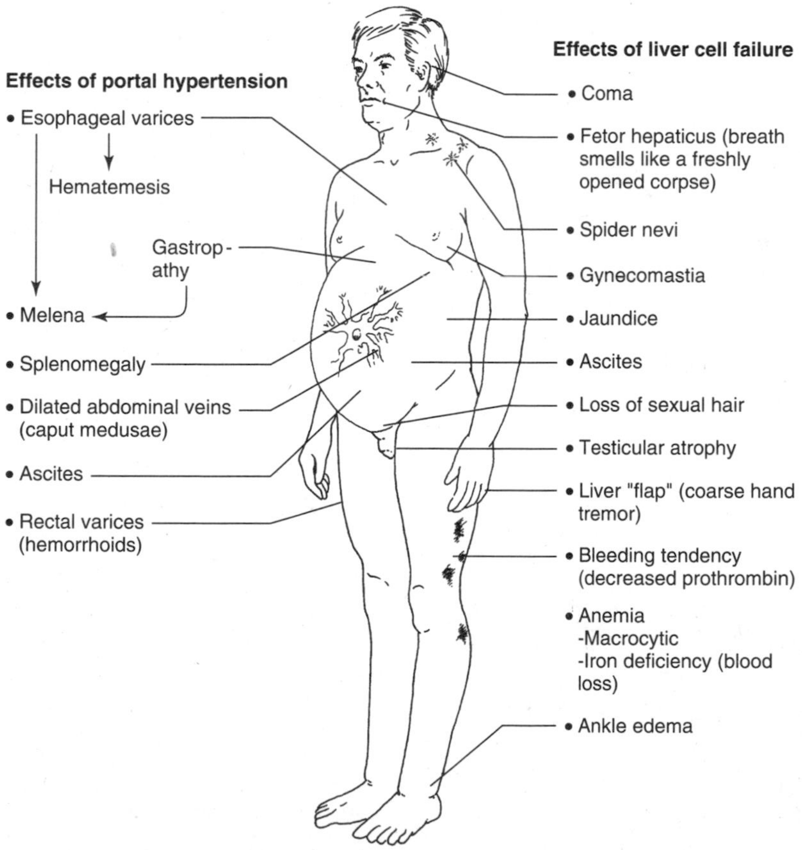

Figure 10–12. Clinical effects of cirrhosis of the liver. (Reproduced, with permission, from Chandrasoma P, Taylor CE: *Concise Pathology,* 2nd ed. Appleton & Lange, 1994.)

sentations of cirrhosis are a consequence of both progressive hepatocellular dysfunction and portal hypertension (Figure 10–12). As with other presentations of liver disease, not all patients with cirrhosis develop life-threatening complications. Indeed, in nearly 40% of cases, cirrhosis is diagnosed at autopsy in patients who did not manifest obvious signs of end-stage liver disease.

Etiology

The causes of cirrhosis are listed in Table 10–1. The initial injury can be due to a wide range of processes. A crucial feature is that the liver injury is not acute and self-limited but rather chronic and progressive. In the United States, alcohol abuse is the most common cause of cirrhosis. In other countries, infectious agents (particularly hepatitis B and hepatitis C) are common causes. Other causes include chronic biliary obstruction, metabolic disorders, chronic congestive heart failure, and primary (autoimmune) biliary cirrhosis.

Pathogenesis

Increased or altered synthesis of collagen and other connective tissue or basement membrane components of the extracellular matrix is implicated in the development of hepatic fibrosis and hence in the pathogenesis of cirrhosis. The role of the extracellular matrix in cellular function is an important area of research, and recent studies suggest that it is involved in modulating the activities of the cells with which it is in contact. Thus, fibrosis may affect not only the physics of blood flow through the liver but also the functions of the cells themselves.

Hepatic fibrosis appears to occur in three situations: (1) as an immune response, (2) as part of the process of wound healing, and (3) in response to agents that induce primary fibrogenesis. HBV and *Schistosoma* species are good examples of agents producing fibrosis on an immunologic basis. Agents such as carbon tetrachloride or hepatitis A that attack and kill hepatocytes directly are examples of agents producing fibrosis as part of wound healing. In both immune responses and wound healing, the fibrosis is triggered indirectly by the effects of cytokines released from invading inflammatory cells. Finally, certain agents such as ethanol and iron may cause primary fibrogenesis by directly increasing collagen gene transcription and thus increasing also the amount of connective tissue secreted by cells.

The actual culprit in all of these mechanisms of increased fibrogenesis may be the fat-storing cells of the hepatic reticuloendothelial system. In response to cytokines, they differentiate from quiescent cells in which vitamin A is stored into myofibroblasts, which lose their vitamin A storage capacity and become actively engaged in extracellular matrix production. It appears that hepatic fibrosis occurs in two stages. The first stage is characterized by a change in extracellular matrix composition from non-cross-linked, non-fibril-forming collagen to collagen that is more dense and subject to cross-link formation. At this stage, liver injury is still reversible. The second stage involves formation of subendothelial collagen cross-links, proliferation of myoepithelial cells, and distortion of hepatic architecture with the appearance of regenerating nodules. This second stage is irreversible. Alterations in the composition of extracellular matrix can mediate changes in cellular functions of hepatocytes and other cells such as lipocytes (Figure 10–10 and Figure 10–13). Thus, the change in collagen balance may play a crucial role in proceeding from reversible to irreversible forms of chronic liver injury by affecting hepatocyte function as well.

Regardless of the possible effects on hepatocyte function, the increased fibrosis markedly alters the nature of blood flow in the liver, resulting in important complications to be discussed below.

The manner in which alcohol causes chronic liver disease and cirrhosis is not well understood. However, chronic alcohol abuse is associated with impaired protein synthesis and secretion, mitochondrial injury, lipid peroxidation, formation of acetaldehyde and its interaction with cellular proteins and membrane lipids, cellular hypoxia, and both cell-mediated and antibody-mediated cytotoxicity. The relative importance of each of these factors in producing cell injury is unknown. Genetic, nutritional, and environmental factors (including simultaneous exposure to other hepatotoxins) also influences the development of liver disease in chronic alcoholics. Finally, acute liver injury (eg, from exposure to alcohol or other toxins) from which a person with a normal liver would fully recover may be sufficient to produce irreversible decompensation (eg, hepatorenal syndrome) in a patient with underlying hepatic cirrhosis.

Pathology

Grossly, the liver may be large or small, but it always has a firm consistency. Liver biopsy is the only method of definitively diagnosing cirrhosis.

Histologically, all forms of cirrhosis are characterized by three findings: (1) marked distortion of hepatic architecture; (2) scarring due to increased deposition of fibrous tissue and collagen; and (3) regenerative nodules surrounded by scar tissue. When the nodules are small (< 3 mm in size) and uniform, the process is termed **micronodular cirrhosis.** In **macronodular cirrhosis,** the nodules are over 3 mm and variable in size. Cirrhosis due to alcohol abuse is usually micronodular but can be macronodular or both micro- and macronodular. Scarring may be most severe in central regions, or dense bands of connective tissue may join portal and central areas.

More specific histopathologic findings may help to establish the cause of cirrhosis. For example, invasion and destruction of bile ducts by granulomas suggests primary (autoimmune) biliary cirrhosis; extensive iron deposition in hepatocytes and bile ducts suggests hemochromatosis; and alcoholic hyalin and infiltration with polymorphonuclear cells suggest alcoholic cirrhosis.

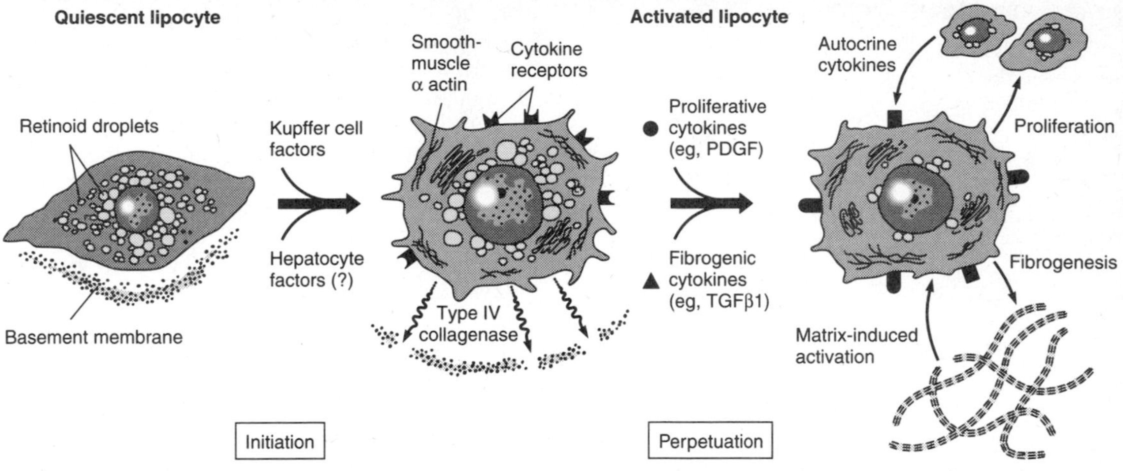

Figure 10–13. Model of lipocyte activation. Current evidence suggests that the process of lipocyte activation is a cascade occurring in at least two stages. Initiation is characterized by cellular enlargement, the expression of smooth muscle α actin, and the induction of cytokine receptors; initiating stimuli may include as yet uncharacterized paracrine factors from Kupffer cells, hepatocytes, or both. Initiation may also include the early disruption of the extracellular matrix through the secretion by lipocytes of type IV collagenase, leading to its eventual replacement with fibril-forming collagens. Perpetuation reflects the subsequent effects of proliferative and fibrogenic cytokines on the cells and the additional stimulation in response to the altered extracellular matrix. (PDGF, platelet-derived growth factor; TGFβ1, transforming growth factor β1.) (Reproduced, with permission, from Friedman SL: The cellular basis of hepatic fibrosis. N Engl J Med 1993;328:1828.)

Clinical Manifestations

The clinical manifestations of progressive hepatocellular dysfunction in cirrhosis are similar to those of acute or chronic hepatitis and include constitutional symptoms and signs: fatigue, loss of vigor, and weight loss; gastrointestinal symptoms and signs: nausea, vomiting, jaundice, and tender hepatomegaly; and extrahepatic symptoms and signs: palmar erythema, spider angiomas, muscle wasting, parotid and lacrimal gland enlargement, gynecomastia and testicular atrophy in men, menstrual irregularities in women, and coagulopathy.

Clinical manifestations of portal hypertension include ascites, portosystemic shunting, encephalopathy, splenomegaly, and esophageal and gastric varices with intermittent hemorrhage (see Table 10–15).

A. Portal Hypertension: Portal hypertension is a rise in intrahepatic vascular resistance. The cirrhotic liver loses the physiologic characteristic of a low-pressure circuit for blood flow seen in the normal liver. The increased blood pressure within the sinusoids is transmitted back to the portal vein. Because the portal vein lacks valves, this elevated pressure is transmitted back to other vascular beds, resulting in splenomegaly, portal-to-systemic shunting, and many of the complications of cirrhosis discussed below.

B. Ascites: Ascites is the presence of excess fluid in the peritoneal cavity. Patients with ascites develop physical examination findings of increasing abdominal girth, a fluid wave, a ballotable liver, and shifting dullness.

The pathogenesis of ascites is complex (Figure 10–14). In brief, the elevated pressure within the sinusoids increases the volume of flow into the lymphatic vessels at the expense of flow into the central vein, both of which drain the space of Disse. Eventually, flow into the hepatic lymphatics exceeds

Table 10–15. Complications of cirrhosis.

Due to portal hypertension with portal-to-systemic shunting
Ascites and increased risk of spontaneous bacterial peritonitis
Increased risk of sepsis
Increased risk of disseminated intravascular coagulation
Splenomegaly with thrombocytopenia
Encephalopathy
Varices
Drug sensitivity
Bile acid deficiency with malabsorption of fat and fat-soluble vitamins
Hyperestrogenemia
Hyperglycemia
Due to loss of hepatocytes
Hypoglycemia
Coagulopathy due to deficient clotting factor synthesis
Peripheral edema due to hypoalbuminemia
Hepatic coma
Other complications
Hepatorenal syndrome
Hepatocellular carcinoma

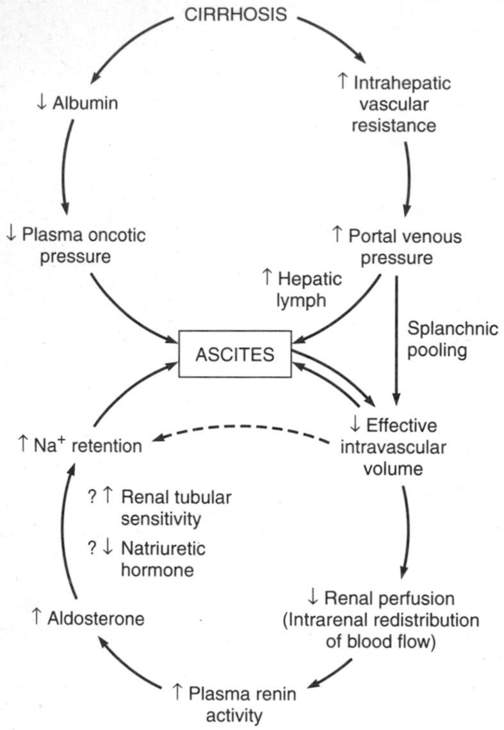

Figure 10–14. Multiple factors involved in development of ascites. Current concepts suggest that the initiating factor may be either primary sodium retention ("overflow"), diminished effective intravascular volume ("underfilling"), or arteriolar vasodilation. The decrease in effective intravascular volume is perhaps due to nitric oxide-mediated splanchnic arteriolar vasodilation. The decrease in renal perfusion is perhaps due to endothelin-mediated renal vasoconstriction. (Modified and reproduced, with permission, from Podolsky DK, Isselbacher KJ: Cirrhosis of the liver. In: *Harrison's Principles of Internal Medicine,* 12th ed. Wilson JD et al [editors]. McGraw-Hill, 1991.)

its capacity for drainage, resulting in overflow of lymphatic fluid into the peritoneal space. Additional factors contributing to the formation of ascites include decreased serum albumin and consequent loss of colloid osmotic pressure within the vascular space and increased retention of sodium and water by the kidney.

In cirrhotic patients with ascites, there is both increased formation and decreased reabsorption of hepatic and splanchnic lymph. In the intestine, increases in portal venous pressure lead to an increase in pressure within the splanchnic capillaries and an increase in fluid loss into the intestinal space. Because the splanchnic capillaries restrict the loss of protein into the interstitial space, however, an oncotic gradient develops between the capillary lumen and the interstitium. This gradient restores most of the excess interstitial fluid to the capillary lumen, the remainder being removed by the intestinal lymphatics. In the liver, however, the discontinuous endothelial lining of the sinusoids does not restrict the loss of protein to the interstitial space; there is little if any oncotic gradient between the sinusoid and the interstitium; and little of the excess fluid entering the interstitium returns to the vascular space. In cirrhosis, large amounts of fluid are lost into the interstitium, which must therefore be returned to the vascular space by the hepatic lymphatics. When the rate of fluid loss into the interstitium exceeds the rate of removal by the lymphatics, the fluid "weeps'' out of the hepatic lymphatics into the peritoneal cavity. Water and protein must then be reabsorbed by the lymphatics of the peritoneum. The maximum amount of ascitic fluid that can be reabsorbed ranges between 800 and 1000 mL/24 h and is influenced by the intra-abdominal pressure and the character of the peritoneum itself.

Retention of excess sodium by the kidney is important in the genesis of ascites. Factors important in the pathogenesis of this sodium retention include increased reabsorption of sodium by both proximal and distal tubules; increased sympathetic tone; reduced renal blood flow resulting from vasoconstriction, leading to increased plasma aldosterone levels; and alterations in the production of prostaglandins and kinins by the kidney. Sodium retention in cirrhosis is "paradoxical" because normally the kidneys retain sodium in the face of volume depletion. Historically, this paradox was explained by the "underfilling" and later the "overflow" hypotheses (see Figure 10–14). Subsequent evidence that intravascular volume is actually expanded in cirrhosis has led to the new view that arteriolar vasodilation triggers sodium retention in this setting. Nitric oxide produced by vascular endothelium may be the mediator of arteriolar vasodilation. Sodium retention may be further exacerbated by intrarenal endothelin-mediated vasoconstriction.

C. Hypoalbuminemia and Peripheral Edema: Progressive worsening of hepatocellular function in cirrhosis can result in a fall in the concentration of albumin and other serum proteins synthesized by the liver. As the concentration of these plasma proteins goes down, the plasma oncotic pressure is lowered, there-by tilting the balance of hemodynamic forces toward the development of both peripheral edema and ascites.

These hemodynamic changes further contribute to an avid sodium-retaining state despite total body water and sodium overload seen by urinalysis in the cirrhotic patient. Serum sodium may be low as a result of superimposed water retention due to antidiuretic hormone release triggered by volume stimuli. A low serum potassium and metabolic alkalosis may be observed as a consequence of elevated aldosterone levels responding to renin release (and angiotensin II release) by the kidneys, which sense afferent intravascular depletion.

D. Spontaneous Bacterial Peritonitis: Spontaneous bacterial peritonitis is the development of infected ascites in the absence of a clear event (such as bowel perforation) that would account for the entry of pathogenic organisms into the peritoneal space. Symptoms and signs include fever, hypotension, abdominal pain or tenderness, decreased or absent bowel sounds, or abrupt onset of hepatic encephalopathy in a patient with ascites.

Patients with large-volume ascites or with very low ascitic fluid protein levels are at increased risk for this complication. Ascitic fluid is an excellent culture medium for a variety of pathogens, including Enterobacteriaceae (chiefly *E coli*), group D streptococci (enterococci), *Streptococcus pneumoniae,* and viridans streptococci. The greater risk in patients with low ascitic fluid protein levels may be due to a low level of opsonic activity in the fluid.

The exact pathogenesis of spontaneous bacterial peritonitis is unknown. Peritonitis may occur because of bacterial seeding of the ascitic fluid via the blood or lymph or by bacteria traversing the gut wall. Enteric organisms may enter the portal venous blood via the portosystemic collaterals, bypassing the reticuloendothelial system of the liver.

E. Gastroesophageal Varices and Bleeding: As blood flow through the liver is progressively impeded, hepatic portal venous pressure rises. In response to the elevated portal venous pressure, there is enlargement of blood vessels that anastomose with the portal vein, such as those on the surface of the bowel and lower esophagus. These enlarged vessels are termed **varices.** Physical examination may reveal enlargement of hemorrhoidal and periumbilical vessels. Gastroesophageal varices are of more significance clinically, however, because of their tendency to rupture. The resulting massive bleeding is often life-threatening, since varices in these sites are not easy to tamponade. Gastrointestinal bleeding from varices and other sources (eg, duodenal ulcer, gastritis) in patients with cirrhosis is often exacerbated by concomitant coagulopathy (see below).

F. Hepatic Encephalopathy: Hepatic encephalopathy is manifested by waxing and waning alterations in mental status that occur as a consequence of advanced decompensated liver disease or portal-to-systemic shunting (see Table 10–16 for a list of common precipitants). Abnormalities range from subtle alterations in mental status to profound obtundation. Cognitive changes include a full spectrum of mental abnormalities, ranging from mild confusion, apathy, agitation, euphoria, restlessness, and reversal of the day-night sleep pattern to somnolence, marked confusion, and even coma. Motor changes range from fine tremor, slowed coordination, and asterixis to decerebrate posturing and flaccidity. **Asterixis** is a phenomenon of intermittent myoelectrical silence manifested by many muscle groups and enhanced by fatigue. It is best demonstrated by asking the patient to flex the wrists with fingers extended ("stop traffic") and then observing a flapping motion of the fingers.

Common precipitants of encephalopathy are onset of gastrointestinal bleeding, increased dietary protein intake, and an increased catabolic rate due to infection (including spontaneous bacterial peritonitis). Similarly, because of compromised "first-pass" clearance of ingested drugs, affected patients are exquisitely sensitive to sedatives and other drugs normally metabolized in the liver.

The pathogenesis of hepatic encephalopathy is poorly understood. One proposed mechanism postulates that the encephalopathy is caused by toxins such as ammonia, derived from metabolic degradation of urea or protein in the gut; glutamine, derived from degradation of ammonia; or mercaptans, derived from degradation of sulfur-containing compounds in the gut. Because of anatomic or functional shunts, these toxins bypass the liver's detoxification processes and produce alterations in mental status. Increased levels of ammonia, glutamine, and mercaptans can be found in the blood and cerebrospinal fluid. However, blood ammonia and spinal fluid glutamine levels correlate poorly with the presence and severity of encephalopathy.

Alternatively, there may be impairment of the normal blood-brain barrier, rendering the central nervous system susceptible to various noxious agents. Increased levels of other substances, including metabolic products such as short-chain fatty acids and endogenous benzodiazepine-like metabolites, have also been found in the blood. Cerebral edema, which is an important accompanying feature in patients with encephalopathy in acute liver disease, is not seen in cirrhotic patients with encephalopathy.

A third proposed mechanism postulates a role for GABA, the principal inhibitory neurotransmitter of the brain. GABA is produced in the gut, and in-

Table 10–16. Common precipitants of hepatic encephalopathy.[1]

Increased nitrogen load
Gastrointestinal bleeding
Excess dietary protein
Azotemia
Constipation
Electrolyte imbalance
Hypokalemia
Alkalosis
Hypoxia
Hypovolemia
Drugs
Opioids, tranquilizers, sedatives
Diuretics
Miscellaneous
Infection
Surgery
Superimposed acute liver disease
Progressive liver disease

[1]Reproduced, with permission, from Podolsky DK, Isselbacher KJ: Cirrhosis of the liver. In: *Harrison's Principles of Internal Medicine,* 12th ed. Wilson JD et al (editors). McGraw-Hill, 1991.

creased levels are found in the blood of patients with liver failure.

A fourth proposal postulates that there is an increased entry of aromatic amino acids into the central nervous system, resulting in increased synthesis of "false" neurotransmitters such as octopamine and decreased synthesis of normal neurotransmitters such as norepinephrine.

G. Coagulopathy: Factors contributing to coagulopathy in cirrhosis include loss of hepatic synthesis of clotting factors, some of which have a half-life of just a few hours. Under these circumstances, a minor or self-limited source of bleeding can become massive.

Hepatocytes are also functionally involved in maintenance of a normal coagulation cascade through the absorption of vitamin K (a fat-soluble vitamin whose absorption is dependent on bile flow), which is necessary for the activation of some clotting factors (II, VII, IX, X). An ominous sign of the severity of liver disease is the development of a coagulopathy that does not respond to parenteral vitamin K, suggesting deficient clotting factor synthesis rather than impaired absorption of vitamin K due to fat malabsorption. Finally, loss of the liver's capacity to remove activated clotting factors and fibrin degradation products may play a role in the increased susceptibility to **disseminated intravascular coagulation,** a syndrome of coagulation factor consumption that results in uncontrolled simultaneous clotting and bleeding.

H. Splenomegaly and Hypersplenism: Enlargement of the spleen is a consequence of elevated portal venous pressure and consequent engorgement of the organ. Thrombocytopenia and hemolytic anemia occur because of sequestering of formed elements of the blood in the spleen, from which they are normally cleared as they age and are damaged.

I. Hepatorenal Syndrome: This disorder is discussed in the section on clinical manifestations of chronic hepatitis.

J. Hepatocellular Carcinoma: Hepatocellular carcinoma occurs in up to 5% of cirrhotic patients. Several etiologic factors have been identified in the development of this tumor: (1) Malignant transformation is heightened in any form of chronic liver disease. (2) The risk of developing hepatocellular carcinoma is increased 100-fold in chronic HBV carriers. (3) Mycotoxins—metabolites of saprophytic fungi—are known hepatic carcinogens and have been proposed to act synergistically with cirrhosis and HBV infection in increasing the risk of liver cell cancer. (4) Hormonal factors have been implicated by experimental studies. The tumor is known to have a male predominance.

K. Miscellaneous Manifestations: Other findings on physical examination of patients with cirrhosis include **spider angiomas** (prominent blood vessels seen in the skin, particularly on the face and trunk), **Dupuytren's contractures** (fibrosis of the palmar fascia), testicular atrophy, **gynecomastia** (enlargement of breast tissue in men), palmar erythema, lacrimal and parotid gland enlargement, and diminished axillary and pubic hair (Figure 10–12). These findings are largely a consequence of estrogen excess due to decreased clearance of endogenous estrogens by the diseased liver combined with decreased hepatic synthesis of steroid hormone-binding globulin. Both of these mechanisms result in tissues receiving higher than normal concentrations of estrogens. In addition, a longer half-life of androgens may allow a greater degree of "peripheral aromatization" (conversion to estrogens by adipose tissue, hair follicles, etc), further increasing estrogen-like effects in patients with cirrhosis. Xanthomas of the eyelids and extensor surfaces of tendons of the wrists and ankles can occur with chronic cholestasis such as occurs in primary biliary cirrhosis. Finally, profound muscle wasting and cachexia in cirrhosis probably reflect diminution of the liver's synthesis of carbohydrate, lipid, and amino acids.

29. What are the defining features of cirrhosis?
30. What are the three categories of hepatic fibrosis? Name one agent causing each.
31. What are the two postulated stages in the development of cirrhosis?
32. What are some ways alcohol may injure the liver?
33. What are the major clinical manifestations of cirrhosis?
34. For each major clinical manifestation of cirrhosis, suggest a reasonable hypothesis to account for its pathogenesis.

REFERENCES

General

Arias I et al (editors): The Liver: *Biology and Pathobiology,* 2nd ed. Raven Press, 1988.

Friedman SL: Seminars in Medicine of the Beth Israel Hospital, Boston: The cellular basis of hepatic fibrosis: Mechanisms and treatment strategies. N Engl J Med 1993;328:1828.

Ganong WF: *Review of Medical Physiology,* 16th ed. Appleton & Lange, 1993.

Wilson J et al (editors): *Harrison's Principles of Internal Medicine,* 12th ed. McGraw-Hill, 1991.

Zakim D, Boyer T (editors): *Hepatology: A Textbook of Liver Disease,* 2nd ed. Saunders, 1990.

Acute Hepatitis

Achord JL: Review of alcoholic hepatitis and its treatment. Am J Gastroenterol 1993;88:1822.

Capocaccia L, Angelico M: Fulminant hepatic failure:

Clinical features, etiology, epidemiology, and current management. Dig Dis Sci 1991;36:775.

Dienstag JL (editor): Viral hepatitis. Semin Liver Dis 1991;11:73.

Kaplowitz N (editor): Recent advances in drug metabolism and hepatotoxicity. Semin Liver Dis 1990;10:235.

Lee WM: Acute liver failure. N Engl J Med 1993; 329:1802.

Lieber CS: Alcoholic liver disease approach. Semin Liver Dis 1993;13:105.

Chronic Hepatitis

Czaja AJ: Chronic active hepatitis: The challenge for a new nomenclature. Ann Intern Med 1993;119:510.

Maddrey WC: Chronic hepatitis. Dis Mon (Feb) 1993;39:53.

Cirrhosis

Forns X et al: Management of ascites and renal failure in cirrhosis. Semin Liver Dis 1994;14:82.

Grossman RJ, Grace ND (editors): Complications of portal hypertension: Esophagogastric varices and ascites. Gastroenterol Clin North Am 1992;21:1.

Runyon BA: Care of patients with ascites. N Engl J Med 1994;330:337.

Tsukuma H et al: Risk factors for hepatocellular carcinoma among patients with chronic liver disease. N Engl J Med 1993;328:1799.

11 Renal Disease

Vishwanath R. Lingappa, MD, PhD

Patients with renal disease who present early in the course of illness typically have abnormalities of urine volume or composition (eg, the presence of red blood cells or abnormal amounts of protein). Later, they manifest systemic signs and symptoms of lost renal function (eg, edema, fluid overload, electrolyte abnormalities). Depending on the nature of the renal disease, they may progress—rapidly or slowly—to display a wide range of chronic complications due to inadequate residual renal function.

Because there are no pain receptors within the substance of the kidney, pain is a prominent presenting complaint only in those renal diseases (eg, nephrolithiasis) in which there is impingement on the ureter or the renal capsule.

Because of the crucial role of the kidney in filtering blood, a wide range of systemic diseases and disease of other organ systems may be manifested most prominently in the kidney. Thus, renal disease is a prominent presentation of long-standing diabetes mellitus, hypertension, and autoimmune disorders such as systemic lupus erythematosus.

Without treatment, renal disease may result in loss of sufficient kidney function to be incompatible with life. However, not all renal disease pursues this inexorable course with its dismal outcome. The consequences of renal disease depend on the extent and nature of the injury and its natural history and time course. Some forms are transient. Even when severe, they may be self-limited and reversible and, if managed properly, may have no permanent ill consequences. Other forms progress eventually to renal failure, either rapidly or slowly, with a host of metabolic and hemodynamic consequences such as loss of renal filtration capacity (eg, disordered regulation of body electrolyte and volume status) as well as loss of nonexcretory renal functions such as the production of erythropoietin (resulting in anemia).

1. What are some important causes of renal disease?
2. What are some consequences of renal failure?

NORMAL STRUCTURE & FUNCTION OF THE KIDNEY

ANATOMY, HISTOLOGY, & CELL BIOLOGY

The kidneys are a pair of encapsulated organs located in the retroperitoneal area (Figure 11–1). A renal artery enters and a renal vein exits from each kidney at the hilum. Approximately 25% of cardiac output goes to the kidneys, where the blood is filtered to remove wastes—in particular urea and nitrogen-containing compounds—and to regulate extracellular electrolytes and intravascular volume. Because renal blood flow is from cortex to medulla and because there is a high rate of metabolic activity in the medulla, the normal oxygen tension in the medulla is lower than in other parts of the kidney. This makes the medulla particularly susceptible to ischemic injury.

The anatomic unit of kidney function is the **nephron,** a structure consisting of a tuft of capillaries termed the **glomerulus,** the site at which blood is filtered, and a **renal tubule** from which water and salts in the filtrate are reclaimed (Figure 11–2). Each kidney has approximately 1 million nephrons.

A glomerulus consists of an **afferent** and an **efferent arteriole** and an intervening tuft of capillaries lined by endothelial cells and covered by epithelial cells that form a continuous layer with those of **Bowman's capsule** and the renal tubule. The space between capillaries in the glomerulus comprises the **mesangium.** Material comprising a basement membrane is located between the capillary and the epithelial cells (Figure 11–2).

The renal tubule itself has a number of different structural regions: the **proximal convoluted tubule,** from which approximately 80% of the electrolytes and water are reclaimed; the **loop of Henle,** where concentration of the urine occurs; and a **distal convoluted tubule** and **collecting duct,** where additional electrolyte and water changes are made in response to hormonal control (Figure 11–3).

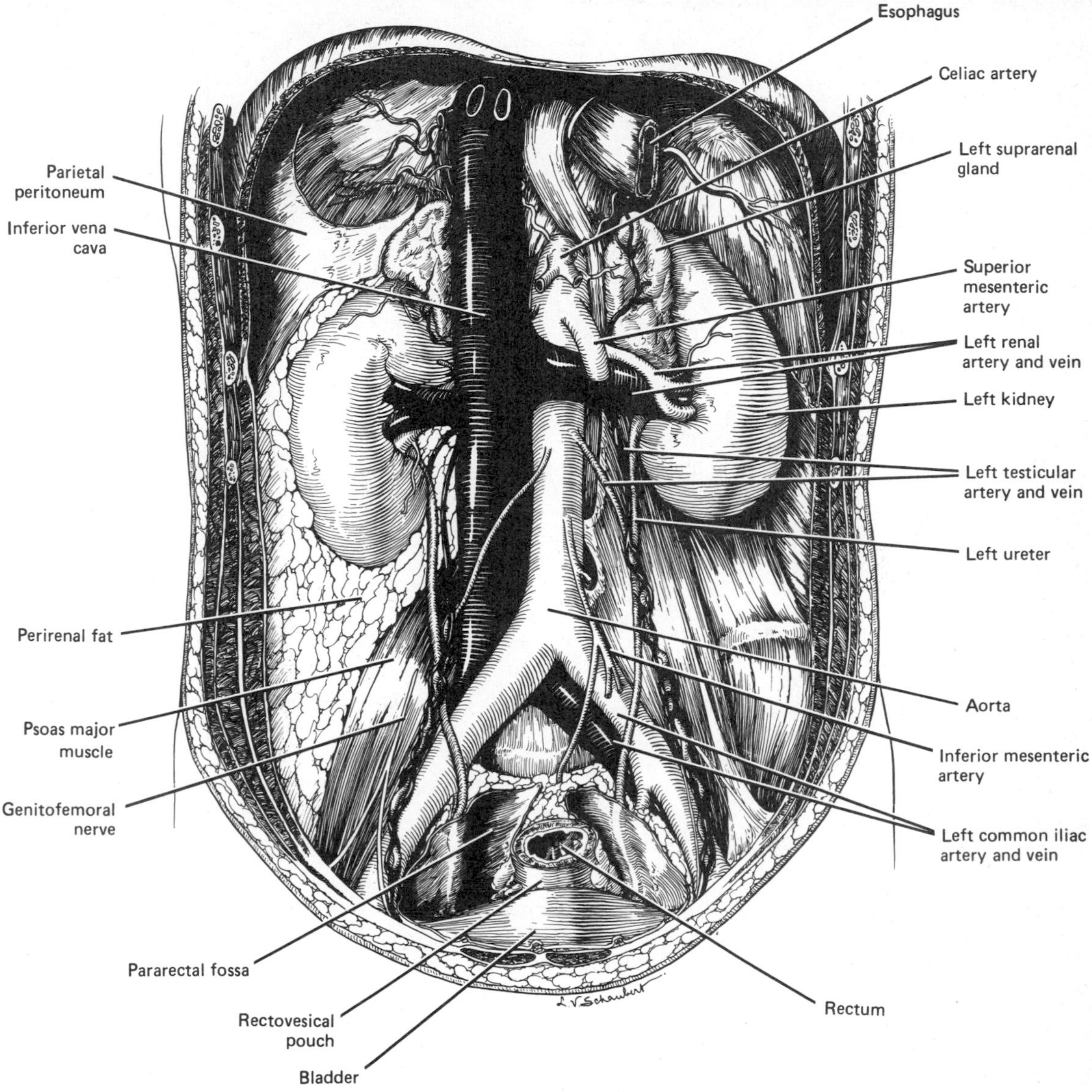

Figure 11–1. Vessels and organs of the peritoneum. (Reproduced, with permission, from Lindner HH: *Clinical Anatomy.* Appleton & Lange, 1989.)

PHYSIOLOGY

Glomerular Filtration & Tubular Resorption

Approximately 120 mL/min of glomerular filtrate are generated in a normal person with two fully functional kidneys. The size cutoff of substances for filtration is about 70 kilodaltons. However, substances smaller than this are often retained, either due to charge effects (eg, albumin) or because they are tightly bound to other proteins to give them a larger effective size (eg, various growth factors and nonprotein hormones).

After filtration at the glomerulus, most of the sodium and with it water—and, under normal conditions, almost all of the potassium and glucose—are actively resorbed from the tubular fluid in the proximal tubule. In addition to absorption, a number of substances are secreted into the tubular fluid through the action of transporters along the renal tubule.

Normally, about 30 mL/min of isotonic filtrate is delivered to the loop of Henle, where a countercurrent multiplier mechanism achieves concentration of

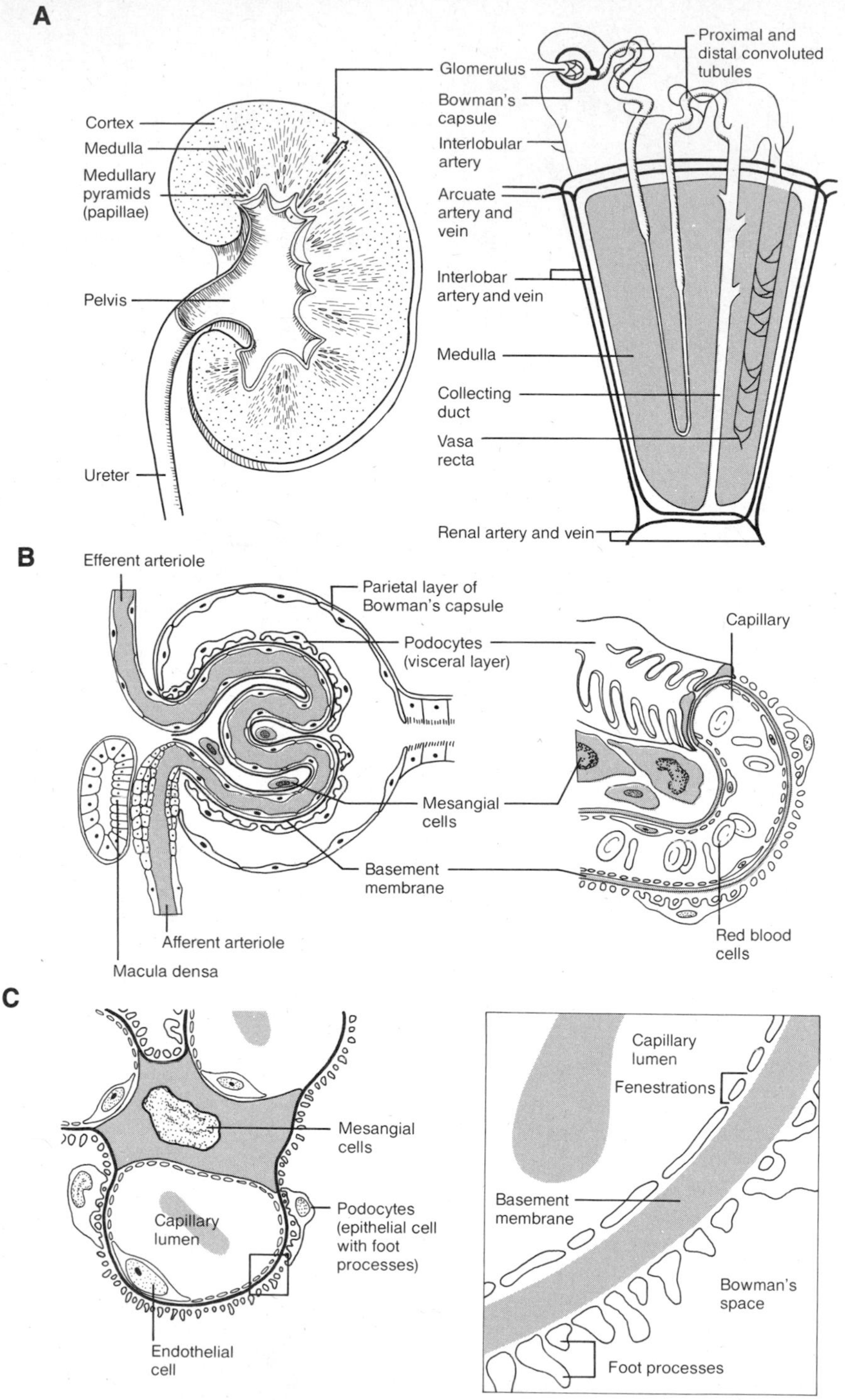

Figure 11–2. Structures of the kidney. **A:** Landmarks of the normal kidney. **B:** Glomerulus and glomerular capillary. **C:** Detailed structure of the glomerulus and the glomerular filtration membrane composed of endothelial cell, basement membrane, and podocyte. (Reproduced, with permission, from Chandrasoma P, Taylor CE: *Concise Pathology,* 2nd ed. Appleton & Lange, 1994.)

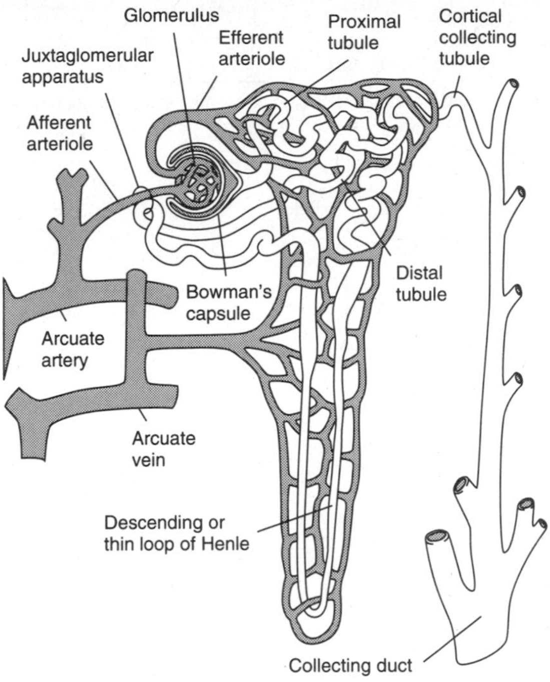

Figure 11–3. The vascular supply of a nephron in the outer part of the cortex. (Reproduced, with permission, from Guyton AC: *Textbook of Medical Physiology,* 8th ed. Saunders, 1991; and from Smith HW: *The Kidney: Structure and Functions in Health and Disease.* Oxford Univ Press, 1951.)

the urine. The loop of Henle passes down into the medulla of the kidney. There active secretion of sodium from the cells in the ascending limb establishes a hypertonic concentration gradient to resabsorb water and chloride from the tubular fluid across the cells of the descending limb.

Under normal circumstances, no more than about 5–10 mL/min are delivered to the collecting tubule. Water absorption in the collecting tubule occurs directly through water channels controlled by **vasopressin** (also known as **antidiuretic hormone [ADH]**). Under the control of aldosterone, sodium resorption from tubular fluid and potassium and hydrogen transport into tubular fluid occur in different types of cells in the renal collecting tubule. Phosphoric and sulfuric acid and other acids are not volatile and therefore cannot be excreted by the lungs. Instead, they must be excreted as salts by the kidney and are thus termed fixed acids. Urinary excretion of fixed acids also occurs at the collecting tubule. Even though it deals with less than a tenth of the total glomerular filtrate, the renal collecting tubule is the site of regulation of urine volume and the site at which water, sodium, acid-base, and potassium balance are achieved. The crucial role of the collecting tubule in regulation of kidney function depends on two features: First, the collecting tubule is under hormonal control—in contrast to the proximal tubule, whose actions are a simple function of volume and composition of tubular fluid and constitutively active transporters; and second, the collecting tubule is the last stop before approximately 1-2 mL/min of the original glomerular filtrate exits into the ureters as urine.

Insight into the functional roles of the proximal and distal renal tubules can be seen in the clinical features of the various forms of renal tubular acidosis (Table 11–1).

Renal Regulation of Blood Pressure

The kidney plays an important role in blood pressure regulation by virtue of its effect on sodium balance, a major determinant of blood pressure. First, the **macula densa** senses the sodium concentration in the proximal tubular fluid (Figure 11–2). Likewise, an associated structure, the **juxtaglomerular apparatus,** assesses the perfusion pressure, an important indicator of intravascular volume status under normal circumstances. Through the action of these two sensors, either low sodium or low perfusion pressure acts as a stimulus to renin release. **Renin,** a protease made in the juxtaglomerular cells, cleaves angiotensinogen in the blood to generate **angiotensin I,** which is then cleaved to **angiotensin II** by **angiotensin-converting enzyme.** Angiotensin II raises blood pressure by triggering vasoconstriction directly and by stimulating aldosterone secretion, resulting in sodium and water retention by the collecting tubule. All of these effects raise proximal tubular sodium concentration and renal perfusion pressure and thus alleviate the initial stimuli for renin release.

Intravascular volume depletion also triggers vasopressin release. Released from the posterior pituitary upon stimulation of receptors in the hypothalamus, vasopressin facilitates vesicular fusion at the collecting renal tubular apical membrane, thereby increasing the number of water channels resulting in reabsorption of free water. Further discussions of water balance and the role of vasopressin are presented in Chapter 18.

Renal Regulation of Calcium Metabolism

The kidney plays a number of important roles in calcium and phosphate homeostasis. First, the kidney is the site of 1α-hydroxylation or 24-hydroxylation of **vitamin D,** thereby activating or inactivating calcium uptake from the gut. Second, the kidney is a site of action of **parathyroid hormone,** resulting in calcium retention and phosphate wasting in the urine. These actions can be thought of as compensation for the fact that mobilization of calcium from bone results in a molar equivalent of phosphate mobilization. The action of the kidney in effect converts this dual effect on calcium and phosphate in bone into a concerted action on calcium balance.

Table 11–1. Characteristics of the different types of renal tubular acidosis.[1,2]

	Type 1 (Distal)	Type 2 (Proximal)	Type 4
Basic defect	Decreased distal acidification, eg, due to H^+-ATPase defect, reduced cortical Na^+ reabsorption, or increased membrane permeability.	Diminished proximal HCO_3^- reabsorption, eg, due to impaired Na^+-K^+ ATPase, Na^+-H^+ exchange, or carbonic anhydrase deficiency	Aldosterone deficiency or resistance
Urine pH during acidemia	>5.3	Variable: >5.3 if above reabsorptive threshold; <5.3 if below	Usually <5.3
Plasma $[HCO_3^-]$, untreated	May be below 10 meq/L	Usually 14–20 meq/L	Usually above 15 meq/L
Fractional excretion of HCO_3^- at normal plasma $[HCO_3^-]$	<3% in adults; may reach 5–10% in young children	>15–20%	<3%
Diagnosis	Response to $NaHCO_3$ or NH_4Cl	Response to $NaHCO_3$	Measure plasma aldosterone concentration
Plasma $[K^+]$	Usually reduced or normal; elevated with voltage defect	Normal or reduced	Elevated
Dose of HCO_3^- to normalize plasma $[HCO_3^-]$, meq/kg per day	1–2 in adults; 4–14 in children	10–15	1–3; may require no alkali if hyperkalemia corrected
Nonelectrolyte complications	Nephrocalcinosis and renal stones	Rickets or osteomalacia	None

[1]Reproduced, with permission, from Rose BD: *Clinical Physiology of Acid-Base and Electrolyte Disorders,* 3rd ed. McGraw-Hill, 1989.
[2]What was once called type 3 RTA is actually a variant of type 1.

Further discussion of the role of the kidney in calcium and phosphate homeostasis is presented in Chapter 17.

Renal Regulation of Erythropoiesis

The kidney is the site of production of the hormone **erythropoietin,** which stimulates bone marrow production and maturation of red blood cells. Thus, patients with end-stage renal disease typically display a profound anemia, with hematocrits in the range of 20–25%, which responds satisfactorily to recombinant erythropoietin injections and poorly to other therapies.

Regulation of Renal Function

There are a variety of physical, hormonal, and neural mechanisms by which the function of the kidney is controlled. The physics of the countercurrent multiplier in the loop of Henle and the hypertonic medullary interstitium allow "automatic" concentration of the urine under normal circumstances. This confers on the normal kidney the ability to maintain homeostasis under widely diverse conditions (by generating either a concentrated or dilute urine, depending on whether the body needs to excrete or conserve salt and water).

Adaptations of the kidney to injury can also be thought of as a form of regulation. Thus, loss of nephrons results in compensatory **glomerular hyperfiltration** and renal hypertrophy. While hyperfiltration may be adaptive for the moment, allowing maintenance of the glomerular filtration rate (GFR), it has been implicated as a common inciting event in further nephron destruction from a variety of causes, including diabetes mellitus. Once glomerular hyperfiltration occurs, an inexorable gradual progression to chronic renal failure is believed to begin.

There are other clinically important adaptations to injury. Poor renal perfusion from any cause results in attempts by the body to improve perfusion through afferent arteriolar vasodilation and efferent arteriolar vasoconstriction in response to hormonal and neural cues. These regulatory effects are reinforced by inputs sensing sodium balance. Alteration of sodium balance is another way to influence blood pressure and hence renal perfusion pressure. At least some cases of essential hypertension whose causes are poorly understood may be due to disordered tubuloglomerular feedback.

Sympathetic innervation by the renal nerves is another influence on renin release, and renal prostaglandins play an important role in vasodilation, especially in patients with chronic poor perfusion. Finally, the kidney is the source of various peptide hormones whose functions are poorly understood, such as the **endothelins,** powerful vasoconstrictors differentially synthesized by vascular endothelium and renal tubular cells in different regions of the nephron.

3. What are the parts of the nephron, and what role do they play in renal function?
4. How is renal function regulated?
5. What are the nonexcretory functions of the kidney?
6. What are the relationships, if any, between each nonexcretory function named above and the kidney's role in fluid, electrolyte, and blood pressure regulation?

OVERVIEW OF RENAL DISEASE

ALTERATIONS OF KIDNEY STRUCTURE & FUNCTION IN DISEASE

Renal disease can be categorized either by the site of the lesion (eg, glomerulopathy versus tubulointerstitial disease) or by the nature of the factors that have led to kidney disease (eg, immunologic, metabolic, infiltrative, infectious, hemodynamic, or toxic).

Certain regions of the kidney are particularly susceptible to certain kinds of injury: (1) The renal medulla is a low oxygen tension environment, which makes it more susceptible to ischemic injury. (2) The glomerulus is the initial filter of blood entering the kidney and thus is a prominent site of injury related to immune complex deposition and complement fixation. (3) Hemodynamic factors regulating blood flow have profound effects on the kidney both because the GFR, a primary determinant of renal function, depends on blood flow and because the kidney is susceptible to hypoxic injury.

One useful organizing scheme that combines a consideration of both the site and the cause of renal disease in approaching patients with new renal failure is to first categorize the cause of the patient's renal failure as prerenal, intrarenal, or postrenal and then to subdivide each of these categories according to specific causes and anatomic locations (Table 11–2).

Prerenal causes of renal failure are those resulting from inadequate blood flow to the kidney, whether due to intravascular volume depletion, structural lesions of the renal arteries, drug effects on renal blood flow, or hypotension from any cause resulting in renal hypoperfusion.

Intrarenal causes are those disorders that result in damage to the nephron directly rather than indirectly as a consequence of inadequate perfusion or obstruction. As mentioned earlier, intrarenal causes include specific disorders of the kidney as well as systemic diseases with prominent manifestations in the kidney. Some of these disorders are manifested as glomerular injury while others involve primarily the tubules. Within each category, disorders can be approached according to their specific cause or their phenotype and manifestations.

Table 11–2. Major causes of kidney disease.[1]

- **Prerenal disease**
  - True volume depletion
    - Gastrointestinal, renal, or sweat losses or bleeding
  - Heart failure
  - Hepatic cirrhosis (including the hepatorenal syndrome)
  - Nephrotic syndrome (particularly after diuretic therapy for edema)
  - Hypotension
  - Nonsteroidal anti-inflammatory drugs
  - Bilateral renal artery stenosis (particularly after therapy with an angiotensin-converting enzyme inhibitor)
- **Intrarenal disease**
  - Vascular disease
    - Acute
      - Vasculitis
      - Malignant hypertension
      - Scleroderma
      - Thromboembolic disease
    - Chronic
      - Nephrosclerosis
  - Glomerular disease
    - Glomerulonephritis
    - Nephrotic syndrome
  - Tubular disease
    - Acute
      - Acute tubular necrosis
      - Multiple myeloma
      - Hypercalcemia
      - Uric acid nephropathy
    - Chronic
      - Polycystic kidney disease
      - Medullary sponge kidney
  - Interstitial disease
    - Acute
      - Pyelonephritis
      - Interstitial nephritis (usually drug-induced)
    - Chronic
      - Pyelonephritis (due primarily to vesicoureteral reflux)
      - Analgesic abuse
- **Postrenal disease**
  - Obstructive uropathy
  - Prostatic disease
  - Malignancy
  - Calculi
  - Congenital abnormalities

[1]Reproduced, with permission, from Rose BD: Diagnostic approach to patient with renal disease. In: *Pathophysiology of Renal Disease,* 2nd ed. McGraw-Hill, 1987.

Postrenal causes are those related to urinary tract obstruction, either due to kidney stones, structural lesions (eg, tumors, prostatic hypertrophy, or strictures) or functional abnormalities (eg, spasm or drug effects).

MANIFESTATIONS OF ALTERED KIDNEY FUNCTION

The major manifestations of altered kidney function are the effects on excretion of urea and on maintenance of sodium, potassium, water, and acid-base balance. Failure to excrete urea adequately, manifested as progressive elevation of BUN and serum creatinine, results in uremia (see Chronic Renal

Failure, below). In the absence of adequate renal clearance mechanisms, ingestion of excess amounts of sodium, potassium, water, or acids results in electrolyte, volume and acid-base abnormalities that can be life-threatening. Furthermore, excess sodium ingestion in a patient with renal failure results in intravascular volume expansion, with complications of hypertension, congestive heart failure, and peripheral edema.

7. What characteristics of various parts of the nephron make it particularly susceptible to certain types of injury?
8. What are the features that distinguish prerenal, intrarenal, and postrenal causes of renal failure?
9. What are the major categories of complications of inadequate renal function?

PATHOPHYSIOLOGY OF SELECTED RENAL DISEASES

ACUTE RENAL FAILURE

Clinical Presentation

Acute renal failure is a heterogeneous group of disorders that have in common the rapid deterioration of renal function resulting in accumulation in the blood of nitrogenous wastes that would normally be excreted in the urine. The patient presents with a rapidly rising blood urea nitrogen and serum creatinine. Depending on the cause and on when the patient comes to medical attention, there may be other presenting features as well (Table 11–3). Thus, diminished urine volume (oliguria) is a common but variable presenting manifestation. Urine volume may be normal early, or indeed at any time with milder forms of acute renal injury. Patients presenting relatively late may display any of the clinical manifestations described below.

Etiology

The major causes of acute renal failure are presented in Table 11–4.

A. Prerenal Causes: Some patients who are dependent on prostaglandin-mediated vasodilation to maintain renal hypoperfusion can develop renal failure simply from ingestion of NSAIDs. Similarly, patients with renal hypoperfusion (eg, due to renal artery stenosis, congestive heart failure, or intrarenal small vessel disease) who are dependent on angiotensin II-mediated vasoconstriction of the efferent renal arteriole to maintain renal perfusion pressure may develop acute renal failure upon ingesting angiotensin-converting enzyme inhibitors.

B. Intrarenal Causes: The intrarenal causes can be further divided into specific **inflammatory diseases** such as vasculitis, glomerulonephritis, and drug-induced injury and **acute tubular necrosis** due to many causes (including ischemia, poisons, and hemolysis).

Notable among intrarenal causes are the toxic effects of aminoglycoside antibiotics and rhabdomyolysis, in which myoglobin, released into the bloodstream after crush injury to muscle, precipitates in the renal tubules. The former may be mitigated by close monitoring of renal dysfunction during antibiotic therapy, especially in elderly patients and those with some degree of underlying renal compromise. The latter may be detected by obtaining a serum creatine kinase level in patients admitted to the hospital with trauma or altered mental status and may be mitigated by maintaining a vigorous alkaline diuresis to prevent myoglobin precipitation in the tubules.

C. Postrenal Causes: The postrenal causes are those that result in urinary tract obstruction, such as renal stones.

Pathology & Pathogenesis

Regardless of their origin, all forms of acute renal failure, if untreated, will result in acute tubular necrosis, with death and sloughing of cells that make up the renal tubule. Depending on the timing of intervention between onset of initial injury and eventual acute tubular necrosis, acute renal failure may be reversible, with either prevention of or recovery from acute tubular necrosis; or irreversible, with permanent partial or complete loss of renal function.

The precise molecular mechanisms responsible for the development of acute tubular necrosis remain unknown. Theories favoring either a tubular or vascular basis have been proposed (Figure 11–4). According to the tubular theory, occlusion of the tubular lumen with cellular debris forms a cast that increases intratubular pressure sufficiently to decrease net filtration pressure. Vascular theories propose that decreased renal perfusion pressure from the combination of afferent arteriolar vasoconstriction and efferent arteriolar vasodilation reduces glomerular perfusion pressure and therefore glomerular filtration. It may be that both mechanisms act to produce acute renal failure, varying in relative importance in different individuals depending on the cause and the time of presentation. Renal damage, whether due to tubular occlusion or vascular hypoperfusion, is potentiated by the hypoxic state of the renal medulla, which increases the risk of ischemia. Recent work has implicated cytokines and endogenous peptides such as endothelins and the regulation of their production as possible explanations for why, subjected to the same toxic insult, some patients develop acute renal failure while others do not and why some with acute renal failure recover while others do not.

Table 11–3. Initial clinical and laboratory data base for defining major syndromes in nephrology.

Syndrome	Important Clues to Diagnosis	Common Findings Not of Diagnostic Value
Acute or rapidly progressive renal failure	Anuria Oliguria Documented recent decline in GFR	Hypertension Hematuria, proteinuria, pyuria, casts Edema
Acute nephritis	Hematuria, red cell casts Azotemia, oliguria Edema, hypertension	Proteinuria, pyuria Circulatory congestion
Chronic renal failure	Azotemia for >3 months Prolonged symptoms or signs of uremia Symptoms or signs of renal osteodystrophy Kidneys reduced in size bilaterally Broad casts in urinary sediment	Hematuria, proteinuria, casts Oliguria, polyuria, nocturia Edema, hypertension Electrolyte disorders
Nephrotic syndrome	Proteinuria >3.5 g/1.73 m^2 per 24 hours Hypoalbuminemia Hyperlipidemia Lipiduria	Casts Edema
Asymptomatic urinary abnormalities	Hematuria Proteinuria (below nephrotic range) Sterile pyuria, casts	
Urinary tract infection	Bacteriuria >10^5 colonies/mL Other infectious agent documented in urine Pyuria, leukocyte casts Frequency, urgency Bladder tenderness, flank tenderness	Hematuria Mild azotemia Mild proteinuria Fever
Renal tubular defects	Electrolyte disorders Polyuria, nocturia Symptoms or signs of renal osteodystrophy Large kidneys Renal transport defects	Hematuria Mild azotemia Mild proteinuria Fever
Hypertension	Systolic/diastolic hypertension	Proteinuria Casts Azotemia
Nephrolithiasis	History of stone passage or removal Stone seen by x-ray Renal colic	Hematuria Pyuria Frequency, urgency
Urinary tract obstruction	Azotemia, oliguria, anuria Polyuria, nocturia, urinary retention Slowing of urinary stream Large prostate, large kidneys Flank tenderness, full bladder after voiding	Hematuria Pyuria Enuresis, dysuria

[1]Reproduced, with permission, from Coe FL, Brenner BM: Approach to the patient with diseases of the kidney and urinary tract. In: *Harrison's Principles of Internal Medicine,* 12th ed. Wilson JD et al (editors). McGraw-Hill, 1991.

Clinical Manifestations

Because symptoms and physical findings of acute renal failure are relatively nonspecific, laboratory studies are of great diagnostic importance. The initial symptoms are typically fatigue and malaise—probably early consequences of loss of the ability to excrete water, salt, and wastes via the kidneys. Later, more profound symptoms and signs of loss of renal water and salt excretory capacity develop: dyspnea, orthopnea, rales, prominent third heart sound (S_3), and peripheral edema. Altered mental status reflects the toxic effect of uremia on the brain, with elevated blood levels of nitrogenous wastes and fixed acids.

The clinical manifestations of acute renal failure depend not only on the cause but also on the point in the natural history of the disease at which the patient comes to medical attention. Patients with renal hypoperfusion (prerenal causes of acute renal failure) first develop **prerenal azotemia** (elevated BUN without tubular necrosis), a direct physiologic consequence of decrease in GFR. With appropriate treatment, renal perfusion can be improved, prerenal

Table 11–4. Major causes of acute renal failure.

Disorder	Examples
Hypovolemia	Volume loss via the skin, gastrointestinal tract, or kidney. Hemorrhage. Sequestration of extracellular fluid (burns, pancreatitis, peritonitis).
Cardiovascular failure	Impaired cardiac output (infarction, tamponade). Vascular pooling (anaphylaxis, sepsis, drugs).
Extrarenal obstruction	Urethral occlusion. Vesical, pelvic, prostatic, or retroperitoneal neoplasms. Surgical accident. Medication. Calculi. Pus, blood clots.
Intrarenal obstruction	Crystals (uric acid, oxalic acid, sulfonamides, methotrexate).
Bladder rupture	Trauma.
Vascular diseases	Vasculitis. Malignant hypertension. Thrombotic thrombocytopenic purpura. Scleroderma. Arterial or venous occlusion.
Glomerulonephritis	Immune complex disease. Anti-GBM disease.
Interstitial nephritis	Drugs. Hypercalcemia. Infections. Idiopathic.
Postischemic	All conditions listed above under hypovolemia and cardiovascular failure.
Pigment-induced	Hemolysis (transfusion reaction, malaria). Rhabdomyolysis (trauma, muscle disease, coma, heat stroke, severe exercise, potassium or phosphate depletion).
Poison-induced	Antibiotics. Contrast material. Anesthetic agents. Heavy metals. Organic solvents.
Pregnancy-related	Septic abortion. Uterine hemorrhage. Eclampsia.

[1]Reproduced, with permission, from Andersen RJ, Schrier RW: Acute renal failure. In: *Harrison's Principles of Internal Medicine,* 12th ed. Wilson JD et al (editors). McGraw-Hill, 1991.

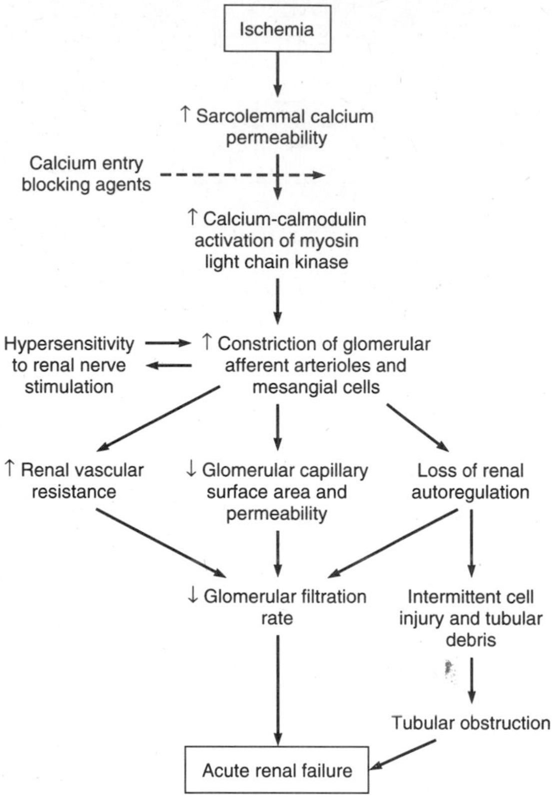

Figure 11–4. Potential pathogenic schema in acute renal failure. (Reproduced, with permission, from Anderson RJ, Schrier RW: Acute renal failure. In: *Harrison's Principles of Internal Medicine,* 12th ed. Wilson JD et al [editors]. McGraw-Hill, 1991.)

azotemia can be readily reversed, and the development of acute tubular necrosis can be prevented. Without treatment, prerenal azotemia may progress to acute tubular necrosis. Recovery, if it occurs, will then follow a protracted course, often requiring supportive dialysis before adequate renal function is regained.

A variety of clinical tests can help determine whether a patient with signs of acute renal failure is in the early phase of prerenal azotemia or has progressed to full-blown acute tubular necrosis. However, the overlap in clinical presentation along the continuum between prerenal azotemia and acute tubular necrosis is such that any one of these tests must be interpreted in the context of other findings and the clinical history.

Perhaps the earliest manifestation of prerenal azotemia is an elevated ratio of BUN to serum creatinine. Normally 10–15:1, this ratio may rise to 20–30:1 in prerenal azotemia, with a normal or near-normal serum creatinine. If the patient proceeds to acute tubular necrosis, this ratio may normalize, but with a progressively elevated serum creatinine. Likewise, a fluctuating but not inexorably rising serum creatinine suggests prerenal azotemia.

Urinalysis may also be useful. There are no typical abnormal findings in simple prerenal azotemia, whereas granular casts, tubular epithelial cells, and epithelial cell casts are found in acute tubular necrosis. Casts are formed when debris in the renal tubules (protein, red cells, or epithelial cells) takes on the cylindric, regular bordered shape of the tubule.

Likewise, since hypovolemia is a stimulus to vasopressin release (see Chapter 18), the urine is maximally concentrated (up to 1500 mosm/L) in prerenal azotemia. However, with progression to acute tubular necrosis, the ability to generate a concentrated urine is lost. Thus, a urine osmolality of less than 350 mosm/L is a typical finding in acute tubular necrosis.

Finally, the fractional excretion of sodium–

$$FE_{Na}\,(\%) = \left(\frac{U_{Na}/P_{Na}}{U_{Cr}/P_{Cr}}\right) \times 100$$

is an important indicator of whether a patient with acute renal failure has progressed from simple prerenal azotemia to frank acute tubular necrosis. In simple prerenal azotemia, over 99% of filtered sodium will be reabsorbed. This value allows accurate identification of sodium retention states (such as prerenal azotemia) even when there is water retention due to vasopressin release. There are, however, some rare conditions in which the FE_{Na} is less than 1% in patients with acute tubular necrosis (Table 11–5).

10. What are the current theories of the development basis of acute tubular necrosis?
11. What clues are helpful in determining whether newly diagnosed renal failure is acute or chronic?
12. What is the natural history of acute renal failure?

CHRONIC RENAL FAILURE

Clinical Presentation

Patients with chronic renal failure and uremia show a constellation of symptoms, signs, and laboratory abnormalities in addition to those observed in acute renal failure. This reflects the long-standing and progressive nature of their renal impairment and its effects on many types of tissues (Table 11–6).

Table 11–5. Causes of acute renal failure in which FE_{Na} may be below 1%.[1]

Prerenal disease
Acute tubular necrosis
10% of nonoliguric cases
Superimposed upon chronic prerenal state
Hepatic cirrhosis
Heart failure
Severe burns
Myoglobinuria or hemoglobinuria
Radiocontrast media
Sepsis
Acute glomerulonephritis or vasculitis
Acute obstructive uropathy
Acute interstitial nephritis

[1]Reproduced, with permission, from Rose BD: Acute renal failure—prerenal disease vs acute tubular necrosis. In: *Pathophysiology of Renal Disease,* 2nd ed. McGraw-Hill, 1987.

Thus, osteodystrophy, neuropathy, bilateral small kidneys shown by abdominal x-ray or ultrasound, and anemia are typical initial findings that suggest a chronic course for a patient newly diagnosed with renal failure on the basis of elevated BUN and serum creatinine.

Etiology

The most common cause of chronic renal failure is diabetes mellitus (see Chapter 16), followed closely by hypertension and glomerulonephritis (Table 11–7). Polycystic kidney disease, obstruction, and infection are among the less common causes of chronic renal failure.

Pathology & Pathogenesis

A. Development of Chronic Renal Failure: As occurs in other organs also (eg, the liver), the pathogenetic features of acute and chronic diseases of the kidney are quite distinctive. Whereas acute injury to the kidney results in death and sloughing of tubular epithelial cells, often followed by their regeneration with reestablishment of normal architecture, chronic injury results in irreversible loss of nephrons. As a result, a greater functional burden is borne by fewer nephrons, manifested as an increase in glomerular filtration pressure and hyperfiltration. For reasons not well understood, this compensatory hyperfiltration—which can be thought of as a form of "hypertension" at the level of the individual nephron—predisposes to fibrosis and scarring **(glomerular sclerosis).** As a result, the rate of nephron destruction and loss increases, thus speeding the progression to **uremia,** the complex of signs and symptoms that occurs when residual renal function is inadequate.

Owing to the tremendous functional reserve of the kidneys, up to 50% of nephrons can be lost without any evidence of functional impairment—which is why individuals with two healthy kidneys are able to donate one for transplantation. When GFR is further reduced to the 30–50% range, some degree of azotemia (elevation of blood levels of products normally excreted by the kidneys) is observed. Nevertheless, patients may be largely asymptomatic because a new steady state is achieved in which blood levels of these products are not high enough to cause overt toxicity. However, even at this apparently stable level of renal function, hyperfiltration-accelerated evolution to endstage chronic renal failure is in progress. Furthermore, since patients with this level of GFR have little functional reserve, they can easily become uremic with any added stress (eg, infection, obstruction, dehydration, or nephrotoxic drugs) or with any catabolic state associated with increased turnover of nitrogen-containing products with reduction in GFR. Below approximately 20% of normal, renal excretory capacity is insufficient to prevent the development of frank uremia.

B. Pathogenesis of Uremia: The pathogenesis of chronic renal failure in part derives from a combination of the toxic effects of (1) retained products normally excreted by the kidneys (eg, urea and other nitrogen-containing products of protein metabolism);

Table 11–6. Clinical abnormalities in uremia.[1,2]

Fluid and electrolyte	**Cardiovascular**
Volume expansion and contraction (I)	Arterial hypertension (I or P)
Hypernatremia and hyponatremia (I)	Congestive heart failure or pulmonary edema (I)
Hyperkalemia and hypokalemia (I)	Pericarditis (I)
Metabolic acidosis (I)	Cardiomyopathy (I or P)
Hypocalcemia (I)	Uremic lung (I)
Bone and mineral	Accelerated atherosclerosis (P or D)
Renal osteodystrophy (I or P)	Hypotension and arrhythmias (D)
Osteomalacia (D)	**Skin**
Metabolic	Skin pallor (I or P)
Carbohydrate intolerance (I)	Hyperpigmentation (I, P, or D)
Hypothermia (I)	Pruritus (P)
Hypertriglyceridemia (P)	Ecchymoses (I or P)
Protein-calorie malnutrition (I or P)	Uremic frost
Impaired growth and development (P)	**Gastrointestinal**
Infertility and sexual dysfunction (P)	Anorexia (I)
Amenorrhea (P)	Nausea and vomiting (I)
Dialysis (amyloid, β_2-microglobulin) arthropathy (D)	Uremic fetor (I)
Neuromuscular	Gastroenteritis (I)
Fatigue (I)	Peptic ulcer (I or P)
Sleep disorders (P)	Gastrointestinal bleeding (I, P, or D)
Impaired mentation (I)	Hepatitis (d)
Lethargy (I)	Refractory ascites on hemodialysis (D)
Asterixis (I)	Peritonitis (D)
Muscular irritability (I)	**Hematologic**
Peripheral neuropathy (I or P)	Normocytic, normochromic anemia (P)
Restless legs syndrome (I or P)	Microcytic (aluminum-induced) anemia
Paralysis (I or P)	Lymphocytopenia (P)
Myoclonus (I)	Bleeding diathesis (I or D)
Seizures (I or P)	Increased susceptibility to infection (I or P)
Coma (I)	Splenomegaly and hypersplenism (P)
Muscle cramps (D)	Leukopenia (D)
Dialysis disequilibrium syndrome (D)	Hypocomplementemia (D)
Dialysis dementia (D)	
Myopathy (P or D)	

[1]Virtually all the abnormalities contained in this table are completely reversed in time by successful renal transplantation. The response of these abnormalities to hemo- or peritoneal dialysis therapy is more variable. (I) denotes an abnormality that usually improves with an optimal program of dialysis and related therapy. (P) denotes an abnormality that tends to persist or even progress, despite an optimal program. (D) denotes an abnormality that develops only after initiation of dialysis therapy.
[2]Reproduced, with permission, from Brenner BM, Lazarus JM: Chronic renal failure. In: *Harrison's Principles of Internal Medicine,* 12th ed. Wilson JD et al (editors). McGraw-Hill, 1991.

(2) normal products such as hormones but now present in increased amounts; and (3) loss of normal products of the kidney (eg, loss of erythropoietin and insulinases).

Excretory failure results also in fluid shifts, with increased intracellular sodium and water and decreased intracellular potassium. These alterations may contribute to subtle alterations in function of a host of enzymes, transport systems, etc.

Table 11–7. Primary diagnoses: Medicare End-Stage Renal Disease Program.[1,2]

Diabetic nephropathy	27.7%
Hypertension	24.5%
Glomerulonephritis	21.2%
Polycystic kidney disease	3.9%
Other, unknown	22.7%

[1]Number of new patients in 1985: 28,944.
[2]From Health Care Financing Administration, Bureau of Data Management and Strategy. Reproduced, with permission, from Brenner BM, Lazarus JM: Chronic renal failure. In: *Harrison's Principles of Internal Medicine,* 12th ed. Wilson JD et al (editors). McGraw-Hill, 1991.

Finally, uremia has a number of effects on metabolism that are currently not well understood, including the following: (1) A decrease in basal body temperature (perhaps due to decreased Na^+-K^+ ATPase activity). (2) Slowed glucose metabolism, in part due to a form of increased peripheral resistance to insulin action. Whether this is specific to uremia or is a consequence of the effects of alterations in potassium, sodium, or acid-base balance has not been determined. (3) Diminished lipoprotein lipase activity with accelerated atherosclerosis.

Clinical Manifestations

A. Sodium Balance and Volume Status: Patients with chronic renal failure typically have some degree of sodium and water excess, reflecting loss of the renal route of salt and water excretion. A moderate degree of sodium and water excess may occur without objective signs of extracellular fluid excess. However, continued excessive salt (sodium) ingestion will contribute to congestive heart failure, hypertension, ascites, and edema. On the other hand, excessive water ingestion contributes to milder symptoms of hyponatremia, peripheral edema, and weight gain. A common recommendation for the patient with chronic renal failure is to avoid excess salt intake and to restrict fluid intake so that it equals urine output plus 500 mL (insensible losses). Further adjustments in volume status can be made either through the use of diuretics or dialysis.

Because these patients also have impaired renal salt and water conservation mechanisms, they are more sensitive to sudden extrarenal sodium and water losses (eg, vomiting, diarrhea, and increased sweating with fever). Under these circumstances, they will more easily develop ECF depletion, further deterioration of renal function (which may not be reversible), and even vascular collapse and shock. The symptoms and signs of dry oral and other mucous membranes, dizziness, syncope, tachycardia, and decreased jugular venous filling suggest progression of volume depletion.

B. Potassium Balance: Hyperkalemia is a serious problem in chronic renal failure for patients whose GFR has fallen below 5 mL/min. Above that GFR level, patients with chronic renal failure generally do not have difficulties in potassium homeostasis because as GFR falls, aldosterone-mediated potassium transport in the collecting tubule increases in a compensatory fashion. However, this means that a patient whose GFR is between 50 mL/min and 5 mL/min is dependent on tubular transport to maintain potassium balance. Treatment with potassium-sparing diuretics, angiotensin-converting enzyme inhibitors, or beta-blockers—drugs that may impair aldosterone-mediated potassium transport—can therefore precipitate dangerous hyperkalemia in a patient with chronic renal failure.

Patients with diabetes mellitus (the leading cause of chronic renal failure) may have a syndrome of **hyporeninemic hypoaldosteronism.** This syndrome, also termed **type IV renal tubular acidosis,** is a condition in which lack of renin production by the kidney diminishes the levels of angiotensin II and therefore impairs aldosterone secretion. As a result, affected patients are unable to compensate for falling GFR by enhancing their aldosterone-mediated potassium transport and therefore have relative difficulty handling potassium. This difficulty is usually manifested as extreme hyperkalemia even before GFR has fallen below 5 mL/min (Table 11–1).

Finally, just as chronic renal failure patients are more susceptible to the effects of sodium or volume overload, so also are they at greater risk of hyperkalemia in the face of sudden loads of potassium from either endogenous sources (eg, hemolysis, infection, trauma) or exogenous sources (eg, stored blood, potassium-rich foods or potassium-containing medications).

C. Metabolic Acidosis: The diminished capacity to excrete acid and generate buffers in chronic renal failure results in metabolic acidosis. In most cases when the GFR is above 20 mL/min, only moderate acidosis will develop before reestablishment of a new steady state of buffer production and consumption. The fall in blood pH in these individuals can usually be corrected with 20–30 mmol (2–3 g) of sodium bicarbonate by mouth daily. However, these patients are highly susceptible to acidosis in the event of a sudden acid load or the onset of disorders that increase the generated acid load.

D. Mineral and Bone: Several disorders of phosphate, calcium, and bone metabolism are observed in chronic renal failure as a result of a complex series of events (Figure 11–5). The key factors in the pathogenesis of these disorders include the following: (1) diminished absorption of calcium from the gut, (2) overproduction of parathyroid hormone, (3) disordered vitamin D metabolism, and (4) chronic metabolic acidosis. All of these factors contribute to enhanced bone resorption. Hyperuricemia is also a common finding in chronic renal failure, though symptomatic gout is relatively rare. Hypophosphatemia and hypermagnesemia can occur through overuse of phosphate binders and magnesium-containing antacids, though hyperphosphatemia is more common. Hyperphosphatemia contributes to the development of hypocalcemia and thus serves as an additional trigger for secondary hyperparathyroidism, elevating blood PTH levels. The elevated blood PTH further depletes bone calcium and contributes to osteomalacia and osteoporosis of chronic renal failure (see below).

E. Cardiovascular and Pulmonary Abnormalities: Congestive heart failure and pulmonary edema are most commonly due to volume and salt overload. However, a poorly understood syndrome involving increased permeability of the alveolar capillary membrane is also observed that can result in pulmonary edema even with normal or only slightly elevated pulmonary capillary wedge pressures.

Hypertension is a common finding in chronic renal failure, usually on the basis of fluid and sodium overload. However, hyperreninemia is a recognized syndrome in which falling renal perfusion triggers the failing kidney to overproduce renin and thereby elevate systemic blood pressure.

Pericarditis resulting from irritation and inflammation of the pericardium by uremic toxins is a complication whose incidence in chronic renal failure is decreasing owing to the aggressive and early institution of renal dialysis.

Accelerated atherosclerosis is a complication seen in chronically dialysed patients with chronic renal failure, resulting in a myriad of complications including myocardial infarction, stroke, and peripheral vascular disease. Cardiovascular risk factors in these patients include hypertension, hyperlipidemia, glucose intolerance, chronic elevated cardiac output, and valvular and myocardial calcification as a consequence of elevated calcium × phosphate product.

F. Hematologic Abnormalities: Patients with chronic renal failure have marked abnormalities in

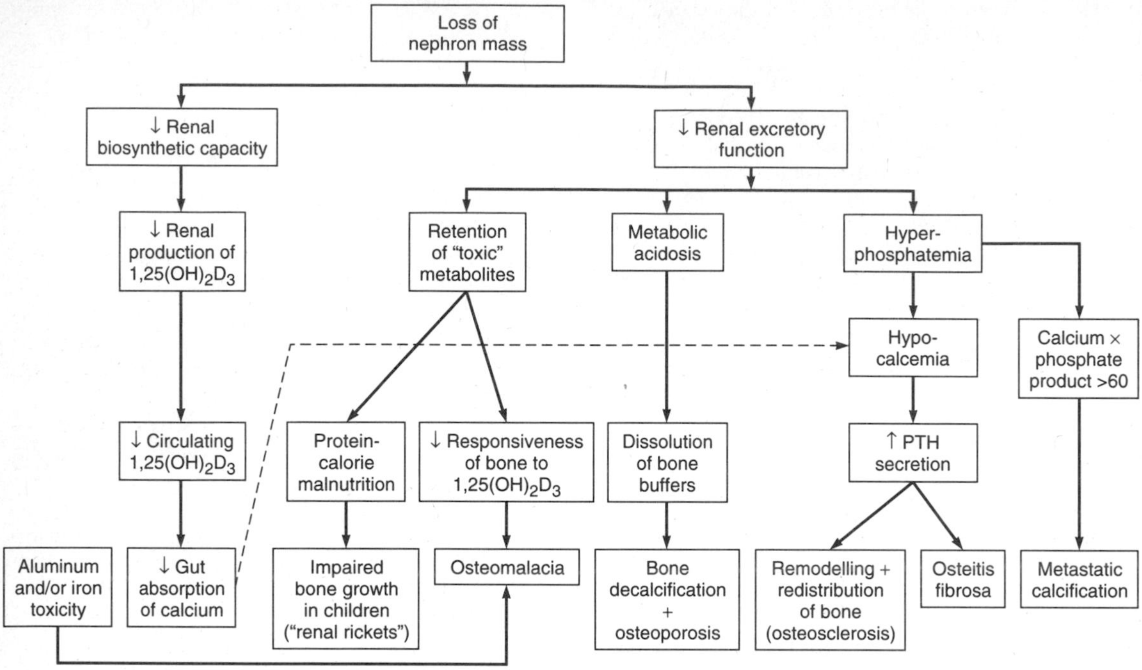

Figure 11–5. Pathogenesis of bone diseases in chronic renal failure. (Reproduced, with permission, from Brenner BM, Lazarus JM: Chronic renal failure. In: *Harrison's Principles of Internal Medicine,* 12th ed. Wilson JD et al [editors]. McGraw-Hill, 1991.)

red blood cell count, white blood cell function, and clotting parameters. Normochromic, normocytic anemia with symptoms of listlessness and easy fatigability and hematocrits typically in the range of 20–25% is a consistent feature. The anemia is believed to be due chiefly to lack of production of erythropoietin and loss of its stimulatory effect on erythropoiesis, since patients with chronic renal failure, regardless of dialysis status, show a dramatic improvement in hematocrit when treated with erythropoietin. Additional causes of anemia may include bone marrow suppressive effects of uremic poisons, bone marrow fibrosis due to elevated blood PTH, toxic effects of aluminum (from phosphate-binding antacids and dialysis solutions), and hemolysis and gastrointestinal blood loss related to dialysis (while the patient is anticoagulated with heparin).

Patients with chronic renal failure display abnormal hemostasis manifested as increased bruising, increased blood loss at surgery, and an increased incidence of spontaneous gastrointestinal and cerebrovascular hemorrhage (including both hemorrhagic strokes and subdural hematomas). Laboratory abnormalities include prolonged bleeding time, decreased platelet factor III, abnormal platelet aggregation and adhesiveness, and impaired prothrombin consumption—none of them reversible even in well-dialysed patients.

Uremia is associated with increased susceptibility to infections, believed to be due to leukocyte suppression by uremic toxins. The suppression seems to be greater for lymphoid cells than neutrophils and seems also to affect chemotaxis, the acute inflammatory response, and delayed hypersensitivity more so than other leukocyte functions. Acidosis, hyperglycemia, malnutrition, and hyperosmolality also are believed to contribute to immunosuppression in chronic renal failure. The invasiveness of dialysis and the use of immunosuppressive drugs in renal transplant patients also contribute to an increased incidence of infections.

G. Neuromuscular Abnormalities: Central nervous system symptoms and signs may range from mild sleep disorders and impairment of mental concentration, loss of memory, errors in judgment, and neuromuscular irritability (manifested as hiccups, cramps, fasciculations, and twitching) to asterixis, myoclonus, stupor, and seizures and coma in end-stage uremia. Asterixis is manifested as involuntary flapping motions seen when the arms are extended and wrists held back to "stop traffic," due to altered nerve conduction in metabolic encephalopathy.

Peripheral neuropathy (sensory greater than motor, lower extremities greater than upper), typified by the "restless legs" syndrome (poorly localized sense of discomfort and involuntary movements of the lower extremities) is a common finding in chronic renal failure and an important indication for institution of dialysis.

Patients receiving dialysis therapy can develop aluminum toxicity, characterized by speech dyspraxia (inability to repeat words), myoclonus, dementia, and seizures. Likewise, aggressive acute dialysis can result in a disequilibrium syndrome characterized by nausea, vomiting, drowsiness, headache, and seizures in a patient with very high BUN levels. Presumably, this is an effect of rapid pH or osmolality change in extracellular fluid, resulting in cerebral edema.

H. Gastrointestinal Abnormalities: Up to 25% of patients with uremia have peptic ulcer disease, perhaps as a consequence of secondary hyperparathyroidism. A variety of other gastrointestinal abnormalities and syndromes are described as well, including uremic gastroenteritis, characterized by mucosal ulcerations with blood loss in the chronic renal failure patient, and a distinctive form of bad breath (uremic fetor) due to degradation of urea to ammonia by enzymes in the saliva.

Nonspecific gastrointestinal findings in uremic patients include anorexia, hiccups, nausea, vomiting, and diverticulosis. Although their precise pathogenesis is unclear, many of these findings improve with dialysis.

I. Endocrine and Metabolic Abnormalities: Women with uremia have low estrogen levels, which perhaps explains the high incidence of amenorrhea and the observation that they rarely are able to carry a pregnancy to term. Regular menses—but not a higher rate of successful pregnancies—typically return with frequent dialysis.

Similarly, low testosterone levels, impotence, oligospermia, and germinal cell dysplasia are common findings in men with chronic renal failure.

Finally, chronic renal failure eliminates the kidney as a site of insulin degradation, thereby increasing the half-life of insulin and typically producing a stabilizing effect on diabetic patients whose blood glucose was previously difficult to control.

J. Dermatologic Abnormalities: Skin changes arise from many of the effects of chronic renal failure already discussed. Patients with chronic renal failure may display pallor due to anemia, skin color changes due to accumulated pigmented metabolites or a gray discoloration due to transfusion-mediated hemochromatosis; ecchymoses and hematomas due to clotting abnormalities; and pruritus and excorations due to calcium deposits from secondary hyperparathyroidism. Finally, when urea concentrations are extremely high, evaporation of sweat leaves a residue of urea termed "uremic frost."

13. What is uremia?
14. What are the most prominent symptoms and signs of uremia?
15. What is the mechanism by which altered sodium, potassium, and volume status develop in chronic renal failure?
16. What are the most common causes of chronic renal failure?

GLOMERULONEPHRITIS & NEPHROTIC SYNDROME

Clinical Presentation

A number of disorders result in structural alterations of the glomerulus and present with some combination of the following findings: hematuria, proteinuria, reduced GFR, and hypertension. Some of these disorders are specific to the kidney, while others are systemic diseases in which the kidney is primarily or prominently involved.

Disorders resulting in glomerular disease, whether manifestations of systemic injury or otherwise, fall into five categories:

(1) **Acute glomerulonephritis,** in which there is an abrupt onset of hematuria and proteinuria with reduced GFR and renal salt and water retention, followed by full recovery of renal function. Patients with acute glomerulonephritis are a subset of those with an intrarenal cause of acute renal failure.

(2) **Rapidly progressive glomerulonephritis,** in which recovery from the acute disorder does not occur. Worsening renal function results in irreversible and complete renal failure over weeks to months. Early in the course of rapidly progressive glomerulonephritis, these patients can be categorized as having a form of acute renal failure. Later, with progression of their renal failure over time, they display all of the features described for chronic renal failure.

(3) **Chronic glomerulonephritis,** in which renal impairment following acute glomerulonephritis progresses slowly over a period of years but which eventually results in chronic renal failure.

(4) **Nephrotic syndrome,** manifested as marked proteinuria, particularly albuminuria (defined as 24-hour urine protein excretion greater than 3.5 g), hypoalbuminemia, edema, hyperlipidemia, and fat bodies in the urine. Nephrotic syndrome may be either isolated (eg, minimal change disease) or part of some other glomerular syndrome (eg, with hematuria and casts).

(5) **Asymptomatic urinary abnormalities,** including hematuria and proteinuria (usually in amounts below what is seen in nephrotic syndrome) but no functional abnormalities associated with reduced GFR, edema, or hypertension. Many patients with

these findings will develop chronic renal failure slowly over decades.

Etiology

Acute glomerulonephritis occurs most typically in the setting of infectious diseases—classically pharyngeal or cutaneous infections with certain "nephritogenic" strains of group A beta-hemolytic streptococci but also other pathogens (Table 11–8).

Rapidly progressive glomerulonephritis appears to be a heterogeneous group of disorders, all of which display pathologic features common to various categories of necrotizing vasculitis (Table 11–9; and see below).

Chronic glomerulonephritis and nephrotic syndrome are also of unclear origin. For some reason, progressive renal deterioration in patients with chronic glomerulonephritis proceeds slowly but inexorably, resulting in chronic renal failure as many as 20 years after initial discovery of an abnormal urinary sediment.

Some cases of nephrotic syndrome are variants of acute glomerulonephritis, rapidly progressive glomerulonephritis, or chronic glomerulonephritis in which massive proteinuria is a presenting feature. Other cases of nephrotic syndrome fall into the category of **minimal change disease,** in which massive proteinuria is the sole laboratory abnormality and progression to end-stage renal disease does not occur.

The most common cause of asymptomatic urinary abnormalities is **IgA nephropathy,** a poorly understood immune complex disease characterized by diffuse mesangial IgA deposition. Other causes are listed in Table 11–10.

Table 11–8. Causes of acute glomerulonephritis.[1,2]

Infectious diseases
- Poststreptococcal glomerulonephritis*
- Nonstreptococcal postinfectious glomerulonephritis
  - Bacterial: infective endocarditis,* "shunt nephritis," sepsis,* pneumococcal pneumonia, typhoid fever, secondary syphilis, meningococcemia
  - Viral: hepatitis B, infectious mononucleosis, mumps, measles, varicella, echovirus, coxsackievirus
  - Parasitic: malaria, toxoplasmosis

Multisystem diseases: systemic lupus erythematosus,* vasculitis,* Henoch-Schönlein purpura,* Goodpasture's syndrome

Primary glomerular diseases: mesangiocapillary glomerulonephritis, Berger's disease (IgA nephropathy),* "pure" mesangial proliferative glomerulonephritis

Miscellaneous: Guillain-Barré syndrome, irradiation of Wilms' tumor, self-administered diphtheria-pertussis-tetanus vaccine, serum sickness

[1]Reproduced, with permission, from Glassock RJ, Brenner BM: The major glomerulopathies. In: *Harrison's Principles of Internal Medicine,* 12th ed. Wilson JD et al (editors). McGraw-Hill, 1991.
[2]Most common causes are marked with asterisks.

Table 11–9. Causes of rapidly progressive glomerulonephritis.[1,2]

Infectious diseases
- Poststreptococcal glomerulonephritis*
- Infective endocarditis*
- Occult visceral sepsis
- Hepatitis B infection (with vasculitis or cryoimmunoglobulinemia)
- Human immunodeficiency virus infection (?)

Multisystem diseases
- Systemic lupus erythematosus*
- Henoch-Schönlein purpura*
- Systemic necrotizing vasculitis (including Wegener's granulomatosis)*
- Goodpasture's syndrome*
- Essential mixed (IgG/IgM) cryoimmunoglobulinemia
- Malignancy
- Relapsing polychondritis
- Rheumatoid arthritis (with vasculitis)

Drugs
- Penicillamine*
- Hydralazine
- Allopurinol (with vasculitis)
- Rifampin

Idiopathic or primary glomerular disease
- Idiopathic crescentic glomerulonephritis*
  - Type I—with linear deposits of immunoglobulin (anti-GBM antibody-mediated)
  - Type II—with granular deposits of immunoglobulin (immune complex-mediated)
  - Type III—with few or no immune deposits of immunoglobulin ("pauci-immune")
  - Anti-neutrophil cytoplasmic antibody-induced, ? "forme fruste" of vasculitis
- Superimposed on another primary glomerular disease
  - Mesangiocapillary (membranoproliferative glomerulonephritis)* (especially type II)
  - Membranous glomerulonephritis*
  - Berger's disease (IgA nephropathy)*

[1]Reproduced, with permission, from Glassock RJ, Brenner BM: The major glomerulopathies. In: *Harrison's Principles of Internal Medicine,* 12th ed. Wilson JD et al (editors). McGraw-Hill, 1991.
[2]Most common causes are marked with asterisks.

Pathology & Pathogenesis

The different forms of glomerulonephritis and nephrotic syndrome probably represent differences in the nature, extent, and specific cause of immune-mediated renal damage. A number of cytokines—in particular transforming growth factor-$\beta 1$ (TGF-$\beta 1$) and platelet-derived growth factor (PDGF)—are synthesized by mesangial cells, inciting an inflammatory reaction in some forms of glomerular disease. Classic associations between the natural history and defining fluorescence and electron microscopic observations have been made (Figure 11–6; Table 11–11). However, because it is not known exactly how the various forms of immune-mediated renal damage occur, each category is described separately with its associated findings.

A. Acute Glomerulonephritis: Postinfectious acute glomerulonephritis is due to immune attack on the infecting organism in which there is cross-reactivity between an antigen of the infecting organism

Table 11–10. Glomerular causes of asymptomatic urinary abnormalities.

Hematuria with or without proteinuria
Primary glomerular diseases
Berger's disease (IgA nephropathy)*
Mesangiocapillary glomerulonephritis
Other primary glomerular hematurias accompanied by "pure" mesangial proliferation, focal and segmental proliferative glomerulonephritis, or other lesions
"Thin basement membrane" disease (?"forme fruste" of Alport's syndrome)
Associated with multisystem or heredofamilial diseases
Alport's syndrome and other "benign" familial hematurias
Fabry's disease
Sickle cell disease
Associated with infections
Resolving poststreptococcal glomerulonephritis*
Other postinfectious glomerulonephritides*
Isolated nonnephrotic proteinuria
Primary glomerular diseases
"Orthostatic" proteinuria*
Focal and segmental glomerulosclerosis*
Membranous glomerulonephritis*
Associated with multisystem or heredofamilial diseases
Diabetes mellitus*
Amyloidosis*
Nail-patella syndrome

[1]Reproduced, with permission, from Glassock RJ, Brenner BM: The major glomerulopathies. In: *Harrison's Principles of Internal Medicine,* 12th ed. Wilson JD et al (editors). McGraw-Hill, 1991.
[2]Most common causes are marked with asterisks.

Table 11–11. Location of electron-dense deposits in glomerular disease.[1]

Subepithelial
Amorphous (epimembranous) deposits
Membranous nephropathy
Systemic lupus erythematosus
Humps
Acute postinfectious glomerulonephritis, eg, poststreptococcal glomerulonephritis, bacterial endocarditis
Intramembranous
Membranous nephropathy
Membranoproliferative glomerulonephritis type II
Subendothelial
Systemic lupus erythematosus
Membranoproliferative glomerulonephritis type I
Less commonly, bacterial endocarditis, IgA nephropathy, Henoch-Schönlein purpura, mixed cryoglobulinemia
Mesangial
Focal glomerulonephritis
IgA nephropathy
Henoch-Schönlein purpura
Systemic lupus erythematosus
Mild or resolving acute postinfectious glomerulonephritis
Subepithelial and subendothelial
Systemic lupus erythematosus
Membranoproliferative glomerulonephritis, type III
Postinfectious glomerulonephritis

[1]Reproduced, with permission, from Rose BD: Pathogenesis, clinical manifestations and diagnosis of glomerular disease. In: *Pathophysiology of Renal Disease.* McGraw-Hill, 1987.

(eg, of group A beta-hemolytic streptococci) and a host antigen. The result is deposition of immune complexes and complement (Figure 11–7; Table 11–12) in glomerular capillaries and the mesangium. Symptoms and signs typically occur 7–10 days after onset of the acute pharyngeal or cutaneous infection and resolve over weeks following treatment of the infection.

B. Rapidly Progressive Glomerulonephritis: Whereas the natural history of most cases of acute glomerulonephritis includes resolution of the underlying renal disease, some cases display—often abruptly—a form of renal disease that rapidly progresses to chronic renal failure over a period of weeks to months. While it is unclear why some patients have this rapid downhill course, a distinctive pathologic feature in such cases is extracapillary cellular proliferation, typically involving 70% of the glomeruli. Gaps and focal discontinuities in the glomerular basement membrane may also be observed. Immunofluorescence studies permit distribution into subgroups correlating with other features of the disease. Five to 20 percent of patients have linear anti-GBM antibody deposits in glomeruli and a tendency to hemoptysis reminiscent of Goodpasture's syndrome. Thirty to 40 percent have granular immunoglobulin deposits and an autoantibody pattern typical of Wegener's granulomatosis (antineutrophil cytoplasmic antibody). The latter patients are typically older, with more systemic constitutional symptoms (Tables 11–13 and 11–14).

C. Chronic Glomerulonephritis: Some patients with acute glomerulonephritis develop chronic renal failure slowly over a period of 5–20 years. Cellular proliferation, either in the mesangium or in the capillary, is a pathologic structural hallmark in some of these cases, while others are notable for obliteration of glomeruli (**sclerosing chronic glomerulonephritis,** which includes both focal and diffuse subsets), and yet others display irregular subepithelial proteinaceous deposits with uniform involvement of individual glomeruli **(membranous glomerulonephritis).**

D. Nephrotic Syndrome: In patients with nephrotic syndrome, the glomerulus may appear intact or only subtly altered, without a cellular infiltrate as a manifestation of inflammation. Immunofluorescence with antibodies to IgG often demonstrates deposition of antigen-antibody complexes in the glomerular basement membrane. In the subset of patients with minimal change disease, in which proteinuria is the sole urinary sediment abnormality and in which (often) no changes can be seen by light microscopy, electron microscopy reveals obliteration of epithelial foot processes (Table 11–15). In animal

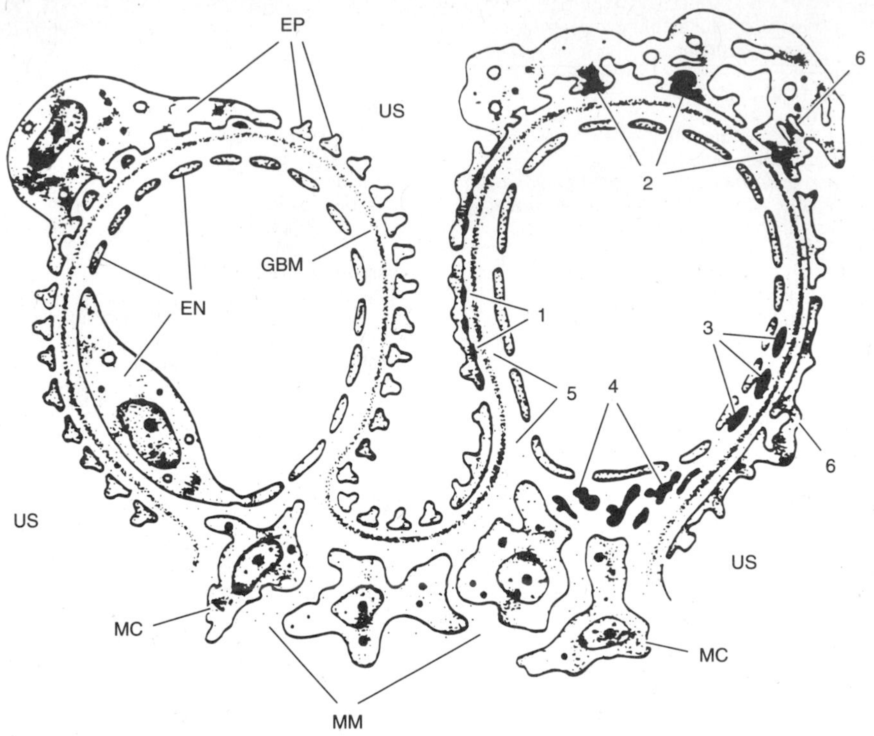

Figure 11–6. Anatomy of a normal glomerular capillary on the left. Note the fenestrated endothelium (EN), glomerular basement membrane (GBM), and the epithelium with its foot processes (EP). The mesangium is composed of mesangial cells (MC) surrounded by extracellular matrix (MM) in direct contact with the endothelium. Ultrafiltration occurs across the glomerular wall and through channels in the mesangial matrix into the urinary space (US). Typical localization of immune deposits and other pathologic changes is depicted on the right. (1) Uniform subepithelial deposits as in membranous nephropathy. (2) Large, irregular subepithelial deposits or "humps" seen in acute postinfectious glomerulonephritis. (3) Subendothelial deposits as in diffuse proliferative lupus glomerulonephritis. (4) Mesangial deposits characteristic of IgA nephropathy. (5) Antibody binding to the glomerular basement membrane (as in Goodpasture's syndrome) does not produce visible deposits, but a smooth linear pattern is seen on immunofluorescence. (6) Effacement of the epithelial foot processes is common in all forms of glomerular injury with proteinuria. (Reproduced, with permission, from Luke RG et al: Nephrology and hypertension. In: *Medical Knowledge Self-Assessment Program IX.* American College of Physicians, 1992.)

Table 11–12. Factors causing and mediators of glomerular injury.[1]

Factors affecting immune complex deposition
Host immune response
Rate of complex clearance
In situ complex formation
Antigenic or complex charge
Renal hemodynamics
Mediators of glomerular damage
Complement
Neutrophils
Macrophages
Platelets
Vasoactive amines
Fibrin
Lymphokines

[1]Modified and reproduced, with permission, from Rose BD: Pathogenesis, clinical manifestations and diagnosis of glomerular disease. In: *Pathophysiology of Renal Disease,* 2nd ed. McGraw-Hill, 1987.

models, T cell-derived "permeability factors," as well as non-complement-fixing antibodies to glomerular epithelial cells, can mimic this process.

Clinical Manifestations

Damage to the glomerular capillary wall results in leakage of red blood cells and proteins, which are normally too large to cross the glomerular capillary, into the renal tubular lumen, giving rise to hematuria and proteinuria.

A fall in GFR results either because glomerular capillaries are infiltrated with inflammatory cells or because contractile cells (eg, mesangial cells) respond to vasoactive substances by restricting blood flow to many glomerular capillaries.

Edema and hypertension are a direct consequence of fluid and salt overload secondary to the fall of GFR in the face of excess consumption of salt and water.

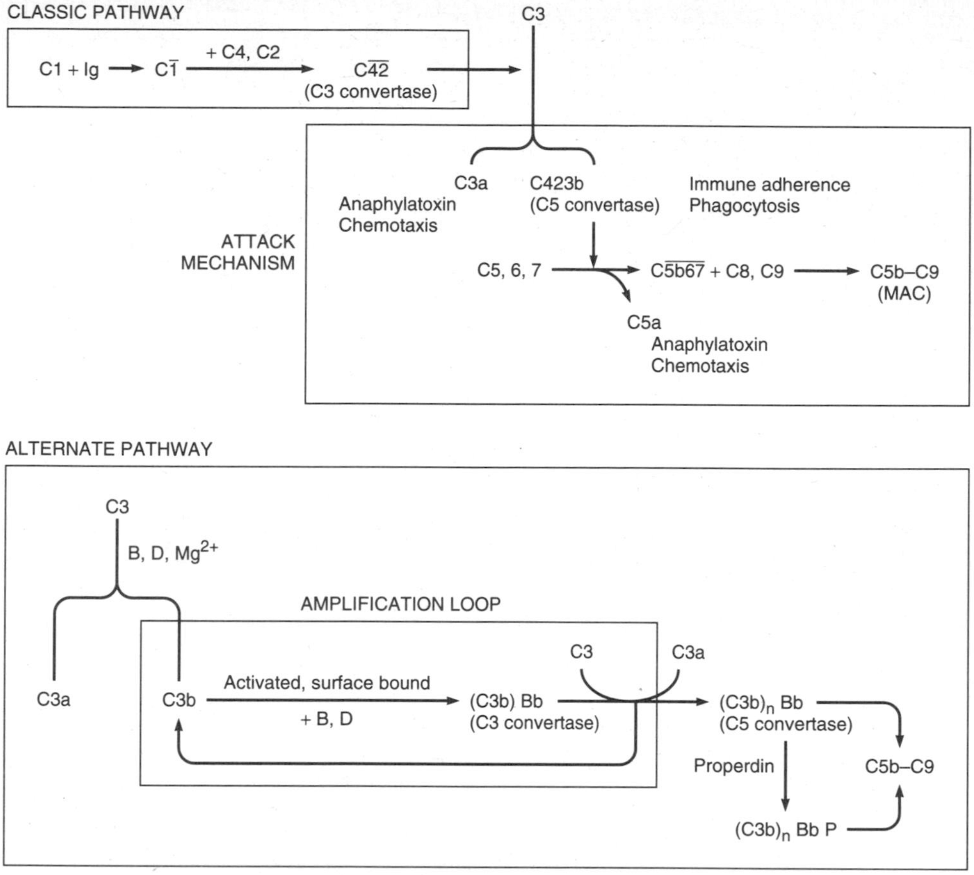

Figure 11–7. Sequence of complement activation and effects of the activated complement components in the classic and alternative pathways. Activated products are indicated by an overbar, while fragments from enzymatic cleavage are indicated by small letters (C3 is cleaved to C3a + C3b). In the classic pathway (*top*), C1 is bound to the Fc receptor on the immunoglobulin (IgG) and reacts with C4 and then C2. These components are cleaved, resulting in the formation of C42, a C3 convertase that cleaves C3 into two components, C3a and C3b. The latter combines with the C3 convertase to form C423b, a C5 convertase which activates the remaining components of the complement cascade, leading to the production of C5b–C9, the membrane attack complex (MAC). In the alternate pathway (*bottom*), C3 is cleaved by factors B, D, and magnesium, independent of C1, C4. and C2. The C3b that is formed is rapidly inactivated unless it is bound by, for example, the cell surface of a microorganism, damaged renal tissue, or IgA. The bound C3b combines with factor B, which is then cleaved by factor D to form C3bBb, the C3 convertase of the alternative pathway. This convertase produces further breakdown of C3, leading to a self-perpetuating cycle known as the amplification loop. As more C3b is generated, $(C3b)_n$Bb is produced, a C5 convertase that activates C5 to C9. Properdin contributes to this process by binding to the C3 and C5 convertases, thereby minimizing their inactivation. (Reproduced, with permission, from Rose BD: Pathogenesis, clinical manifestations, and diagnosis of glomerular disease. In: *Pathophysiology of Renal Disease,* 2nd ed. McGraw-Hill, 1987.)

A transient fall in serum complement is observed as a result of immune complex and complement deposition in the glomerulus.

An elevation of titer of antibody to streptococcal antigens is observed in cases associated with group A beta-hemolytic streptococcal infections. Another characteristic of the clinical course in poststreptococcal acute glomerulonephritis is a lag between clinical signs of infection and the development of clinical signs of nephritis.

Patients with the nephrotic syndrome have profoundly decreased plasma oncotic pressures and therefore have activated the renin-angiotensin-aldosterone system, the sympathetic nervous system, and the secretion of vasopressin and have altered the renal response to atrial natriuretic peptide. Nevertheless,

Table 11–13. Serologic findings in selected multisystem diseases.[1]

Disease	C3	Ig	FANA	Anti-dsDNA	Anti-GBM	Cryo-Ig	CIC	ANCA
Systemic lupus erythematosus	↓↓	↑ IgG	+++	++	–	++	+++	±
Goodpasture's syndrome	–	–	–	–	+++	–	±	–
Henoch-Schönlein purpura	–	↑ IgA	–	–	–	±	++	–
Polyarteritis nodosa	↓↑	↑ IgG	+	±	–	++	+++	+++
Wegener's granulomatosis	↓↑	↑ IgA, IgE	–	–	–	±	++	+++
Cryoimmunoglobulinemia	↓	±	–	–	–	+++	++	–
Multiple myeloma	–	↓↑ IgG, IgA, IgD, IgE	–	–	–	+	±	–
Waldenström's macroglobulinemia	–	↑ IgM	–	–	–	–	–	–
Amyloidosis	–	± Ig	–	–	–	–	–	–

Key: – = normal; + = occasionally slightly abnormal; ++ = often abnormal; +++ = severely abnormal; ↑ = increase; ↓ = decrease; ± = variable; ↑↓ = variable increase or decrease in serum level; C3 = C3 component of complement; Ig = immunoglobulin levels; FANA = fluorescent antinuclear antibody assay; anti-dsDNA = antibody to double-stranded (native) DNA; anti-GBM = antibody to glomerular basement membrane antigens; cryo-Ig = cryoimmunoglobulin; CIC = circulating immune complexes; ANCA = antineutrophil cytoplasmic antibody.

[1]Reproduced, with permission, from Glassock RJ, Brenner BM: Glomerulopathies associated with multisystem diseases. In: *Harrison's Principles of Internal Medicine,* 12th ed. Wilson JD et al (editors). McGraw-Hill, 1991.

they may develop signs of intravascular volume depletion, including syncope, shock, and acute renal failure.

Hyperlipidemia associated with nephrotic syndrome appears to be a result of decreased plasma oncotic pressure, which stimulates hepatic VLDL synthesis and secretion.

Loss of other plasma proteins besides albumin in nephrotic syndrome may present as any of the following: (1) A defect in bacterial opsonization and thus increased susceptibility to infections (eg, due to loss of IgG). (2) Hypercoagulability (eg, due to antithrombin III deficiency, reduced levels of protein C and protein S, hyperfibrinogenemia, and hyperlipidemia). (3) Vitamin D deficiency state and secondary hyperparathyroidism (eg, due to loss of vitamin D-binding proteins). (4) Altered thyroid function tests without any true thyroid abnormality (due to reduced levels of thyroxine-binding globulin).

Table 11–14. Serum complement profile and serology in acute glomerulonephritis.[1]

Type of Glomerulonephritis	Profile[2]	Serology
Poststreptococcal	Low, alternative	Antistreptococcal antibodies
Other postinfectious[3]	Low, classic	Blood or other cultures
Systemic lupus erythematosus	Low, classic	Antinuclear, anti-dsDNA, anti-Sm antibodies
Membranoproliferative		
Type I	Low, classic	Idiopathic, none; secondary, various
Type II	Low, alternative	C3 nephritic factor
Essential mixed cryoglobulinemia	Low, classic	Rheumatoid factor, IgG and IgM cryoglobulins
Anti-GBM (Goodpasture's syndrome)	Normal	Anti-GBM antibodies
Wegener's granulomatosis	Normal	Antineutrophil cytoplasmic antibodies
Microscopic polyarteritis	Normal	Antineutrophil cytoplasmic antibodies

[1]Reproduced, with permission, from Luke RG et al: Nephrology and hypertension: Serum complement profile and serology in acute glomerulonephritis. In: *Medical Knowledge Self-Assessment Program IX.* American College of Physicians, 1992.

[2]Pathway of complement activation: classic = low C2, C4, and C3; alternative = low C3, normal C2 and C4.

[3]Especially chronic bacteremia, eg, infective endocarditis, infected ventriculoatrial shunt.

Table 11–15. Clinical and histologic features of idiopathic nephrotic syndrome.[1]

Glomerular Disease	Distinguishing Clinical and Laboratory Findings	Characteristic Morphologic Features
Minimal change disease	Commonest cause in children (75%); steroid- or cyclophosphamide-sensitive (80% of cases); nonprogressive; normal renal function; scant hematuria.	**LM:** normal **IF:** negative to trace IgM **EM:** podocyte effacement; no immune deposits
Focal and segmental glomerulosclerosis	Early-onset hypertension; microscopic hematuria; progressive renal failure (75% of cases).	**LM:** early, segmental sclerosis in some glomeruli with tubular atrophy; late, sclerosis of most glomeruli **IF:** focal and segmental IgM, C3 **EM:** Foot process fusion, sclerosis, hyalin
Membranous nephropathy	Commonest cause in adults (40–50%); peak incidence fourth and sixth decades; male : female 2–3 : 1; microscopic hematuria (55%); early hypertension (30%); spontaneous remission (20%); progressive renal failure (30–40%).	**LM:** early, normal; late, GBM thickening **IF:** granular IgG and C3 **EM:** subepithelial deposits and GBM expansion
Membranoproliferative glomerulonephritis	Peak incidence second and third decades; mixed nephrotic-nephritic features; slowly progressive in most, rapid in some; hypocomplementemia.	**LM:** hypercellular glomeruli with duplicated GBM ("tramtracks") **IF:** type I, diffuse C3, variable IgG and IgM; type II, C3 capillary wall and mesangial nodules **EM:** type I, subendothelial immune deposits; type II, dense GBM

Key: LM = light microscopy; IF = immunofluorescence; EM = electron microscopy; GBM = glomerular basement membrane
[1]Reproduced, with permission, from Glassock RJ, Brenner BM: The major glomerulopathies. In: *Harrison's Principles of Internal Medicine,* 12th ed. Wilson JD et al (editors). McGraw-Hill, 1991; and from Luke RG et al: Nephrology and hypertension: Clinical and histologic features of idiopathic nephrotic syndrome. In: *Medical Knowledge Self-Assessment Program IX.* American College of Physicians, 1992.

17. What are the categories of glomerulonephritis and their common and distinctive features?
18. What are the pathophysiologic consequences of nephrotic syndrome?

RENAL STONES

Clinical Presentation

Patients with renal stones present with flank pain and hematuria with or without fever. Depending on the level of the stone and the patient's underlying anatomy (eg, if there is only a single functioning kidney or significant preexisting renal disease), the presentation may be complicated by obstruction (Tables 11–16 and 11–17) with decreased or absent urine production.

Etiology

A variety of disorders may result in the development of renal stones (Table 11–18). Most cases of calcium stones are due to idiopathic hypercalciuria, with hyperuricosuria and hyperparathyroidism as other major causes. Uric acid stones are typically caused by hyperuricosuria, especially in patients with a history of gout or excessive purine intake (eg, a diet high in organ meat products). Defective amino acid transport, as occurs in cystinuria, can result in stone formation. Finally, struvite stones, made up of magnesium, ammonium, and phosphate salts, are a result of chronic or recurrent urinary tract infection by urease-producing organisms (typically *Proteus*).

Pathology & Pathogenesis

Renal stones are a result of alterations in the dynamics of solubility of various substances in urine such that there is nucleation and precipitation. Diet, urine pH, and activity are parameters that can upset the balance between water conservation and excretion of supersaturated solutes and thereby precipitate stone formation. Stone formation per se within the renal pelvis is painless until a fragment breaks off and travels down the ureter, precipitating renal colic. Hematuria and renal damage can occur in the absence of pain.

Clinical Manifestations

The pain, hematuria, and even ureteral obstruction caused by a renal stone is self-limited. Passage of the stone usually requires only fluids, bed rest, and analgesia. The major complications are (1) hydronephro-

Table 11–16. Common mechanical causes of urinary tract obstruction.[1]

Ureter	Bladder Outlet	Urethra
Ureteropelvic junction narrowing or obstruction Ureterovesical junction narrowing or obstruction Ureterocele Retrocaval ureter	Bladder neck obstruction Ureterocele	Posterior urethral valves Anterior urethral valves Stricture Meatal stenosis Phimosis
Calculi Inflammation Trauma Sloughed papillae Tumor Blood clots Uric acid crystals	Benign prostatic hypertrophy Cancer of prostate Cancer of bladder Calculi Diabetic neuropathy Spinal cord disease	Stricture Tumor Calculi Trauma Phimosis
Pregnant uterus Retroperitoneal fibrosis Aortic aneurysm Uterine leiomyomas Carcinoma of uterus, prostate, bladder, colon, rectum Retroperitoneal lymphoma Accidental surgical ligation	Carcinomas of cervix, colon Trauma	Trauma

[1]Reproduced, with permission, from Brenner BM, Milford EL, Seifter JL: Urinary tract obstruction. In: *Harrison's Principles of Internal Medicine,* 12th ed. Wilson JD et al (editors). McGraw-Hill, 1991.

sis and permanent renal damage due to complete obstruction of a ureter, with resulting buildup of pressure and backup of urine; (2) infection or abscess formation behind a partially or completely obstructing stone, which can rapidly destroy the involved kidney; (3) renal damage subsequent to repeated kidney stones; and (4) hypertension due to increased renin production by the obstructed kidney.

19. How do patients with renal stones present?
20. Why do renal stones form?
21. What are the common categories of renal stones (by composition)?

Table 11–17. Pathophysiology of bilateral ureteral obstruction.[1]

Hemodynamic Effects	Tubular Effects	Clinical Features
↑ Renal blood flow ↓ GFR ↓ Medullary blood flow ↑ Vasodilator prostaglandins	↑ Ureteral and tubular pressures ↑ Reabsorption of Na^+, urea, and water	Pain (capsule distention) Azotemia Oliguria
↓ Renal blood flow ↓ ↓ GFR ↑ Vasoconstrictor prostaglandins ↑ Renin-angiotensin production	↓ Medullary osmolality ↓ Concentrating ability Structural damage; parenchymal atrophy ↓ Transport functions for Na^+, K^+, H^+	Azotemia Hypertension ADH-insensitive polyuria Natriuresis Hyperkalemic, hyperchloremic acidosis
Slow ↑ in GFR (variable)	↓ Tubular pressure ↑ Solute load per nephron (urea, NaCl) Natriuretic factors present	Postobstructive diuresis Potential for volume depletion and electrolyte imbalance (↓ Na^+, K^+, PO_4^{3-}, Mg^{2+} excretion)

[1]Reproduced, with permission, from Brenner BM, Milford EL, Seifter JL: Urinary tract obstruction. In: *Harrison's Principles of Internal Medicine,* 12th ed. Wilson JD et al (editors). McGraw-Hill, 1991.

Table 11–18. Major causes of renal stones.[1]

Stone Type and Causes	All Stones (%)	Occurrence of Specific Causes[2]	M:F Ratio	Etiology	Diagnosis	Treatment[4]
Calcium stones	75–85%		2:1 to 3:1			
Idiopathic hypercalciuria		50–55%	2:1	Hereditary (?)	Normocalcemia, unexplained hypercalciuria[3]	Thiazide diuretic agents
Hyperuricosuria		20%	4:1	Diet	Urine uric acid >750 mg/24 h (women), >800 mg/24 h (men)	Allopurinol or diet
Primary hyperparathyroidism		5%	3:10	Neoplasia	Unexplained hypercalcemia	Surgery
Distal renal tubular acidosis		Rare	1:1	Hereditary	Hyperchloremic acidosis, minimum urine pH >5.5	Alkali replacement
Intestinal hyperoxaluria		≈1–2%	1:1	Bowel surgery	Urine oxalate >50 mg/24 h	Cholestyramine or oral calcium loading
Hereditary hyperoxaluria		Rare	1:1	Hereditary	Urine oxalate and glycolic or L-glyceric acid increased	Fluids and pyridoxine
Idiopathic stone disease		20%	2:1	Unknown	None of the above	Oral phosphate, fluids
Uric acid stones	5–8%					
Gout		≈50%	3:1 to 4:1	Hereditary	Clinical diagnosis	Alkali to raise urine pH
Idiopathic		≈50%	1:1	Hereditary (?)	Uric acid stones, no gout	Allopurinol if daily urine uric acid above 1000 mg
Dehydration		?	1:1	Intestinal, habit	History, intestinal fluid loss	Alkali, fluids, reversal of cause
Lesch-Nyhan syndrome		Rare	Men	Hereditary	Reduced hypoxanthine-guanine phosphoribosyl transferase level	Allopurinol
Malignant tumors		Rare	1:1	Neoplasia	Clinical diagnosis	Allopurinol
Cystine stones	1%		1:1	Hereditary	Stone type; elevated cystine excretion	Massive fluids, alkali, penicillamine if needed
Struvite stones	10–15%		2:10	Infection	Stone type	Antimicrobial agents and judicious surgery

[1]Reproduced, with permission, from Coe FL, Favus MJ: Nephrolithiasis. In: *Harrison's Principles of Internal Medicine,* 12th ed. Wilson JD et al (editors). McGraw-Hill, 1991.
[2]Values are percentages of patients within each category of stone who display each specific cause.
[3]Urine calcium above 300 mg/24 h (men), 250 mg/24 h (women), or 4 mg/kg/24 h either sex. Hyperthyroidism, Cushing's syndrome, sarcoidosis, malignant tumors, immobilization, vitamin D intoxication, rapidly progressive bone disease, and Paget's disease all cause hypercalciuria and must be excluded in diagnosis of idiopathic hypercalciuria.
[4]Besides fluids, which are a mainstay of therapy in all forms of stone disease.

REFERENCES

General

Rose BD: *Pathophysiology of Renal Disease,* 2nd ed. McGraw-Hill, 1987.

Rose BDF: *Clinical Physiology of Acid-Base Disorders,* 3rd ed. McGraw-Hill, 1989.

Klahr S, Schreiner G, Ichikawa I: The progression of renal disease. N Engl J Med 1988;318:1657.

Marsen TA et al: Renal actions of endothelin: Linking cellular signalling pathways to kidney disease. Kidney Int 1994; 45:336.

Acute Renal Failure

Anderson RJ: Prevention and management of acute renal failure. Hosp Pract (Off Ed) 1993;(Aug 15): 61.

Davidman M et al: Iatrogenic renal disease. Arch Intern Med 1991;151:1809.

Gurwitz JH et al: Nonsteroidal anti-inflammatory drug-associated azotemia in the very old. JAMA 1990; 264:471.

Turney JH: Acute renal failure: Some progress? N Engl J Med 1994;331:1372.

Chronic Renal Failure

Ihle BU et al: The effect of protein restriction on the progression of renal insufficiency. N Engl J Med 1989;321:1773.

Eschbach JW: The anemia of chronic renal failure: Pathophysiology and the effects of recombinant erythropoietin. Kidney Int 1989;35:134.

Seney FD Jr, Burns DK, Silva FG: AIDS and the kidney. Am J Kidney Dis 1990;16:1.

Glomerulonephritis and Nephrotic Syndrome

Bernard DB: Extrarenal complications of the nephrotic syndrome. Kidney Int 1988;33:1184.

Couser WG: New insights into mechanisms of immune glomerular injury. West J Med 1994;160:440.

Renal Stones

Coe FL, Parks JH: Pathophysiology of kidney stones and strategies for treatment. Hosp Pract (Off Ed) 1988;23:145.

Thyroid Disease

12

Stephen J. McPhee, MD

The thyroid gland synthesizes the hormones **thyroxine (T_4)** and **triiodothyronine (T_3),** iodine-containing amino acids that regulate the body's metabolic rate. Adequate levels of thyroid hormone are necessary in infants for normal development of the central nervous system; in children for normal skeletal growth and maturation; and in adults for normal function of multiple organ systems. Thyroid dysfunction is one of the most common disorders encountered in clinical practice. While abnormally high or low levels of thyroid hormones may be tolerated for long periods of time, usually there are symptoms and signs of thyroid dysfunction.

NORMAL STRUCTURE & FUNCTION

ANATOMY

The normal thyroid gland is a firm, reddish brown, smooth gland consisting of two lateral lobes and a connecting central isthmus (Figure 12–1). A pyramidal lobe of variable size may extend upward from the isthmus. The normal weight of the thyroid ranges from 30 g to 40 g. The gland is surrounded by an adherent fibrous capsule from which multiple fibrous projections extend deeply into its structure, dividing it into many small lobules. The thyroid is highly vascular and has one of the highest rates of blood flow per gram of tissue of any organ.

HISTOLOGY

Histologically, the thyroid gland consists of many closely packed acini, called **follicles,** each surrounded by capillaries and stroma. Each follicle is roughly spherical, lined by a single layer of cuboidal epithelial cells, and filled with **colloid,** a proteinaceous material composed mainly of **thyroglobulin** and stored thyroid hormones. When the gland is inactive, the follicles are large, the lining cells are flat, and the colloid is abundant. When the gland is active, the follicles are small, the lining cells are cuboidal or columnar, the colloid is scanty, and its edges are scalloped, forming **"reabsorption lacunae"** (Figure 12–2). Scattered between follicles are the **parafollicular cells (C cells),** which secrete **calcitonin,** a hormone that inhibits bone resorption and lowers the plasma calcium level (see Chapter 17).

The ultrastructure of a follicular epithelial cell is diagrammed in Figure 12–3. The cells vary in appearance with the degree of gland activity. The follicular cell rests on a basal lamina. The nucleus is round and centrally located. The cytoplasm contains mitochondria, rough endoplasmic reticulum, and ribosomes. The apex has a discrete Golgi apparatus, small secretory granules containing colloid, and abundant lysosomes and phagosomes. At the apex, the cell membrane is folded into microvilli.

PHYSIOLOGY

Formation & Secretion of Thyroid Hormones

A. T4, T3, Thyroglobulin: Thyroid follicular cells have three functions: (1) to collect and transport iodine to the colloid; (2) to synthesize **thyroglobulin,** a glycoprotein (MW 660,000) made up of two subunits and containing many tyrosine residues, and secrete it into the colloid; and (3) to release thyroid hormones from thyroglobulin and secrete them into the circulation. The structures of the two thyroid hormones, T_3 and T_4, are shown in Figure 12–4. T_3 and T_4 are synthesized in the colloid by iodination and condensation of tyrosine molecules bound together in thyroglobulin.

B. Iodine Metabolism and Trapping: For normal thyroid hormone synthesis, an adult requires a minimum daily intake of 150 μg of iodine. In the USA, the average intake is about 500 μg/d. Iodine ingested in food is first converted to **iodide,** which is absorbed and taken up by the thyroid. The follicular cells actively transport iodide from the circulation to the colloid ("iodide trapping," or "iodide pump").

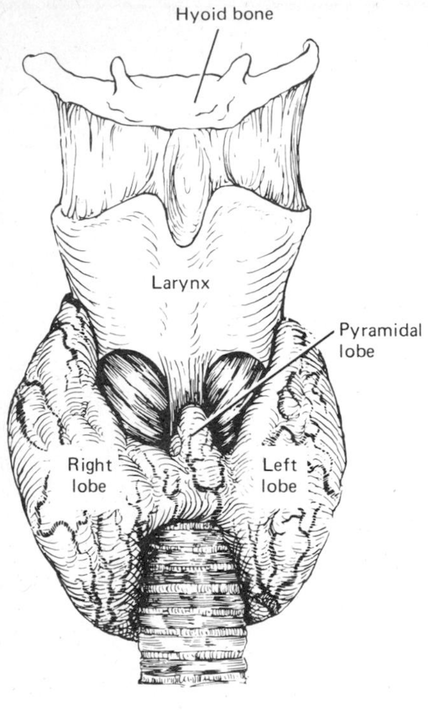

Figure 12–1. The human thyroid. (Reproduced, with permission, from Ganong WF: *Review of Medical Physiology,* 16th ed. Appleton & Lange, 1993.)

This active transport mechanism depends on Na^+-K^+ ATPase for energy; it is stimulated by thyroid-stimulating hormone (TSH). At the normal rate of thyroid hormone synthesis, about 120 μg/d of iodide enters the thyroid. About 80 μg/d is secreted in T_3 and T_4 and the rest diffuses into the extracellular fluid and is excreted in the urine.

C. Thyroid Hormone Synthesis and Secretion: Thyroid hormones are synthesized in the colloid, near the apical cell membrane of the follicular cells. Catalyzed by the enzyme thyroidal peroxidase, iodide in the thyroid cell is oxidized to iodine. The iodine enters the colloid and is rapidly bound (at the 3 position) to tyrosine molecules attached to thyroglobulin, forming **monoiodotyrosine (MIT).** MIT is next iodinated (at the 5 position) to form **diiodotyrosine (DIT).** Two DIT molecules then condense in an oxidative process ("coupling reaction") to form one **thyroxine (T_4)** molecule. **T_3** is probably formed by condensation of MIT with DIT. Figure 12–4 shows the structures of MIT, DIT, T_4, and T_3. In the normal thyroid, the average distribution of iodinated compounds is 23% MIT, 33% DIT, 35% T_4, and 7% T_3. Reverse T_3, formed by 5-deiodination of the inner ring of T_4, is metabolically inert.

The thyroid secretes about 80 μg (103 nmol) of T_4 and 4 μg (7 nmol) of T_3 per day. Upon stimulation by TSH, the folds of the apical cell membrane (lamellipodia) encircle some colloid and bring it into the cytoplasm by endocytosis, forming **endosomes.** The latter fuse with lysosomes containing proteases that break peptide bonds between the iodinated residues and thyroglobulin, releasing T_4, T_3, DIT, and MIT into the cytoplasm. The free T_4 and T_3 then cross the cell membrane and enter adjacent capillaries. The MIT and DIT are enzymatically degraded in the cell by thyroid deiodinase (iodotyrosine dehalogenase) to iodine and tyrosine, which are reused in colloid synthesis.

D. Thyroid Hormone Transport and Metabolism: The normal plasma level of T_4 is approximately 8 μg/dL (103 nmol/L) (range: 5–12 μg/dL or 65–156 nmol/L), and the normal plasma level of T_3 is approximately 0.15 μg/dL (2.3 nmol/L) (range: 0.08–0.22 μg/dL or 1.2–3.3 nmol/L). Both hormones are bound to plasma proteins, including albumin, **transthyretin** (formerly called thyroxine-binding prealbumin [TBPA], and **thyroxine-binding globulin (TBG).** The thyroid hormone-binding proteins serve mainly to transport T_4 and T_3 in the serum and to facilitate uniform distribution of hormones within tissues.

Physiologically, it is the free (unbound) T_4 and T_3 in plasma which are active and which inhibit pituitary secretion of TSH. The free T_4 and T_3 are in equilibrium with the protein-bound hormones in plasma and tissue. Tissue uptake of the free hormones is proportionate to their plasma concentrations.

Almost all (99.98%) of the circulating T_4 is bound to TBG (thyroxine-binding globulin) and other plasma proteins, so that the free T_4 level is approximately 2 ng/dL and the biologic half-life of T_4 is long (about 6–7 days). Somewhat less T_3 (99.8%) is protein-bound, so a somewhat larger percentage of the T_3 is free. Because of this, the half-life of T_3 is shorter (about 30 hours), T_3 acts more rapidly than T_4, and T_3 is three to five times more potent on a molar basis than T_4.

T_4 and T_3 are metabolized in the liver, the kidneys, and many other tissues by deiodination and by conjugation to **glucuronides**. Normally, one-third of circulating T_4 is deiodinated to T_3, and 45% is converted to the inactive **reverse triiodothyronine (RT_3).** About 87% of circulating T_3 derives from peripheral conversion of T_4 to T_3 and only 13% from thyroid secretion. Both T_4 and T_3 are conjugated to glucuronides in the liver and excreted into the bile. Upon passage into the intestine, the conjugates are hydrolyzed, and some T_4 and T_3 are reabsorbed (enterohepatic circulation) and some are excreted in the stool.

Regulation of Thyroid Secretion

Thyroid hormone secretion is stimulated by pituitary **thyroid-stimulating hormone (TSH, thyrotropin).** Pituitary TSH secretion is in turn stimulated by **thyrotropin-releasing hormone (TRH),** a

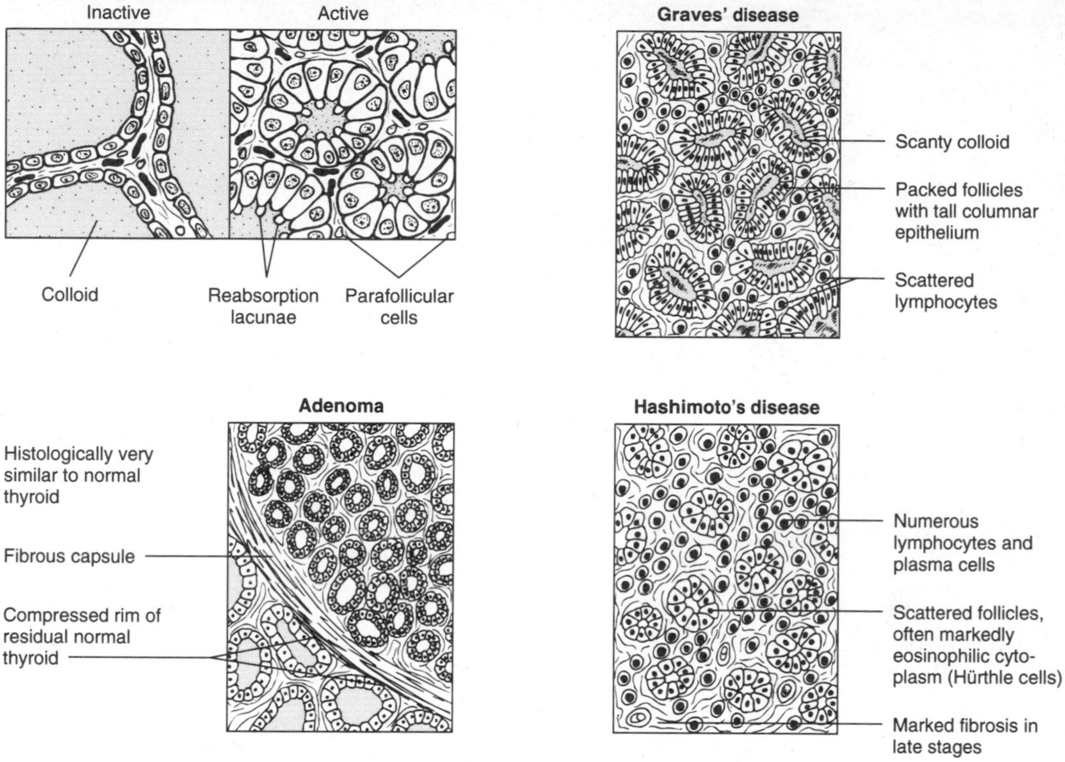

Figure 12–2. Normal and abnormal thyroid histology. (Reproduced, with permission, from Ganong WF: *Review of Medical Physiology,* 16th ed. Appleton & Lange, 1993; from Chandrasoma P, Taylor CE: *Concise Pathology,* 2nd ed. Appleton & Lange, 1994; and from Greenspan FS, Baxter JD: *Basic and Clinical Endocrinology,* 4th ed. Appleton & Lange, 1994.)

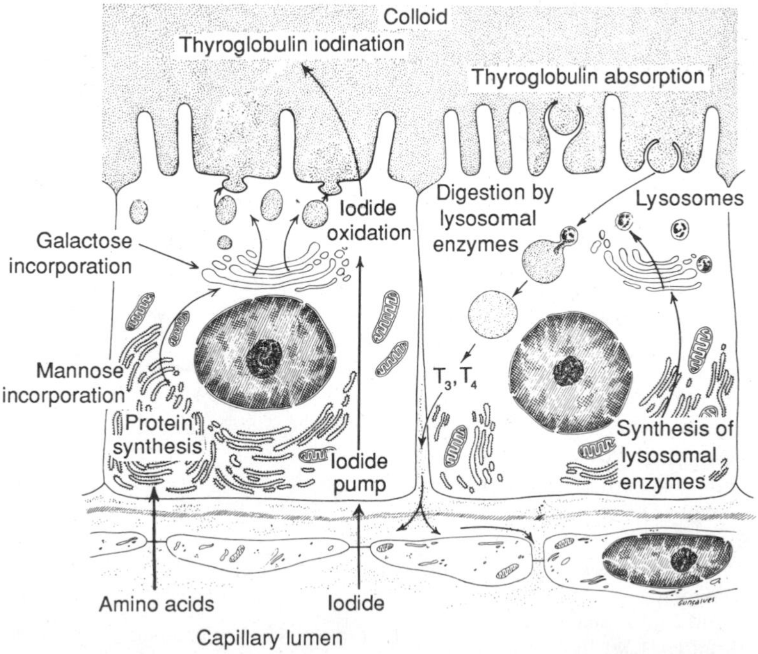

Figure 12–3. Thyroid cell ultrastructure (schematic). The processes of synthesis and iodination of thyroglobulin are shown on the left and its reabsorption and digestion on the right. (Reproduced, with permission, from Junqueira LC, Carneiro J, Kelley R: *Basic Histology,* 7th ed. Appleton & Lange, 1992.)

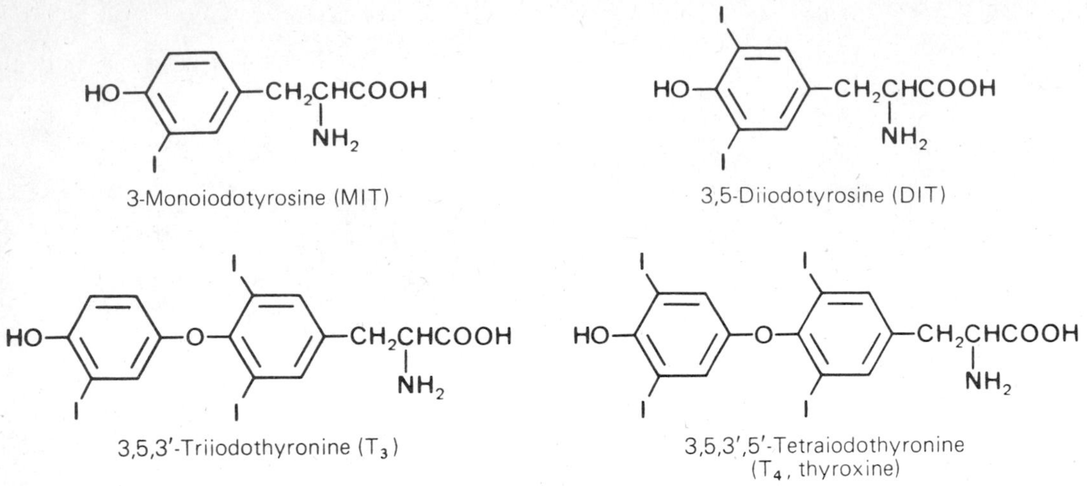

Figure 12–4. MIT, DIT, T_3, and T_4. RT_3 is 3,3′,5′-triiodothyronine. (Reproduced, with permission, from Junqueira LC, Carneiro J, Kelley R: *Basic Histology,* 7th ed. Appleton & Lange, 1992.)

tripeptide secreted by the hypothalamus that also increases the biologic activity of TSH, apparently by altering its glycosylation.

TSH is a two-subunit glycoprotein containing 211 amino acids. The alpha subunit is identical to that of pituitary follicle-stimulating hormone (FSH) and luteinizing hormone (LH) and placental human chorionic gonadotropin (hCG). The beta subunit confers the specific binding properties and biologic activity of TSH. The gene encoding for the alpha subunit is located on chromosome 6, and the gene for the beta subunit is on chromosome 1.

TSH has a biologic half-life of about 60 minutes. The average plasma level of TSH is 2 μU/mL (normal range: 0.4–4.8 μU/mL). Normal TSH secretion exhibits a circadian pattern, rising in the afternoon and evening, peaking after midnight, and declining during the day.

Circulating free T_4 and T_3 inhibit TSH secretion by the pituitary both directly and indirectly, by regulating biosynthesis of TRH in the hypothalamus. TSH secretion is inhibited by stress, perhaps via glucocorticoid inhibition of TRH secretion. In infants—but not in adults—TSH secretion is increased by cold and inhibited by warmth. Dopamine and somatostatin inhibit pituitary secretion of TSH experimentally, but whether they do so physiologically is unknown. In animals, there is a pituitary-specific form of the thyroid hormone receptor that may be selectively regulated by thyroid hormone. Figure 12–5 illustrates the hypothalamic-pituitary-thyroid axis and various stimulatory and inhibitory factors.

When TSH is secreted or administered, it binds to a specific **TSH receptor (TSH-R)** in the thyroid cell membrane, activating the GTP-binding (G_s) protein-adenylyl cyclase-cAMP cascades. The increase in intracellular cAMP mediates immediate increases in uptake and transport of iodide, iodination of thyroglobulin, and synthesis of iodotyrosines, T_3 and T_4. Within a few hours, there is an increase in mRNA for thyroglobulin and thyroidal peroxidase, enhanced lysosomal activity, increased secretion of thyroglob-

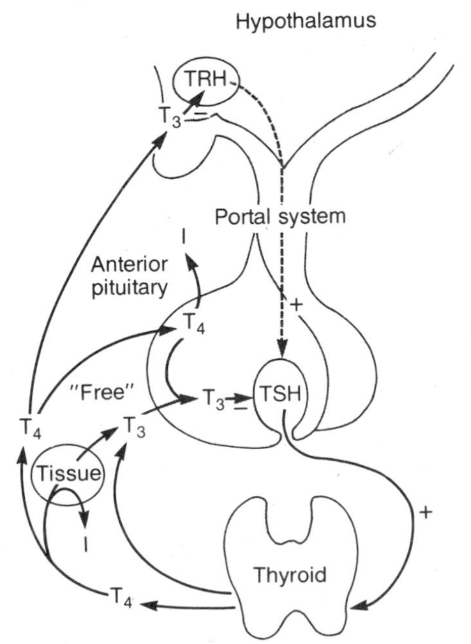

Figure 12–5. Hypothalamic-pituitary-thyroid axis. (Reproduced, with permission, from Greenspan FS: The thyroid. In: *Basic and Clinical Endocrinology,* 4th ed. Greenspan FS, Baxter JD [editors]. Appleton & Lange, 1994.)

ulin into colloid, more endocytosis of colloid, and increased secretion of T_4 and T_3 from the gland.

TSH binding to TSH-R also stimulates membrane phospholipase C, which leads to thyroid cell hypertrophy. With chronic TSH stimulation, the entire gland hypertrophies, increases in vascularity and becomes a **goiter.**

The TSH receptor (TSH-R) has been cloned. It is a single-chain glycoprotein composed of 744 amino acids. Two specific amino acid sequences are thought to represent different binding sites for TSH and for the **TSH receptor-stimulating antibody (TSH-R [stim] Ab)** found in Graves' disease (see below).

The amount of thyroid hormone needed to maintain normal organ system function in thyroidectomized individuals is defined as the amount necessary to maintain the plasma TSH within the normal range (0.5–5.0 μU/mL). About 80% of orally administered levothyroxine is absorbed from the gastrointestinal tract, and 100–150 μg/d usually maintains a normal plasma TSH.

Mechanism of Action of Thyroid Hormones

Thyroid hormones enter cells either by passive diffusion or specific transport through the cell membrane and cytoplasm. Within the cell cytoplasm, T_4 is converted to T_3. The nuclear receptor for T_3 has been cloned and found to be similar to the nuclear receptors for glucocorticoids, mineralocorticoids, estrogens, progestins, vitamin D_3, and retinoic acid. For reasons that are presently unclear, at least two different T_3 receptors, coded by different genes, exist in human tissues. The two biologically active human thyroid hormone receptors (hTR) are labeled hTR-α1 and hTR-β1. The gene for the alpha form is on chromosome 17 and that for the beta form is on chromosome 3. The two different receptor forms may help to explain both the normal variation in thyroid hormone responsiveness of various organs and the selective tissue abnormalities found in various thyroid resistance syndromes. Point mutations in the hTR-β1 gene result in abnormal T_3 receptors and the syndrome of **generalized resistance to thyroid hormone (Refetoff's syndrome).**

When the T_3-receptor complex binds to DNA, it increases expression of specific genes, with the induction of messenger RNAs. A wide variety of enzymes must be produced to account for the many effects of thyroid hormones on cell function.

Effects of Thyroid Hormones

The effects of thyroid hormones in various organs are summarized in Table 12–1. Thyroid hormones increase the activity of membrane-bound Na^+-K^+ ATPase, and increase heat production, and stimulate oxygen consumption ("calorigenesis"). Thyroid hormones also affect tissue growth and maturation, help regulate lipid metabolism, and increase intestinal absorption of carbohydrates.

The effects of T_4 and T_3 and of the catecholamines epinephrine and norepinephrine are closely interrelated. Both increase the metabolic rate and stimulate the nervous system and heart. In humans, the transcriptional effects of T_3 include production of increased β-adrenergic receptors, and in animals, incubation of thyroid cells in a medium containing TSH increases the number of α_1-adrenergic receptors, presumably by inducing their biosynthesis.

OVERVIEW OF THYROID DISEASE

The symptoms and signs of thyroid disease in humans are predictable consequences of the physiologic effects of thyroid hormones discussed above. The clinician commonly encounters patients with one of five types of thyroid dysfunction: (1) **hyperthyroidism** (thyrotoxicosis), caused by an excess of thyroid hormone; (2) **hypothyroidism** (myxedema), caused by a deficiency of thyroid hormone; (3) **goiter,** a diffuse enlargement of the thyroid gland, caused by prolonged elevation of TSH; (4) **thyroid nodule,** a focal enlargement of a portion of the gland, caused by a benign or malignant neoplasm; and (5) **abnormal thyroid function tests in a clinically euthyroid patient,** caused by alterations in transport or metabolism of thyroid hormone.

Several laboratory tests are useful in the initial evaluation of patients suspected of thyroid dysfunction. The first is the **free thyroxine index (FT_4I),** the product of the total plasma T_4 (TT_4) and the T_4 resin uptake (RT_4U) ($FT_4I = TT_4 \times RT_4U$). The TT_4 by itself often reflects the functional state of the thyroid, but it may be misleading when there are alterations in hormone-binding proteins. The RT_4U is an indicator of thyroid-binding globulin level and serves to correct for such alterations. Some laboratories measure T_3 resin uptake (RT_3U).

The second is the plasma TSH level, which is below normal in hyperthyroidism and above normal in hypothyroidism (except in pituitary or hypothalamic disease).

Finally, a variety of thyroid autoantibodies are detectable in thyroid dysfunction, including (1) **thyroglobulin antibody (Tg Ab);** (2) **thyroidal peroxidase antibody (TPO Ab),** formerly termed antimicrosomal antibody; and (3) **TSH receptor antibody,** either **stimulating (TSH-R [stim] Ab)** or **blocking (TSH-R [block] Ab).** Thyroglobulin and thyroidal peroxidase antibodies are found in both hypothyroidism due to Hashimoto's thyroiditis and hyperthyroidism due to Graves' disease (see below).

Table 12–1. Physiologic effects of thyroid hormones.

Target Tissue	Effect	Mechanism
Heart	Chronotropic	Increase number and affinity of beta-adrenergic receptors.
	Inotropic	Enhance responses to circulating catecholamines. Increase proportion of alpha myosin heavy chain (with higher ATPase activity).
Adipose tissue	Catabolic	Stimulate lipolysis.
Muscle	Catabolic	Increase protein breakdown.
Bone	Developmental	Promote normal growth and skeletal development.
Nervous system	Developmental	Promote normal brain development.
Gut	Metabolic	Increase rate of carbohydrate absorption.
Lipoprotein	Metabolic	Stimulate formation of LDL receptors.
Other	Calorigenic	Stimulate oxygen consumption by metabolically active tissues (exceptions: adult brain, testes, uterus, lymph nodes, spleen, anterior pituitary). Increase metabolic rate.

TSH-R [stim] Ab is characteristic of hyperthyroidism due to Graves' disease. Detection of TSH-R [block] Ab in maternal serum is predictive of congenital hypothyroidism in newborns of mothers with autoimmune thyroid disease.

Other tests such as the radioactive iodine uptake (RAIU) and thyrotropin-releasing hormone (TRH) test are discussed below.

1. Describe a thyroid follicle and its change with activity versus inactivity of the gland.
2. What forms of thyroid hormone does the thyroid gland secrete? In what amounts each day? What are the normal proportions of the different forms?
3. To what is thyroid hormone bound during its transport in plasma?
4. How are thyroid hormone levels regulated?
5. What is the mechanism of action of thyroid hormone?
6. What are the most prominent organ system-specific effects of thyroid hormone?

PATHOPHYSIOLOGY OF SELECTED THYROID DISEASES

The pathogenesis of most thyroid diseases probably involves an autoimmune process with sensitization of the host's own lymphocytes to various thyroidal antigens. Three major thyroidal antigens have been documented: thyroglobulin (Tg), thyroidal peroxidase (TPO), and the TSH receptor (TSH-R). Both environmental factors (eg, viral or bacterial infection or high iodine intake) and genetic factors (eg, defect in suppressor T lymphocytes) may be responsible for initiating autoimmune thyroid disease.

HYPERTHYROIDISM

Etiology

The causes of hyperthyroidism are listed in Table 12–2. Most commonly, thyroid hormone overproduction is due to Graves' disease. In Graves' disease, the TSH receptor autoantibody TSH-R [stim] Ab stimulates the thyroid follicular cells to produce excessive amounts of T_4 and T_3. Less commonly, patients with multinodular goiter may become thyrotoxic if given inorganic iodine (eg, potassium iodide) or organic iodine compounds (eg, the antiarrhythmic drug amiodarone, which contains 37% iodine by weight). Patients from regions of endemic goiter may develop thyrotoxicosis when given iodine supplementation (jodbasedow phenomenon). Large follicular adenomas (> 3 cm in diameter) may produce excessive thyroid hormone.

Occasionally, TSH overproduction (eg, from a pituitary adenoma) may cause excessive thyroid hormone production. The diagnosis is suggested by clinically evident hyperthyroidism with *elevated* serum TSH levels that fail to increase after TRH administration. Neuroradiologic procedures such as CT scans or MRI of the sella turcica confirm the presence of a pituitary tumor. Even more rarely, hyperthyroidism results from TSH overproduction due to pituitary (but not peripheral tissue) resistance to the suppressive effects of T_4 and T_3. The diagnosis is suggested by finding elevated serum T_4 and T_3 levels with an inappropriately normal serum TSH level.

Hypothalamic disease, resulting in excessive TRH production, is also quite rare. The diagnosis should be suspected when serum T_4 and T_3 are elevated with a paradoxically elevated serum TSH.

Table 12–2. Hyperthyroidism: Causes and pathogenetic mechanisms.

Etiologic Classification	Pathogenetic Mechanism
A. Thyroid hormone overproduction	
1. Graves' disease	Thyroid stimulating hormone receptor-stimulating antibody (TSH-R [stim])
2. Toxic multinodular goiter	Autonomous hyperfunction
3. Follicular adenoma	Autonomous hyperfunction
4. Pituitary adenoma	TSH hypersecretion (rare)
5. Pituitary insensitivity	Resistance to thyroid hormone (rare)
6. Hypothalamic disease	Excess TRH production (rare)
7. Germ cell tumors: choriocarcinoma, hydatidiform mole	hCG stimulation
8. Struma ovarii (ovarian teratoma)	Functioning thyroid elements
9. Metastatic follicular thyroid carcinoma	Functioning metastases
B. Thyroid gland destruction	
1. Lymphocytic thyroiditis	Release of stored hormone
2. Granulomatous (subacute) thyroiditis	Release of stored hormone
3. Hashimoto's thyroiditis	Transient release of stored hormone
C. Other	
1. Thyrotoxicosis medicamentosa, thyrotoxicosis factitia	Ingestion of excessive exogenous thyroid hormone

Hyperthyroidism may be precipitated by germ cell tumors (choriocarcinoma and hydatidiform mole), which secrete large quantities of human chorionic gonadotropin (hCG). The large quantities of hCG secreted by these tumors bind to the follicular cell TSH receptor and stimulate overproduction of thyroid hormone. Rarely, hyperthyroidism can be produced by ovarian teratomas containing thyroid elements (struma ovarii). Patients with large metastases from follicular thyroid carcinomas may produce excess thyroid hormone, particularly following iodide administration.

Transient hyperthyroidism is occasionally observed in patients with lymphocytic granulomatous (subacute) thyroiditis (Hashimoto's thyroiditis). In such cases, the hyperthyroidism is due to destruction of the thyroid with release of stored hormone.

Finally, patients who consume excessive amounts of exogenous thyroid hormone (accidentally or deliberately) may present with symptoms, signs, and laboratory findings of hyperthyroidism.

Pathogenesis

Whatever the cause of hyperthyroidism, serum thyroid hormones are elevated. The free T_3 index is elevated. The free thyroxine index (FT_4I) is also typically elevated, but in about 5–10% of patients, T_4 secretion is normal while T_3 levels are high (so-called **T_3 toxicosis**). Total serum T_4 and T_3 levels are not always reliable because of variations in concentrations of thyroid-hormone binding proteins.

Hyperthyroidism due to Graves' disease is characterized by a suppressed serum TSH level as determined by sensitive immunoenzymometric or immunoradiometric assays. However, TSH levels may also be suppressed in some psychiatric and other nonthyroidal illnesses. In the rare TSH-secreting pituitary adenomas (so-called **secondary hyperthyroidism**) and in hypothalamic disease with excessive TRH production (so-called **tertiary hyperthyroidism**), hyperthyroidism is accompanied by TSH elevations.

The radioactive iodine (RAI) uptake of the thyroid gland at 4, 6, or 24 hours is increased when the gland produces an excess of hormone (eg, Graves' disease); it is decreased when the gland is leaking stored hormone (eg, painless thyroiditis), when hormone is produced elsewhere (eg, struma ovarii), or when excessive exogenous thyroid hormone is being ingested (eg, factitious hyperthyroidism).

The TRH test is sometimes helpful in diagnosis of patients who appear hyperthyroid but have high-normal serum T_4 and T_3 levels. In normal individuals, administration of TRH (500 μg intravenously) produces an increase in serum TSH of at least 6 mU/L within 15–30 minutes. In hyperthyroid individuals, TSH secretion is suppressed and TRH administration fails to induce a rise in the TSH level (Figure 12–6).

Graves' Disease

A. Pathology: Graves' disease is the most common cause of hyperthyroidism. In this condition, the thyroid gland is symmetrically enlarged and its vascularity markedly increased. The gland may double or triple in weight. Microscopically, the follicular epithelial cells are columnar in appearance and increased in number and size. The follicles are small and closely packed together. The colloid is scanty, with the edges scalloped in appearance secondary to the rapid proteolysis of thyroglobulin. The gland's interstitium is diffusely infiltrated with lymphocytes and may contain lymphoid follicles with germinal centers.

B. Pathogenesis: The serum of patients with Graves' disease contains TSH-R [stim] Ab, an antibody directed against the TSH receptor site in the

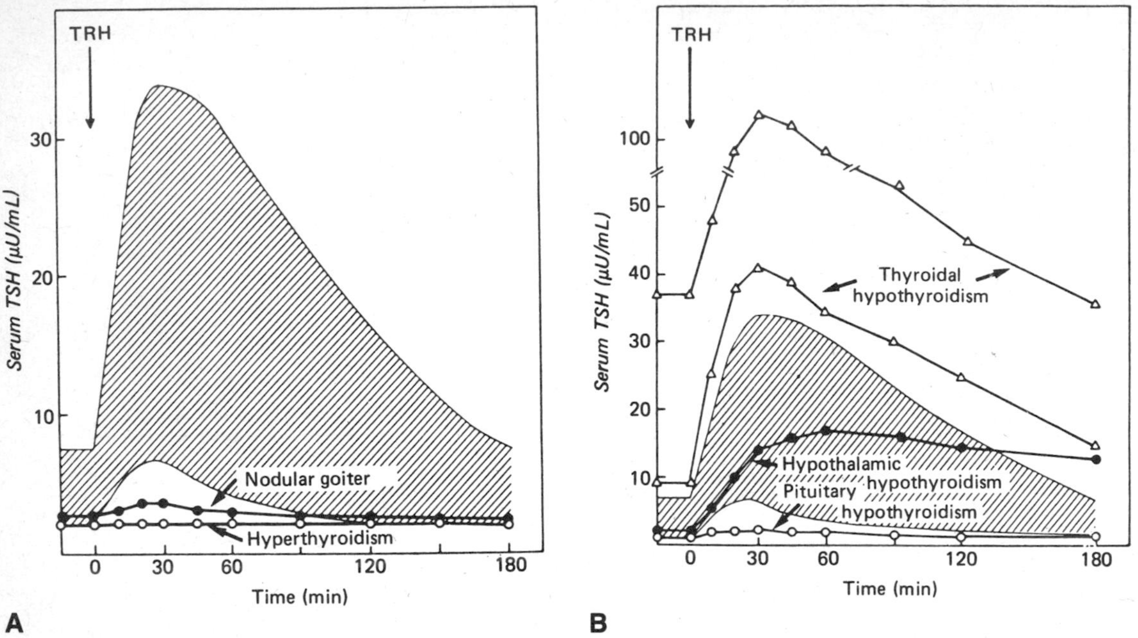

Figure 12–6. TRH stimulation test in euthyroid (shaded), hyperthyroid (***A***), and hypothyroid patients (***B***). (Reproduced, with permission, from Utiger RO: Tests of the hypothalamic-pituitary-thyroid axis. In: *The Thyroid,* 4th ed. Werner SC, Ingbar SH [editors]. Harper & Row, 1978.)

thyroid follicular epithelial membrane. This antibody was formerly called long-acting thyroid stimulator (LATS) or thyroid-stimulating immunoglobulin (TSI). When it binds to the cell membrane TSH receptors, TSH-R [stim] Ab stimulates hormone synthesis and secretion in a manner analagous to TSH. While serum levels of TSH-R [stim] Ab correlate only roughly (if at all) with disease severity, its presence can be helpful diagnostically, and its disappearance can be helpful in deciding when antithyroid drug therapy can be withdrawn without precipitating a relapse.

The genesis of TSH-R [stim] Ab in patients with Graves' disease is uncertain. However, Graves' disease is familial. In Caucasians, it is associated with the HLA-B8 and HLA-DR3 histocompatibility antigens; in Asians, with HLA-Bw46 and HLA-B5; and in blacks, with HLA-B17. Furthermore, patients with Graves' disease frequently suffer from other autoimmune disorders (Table 12–3). The precipitating cause of this antibody production is unknown. One theory of the pathogenesis of Graves' disease is a defect of suppressor T lymphocytes, which allows helper T lymphocytes to stimulate B lymphocytes to secrete antibodies directed against follicular cell membrane antigens, including the TSH receptor (Figure 12–7).

A second group of autoantibodies has been identified that stimulate the growth of thyroid epithelial cells and produce the goiter of Graves' disease. In rats, this thyroid growth-promoting IgG and TSH-receptor antibody appear to be identical.

Finally, moderate titers of other autoantibodies (thyroidal peroxidase antibody and TSH-R [block] Ab) can be found in patients with Graves' disease. Their significance is uncertain. In some cases, TSH-R [block] Ab) appears following ^{131}I radioiodine therapy of Graves' disease.

Patients with hyperthyroidism from Graves' disease may later develop hypothyroidism by one of several mechanisms: (1) thyroid ablation by surgery or ^{131}I radiation treatment; (2) autoimmune thyroiditis, leading to thyroid destruction; and (3) development of antibodies that block TSH stimulation (TSH-R [block] Ab).

7. What are the five categories of thyroid dysfunction most commonly observed in patients?
8. What are seven different physiologic mechanisms by which a patient might develop hyperthyroidism?
9. What are the most useful initial tests of thyroid function in hyperthyroidism? What results would you expect compared to normal?
10. How can a radioactive iodine scan help make the diagnosis of hyperthyroidism?
11. Describe the mechanism of hyperthyroidism in Graves' disease?

Table 12–3. Autoimmune disorders associated with Graves' disease and Hashimoto's thyroiditis.

A. Endocrine disorders
Diabetes mellitus
Hypoadrenalism, autoimmune (Addison's disease)
Orchitis or oophoritis, autoimmune
Hypoparathyroidism, idiopathic
B. Nonendocrine disorders
Pernicious anemia
Vitiligo
Systemic lupus erythematosus
Rheumatoid arthritis
Immune thrombocytopenic purpura
Myasthenia gravis
Sjögren's syndrome
Primary biliary cirrhosis
Chronic active hepatitis

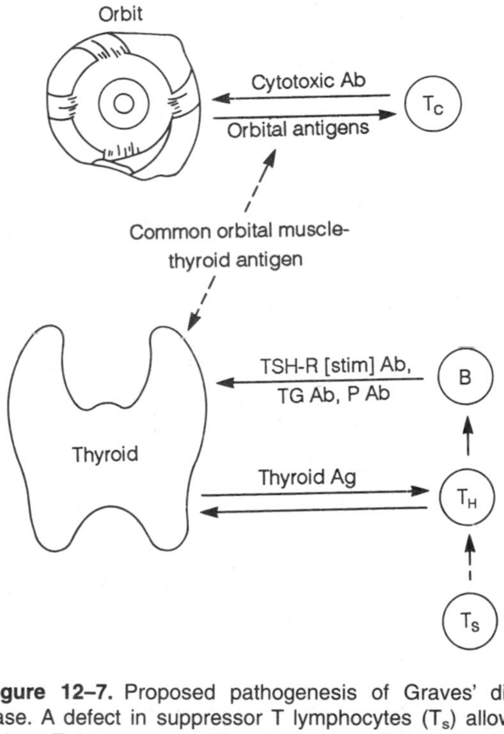

Figure 12–7. Proposed pathogenesis of Graves' disease. A defect in suppressor T lymphocytes (T_S) allows helper T lymphocytes (T_H to stimulate B lymphocytes (B) to synthesize thyroid autoantibodies. The thyroid receptor-stimulating antibody (TSH-R [stim] Ab) is the driving force for thyrotoxicosis. Inflammation of the orbital muscles may be due to sensitization of cytotoxic T lymphocytes (T_C), or killer cells, to orbital antigens linked to an antigen in the thyroid. What triggers this immunologic cascade is not known. (Tg Ab, thyroglobulin antibody; P Ab, peroxidase or microsomal antibody; Ag, antigen; Ab, antibody.) (Reproduced, with permission, from Greenspan FS, Baxter JD: *Basic and Clinical Endocrinology,* 4th ed. Appleton & Lange, 1994.)

Clinical Manifestations

The clinical consequences of thyroid hormone excess (Table 12–4) are exaggerated expressions of the physiologic activity of T_3 and T_4.

An excess of thyroid hormone causes enough extra heat production to result in a slight rise in body temperature and to activate heat-dissipating mechanisms, including cutaneous vasodilation and a decrease in peripheral vascular resistance and increased sweating. The increased basal metabolic rate leads to weight loss, especially in older patients with poor appetite. In younger patients, food intake typically increases, and some patients have seemingly insatiable appetites.

The apparent increased catecholamine effect of hyperthyroidism is probably multifactorial in origin. Thyroid hormones increase beta-adrenergic receptors in many tissues, including heart muscle, skeletal muscle, adipose tissue, and lymphocytes. They also decrease alpha-adrenergic receptors in heart muscle and may amplify catecholamine action at a postreceptor site. Thus, thyrotoxicosis is characterized by an increased metabolic and hemodynamic sensitivity of the tissues to catecholamines. However, circulating catecholamine levels are normal. Drugs that block beta-adrenergic receptors (eg, propranolol) and sympathectomy reduce or eliminate the tachycardia, arrhythmias, sweating, and tremor of hyperthyroidism.

Thyroid hormone excess causes rapid mentation, nervousness, irritability, emotional lability, restlessness, and even mania and psychosis. Patients complain of poor concentration and reduced performance at work or in school. Tremor is common and deep tendon reflexes are brisk, with a rapid relaxation

Table 12–4. Clinical findings in hyperthyroidism (thyrotoxicosis).

Symptoms
1. Alertness, emotional lability, nervousness, irritability
2. Poor concentration
3. Muscular weakness, fatigability
4. Palpitations
5. Voracious appetite, weight loss
6. Hyperdefecation (increased frequency of bowel movements)
7. Heat intolerance
Signs
1. Hyperkinesia, rapid speech
2. Proximal muscle (quadriceps) weakness, fine tremor
3. Fine, moist skin; fine, abundant hair; onycholysis
4. Lid lag, stare, chemosis, periorbital edema, proptosis
5. Accentuated first heart sound, tachycardia, atrial fibrillation (resistant to digitalis), widened pulse pressure, dyspnea
Laboratory findings
1. Elevated serum total T_4, elevated resin T_3 or T_4 uptake, elevated free thyroxine index
2. Suppressed serum TSH level
3. Increased radioiodine uptake by thyroid gland (some causes)
4. Increased basal metabolic rate (BMR)
5. Decreased serum cholesterol level

phase. Muscle weakness and atrophy (**thyrotoxic myopathy**) commonly develops in hyperthyroidism, particularly if severe and prolonged. Proximal muscle weakness may interfere with walking, climbing, rising from a deep knee bend, or weight lifting. Such muscle weakness may be due to increased protein catabolism and muscle wasting, to decreased muscle efficiency, or to changes in myosin. Despite an increased number of beta-adrenergic receptors in muscle, the increased proteolysis is apparently not mediated by beta receptors, and muscle weakness and wasting are not affected by beta-adrenergic blockers. Myasthenia gravis or periodic paralysis may accompany hyperthyroidism.

Vital capacity and respiratory muscle strength are reduced. Extreme muscle weakness may cause respiratory failure.

Cardiac output is increased, peripheral vascular resistance is lower, heart rate is increased, pulse pressure is increased, and circulation time is shortened in the hyperthyroid state. Tachycardia, usually supraventricular, is frequent and thought to be related to the direct effects of thyroid hormone on the cardiac conducting system. Atrial fibrillation may occur, particularly in elderly patients. Continuous 24-hour electrocardiographic monitoring of thyrotoxic patients shows persistent tachycardia but preservation of the normal circadian rhythm of the heart rate, suggesting that normal adrenergic responsiveness persists. Myocardial calcium uptake is increased in thyrotoxic rats; in humans, calcium channel-blocking agents (eg, diltiazem) can decrease the heart rate, the number of premature ventricular beats, and the number of bouts of supraventricular tachycardia, paroxysmal atrial fibrillation, and ventricular tachycardia. Long-standing hyperthyroidism may lead to cardiomegaly and a "high-output" congestive heart failure. Flow murmurs are common and extracardiac sounds occur, generated by the hyperdynamic heart.

Hyperthyroidism leads to increased hepatic gluconeogenesis, enhanced carbohydrate absorption, and increased insulin degradation. In nondiabetic patients, after ingestion of carbohydrate, the blood glucose rises rapidly, sometimes causing glycosuria, then falls rapidly. There may be an adaptive increase in insulin secretion, perhaps explaining the normal glycemic, glycogenolytic, glycolytic, and ketogenic sensitivity to epinephrine. Diabetic patients have an increased insulin requirement in the hyperthyroid state.

Metabolically, the total plasma cholesterol is usually low, related to an increase in the number of hepatic LDL receptors. Lipolysis is increased, and adipocytes show an increase in beta-adrenergic receptor density and increased responsiveness to catecholamines. With the rise in metabolic rate, there is an increased need for vitamins; if dietary sources are inadequate, vitamin deficiency syndromes may occur. Bone resorption exceeds bone formation in hyperthyroidism, leading to hypercalciuria and sometimes hypercalcemia. Long-standing hyperthyroidism may lead to osteopenia.

There is an increase in frequency of bowel movements (hyperdefecation) due to more rapid gastrointestinal motility. Accelerated small bowel transit may be caused by increased frequency of bowel contractions and of giant migrating contractions. In severe thyrotoxicosis, abnormal liver function tests may be observed, reflecting malnutrition.

In women, hyperthyroidism may lead to oligomenorrhea and decreased fertility. In the follicular phase of the menstrual cycle, there is also an increased basal plasma LH and an increased LH and FSH response to GnRH (Chapter 19). There is also an increase in sex hormone-binding globulin, leading to increased levels of total estradiol. In men, hyperthyroidism may cause decreased fertility and impotence from altered steroid hormone metabolism. Serum levels of total testosterone, total estradiol, sex hormone-binding globulin, LH, and FSH and gonadotropin response to GnRH are significantly greater than normal. However, the ratio of free testosterone to free estradiol is lower than normal. Mean sperm counts are normal, but the percentage of forward progressive sperm motility is lower than normal (Chapter 20). These hormone and semen abnormalities are reversible with successful treatment of the hyperthyroidism. Gynecomastia may occur despite high normal serum testosterone levels secondary to increased peripheral conversion of androgens to estrogens (Chapter 20).

There is an increased plasma concentration of atrial natriuretic peptide (ANP) and its precursors. The plasma ANP concentration correlates with the serum thyroxine level and heart rate and decreases to normal with successful antithyroid therapy.

The wide-eyed stare of hyperthyroid patients may be due to increased sympathetic tone. In Graves' disease, about 70% of patients develop proptosis due to infiltration of orbital soft tissues and extraocular muscles with lymphocytes, mucopolysaccharides, and edema fluid (Figure 12–8). This may lead to fibrosis of the extraocular muscles, restricted ocular motility, and diplopia. In severe Graves' ophthalmopathy, pressure on the optic nerve or keratitis due to corneal exposure may lead to blindness. The pathogenesis of Graves' ophthalmopathy may involve cytotoxic lymphocytes (killer cells) and cytotoxic antibodies to an antigen common to orbital fibroblasts, orbital muscle, and thyroid tissue (Figure 12–7). It is postulated that cytokines released from these sensitized lymphocytes cause inflammation of orbital tissues, resulting in the proptosis, diplopia, and edema.

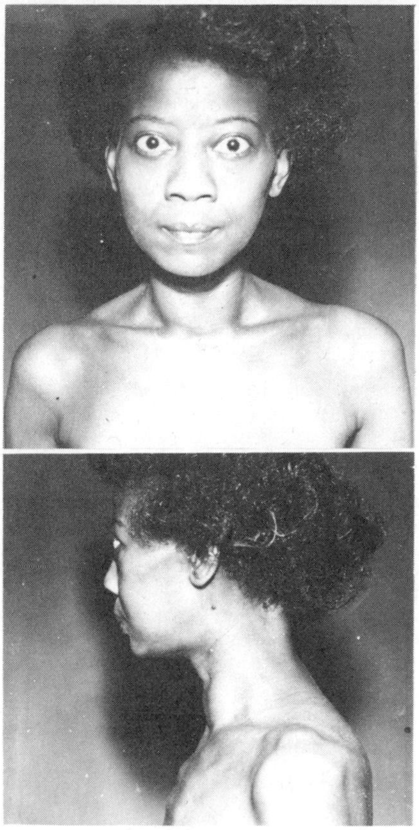

Figure 12–8. Graves' disease. (Courtesy of PH Forsham.)

The skin is warm, sweaty, and velvety in texture. There may be onycholysis (ie, retraction of the nail from the nail plate). In Graves' disease, the pretibial skin may become thickened, resembling an orange peel (**pretibial myxedema** or **thyrotoxic dermopathy**). The dermopathy is usually a late manifestation of Graves' disease, and affected patients invariably have ophthalmopathy. The most common form of the dermopathy is nonpitting edema, but nodular, plaque-like, and even polypoid forms also occur. The pathogenesis of thyroid dermopathy may also involve lymphocyte cytokine stimulation of fibroblasts. Thyroid dermopathy is associated with a very high serum titer of TSH-R [stim] Ab.

Untreated hyperthyroidism may decompensate into a state called **thyroid storm.** Patients so affected have tachycardia, fever, agitation, nausea, vomiting, diarrhea, and restlessness or psychosis. The condition is usually precipitated by an intercurrent illness or by a surgical emergency.

12. Describe the physiologic consequences of hyperthyroidism and identify their mechanism (as is best known) on the following systems:
    - Heart
    - Liver
    - Lungs
    - GI tract
    - Kidney
    - Eyes
    - Skin
    - Brain
    - Bone
    - Reproductive system

HYPOTHYROIDISM

Etiology

The causes of hypothyroidism are listed in Table 12–5. The most common cause is Hashimoto's thyroiditis, which probably results from an autoimmune destruction of the thyroid, though the precipitating cause and exact mechanism of the autoimmunity and subsequent destruction are unknown. Hypothyroidism may also be caused by lymphocytic thyroiditis following a transient period of hyperthyroidism. Thyroid ablation, whether by surgical resection or by therapeutic radiation, commonly results in hypothyroidism.

Diseases of the pituitary or hypothalamus may cause diminished TSH secretion, producing hypothyroidism as a secondary or tertiary result. In some cases of hypothyroidism caused by hypothalamic disease, the TSH secreted by the pituitary lacks biologic activity and exhibits impaired binding to its receptor. This defect can be reversed by administration of TRH. Thus, TRH may regulate not only the secretion of TSH but also the specific molecular and conformational features that enable it to act at its receptor.

Finally, a host of drugs, including the thioamide antithyroid medications propylthiouracil and methimazole, may produce hypothyroidism. The thioamides inhibit thyroid peroxidase and block the synthesis of thyroid hormone. In addition, propylthiouracil (but not methimazole) blocks the peripheral conversion of T_4 to T_3. Lithium is concentrated by the thyroid and inhibits the release of hormone from the gland. Most patients treated with lithium compensate by increasing TSH secretion, but some become hypothyroid.

Pathogenesis

Hypothyroidism is characterized by abnormally low serum T_4 and T_3 levels. The free T_4 index is always depressed. The serum TSH level is elevated in

Table 12–5. Hypothyroidism: Causes and pathogenetic mechanisms.

Etiologic Classification	Pathogenetic Mechanism
A. Congenital	Aplasia or hypoplasia of thyroid gland Defects in hormone biosynthesis or action
B. Acquired	
1. Hashimoto's thyroiditis	Autoimmune destruction
2. Severe iodine deficiency	Diminished hormone synthesis, release
3. Lymphocytic thyroiditis	Diminished hormone synthesis, release
4. Thyroid ablation	Diminished hormone synthesis, release
a. Thyroid surgery	
b. ^{131}I radiation treatment of hyperthyroidism	
c. External beam radiation therapy of head and neck cancer	
5. Drugs	Diminished hormone synthesis, release
a. Iodine, inorganic	
b. Iodine, organic (amiodarone)	
c. Thioamides (propylthiouracil,[1] methimazole)	
d. Potassium perchlorate	
e. Thiocyanate	
f. Lithium	
6. Hypopituitarism	Deficient TSH secretion
7. Hypothalamic disease	Deficient TRH secretion

[1] Also blocks peripheral conversion of T_4 to T_3.

hypothyroidism (except in cases of pituitary or hypothalamic disease). Marked elevations of serum TSH (> 20 μU/mL) are found in frank hypothyroidism. Modest TSH elevations (5–20 μU/mL) may be found in euthyroid individuals with normal serum T_4 and T_3 levels and indicate impaired thyroid reserve and incipient hypothyroidism. In patients with primary hypothyroidism (end-organ failure), the nocturnal TSH surge is intact. In patients with central (pituitary or hypothalamic) hypothyroidism, the serum TSH level is low and the normal nocturnal TSH surge is absent.

In hypothyroidism due to end-organ failure, administration of TRH produces a prompt rise in the TSH level, the magnitude of which is proportionate to the baseline serum TSH level (Figure 12–6). However, the TRH test is not usually performed in patients with primary hypothyroidism, since the elevated basal serum TSH level suffices to make the diagnosis. The test is useful in the clinically hypothyroid patient with an unexpectedly low serum TSH level in establishing a central (pituitary or hypothalamic) origin. Pituitary disease is suggested by the failure of TSH to rise following TRH administration; hypothalamic disease is suggested by a delayed TSH response (at 60 minutes, rather than 30 minutes) with a normal increment.

As in euthyroid patients (see below), hypothyroid patients subjected to caloric restriction—both those treated with T_4 and those not treated—exhibit decreased serum T_3 concentrations but no alterations in basal or TRH-stimulated TSH secretion.

Hashimoto's Thyroiditis

A. Pathology: In the early stages of Hashimoto's thyroiditis, the gland is diffusely enlarged, firm, rubbery, and nodular. As the disease progresses, the gland becomes smaller. In the late stages, the gland is atrophic and fibrotic, weighing as little as 10–20 g. Microscopically, there is destruction of thyroid follicles and lymphocytic infiltration with lymphoid follicles present. The surviving thyroid follicular epithelial cells are large, with abundant pink cytoplasm (Hürthle cells). As the disease progresses, there is an increasing amount of fibrosis.

B. Pathogenesis: The pathogenesis of Hashimoto's thyroiditis is unclear. Again, it is possible that a defect in suppressor T lymphocytes allows helper T lymphocytes to interact with specific antigens on the thyroid follicular cell membrane. Once these lymphocytes become sensitized to thyroidal antigens, autoantibodies are formed that react with these antigens. Cytokine release and inflammation then cause glandular destruction. The most important thyroid autoantibodies in Hashimoto's thyroiditis are thyroglobulin antibody (Tg Ab), thyroidal peroxidase antibody (TPO Ab) (formerly termed antimicrosomal antibody), and the TSH receptor blocking antibody (TSH-R [block] Ab). During the early phases, Tg Ab is markedly elevated and TPO Ab only slightly elevated. Later, Tg Ab may disappear, but TPO Ab persists for many years. TSH-R [block] Ab is found in patients with atrophic thyroiditis and myxedema and in mothers who give birth to infants with no detectable thyroid tissue **(athyreotic cretins).** Serum levels of these antibodies do not correlate with the severity of the hypothyroidism, but their presence is helpful in diagnosis. In general, high antibody titers are diagnostic of Hashimoto's thyroiditis; moderate titers are seen in Graves' disease, multinodular goiter, and thyroid neoplasm; and low titers are found in the elderly.

Patients with Hashimoto's thyroiditis have an increased frequency of the HLA-DR5 histocompatibility antigen, and the disease is associated with a host of other autoimmune diseases (Table 12–3). A **polyglandular failure syndrome** has been defined in which two or more endocrine disorders mediated by autoimmune mechanisms occur. Affected patients frequently have circulating organ- and cell-specific autoantibodies that lead to organ hypofunction.

13. What are some drugs that cause hypothyroidism?
14. What are the most useful initial tests of thyroid function in hypothyroidism? What results would you expect compared to normal?
15. What are the key physical and pathophysiologic findings in Hashimoto's thyroiditis?

Table 12–6. Clinical findings in adult hypothyroidism (myxedema).

Symptoms
1. Slow thinking
2. Lethargy, decreased vigor
3. Dry skin; thickened hair; hair loss; broken nails
4. Diminished food intake; weight gain
5. Constipation
6. Menorrhagia; diminished libido
7. Cold intolerance

Signs
1. Round puffy face; slow speech; hoarseness
2. Hypokinesia; generalized muscle weakness; delayed relaxation of deep tendon reflexes
3. Cold, dry, thick, scaling skin; dry, coarse, brittle hair; dry, longitudinally ridged nails
4. Periorbital edema
5. Normal or faint cardiac impulse; indistinct heart sounds; cardiac enlargement; bradycardia
6. Ascites; pericardial effusion; ankle edema
7. Mental clouding, depression

Laboratory findings
1. Decreased serum total T_4 and T_3; decreased T_3 and T_4 resin uptake; decreased free thyroxine index
2. Increased serum TSH level
3. Decreased radioiodine uptake by thyroid gland
4. Diminished basal metabolic rate (BMR)
5. Macrocytic anemia
6. Elevated serum cholesterol level
7. Elevated serum CK level
8. Decreased circulation time, low voltage of QRS complex on ECG

Clinical Manifestations

The clinical consequences of thyroid hormone deficiency are summarized in Table 12–6.

Hypothermia is common, and the patient may complain of cold intolerance. The decreased basal metabolic rate leads to weight gain despite reduced food intake.

Thyroid hormones are required for normal development of the nervous system. In hypothyroid infants, synapses develop abnormally, myelination is defective, and mental retardation occurs. Hypothyroid adults have slowed mentation, forgetfulness, decreased hearing, and ataxia. Some patients have severe mental symptoms, including reversible dementia or overt psychosis ("myxedema madness''). The cerebrospinal fluid protein level is abnormally high. However, cerebral blood flow and oxygen consumption are normal. Deep tendon reflexes are sluggish, with a slowed ("hung-up'') relaxation phase. Paresthesias are common, often caused by compression neuropathies due to accumulation of myxedema (carpal tunnel syndrome and tarsal tunnel syndrome).

Hypothyroidism is associated with muscle weakness, cramps, and stiffness. The serum creatine kinase (CK) level may be elevated. The pathophysiology of the muscle disease in hypothyroidism is poorly understood. Study of the bioenergetic abnormalities in hypothyroid muscle suggests a hormone-dependent, reversible mitochondrial impairment. Changes in energy metabolism are not found in hyperthyroid muscle.

Patients rendered acutely hypothyroid by total thyroidectomy exhibit a decreased cardiac output, decreased stroke volume, decreased diastolic volume at rest, and an increased peripheral resistance. However, the pulmonary capillary wedge pressure, right atrial pressure, heart rate, left ventricular ejection fraction, and left ventricular systolic pressure-volume relation (a measure of contractility) are not significantly different from the euthyroid state. Thus, in early hypothyroidism, alterations in cardiac performance are probably primarily related to changes in loading conditions and exercise-related heart rate rather than to changes in myocardial contractility.

In chronic hypothyroidism, echocardiography shows bradycardia and features that suggest cardiomyopathy, including increased thickening of the intraventricular septum and ventricular wall, decreased regional wall motion, and decreased global left ventricular function. These changes may be due to deposition of excessive mucopolysaccharides in the interstitium between myocardial fibers, leading to fiber degeneration, decreased contractility, low cardiac output, cardiac enlargement, and congestive heart failure. Pericardial effusion (with high protein content) may lead to findings of decreased electrocardiographic voltage and flattened T waves and dependent edema, but cardiac tamponade is rare.

Hypothyroid patients exhibit decreased ventilatory responses to hypercapnia and hypoxia. There is a high incidence of sleep apnea in untreated hypothyroidism; such patients sometimes demonstrate myopathy of upper airway muscles. Weakness of the diaphragm also occurs frequently and, when severe, can cause chronic alveolar hypoventilation (CO_2 retention). Pleural effusions (with high protein content) may accumulate.

Metabolically, in hypothyroidism, the plasma cholesterol and triglyceride levels increase, related to decreased lipoprotein lipase activity and decreased formation of hepatic LDL receptors. In hypothyroid children, bone growth is slowed and skeletal maturation (closure of epiphyses) is delayed. Pituitary secretion of growth hormone may also be depressed because thyroid hormone is needed for its synthesis. Hypothyroid animals demonstrate decreased width of epiphysial growth plate and articular cartilage and decreased volume of epiphysial and metaphysial trabecular bone. These changes are not solely due to lack of pituitary growth hormone, since administering exogenous growth hormone does not restore normal cartilage morphology or bone remodeling, whereas administering T_4 does. If unrecognized, prolonged juvenile hypothyroidism results in a permanent height deficit.

A normochromic, normocytic anemia may occur as a result of decreased erythropoiesis. Alternatively, a moderate macrocytic anemia can occur as a result of decreased absorption of cyanocobalamin (vitamin B_{12}) from the intestine and diminished bone marrow metabolism. Frank megaloblastic anemia suggests coexistent pernicious anemia.

Constipation is common and reflects slowed gastrointestinal motility. Achlorhydria occurs when hypothyroidism is associated with pernicious anemia. Ascitic fluid with high protein content may accumulate.

The skin in hypothyroidism is dry and cool. Normally, the skin contains a variety of proteins complexed with polysaccharides, chondroitin sulfuric acid, and hyaluronic acid. In hypothyroidism, these complexes accumulate, promoting sodium and water retention and producing a characteristic diffuse, nonpitting puffiness of the skin (myxedema). The patient's face appears puffy, with coarse features (Figure 12–9). Similar accumulation of mucopolysaccharides in the larynx may lead to hoarseness. The hair is brittle and lacking in luster, and there is frequently loss of body hair, particularly over the scalp and lateral eyebrows. If thyroid hormone is administered, the protein complexes are mobilized, a diuresis ensues, and myxedema resolves.

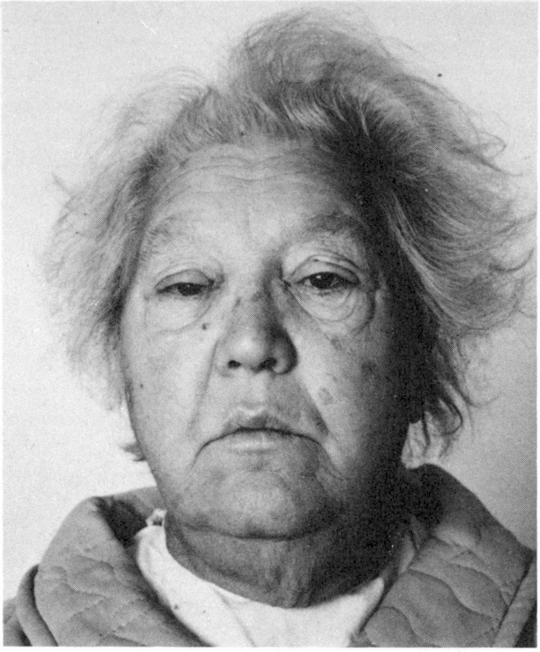

Figure 12–9. Myxedema. (Reproduced, with permission, from Greenspan FS: The thyroid. In: *Basic and Clinical Endocrinology,* 4th ed. Greenspan FS, Baxter JD [editors]. Appleton & Lange, 1994.)

Carotenemia (manifested as yellow-orange discoloration of the skin) may occur in hypothyroidism because thyroid hormones are needed for hepatic conversion of carotene to vitamin A. In the absence of sufficient hormone, carotene accumulates in the bloodstream and skin.

In women, hypothyroidism may lead to menorrhagia from anovulatory cycles. Alternatively, menses may become scanty or disappear secondary to diminished secretion of gonadotropins. Since thyroid hormone normally has an inhibitory effect on prolactin secretion, hypothyroid patients may exhibit hyperprolactinemia, with galactorrhea and amenorrhea. In men, hypothyroidism can cause infertility and gynecomastia from enhanced release of prolactin. Hyperprolactinemia occurs because TRH stimulates prolactin release.

There is reduced renal blood flow and a decreased glomerular filtration rate. The vasoconstriction may be due to decreased concentrations of plasma ANP. The consequent reduced ability to excrete a water load may cause hyponatremia. However, the serum creatinine level is usually normal.

Long-standing severe untreated hypothyroidism may lead to a state called **myxedema coma.** Affected patients have typical myxedematous facies and skin, bradycardia, hypothermia, alveolar hypoventilation, and severe obtundation or coma. This condition is usually precipitated by an intercurrent illness such as an infection or stroke or by a medication such as a sedative-hypnotic. The mortality rate approaches 100% unless myxedema coma is recognized and treated promptly.

16. What are the effects of hypothyroidism on?—
    - Nervous system
    - Muscle
    - Cardiovascular system
    - Lungs
    - Liver
    - Blood
    - GI tract
    - Skin
    - Reproductive system
    - Kidney

GOITER

Etiology

Diffuse thyroid enlargement most commonly results from prolonged stimulation by TSH (or a TSH-like agent). Such stimulation may be the result of one of the causes of hypothyroidism (eg, TSH in Hashimoto's thyroiditis) or of hyperthyroidism (eg, TSH-R [stim] Ab in Graves' disease, hCG in germ cell tumors, or TSH in pituitary adenoma). Alternatively, goiter may occur in a clinically euthyroid patient. Table 12–7 lists the causes and pathogenetic mechanisms.

Iodine deficiency is the most common cause of goiter in developing nations. A diet that contains less than 10 μg/d of iodine hinders the synthesis of thyroid hormone, resulting in an elevated TSH level and thyroid hypertrophy. Iodination of salt has eliminated this problem in much of the developed world.

Table 12–7. Goiter: Causes and pathogenetic mechanisms.

Causes	Pathogenetic Mechanism
A. Goiter associated with hypothyroidism or euthyroidism:	Elevation of serum TSH
1. Iodine deficiency	Interferes with hormone biosynthesis
2. Iodine excess	Blocks secretion of hormone
3. Goitrogen in diet or drinking water	Interferes with hormone biosynthesis
4. Goitrogenic medication	Interferes with hormone biosynthesis
a. Thioamides: propylthiouracil, methimazole, carbamizole	
b. Thiocyanates: nitroprusside	
c. Aniline derivatives: sulfonylureas, sulfonamides, aminosalicylic acid, phenylbutazone, aminoglutethimide	
d. Lithium	Blocks secretion of hormone
5. Congenital	Various defects in hormone biosynthesis
a. Defective transport of iodide	
b. Defective organification of iodide due to absence or reduction of peroxidase or production of an abnormal peroxidase	
c. Synthesis of an abnormal thyroglobulin	
d. Abnormal interrelationships of iodotyrosine	
e. Impaired proteolysis of thyroglobulin	
f. Defective deiodination of iodotyrosine	
6. Pituitary and peripheral resistance to thyroid hormone	Receptor or postreceptor abnormality
B. Goiter associated with hyperthyroidism:	
1. Graves' disease	TSH-R [stim] Ab stimulation of gland
2. Toxic multinodular goiter	Autonomous hyperfunction
3. Germ cell tumor	hCG stimulation of gland
4. Pituitary adenoma	TSH overproduction
5. Thyroiditis	Enlargement due to "injury," infiltration, and edema

A goiter may also develop from ingestion of **goitrogens** (factors that block thyroid hormone synthesis) either in food or in medication. Dietary goitrogens are found in vegetables of the Brassicaceae family (rutabagas, cabbage, turnips, cassava, etc). A goitrogenic hydrocarbon has been found in the water supply in some locations. Medications that act as goitrogens include thioamides and thiocyanates (propylthiouracil, methimazole, nitroprusside, etc), sulfonylureas, and lithium. Lithium inhibits thyroid hormone release and perhaps also iodide organification. Most patients compensate by increasing TSH production and, despite the enlarged gland, remain clinically euthyroid.

A congenital goiter associated with hypothyroidism **(sporadic cretinism)** may occur as a result of a defect in any of the steps of thyroid hormone synthesis (Table 12–7). All of these defects are rare.

Goiter with hyperthyroidism is usually due to Graves' disease. In Graves' disease, the gland is enlarged because of stimulation by TSH-R [stim] Ab and other antibodies rather than by TSH.

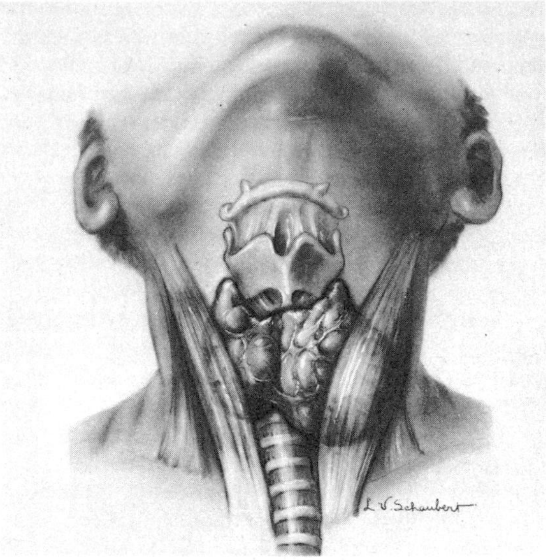

Figure 12–10. Goiter. (Reproduced, with permission, from Greenspan FS: The thyroid. In: *Basic and Clinical Endocrinology,* 4th ed. Greenspan FS, Baxter JD [editors]. Appleton & Lange, 1994.)

Pathogenesis & Pathology

In goiter due to impaired thyroid hormone synthesis, there is a progressive fall in serum T_4 and a progressive rise in serum TSH. As the TSH increases, iodine turnover by the gland is accelerated and the ratio of T_3 secretion relative to T_4 secretion is increased. Consequently, the serum T_3 may be normal or increased, and the patient may remain clinically euthyroid. If there is more marked impairment of hormone synthesis, goiter formation is associated with a low T_4, low T_3, and elevated TSH, and the patient becomes clinically hypothyroid.

In the early stages, there is diffuse enlargement of the gland, with cellular hyperplasia caused by the TSH stimulation. Later, there are enlarged follicles with flattened follicular epithelial cells and accumulation of thyroglobulin. This accumulation occurs particularly in iodine deficiency goiter, perhaps because poorly iodinated thyroglobulin is less easily digested by proteases. As TSH stimulation continues, multiple nodules may develop in some areas and atrophy and fibrosis in others, producing a multinodular goiter (Figure 12–10).

In patients with severe iodine deficiency or inherited metabolic defects, a nontoxic goiter develops because impaired hormone synthesis leads to an appropriate increase in TSH secretion. The elevation in serum TSH level results in diffuse thyroid hyperplasia. If TSH stimulation is prolonged, the diffuse hyperplasia is followed by focal hyperplasia with necrosis, hemorrhage, and formation of nodules. These nodules often vary from "hot" nodules that can trap iodine and synthesize thyroglobulin to "cold" ones that cannot. In early goiters, the hyperplasia is TSH-dependent, but in later stages the nodules become TSH-independent, or **autonomous nodules.** Thus, over a period of time there may be a transition from a nontoxic, TSH-dependent, diffuse hyperplasia to a toxic or nontoxic, TSH-independent, multinodular goiter.

The exact mechanism underlying this transition to autonomous growth and function is unknown. However, mutations of the *gsp* oncogene have been found in nodules from many patients with multinodular goiter. Such mutations presumably occur during TSH-induced cell division. The *gsp* oncogene is responsible for activation of regulatory GTP-binding (G_s) protein in the follicular cell membrane. Chronic activation of this protein and its effector, adenylyl cyclase, is postulated to result in thyroid cell proliferation, hyperfunction, and independence from TSH.

Clinical Manifestations

With decades of TSH stimulation, enormous hypertrophy and enlargement of the gland can occur. The enlarged gland may weigh 1–5 kg and may produce respiratory difficulties secondary to obstruction of the trachea or dysphagia secondary to obstruction of the esophagus. More modest enlargements pose cosmetic problems.

Some patients with multinodular goiter also develop hyperthyroidism late in life **(Plummer's disease),** particularly following administration of iodide or iodine-containing drugs.

THYROID NODULE & NEOPLASMS

Tumors of the thyroid usually present as a solitary mass in the neck. The commonest neoplasm, accounting for 30% of all solitary thyroid nodules, is the **follicular adenoma.** It is a solitary, firm, gray or red nodule, up to 5 cm in diameter, completely surrounded by a fibrous capsule. The surrounding normal thyroid tissue is compressed by the adenoma. Microscopically, the adenoma consists of normal-appearing follicles of varying size, sometimes associated with hemorrhage, fibrosis, calcification, and cystic degeneration (Figure 12–2). Occasionally, only ribbons of follicular cells are present, without true follicles. Malignant change probably occurs in less than 10% of follicular adenomas.

Thyroid cancers are infrequent. Most are derived from the follicular epithelium and, depending on their microscopic appearance, are classified as **papillary** or **follicular carcinoma.** Most papillary and follicular cancers pursue a prolonged clinical course (15–20 years). Papillary carcinoma typically metastasizes to regional lymph nodes in the neck, while follicular cancer tends to spread via the bloodstream to distant sites such as bone or lung. **Medullary carcinoma** is an uncommon neoplasm of the C cells (parafollicular cells) of the thyroid that produce calcitonin (see Chapter 17).

ALTERATIONS IN HORMONE TRANSPORT & METABOLISM

Increases & Decreases in Hormone-Binding Proteins

Sustained increases or decreases in the concentration of TBG and other thyroid-binding proteins in the plasma are produced by several normal and disordered physiologic states and medications. These are summarized in Table 12–8. For example, TBG levels are elevated during pregnancy and by estrogen and oral contraceptive therapy. TBG levels are depressed in the nephrotic syndrome and by glucocorticoid, androgen, and antiestrogen (danazol) therapy.

When a sustained increase in the concentration of TBG and other binding proteins occurs, the concentration of free thyroid hormones falls temporarily. This fall stimulates TSH secretion, which then results in an increase in the production of free hormone. Eventually, a new equilibrium is reached in which the levels of total plasma T_4 and T_3 are elevated, but the concentrations of free hormones, the rate of hormone degradation, and the rate of TSH secretion are normal. Therefore, individuals manifesting sustained increases in TBG and other binding proteins remain euthyroid. When a sustained decrease in the concentration of TBG and other binding proteins occurs, equivalent changes occur in the opposite direction, and again the individuals remain euthyroid.

Abnormal Hormone-Binding Proteins

Changes in serum concentrations of the hormone-binding proteins transthyretin or albumin alone usually do not cause significant changes in thyroid hormone levels. However, several unusual syndromes of **familial euthyroid hyperthyroxinemia** have been described. In the first, a familial syndrome called **euthyroid dysalbuminemic hyperthyroxinemia,** there is abnormal binding of T_4 (but not T_3) to albumin. In the second, there is an increased serum level of transthyretin. In the third, there are alterations in transthyretin, a tetrameric protein that transports 15–20% of circulating T_4. The alterations in

Table 12–8. Effects of normal and disordered physiologic states and medications on plasma thyroid-binding proteins and thyroid hormone levels.[1]

Condition	Concentrations of Binding Proteins	Total Plasma T_4, T_3, RT_3	Free Plasma T_4, T_3, RT_3	Plasma TSH	Clinical State
Hyperthyroidism	Normal	High	High	Low	Hyperthyroid
Hypothyroidism	Normal	Low	Low	High	Hypothyroid
Drugs (estrogens, methadone, heroin, perphenazine, clofibrate), pregnancy, acute and chronic hepatitis, acute intermittent porphyria, estrogen-producing tumors, idiopathic, hereditary	High	High	Normal	Normal	Euthyroid
Drugs (glucocorticoids, androgens, danazol, asparaginase), acromegaly, nephrotic syndrome, hypoproteinemia, chronic liver disease (cirrhosis), testosterone-producing tumors, hereditary	Low	Low	Normal	Normal	Euthyroid

[1] Modified, with permission, from Ganong WF: *Review of Medical Physiology,* 16th ed. Appleton & Lange, 1993.

transthyretin structure produced by different point mutations can markedly increase its affinity for T_4 and produce euthyroid hyperthyroxinemia. In some families, these mutations in transthyretin are transmitted by autosomal dominant inheritance. In all three of these syndromes, total T_4 is elevated, but free T_4 is normal and the patients are euthyroid. Finally, a fourth syndrome has also been described in which there is both pituitary and peripheral resistance to thyroid hormone. As noted above, this condition may be due to point mutations in the human thyroid receptor (hTR-β1) gene, resulting in abnormal nuclear T_3 receptors.

Effects of Nonthyroidal Illness & Drugs

Several nonthyroidal illnesses and various drugs inhibit the 5′-deiodinase that converts T_4 to T_3, resulting in a fall in plasma T_3. Illnesses that depress 5′-deiodinase include severe burns or trauma, surgery, advanced cancer, cirrhosis, renal failure, myocardial infarction, prolonged fever, and caloric deprivation (fasting, anorexia nervosa, malnutrition). The decreased serum T_3 in nonthyroidal illness is thought to be an adaptive physiologic change, enabling the sick patient to conserve energy and protein. Drugs which depress 5′-deiodinase include glucocorticoids, propranolol, amiodarone, propylthiouracil, and cholecystography dyes (eg, ipodate, iopanoic acid).

Since T_3 is the major active thyroid hormone at the tissue level, it is surprising that patients with mild to moderate nonthyroidal illness exhibit normal TSH levels despite low T_3 levels and do not appear hypothyroid. However, such patients retain the ability to respond to a further reduction (or to an increase) in serum T_3 by increasing (or decreasing) pituitary TSH secretion. Patients with severe illness (eg, patients undergoing bone marrow transplantation for leukemia) may manifest impaired TSH secretion. Such patients have low serum T_3 levels resulting both from decreased secretion of T_3 by the gland and decreased peripheral conversion of T_4 to T_3.

The low T_3 state generally disappears with recovery from the illness or cessation of the drug. In the meantime, the clinician may find it difficult to decide whether an individual patient's serum T_3 level is low because of underlying illness or medication or because of mild hypothyroidism.

Most patients with nonthyroidal illness have low serum T_3 levels related to the decreased peripheral conversion of T_4 to T_3. However, in some patients, the primary cause of the low serum T_3 is reduced secretion of T_4 by the gland. In others, the binding of T_4 and T_3 by serum thyroid-binding proteins is impaired, both because of the decreased concentrations of thyroid-binding proteins (Table 12–8) and the presence of circulating inhibitors of binding.

17. What is a goiter?
18. What are the causes and mechanisms of goiter formation?
19. What is the basis for transition from nontoxic, TSH-dependent diffuse hyperplasia to a toxic or nontoxic TSH-independent multinodular goiter?
20. How large can the thyroid gland become with decades of stimulation?
21. What are the different types of thyroid cancer and their characteristics?
22. What are some physiologic and pathophysiologic conditions in which thyroid metabolism is altered? How and with what effects?
23. What is the overall thyroid status of a patient with a sustained decrease in thyroid-binding globulin?
24. What are some of the factors which depress 5′-deiodinase activity?
25. How does nonthyroidal illness typically affect thyroid hormone levels?

REFERENCES

General

Braverman LE, Utiger RD (editors): *Werner and Ingbar's The Thyroid: A Fundamental and Clinical Text,* 6th ed. Lippincott, 1991.

Brent GA, Moore DD, Larsen PR: Thyroid hormone regulation of gene expression. Annu Rev Physiol 1991;53:17.

Greenspan FS: The thyroid gland. In: *Basic and Clinical Endocrinology,* 4th ed. Greenspan FS, Baxter JD (editors). Appleton & Lange, 1994.

Larsen PR, Ingbar SH: The thyroid gland. In: *Williams Textbook of Endocrinology,* 8th ed. Wilson JD, Foster DW (editors). Saunders, 1992.

Magner JA: Thyroid-stimulating hormone: Biosynthesis, cell biology and bioactivity. Endocr Rev 1990;11:354.

Shepard AR, Eberhardt NL: Molecular mechanisms of thyroid hormone action. Clin Lab Med 1993;13:531.

Volpé R: Autoimmunity causing thyroid dysfunction. Endocrinol Metab Clin North Am 1991;20:565.

Hyperthyroidism

Bahn RS, Heufelder AE: Pathogenesis of Graves' ophthalmopathy. N Engl J Med 1993;329:1468.

Burch HB, Wartofsky L: Life-threatening thyrotoxicosis: Thyroid storm. Endocrinol Metab Clin North Am 1993;22:263.

Fatourechi V, Pajouhi M, Fransway AF: Dermopathy of Graves' disease (pretibial myxedema): Review of 150 cases. Medicine 1994;73:1.

Levey GS, Klein I: Catecholamine-thyroid hormone interactions and the cardiovascular manifestations of hyperthyroidism. Am J Med 1990;88:642.

McDougall IR: Graves' disease: Current concepts. Med Clin North Am 1991;75:79.

Weetman AP: Extrathyroidal complications of Graves' disease. Q J Med 1993;86:473.

Hypothyroidism

Myerson J et al: Polyglandular autoimmune syndrome: Current concepts. Can Med Assoc J 1988; 138:605.

Rapoport B: Pathophysiology of Hashimoto's thyroiditis and hypothyroidism. Annu Rev Med 1991;42:91.

Sharma AT, Paliwal RK, Pendse AK: Hashimoto's thyroiditis: A clinical review. J Postgrad Med 1990; 36:87.

Weetman AP: Autoimmune thyroiditis: Predisposition and pathogenesis. Clin Endocrinol 1992;36:307.

Goiter

Boyages SC: Iodine deficiency disorders. J Clin Endocrinol Metab 1993;77:587.

Fenzi G et al: Clinical approach to goiter. Baillieres Clin Endocrinol Metab 1988;23:671.

Greenspan FS: The problem of nodular goiter. Med Clin North Am 1991;75:195.

Lamberg BA: Endemic goiter-iodine deficiency disorders. Ann Med 1991;23:367.

Thyroid Nodule & Neoplasm

Hay ID: Papillary thyroid carcinoma. Endocrinol Metab Clin North Am 1990;19:545.

Kaplan M: Thyroid carcinoma. Endocrinol Metab Clin North Am 1990;19:469.

Matsuo K et al: The thyrotropin receptor (TSH-R) is not an oncogene for thyroid tumors: Structural studies of the TSH-R and the alpha-subunit of G_s in human thyroid neoplasms. J Clin Endocrinol Metab 1993;76:1446.

Mazzaferri E: Management of a solitary thyroid nodule. N Engl J Med 1993;328:553.

Nelkin BD et al: The molecular biology of medullary thyroid carcinoma: A model for cancer development and progression. JAMA 1989;261:3130.

Alterations in Hormone Transport and Metabolism

Howland RH: Thyroid dysfunction in refractory depression: Implications for pathophysiology and treatment. J Clin Psychiatry 1993;54:47.

Lever EG, Medeiros-Neto GA, DeGroot LJ: Inherited disorders of thyroid metabolism. Endocr Rev 1983; 4:213.

Moses AC et al: A point mutation in transthyretin increases affinity for thyroxine and produces euthyroid hyperthyroxinemia. J Clin Invest 1990;86:2025.

Rosen HN et al: Thyroxine interactions with transthyretin: A comparison of 10 different naturally occurring human transthyretin variants. J Clin Endocrinol Metab 1993;77:370.

Weiss RE, Refetoff S: Thyroid hormone resistance. Annu Rev Med 1992;43:363.

13 Disorders of the Adrenal Cortex

Stephen J. McPhee, MD

The adrenal gland is actually two endocrine organs, one wrapped around the other. The outer **adrenal cortex** secretes many different steroid hormones, including glucocorticoids such as cortisol, mineralocorticoids such as aldosterone, and sex hormones, chiefly androgens. The glucocorticoids help to regulate carbohydrate, protein, and fat metabolism. The mineralocorticoids help to regulate sodium and potassium balance and extracellular fluid volume. The glucocorticoids and mineralocorticoids are essential for survival, but the adrenal androgens have only a minor role in reproductive function. The inner **adrenal medulla,** discussed in the next chapter, secretes catecholamines (epinephrine, norepinephrine, and dopamine). The catecholamines help prepare the individual to deal with emergency situations.

The major disorders of the adrenal cortex (Table 13–1) are characterized by excessive or deficient secretion of each type of adrenal hormone: **hypercortisolism (Cushing's syndrome), adrenal insufficiency (Addison's disease), hyperaldosteronism (Conn's syndrome), hypoaldosteronism,** and **androgen excess (adrenogenital syndrome).**

NORMAL STRUCTURE & FUNCTION OF THE ADRENAL CORTEX

ANATOMY

The adrenal glands are paired organs located in the retroperitoneal area near the superior poles of the kidneys (Figure 13–1). They are flattened, crescent-shaped structures about 3–6 cm long, 1–3 cm wide, and 4–10 mm thick. Together, they normally weigh about 7–20 g. They are covered by tight fibrous capsules and surrounded by fat. The blood flow to the adrenals is copious.

Grossly, each gland consists of two concentric layers: the yellow peripheral layer is the **adrenal cortex,** and the reddish-brown central layer is the **adrenal medulla.** Adrenal cortical tissue is sometimes found at other sites, usually near the kidney or along the path taken by the gonads during their embryonic descent (Figure 13–1).

HISTOLOGY

The adrenal cortex can be subdivided into three concentric layers, not sharply defined, each with a different cellular appearance: the zona glomerulosa, the zona fasciculata, and the zona reticularis (Figure 13–2). The **zona glomerulosa** is the outermost layer, situated immediately beneath the capsule. Zona glomerulosa cells are columnar or pyramidal in appearance and are arranged in closely packed, rounded or arched clusters surrounded by capillaries. They secrete **mineralocorticoids,** primarily **aldosterone. The zona fasciculata** is the middle layer of cortex. Zona fasciculata cells are polyhedral in shape and arranged in straight cords or columns, one or two cells thick, running at right angles to the capsule with capillaries between them. The **zona reticularis,** the innermost layer of the cortex, lies between the zona fasciculata and the adrenal medulla; it accounts for 7% of the mass of the adrenal gland. Zona reticularis cells are smaller than the other two types and are arranged in irregular cords or interlaced in a network. Zona fasciculata and zona reticularis cells secrete both **glucocorticoids,** primarily **cortisol** and **corticosterone,** and **sex hormones,** primarily **androgens** such as **dehydroepiandrosterone.** The ultrastructure of all three types of adrenocortical cells is similar to that of other steroid-synthesizing cells in the body. The steroid hormones produced are low-molecular-weight lipid-soluble molecules able to diffuse freely across cell membranes.

PHYSIOLOGY OF NORMAL ADRENAL CORTEX

1. GLUCOCORTICOIDS

Glucocorticoid Synthesis, Protein Binding, & Metabolism

The glucocorticoids help regulate the metabolism of carbohydrates, proteins, and fat. They act on virtually all cells of the body.

Table 13–1. Principal diseases of the adrenal glands.

A. Hyperfunction of cortex
1. Bilateral hyperplasia
ACTH excess (mainly zona fasciculata and reticularis)
Enzyme deficiencies
2. Adenoma
Primary hyperaldosteronism (Conn's syndrome) (zona glomerulosa)
Hypercortisolism (Cushing's syndrome) (zona fasciculata)
Virilization (zona reticularis)
3. Carcinoma
Cushing's syndrome
Virilization
Feminization (rare)
B. Hypofunction of cortex
1. Bilateral adrenal gland destruction (Addison's disease)
Autoimmune
Infection
Tuberculosis
Histoplasmosis
AIDS-related (CMV, disseminated *Mycobacterium avium* complex)
Ischemia, shock
Bacteremia (meningococcus, *Pseudomonas*)
Hemorrhage, anticoagulation
Metastatic tumor (lung carcinoma, other carcinomas, Kaposi's sarcoma)
C. Hyperfunction of medulla
1. Pheochromocytoma
2. Hyperplasia (rare)
3. Other: ganglioneuroma, neuroblastoma
D. Hypofunction of medulla

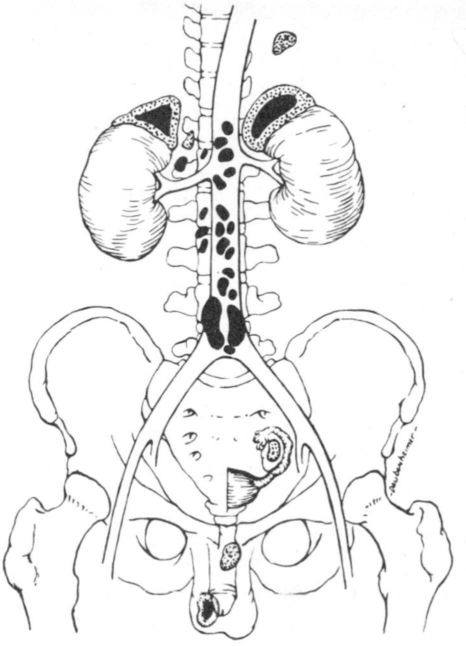

Figure 13–1. Human adrenal glands. Adrenocortical tissue is stippled; adrenal medullary tissue is black. Note location of adrenal at superior pole of each kidney. Also shown are extra-adrenal sites at which cortical and medullary tissue is sometimes found. (Reproduced, with permission, from Forsham PH: The adrenal cortex. In: *Textbook of Endocrinology,* 4th ed. Williams RH [editor]. Saunders, 1968.)

A. Synthesis and Binding to Plasma Proteins: The major glucocorticoids secreted by the adrenal cortex are cortisol and corticosterone. Biosynthetic pathways for these hormones are illustrated in Figure 13–3.

Both cortisol and corticosterone are secreted in an unbound state but circulate bound to plasma proteins. They bind mainly to **corticosteroid-binding globulin (CBG)** (or **transcortin**) and to a lesser extent to albumin. Protein binding serves mainly to distribute and deliver the hormones to target tissues, but it may also delay their metabolic clearance and prevent marked fluctuations of glucocorticoid levels during episodic secretion by the gland.

B. Corticosteroid-Binding Globulin (CBG): CBG (MW about 50,000) is an α-globulin synthesized in the liver. Its production is increased by pregnancy, estrogen or oral contraceptive therapy, hyperthyroidism, diabetes, certain hematologic disorders, and familial CBG excess. When the CBG level rises, more cortisol is bound, and the free cortisol level falls temporarily. This fall stimulates pituitary ACTH secretion and more adrenal cortisol production. Eventually, the free cortisol level and the ACTH secretion return to normal, but with an elevated level of protein-bound cortisol. CBG production is decreased in cirrhosis, nephrotic syndrome, hypothyroidism, multiple myeloma, and familial CBG deficiency. When the CBG level falls, changes in the opposite direction occur.

C. Free and Bound Glucocorticoid: Normally, about 90% of the circulating cortisol is bound to CBG and 10% is free (unbound). The bound hormone is inactive. The free hormone is physiologically active. The normal total plasma cortisol is 13.5 μg/dL (375 nmol/L), and the normal plasma free cortisol level is approximately 0.5 μg/dL. Because cortisol is protein-bound to a greater degree than corticosterone, its half-life in the circulation is longer (about 60–90 minutes) than that of corticosterone (about 50 minutes).

D. Metabolism: The glucocorticoids are metabolized in the liver and conjugated to glucuronide or sulfate groups. The inactive conjugated metabolites are excreted in the urine and stool. The metabolism of cortisol is decreased in infancy, old age, pregnancy, chronic liver disease, hypothyroidism, anorexia nervosa, surgery, starvation, and other major physiologic stress. Catabolism of cortisol is increased in thyrotoxicosis. Because of its avid protein

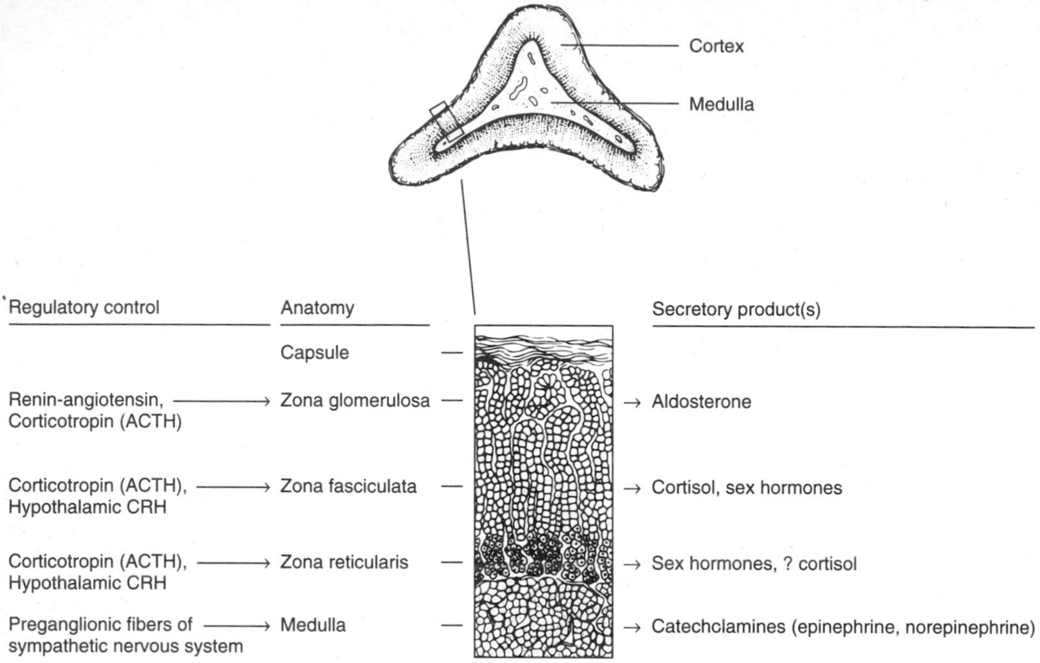

Figure 13–2. Anatomy, regulatory control, and secretory products of the adrenal gland. (Modified and reproduced, with permission, from Chandrasoma P, Taylor CE: *Concise Pathology,* 2nd ed. Appleton & Lange, 1994.)

binding and extensive metabolism before excretion, less than 1% of secreted cortisol appears in the urine as free cortisol.

Regulation of Secretion

A. Adrenocorticotropic Hormone (ACTH) and Corticotropin Releasing Hormone (CRH): Glucocorticoid secretion is regulated primarily by ACTH. **ACTH** is a 39-amino-acid polypeptide secreted by the anterior pituitary. Its half-life in the circulation is very short (about 10 minutes). The site of its catabolism is unknown. ACTH regulates both basal secretion of glucocorticoids and increased secretion provoked by stress.

ACTH, in turn, is regulated by the central nervous system and hypothalamus via **corticotropin-releasing hormone (CRH).** CRH is a 41-amino-acid polypeptide secreted in the median eminence of the hypothalamus and transported in the portal-hypophysial vessels to the anterior pituitary. There, within minutes, CRH causes a marked increase in ACTH secretion. This in turn leads to a transient increase in cortisol secretion by the adrenal (Figures 13–4 and 13–12).

The control of ACTH and CRH secretion involves three components: episodic secretion and diurnal rhythm of ACTH, stress responses of the hypothalamic-pituitary-adrenal axis, and negative feedback inhibition of ACTH secretion by cortisol.

B. Episodic and Diurnal Rhythm of ACTH Secretion: ACTH is secreted in episodic bursts throughout the day, following a diurnal (circadian) rhythm, with bursts most frequent in the early morning and least frequent in the evening (Figure 13–5). The peak level of cortisol in the plasma normally occurs between 6:00 and 8:00 AM (during sleep, just before awakening) and the nadir at around 12:00 PM. The diurnal rhythm of ACTH secretion persists in patients with adrenal insufficiency who are receiving maintenance doses of glucocorticoids but is lost in Cushing's syndrome. The diurnal rhythm is also altered by changes in patterns of sleep, light-dark exposure, or food intake; physical stress such as major illness, surgery, trauma, or starvation; psychologic stress, including severe anxiety, depression, and mania; central nervous system and pituitary disorders; liver disease and other conditions that affect cortisol metabolism; chronic renal failure; alcoholism; and antiserotonergic drugs such as cyproheptadine.

Normally, the morning plasma ACTH concentration is about 25 pg/mL (5.5 pmol/L). Plasma ACTH and cortisol values in various normal and abnormal states are shown in Figure 13–6.

C. Stress Response: Plasma ACTH and cortisol secretion are also triggered by various forms of stress. Emotional stress (such as fear and anxiety) and bodily injury (such as surgery or hypoglycemia) release CRH from the hypothalamus and thus ACTH

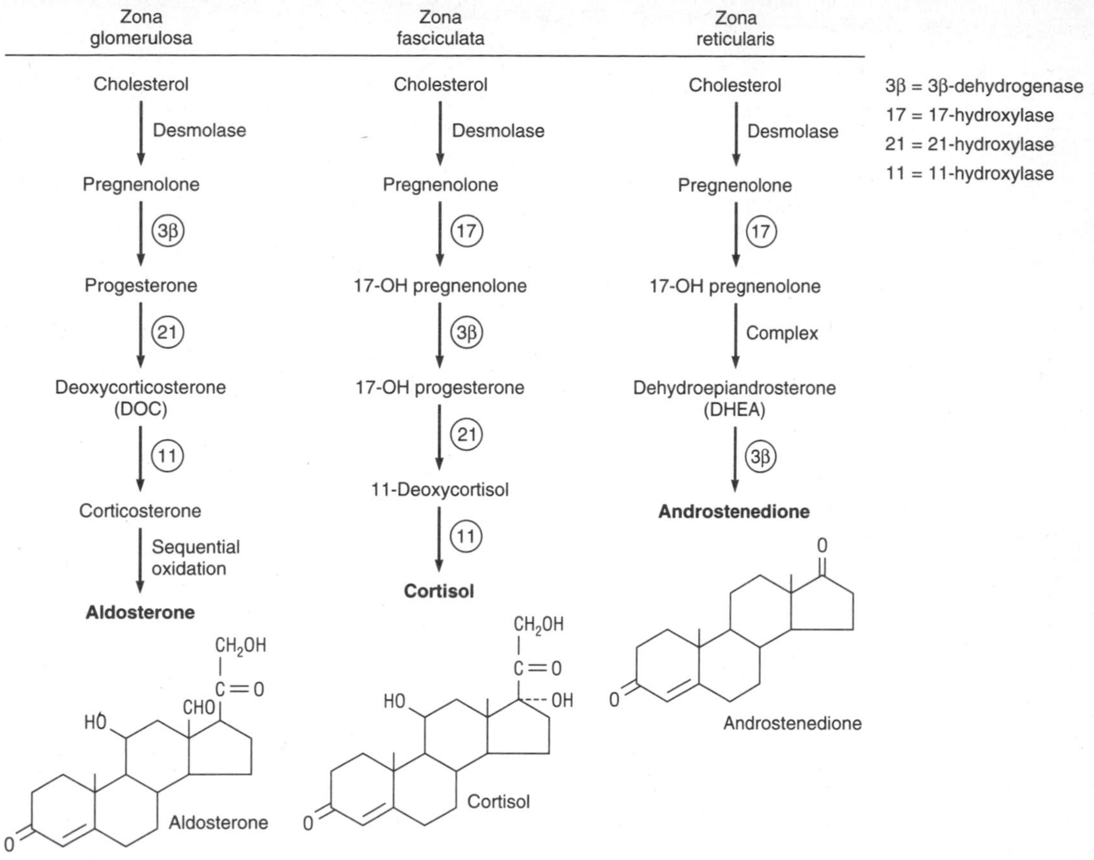

Figure 13–3. Simplified pathways of steroid synthesis in the different zones of the adrenal cortex. Note the differences in the types of enzyme necessary and the different order of enzymatic reactions in the different zones.

from the pituitary. This, in turn, results in a transient increase in cortisol secretion (Figure 13–7). If the stress is prolonged, it may abolish the normal diurnal rhythm of ACTH and cortisol secretion.

The stress response of plasma ACTH and cortisol is abolished in Cushing's syndrome but is exaggerated following adrenalectomy. The circulating catecholamines, epinephrine and norepinephrine, do not increase ACTH secretion.

D. Negative Feedback: ACTH secretion is inhibited in a negative feedback fashion by high circulating levels of free cortisol. This feedback inhibition occurs at both the pituitary and the hypothalamus (Figure 13–4).

A rising level of plasma cortisol inhibits release of ACTH from the pituitary, both by inhibiting CRH release from the hypothalamus and by interfering with the stimulatory action of CRH on the pituitary. The fall in plasma ACTH leads to a decline in adrenal secretion of cortisol. Conversely, a drop in plasma cortisol level stimulates ACTH secretion. In chronic adrenal insufficiency, there is a marked increase in the rate of ACTH synthesis and secretion.

ACTH secretion is also inhibited by chronic treatment with exogenous corticosteroids in proportion to their glucocorticoid potency. When prolonged corticosteroid treatment is stopped, the adrenal is atrophic and unresponsive and the patient is at risk for acute adrenal insufficiency. The pituitary may not be able to secrete normal amounts of ACTH for as long as a month, presumably due to diminished ACTH synthesis. Thereafter, there is a slow rise in ACTH to higher than normal levels (Figure 13–8). The higher than normal level of ACTH in turn stimulates adrenal glucocorticoid output, and feedback inhibition gradually reduces the ACTH level to normal. The risk of acute adrenal insufficiency following sudden cessation of corticosteroid therapy can be avoided by slowly tapering the corticosteroid dosage over a long period of time (or by switching to alternate-day steroid regimens before tapering).

E. Effects of ACTH on the Adrenal: Circulating ACTH binds to high-affinity receptors on adrenocortical cell membranes, activating adenylyl cyclase, increasing intracellular cAMP, and promoting synthesis of the enzyme that converts cholesterol to steroid

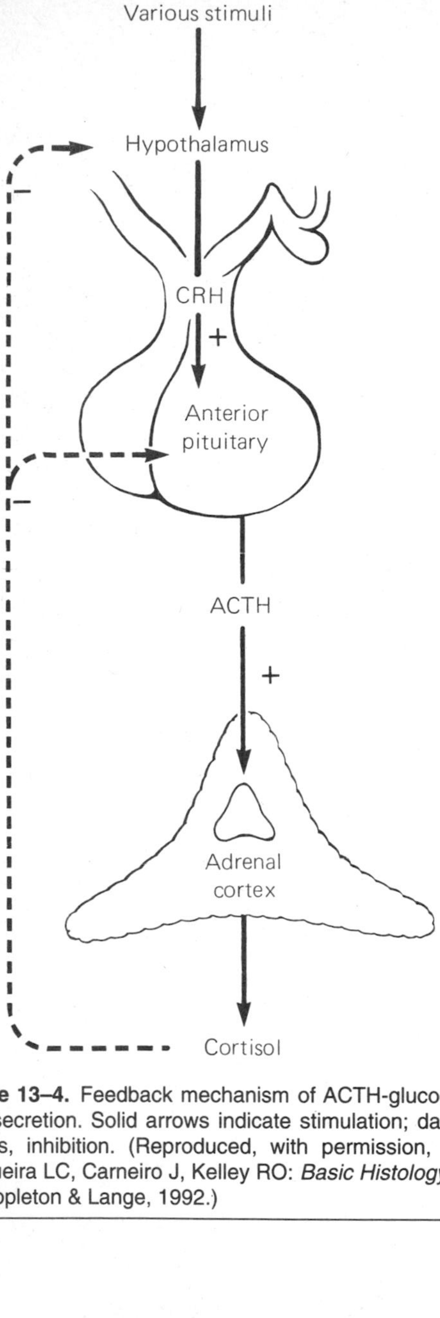

Figure 13–4. Feedback mechanism of ACTH-glucocorticoid secretion. Solid arrows indicate stimulation; dashed arrows, inhibition. (Reproduced, with permission, from Junqueira LC, Carneiro J, Kelley RO: *Basic Histology,* 7th ed. Appleton & Lange, 1992.)

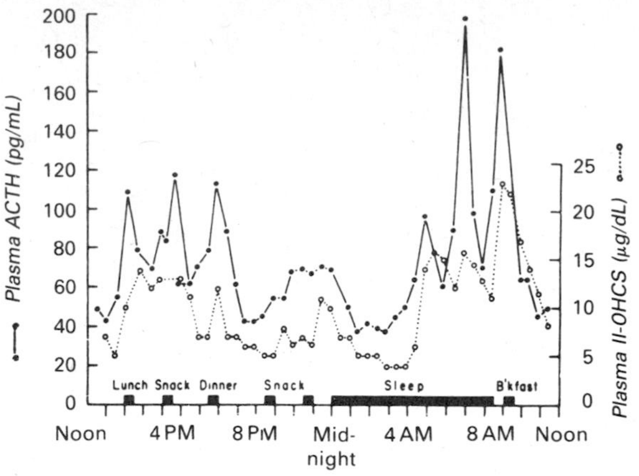

Figure 13–5. Fluctuations in plasma ACTH and glucocorticoids (11-OHCS) throughout the day. Note the greater ACTH and glucocorticoid rises in the morning before awakening. (Reproduced, with permission, from Krieger DT et al: Characterization of the normal temporal pattern of plasma corticosteroid levels. J Clin Endocrinol Metab 1971;32:266.)

hormone precursors. Increased glucocorticoid synthesis and secretion result within minutes.

Prolonged hypersecretion or administration of ACTH causes adrenocortical hyperplasia and hypertrophy. Conversely, prolonged ACTH deficiency results in adrenocortical atrophy.

Mechanism of Action

The physiologic effects of glucocorticoids in various tissues are the result of their binding to cytosolic glucocorticoid receptors. The hormone-receptor complexes then enter the nucleus, bind to nuclear DNA, and promote the transcription of DNA, the production of mRNAs, and the synthesis of proteins. The enzymes and other proteins thus produced mediate the glucocorticoid response, which may be inhibitory or stimulatory depending on the tissue involved. The cytosolic glucocorticoid receptors present in virtually all tissues are quite similar. However, the proteins produced vary widely as a result of the expression of different genes in specific target tissue cells. The regulation of this expression is not well understood.

Effects

The physiologic effects of glucocorticoids on target tissues are summarized in Table 13–2. In most tissues, glucocorticoids inhibit synthesis of DNA, RNA, and protein and have a catabolic effect, promoting degradation of protein and fat to provide substrate for intermediary metabolism. In the liver, however, glucocorticoids have a synthetic effect, promoting the uptake and use of carbohydrates (in synthesis of glucose and glycogen), amino acids (in synthesis of RNA and protein enzymes), and fatty acids (as an energy source).

During fasting, glucocorticoids help to maintain plasma glucose levels by several mechanisms (Table 13–2). In peripheral tissues, glucocorticoids antagonize the effects of insulin. The brain and heart are spared this antagonism, and the extra supply of glucose helps these vital organs to cope with stress. In diabetics, the insulin antagonism may worsen control of blood sugar, raise plasma lipid levels, and increase

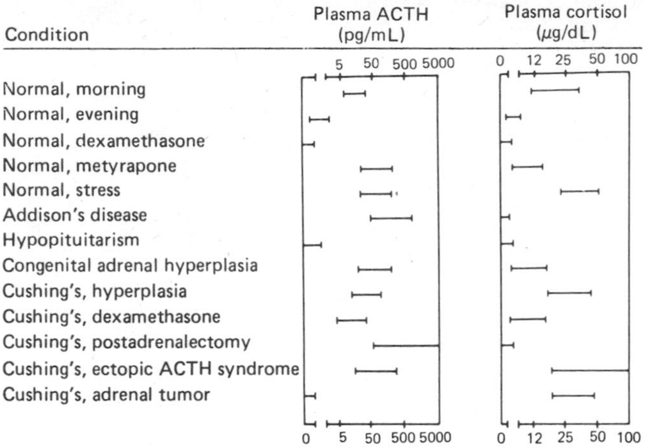

Figure 13–6. Plasma concentrations of ACTH and cortisol in various clinical states. (Reproduced, with permission, from Liddle G: The adrenal cortex. In: *Textbook of Endocrinology,* 5th ed. Williams RH [editor]. Saunders, 1974.)

the formation of ketone bodies. However, in nondiabetics, the rise in blood glucose stimulates a compensatory increase in insulin secretion that prevents these sequelae.

Small amounts of glucocorticoids must be present for other metabolic processes to occur **(permissive action).** For example, glucocorticoids must be present for catecholamines to produce their calorigenic, lipolytic, pressor, and bronchodilator effects and for glucagon to increase hepatic gluconeogenesis.

Glucocorticoids are also required to resist various stresses. Indeed, the increased secretion of pituitary ACTH and consequent increase in circulating glucocorticoids following injury is essential to survival. Hypophysectomized or adrenalectomized individuals treated with only maintenance doses of glucocorticoids may die when exposed to such stress. The reasons for this are unclear but may be related to interactions between glucocorticoids and catecholamines in maintaining vascular reactivity and in mobilizing free fatty acids as an emergency energy supply.

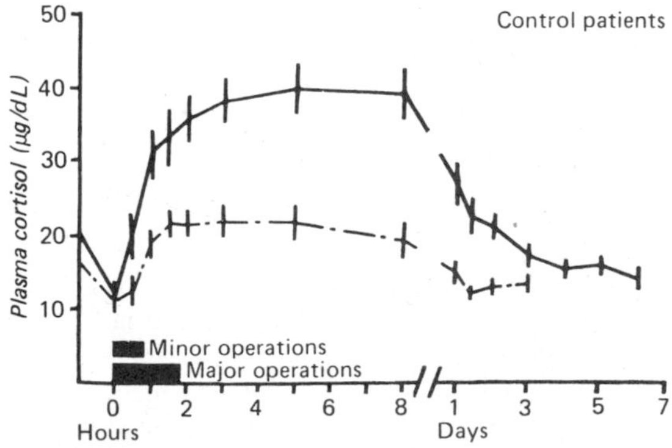

Figure 13–7. Plasma cortisol responses to major surgery (continuous line) and minor surgery (broken line) in normal subjects. Mean values and standard errors for 20 patients are shown in each case. (Reproduced, with permission, from Plumpton FS, Besser GM, Cole P: Anesthesia 1969;24:3).

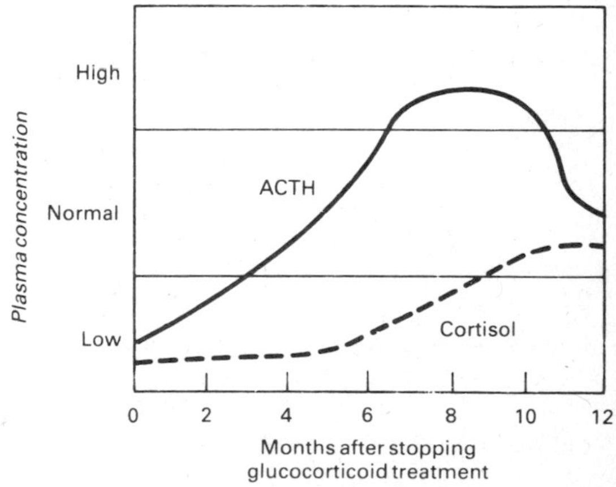

Figure 13–8. Pattern of plasma ACTH and cortisol values in patients recovering from prior long-term daily treatment with large doses of glucocorticoids. (Courtesy of R Ney. Reproduced, with permission, from Ganong WF: *Review of Medical Physiology,* 16th ed. Appleton & Lange, 1993.)

Table 13–2. Physiologic effects of glucocorticoids.

Target Tissue	Effect	Mechanism
Liver	Synthetic	Increase gluconeogenesis Increase glycogen synthesis, storage Increase glucose-6-phosphatase activity Increase blood glucose
Muscle	Catabolic	Inhibit glucose uptake and metabolism Decrease protein synthesis Increase release of amino acids, lactate
Fat	Lipolytic	Stimulate lipolysis Increase release of FFAs and glycerol
Immune system	Suppression	Reduce number of circulating lymphocytes, monocytes, eosinophils, basophils Inhibit T-lymphocyte production of interleukin-2 Interfere with antigen processing, antibody production and clearance
	Anti-inflammatory	Decrease migration of neutrophils, monocytes, lymphocytes to sites of injury
	Other	Stimulate release of neutrophils from marrow Interfere with neutrophil migration out of vascular compartment
Cardiovascular		Increase cardiac output Increase peripheral vascular tone
Renal		Increase glomerular filtration rate Aid in regulating water, electrolyte balance
Other	Insulin antagonism Permissive action Resistance to stress	Increase blood glucose

1. What are the histologic layers of the adrenal cortex, and what steroids does each secrete?
2. What three roles are proposed for steroid-binding proteins?
3. In what conditions are corticosteroid-binding globulin increased? Decreased?
4. In what conditions is cortisol metabolism increased? Decreased?
5. Describe the diurnal rhythm of ACTH secretion, and name the conditions in which it is altered.
6. What stress responses trigger ACTH secretion?
7. Describe the negative feedback control of the hypothalamic-pituitary-adrenal axis.
8. Describe the major physiologic effects of glucocorticoids.

2. MINERALOCORTICOIDS

Synthesis, Protein Binding, & Metabolism

The primary function of the mineralocorticoids is to regulate sodium excretion and maintain a normal intravascular volume. However, other factors affect sodium excretion besides the mineralocorticoids, such as the glomerular filtration rate, atrial natriuretic peptide, the presence of an osmotic diuretic, and changes in tubular reabsorption of sodium.

A. Synthesis: Aldosterone is the principal mineralocorticoid secreted by the adrenal. Corticosterone and deoxycorticosterone also have minor mineralocorticoid effects. Their biosynthetic pathways are depicted in Figure 13–3.

B. Protein Binding: Aldosterone is bound to plasma proteins (albumin and corticosteroid-binding globulin) only to a slight extent. The amount of aldosterone secreted under normal circumstances is small (about 0.15 mg/24 h). The normal average plasma concentration of (free and bound) aldosterone is 0.006 μg/dL (0.17 nmol/L). Free (unbound) aldosterone comprises 30–40% of the total.

C. Metabolism: The half-life of aldosterone is short (about 20–30 minutes). Aldosterone is catabolized principally in the liver, and its metabolites are excreted in the urine. Less than 1% of secreted aldosterone is excreted in urine in the free form.

Regulation of Mineralocorticoid Secretion

Aldosterone secretion is regulated primarily by the renin-angiotensin system, but also by pituitary ACTH and by the plasma electrolytes, sodium and potassium.

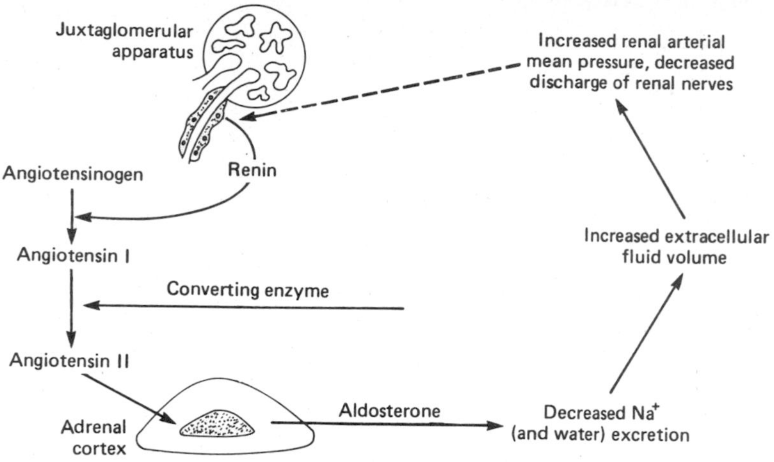

Figure 13–9. Feedback mechanism regulating aldosterone secretion. The dashed arrow indicates inhibition. (Redrawn and reproduced, with permission, from Ganong WF: *Review of Medical Physiology,* 16th ed. Appleton & Lange, 1993.)

A. Regulation by Renin-Angiotensin System: The **renin-angiotensin system** regulates aldosterone secretion in a feedback fashion (Figure 13–9). **Renin** is a proteolytic enzyme (MW about 40,000) produced by the juxtaglomerular cells of the kidney in response to changes in renal perfusion pressure and to reflex increases in renal nerve discharge. Once in the circulation, renin acts on **angiotensinogen,** an α_2-globulin produced in the liver, to form **angiotensin I,** a decapeptide. In the lung, angiotensin I is converted by angiotensin-converting enzyme (ACE) to **angiotensin II,** an octapeptide. Angiotensin II binds to zona glomerulosa cell membrane receptors and stimulates synthesis and secretion of aldosterone. The aldosterone promotes sodium and water retention, causing plasma volume expansion, which then shuts off renin secretion. In the supine state, there is a diurnal rhythm of aldosterone and renin secretion, with the highest values in the early morning before awakening.

The physiologic stimuli for the renin-angiotensin system to increase aldosterone secretion are factors which reduce renal perfusion and include extracellular fluid volume depletion, dietary sodium restriction and decreases in intra-arterial vascular volume (eg, due to hemorrhage or upright posture). Less commonly, certain disease states cause reduced renal perfusion, including renal artery stenosis, salt-losing disorders, congestive heart failure, and hypoproteinemic states (cirrhosis of the liver, or nephrotic syndrome). These disease states are said to cause a **secondary hyperaldosteronism.**)

B. Regulation by ACTH: ACTH also stimulates mineralocorticoid output. Quantitatively more ACTH is needed to stimulate mineralocorticoid than glucocorticoid secretion, but the amount required is still within the range of normal ACTH secretion. The effect of ACTH on aldosterone secretion is transient, however. Even if ACTH secretion remains elevated, aldosterone production declines to normal within 48 hours, perhaps because renin secretion decreases in response to hypervolemia.

C. Regulation by Plasma Electrolytes: An increase in plasma potassium concentration—or a fall in plasma sodium—stimulates aldosterone release. Conversely, a fall in plasma potassium level—or a rise in plasma sodium—inhibits its release. While minor changes of plasma potassium (1 meq/L or less) have an effect, major changes in plasma sodium (drops of about 20 meq/L) are needed to stimulate aldosterone secretion. Sodium depletion increases the affinity and number of angiotensin II receptors on adrenocortical cells.

Mechanism of Action

The mechanism of action of aldosterone is complex and incompletely understood.

Aldosterone, like other steroid hormones, acts by binding to a mineralocorticoid receptor in the cytosol. The steroid-receptor complex then moves into the nucleus of the target cell and increases transcription of DNA, induction of mRNA, and stimulation of protein synthesis by ribosomes. This protein acts to increase active transport of sodium via the sodium pump (Figure 13–10).

In addition, functional studies have been conducted on extrarenal, nonepithelial cells such as smooth muscle cells and circulating mononuclear leukocytes. High-affinity binding sites for aldosterone have been found in mononuclear leukocytes.

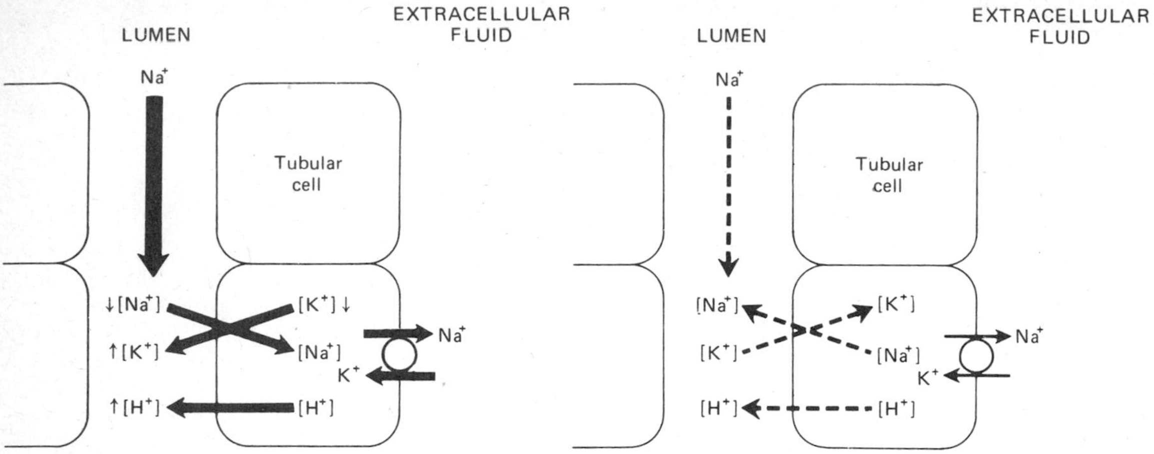

Figure 13–10. Mineralocorticoid action. On the left, high sodium intakes and high tubular sodium with increased mineralocorticoid action lead to K^+ and H^+ secretion and Na^+ movement into extracellular fluid. On the right, similar amounts of mineralocorticoid are ineffective when tubular sodium is reduced. (Reproduced, with permission, from Greenspan FS, Baxter JD: *Basic and Clinical Endocrinology,* 4th ed. Appleton & Lange, 1994.)

In these cells, aldosterone produces effects in vitro on intracellular sodium, potassium, and calcium concentrations and cell volume. These effects on transmembrane electrolyte movements are quite rapid, with onset within 1–2 minutes. These have been shown to involve activation of the cell membrane sodium-proton exchanger at very low physiologic concentrations of aldosterone. The inositol 1,4,5-trisphosphate-calcium messenger cascade, which responds over the same rapid time course, may also be involved. The rapid response of the sodium-proton exchanger of the cell membrane cannot be explained by a mechanism of action involving the interaction of a steroid receptor complex with nuclear DNA, since it is too fast. Instead, the rapid direct membrane effects of aldosterone might indicate distinct membrane receptors with a high affinity for aldosterone. Genomic mechanisms are presumably responsible for later effects of aldosterone.

Effects

The target cells for the mineralocorticoids are the kidney, colon, duodenum, salivary glands, and sweat glands. In the distal renal tubules and collecting ducts, aldosterone acts to promote the exchange of sodium ions for potassium and hydrogen ions, causing sodium retention, potassium diuresis, and increased urine acidity (Figure 13–10). Elsewhere, it acts to increase the reabsorption of sodium from the colonic fluid, saliva, and sweat. The mineralocorticoids may also increase potassium and decrease sodium concentrations in muscle and brain cells.

9. How is aldosterone secretion regulated?
10. How does ACTH affect aldosterone secretion differently than glucocorticoid secretion?
11. What are the effects of aldosterone, and on which tissues does it act?

PATHOPHYSIOLOGY OF SELECTED ADRENOCORTICAL DISORDERS

Characteristic syndromes are produced by excessive or deficient secretion of each type of adrenal hormone. Excessive glucocorticoid secretion **(Cushing's syndrome)** results in a moon-faced, plethoric appearance, with truncal obesity, purple abdominal striae, hypertension, osteoporosis, mental aberrations, protein depletion, and glucose intolerance or frank diabetes mellitus.

Excessive mineralocorticoid secretion **(Conn's syndrome)** leads to sodium retention, usually without edema, and potassium depletion, resulting in hypertension, muscle weakness, polyuria, hypokalemia, metabolic alkalosis, and sometimes hypocalcemia and tetany.

Excessive androgen secretion causes masculinization (adrenogenital syndrome) and precocious pseudopuberty or female pseudohermaphroditism.

Rare estrogen-secreting adrenal tumors may cause feminization.

Deficient glucocorticoid secretion due to autoimmune or other destruction of the adrenal glands **(Addison's disease)** causes symptoms of weakness, fatigue, malaise, anorexia, nausea and vomiting, weight loss, hypotension, hypoglycemia, and marked intolerance of physiologic stress (eg, infection). Elevation of plasma ACTH may produce hyperpigmentation.

Associated mineralocorticoid deficiency leads to renal sodium wasting and potassium retention and can produce manifestations of severe dehydration, hypotension, decreased cardiac size, hyponatremia, hyperkalemia, and metabolic acidosis. Deficient mineralocorticoid secretion also occurs in patients with renal disease and low circulating renin levels **(hyporeninemic hypoaldosteronism).**

CUSHING'S SYNDROME

Cushing's syndrome is the clinical condition resulting from chronic exposure to excessive circulating levels of glucocorticoids (Figure 13–11). It is also called **hyperadrenocorticalism, hyperadrenal corticalism,** or **hypercortisolism. Cushing's disease,** the most common cause of the syndrome, is caused by pituitary hypersecretion of ACTH, leading to bilateral adrenal hyperplasia.

Etiology

Cushing's syndrome may occur either spontaneously or as the result of chronic corticosteroid administration (iatrogenic Cushing's syndrome). The causes of Cushing's syndrome are summarized in Table 13–3.

A. Cushing's Disease: Cushing's disease is the most common cause of noniatrogenic Cushing's syndrome. Over 90% of patients with Cushing's disease have a pituitary adenoma causing excessive secretion of ACTH (Figure 13–12). Such adenomas are located in the anterior pituitary, are usually less than 10 mm in diameter **(microadenomas),** and are composed of basophilic corticotroph cells containing ACTH in secretory granules.

Less commonly, patients with Cushing's disease have **diffuse hyperplasia** of pituitary corticotroph

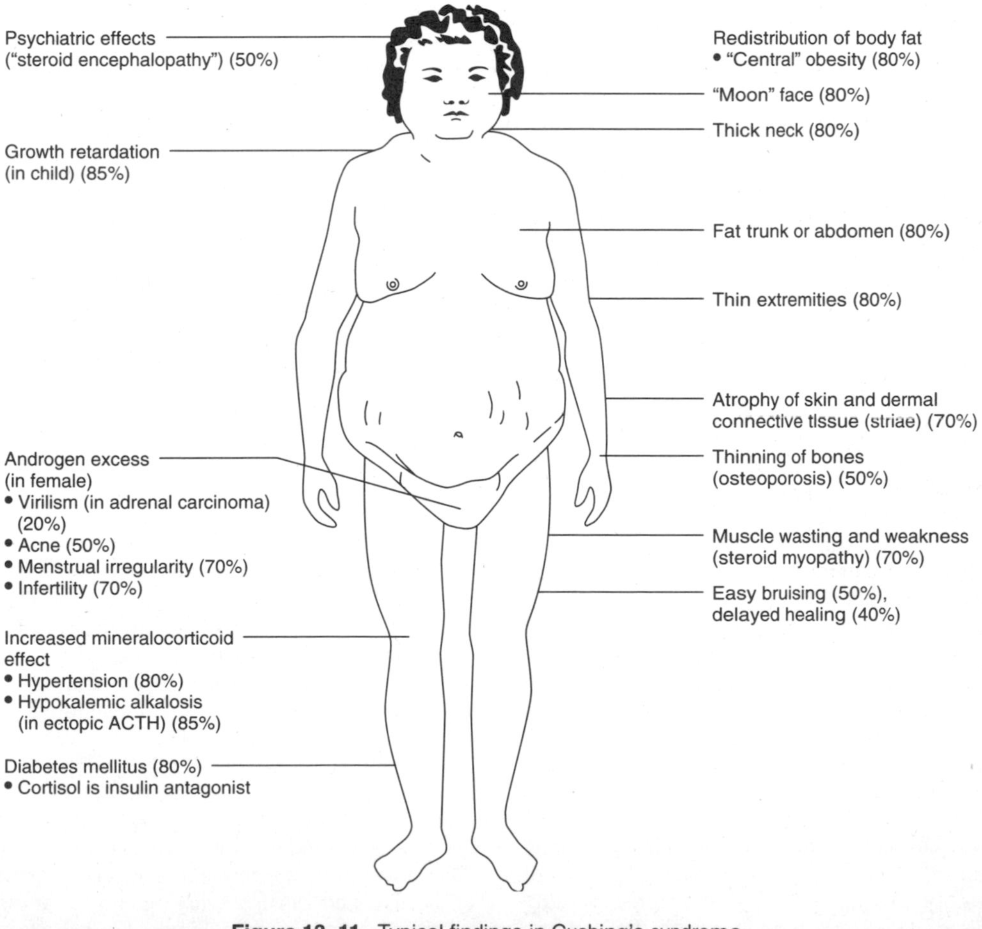

Figure 13–11. Typical findings in Cushing's syndrome.

Table 13–3. Causes of Cushing's syndrome.

NONIATROGENIC

ACTH-Dependent

1. **Cushing's disease (ACTH-secreting pituitary adenoma):**
   - *Epidemiology:* 68% of cases of noniatrogenic Cushing's syndrome. More common in women (F : M ratio of approximately 8:1). Age at diagnosis usually 20–40 years.
   - *Clinical features:* Hyperpigmentation and hypokalemic alkalosis are rare; androgenic manifestations limited to acne and hirsutism. Secretion of cortisol and adrenal androgens is only moderately increased.
   - *Course:* Slow progression over several years.
2. **Ectopic ACTH syndrome:**
   - *Epidemiology:* 15% of cases of spontaneous Cushing's syndrome. More common in men (M : F ratio of approximately 3:1). Age at diagnosis usually 40–60 years. Occurs in 0.5–2% of patients with small cell carcinoma of lung (about 50% of all cases). Other tumors responsible: thymoma; pancreatic islet-cell tumors; carcinoid tumors of lung, gut, pancreas or ovary; medullary thyroid carcinoma; pheochromocytoma.
   - *Clinical features:* Frequently limited to weakness, hypertension, and glucose intolerance, due to the rapid onset of hypercortisolism. Weight loss and anemia are common effects of malignancy. Primary tumor usually apparent. Hyperpigmentation, hypokalemia, and alkalosis may occur from the mineralocorticoid effects of cortisol and other steroids secreted.
   - *Course:* With underlying carcinoma, hypercortisolism is of rapid onset, steroid hypersecretion is frequently severe, with equally elevated levels of glucocorticoids, androgens, and deoxycorticosterone (DOC). With underlying benign tumor, more slowly progressive course.

ACTH-Independent

3. **Functioning adrenocortical tumor:**
   - *Epidemiology:* 17% of cases of Cushing's syndrome. Adrenal adenoma in 9%, adrenal carcinoma in 8%. More common in women. Adrenal carcinoma occurs in about 2 per million population per year. Age at diagnosis usually 35–40 years.
   - *Clinical features and course:* Adenoma: Onset is gradual. Usually secretes only cortisol. Hypercortisolism is mild to moderate. Androgenic effects absent. Carcinoma: Rapid onset, rapidly progressive. Marked elevations of glucocorticoids, androgens, and mineralocorticoids. Hypokalemia, abdominal pain, abdominal masses, hepatic and pulmonary metastases.

IATROGENIC

4. **Exogenous glucocorticoid administration:** Glucocorticoid administered in high doses in the treatment of nonendocrine disorders.

cells responsible for ACTH hypersecretion. The hyperplasia is probably due to hypersecretion of CRH by the hypothalamus.

In Cushing's disease, the chronic ACTH hypersecretion causes bilateral hyperplasia of the adrenal cortex. Combined adrenal weights (normal: 8–10 g) range from 12 g to 24 g.

B. Ectopic ACTH Syndrome: In the **ectopic ACTH syndrome,** a nonpituitary tumor synthesizes and hypersecretes biologically active ACTH or an ACTH-like peptide (or CRH) (Figure 13–12). The neoplasm most frequently responsible is small-cell carcinoma of the lung. Other associated tumors are listed in Table 13–3.

Chronic ACTH hypersecretion causes marked bilateral adrenocortical hyperplasia, with combined adrenal weights ranging from 24 g to 50 g or more. Pituitary corticotroph cells are suppressed by high circulating cortisol levels and have a decreased ACTH content.

C. Functioning Adrenocortical Tumors: Both **adrenocortical adenomas** and **carcinomas** may cause Cushing's syndrome by elaborating cortisol autonomously (Figure 13–12). Adenomas usually range in size from 1 cm to 6 cm, weigh 10–70 g, are encapsulated, and consist predominantly of zona fasciculata cells. Carcinomas (rare) are usually large, weighing 100 g to several kilograms, and often palpable as an abdominal mass. Grossly, they are highly vascular, with areas of necrosis, hemorrhage, cystic degeneration, and calcification. They are highly malignant lesions, tending to invade adrenal capsule and blood vessels and to metastasize to the kidney, retroperitoneum, liver, and lung.

Pathogenesis

Both Cushing's disease and ectopic ACTH syndrome are characterized by chronic ACTH hypersecretion and increased secretion of cortisol. On the other hand, glucocorticoid-secreting adrenocortical adenomas and carcinomas are characterized by autonomous secretion of cortisol and suppression of pituitary ACTH (Figures 13–12 and 13–13).

A. Cushing's Disease: In Cushing's disease, there is a persistent overproduction of ACTH by the pituitary adenoma. The ACTH hypersecretion is episodic and random; the normal diurnal rhythm of ACTH and cortisol secretion is absent. Plasma levels of ACTH and cortisol vary and may at times be within the normal range (Figure 13–13). However, a

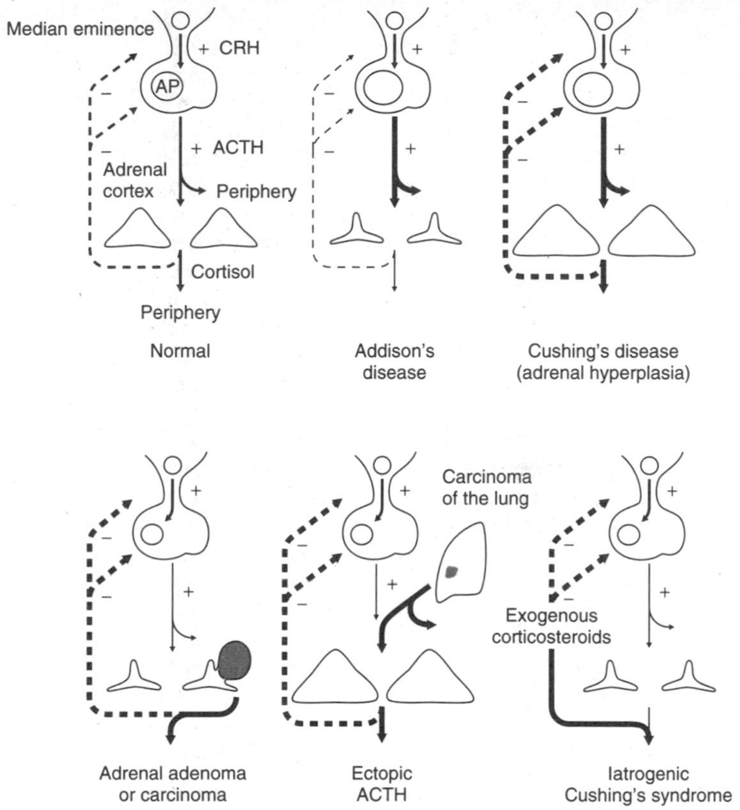

Figure 13–12. Hypothalamic, pituitary, and adrenal cortical relationships. Solid arrows indicate stimulation; dashed arrows, inhibition. **Normal:** Corticotropin-releasing hormone (CRH) elaborated by the median eminence (ME) of the hypothalamus stimulates secretion of adrenocorticotropic hormone (ACTH) by the anterior pituitary (AP). ACTH triggers the synthesis and release of cortisol, the principal glucocorticoid of the adrenal cortex (AC). A rising level of cortisol inhibits the stimulatory action of CRH on ACTH release (or cortisol may inhibit CRH release), completing a negative feedback loop. **Addison's disease:** In primary destructive disease of the adrenal cortex, the level of plasma cortisol is very low, and the effect of CRH on the anterior pituitary proceeds without inhibition, causing a marked increase in the secretion of ACTH. High levels of ACTH produce characteristic skin pigmentary changes. **Cushing's disease (adrenal hyperplasia):** The primary lesion may be at the level of the pituitary or hypothalamus. In either case, production of ACTH and cortisol is excessive. The former causes bilateral adrenal hyperplasia and the latter causes clinical manifestations of hypercortisolism. Cells of the anterior pituitary are relatively resistant to the high levels of circulating cortisol. **Adrenal adenoma or carcinoma:** An adenoma or carcinoma of the adrenal cortex may produce cortisol autonomously. When the rate of production exceeds physiologic quantities, Cushing's syndrome results; the effect of CRH on the anterior pituitary is inhibited by the high levels of circulating cortisol, with resultant diminished ACTH secretion and atrophy of normal adrenal tissue. **Ectopic ACTH:** In this syndrome, ACTH or an ACTH-like peptide is elaborated by a tumor such as carcinoma of the lung. The adrenals are stimulated; circulating cortisol is increased; and ACTH secretion inhibited. Tumors elaborating CRH have also been reported. **Iatrogenic Cushing's syndrome:** Exogenous corticosteroid administration in excess of physiologic quantities of cortisol leads directly to peripheral manifestations of hypercortisolism and inhibits the effect of CRH on the anterior pituitary, with resultant diminished ACTH secretion, diminished cortisol production, and atrophy of normal adrenal tissue. (Modified and reproduced, with permission, from Burns TW, Carlson HE: Endocrinology. In: *Pathologic Physiology: Mechanisms of Disease.* Sodeman WA, Sodeman TM [editors] Saunders, 1985.)

24-hour urine free cortisol measurement confirms hypercortisolism. The excessive cortisol does not suppress ACTH secretion by the pituitary adenoma.

Despite ACTH hypersecretion, the pituitary and adrenals fail to respond normally to stress. Stimuli such as hypoglycemia or surgery fail to increase ACTH and cortisol secretion, probably because chronic hypercortisolism has suppressed CRH secretion by the hypothalamus. Hypercortisolism also inhibits other normal pituitary and hypothalamic functions, affecting thyrotropin, growth hormone, and gonadotropin release.

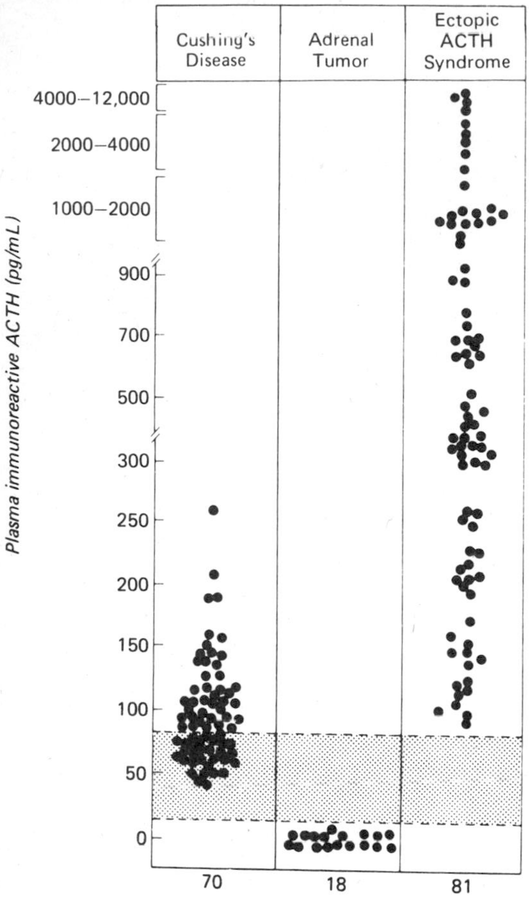

Figure 13–13. Basal plasma ACTH concentrations in patients with various types of noniatrogenic Cushing's syndrome. (Reproduced, with permission, from Scott AP et al: Pituitary adrenocorticotropin and the melanocyte stimulating hormones. In: *Peptide Hormones.* Parsons JA [editor]. University Park Press, 1979.)

Surgical removal of the ACTH-producing adenoma reverses these abnormalities.

B. Ectopic ACTH Syndrome: In the ectopic ACTH syndrome, hypersecretion of ACTH and cortisol is random and episodic and quantitatively greater than in patients with Cushing's disease (Figure 13–13). Indeed, plasma levels and urinary excretion of cortisol, adrenal androgens, and other steroids are often markedly elevated. Ectopic ACTH secretion by tumors is not suppressible by exogenous glucocorticoids such as dexamethasone (Figure 13–14).

C. Adrenal Tumors: Primary adrenal adenomas and carcinomas are not under hypothalamic-pituitary control and thus autonomously hypersecrete cortisol. The hypercortisolism suppresses pituitary ACTH production, resulting in atrophy of the uninvolved adrenal cortex (Figure 13–12). Steroid secretion is random and episodic and usually is not suppressible by dexamethasone.

Clinical Manifestations

The clinical manifestations of Cushing's syndrome (Figure 13–11) are predictable consequences of the physiologic effects of cortisol discussed above and in Table 13–2.

Cortisol excess promotes synthesis of glucose in the liver from amino acids liberated by protein catabolism. Cortisol also antagonizes the action of insulin in transporting glucose into cells. Both actions lead to glucose intolerance. Thirst and polyuria signal hyperglycemia. Overt diabetes mellitus occurs in about 10–15% of patients with Cushing's syndrome. The diabetes is characterized by insulin resistance, ketosis, and hyperlipidemia, but acidosis and microvascular complications are rare.

With chronic cortisol excess, muscle wasting occurs as a result of excess protein catabolism. Proximal muscle weakness, usually most prominent in the lower extremities, occurs in about 60% of cases.

Obesity and redistribution of body fat are probably the most recognizable features of Cushing's syndrome. Weight gain is often the initial symptom. The obesity is centralized, with relative sparing of the extremities. The redistribution of adipose tissue affects mainly the face, neck, trunk, and abdomen, producing the characteristic "moon" facies, "buffalo hump," supraclavicular fat pads, truncal obesity, and abdominal striae. The reason for the abnormal fat redistribution is unknown.

Given the known lipolytic effects of glucocorticoids, the increased fat deposition caused by glucocorticoid excess seems paradoxical. It may be explained by the increase in appetite or by the lipogenic effects of the hyperinsulinemia the cortisol excess causes.

Glucocorticoid excess inhibits fibroblasts, leading to loss of collagen and connective tissue. Thinning of the skin, abdominal striae, easy bruisability, poor wound healing, and frequent skin infections are the result. Atrophy leads to a translucent appearance of the skin. Prominent reddish-purple **striae** occur in 50–70% of patients, most commonly over the abdominal wall, breasts, hips, buttocks, thighs, and axillas. The striae result from increased subcutaneous fat deposition, which stretches the thin skin and ruptures the subdermal tissues. These striae are depressed below the skin surface because of loss of underlying connective tissue and are wider (not infrequently 0.5–2 cm) than the pinkish-white striae of pregnancy or rapid weight gain. Easy bruisability occurs in about 40% of cases. Wound healing is delayed, and surgical incisions sometimes undergo dehiscence. Fungal infections of the skin and mucous membranes are frequent, including tinea versicolor, seborrheic dermatitis, onychomycosis, and oral candidiasis.

In the ectopic ACTH syndrome, hyperpigmentation of the skin occurs owing to the markedly elevated level of circulating ACTH, which has some melanocyte-stimulating hormone (MSH)-like activity. However, hyperpigmentation is rare in Cushing's disease or adrenal tumors.

Hirsutism from increased secretion of adrenal androgens occurs in about 80% of female patients over the face, abdomen, breasts, chest, and upper thighs. Acne often accompanies the hirsutism.

While the physiologic role of glucocorticoids in bone and calcium metabolism is not well understood, excessive glucocorticoid production inhibits bone formation and accelerates bone resorption (see Chapter 17). Glucocorticoids directly inhibit bone formation by decreasing cell proliferation and synthesis of RNA, protein, collagen, and hyaluronic acid. They directly stimulate osteoclasts, leading to osteolysis and increased urinary hydroxyproline excretion. They potentiate the actions of PTH and 1,25-$(OH)_2$ vitamin D on bone.

Furthermore, glucocorticoid excess decreases intestinal calcium absorption and increases urinary calcium excretion (hypercalciuria), resulting in a negative calcium balance. To maintain normal serum calcium levels, there is a secondary increase in PTH secretion, accelerating bone resorption. Glucocorticoids may also directly stimulate PTH secretion.

As a result of the hypercalciuria, kidney stones occur in about 15% of patients. Such patients may present with renal colic. Glucocorticoids also reduce the renal tubular reabsorption of phosphate, leading to phosphaturia and reduced serum phosphorus concentrations.

The combination of decreased bone formation and increased bone resorption ultimately leads to a generalized loss in bone mass **(osteoporosis)** and an increased risk of bony fracture. Osteoporosis is present in most patients; back pain is an initial complaint in 58% of cases. X-rays frequently reveal vertebral compression fractures (16–22% of cases) and rib fractures.

Glucocorticoid excess alters the normal inflammatory response to infection or injury by several mechanisms. Glucocorticoids inhibit the action of phospholipase A_2 in releasing arachidonic acid from tissue phospholipids, thereby reducing formation of leukotrienes (powerful mediators of inflammation), thromboxanes, prostaglandins, and prostacyclin. They stabilize lysosomal membranes, inhibiting the release of interleukin-1 (endogenous pyrogen) from granulocytes. They suppress antibody formation and inhibit the accumulation and migration of polymorphonuclear neutrophils to sites of inflammation. They inhibit fibroblastic activity, preventing the walling off of bacterial and other infections. And they decrease local swelling and block the systemic effects of bacterial toxins.

Glucocorticoid excess also suppresses manifestations of allergic disorders that are due to the release of histamine from tissues.

Hypertension occurs in about 75–85% of patients with spontaneous Cushing's syndrome. The exact pathogenesis of the hypertension is unclear. It may be related to salt and water retention from the mineralocorticoid effects of the excess glucocorticoid. It may be due to increased secretion of angiotensinogen or deoxycorticosterone. Or it may be due to a direct effect of glucocorticoids on blood vessels.

Gonadal dysfunction occurs commonly in Cushing's syndrome and is the result of increased secretion of adrenal androgens (in females) and cortisol (in males and females). In premenopausal women, the androgens may cause hirsutism, acne, amenorrhea and infertility. The high levels of cortisol can suppress pituitary LH secretion. In men, this results in decreased testosterone secretion by the testis, for which the increased adrenal secretion of weak androgens does not compensate. Symptoms of decreased libido, loss of body hair, soft testes, and impotence ensue.

Excess glucocorticoids frequently produce mental symptoms, including euphoria, increased appetite, irritability, emotional lability, decreased libido, anxiety, and depression. Many patients experience impaired cognitive function, with poor concentration and poor memory, and disordered sleep, with decreased REM sleep and early morning awakening. Severe psychologic disturbances occur less commonly and include severe depression, frank psychosis with delusions, hallucinations, paranoia, or hyperkinetic, even manic behavior. Glucocorticoid excess also accelerates the basic electroencephalographic rhythm. The pathogenesis of these central nervous system effects is not well understood.

Glucocorticoid excess inhibits growth in children, in part by directly inhibiting bone cells and in part by decreasing growth hormone and TSH secretion and somatomedin generation.

Routine laboratory tests in Cushing's syndrome usually demonstrate a high normal hemoglobin, hematocrit, and red cell number. Polycythemia occurs rarely, secondary to androgen excess. The total white blood cell count is usually normal; however, the percentages of lymphocytes and eosinophils and the total lymphocyte and eosinophil counts are frequently subnormal.

Serum electrolytes are usually normal. Hypokalemic metabolic alkalosis sometimes occurs as a result of mineralocorticoid hypersecretion in patients with ectopic ACTH syndrome or adrenocortical carcinoma. Fasting hyperglycemia occurs in about 10–15% of patients; postprandial hyperglycemia and glucosuria are more common. Most patients with Cushing's syndrome have secondary hyperinsulinemia and abnormal glucose tolerance tests. The serum calcium is generally normal; the serum phosphorus is low normal or slightly low. Hypercalciuria can be demonstrated in 40% of cases.

Routine x-rays may reveal cardiomegaly due to hypertensive or atherosclerotic heart disease, vertebral compression fractures, rib fractures, and renal calculi.

The ECG may show left ventricular hypertrophy (LVH) from hypertension, ischemia, or ST–T wave changes from electrolyte disturbances (eg, flattening of T waves from hypokalemia).

Diagnosis

Suspected hypercortisolism can be investigated by several approaches (Table 13–4; Figure 13–14).

Measurement of free cortisol in a 24-hour urine specimen collected on an outpatient basis demonstrates excessive excretion of cortisol (24-hour urinary free cortisol levels > 150 μg/24 h). Urinary free cortisol values are rarely normal in Cushing's syndrome.

Performance of an overnight 1-mg dexamethasone suppression test will demonstrate lack of the normal suppression of adrenal cortisol production by exogenous corticosteroid (dexamethasone). The overnight dexamethasone suppression test is accomplished by prescribing 1 mg of dexamethasone at 11:00 PM, and then obtaining a plasma cortisol level at 8:00 AM the following morning. In normal individuals, the dexamethasone suppresses the early morning surge in cortisol, resulting in plasma cortisol levels of less than 5 μg/dL (0.14 μmol/L); in Cushing's syndrome, cortisol secretion is not suppressed, and values are greater than 10 μg/dL (0.28 μmol/L).

If the overnight dexamethasone suppression test is normal, the diagnosis is very unlikely; if the urine free cortisol is also normal, Cushing's syndrome is excluded. If both tests are abnormal, hypercortisolism is present and the diagnosis of Cushing's syndrome can be considered established if conditions causing false positives are excluded (acute or chronic illness, obesity, high-estrogen states, drugs, alcoholism, and depression).

In patients with equivocal or borderline results, a 2-day low-dose dexamethasone suppression test is often performed. Normal responses to this test exclude the diagnosis of Cushing's syndrome. Normal responses are an 8:00 AM plasma cortisol less than 5 μg/dL (0.14 μmol/L); a 24-hour urinary free cortisol less than 25 μg/24 h (69 nmol/24 h); and a 24-hour urinary 17-hydroxycorticosteroid level less than 4 mg/24 h (11.2 μmol/24 h) or 1 mg/g creatinine (0.3 mmol/mol creatinine).

Confirmation of the diagnosis of Cushing's syndrome entails a more prolonged dexamethasone suppression test.

Table 13–4. Laboratory diagnosis of Cushing's syndrome.[1]

STEP A: ESTABLISHMENT OF PRESENCE OF HYPERCORTISOLISM

- Overnight dexamethasone suppression: Plasma cortisol > 5 μg/dL (140 nmol/L in an 8 AM sample after 1 mg of dexamethasone at 11 PM (best screening test)
- Urinary 24-hour free cortisol level > 100 μg/d (275 nmol/d) (very good screening test)
- Low-dose 2-day dexamethasone suppression: Failure to suppress plasma cortisol to <5 μg/dL (140 nmol/L) = Cushing's syndrome (definitive diagnostic test)

STEP B: DIFFERENTIAL DIAGNOSIS OF CUSHING'S SYNDROME

	Plasma ACTH	Suppression With High-Dose Dexamethasone[2]	CT Scan Findings
Cushing's disease = pituitary-induced adrenal hyperplasia	Elevated	Yes[3]	Pituitary adenoma may be small; bilateral adrenal hyperplasia
Adrenal adenoma	Low	No	Adrenal neoplasm: small
Adrenal carcinoma	Low	No	Adrenal neoplasm: large
Ectopic ACTH production	Very high	No	Bilateral adrenal hyperplasia; normal pituitary; some other malignant neoplasm

[1] Modified from Chandrasoma P, Taylor CR: *Concise Pathology,* 2nd ed. Appleton & Lange, 1994.
[2] Dexamethasone is a synthetic glucocorticoid that suppresses ACTH secretion. At low doses (eg, 1 mg at 11 PM), suppression is not adequate to decrease excess cortisol secretion in any patient with Cushing's syndrome. At high doses (eg, 8 mg at 11 PM), it suppresses excessive ACTH secretion by pituitary adenomas.
[3] Rarely, pituitary adenomas do not suppress; pituitary venous sampling is indicated in cases where an ectopic ACTH-producing neoplasm is not found.

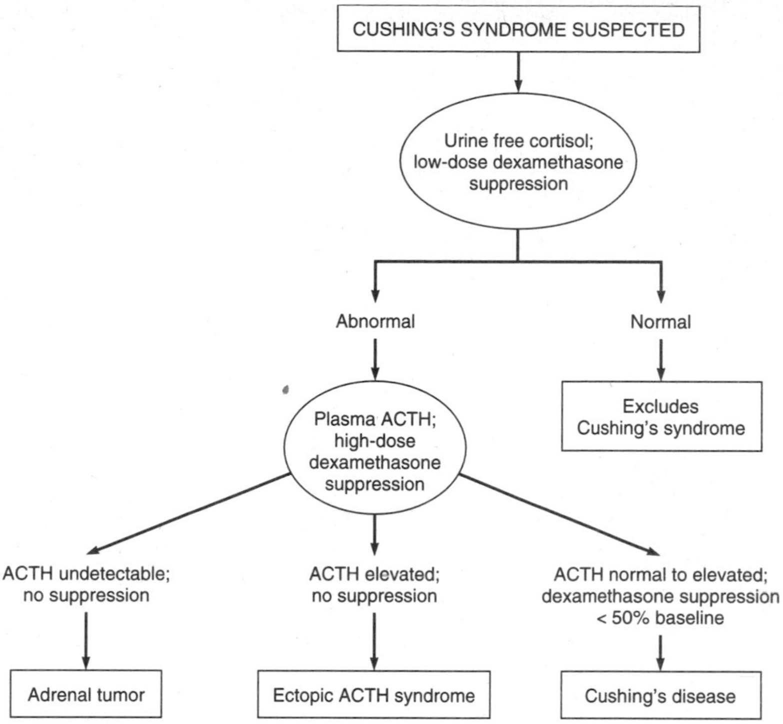

Figure 13–14. Diagnostic evaluation of Cushing's syndrome and procedures for determining the cause. Boxes enclose clinical decisions, and ovals enclose diagnostic tests. (Redrawn and reproduced, with permission, from Baxter JD, Tyrrell JB: The adrenal cortex. In: *Endocrinology and Metabolism.* Felig P et al [editors]. 2nd ed. McGraw-Hill, 1987.)

12. What are the signs and symptoms of excess of each class of adrenal steroids?
13. What are the signs and symptoms of deficiency of each class of adrenal steroids?
14. What are the major causes of Cushing's syndrome?
15. How is the regulation of glucocorticoid secretion altered in patients with Cushing's disease? With ectopic ACTH secretion? With autonomous adrenal tumors?
16. What are the signs and symptoms of glucocorticoid excess?
17. Suggest some different ways to make the diagnosis of Cushing's disease in a patient with suggestive signs and symptoms.

ADRENOCORTICAL INSUFFICIENCY

Adrenocortical insufficiency generally occurs either because of destruction or dysfunction of the adrenal cortex **(primary adrenocortical insufficiency)** or because of deficient pituitary ACTH secretion **(secondary adrenocortical insufficiency)**. However, congenital defects in any one of several enzymes occurring as an "inborn error of metabolism'' can lead to deficient cortisol secretion. Enzyme deficiencies can also result from treatment with various drugs, such as metyrapone, amphenone, and mitotane.

The causes of adrenocortical insufficiency are shown in Table 13–5. No matter what the origin, the clinical manifestations of adrenocortical insufficiency are a consequence of deficiencies of cortisol, aldosterone, and (in women) androgenic steroids.

Etiology

A. Primary Adrenocortical Insufficiency: Primary adrenocortical insufficiency (Addison's disease) is most often due to autoimmune destruction of the adrenal cortex (about 80% of cases). In the past, tuberculosis involving the adrenals was the most common cause, but it now accounts for about 20% of cases. Less common causes include adrenal hemorrhage or infarction, other granulomatous disease such as histoplasmosis, metastatic carcinoma, and AIDS-related (cytomegalovirus) adrenalitis.

Primary adrenal insufficiency is rare, with reported

Table 13–5. Causes of adrenocortical insufficiency.[1]

I. Primary adrenocortical insufficiency (Addison's disease)
Major causes
Autoimmune (about 80%)
Tuberculosis (about 20%)
Uncommon causes
Adrenal hemorrhage and infarction
Fungal and other granulomatous infections
Metastatic and lymphomatous replacement
AIDS-related CMV adrenalitis
Amyloidosis
Sarcoidosis
Hemochromatosis
Radiation therapy
Surgical adrenalectomy
Enzyme inhibitors (metyrapone, aminoglutethimide, trilostane, ketoconazole)
Cytotoxic agents (mitotane)
Congenital defects (enzyme defects, adrenal hypoplasia, familial glucocorticoid deficiency)
II. Secondary adrenocortical insufficiency
Major cause
Chronic exogenous glucocorticoid therapy
Uncommon causes
Pituitary tumor
Hypothalamic tumor

[1] Modified and reproduced, with permission, from Baxter JD, Tyrell JB, in: *Endocrinology and Metabolism.* Felig P et al (editors). McGraw-Hill, 1981; and from Greenspan FS, Baxter JD (editors): *Basic and Clinical Endocrinology,* 4th ed. Appleton & Lange, 1994.

prevalence rates of 39–60 cases per million population. However, as the number of patients with AIDS increases and as patients with malignancies live longer, more cases of adrenocortical insufficiency may be encountered. Addison's disease is somewhat more common in women, with a female:male ratio of 1.25:1, and usually occurs in the third to fifth decades.

1. Autoimmune adrenocortical insufficiency– Autoimmune destruction of the adrenal glands is thought to be related to generation of **antiadrenal antibodies**. Circulating adrenal autoantibodies can be detected in over 60% of patients with autoimmune adrenal insufficiency. Autoantibodies to other tissue antigens are frequently found as well. Thyroid antibodies have been found in 45%, gastric anti-parietal cell antibodies in 30%, intrinsic factor antibodies in 9%, parathyroid antibodies in 26%, gonadal antibodies in 17%, and islet cell antibodies in 8%.

Autoimmune adrenocortical insufficiency is frequently associated with other autoimmune endocrine disorders. Clinical hyperthyroidism occurs in 7%, Hashimoto's thyroiditis with goiter in 9%, and up to 80% of patients have subclinical thyroiditis with lymphocytic infiltration of the thyroid and raised TSH levels. Ovarian failure occurs in approximately 25% of female patients, but testicular failure occurs in less than 5% of males. Diabetes mellitus (usually type I) occurs in about 12% and hypoparathyroidism in 6%. Two distinct polyglandular syndromes involving the adrenal glands have been described. One syndrome includes adrenocortical insufficiency, Hashimoto's thyroiditis, and insulin-dependent diabetes mellitus (Schmidt's syndrome). The other includes adrenocortical insufficiency, hypoparathyroidism, and chronic mucocutaneous candidiasis. There is also an increased incidence of other nonendocrine immunologic disorders, including alopecia, vitiligo, pernicious anemia, chronic hepatitis, and gastrointestinal malabsorption.

Pathologically, the adrenal glands are small and atrophic, and the capsule is thickened. There is an intense lymphocytic infiltration of the adrenal cortex. Cortical cells are degenerating or absent and are surrounded by fibrous stroma and lymphocytes. The adrenal medulla is preserved.

2. Adrenal tuberculosis–Tuberculosis causes adrenal failure by total or near-total destruction of both glands. Such destruction usually occurs gradually and produces a picture of chronic adrenal insufficiency. Adrenal tuberculosis usually results from hematogenous spread of systemic tuberculous infection (lung, gastrointestinal tract, or kidney) to the adrenal cortex. Pathologically, the adrenal is replaced with caseous necrosis; both cortical and medullary tissue is destroyed. Calcification of the adrenals can be detected radiographically in about 50% of cases.

3. Bilateral adrenal hemorrhage–Bilateral adrenal hemorrhage leads to rapid destruction of the adrenals and precipitates acute adrenal insufficiency. In children, hemorrhage is usually related to fulminant meningococcal septicemia (**Waterhouse-Friderichsen syndrome**) or *Pseudomonas* septicemia. In adults, hemorrhage is related to anticoagulant therapy of other disorders in one-third of cases. Other causes in adults include septicemia, coagulation disorders, adrenal vein thrombosis, adrenal metastases, trauma, abdominal surgery, and obstetric complications.

Pathologically, the adrenal glands are often massively enlarged. The inner cortex and medulla are almost entirely replaced by hematomas. There is ischemic necrosis of the outer cortex, and only a thin rim of subcapsular cortical cells survives. There is often thrombosis of the adrenal veins. In surviving patients, the hematomas may later calcify.

4. Adrenal metastases–Metastases to the adrenals occur frequently from lung, breast, and stomach carcinomas, melanoma, lymphoma, and many other malignancies. However, metastatic disease seldom produces adrenal insufficiency because over 80–90% of the adrenal must be destroyed before overt adrenal insufficiency develops. On pathologic examination, the adrenal glands are often massively enlarged.

5. AIDS-related adrenal insufficiency–The adrenal gland is commonly affected in AIDS, often by opportunistic infection (especially cytomegalovirus, disseminated *Mycobacterium avium* complex, or *Cryptococcus*) or by Kaposi's sarcoma. Although pathologic involvement of the adrenal glands is frequent, clinical adrenal insufficiency is uncommon. In some cases, adrenal necrosis is related to the presence of CMV inclusion bodies, is usually limited in extent to less than 50–70% of the gland, and may be restricted to the medulla.

Ketoconazole, an antifungal agent frequently used in AIDS patients, interferes with steroid synthesis by the adrenals and gonads. Ketoconazole-related adrenal insufficiency is usually dose-related and reversible, but it may occur with low doses and may be persistent.

6. Familial glucocorticoid deficiency–A familial syndrome of glucocorticoid deficiency has been described related to **hereditary adrenocortical unresponsiveness to ACTH**. This unresponsiveness causes both decreased adrenal secretion of glucocorticoids and androgens and increased pituitary secretion of ACTH. The diagnosis is suggested when cortisol secretion does not respond to either endogenous or exogenous ACTH stimulation. On histologic examination, there is preservation of the zona glomerulosa but degeneration of the zona fasciculata and zona reticularis.

B. Secondary Adrenocortical Insufficiency: Secondary adrenocortical insufficiency most commonly results from ACTH deficiency due to chronic exogenous glucocorticoid therapy. ACTH deficiency also rarely results from pituitary and hypothalamic tumors.

Pathogenesis

A. Primary Adrenocortical Insufficiency: Primary adrenocortical insufficiency becomes clinically apparent following destruction of more than 90% of both adrenal cortices. Gradual adrenocortical destruction, such as occurs in the autoimmune, tuberculous, and other invasive forms, results initially in a decreased adrenal reserve. Basal glucocorticoid secretion is normal but does not increase in response to stress and surgery; trauma or infection can precipitate acute adrenal crisis. With further loss of cortical tissue, even basal secretion of glucocorticoids and mineralocorticoids becomes deficient, leading to the clinical manifestations of chronic adrenal insufficiency. The fall in plasma cortisol reduces the feedback inhibition of pituitary ACTH secretion (Figure 13–12), and the plasma level of ACTH rises (Figure 13–15).

Rapid adrenocortical destruction such as occurs in septicemia or adrenal hemorrhage results in sudden loss of both glucocorticoid and mineralocorticoid secretion, leading to acute adrenal crisis.

B. Secondary Adrenocortical Insufficiency: Secondary adrenocortical insufficiency occurs when large doses of glucocorticoids are given for their anti-inflammatory and immunosuppressive effects in treatment of asthma, rheumatoid arthritis, ulcerative colitis, and other diseases. If such treatment is extended beyond 4–5 weeks, it produces prolonged suppression of CRH, ACTH, and endogenous cortisol secretion (Figure 13–12). Should the exogenous steroid treatment be abruptly discontinued, the hypothalamus and pituitary are unable to respond normally to the reduction in level of circulating glucocorticoid. The patient may develop symptoms and signs of chronic adrenocortical insufficiency or, if subjected to stress, acute adrenal crisis. The prolonged suppression of the hypothalamic-pituitary-adrenal axis can be avoided by using alternate-day steroid regimens whenever possible.

ACTH deficiency is the primary problem in secondary adrenocortical insufficiency. The ACTH deficiency leads to diminished cortisol and adrenal androgen secretion, but aldosterone secretion generally remains normal. In the early stages, there is a decreased pituitary ACTH reserve. Basal ACTH and cortisol secretion may be normal but do not increase in response to stress. With progression, there is further loss of ACTH secretion, atrophy of the adrenal cortex, and decreased basal cortisol secretion. At this stage, there is decreased responsiveness not only of

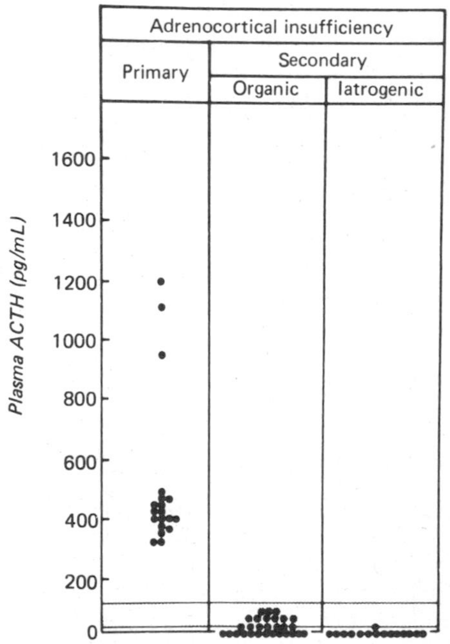

Figure 13–15. Basal plasma ACTH levels in primary and secondary adrenocortical insufficiency. (Reproduced, with permission, from Irvine WJ, Toft AD, Feek CM: Addison's disease. In: *The Adrenal Gland.* James VHT [editor]. Raven Press, 1979.)

pituitary ACTH to stress but also of adrenal cortisol to stimulation with exogenous ACTH.

Clinical Manifestations

The clinical manifestations of glucocorticoid deficiency are nonspecific symptoms: weakness, lethargy, easy fatigability, anorexia, nausea, and occasionally vomiting. Hypoglycemia occurs occasionally. In primary adrenal insufficiency, hyperpigmentation of skin and mucous membranes also occurs. In secondary adrenal insufficiency, hyperpigmentation does not occur, but arthralgias and myalgias may occur.

Other clinical features of adrenocortical insufficiency are listed in Table 13–6 and detailed below.

Impaired gluconeogenesis predisposes to hypoglycemia. Severe hypoglycemia may occur spontaneously in children. In adults, the blood glucose level is normal provided there is adequate intake of calories, but fasting causes severe (and potentially fatal) hypoglycemia. In acute adrenal crisis, hypoglycemia may also be provoked by fever, infection, or nausea and vomiting.

In primary adrenal insufficiency, the persistently low or absent plasma cortisol level results in marked hypersecretion of ACTH by the pituitary. Because ACTH has intrinsic melanocyte-stimulating hormone (MSH) activity, a variety of pigmentary changes can occur. These include generalized hyperpigmentation (diffuse darkening of the skin); increased pigmentation of skin creases, nail beds, nipples, areolae, pressure points (such as the knuckles, toes, elbows, and knees), and scars formed after the onset of ACTH excess; increased tanning and freckling of sun-exposed areas; and hyperpigmentation of the buccal mucosa, the gums, and the perivaginal and perianal areas.

Vitiligo occurs in 4–17% of patients with the autoimmune form of adrenal insufficiency but is rare in insufficiency due to other causes.

In primary adrenal insufficiency, aldosterone deficiency results in unregulated renal loss of sodium and retention of potassium, causing hypovolemia and hyperkalemia. The hypovolemia in turn leads to prerenal azotemia and hypotension. Salt craving has been documented in about 20% of patients with adrenal insufficiency.

Patients may also be unable to excrete a water load. Hyponatremia may develop, reflecting retention of water in excess of sodium. The defective water excretion is probably related to increases in posterior pituitary vasopressin secretion that are reduced by glucocorticoid administration. In addition, the glomerular filtration rate (GFR) is low. Treatment with mineralocorticoids raises the GFR by restoring plasma volume, and treatment with glucocorticoids improves the GFR even further.

The inability to excrete a water load may predispose to water intoxication. A dramatic example of this sometimes occurs when untreated patients with adrenal insufficiency are given a glucose infusion and subsequently develop high fever **("glucose fever")**, collapse, and death. The pathogenesis of this condition is thought to be related to metabolism of the glucose and release of free water to dilute plasma. This dilution results in an osmotic gradient between plasma and cells of the hypothalamic thermoregulatory center which causes them to swell and malfunction.

In secondary adrenal insufficiency, aldosterone secretion by the zona glomerulosa is usually preserved. Thus, clinical manifestations of mineralocorticoid deficiency, such as volume depletion, dehydration, hypotension, and electrolyte abnormalities, generally do not occur. Hyponatremia may occur as a result of inability to excrete a water load but is not accompanied by hyperkalemia.

Hypotension occurs in about 90% of patients. It frequently causes orthostatic symptoms and occasionally syncope or recumbent hypotension. Hyperkalemia may cause cardiac arrhythmias, which are sometimes lethal. Refractory shock may occur in glucocorticoid-deficient individuals who are subjected to stress. Vascular smooth muscle becomes unresponsive to circulating epinephrine and norepinephrine, and capillaries dilate and become permeable. These effects impair vascular compensation for hypovolemia and promote vascular collapse.

Cortisol deficiency commonly results in loss of appetite, weight loss, and gastrointestinal disturbances. Weight loss is common and, in chronic cases, may be profound (15 kg or more). Nausea and vomiting occur in most patients; diarrhea is less frequent. Such gastrointestinal symptoms often intensify during acute adrenal crisis.

In women with adrenal insufficiency, loss of pubic and axillary hair may occur as a result of decreased secretion of adrenal androgens. Amenorrhea occurs commonly—in most cases related to weight loss and chronic illness but sometimes due to ovarian failure.

Central nervous system consequences of adrenal insufficiency include personality changes (irritability, apprehension, inability to concentrate, and emotional

Table 13–6. Clinical features of adrenocortical insufficiency.[1]

Weakness, fatigue, anorexia, weight loss	100%
Hyperpigmentation	92%
Hypotension	88%
Gastrointestinal disturbances	56%
Salt craving	19%
Postural symptoms	12%

[1] Modified and reproduced, with permission, from Baxter JD, Tyrell JB, in: *Endocrinology and Metabolism.* Felig P et al (editors). McGraw-Hill, 1981; and from Greenspan FS, Baxter JD: *Basic and Clinical Endocrinology.* Appleton & Lange, 1994.

Table 13–7. Typical plasma electrolyte levels in normal humans and in patients with adrenocortical diseases.

	Na^+ (meq/L)	K^+ (meq/L)	Cl^- (meq/L)	HCO_3^- (meq/L)
Normal	142	4.5	105	25
Adrenal insufficiency	120	6.7	85	45
Primary hyperaldosteronism	145	2.4	96	41
Hypoaldosteronism	145	6.7	105	25

[1] Modified and reproduced, with permission, from Ganong WF: *Review of Medical Physiology,* 16th ed. Appleton & Lange, 1993.

lability), increased sensitivity to olfactory and gustatory stimuli, and the appearance of electroencephalographic waves slower than the normal alpha rhythm.

Patients with **acute adrenal crisis** have symptoms of high fever, weakness, apathy, and confusion. Anorexia, nausea, and vomiting may lead to volume depletion and dehydration. Abdominal pain may mimic that of acute abdominal process. Hyponatremia, hyperkalemia, lymphocytosis, eosinophilia, and hypoglycemia occur frequently. Acute adrenal crisis can occur in patients with undiagnosed ACTH deficiency or in patients receiving corticosteroids who are not given increased steroid dosage during periods of stress. Precipitants include infection, trauma, surgery, and dehydration. If unrecognized and untreated, coma, severe hypotension, or shock unresponsive to vasopressors may rapidly lead to death.

Laboratory findings in primary adrenocortical insufficiency include hyponatremia, hyperkalemia, hypoglycemia, and mild azotemia (Table 13–7). The hyponatremia and hyperkalemia are manifestations of mineralocorticoid deficiency. The azotemia, with elevations of BUN and serum creatinine, is due to volume depletion and dehydration. Mild acidosis is frequently present. Hypercalcemia of mild to moderate degree occurs infrequently.

In secondary adrenocortical insufficiency, mineralocorticoid secretion is usually normal. Thus, serum sodium, potassium, creatinine, BUN, and bicarbonate are usually normal. Plasma glucose may be low, though severe hypoglycemia is unusual.

Hematologic manifestations of adrenal insufficiency include normocytic, normochromic anemia, neutropenia, lymphocytosis, monocytosis, and eosinophilia. Abdominal x-rays demonstrate adrenal calcification in about 50% of patients with Addison's disease due to adrenal tuberculosis and in a smaller percentage of patients with bilateral adrenal hemorrhage. CT scans detect adrenal calcification even more frequently in such cases and may also reveal bilateral adrenal enlargement in cases of adrenal hemorrhage; tuberculous, fungal, or cytomegalovirus infection; metastases; and other infiltrative diseases. Electrocardiographic findings include low voltage, a vertical QRS axis, and nonspecific ST–T wave changes related to electrolyte abnormalities (eg, peak T waves from hyperkalemia).

Diagnosis

A. Primary Adrenal Insufficiency: To establish the diagnosis of primary adrenal insufficiency, the physician must demonstrate a low level of plasma cortisol (< 3 μg/dL; 84 nmol/L) and an inability of the adrenal glands to respond normally to ACTH stimulation. This is usually done by performing an ACTH stimulation test (Figure 13–16). To do so, the physician obtains an 8:00 AM plasma cortisol, then administers 250 μg of synthetic ACTH (cosyntropin) intravenously or intramuscularly. Repeat plasma cortisol levels are obtained 60 and 120 minutes later. Normal subjects have a normal 8:00 AM plasma cortisol and usually a twofold or greater increase in plasma cortisol following cosyntropin. In Addison's disease, there is a low 8:00 AM plasma cortisol and virtually no increase in plasma cortisol following cosyntropin. Because making a diagnosis of adrenal insufficiency implies lifelong therapy with exogenous glucocorticoids, the physician must confirm the diagnosis. This is usually done with a more prolonged ACTH stimulation test, by determining the response of the urinary 17-hydroxycorticosteroids to ACTH that is injected daily over a 3- to 5-day period.

B. Secondary Adrenocortical Insufficiency: The diagnosis of ACTH deficiency due to exogenous glucocorticoids is suggested by obtaining a history of chronic glucocorticoid therapy or by finding cushingoid features on physical examination. Hypothalamic or pituitary tumors leading to ACTH deficiency usually produce symptoms and signs of other endocrinopathies. Deficient secretion of other pituitary hormones such as LH and FSH or TSH may produce hypogonadism or hypothyroidism. Excessive secre-

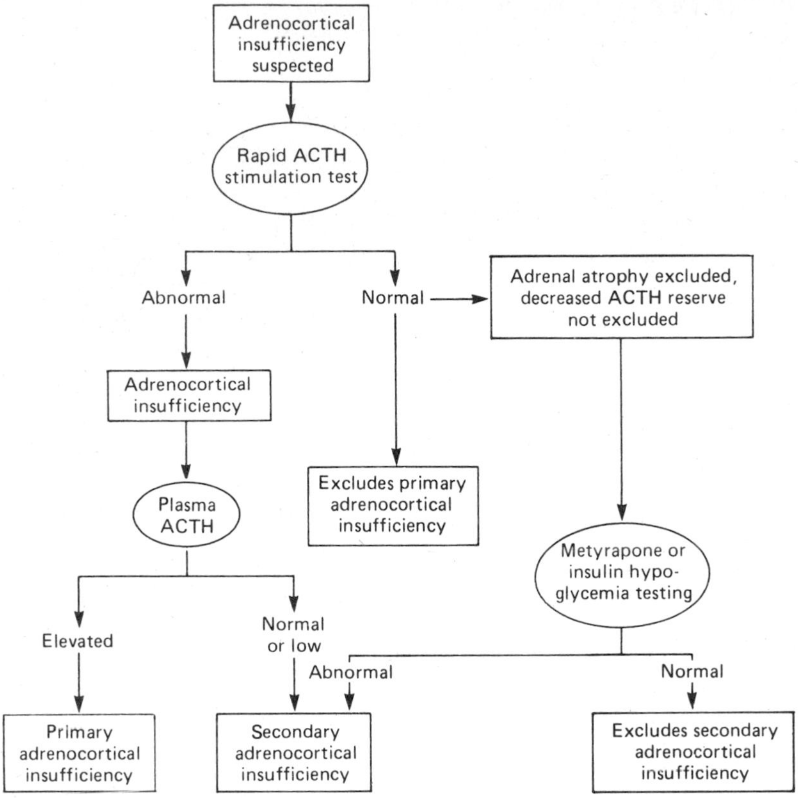

Figure 13–16. Diagnostic evaluation of suspected primary or secondary adrenocortical insufficiency. Boxes enclose clinical decisions, and ovals enclose diagnostic tests. (Redrawn and reproduced, with permission, from Baxter JD, Tyrrell JB: The adrenal cortex. In: *Endocrinology and Metabolism.* Felig P et al [editors]. McGraw-Hill, 1981.)

tion of growth hormone or prolactin from a pituitary adenoma may produce acromegaly or amenorrhea and galactorrhea.

18. What are the major causes of glucocorticoid deficiency?
19. With what other autoimmune disorders is autoimmune adrenal failure associated?
20. What are the major causes of adrenal hemorrhage?
21. What are the clinical signs and symptoms of adrenal failure?
22. Name some different ways to make the diagnosis of adrenal insufficiency in a patient with suggestive signs and symptoms.

HYPERALDOSTERONISM (EXCESSIVE PRODUCTION OF MINERALOCORTICOIDS)

Primary hyperaldosteronism occurs because of excessive unregulated secretion of aldosterone by the adrenal cortex. **Secondary hyperaldosteronism** occurs because of excessive secretion of renin by the juxtaglomerular apparatus of the kidney.

Etiology

The causes of hyperaldosteronism are listed in Table 13–8.

A. Primary Hyperaldosteronism: Primary hyperaldosteronism (Conn's syndrome) is rare and most commonly results from an aldosterone-secreting tumor of the adrenal cortex, usually a solitary **adenoma** (Figure 13–17). Bilateral tumors are un-

Table 13–8. Causes of hyperaldosteronism.

- **Primary hyperaldosteronism (Conn's syndrome)**
  - Aldosterone-secreting adrenocortical adenoma
  - Bilateral hyperplasia of zona glomerulosa
  - Aldosterone-secreting adrenocortical carcinoma (rare)
  - Idiopathic
- **Secondary hyperaldosteronism**
  - Renal ischemia
    - Renal artery stenosis
    - Malignant hypertension
  - Decreased intravascular volume
    - Congestive heart failure
    - Chronic diuretic or laxative use
    - Hypoproteinemic states (cirrhosis, nephrotic syndrome)
  - Sodium-wasting disorders
    - Chronic renal failure
    - Renal tubular acidosis
  - Juxtaglomerular cell hyperplasia (Bartter's syndrome)
  - Surreptitious vomiting or diuretic ingestion (pseudo-Bartter's syndrome)
  - Oral contraceptives
  - Renin-secreting tumors (rare)

usual. Small satellite adenomas are sometimes found. Adenomas are readily identified by their characteristic golden-yellow color. The adjacent adrenal cortex may be compressed. Adenomas producing excessive aldosterone are indistinguishable from those producing excessive cortisol except that they tend to be smaller (usually < 2 cm in diameter).

Bilateral adrenal hyperplasia accounts for most of the remaining cases of primary hyperaldosteronism. Affected patients have bilateral hyperplasia of the zona glomerulosa.

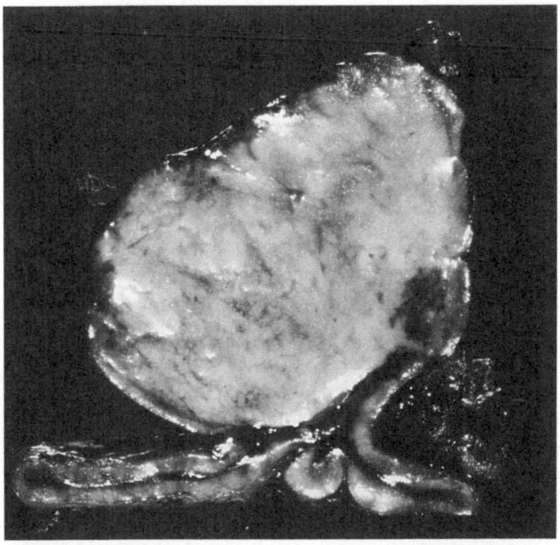

Figure 13–17. Cross section of adrenal, showing an adrenocortical adenoma in a patient with primary hyperaldosteronism. The gross and microscopic features do not permit differentiation of aldosterone- and cortisol-secreting adenomas in most cases. (Reproduced, with permission, from Chandrasoma P, Taylor CE: *Concise Pathology.* Appleton & Lange, 1991.)

Adrenocortical carcinomas producing only aldosterone are extremely rare. Such tumors are generally large, and there is no diurnal rhythm in aldosterone production.

In some cases, no definite abnormality is detected in the gland despite evident hyperaldosteronism.

B. Secondary Hyperaldosteronism: Secondary hyperaldosteronism is common. It results from excessive renin production by the juxtaglomerular apparatus of the kidney. The high renin output occurs in response to (1) renal ischemia (eg, renal artery stenosis or malignant hypertension); (2) decreased intravascular volume (eg, congestive heart failure, cirrhosis, nephrotic syndrome, or laxative or diuretic abuse); (3) sodium-wasting disorders (eg, chronic renal failure or renal tubular acidosis); (4) hyperplasia of the juxtaglomerular apparatus (Bartter's syndrome); or (5) renin-secreting tumors. In these states, stimulation of the zona glomerulosa by the renin-angiotensin system leads to increased aldosterone production.

Pathologically, in secondary hyperaldosteronism, the adrenals appear grossly normal; microscopically, there may be hyperplasia of the zona glomerulosa.

Regulation of Mineralocorticoid Secretion in Hyperaldosteronism

In primary hyperaldosteronism, there is a primary (autonomous) increase in aldosterone production by the abnormal zona glomerulosa tissue (adenoma or hyperplasia). However, circulating levels of aldosterone are still modulated to some extent by variations in ACTH secretion. The chronic aldosterone excess results in expansion of the extracellular fluid volume and plasma volume. In turn, this expansion is registered by stretch receptors of the juxtaglomerular apparatus and sodium flux at the macula densa, leading to suppression of renin production.

Patients with secondary hyperaldosteronism also produce excessively large amounts of aldosterone, but in contrast to primary hyperaldosteronism, have elevated plasma renin activity.

Clinical Consequences of Mineralocorticoid Excess

The major consequences of chronic aldosterone excess are sodium retention and potassium and hydrogen ion wasting by the kidney.

The excess aldosterone initially stimulates sodium reabsorption by the proximal renal tubules, causing the extracellular fluid volume to expand and the blood pressure to rise. When the extracellular fluid expansion reaches a certain point, however, sodium excretion resumes despite the continued action of aldosterone on the renal tubule. This **"escape" phenomenon** is probably due to increased secretion of **atrial natriuretic peptide.** Because the escape phenomenon causes the excretion of excess salt, affected patients are not edematous. Such escape from the action of aldosterone does not occur in the distal tubules, thus enabling potassium depletion and alkalosis to develop. Affected patients are not markedly hypernatremic because water is retained along with the sodium ions.

The chronic aldosterone excess also produces a prolonged potassium diuresis. Total body potassium stores are depleted, and hypokalemia develops. Patients may complain of tiredness, loss of stamina, weakness, nocturia, and lassitude—all symptoms of potassium depletion. Prolonged potassium depletion damages the kidney **(hypokalemic nephropathy),** causing resistance to antidiuretic hormone (vasopressin). The resultant loss of concentrating ability causes thirst and polyuria (especially nocturnal).

When the potassium loss is marked, intracellular potassium ions are replaced by sodium and hydrogen ions. The intracellular movement of hydrogen ion, along with increased renal secretion of hydrogen ion instead of potassium ion, causes metabolic alkalosis to develop.

Hypertension—related to sodium retention and expansion of plasma volume—is a characteristic finding. Hypertension can range from borderline to severe, but it is usually mild or moderate. Accelerated (malignant) hypertension is extremely rare. Because the hypertension is sustained, however, it may produce left ventricular hypertrophy and retinopathy.

Severely potassium-depleted patients may develop blunting of baroreceptor function, manifested by postural falls in blood pressure without reflex tachycardia. The heart may be mildly enlarged as a result of plasma volume expansion and left ventricular hypertrophy.

The potassium depletion causes a minor but detectable degree of carbohydrate intolerance (demonstrated by an abnormal glucose tolerance test). The decrease in glucose tolerance is corrected following potassium repletion.

In addition, the alkalosis accompanying severe potassium depletion may lower the plasma ionized calcium to the point where latent or frank tetany occurs (see Chapter 17). The hypokalemia may cause severe muscle weakness, muscle cramps, and intestinal atony. Paresthesias may develop as a result of the hypokalemia and alkalosis. A positive Trousseau or Chvostek sign is suggestive of alkalosis and hypocalcemia (see Chapter 15).

Laboratory findings in hyperaldosteronism include hypokalemia and alkalosis (Table 13–7). Typically, the serum potassium is below 3.6 meq/L (3.6 mmol/L), serum sodium is normal or slightly elevated, serum bicarbonate is increased, and serum chloride is decreased (hypokalemic, hypochloremic metabolic alkalosis). Urinary electrolytes show an inappropriately large amount of potassium in the urine.

The hematocrit may be reduced because of hemodilution by the expanded plasma volume. Affected patients may fail to concentrate urine (nephrogenic diabetes insipidus) and may have abnormal glucose tolerance tests.

The plasma renin level is suppressed in primary hyperaldosteronism and elevated in secondary hyperaldosteronism. Adrenal cortisol production is normal or low.

The ECG may show changes of modest left ventricular hypertrophy and potassium depletion (flattening of T waves and appearance of U waves).

Diagnosis of Hyperaldosteronism

A. Primary Hyperaldosteronism: The diagnosis of primary hyperaldosteronism is usually suggested by finding hypokalemia in an untreated patient with hypertension (ie, one not taking diuretics). Thus, screening such patients for hyperaldosteronism is most easily accomplished by determining the serum potassium level (Table 13–7). However, a low-sodium intake, by diminishing renal potassium loss, may mask total body potassium depletion. In patients with normal renal function, dietary salt loading will unmask hypokalemia as a manifestation of total body potassium depletion. Thus, finding a low serum potassium in a hypertensive patient on a high-salt intake and not receiving diuretics warrants further evaluation for hyperaldosteronism.

If hypokalemia is documented, the next step should be to assess the renin-angiotensin system by determining the random **plasma renin activity.** If the random plasma renin activity level is low, primary hyperaldosteronism is likely. However, if plasma renin activity is normal or high, it is very unlikely. If the renin activity is high, secondary hyperaldosteronism must be considered.

Subsequent workup entails measuring the 24-hour urinary aldosterone excretion and the plasma aldosterone level with the patient on a diet containing more than 120 meq of sodium per day. The urinary aldosterone excretion exceeds 14 μg/d, and the plasma aldosterone is usually greater than 90 pg/mL in primary hyperaldosteronism.

Measurement of the plasma aldosterone level can also help to differentiate between **adrenal adenoma** and **adrenal hyperplasia.** This distinction is important because surgery is indicated for treatment of adenoma but not hyperplasia. It is made by examining both the degree of plasma aldosterone elevation and its response to assumption of the upright posture. First, the 8:00 AM plasma aldosterone level is measured after the patient has been given at least 4 days of high sodium intake (exceeding 120 meq daily) and has been supine overnight (at least 6 hours). A plasma aldosterone level of greater than 20 ng/dL (555 pmol/L) indicates adrenal adenoma, and less than 20 ng/dL usually indicates hyperplasia. Then, after the patient has been erect for 2–4 hours, the plasma aldosterone level is again measured. Normally, the upright posture stimulates the renin-angiotensin system, causing a rise in plasma aldosterone. In most patients with adrenal hyperplasia, the erect plasma aldosterone level rises, owing to an enhanced sensitivity of the hyperplastic gland to the increased renin and angiotensin. In contrast, in most patients with adrenal adenoma, the erect plasma aldosterone level shows either no change or a decrease, due to profound suppression of renin by the high circulating aldosterone level and to a decreased number and affinity of angiotensin II receptors in the adenoma tissue.

B. Secondary Hyperaldosteronism: Patients with secondary hyperaldosteronism due to malignant hypertension, renal artery stenosis, or chronic renal disease also excrete large amounts of aldosterone but—in contrast to primary hyperaldosteronism—have elevated plasma renin activity.

23. What are the causes of hyperaldosteronism?
24. What are the presenting signs and symptoms of a patient with hyperaldosteronism?
25. How is the diagnosis of hyperaldosteronism made?

HYPOALDOSTERONISM (DEFICIENT PRODUCTION OF MINERALOCORTICOIDS)

Primary mineralocorticoid deficiency (hypoaldosteronism) may result either from destruction of adrenocortical tissue or from defective mineralocorticoid synthesis. Hypoaldosteronism is characterized by sodium loss, with hyponatremia, hypovolemia, and hypotension, and impaired secretion of both potassium and hydrogen ion in the renal tubule, resulting in hyperkalemia and metabolic acidosis. Renin activity is typically increased.

A **secondary mineralocorticoid deficiency** may occur when renin production is suppressed or deficient. Renin production may be suppressed by the sodium retention and volume expansion resulting from exogenous mineralocorticoids (fludrocortisone acetate) or mineralocorticoid-like substances (licorice). When this happens, hypertension, hypokalemia, and metabolic alkalosis result. When renin production is deficient and unable to stimulate mineralocorticoid production, sodium loss, hyperkalemia, and metabolic acidosis occur.

Etiology

Acute and chronic adrenocortical insufficiency are discussed above. In long-standing **hypopituitarism,** atrophy of the zona glomerulosa occurs, and the increase in aldosterone secretion normally produced by surgery or other stress is absent. **Hyporeninemic hypoaldosteronism (type IV renal tubular acidosis)** is a disorder characterized by hyperkalemia and acidosis in association with (usually mild) chronic renal insufficiency. Typically, affected individuals are men in the fifth to seventh decades of life who have underlying pyelonephritis, diabetes mellitus, or gout. The chronic renal insufficiency is usually not severe enough to account for the hyperkalemia. Plasma and urinary aldosterone levels and plasma renin activity are consistently low and unresponsive to stimulation by ACTH administration, upright posture, dietary sodium restriction, or furosemide administration. The syndrome is thought to be due to impairment of the juxtaglomerular apparatus associated with the underlying renal disease. Finally, two genetic disorders may produce the symptoms and signs of hypoaldosteronism. In **congenital adrenal hypoplasia,** there are enzymatic abnormalities in mineralocorticoid biosynthesis. Aldosterone levels are low. In **pseudohypoaldosteronism,** there is renal tubular resistance to mineralocorticoid hormones, presumably due to a deficiency of mineralocorticoid hormone receptors. Affected patients manifest symptoms and signs of hypoaldosteronism, but aldosterone levels are high.

Clinical Consequences of Mineralocorticoid Deficiency

Patients undergoing bilateral adrenalectomy, if not given mineralocorticoid replacement therapy, will develop profound urinary sodium losses resulting in hypovolemia, hypotension, and, eventually, shock and death. In adrenal insufficiency, these changes can be delayed by increasing the dietary salt intake. However, the amount of dietary salt needed to prevent them entirely is so large that collapse and death are inevitable unless mineralocorticoid treatment is also initiated. Secretion of both potassium and hydrogen ion are impaired in the renal tubule, resulting in hyperkalemia and metabolic acidosis (Table 13–7).

DISORDERS OF ADRENAL ANDROGEN PRODUCTION

The adrenal cortex also secretes androgens, principally **androstenedione** and **dehydroepiandrostenedione (DHEA).** In general, the secretion of adrenal androgens parallels that of cortisol. ACTH is the major factor regulating androgen production by the adrenal cortex. The adrenal androgens are secreted in an unbound state but circulate weakly bound to plasma proteins, chiefly albumin. They are metabolized either by degradation and inactivation or by peripheral conversion to the more potent androgens testosterone and dihydrotestosterone. The androgen metabolites are conjugated either as glucuronides or sulfates and excreted in the urine.

Dehydroepiandrosterone has both masculinizing and anabolic effects. However, it is less than one-fifth as potent as the androgens produced by the testis and is secreted in very small quantities. Consequently, it has very little physiologic effect under normal conditions. The androgenic steroids are thought to be required for the maintenance of libido and the capacity to achieve orgasm in the female, perhaps through a tropic action on the clitoris.

Excessive secretion of adrenal androgens may occur as an associated phenomenon with Cushing's syndrome, particularly that due to adrenocortical neoplasms (particularly carcinomas). Or it may be congenital, resulting from one of several enzymatic defects in steroid metabolism (such as **congenital adrenal hyperplasia** caused by 21-hydroxylase, 11-hydroxylase, 17-hydroxylase, or 3β-dehydrogenase deficiency [Figure 13–3]). Excessive production of adrenal androgens has little effect in mature males but may cause hirsutism in mature females. It may result in precocious pseudopuberty in prepubertal boys and in masculinization in prepubertal girls.

Deficiency of adrenal sex hormones usually has little effect in the presence of normal testes or ovaries. In mature women, minor menstrual abnormalities may occur.

26. What are the causes of hypoaldosteronism?
27. What are the clinical manifestations of hypoaldosteronism?
28. What is the effect of excess or deficiency of adrenal androgens on otherwise normal adult men and women (ie, individuals with normal gonads)?

REFERENCES

General

Baxter JD, Tyrell JB: The adrenal cortex. In: *Endocrinology and Metabolism,* 2nd ed. Felig P et al (editors). McGraw-Hill, 1987.

Besser GM, Rees LH: The pituitary-adrenocortical axis. Clin Endocrinol Metab 1985;14:765.

Buckingham JC, Smith T, Loxley HD: Control of adrenocortical hormone secretion. In: *The Adrenal Gland,* 2nd ed. James VHT (editor). Raven Press, 1992.

Fraser R: Biosynthesis of adrenocortical steroids. In: *The Adrenal Gland,* 2nd ed. James VHT (editor). Raven Press, 1992.

Hale AC, Rees LH: ACTH and related peptides. In: *Endocrinology,* 2nd ed. DeGroot LJ et al (editors). Saunders, 1989.

Taylor AL, Fishman LM: Corticotropin-releasing hormone. N Engl J Med 1988;319:213.

Tyrell JB, Aron DC, Forsham PH: Glucocorticoids and adrenal androgens. In: *Basic and Clinical Endocrinology,* 4th ed. Greenspan FS, Baxter JD (editors). Appleton & Lange, 1994.

Cushing's Syndrome

Aiba M et al: Adrenocorticotropic hormone-independent bilateral adrenocortical macronodular hyperplasia as a distinct subtype of Cushing's syndrome. Am J Clin Pathol 1991;96:334.

Delisle L et al: Ectopic corticotropin syndrome and small-cell carcinoma of the lung: Clinical features, outcome and complications. Arch Intern Med 1993;153:746.

Findling JW: Cushing's syndromes: An enlarging clinical spectrum. (Editorial.) N Engl J Med 1989; 321:1677.

Kaye TB, Crapo L: The Cushing's syndrome: An update on diagnostic tests. Ann Intern Med 1990;112:434.

Kovacs K: The pathology of Cushing's disease. J Steroid Biochem Mol Biol 1993;45:179.

Luton J-P et al: Clinical features of adrenocortical carcinoma, prognostic factors, and the effect of mitotane therapy. N Engl J Med 1990;322:1195.

Trainer PJ, Grossman A: The diagnosis and differential diagnosis of Cushing's syndrome. Clin Endocrinol 1991;34:317.

Zeiger MA et al: Primary bilateral adrenocortical causes of Cushing's syndrome. Surgery 1991;110:1106.

Adrenocortical Insufficiency

Aron DC: Endocrine complications of the acquired immunodeficiency syndrome. Arch Intern Med 1989; 149:330.

Burke CW: Adrenocortical insufficiency. Clin Endocrinol Metab 1985;14:947.

Chin R: Adrenal crisis. Crit Care Clin 1991;7:23.

Mansell P et al: Secondary adrenocortical insufficiency. Br Med J 1993:307:253.

Werbel SS, Ober KP: Acute adrenal insufficiency. Endocrinol Metab Clin North Am 1993;22:303.

Hyperaldosteronism

Antonipillai I, Horton A: Paracrine regulation of the renin-aldosterone system. J Steroid Biochem Mol Biol 1993;45:27.

Baxter JD et al: The endocrinology of hypertension. In: *Endocrinology and Metabolism,* 2nd ed. Felig P et al (editors). McGraw-Hill, 1987.

Biglieri EG : The spectrum of mineralocorticoid hypertension. Hypertension 1991;18:251.

Biglieri EG, Kater CE, Ramsay DJ: Endocrine hypertension. In: *Basic and Clinical Endocrinology,* 4th ed.

Greenspan FS, Baxter JD (editors). Appleton & Lange, 1994.
Gleason PE et al: Evaluation of diagnostic tests in the differential diagnosis of primary aldosteronism: unilateral adenoma versus bilateral micronodular hyperplasia. J Urol 1993;150(5 Part 1):1365.
Melby JC: Diagnosis of hyperaldosteronism. Endocrinol Metab Clin North Am 1991;20:247.

Hypoaldosteronism

Holland OB: Hypoaldosteronism: Disease or normal response? (Editorial.) N Engl J Med 1991;324:488.
Polsky FI, Roque D, Hill PE: Hyporeninemic hypoaldosteronism complicating primary autonomic insufficiency. West J Med 1993;159:185.
Williams GH: Hyporeninemic hypoaldosteronism. (Editorial.) N Engl J Med 1986;314:1041.

14 Disorders of the Adrenal Medulla

Stephen J. McPhee, MD

The **adrenal medulla** secretes catecholamines (epinephrine, norepinephrine, and dopamine). The catecholamines help prepare the individual to deal with emergency situations. The major disorder of the adrenal medulla is **pheochromocytoma,** a neoplasm characterized by excessive catecholamine secretion.

NORMAL STRUCTURE & FUNCTION OF THE ADRENAL MEDULLA

ANATOMY

The adrenal medulla is the reddish-brown central layer of the adrenal gland (Figure 13-2). Accessory medullary tissue is sometimes located in the retroperitoneum near the sympathetic ganglia or along the abdominal aorta (paraganglia) (Figure 14–1).

HISTOLOGY

The adrenal medulla is made up of polyhedral cells arranged in cords or clumps. Embryologically, the adrenal medullary cells derive from neural crest cells. Medullary cells are innervated by cholinergic preganglionic nerve fibers that reach the gland via the splanchnic nerves. Medullary parenchymal cells accumulate and store their hormone products in prominent, dense secretory granules, 150–350 nm in diameter. Histologically, these cells and granules have a high affinity for chromium salts **(chromaffin reaction)** and thus are called **chromaffin cells** and **chromaffin granules.** The granules contain the catecholamines epinephrine and norepinephrine. Morphologically, two types of medullary cells can be distinguished: epinephrine-secreting cells have larger, less dense granules, and norepinephrine-secreting cells have smaller, very dense granules. Separate dopamine-secreting cells have not been identified. Ninety percent of medullary cells are the epinephrine-secreting type and 10% the norepinephrine-secreting type.

PHYSIOLOGY

The catecholamines help to regulate metabolism, contractility of cardiac and smooth muscle, and neurotransmission.

Formation, Secretion, & Metabolism of Catecholamines

The adrenal medulla secretes three catecholamines: epinephrine, norepinephrine, and dopamine. The major biosynthetic pathways and hormonal intermediates for the catecholamines are shown in Figure 14–2. In humans, most (80%) of the catecholamine output of the adrenal medulla is epinephrine. Norepinephrine is principally found in nerve endings of the sympathetic nervous system and in the central nervous system, where it functions as a major neurotransmitter.

Under normal circumstances, only small quantities of epinephrine and norepinephrine are secreted by the adrenal medulla. Larger quantities are secreted in response to stimuli causing intense emotional reactions (eg, fright). Secretion occurs following release of acetylcholine from the preganglionic neurons that innervate the medullary cells.

About 70% of the epinephrine and norepinephrine and 95% of the dopamine found in plasma are conjugated to sulfate and inactive. In the supine state, the normal plasma level of free epinephrine is about 30 pg/mL (0.16 nmol/L); there is a 50–100% increase upon standing. The normal plasma level of free norepinephrine is about 300 pg/mL (1.8 nmol/L), and the plasma free dopamine level is about 35 pg/mL (0.23 nmol/L).

In the circulation, the catecholamines have a short half-life of about 2 minutes. They are metabolized primarily by methoxylation to metanephrine and normetanephrine and by oxidation to 3-methoxy-4-hydroxymandelic acid (vanillylmandelic acid [VMA]) and excreted in the urine as free or conju-

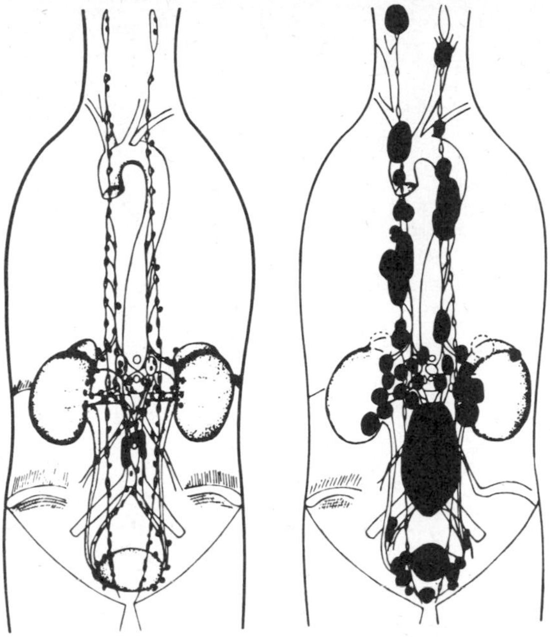

Figure 14–1. ***Left:*** Anatomic distribution of extra-adrenal chromaffin tissue in the newborn. ***Right:*** Locations of extra-adrenal pheochromocytomas reported before 1965. (Reproduced, with permission, from Coupland R: *The Natural History of the Chromaffin Cell.* Longman, Green, 1965.)

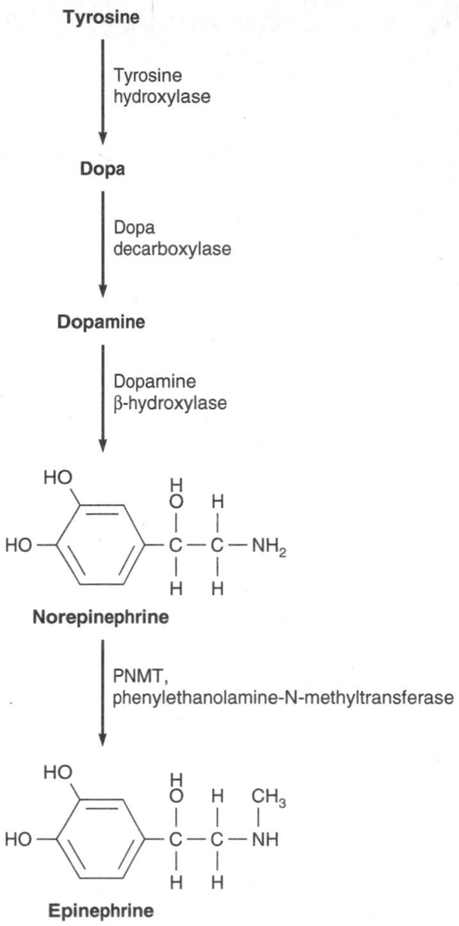

Figure 14–2. Biosynthesis of catecholamines. (Reproduced, with permission, from Greenspan FS, Baxter JD: *Basic and Clinical Endocrinology,* 4th ed. Appleton & Lange, 1994.)

gated metanephrine and normetanephrine (about 50%) and as VMA (about 35%). Normally, only very small quantities of free epinephrine (about 6 μg/d) and norepinephrine (about 30 μg/d) are excreted, but about 700 μg of VMA is excreted daily.

Regulation of Catecholamine Secretion

Physiologic stimuli affect medullary secretion through the nervous system. Medullary cells secrete catecholamines following release of acetylcholine from the preganglionic neurons that innervate them. Catecholamine secretion is low in the basal state and is reduced even further during sleep. In emergency situations, there is increased adrenal catecholamine secretion as part of a generalized sympathetic discharge to prepare the individual for stress ("fight or flight'' response). Hypoglycemia and certain drugs are also potent stimuli to catecholamine secretion.

Mechanism of Action of Catecholamines

The effects of epinephrine and norepinephrine are mediated by their actions on two classes of receptors: alpha- and beta-adrenergic receptors (Table 14–1). Alpha receptors are subdivided into α_1 and α_2 receptors, and beta receptors, into β_1 and β_2 receptors. Alpha$_1$ receptors mediate smooth muscle contraction in blood vessels and the genitourinary tract and increase glycogenolysis. Alpha$_2$ receptors mediate smooth muscle relaxation in the gastrointestinal tract and vasoconstriction of some blood vessels and decrease lipolysis, renin release, platelet aggregation, and insulin secretion. Beta$_1$ receptors mediate an increased rate and force of myocardial contraction and stimulate lipolysis and renin release. Beta$_2$ receptors mediate smooth muscle relaxation in the bronchi, blood vessels, genitourinary tract, and gastrointestinal tract and increase hepatic gluconeogenesis and glycogenolysis, muscle glycogenolysis, and release of insulin and glucagon.

Table 14–1. Physiologic effects of catecholamines on adrenergic receptors of selected tissues.[1]

Organ or Tissue	Adrenergic Receptor	Effect
Heart (myocardium)	β_1	Increased force of contraction (inotropic) Increased rate of contraction (chronotropic) Increased excitability (predisposes to arrhythmia)
Blood vessels	α β	Vasoconstriction, hypertension Vasodilation
Kidney	β	Increased renin release
Gut	α, β	Decreased motility and increased sphincter tone
Pancreas	α β	Decreased insulin release Decreased glucagon release Increased insulin release Increased glucagon release
Liver	α, β	Increased gluconeogenesis Increased glycogenolysis Release of potassium
Adipose tissue	α β	Decreased lipolysis Increased lipolysis
Skin (apocrine glands on hands, axillas, etc)	α	Increased sweating
Lung	β_2	Dilation of bronchi and bronchioles
Uterus	α β_2	Contraction Relaxation
Skeletal muscle	β_2 β	Vasodilation Increased glycogenolysis Increased release of lactic acid
Central nervous system	α	Increased alertness, anxiety, fear
Most tissues	β	Increased calorigenesis Increased metabolic rate

[1] Modified and reproduced, with permission, from Greenspan FS, Baxter JD (editors): *Basic and Clinical Endocrinology,* 4th ed. Appleton & Lange, 1994; and from Ganong WF: *Review of Medical Physiology,* 15th ed. Appleton & Lange, 1991.

Effects of Catecholamines

The catecholamines have been termed the hormones of "fight or flight" because their effects on the heart, blood vessels, smooth muscle, and metabolism assist the organism in responding to stress. The principal physiologic effects of the catecholamines are shown in Table 14–1.

In the peripheral circulation, norepinephrine produces vasoconstriction in most organs (via α_1 receptors). Epinephrine produces vasodilation via β_2 receptors in skeletal muscle and liver and vasoconstriction elsewhere. The former usually outweighs the latter, and for that reason total peripheral resistance usually falls.

Norepinephrine causes both systolic and diastolic blood pressures to rise. The rise in blood pressure stimulates the carotid and aortic baroreceptors, resulting in reflex bradycardia and a fall in cardiac output. Epinephrine, however, causes a widening of pulse pressure but does not stimulate the baroreceptors to the same degree, so the pulse rises and the cardiac output increases.

The effects on metabolism include effects on glycogenolysis, lipolysis, and insulin secretion, mediated by both alpha- and beta-adrenergic receptors. These metabolic effects result primarily from the action of epinephrine on four target tissues: liver, muscle, pancreas, and adipose tissue (see Table 14–1).

The result is an increase in the levels of circulating glucose and free fatty acids. The increased supply of these two substances guarantees an adequate supply of metabolic fuel to the nervous system and muscle during physiologic stress.

The amount of circulating plasma epinephrine and norepinephrine that is needed to produce these various effects has been determined by infusing the catecholamines into resting subjects. For norepinephrine, the threshold for the cardiovascular and metabolic effects is about 1500 pg/mL, or about five times the basal level. In normal individuals, the plasma norepinephrine level rarely exceeds this threshold. However, for epinephrine, the threshold for tachycardia occurs at a plasma level of about 50 pg/mL, or about twice the basal level. The threshold for increased systolic blood pressure and lipolysis is at about 75 pg/mL; for hyperglycemia and increased plasma lactate, about 150 pg/mL; and for the alpha-mediated increase in insulin secretion, about 40 pg/mL. In normal individuals, plasma epinephrine levels often exceed these thresholds.

The physiologic effect of circulating dopamine is unknown. Centrally, dopamine acts to inhibit prolactin secretion. Peripherally, in small doses, injected dopamine produces renal vasodilation, probably by binding to a specific dopaminergic receptor. In moderate doses, it also produces vasodilation of the mesenteric circulation and vasoconstriction elsewhere. It has a positive inotropic effect on the heart, mediated by action on the β_1-adrenergic receptors. Moderate to large doses of dopamine increase the systolic blood pressure without affecting diastolic pressure.

1. What is the embryologic origin of the cells of the adrenal medulla?
2. What fibers innervate the adrenal medulla?
3. Which catecholamines are secreted by the adrenal medulla? Of these, which is the major product?
4. What are the major physiologic stimuli of catecholamine secretion?
5. What are the subtypes and distribution of catecholamine receptors?
6. What physiologic processes do each subtype of catecholamine receptor control, and how do catecholamines affect the physiologic process?

OVERVIEW OF ADRENAL MEDULLARY DISORDERS

Pheochromocytoma is an uncommon tumor of adrenal medullary tissue that causes production of excessive amounts of catecholamines. Patients typically present with episodic (or sustained) hypertension or with a syndrome characterized by palpitations, tachycardia, chest pain, headache, anxiety, blanching, excessive sweating, hyperglycemia, and glucosuria.

Two unusual catecholamine deficiency states have also been described. **Sympathetic neural failure** is caused by deficient production of norepinephrine, and **adrenomedullary failure** is caused by deficient production of epinephrine.

PATHOPHYSIOLOGY OF SELECTED DISORDERS OF THE ADRENAL MEDULLA

PHEOCHROMOCYTOMA

Pheochromocytomas are neoplasms of the chromaffin cells of the adrenal medulla or extramedullary sites. These tumors secrete excessive amounts of epinephrine, norepinephrine, or both. Most pheochromocytomas secrete norepinephrine and cause episodic (or sustained) hypertension. Pheochromocytomas that secrete epinephrine cause hypertension less often; more often, they produce episodic hyperglycemia, glucosuria, and other metabolic effects.

Table 14–2 summarizes the clinical features of pheochromocytoma. Pheochromocytomas are uncommon, probably found in less than 0.1% of all patients with hypertension and in approximately two individuals per million population. Pheochromocytomas occur in both sexes and in all age groups but are most often diagnosed in the fourth or fifth decades. The diagnosis is important because sudden release of catecholamines from these tumors during surgery or obstetric delivery may prove fatal. Pheochromocytoma is sometimes called "the 10% tumor" because 10% occur in extra-adrenal paraganglia, 10% are multiple, and 10% are malignant (Table 14–2).

Etiology

Pheochromocytomas usually occur sporadically but may also occur in familial distribution with an

Table 14–2. Clinical features of pheochromocytoma.[1]

Epidemiology	Adults; both sexes; all ages, especially 30–50 years
Biologic behavior	90% benign; 10% malignant
Secretion	High levels of catecholamines; most secrete norepinephrine
Clinical presentation	Episodic or sustained hypertension, sweating, palpitations, hyperglycemia, glycosuria
Macroscopic features	Mass, often hemorrhagic; 10% bilateral; 10% extra-adrenal
Microscopic features	Nests of large cells, vascular stroma

[1] Modified from Chandrasoma P, Taylor CR (editors): *Concise Pathology,* 2nd ed. Appleton & Lange, 1994.

autosomal dominant pattern of inheritance. Patients with neurofibromatosis (Recklinghausen's disease) also have an increased incidence of pheochromocytoma. More commonly, pheochromocytomas occur in association with other endocrine tumors. In the syndrome called multiple endocrine neoplasia (MEN) type 2a (Sipple's syndrome), pheochromocytomas occur in association with calcitonin-producing adenomas of the thyroid, parathyroid hormone-producing adenomas of the parathyroid, or pituitary adenomas. In MEN 2b, pheochromocytomas occur in association with numerous oral mucosal neuromas. About 50% of patients with MEN 2a and 2b have bilateral pheochromocytomas.

Almost all pheochromocytomas (over 95%) occur in the abdomen, and most of these (85%) are in the adrenal medulla. Extra-adrenal pheochromocytomas are found in the perirenal area, the organ of Zuckerkandl, the urinary bladder, the heart, the neck, and the posterior mediastinum (Figure 14–1). About 10% of pheochromocytomas are multicentric, most commonly occurring in both adrenal glands and less commonly in the extra-adrenal paraganglia.

Grossly, pheochromocytomas are generally well-circumscribed but vary in size, with weights ranging from under 1 g to several kilograms (Figure 14–3). They are highly vascular tumors and frequently have cystic, necrotic, or hemorrhagic areas. Microscopically, the tumor consists of large pleomorphic cells arranged in sheets separated by a highly vascular stroma. In the cytoplasm, there are catecholamine-containing storage granules similar to those in normal adrenal medullary cells. Mitoses are rare, but tumor invasion of the adrenal capsule and blood vessels is common even in benign pheochromocytomas. About 10% of pheochromocytomas are malignant. Malignancy is established only when metastasis is found in a site where chromaffin cells are not usually demonstrated (eg, liver, lung, bone, or brain).

Very rarely, a pathologic picture of diffuse adrenal medullary hyperplasia is found in the syndrome of multiple endocrine neoplasia.

Pathogenesis

Most pheochromocytomas release predominantly norepinephrine, but most also release epinephrine. Rarely, a pheochromocytoma releases only epinephrine, or epinephrine predominantly.

In about half of patients with pheochromocytoma, clinical manifestations vary in intensity and occur in an episodic or paroxysmal fashion. The paroxysms are related to sudden catecholamine discharge from the tumor. The sudden catecholamine excess causes hypertension, palpitations, tachycardia, chest pain, headache, anxiety, blanching, and excessive sweating. Such paroxysms usually occur several times a week but may occur only once every few months or up to 25 times daily. Paroxysms typically last for 15 minutes or less but may last for days. As time passes, the paroxysms usually become more frequent but generally do not change in character. A typical paroxysm may be produced by activities that compress the tumor (eg, bending, lifting, exercise, defecation, eating, or deep palpation of the abdomen) and by emotional distress or anxiety.

Other patients have persistently secreting tumors and more chronic symptoms, including sustained hypertension. However, such patients also usually experience paroxysms related to transient increases in catecholamine release.

Clinical Manifestations

The clinical manifestations of pheochromocytoma are due to increased secretion of epinephrine and norepinephrine. Commonly reported manifestations are listed in Table 14–3.

The most common presenting feature of pheochromocytoma is hypertension. In many cases, hypertension is sustained but the blood pressure shows marked fluctuations with peak pressures occurring during symptomatic paroxysms. During a hypertensive episode, the systolic blood pressure can rise to as high as 300 mm Hg. In other cases, hypertension is truly intermittent. The blood pressure elevation caused by the catecholamine excess results from several mechanisms: β_1 receptor-mediated increases in cardiac output and in renin release, leading to increased circulating levels of angiotensin II; and alpha receptor-mediated vasoconstriction of arterioles, leading to an increase in peripheral resistance.

Peripheral vasoconstriction, mediated by alpha receptors, causes both facial pallor and cool, moist hands and feet. Chronic vasoconstriction of the arterial and venous beds leads to a reduction in plasma volume and predisposes to postural hypotension.

If unrecognized and untreated, pheochromocytoma may be complicated by hypertensive retinopathy,

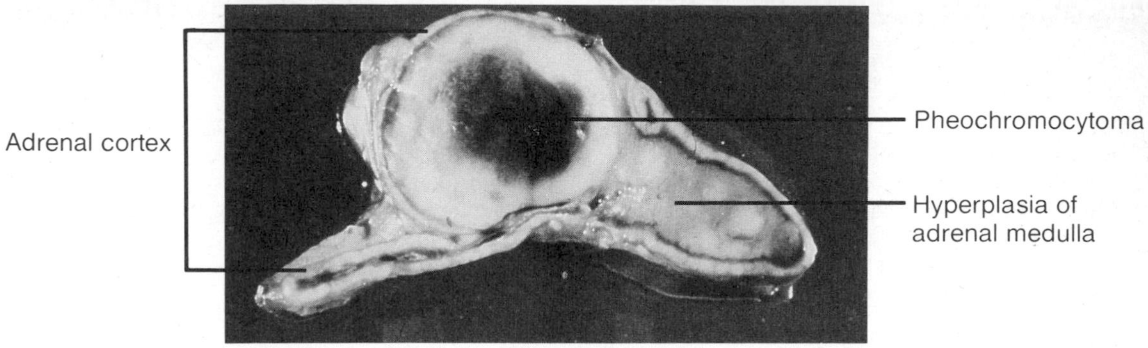

Figure 14–3. Cross section of adrenal, showing a pheochromocytoma associated with hyperplasia of the medulla in a patient with multiple endocrine neoplasia type 2a. He also had a medullary carcinoma of the thyroid and a large pheochromocytoma in the opposite adrenal. (Reproduced, with permission, from Chandrasoma P, Taylor CE: *Concise Pathology,* 2nd ed. Appleton & Lange, 1994.)

nephropathy, myocarditis, myocardial infarction, congestive heart failure, and stroke.

The metabolic effects of excessive circulating catecholamines increase both blood glucose and free fatty acid levels. Increased glycolysis and glycogenolysis, combined with an alpha receptor-mediated inhibition of insulin release, cause the increase in blood sugar levels. Glucose intolerance is common, and diabetes mellitus may occur.

An increase in metabolic rate may cause weight loss (or, in children, lack of weight gain), and impaired heat loss from peripheral vasoconstriction may cause a rise in temperature, heat intolerance, flushing, or increased sweating.

During paroxysms, patients may experience marked anxiety, and when episodes are prolonged or severe, there may be visual disturbances, paresthesias, or seizures. A feeling of fatigue or exhaustion usually follows these episodes. Untreated patients with pheochromocytomas frequently die of cerebral hemorrhage.

Somewhat different clinical manifestations occur with predominantly epinephrine-releasing pheochromocytomas. Symptoms and signs include hypotension, prominent tachycardia, cardiac arrhythmias, and noncardiogenic pulmonary edema.

Pheochromocytoma is diagnosed by demonstrating abnormally high concentrations of catecholamines or their breakdown products in the urine or plasma. A reliable assay showing increased plasma or urine levels of epinephrine or norepinephrine or their metabolites (metanephrines or VMA) is usually sufficient to establish the diagnosis. For outpatients, the best screening tests are 24-hour urinary metanephrines or VMA, one or both of which are elevated in almost all cases. For inpatients, plasma catecholamine levels may be determined from samples obtained while the patient is supine. If the patient has paroxysmal symptoms, sampling of blood or timed urine collections during an episode may be needed to establish the diagnosis.

Administration of glucagon can precipitate a paroxysm, but this maneuver is not generally recommended. On the other hand, administration of the antihypertensive agent clonidine can be used to differentiate essential hypertension from hypertension due to pheochromocytoma. This potent α_2 agonist stimulates alpha receptors in the brain, reducing sympathetic outflow and blood pressure. A dose of 0.3 mg is given orally, and blood pressure and plasma catecholamine levels are determined periodically over the next 3 hours. Essential hypertension is dependent on centrally mediated catecholamine release. Administering clonidine normally suppresses sympathetic nervous system activity and substan-

Table 14–3. Common symptoms in patients with pheochromocytoma.[1]

Symptoms during or following paroxysms
Headache
Sweating
Palpitations, tachycardia
Chest pain
Anxiety, fear of impending death
Tremor
Fatigue or exhaustion
Nausea, vomiting
Abdominal pain
Visual disturbances
Symptoms between paroxysms
Increased sweating
Cold hands and feet
Weight loss
Constipation

[1] Modified and reproduced, with permission, from Greenspan FS, Baxter JD (editors): *Basic and Clinical Endocrinology,* 4th ed. Appleton & Lange, 1994.

tially lowers plasma norepinephrine levels, reducing blood pressure. But in patients with pheochromocytoma, the drug has little or no effect on the plasma catecholamine levels because these tumors, which are not thought to be innervated, behave autonomously. Thus, the blood pressure remains unchanged.

When a diagnosis of pheochromocytoma is made, the next step is to localize the neoplasm or neoplasms radiographically to permit surgical removal.

7. Why is pheocromocytoma called the "10% tumor"?
8. What are the symptoms and signs of pheochromocytoma?
9. What are some complications of untreated pheochromocytoma?
10. What are the metabolic and neurologic effects of pheochromocytoma?
11. How is the diagnosis of pheochromocytoma made?

ADRENAL MEDULLARY HYPOFUNCTION

Bilateral adrenalectomy obviously entails loss of the adrenal medulla. Yet individuals undergoing bilateral adrenalectomy suffer no clinically significant disability, provided they receive glucocorticoid replacement and have an otherwise intact sympathetic nervous system.

Sympathetic neural failure, caused by deficient production of norepinephrine, presents clinically as orthostatic (postural) hypotension. **Adrenomedullary failure,** caused by deficient production of epinephrine, usually causes little or no disability. However, in some patients with insulin-dependent diabetes mellitus, adrenomedullary failure is associated with glucagon deficiency. In these patients, the combined defect can result in episodic hypoglycemia.

Patients with generalized **autonomic insufficiency** may have deficient adrenal medullary secretion of norepinephrine and epinephrine. Such patients usually present with orthostatic hypotension and may have defects in responding to severe physiologic stress, such as in recovery from insulin-induced hypoglycemia. Generalized autonomic insufficiency is associated with a variety of other disorders (Table 14–4).

Table 14–4. Disorders associated with adrenal medullary hypofunction.[1]

Insulin-dependent diabetes mellitus
Familial dysautonomia
Shy-Drager syndrome
Parkinson's disease
Tabes dorsalis
Syringomyelia
Cerebrovascular disease
Idiopathic orthostatic hypotension
Sympathectomy
Drugs: antihypertensives, antidepressants

[1] Modified and reproduced, with permission, from Greenspan FS, Baxter JD (editors): *Basic and Clinical Endocrinology,* 4th ed. Appleton & Lange, 1994.

REFERENCES

General

Goldfien A: Adrenal medulla. In: *Basic and Clinical Endocrinology,* 4th ed. Greenspan FS, Baxter JD (editors). Appleton & Lange, 1994.

Trendelenburg U, Weiner N (editors): Catecholamines. Vol 90 of *Handbook of Experimental Pharmacology.* Springer, 1988.

Pheochromocytoma

Benowitz NL: Pheochromocytoma. Adv Intern Med 1990;35:195.

Cryer PE: Pheochromocytoma. West J Med 1992; 156:399.

Graham PE et al: Laboratory diagnosis of pheochromocytoma: Which analyses should we measure? Ann Clin Biochem 1993;30(Part 2):129.

Kazantsev GB, Prinz RA: Functioning tumors of the adrenal gland. Compr Ther 1993;19:232.

Sjoberg RJ, Simcic KJ, Kidd GS: The clonidine suppression test for pheochromocytoma: A review of its utility and pitfalls. Arch Intern Med 1992;152:1193.

Multiple Endocrine Neoplasia

Casanova S et al: Pheaochromocytoma in multiple endocrine neoplasia type 2A: Survey of 100 cases. Clin Endocrinol 1993;38:531.

Neumann HPH et al: Pheochromocytomas, multiple endocrine neoplasia type 2, and von Hippel-Lindau disease. N Engl J Med 1993;329:1531.

Adrenal Medullary Hypofunction

Cryer PE: Decreased sympathochromaffin activity in IDDM. Diabetes 1989;38:405.

Disorders of the Exocrine Pancreas 15

Stephen J. McPhee, MD

The pancreas is a gland with both exocrine and endocrine functions. The exocrine pancreas contains **acini** that secrete pancreatic juice into the duodenum through the pancreatic ducts. Pancreatic juice contains a number of enzymes, some of which are initially made in an inactive form. Once activated, these enzymes help to digest food and prepare it for absorption in the intestine. Disorders interfering with normal pancreatic enzyme activity (pancreatic insufficiency) cause maldigestion of fat and steatorrhea (fatty stools). Dysfunction of the exocrine pancreas results from inflammation (acute pancreatitis, chronic pancreatitis), neoplasm (pancreatic carcinoma), or duct obstruction by stones or abnormally viscid mucus (cystic fibrosis).

The endocrine pancreas is composed of the **islets of Langerhans.** The islets are distributed throughout the pancreas and contain several different hormone-producing cells. The islet cells manufacture hormones such as insulin that are important in nutrient absorption, storage, and metabolism. Dysfunction of the endocrine pancreas causes diabetes mellitus (see Chapter 16).

Both exocrine and endocrine pancreatic dysfunction occur together in some patients.

NORMAL STRUCTURE & FUNCTION OF THE EXOCRINE PANCREAS

ANATOMY

The pancreas is a solid organ that lies transversely across the posterior abdominal wall deep within the epigastrium. It is firmly fixed in the retroperitoneum in front of the abdominal aorta and the first and second lumbar vertebrae. Thus, the pain of acute or chronic pancreatitis is situated deep in the epigastric region and frequently radiates to the back.

Normally, the pancreas measures about 15 cm long, though it weighs less than 110 g. The organ is covered by a thin capsule of connective tissue that sends septa into it, separating it into lobules (Figure 15–1).

The pancreas can be divided into four parts: a head—including the uncinate process—a neck, a body, and a tail. The head lies in the curved space between the first, second, and third portions of the duodenum. The uncinate process is that portion of the head which extends to the left behind the superior mesenteric vessels. The neck connects the head and body. The body is situated horizontally in the retroperitoneal space with the tail extending toward the hilum of the spleen.

The exocrine pancreas is drained by a major central duct called the **duct of Wirsung,** which runs the length of the gland. This duct is normally about 3–4 mm in diameter. In most individuals, the pancreatic duct enters the duodenum at the duodenal papilla alongside the common bile duct. The sphincter of Oddi surrounds both ducts. In about one-third of individuals, the duct of Wirsung and the common bile duct join to form a common channel before terminating at the **ampulla of Vater** (Figure 15–1).

Many individuals also have a separate accessory pancreatic duct called the **duct of Santorini** that runs from the head and body of the gland to enter the duodenum about 2 cm proximal to the duodenal papilla. Occasionally, the accessory duct joins with the major pancreatic duct.

HISTOLOGY

The exocrine pancreas consists of clusters of acini, or **lobules,** which are drained by ductules. The islets of Langerhans of the endocrine pancreas are clusters of a few hundred cells each located between the lobules.

Each pancreatic acinus is composed of several acinar cells surrounding a lumen (Figure 15–2). The acinar cells synthesize and secrete enzymes. On histologic examination, acinar cells are typical protein-secreting cells. They are pyramidal epithelial cells arranged in rows. Their apexes join to form the lumen of the acinus. Granules containing digestive en-

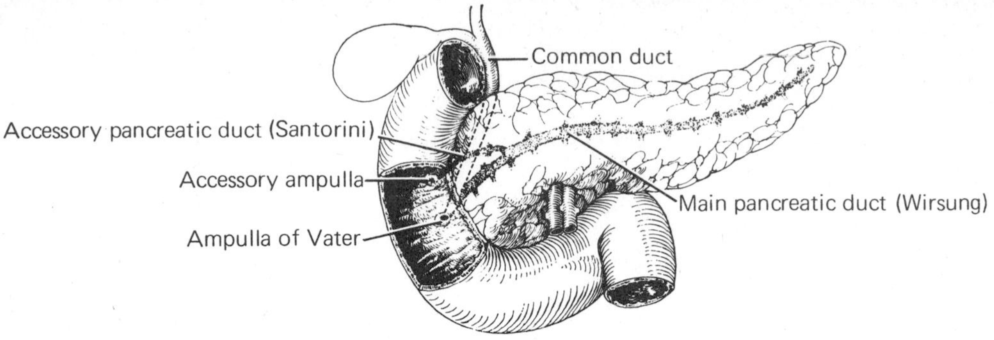

Figure 15–1. Anatomy of the pancreas. (Courtesy of W Silen.) (Reproduced, with permission, from Way LW [editor]: *Current Surgical Diagnosis & Treatment,* 10th ed. Appleton & Lange, 1994.)

zymes called **zymogen granules** are found in the acinar cells. These granules are discharged by exocytosis from the apexes of the cells into the lumen. The number of zymogen granules in the cells varies, with more being found during fasting and fewer after a meal.

PHYSIOLOGY

Composition of Pancreatic Juice

About 1500 mL of pancreatic juice is secreted each day. Pancreatic juice contains water, ions, and a variety of proteins. The principal ions in pancreatic juice are HCO_3^-, Cl^-, Na^+, and K^+. Of these, HCO_3^- is particularly important. At maximum flow rates, the concentration of HCO_3^- in pancreatic juice may reach 150 meq/L (versus 24 meq/L in plasma), and the pH of the juice may reach 8.3. The alkaline nature of pancreatic juice plays a major role in neutralizing the gastric acid entering the duodenum with ingested food (chyme) from the stomach. The pH of the duodenal contents rises to 6.0–7.0, and by the time the chyme reaches the jejunum, its pH is nearly neutral.

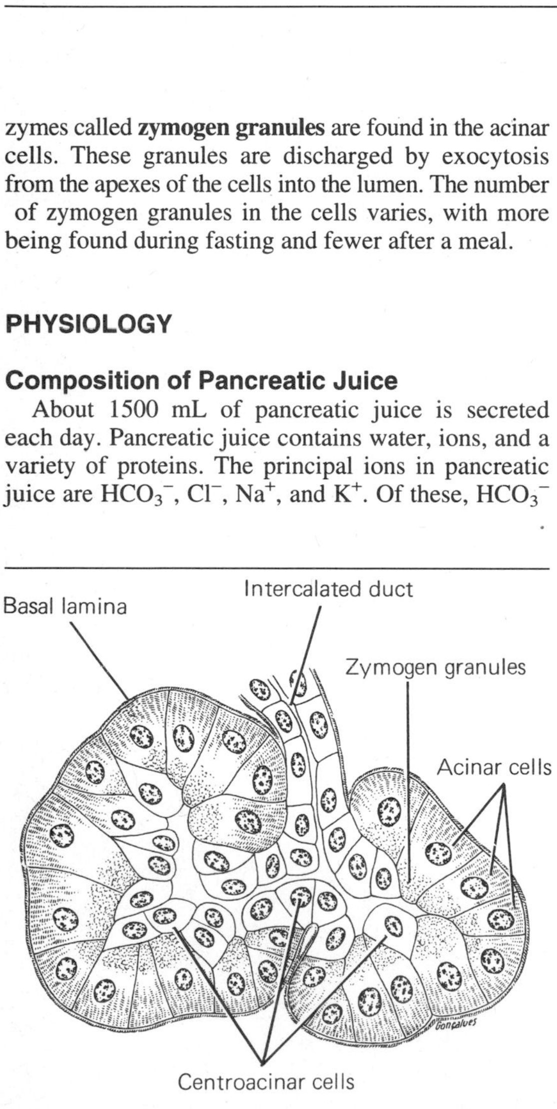

Figure 15–2. Schematic drawing of the pancreatic acini. Acinar cells are pyramidal in shape, with zymogen granules at their apexes. (Reproduced, with permission, from Junqueira LC, Carneiro J, Kelley RO: *Basic Histology,* 7th ed. Appleton & Lange, 1992.)

Most of the proteins in pancreatic juice are enzymes and proenzymes (enzyme precursors that require some structural change to render them active). These enzymes aid in the intraluminal phase of digestion and absorption of fats, carbohydrates, and proteins. The rest of the proteins in pancreatic juice are plasma proteins, mucoproteins, and trypsin inhibitors (see below).

Some of the pancreatic enzymes (lipase, amylase, deoxyribonuclease and ribonuclease) are secreted by the acinar cells in their active forms. The remaining enzymes are secreted as inactive proenzymes or **zymogens** (trypsinogen, chymotrypsinogen, proelastase, procarboxypeptidase, and phospholipase A_2) that are activated in the lumen of the proximal intestine. Activation of zymogens within the acinar cell might otherwise lead to acute pancreatitis and pancreatic autodigestion.

When the pancreatic juice enters the duodenum, trypsinogen is converted to the active form trypsin by an enzyme found in the intestinal brush border called enteropeptidase (or enterokinase). Trypsin then converts the remaining proenzymes into active enzymes, eg, chymotrypsinogen into chymotrypsin. Trypsin can also activate its own precursor, trypsinogen, producing the potential for an autocatalytic chain reaction. It is thus not surprising that pancreatic juice normally contains a trypsin inhibitor so that this autocatalytic reaction does not occur under normal circumstances.

Regulation of Secretion of Pancreatic Juice

Between and after meals, pancreatic secretion is regulated by hormonal and neural actions and by neurohumoral interactions.

Secretion of pancreatic juice is controlled primarily by two different hormones—**secretin** and **cholecystokinin (CCK)**—that are produced by specialized enteroendocrine cells of the duodenal mucosa.

Secretion of secretin is triggered by gastric acid and by the products of protein digestion when they enter the duodenum. Secretin acts chiefly on the pancreatic duct cells to cause an outpouring of very alkaline pancreatic juice. In response to secretin, the pancreas produces a large volume of watery fluid rich in bicarbonate content but with little enzyme activity.

Secretion of CCK is triggered by the products of protein and fat digestion (peptides, amino acids and fatty acids) when they enter the duodenum. CCK acts chiefly on the acinar cells to cause release of enzymes from zymogen granules. Thus, in response to CCK, the pancreas secretes a small volume of juice low in bicarbonate but very high in enzyme content. In addition, CCK increases the secretion of enteropeptidase (enterokinase) from other endocrine cells of the duodenal mucosa. The integrated action of both secretin and CCK produces abundant secretion of enzyme-rich, alkaline pancreatic juice.

The secretion of pancreatic juice is also controlled in part by a reflex mechanism. Acetylcholine released by the vagus nerve acts like CCK on acinar cells to cause discharge of zymogen granules. Thus, stimulation of the vagus nerve causes production of a small volume of pancreatic juice rich in enzymes.

Digestive Functions of Pancreatic Juice

The secretion of pancreatic juice aids digestion in several ways. The large amount of bicarbonate in the juice helps to neutralize the acidic chyme from the stomach so that the pancreatic enzymes can function optimally in a neutral pH range.

In addition, each of the enzymes has an important digestive function. In digesting carbohydrates, pancreatic **amylase** splits straight-chain glucose polysaccharides (so-called amyloses in starch) into smaller sugars, maltose and maltotriose. In digesting fat, pancreatic **lipase** splits triglycerides into fatty acids and monoglyceride. **Phospholipase A_2** splits a fatty acid off from lecithin to form lysolecithin. **Ribonuclease** and **deoxyribonuclease** attack the nucleic acids. The remaining enzymes help to digest proteins. **Trypsin, chymotrypsin,** and **elastase** are endopeptidases; that is, they cleave peptide bonds in the middle of polypeptide chains. **Carboxypeptidase** is an exopeptidase; that is, it splits peptide bonds adjacent to the carboxyl end of peptide chains. Together, these proteases break down proteins into oligopeptides and free amino acids.

1. What histologic features allow the pancreas to secrete digestive enzymes into the gastrointestinal tract?
2. What is the volume, composition, and function of pancreatic juice?
3. What are the neural and hormonal controls over exocrine pancreatic function?
4. Why does trypsinogen not self-activate before arriving in the duodenum?

PATHOPHYSIOLOGY OF SELECTED EXOCRINE PANCREATIC DISORDERS

ACUTE PANCREATITIS

Clinical Presentations

Acute pancreatitis is a clinical syndrome resulting from acute inflammation and destructive autodigestion of the pancreas and peripancreatic tissues. Clinically, acute pancreatitis is a common and important cause of acute upper abdominal pain, nausea, vomiting, and fever. Laboratory findings of marked elevations of serum amylase and lipase help to differentiate it from other entities causing these symptoms. The severity of inflammation varies, and the prognosis ranges from mild, self-limited illness lasting 1–2 days to death from pancreatic necrosis, hemorrhage, or sepsis. Acute pancreatitis often recurs (relapsing acute pancreatitis). With repeated attacks, the gland may eventually be permanently damaged, resulting in chronic pancreatitis.

Etiology

Acute pancreatitis has many causes (Table 15–1), but in none of them is the exact mechanism of damage to the gland clearly understood. However, in all there is escape of activated proteolytic enzymes from the ducts, leading to tissue injury, inflammation, necrosis, and in some cases infection.

The two most common conditions associated with acute pancreatitis are alcohol abuse and biliary tract disease.

Alcohol abuse is a common cause of acute pancreatitis in the USA, accounting for 65% of cases in some series. Acute pancreatitis usually occurs following an episode of heavy drinking. The exact mechanism by which alcohol damages the gland is not clear. Alcohol may have a direct toxic effect on pancreatic acinar cells or may cause inflammation of the sphincter of Oddi, leading to retention of hydrolytic enzymes in the pancreatic duct and acini. Alternatively, alcohol may cause decreased tone at the sphincter of Oddi, predisposing to reflux of bile or duodenal contents into the pancreatic duct and leading to parenchymal injury.

In patients who do not drink alcohol, about 50% of cases of acute pancreatitis are associated with biliary tract disease. In such cases, the hypothesized mechanism is obstruction of the common bile duct and the main pancreatic duct when a gallstone becomes lodged at the ampulla of Vater. Reflux of bile or duodenal contents into the pancreatic duct leads to parenchymal injury. Others have proposed that bacterial toxins or free bile acids travel via lymphatics from the gallbladder to the pancreas, giving rise to inflammation. In either case, acute pancreatitis associated with biliary tract disease is more common in women because gallstones are more common in women.

Acute pancreatitis may result from a variety of infectious agents, including viruses (mumps virus, coxsackievirus, hepatitis A virus, or cytomegalovirus) and bacteria (*Salmonella typhi* or hemolytic streptococci).

Blunt or penetrating trauma and other injuries may cause acute pancreatitis. Pancreatitis sometimes occurs following surgical procedures near the pancreas (duodenal stump syndrome; pancreatic tail syndrome following splenectomy). Infarction of the pancreas may result from occlusion of vessels supplying the gland. Shock and hypothermia may cause decreased perfusion, resulting in cellular degeneration and release of pancreatic enzymes. Radiation therapy of retroperitoneal malignant neoplasms can sometimes cause acute pancreatitis.

Marked hypercalcemia, such as that associated with hyperparathyroidism, sarcoidosis, hypervitaminosis D, or multiple myeloma, causes acute pancreatitis in about 10% of cases. Two mechanisms have been hypothesized. The high plasma calcium concentration may cause calcium to precipitate in the pancreatic duct, leading to ductal obstruction. Alternatively, hypercalcemia may stimulate activation of trypsinogen in the pancreatic duct.

Pancreatitis is also associated with hyperlipidemia, particularly those types characterized by increased plasma levels of chylomicrons (types I, IV, and V). In these cases, it is postulated that free fatty acids liberated by the action of pancreatic lipase cause gland

Table 15–1. Causes of acute pancreatitis.

A. Alcohol ingestion (acute and chronic alcoholism)
B. Biliary tract disease
C. Trauma
   1. Blunt abdominal trauma
   2. Post-operative
   3. Post-endoscopic retrograde cannulation of pancreatic duct, injection of pancreatic duct
   4. Post-electric shock
D. Infections
   1. Viral: Mumps, rubella, cocksackievirus B, echovirus, viral hepatitis A, B, and C, adenovirus, cytomegalovirus, varicella, Epstein-Barr virus, human immunodeficiency virus
   2. Bacterial: *Mycoplasma pneumoniae, Salmonella typhi,* group A streptococci (scarlet fever), staphylococci, actinomycosis, *Mycobacterium tuberculosis, Mycobacterium avium* complex, *Legionella, Campylobacter jejuni, Leptospira icterohaemorrhagiae*
   3. Parasitic: *Ascaris lumbricoides,* hydatid cyst, *Clonorchis sinensis*
E. Metabolic
   1. Hyperlipidemia, apolipoprotein CII deficiency syndrome, hypertriglyceridemia
   2. Hypercalcemia, eg, hyperparathyroidism
   3. Uremia
   4. Post-renal transplant
   5. Pregnancy, eclampsia
   6. Hemochromatosis, hemosiderosis
   7. Malnutrition: kwashiorkor, sprue, postgastrectomy, Whipple's disease
   8. Diabetic ketoacidosis
F. Hereditary
   1. Familial pancreatitis
   2. Cystic fibrosis
G. Drugs
   1. Definite association
      a. Immunosuppressives: azathioprine, mercaptopurine
      b. Diuretics: thiazides, furosemide
      c. Antimicrobials: sulfonamides, tetracyclines, pentamidine, didanosine, metronidazole, erythromycin
      d. Steroids: estrogens, oral contraceptives, corticosteroids, ACTH
      e. Miscellaneous: valproic acid, phenformin, intravenous lipid infusion
   2. Probable association
      a. Immunosuppressives: asparaginase
      b. Diuretics: ethacrynic acid, chlorthalidone
      c. Miscellaneous: procainamide
   3. Possible association
      a. Antimicrobials: isoniazid, rifampin, nitrofurantoin
      b. Analgesics: acetaminophen, propoxyphene, salicylates, sulindac, other NSAIDs
      c. Miscellaneous: methyldopa
H. Poisons and toxins
   1. Venom: scorpion, *T trinitatis*
   2. Inorganic: zinc, cobalt, mercuric chloride, saccharated iron oxide
   3. Organic: Methanol, organophosphates
I. Vascular
   1. Vasculitis: systemic lupus erythematosus, polyarteritis nodosa, malignant hypertension, thrombotic thrombocytopenic purpura
   2. Shock, hypoperfusion, myocardial or mesenteric infarction
   3. Atheromatous embolism
J. Mechanical
   1. Pancreas divisum with accessory duct obstruction
   2. Ampulla of Vater stenosis, tumor, obstruction (regional enteritis, duodenal diverticulum, duodenal surgery, worms, foreign bodies)
   3. Choledochocele
   4. Penetrating duodenal ulcer
   5. Pancreatic carcinoma
K. Idiopathic

inflammation and injury. Alcohol abuse or oral contraceptive use increases the risk of acute pancreatitis in patients with hyperlipidemia.

A variety of drugs have been associated with pancreatitis, including corticosteroids, thiazide diuretics, immunosuppressants, and cancer chemotherapeutic agents.

Rarely, acute pancreatitis may be familial, occurring with an autosomal dominant inheritance pattern.

In about 25% of cases of acute pancreatitis, no etiologic factor can be identified. It is thought that idiopathic acute pancreatitis is often caused by occult biliary microlithiasis.

Pathology & Pathogenesis

The symptoms, signs, laboratory findings and complications of acute pancreatitis can all be explained on the basis of the pathologic damage to the ductules, acini, and islets of the pancreas. However, both the degree of damage and the clinical consequences are quite variable.

When the damage is limited in extent, the pathologic features consist of mild to marked swelling of the gland, especially the acini, and mild to marked infiltration with polymorphonuclear neutrophils. However, damage to tissue is usually only minimal to moderate, and there is no hemorrhage. In some cases, suppuration may be found along with edema, and this may result in tissue necrosis and abscess formation. In severe cases, massive necrosis and liquefaction of the pancreas occurs, predisposing to pancreatic abscess formation. Vascular necrosis and disruption may occur, resulting in hemorrhage. Hemorrhagic pancreatitis, which usually involves the entire gland, is the most serious form of pancreatitis.

In addition, a brownish serous fluid is often found in the peritoneal cavity ("pancreatic ascites"). This fluid contains blood, fat globules ("chicken broth"), and high levels of amylase and other pancreatic enzymes. Fat necrosis may occur in and around the pancreas, omentum, and mesentery, appearing as chalky white foci that may later calcify.

The mechanism by which enzymes and bioactive substances become activated within the pancreas is a major unanswered question in acute pancreatitis. The early initiating events probably occur at a membrane or intracellular level.

A recently proposed theory of the pathogenesis of alcoholic pancreatitis emphasizes disordered agonist-receptor interaction on the membrane of pancreatic acinar cells. According to this theory, alcohol induces alterations in the control of exocrine pancreatic secretion which in turn result in hyperstimulation of pancreatic acinar cells and their muscarinic receptors. This hyperstimulation mimics the mechanism of acute pancreatitis caused by scorpion sting, anti-acetylcholinesterase-containing insecticide poisoning, or administration of supramaximal doses of secretagogues such as acetylcholine and CCK.

Other recent studies suggest that lysosomal enzymes within the pancreatic acinar cell may play an important role. Morphologic studies during the first 24 hours after ligation of the pancreatic duct in animals indicate that the earliest lesions occur in acinar cells. Digestive enzyme zymogens and lysosomal hydrolases such as cathepsin B become localized together, suggesting that intra-acinar cell activation of the zymogens by lysosomal hydrolases may be an important initiating event.

The pathologic changes all result from the action of activated pancreatic enzymes on the pancreas and surrounding tissues. In a manner still not understood, small amounts of trypsin escape from the duct system into the pancreatic parenchyma to initiate pancreatitis, perhaps through inhibition of the trypsin inhibitor. Once there, trypsin activates the proenzymes of chymotrypsin, elastase, and phospholipase A_2, and the activated enzymes cause damage in several ways (Figure 15–3). For example, chymotrypsin activation leads to edema and vascular damage. Similarly, elastase, once activated from proelastase, digests the elastin in blood vessel walls and causes vascular injury and hemorrhage; damage to peripancreatic blood vessels can lead to hemorrhagic pancreatitis. Phospholipase A_2 splits a fatty acid off lecithin, forming lysolecithin, which is cytotoxic to erythrocytes and damages cell membranes. Formation of lysolecithin from the lecithin in bile may contribute to disruption of the pancreas and necrosis of surrounding fat. Phospholipase A_2 also liberates arachidonic acid, which is then converted to prostaglandins, leukotrienes, and other mediators of inflammation, contributing to coagulation necrosis.

Pancreatic lipase, released directly as a result of pancreatic acinar cell damage, acts enzymatically on surrounding adipose tissue, causing fat necrosis (Figure 15–3).

Furthermore, trypsin and chymotrypsin activate kinins, complement, coagulation factors, and plasmin, leading to edema, inflammation, thrombosis, and hemorrhage within the gland. For example, trypsin activation of the kallikrein-kinin system leads to the release of bradykinin and kallidin, causing vasodilation, increased vascular permeability, edema, and inflammation (Figure 15–3).

Finally, the activated pancreatic enzymes enter the bloodstream and may produce effects elsewhere in the body. Circulating phospholipases interfere with the normal function of pulmonary surfactant, contributing to the development of an acute respiratory distress syndrome in some patients with acute pancreatitis. Elevated serum lipase levels are sometimes associated with fat necrosis outside of the abdomen.

Clinical Manifestations

The major clinical consequences—symptoms, signs and complications—of acute pancreatitis (Table 15–2) are readily explained by pathologic de-

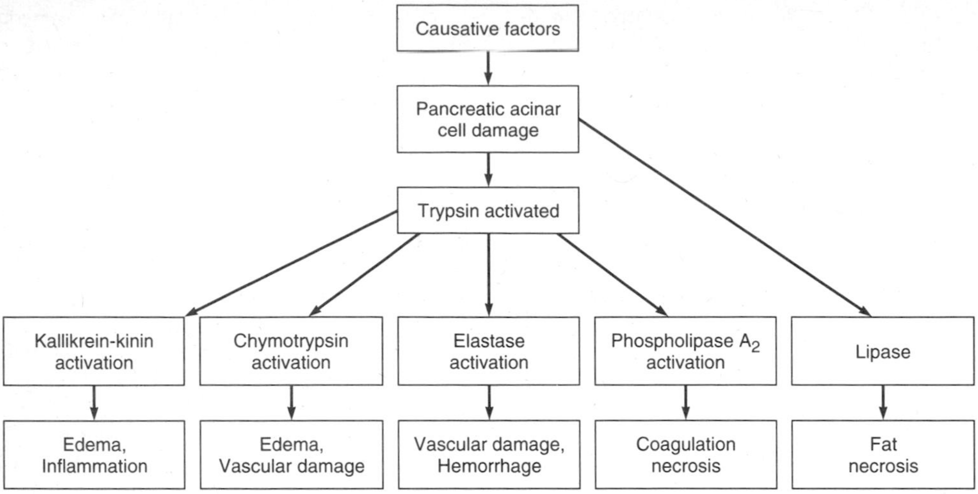

Figure 15–3. Hypothesized pathogenesis of acute pancreatitis. (Reproduced with permission from Marshall JB: Acute pancreatitis: A review with an emphasis on new developments. Arch Intern Med 1993;153:1185.)

struction of ductules, acini, and islets of the pancreas. The extent of damage is highly variable from patient to patient, as are the clinical manifestations, ranging from mild episodes of epigastric pain, nausea, and vomiting to severe (sometimes fatal) episodes of peritonitis, shock, and cyanosis.

The diagnosis of pancreatitis is primarily a clinical one. Distinguishing pancreatitis from other, potentially lethal causes of abdominal pain and identifying those patients with severe pancreatitis who may develop serious complications from the remote systemic effects of the disease are major diagnostic concerns.

Computed tomography is useful in diagnosis (Figure 15–4). It is particularly useful in distinguishing between edematous and necrotizing forms and providing prognostic information by detecting extrapancreatic involvement.

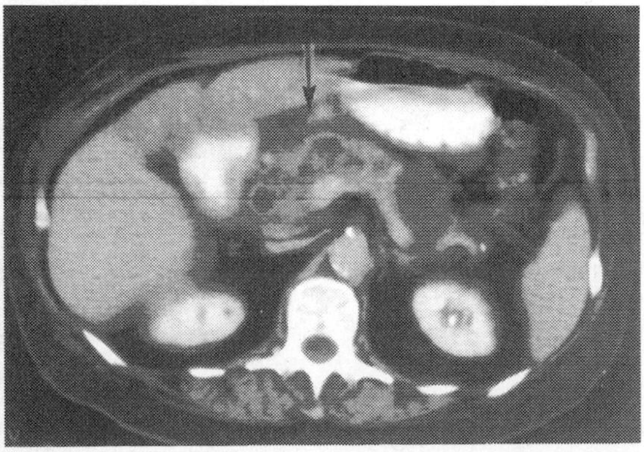

Figure 15–4. Acute pancreatitis on CT. (Courtesy of Henry I. Goldberg, MD, Department of Radiology, University of California, San Francisco.)

Table 15–2. Clinical manifestations and complications of acute pancreatitis.

A. Pancreas
   1. Edema, inflammation, local fat necrosis
   2. Necrosis, hemorrhage
   3. Phlegmon
   4. Pseudocyst: pain, rupture, hemorrhage, infection, obstruction of gastrointestinal tract (stomach, duodenum, colon)
   5. Abscess

B. Contiguous organs
   1. Extension of inflammation, fat necrosis, hemorrhage into peritoneum and retroperitoneum
   2. Thrombosis of adjacent blood vessels
   3. Ileus, bowel obstruction, perforation, infarction
   4. Pancreatic ascites: disruption of main pancreatic duct, leaking pseudocyst
   5. Obstructive jaundice

C. Systemic
   1. Cardiovascular: shock, hypovolemia, peripheral vasodilation, pericardial effusion, nonspecific ECG changes, sudden death
   2. Pulmonary: pleural effusion, pulmonary edema, acute respiratory distress syndrome, atelectasis, pneumonitis, mediastinal abscess
   3. Renal: renal failure, acute tubular necrosis, renal artery or vein thrombosis
   4. Hematologic: disseminated intravascular coagulation (DIC)
   5. Metabolic: hypocalcemia, hypoglycemia, hyperglycemia, hypertriglyceridemia
   6. Gastrointestinal: erosive gastritis, peptic ulcer, hemorrhage, bowel obstruction, portal vein thrombosis, variceal hemorrhage
   7. Nervous system: encephalopathy, retinopathy (sudden blindness), psychosis, fat emboli
   8. Distant fat necrosis (skin, bones, joints)

A. Pain: Patients with acute pancreatitis usually present with severe, constant, deep epigastric pain, often radiating to the back and flanks. The pain is thought to derive in part from stretching of the pancreatic capsule by distended ductules and parenchymal edema, inflammatory exudate, digested proteins and lipids, and hemorrhage. In addition, these materials may seep out of the parenchyma into the retroperitoneum and lesser sac, where they irritate retroperitoneal and peritoneal sensory nerve endings and produce intense back and flank pain. The clinical findings of generalized peritonitis may follow.

B. Nausea, Vomiting, and Ileus: Stretching of the pancreatic capsule may also produce nausea and vomiting. Increasing abdominal pain, peritoneal irritation, and electrolyte imbalance (especially hypokalemia) may cause a paralytic ileus with marked abdominal distention. If gastric motility is inhibited and the gastroesophageal sphincter is relaxed, there may be emesis. Both small and large bowel often dilate during an acute attack. Sometimes only a localized segment of bowel dilates. For example, there may be localized dilation of a segment of jejunum overlying the pancreas. In such cases, a plain x-ray of the abdomen shows thickening of the valvulae conniventes and air-fluid levels ("sentinel loop"). In other cases, there may be segmental dilation of a portion of the overlying transverse colon. The x-ray shows a sharply demarcated area of localized colonic dilation and edema ("colon cut-off sign").

C. Fever: Almost two-thirds of patients with acute pancreatitis develop fever. The pathophysiologic mechanism responsible for fever involves the extensive tissue injury, inflammation, and necrosis and the release of endogenous pyrogens, principally interleukin-1, from polymorphonuclear leukocytes into the circulation. In most cases of acute pancreatitis, fever does not indicate a bacterial infection. However, persistent fever beyond the fourth or fifth day of illness--or spiking temperatures to 40 °C or more—may signify development of infectious complications such as pancreatic abscess or ascending cholangitis.

D. Shock: Hypovolemia, hypotension, and shock may occur as a result of several interrelated factors. Hypovolemia results from massive exudation of plasma and hemorrhage into the retroperitoneal space and from accumulation of fluid in the gut due to ileus. Hypotension and shock may also result from release of kinins into the general circulation. For example, activation during acute inflammation of the proteolytic enzyme kallikrein results in peripheral vasodilation via liberation of the vasoactive peptides, bradykinin and kallidin. This vasodilation causes the pulse rate to rise and the blood pressure to fall. The contracted intravascular volume combined with the hypotension may lead to myocardial and cerebral ischemia, respiratory failure, and decreased urinary output or renal failure due to acute tubular necrosis.

E. Hyperamylasemia and Hyperlipasemia: The cardinal laboratory finding in acute pancreatitis is elevation of the serum amylase level, often up to 10–20 times normal. The elevation occurs almost immediately (within hours), but amylase concentration usually returns to normal within 48–72 hours even if symptoms continue. The sensitivity of the serum amylase for acute pancreatitis is estimated to be 70–95%, meaning that 5–30% of patients with acute pancreatitis have normal or minimally elevated serum amylase values. In addition, the specificity of the test is considerably lower. An elevated serum amylase can be found in a variety of other conditions.

The serum amylase concentration reflects the steady state between the rates of amylase entry into and removal from the blood. Hyperamylasemia can result from either an increased rate of entry or a decreased metabolic clearance of amylase from the circulation. The pancreas and salivary glands have much higher concentrations of amylase than any other organs and probably contribute almost all of the serum amylase activity in normal persons. Amylase of pancreatic origin can now be distinguished from that of salivary origin by a variety of techniques. Pancreatic hyperamylasemia results from injuries to the pancreas, ranging from minor (cannulation of the pancreatic duct) to severe (pancreatitis). In addition, injuries to the bowel wall (infarction or perforation) cause pancreatic hyperamylasemia due to enhanced absorption of amylase from the intestinal lumen. Salivary hyperamylasemia is observed in salivary gland diseases, such as mumps parotitis, but also (inexplicably) in a host of unrelated conditions such as chronic alcoholism, postoperative states (particularly following coronary artery bypass graft surgery), lactic acidosis, anorexia nervosa or bulimia nervosa, and certain malignancies. Hyperamylasemia can also result from decreased metabolic clearance of amylase due to renal failure or macroamylasemia (a condition in which there is an abnormally high-molecular-weight amylase in the serum).

Patients with marked elevations of serum amylase (more than three times the upper limit of normal) usually have acute pancreatitis. Patients with lesser elevations of serum amylase often have other conditions.

Determination of serum lipase activity is often helpful diagnostically. In acute pancreatitis, the serum lipase level is elevated, usually about 72 hours after onset of symptoms. The serum lipase measurement may be a better diagnostic test than serum amylase, because it is as simple to perform and as sensitive as the amylase assay but more specific for acute pancreatitis.

F. Coagulopathy: Tissue factor release and expression during proteolysis may cause activation of the plasma coagulation cascade and may lead to disseminated intravascular coagulation (DIC). In other cases, hypercoagulability of the blood is thought to be due to elevated concentrations of several coagulation factors, including factor VIII, fibrinogen, and perhaps factor V. Clinically affected patients may present with hemorrhagic discoloration (purpura) in the subcutaneous tissues around the umbilicus (Cullen's sign) or in the flanks (Grey Turner's sign).

G. Pleuropulmonary Complications: Pleuropulmonary complications of acute pancreatitis include pleural effusion, pulmonary edema, and respiratory failure (acute respiratory distress syndrome [ARDS]). Quite often, acute pancreatitis is accompanied by a small (usually left-sided) pleural effusion. The effusion may be secondary to a direct effect of the inflamed, swollen pancreas on the pleura abutting the diaphragm or to tracking of exudative fluid from the pancreatic bed retroperitoneally into the pleural cavity through defects in the diaphragm. Characteristically, the pleural fluid is an exudate with high protein, LDH, and amylase levels. The effusion may contribute to segmental atelectasis of the lower lobes, leading to ventilation/perfusion mismatch and hypoxia. Pulmonary edema may occur and is attributed to the effects of circulating activated proteolytic enzymes on the pulmonary capillaries, leading to transudation of fluid into the alveoli. The most dreaded pulmonary complication is the development of ARDS. This is most often seen 3–7 days after the onset of severe hemorrhagic pancreatitis and is thought to be related to hypotension ("shock lung").

H. Jaundice: Jaundice (hyperbilirubinemia) and bilirubinuria occur in about one-fifth of patients with acute pancreatitis. Several factors undoubtedly contribute. A gallstone underlying the pancreatitis may cause transient common bile duct obstruction. Partial obstruction of the common bile duct may also result from swelling of the head of the pancreas. In other cases, more protracted and severe jaundice may result from compression of the common bile duct by inflammatory **pseudocysts,** non-epithelium-lined cavities that contain plasma, blood, pus, and pancreatic juice (see below).

I. Hypocalcemia: In severe cases of acute pancreatitis, the serum calcium level may fall precipitously, occasionally to levels low enough to cause frank tetany, a state of neuromuscular irritability, clinically manifested by positive Chvostek and Trousseau signs. (Chvostek's sign is the finding of unilateral facial spasm elicited by a slight tap over the facial nerve; Trousseau's sign is the finding of unilateral carpal spasm elicited by compression of the upper arm by a tourniquet or blood pressure cuff.) Most often, this occurs between the third and tenth day of illness. Several factors contribute to the decline in serum calcium. Lipolysis of the peripancreatic, retroperitoneal, and mesenteric fat releases free fatty acids that combine with ionized calcium to form soaps. With the ensuing rapid fall in serum calcium, the parathyroid glands are unable to respond quickly and adequately enough to compensate for the hypocalcemia. If there is associated hypomagnesemia, the hypocalcemia may prove to be both severe and refractory, since normal serum magnesium concentrations are required for normal parathyroid function. Severe hypocalcemia is clinically manifested by tetany, stupor, seizures, and even coma.

J. Acidosis: Metabolic acidosis occurs in many patients with severe acute pancreatitis. The acidosis is primarily a lactic acidosis resulting from hypotension and shock. However, in patients with extensive pancreatic necrosis and hemorrhage, there may be destruction or dysfunction of the pancreatic islets, causing deficient insulin production and acute diabetic ketoacidosis. Hyperglycemia is seen in about 25% of patients and transient glycosuria in about 10%.

K. Hyperkalemia and Hypokalemia: The initial phase of acute pancreatitis, marked by acute inflammation and tissue necrosis, often causes release of large amounts of potassium into the circulation. This release, combined with hypovolemia and acidosis, often results in hyperkalemia. Later, following fluid repletion and correction of acidosis, the serum potassium may fall to dangerously low levels.

L. Hyperlipidemia: Acute attacks of pancreatitis, particularly when caused by alcohol abuse, are often accompanied by marked hyperlipidemia. The mechanism is thought to relate to decreased release and activity of the endothelial and plasma enzyme lipoprotein lipase.

M. Pancreatic Phlegmon, Pseudocysts, Ascites, or Abscess: Other complications of acute pancreatitis are listed in Table 15–2 and include pancreatic phlegmon, pseudocysts, abscess, or ascites.

A pancreatic **phlegmon** is a solid mass of inflamed pancreatic tissue, detectable by CT or MRI, that usually resolves spontaneously.

Pancreatic abscess occurs when there is bacterial infection of necrotic tissue in and around the inflamed pancreas. It is a life-threatening complication of acute pancreatitis, occurring in 3–7% of patients, usually 2–4 weeks after the onset of symptoms.

Inflammatory **pseudocysts** are so called because they are non-epithelium-lined cavities that contain plasma, blood, pus and pancreatic juice. They generally occur after recovery from the acute attack and are the result of both parenchymal destruction and ductal obstruction. Some acini continue to secrete pancreatic juice, but because the juice is unable to drain normally, it collects in an area of necrotic tissue, forming the ill-defined pseudocyst (Figure 15–5). As more juice is secreted, the cyst may grow progressively larger and may cause compression of nearby structures such as the portal vein (producing portal hypertension), common bile duct (producing jaundice or cholangitis), or gut (producing gastric outlet or bowel obstruction). Less commonly, the pseudocyst will erode through the bowel wall and rupture into the gut, causing gastrointestinal hemorrhage.

Table 15–3. Adverse prognostic signs in acute pancreatitis: Ranson's criteria of severity of acute pancreatitis.

Criteria present at diagnosis or admission	
Age over 55 years	
White blood cell count > 16,000/μL	
Blood glucose > 200 mg/dL	
Serum LDH > 350 IU/L	
AST (SGOT) > 250 IU/L	
Criteria developing during first 48 hours	
Hematocrit fall > 10%	
BUN rise > 5 mg/dL	
Serum calcium < 8 mg/dL	
Arterial Po_2 < 60 mm Hg	
Base deficit > 4 meq/L	
Estimated fluid sequestration > 6 L	
Mortality rates correlate with number of criteria present	
Number of Criteria	*Mortality Rate*
0–2	1%
3–4	16%
5–6	40%
7–8	100%

Modified from Way LW (editor): *Current Surgical Diagnosis & Treatment,* 10th ed. Appleton & Lange, 1994.

Pancreatic ascites occurs when a direct connection develops between a pancreatic pseudocyst and the peritoneal cavity. Given its origin, it is not surprising that the ascitic fluid resembles pancreatic juice, characteristically an exudate with high protein and extremely high amylase levels. Because pancreatic ascites often proves to be refractory to nonsurgical management, surgical treatment is usually required.

Course & Prognosis

The severity of acute pancreatitis can be estimated by various methods: clinical assessment, biochemical tests, Ranson's prognostic criteria, peritoneal lavage, and computed tomography. Table 15–3 lists Ranson's criteria, adverse prognostic signs that correlate with morbidity and mortality in acute pancreatitis.

Most patients with acute pancreatitis recover completely with supportive medical management. The pancreas then regenerates and returns to normal except for some mild residual scarring. Diabetes mellitus almost never occurs after a single attack of pancreatitis. However, in some cases, one or more pancreatic pseudocysts form in the weeks to months following recovery.

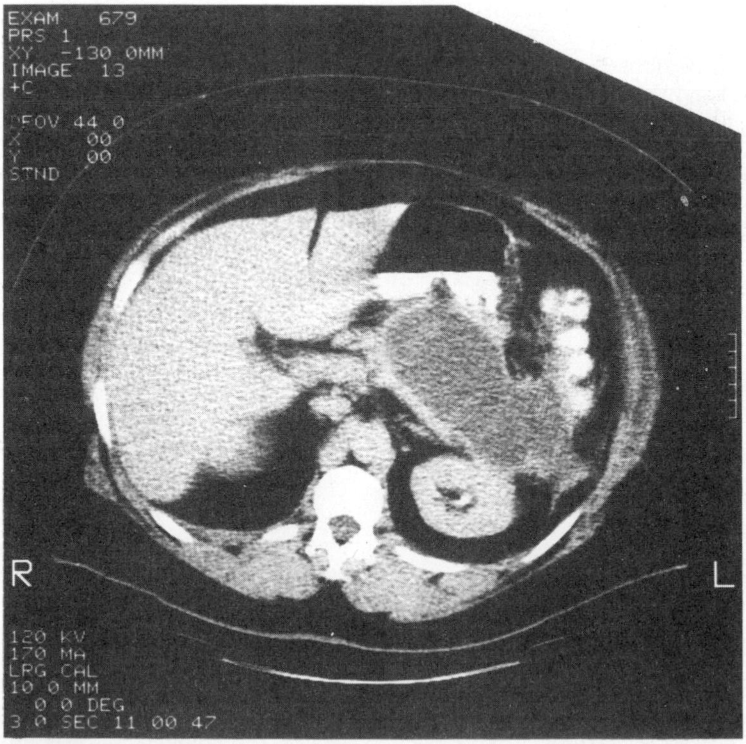

Figure 15–5. Pancreatic pseudocyst on CT. (Reproduced, with permission, from Way LW [editor]: *Current Surgical Diagnosis & Treatment,* 10th ed. Appleton & Lange, 1994.)

A minority of patients develop severe pancreatitis and may die as a consequence of severe hemorrhage, shock, DIC, ARDS, or septic pancreatic abscess.

5. What are the presenting signs and symptoms of acute pancreatitis?
6. What are the most common causes of acute pancreatitis?
7. Which drugs are commonly associated with pancreatitis?
8. What is the pathophysiologic mechanism by which hemorrhagic pancreatitis occurs?
9. What are the complications of severe pancreatitis?
10. What are the pathophysiologic mechanisms by which each of the complications of severe pancreatitis occurs?

CHRONIC PANCREATITIS

Clinical Presentations

Chronic pancreatitis is a recurrent, sometimes relapsing disorder, causing severe abdominal pain, exocrine and endocrine pancreatic insufficiency, severe duct abnormalities, and pancreatic calcifications. In chronic pancreatitis, there is chronic inflammation of the parenchyma, leading to progressive destruction of the acini, stenosis and dilation of the ductules, and fibrosis of the gland. Eventually, there is impairment of the gland's exocrine functions (see Pancreatic Insufficiency, below) and sometimes of its endocrine functions as well (Chapter 16).

Etiology

Chronic pancreatitis frequently results from recurrent attacks of acute pancreatitis. The two major causes of chronic pancreatitis are chronic alcoholism and biliary tract calculi (Table 15–4). Overall, chronic alcoholism accounts for about 40% of cases and gallstones for about 20%. Some cases are due to cystic fibrosis (mucoviscidosis) (see Chapter 2). In many cases, no cause can be identified. The incidence of chronic pancreatitis has been increasing recently for unknown reasons.

Table 15–4. Causes of chronic pancreatitis.

Alcohol abuse
Gallstones
Tropical (malnutrition)
Hyperparathyroidism
Hyperlipidemia
Trauma
Hereditary
Pancreas divisum

Table 15–5. Clinical manifestations of chronic pancreatitis.

Abdominal pain
Nausea
Vomiting
Weight loss
Malabsorption
Hyperglycemia
Jaundice

Pathology & Pathogenesis

As noted above, in acute pancreatitis, peripancreatic and intrapancreatic fat necrosis is the key pathologic finding. In resolving acute pancreatitis, there is organization of fat necrosis with early perilobular fibrosis or peripancreatic pseudocysts. However, if acute pancreatitis is severe, affecting the intrapancreatic fat deposits, it may evolve into chronic pancreatitis. In the early stage of chronic pancreatitis, pseudocysts are present in half (52%), and there is a focally accentuated fibrosis of the perilobular and, to a lesser degree, intralobular type. Marked fibrosis, ductal distortions, and the presence of intraductal calculi are the main features of advanced chronic pancreatitis. Pseudocysts are less frequent (36%).

Thus, pathologically, chronic pancreatitis is characterized by scarring and shrinkage of the pancreas due to fibrosis and atrophy of acini and by stenosis and dilation of ductules. Grossly, the process may be localized, most often involving the head and body of the gland, or it may be diffuse. The ductules and ducts are often filled with inspissated secretions or calculi. The gland may be rock hard as a result of diffuse sclerosis and calcification, and biopsy may be required to differentiate chronic pancreatitis from pancreatic carcinoma (see Carcinoma of the Pancreas, below). Microscopically, there is loss of acini, dilation of ductules, marked fibrosis, and a lymphocytic infiltrate. The islets of Langerhans are usually well preserved.

Satisfactory animal models for human chronic pancreatitis have not yet been produced. One theory of the pathogenesis of chronic pancreatitis postulates aberrant effects of mixed-function oxidases, with induction of cytochrome P450, and lipid peroxidation by free radicals of oxygen.

Clinical Manifestations

The clinical manifestations of chronic pancreatitis are listed in Table 15–5. The major symptom of chronic pancreatitis is severe abdominal pain that can be either constant or intermittent. The pain is thought to derive either from dilation of the duct system, causing ductal and parenchymal hypertension, or from inflammation of the parenchyma, causing pancreatic ischemia. Patients may have recurrent attacks of severe abdominal pain, vomiting, and elevation of serum amylase (chronic relapsing pancreatitis).

Impairment of exocrine function is manifested by pancreatic insufficiency (see below). There is a direct correlation between severity of histologic findings and exocrine pancreatic function as estimated by the CCK-secretin test. In this test, measurements are made of pancreatic juice volume, amylase output, and bicarbonate concentration in the basal state, then 30 minutes after intravenous injection of CCK, and then 60 minutes after intravenous administration of secretin.

Failure to secrete pancreatic juice results in malabsorption of fat (steatorrhea) and fat-soluble vitamins and in weight loss. Endocrine dysfunction produces hyperglycemia, glycosuria, and frank diabetes mellitus in approximately 30–40% of cases of longstanding chronic pancreatitis.

About 5% of patients develop severe sclerosing pancreatitis involving the head of the pancreas, leading to obstruction of the common bile and pancreatic ducts. Common bile duct obstruction results in profound and persistent jaundice, resembling that produced by pancreatic carcinoma.

The diagnosis of chronic pancreatitis is based mainly on symptoms and signs. The serum amylase is elevated in only a minority of cases. In the remaining cases, the amylase level is normal, probably because there is little residual pancreatic tissue. A finding of pancreatic calcifications on abdominal x-ray often suggests the diagnosis.

In patients followed for more than 10 years, the mortality rate is 22%, with pancreatitis-induced complications accounting for 13% of the deaths. The major causes of death are alcoholic liver disease, postoperative complications, and cancer. Pancreatic carcinoma occurs in 3% and extrapancreatic carcinoma in 4%.

Table 15–6. Causes of pancreatic insufficiency.

Primary
- A. Acquired decreased enzyme secretion
  - Chronic pancreatitis (alcohol abuse, trauma, hereditary, idiopathic)
  - Pancreatic, ampullary and duodenal neoplasms
  - Pancreatic resection
  - Severe protein-calorie malnutrition, hypoalbuminemia
- B. Congenital decreased enzyme secretion
  - Cystic fibrosis
  - Hemochromatosis
  - Shwachman's syndrome (pancreatic insufficiency with anemia, neutropenia, and bony abnormalities)
  - Enzyme deficiencies (trypsinogen, enterokinase, amylase, lipase, proteases, α_1-antiprotease deficiency)

Secondary
- A. Intraluminal enzyme destruction: Gastrinoma (Zollinger-Ellison syndrome)
- B. Decreased pancreatic stimulation: Small intestinal mucosal disease (nontropical sprue)
- C. Mistiming of enzyme secretion: Gastric surgery
  1. Subtotal gastrectomy with Billroth I anastomosis
  2. Subtotal gastrectomy with Billroth II anastomosis
  3. Truncal vagotomy and pyloroplasty

Table 15–7. Clinical manifestations of pancreatic insufficiency.[1]

Symptoms and Signs	Percentage
Weight loss	90%
Steatorrhea (stool fat > 6 g/d)	48%
Edema, ascites	12%
Weakness	7%
Hypoproteinemia	14%
Malabsorption of vitamin B_{12}	40%

[1]Modified from Evans WB, Wollaeger EE: Incidence and severity of nutritional deficiency states in chronic exocrine pancreatic insufficiency: Comparison with nontropical sprue. Am J Dig Dis 1966;11:594.

PANCREATIC INSUFFICIENCY

Clinical Presentations

Pancreatic exocrine insufficiency is the syndrome of maldigestion resulting from disorders interfering with effective pancreatic enzyme activity. Because pancreatic lipase is essential for fat digestion, its absence leads to steatorrhea, the occurrence of greasy, bulky, light-colored stools. On the other hand, while pancreatic amylase and trypsin are important for carbohydrate and protein digestion, other enzymes in gastric and intestinal juice can usually compensate for their loss. Thus, patients with pancreatic insufficiency seldom present with maldigestion of carbohydrate and protein (nitrogen loss).

Etiology

Pancreatic insufficiency usually results from chronic pancreatitis in adults or cystic fibrosis (mucoviscidosis) in children (Table 15–6). In some cases it is a consequence of pancreatic resection or carcinoma of the pancreas. Each of these conditions markedly reduces the amount of pancreatic enzymes secreted, often to less than 5% of normal.

Less commonly, pancreatic insufficiency results from disease states that cause hypersecretion of gastric acid. For example, excessive gastrin secretion from a gastrinoma (an islet cell neoplasm composed of G cells) leads to continuous hypersecretion of gastric acid and a very low pH of gastric juice. In affected patients, the excess gastric acid overwhelms the normal pancreatic bicarbonate production and results in an abnormally acidic pH in the duodenum. This acid pH, in turn, causes decreased activity of otherwise adequate amounts of pancreatic enzymes.

Pathology & Pathogenesis

Normally, the activities of the various pancreatic enzymes decrease during their passage from the duodenum to the terminal ileum. However, the degradation rates of individual enzymes vary, with lipase activity lost most rapidly and protease and amylase activity lost more slowly. Lipase activity is usually destroyed by proteolysis, mainly by the action of chymotrypsin. This mechanism persists in patients with pancreatic insufficiency, helping to explain why fat malabsorption develops earlier than protein or starch malabsorption.

Normal fat digestion begins in the duodenum, where pancreatic lipase hydrolyzes triglycerides into free fatty acids and monoglycerides and bile salts permit micellar solubilization of the fatty acids and monoglycerides.

Patients with destruction of the exocrine pancreas develop impaired digestion and absorption of fat. Clinically, fat malabsorption is manifested as steatorrhea. While the steatorrhea is mostly caused by the deficiency of pancreatic lipase, the absence of pancreatic bicarbonate secretion also contributes to its occurrence. Without bicarbonate, acidic chyme from the stomach inhibits the activity of pancreatic lipase and causes the precipitation of bile salts. Deficiency of bile salts in turn causes failure of micelle formation and interference with fat absorption.

Finally, chronic alcohol intake interferes with both of the major mechanisms regulating exocrine pancreatic secretion: the cholinergic and the CCK pathways.

Clinical Manifestations

The symptoms and signs (Table 15–7) exhibited by patients with pancreatic insufficiency vary to some extent with the underlying disease. For example, patients with chronic pancreatitis often have persistent symptoms of abdominal pain, anorexia, nausea, and vomiting. In severe cases of chronic pancreatitis, calcification of the gland and loss of islet cells leading to diabetes mellitus may ensue (see Chronic Pancreatitis, above). In addition, the clinical manifestations of malabsorption depend both on what is being malabsorbed and on how long the process has been occurring.

A. Steatorrhea: Patients with steatorrhea usually describe their stools as voluminous or bulky, foul-smelling, greasy, frothy, pale yellow, and floating. However, significant steatorrhea may occur without any of these characteristics. It can be documented by collecting all stools for 3 days and determining the average daily fecal fat excretion. An abnormal fat excretion is more than 7 g of fat per day.

B. Diarrhea: In patients with fat malabsorption, diarrhea may result from the cathartic action of hydroxylated fatty acids. These fatty acids inhibit the absorption of sodium and water by the colon. Less commonly, watery diarrhea, abdominal cramping, and bloating are due to carbohydrate malabsorption. Indeed, because salivary amylase production remains undisturbed and because pancreatic amylase production must be markedly reduced before intraluminal starch digestion is slowed, symptomatic carbohydrate malabsorption is uncommon in pancreatic insufficiency.

C. Hypocalcemia: Hypocalcemia, hypophosphatemia, tetany, osteomalacia, and osteoporosis can occur both from deficiency of the fat-soluble vitamin D and from the binding of dietary calcium to unabsorbed fatty acids, forming insoluble calcium-fat complexes (soaps) in the gut.

D. Nephrolithiasis: The formation of insoluble calcium soaps in the gut also prevents the normal binding of dietary oxalate to calcium. Dietary oxalate remains in solution and is absorbed from the colon, causing hyperoxaluria and predisposing to nephrolithiasis.

E. Vitamin B_{12} Deficiency: About 40% of patients with pancreatic insufficiency demonstrate malabsorption of vitamin B_{12} (cobalamin), though clinical manifestations of vitamin B_{12} deficiency (anemia, subacute combined degeneration of the spinal cord, and dementia) are rare. The malabsorption of vitamin B_{12} appears to result from reduced degradation by pancreatic proteases of the normal complexes of vitamin B_{12} and its binding protein (R protein), resulting in less free vitamin B_{12} to bind to intrinsic factor in the small intestine.

F. Weight Loss: Long-standing malabsorption leads to protein catabolism and consequent weight loss, muscle wasting, fatigue, and edema. At times weight loss occurs in patients with chronic pancreatitis because eating exacerbates their abdominal pain or because narcotics used to control pain cause anorexia. In patients who develop diabetes mellitus, weight loss may be due to glycosuria. Weight loss may also be due to patients' prolonged fasting during repeated hospitalizations.

11. How is chronic pancreatitis different from acute pancreatitis in terms of symptoms and signs?
12. What are the symptoms and signs of pancreatic insufficiency?

CARCINOMA OF THE PANCREAS

Epidemiology & Etiology

Pancreatic carcinoma is increasing in incidence, and the reason is obscure. In 1990, there were approximately 28,100 new cases of pancreatic cancer in the United States. The disease accounts for approximately 6% of cancer deaths and is the fourth leading cause of cancer death in the USA. Pancreatic cancer usually occurs after age 50 and increases in incidence with age. It is somewhat more frequent in men than in women. It is rarely curable; even with surgical resection, the 5-year survival rate is little more than 5%.

The cause is unknown. The disease is six times more common in diabetic than nondiabetic women (but not in diabetic men) and two and a half to five times more common in cigarette smokers. The role of dietary factors (decaffeinated coffee, high fat intake, and alcohol use) is much debated. There is an increased incidence of pancreatic cancer among patients with hereditary pancreatitis, particularly among those who develop pancreatic calcifications.

Pathology

Carcinomas occur more often in the head (70%) and body (20%) than in the tail (10%) of the pancreas. Virtually all (99%) pancreatic carcinomas originate in ductular cells and only a few (1%) in acinar cells.

Grossly, pancreatic cancer presents as an indurated, infiltrating tumor that obstructs the pancreatic duct and thus frequently causes inflammation of the distal gland. Carcinomas of the head of the pancreas tend to obstruct the common bile duct early in their course, leading to jaundice and—if the tumor is a large one—to widening of the duodenal C loop on contrast x-ray or imaging studies. Tumors of the body and tail tend to present later in their course and thus to be very large when found. Pancreatic cancer frequently causes marked fibrosis in adjacent areas (desmoplastic reaction).

Microscopically, almost all pancreatic cancers (90%) are adenocarcinomas; the remainder are adenosquamous carcinomas, anaplastic carcinomas, and acinar cell carcinomas. Pancreatic cancer tends to spread into surrounding tissues, invading neighboring organs along the perineural fascia, causing severe pain, and via the lymphatics and bloodstream, causing metastases in regional lymph nodes, liver, and other distant sites.

In evaluating patients who are suspected of having pancreatic cancer, ultrasound is very useful both in detecting tumors and in evaluating their extent. If ultrasound fails to provide the information being sought, CT is performed. For patients with an equivocal or inconclusive ultrasound or CT examination, endoscopic retrograde cannulation of the pancreatic duct (ERCP) is recommended. Percutaneous fine-needle aspiration (FNA) biopsy is used to confirm the diagnosis, particularly in patients with cancer of the body or tail of the pancreas, and to evaluate patients with suspected metastases. Angiography is often performed preoperatively to delineate the regional vascular anatomy and to look for major vascular invasion by tumor, a sign of unresectability.

Clinical Manifestations

The clinical manifestations of pancreatic cancer (Table 15–8) vary both with location and with histologic type of tumor.

Patients with carcinoma of the head of the pancreas usually present with painless, progressive jaundice due to common bile duct obstruction. Sometimes the obstruction caused by carcinoma in the head of the pancreas is signaled by the presence of both jaundice and a dilated gallbladder palpable in the right upper quadrant **(Courvoisier's law).** (Courvoisier's law states that palpable enlargement of the gallbladder in a patient with jaundice is caused by carcinoma of the head of the pancreas and not by gallstones in the common bile duct, because with gallstones the gallbladder is usually scarred from inflammation and does not become distended.)

Patients with carcinoma of the body or tail of the pancreas usually present with epigastric abdominal pain, profound weight loss, an abdominal mass, and anemia. These patients usually present at later stages and more often have distant metastases, particularly in the liver.

Adenocarcinomas of the pancreas are sometimes associated with superficial thrombophlebitis or disseminated intravascular coagulation, thought to be related to thromboplastins in the mucinous secretions of the adenocarcinoma. The uncommon acinar cell carcinomas sometimes secrete lipase into the circulation, causing fat necrosis in subcutaneous tissues (manifested as skin rashes) and bone marrow (manifested as lytic bone lesions) throughout the body.

A variety of tumor markers, such as carcinoembry-

Table 15–8. Clinical manifestations of pancreatic carcinoma.

	Percentage
Symptoms and Signs[1]	
Abdominal pain	73–74%
Anorexia	70%
Weight loss	60–74%
Jaundice[2]	65–72%
Diarrhea	27%
Weakness	21%
Palpable gallbladder	9%
Constipation	8%
Hematemesis or melena	7%
Vomiting	6%
Abdominal mass	1–38%
Migratory thrombophlebitis	$<1\%$
Abnormal laboratory tests[3]	
↑ Alkaline phosphatase	82%
↑ 5′-Nucleotidase	71%
↑ LDH	69%
↑ AST	64%
↑ Bilirubin	55%
↑ Amylase	17%
↑ α-Fetoprotein	6%
↑ Carcinoembryonic antigen (CEA)	57%
↓ Albumin	60%

[1]Modified from Anderson A, Bergdahl L: Carcinoma of the pancreas. Am Surg 1976;42:173; and from Hines LH, Burns RP: Ten years' experience treating pancreatic and periampullary cancer. Am Surg 1976;42:442.
[2]With carcinoma of the head of the pancreas.
[3]Modified from Fitzgerald PJ et al: The value of diagnostic aids in detecting pancreas cancer. Cancer 1978;41:868.

onic antigen (CEA), alpha-fetoprotein, pancreatic oncofetal antigen, and galactosyl transferase II, can be found in the serum of patients with pancreatic cancer. However, none of these tumor markers have sufficient specificity or predictive value to be useful in screening for the disease. Measurements of serum amylase or lipase are not helpful in diagnosis.

13. What are the risk factors for pancreatic cancer?
14. What are common symptoms and signs of pancreatic cancer?
15. How can you make the diagnosis of pancreatic cancer in a patient with suggestive symptoms and signs?

REFERENCES

General

Chandrasoma P, Taylor CR: *Concise Pathology*, 2nd ed. Appleton & Lange, 1995.

Chey WY: Regulation of pancreatic exocrine secretion. Int J Pancreatol 1991;9:7.

Thoeni RF, Blankenberg F: Pancreatic imaging: computed tomography and magnetic resonance imaging. Radiol Clin North Am 1993;31:1085.

Acute Pancreatitis

Agarwal N, Pitchumoni CS: Assessment of severity in acute pancreatitis. Am J Gastroenterol 1991;86:1385.

Bilchik AJ et al: Experimental models of acute pancreatitis. J Surg Res 1990;48:639.

Steer ML: How and where does acute pancreatitis begin? Arch Surg 1992;127:1350.

Steinberg W, Tenner S: Acute pancreatitis. (Medical Progress.) N Engl J Med 1994;330:1198.

Chronic Pancreatitis

Hayakawa T et al: Relationship between pancreatic exocrine function and histological changes in chronic pancreatitis. Am J Gastroenterol 1992;87:1170.

Karanjia ND, Reber HA: The cause and management of the pain of chronic pancreatitis. Gastroenterol Clin North Am 1990;19:895.

Lankisch PG et al: Natural course in chronic pancreatitis: Pain, exocrine and endocrine pancreatic insufficiency and prognosis of the disease. Digestion 1993;54:148.

Pancreatic Insufficiency

Durie PR, Forstner GG: Pathophysiology of the exocrine pancreas in cystic fibrosis. J R Soc Med 1989;82(Suppl 16):2.

Goldberg DM, Durie PR: Biochemical tests in the diagnosis of chronic pancreatitis and in the evaluation of pancreatic insufficiency. Clin Biochem 1993;26:253.

Layer P, Groger G: Fate of pancreatic enzymes in the human intestinal lumen in health and pancreatic insufficiency. Digestion 1993;54(Suppl):10.

Pancreatic Carcinoma

Alvarez C et al: Cost-benefit analysis of the work-up for pancreatic cancer. Am J Surg 1993;165:53.

Brambs HJ, Claussen CD: Pancreatic and ampullary carcinoma: Ultrasound, computed tomography, magnetic resonance imaging and angiography. Endoscopy 1993;25:58.

Warshaw AL, Fernandez-del Castillo C: Pancreatic carcinoma. N Engl J Med 1992;326:455.

Disorders of the Endocrine Pancreas

16

Janet L. Funk, MD, & Kenneth R. Feingold, MD

Insulin and **glucagon,** the two key hormones that orchestrate fuel storage and utilization, are produced by the islet cells in the pancreas. **Islet cells** are distributed in clusters throughout the exocrine pancreas. Taken all together, they comprise the endocrine pancreas. **Diabetes mellitus,** a heterogeneous disorder that affects 4% of the population and almost 20% of individuals between the ages of 65 and 74, is the most common disease associated with disordered secretion of hormones of the endocrine pancreas. Pancreatic tumors that secrete excessive amounts of specific islet cell hormones are far less common, but their clinical presentations underscore the important regulatory roles of each of the hormones secreted by the endocrine pancreas.

NORMAL STRUCTURE & FUNCTION OF THE PANCREATIC ISLETS

ANATOMY & HISTOLOGY

The endocrine pancreas is composed of nests of cells called the **islets of Langerhans** which are distributed throughout the exocrine pancreas. There are over 1 million islets in the human pancreas, many of which contain several hundred cells. The endocrine pancreas has great reserve capacity; over 70% of the cells must be lost before dysfunction occurs. There are four cell types within the islets, each of which produces a different major secretory product (Table 16–1). The insulin-secreting **B cells** (β cells) are located in the central portion of the islets and are the predominant cell type (80% of cells) (Figure 16–1). The glucagon-secreting **A cells** (20% of the islet cells) are located mainly in the periphery. The **D cells,** which secrete somatostatin, are located between these two cell types and are few in number. The pancreatic polypeptide-secreting **F cells** are located mainly in the islets in the posterior lobe of the head of the pancreas, a region embryonically derived from the ventral rather than the dorsal bud and which therefore receives a different blood supply.

The islets are much more highly vascularized than the exocrine pancreatic tissues. Blood flow is thought to proceed from the center of the islet to the periphery, thereby allowing insulin produced by the central B cells to inhibit glucagon release by the peripheral A cells. Blood from the islets then drains into the hepatic portal vein. Thus, the islet cell secretory products pass directly into the liver, a major site of action of glucagon and insulin, before proceeding into the systemic circulation.

The islets are also abundantly innervated. Both parasympathetic and sympathetic axons enter the islets and either directly contact cells or terminate in the interstitial space between the cells. Neural regulation of islet cell hormone release, both directly through the sympathetic fibers and indirectly through stimulation of catecholamine release by the adrenal medulla, plays a key role in glucose homeostasis during stress.

1. What percentage of islets must be lost before endocrine pancreatic dysfunction becomes manifest?
2. Describe the histologic and vascular organization of an islet of Langerhans.

PHYSIOLOGY

1. INSULIN

Synthesis & Metabolism

Insulin is a protein composed of two peptide chains (A and B chains) that are connected by two disulfide bonds (Figure 16–2). The precursor of insulin, **preproinsulin** (MW 11,500), is synthesized in the endoplasmic reticulum of B cells, where it is promptly cleaved by microsomal enzymes to form proinsulin (MW 9000). **Proinsulin,** which consists of the A and B chains joined by a 31-amino-acid **C peptide,** is transported to the Golgi apparatus, where it is packaged into secretory vesicles. While in the

Table 16–1. Cell types in pancreatic islets of Langerhans.[1]

Cell Types	Secretory Products
A cell (α)	Glucagon, proglucagon, glucagon-like peptides (GLP-1 and GLP-2)
B cell (β)	Insulin, C peptide, proinsulin, amylin, γ-aminobutyric acid (GABA)
D cell (δ)	Somatostatin
F cell (PP cell)	Pancreatic polypeptide

[1] Modified and reproduced, with permission, from Greenspan FS, Baxter JD: *Basic & Clinical Endocrinology,* 4th ed. Appleton & Lange, 1994.

secretory vesicle, proinsulin is cleaved at two sites to form insulin (51 amino acids; MW 5808) and the biologically inactive C peptide fragment (Figure 16–2). Secretion of insulin is therefore accompanied by an equimolar secretion of C peptide and also by small amounts of proinsulin that escape cleavage.

Human insulin differs by only one or three amino acids from pork and beef insulin, respectively. These preparations of the hormone were used to treat diabetes prior to the availability of recombinant human insulin. Insulin has a circulatory half-life of 3–5 minutes and is catabolized in both the liver and the kidney. The liver catabolizes approximately 50% of insulin on its first pass through the liver after it is secreted from the pancreas into the portal vein. In contrast, both C peptide and proinsulin are catabolized only by the kidney and therefore have half-lives three to four times longer than that of insulin itself.

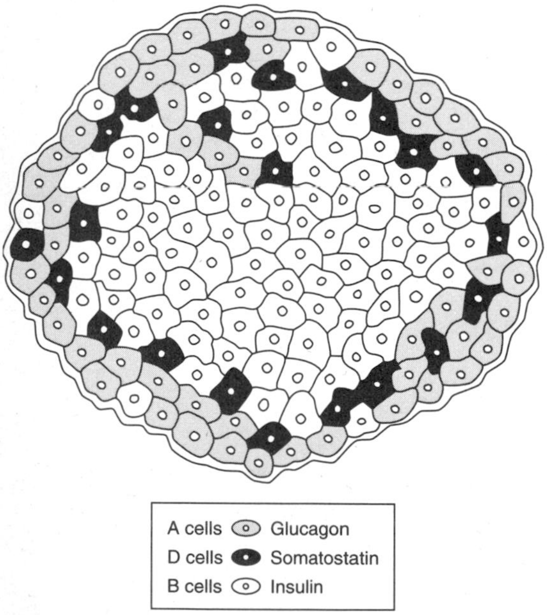

Figure 16–1. Schematic representation of a normal rat islet showing the topographical relationships of the major cell types. (Reproduced, with permission, from Orci L, Unger RH: Functional subdivision of islets of Langerhans and possible role of D cells. Lancet 1975;2:1243.)

Regulation of Secretion

Glucose is the primary physiologic stimulant of insulin release (Figure 16–3). Glucose enters B cells via a **glucose transporter (GLUT 2)** that has a low affinity for glucose, thereby allowing a graded response to glucose uptake. Once in the cell, it is thought that the metabolism of glucose—rather than glucose itself—stimulates insulin secretion. **Glucokinase,** an enzyme with low affinity for glucose whose activity is regulated by glucose, controls the first step in glucose metabolism—phosphorylation of glucose to form glucose 6-phosphate. It is thought that this enzyme may function as the **"glucose sensor"** in B cells. Metabolic coupling factors produced via glucose metabolism, such as ATP, then inhibit potassium efflux from the B cell. This depolarizes the cell and allows calcium to enter. Insulin-containing secretory vesicles are thought to be attached to microtubules that contract in response to calcium, thereby causing the vesicles to be secreted.

Although glucose is the most potent stimulator of insulin release, other factors such as amino acids ingested with a meal or vagal stimulation can cause insulin release (Table 16–2). Glucose-induced insulin secretion can also be enhanced by several enteric hormones. Insulin secretion is inhibited by catecholamines and by somatostatin.

Mechanism of Action

Insulin exerts its effects by binding to **insulin receptors** present on the surfaces of target cells (Figure 16–4). Insulin receptors are present in liver, muscle, and fat—the classic insulin-sensitive tissues responsible for fuel homeostasis. In addition, insulin can mediate other effects in nonclassic target tissues, such as the ovary, via interaction with insulin receptors or by cross-reactivity with insulin-like growth factor-1 (IGF-1) receptors. Binding of insulin to its receptor causes activation of a tyrosine kinase region of the receptor and autophosphorylation of the receptor. The exact sequence of events following phosphorylation of the receptor remains unknown. However, it is generally thought that binding of insulin to its receptor initiates a phosphorylation cascade within the cell—either directly via the tyrosine kinase or through the activation of other intermediates—that ultimately mediates changes in the proteins responsible for the biologic effects of insulin.

Effects

Insulin plays a major role in fuel homeostasis (Table 16–3). Insulin mediates these changes in fuel

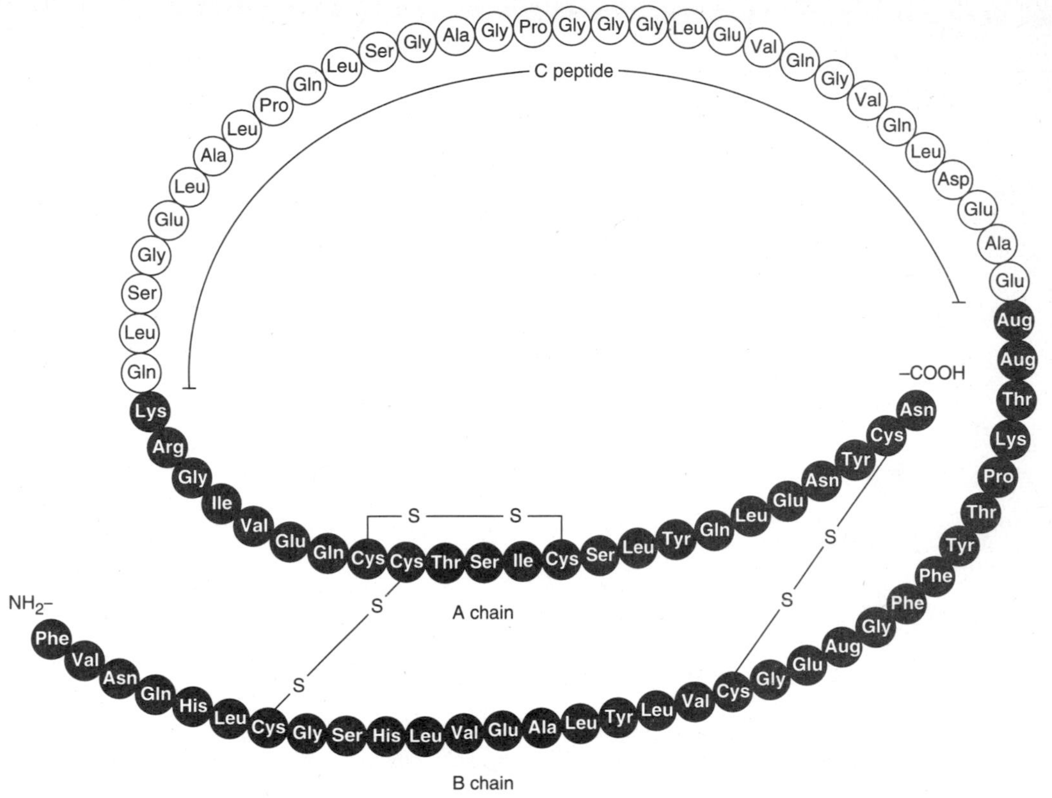

Figure 16–2. Amino acid sequence and covalent structure of human proinsulin. (Reproduced, with permission, from Kohler PO, Jordan RM [editors]: *Clinical Endocrinology.* Wiley, 1986.)

metabolism through its effects on three main tissues: liver, muscle, and fat. In these tissues, insulin promotes fuel storage (anabolism) and prevents the breakdown and release of fuel that has already been stored (catabolism). The complete action of insulin or the overproduction of insulin is incompatible with life.

In the liver, insulin promotes fuel storage by stimulation of glycogen synthesis and storage. Insulin inhibits hepatic glucose output by inhibiting gluconeogenesis (glucose synthesis) and glycogenolysis (glycogen breakdown). By also stimulating glycolysis (metabolism of glucose to pyruvate), insulin promotes the formation of precursors for fatty acid synthesis. Moreover, insulin stimulates lipogenesis, leading to the increased synthesis of very low density lipoproteins (VLDL), particles that deliver triglycerides to fat tissue for storage. Insulin also inhibits fatty acid oxidation and the production of ketone bodies (ketogenesis), an alternative fuel produced only in the liver that can be used by the brain when glucose is not available.

While hepatic uptake of glucose is not regulated by insulin, insulin does stimulate glucose uptake both in muscle and in fat by causing the rapid translocation of an insulin-sensitive glucose transporter (GLUT 4) to the surface of these cells. Uptake of glucose by muscle accounts for the vast majority (85%) of insulin-stimulated glucose disposal. In muscle, insulin promotes the storage of glucose by stimulating glycogen synthesis and inhibiting glycogen catabolism. Insulin also stimulates protein synthesis in muscle.

Insulin stimulates fat storage by stimulating lipoprotein lipase, the enzyme that hydrolyses the triglycerides carried in VLDL and other triglyceride-rich lipoproteins to fatty acids, which can then be taken up by fat cells. Increased glucose uptake caused by up-regulation of the GLUT 4 transporter also aids in fat storage since this increases the levels of α-glycerol phosphate, an intermediate in the esterification of free fatty acids, which are then stored as triglycerides. Insulin also inhibits lipolysis, preventing the release of fatty acids, a potential substrate for hepatic ketone body synthesis, from fat cells. Insulin exerts this effect by decreasing the activity of hormone-sensitive lipase, the enzyme that hydrolyzes stored triglycerides to releasable fatty acids. Together, these changes result in increased fat storage.

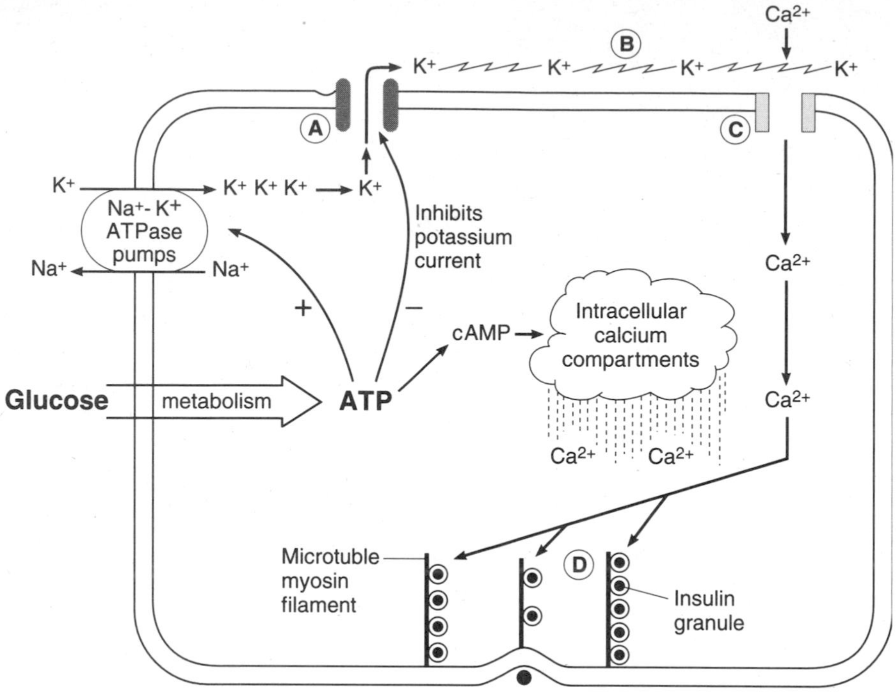

Figure 16–3. Schematic diagram of glucose-stimulated insulin release from B cell. Potassium (K^+) efflux (**A**) polarizes the B cell membrane and prevents calcium entry by closing a voltage-dependent calcium channel (**B**). When glucose is taken up by B cells, the metabolism of glucose is thought to inhibit potassium efflux, thus depolarizing the cell and allowing calcium (Ca^{2+}) entry (**C**). Calcium stimulates the secretion of insulin-containing vesicles (**D**). (Reproduced, with permission, from Greenspan FS, Baxter JD: Basic and Clinical Endocrinology, 4th ed. Appleton & Lange, 1994.)

3. How does human insulin differ from pork and beef insulin?
4. What is the half-life of insulin? How is it catabolized? What percentage is extracted on first pass through the liver?
5. How do the half-lives of C peptide and proinsulin compare with that of insulin?
6. What is the primary stimulant of insulin secretion? What are some other stimulants of insulin secretion?
7. What characteristic of the B cell glucose transporter (GLUT 2) allows a graded response to glucose?
8. What is the probable "glucose sensor" in the B cell?
9. What are the major inhibitors of insulin secretion?
10. What are the current thoughts on the mechanisms of insulin action?
11. Which tissues are insulin-dependent for glucose uptake?
12. What are three ways in which insulin stimulates fat storage?

2. GLUCAGON

Synthesis & Metabolism

Glucagon, a 29-amino-acid-peptide, is synthesized in the A cells of the pancreatic islets. It is derived from a much larger precursor protein, **preproglucagon.** This precursor molecule is proteolytically processed to form several biologically active peptides, similar to the way that the processing of proopiomelanocortin leads to the formation of ACTH, endorphins, and other active peptides (Figure 16–5). Preproglucagon and a smaller precursor protein, **proglucagon,** are synthesized in the pancreas, gastrointestinal tract, and brain. However, only the A cells of the pancreas have been shown to be cabable of forming glucagon from the cleavage of glucagon-like precursor molecules. Other biologically active peptides derived from preproglucagon, such as **glucagon-like peptides (GLP-1 and GLP-2)** and **glucagon-like immunoreactivity** peptides **(GLI-1 and GLI-2),** are primarily synthesized by the gastrointestinal tract in response to a meal. Of these peptides, a metabolite of GLP-1 is a more potent stimulator of insulin secretion than is glucagon, and GLI-2

Table 16–2. Regulation of islet cell hormone release.

	B Cell Insulin Release	D Cell Somatostatin Release	A Cell Glucagon Release
Nutrients			
Glucose	↑	↑	↓
Amino acids	↑	↑	↑
Fatty acids	—	—	↓
Ketones	—	—	↓
Hormones			
Enteric hormones	↑	↑	↑
Insulin	↓	↓?	↓
GABA	—	—	↓
Somatostatin	↓	↓	↓
Glucagon	↑	↑	—
Cortisol	—	—	↑
Catecholamines	↓ (α-adrenergic)	—	↑ (β-adrenergic)
Neural			
Vagal	↑	—	↑
Beta-adrenergic	↑	—	↑
Alpha-adrenergic	↓	—	↓

Key: ↑ = increased; ↓ = decreased; — = no effect or no known effect

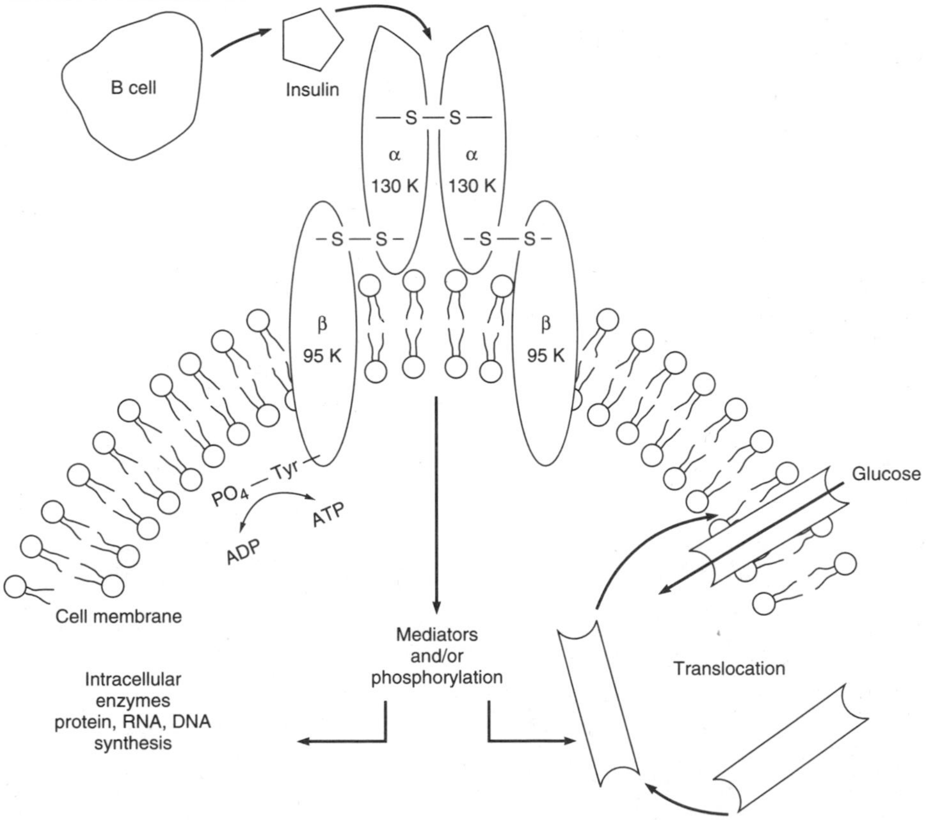

Figure 16–4. Model of insulin receptor. The insulin receptor is composed of two α and two β subunits linked by disulfide bonds. Binding of insulin to the extracellular α subunits activates a tyrosine kinase present in the cytoplasmic domain of the β subunit. The activated kinase autophosphorylates specific tyrosine residues in the β subunit. Kinase activation is a critical initial step in the poorly defined cascade of events that leads to the biologic effects of insulin, such as the translocation of glucose transporters to the cell surface. (Reproduced, with permission, from Rifkin H, Porte D Jr: In: *Ellenberg and Rifkin's Diabetes Mellitus: Theory and Practice,* 4th ed. Elsevier, 1990.)

Table 16–3. Hormonal regulation of fuel homeostasis.

	Insulin	Somatostatin	Glucagon	Catecholamines	Cortisol	Growth Hormone
PANCREAS						
Secretion of—						
Insulin (B cell)	↓	↓	↑	↓		
Glucagon (A cell)	↓	↓		↑	↑	↑
Somatostatin (D cell)	(↓?)	↓	↑			
LIVER						
Fuel storage						
Glycogenesis	↑		↓			
Lipid synthesis	↑		↓			
Fuel breakdown						
Glycogenolysis	↓		↑	↑		↑
Gluconeogenesis	↓		↑	↑	↑	↑
Fatty acid oxidation or ketogenesis	↓		↑			
MUSCLE						
Fuel storage						
Glucose uptake or glycogenesis	↑			↓	↓	↓
Fuel breakdown						
Protein catabolism	↓				↑	
ADIPOSE TISSUE						
Fuel storage						
Lipoprotein lipolysis	↑					
Fatty acid esterification	↑					
Fuel breakdown						
Lipolysis of stored fat	↓			↑	↑	↑

Key: ↑ = increased, ↓ = decreased

is capable of binding to the glucagon receptor, though it has only 10% of the potency of glucagon. The physiologic roles of these nonglucagon peptides are not well understood.

The circulatory half-life of glucagon is 3–6 minutes. Like insulin, glucagon is metabolized in the liver and the kidney. However, the liver accounts for only 25% of glucagon clearance.

Regulation of Secretion

In contrast to the stimulation of insulin secretion by glucose, glucagon secretion is inhibited by glu-

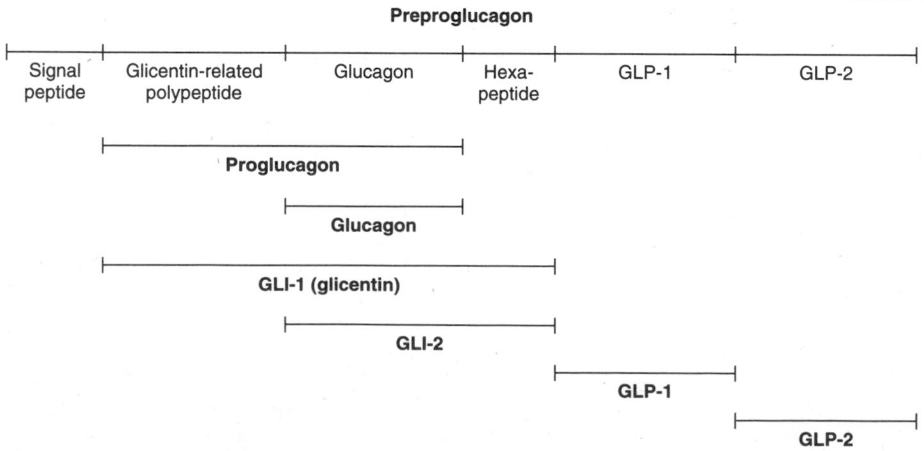

Figure 16–5. Preproglucagon peptide products.

cose (Table 16–2). It is not known whether glucose has a direct inhibitory effect on the A cell or whether its effect is mediated by the stimulation of insulin and somatostatin by B and D cells. Another B cell secretory product, **γ-aminobutyric acid (GABA)** is also thought to inhibit glucagon release. Like insulin, glucagon secretion is stimulated by amino acids, an important regulatory feature in the metabolism of protein meals. In contrast, fatty acids and ketones inhibit glucagon secretion. Counterregulatory hormones such as catecholamines (via a predominating beta-adrenergic effect) and cortisol stimulate glucagon release.

Mechanism of Action

The liver is the major target organ for glucagon action. Glucagon binds to a glucagon receptor present on the cell surface of hepatocytes. Binding of glucagon promotes interaction of the receptor with a stimulatory G protein, which in turn activates adenylyl cyclase. cAMP, generated by adenylyl cyclase, activates protein kinase A, which then phosphorylates enzymes responsible for the biologic activity of glucagon in the liver. There is also some evidence that the glucagon receptor may act via an adenylyl cyclase-independent mechanism by stimulation of phospholipase C.

Effects

Unlike insulin, which regulates fuel homeostasis through its effects on the liver, muscle, and fat, glucagon only affects metabolism by its action in the liver (Table 16–3). Glucagon is known as a **counterregulatory hormone**—one that counters the effects of insulin by acting in a catabolic fashion to maintain serum glucose levels. Glucagon maintains serum glucose levels by stimulating hepatic glucose output. This occurs by stimulating both the breakdown of hepatic glycogen stores (glycogenolysis) and hepatic glucose synthesis (gluconeogenesis). Glucagon also stimulates fatty acid oxidation and ketogenesis, thus providing an alternative fuel (ketone bodies) that can be used by the brain when glucose is not available. Lastly, glucagon stimulates hepatic uptake of amino acids which are then used to fuel gluconeogenesis.

3. SOMATOSTATIN

Synthesis, Metabolism, & Regulation of Secretion

Like glucagon, **somatostatin** is formed by the proteolytic cleavage of a preprohormone that is synthesized in the pancreas, the gastrointestinal tract, and the brain as well as in other tissues. Unlike glucagon, however, all of these tissues have the ability to cleave the preprohormone and prohormone precursors to form somatostatin, a 14-amino-acid peptide. In fact, somatostatin was initially discovered in the hypothalamus as the factor responsible for the inhibition of growth hormone release. Only later was it appreciated that D cells of the pancreas also secrete somatostatin. Unlike most prohormones, **prosomatostatin,** a 28-amino-acid hormone that is present in significant amounts in the gastrointestinal tract, is more potent than somatostatin. **Octreotide,** a synthetic 8-amino-acid analogue of somatostatin that is used clinically, is also more potent than somatostatin. The half-life of somatostatin (< 3 minutes) is shorter than that of insulin or glucagon.

The same secretagogues that stimulate insulin secretion also stimulate somatostatin (Table 16–2). These include glucose, amino acids, enteric hormones, and glucagon.

Mechanism of Action & Effects

Somatostatin release by both the gastrointestinal tract and the pancreas contributes to circulating levels of this hormone (Table 16–3). However, it is thought that the biologic effects of somatostatin may be due to its paracrine actions at both of these sites of production. In the gastrointestinal tract, somatostatin retards the absorption of nutrients through multiple mechanisms, including the inhibition of gut motility, the inhibition of several enteric peptides, and the inhibition of pancreatic exocrine function. In the endocrine pancreas, somatostatin is thought to act via paracrine effects on the other islet cells, inhibiting the release of insulin from B cells and glucagon from A cells. In addition, somatostatin acts in an autocrine fashion to inhibit its own release from D cells.

4. PANCREATIC POLYPEPTIDE

Little is known about the biosynthesis and physiologic function of **pancreatic peptide (PP).** This 36-amino-acid peptide is produced by the F cells in the islets of the posterior lobe of the head of the pancreas. PP is released in response to a mixed meal, an effect that appears to be mediated by protein and vagal stimulation.

13. What are some important stimuli and inhibitors of glucagon secretion?
14. What is the major target organ for glucagon? What are the mechanisms of glucagon action?
15. What metabolic pathways are sensitive to glucagon, and how are they affected?
16. What hormone antagonizes glucagon's effect on metabolic pathways?
17. Where else in the body besides the islets of Langerhans is glucagon made?
18. What is the role of somatostatin in the islets of Langerhans?

5. HORMONAL CONTROL OF CARBOHYDRATE METABOLISM

Carbohydrate metabolism is controlled by the relative amounts of insulin and glucagon that are produced by the endocrine pancreas (Table 16–3; Figure 16–6). When plasma glucose levels are high, plasma glucagon levels are suppressed and the actions of insulin predominate. Fuel storage is promoted by insulin stimulation of glycogen storage in the liver; glucose uptake, glycogen synthesis, and protein synthesis by muscle; and fat storage by adipose tissue. Insulin inhibits the mobilization of substrates from peripheral tissues and opposes any effects of glucagon on the stimulation of hepatic glucose output.

In contrast, when glucose levels are low, plasma insulin levels are suppressed and the effects of glucagon predominate in the liver (ie, increased hepatic glucose output and ketone body formation). In the absence of insulin, muscle glucose uptake is markedly decreased; muscle protein is catabolized; and fat is mobilized from adipose tissue. Therefore, with insulinopenia, glucose loads cannot be cleared, and substrates for hepatic gluconeogenesis (amino acids, glycerol) and ketogenesis (fatty acids)—processes that are stimulated by glucagon—are increased.

Fasting State

After an overnight fast, blood glucose is maintained by the liver, which produces glucose at the same rate at which it is utilized by resting tissues (Table 16–4). Glucose uptake and utilization occur predominantly in tissues that do not require insulin for glucose uptake, such as the brain. Hepatic glucose output is stimulated by glucagon and is primarily due to glycogenolysis. The low levels of insulin that are present (basal secretion of 0.25–1.0 unit/h) allow the release of fatty acids from fat to provide fuel for muscles (fatty acid oxidation) and substrate for hepatic ketogenesis. However, these levels of insulin are sufficient to prevent excessive lipolysis, ketogenesis, and gluconeogenesis, thus preventing hyperglycemia and ketoacidosis.

With prolonged fasting (> 24–60 hours), liver glycogen stores are depleted. Glucagon levels rise slightly, and insulin levels decline further. Gluconeogenesis becomes the predominant source of hepatic glucose production, utilizing substrates such as amino acids that are mobilized from the periphery at a greater rate. With starvation, a switch occurs from gluconeogenesis to the production of ketones, an alternative fuel source for the brain. In this manner, survival is prolonged as muscle protein is conserved in favor of increased mobilization of fatty acids from adipose tissue, a process made possible by insulinopenia. The liver then converts fatty acids to ketone bodies, a process that is stimulated by glucagon.

Table 16–4. Insulin : glucagon (I : G) molar ratios in blood in various conditions.[1]

Condition	Hepatic Glucose Storage (S) or Production (P)[2]	I : G
Glucose availability		
Large carbohydrate meal	++++ (S)	70
IV glucose	++ (S)	25
Small meal	+ (S)	7
Glucose need		
Overnight fast	+ (P)	2.3
Low-carbohydrate diet	++ (P)	1.8
Starvation	++++ (P)	0.4

[1] Courtesy of RH Unger. Reproduced, with permission, from Ganong WF: *Review of Medical Physiology,* 16th ed. Appleton & Lange, 1993.

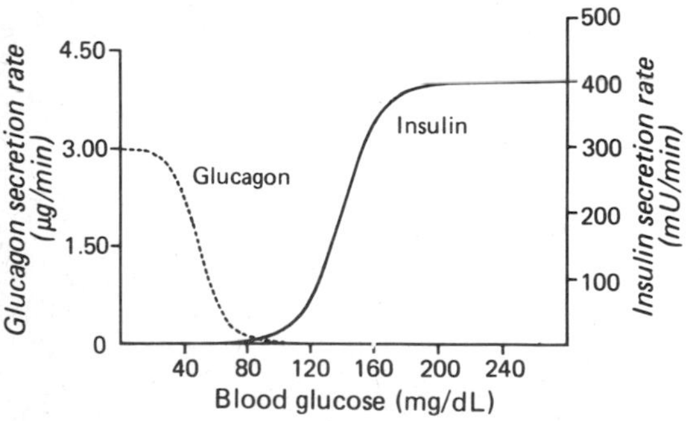

Figure 16–6. Mean rates of insulin and glucagon delivery from an artificial pancreas at various blood glucose levels. The device was programmed to establish and maintain normal blood glucose in insulin-requiring diabetic humans, and the values for hormone output approximate the output of the normal human pancreas. The shape of the insulin curve also resembles the insulin response of incubated B cells to graded concentrations of glucose. (Reproduced, with permission, from Mariles EB et al: Normalization of glycemia in diabetics during meals with insulin and glucagon delivery by the artificial pancreas. Diabetes 1977; 26:663.)

Fed State

With ingestion of a carbohydrate load, insulin secretion is stimulated and glucagon is suppressed (Table 16–4). Hepatic glucose production and ketogenesis are suppressed by the high ratio of insulin to glucagon. Insulin stimulates hepatic glycogen storage. Insulin-mediated glucose uptake, which occurs primarily in muscle, is also stimulated, as is muscle glycogen synthesis. Fat storage occurs in adipose tissue.

With ingestion of a protein meal, both insulin and glucagon are stimulated. In this way, insulin stimulates amino acid uptake and protein formation by muscle. However, stimulation of hepatic glucose output by glucagon counterbalances the tendency of insulin to cause hypoglycemia.

Conditions of Stress

During severe stress, when fuel delivery to the brain is in jeopardy, **counterregulatory hormones**—in addition to glucagon—act synergistically to maintain blood glucose levels by maximizing hepatic output of glucose and peripheral mobilization of substrates and by minimizing fuel storage (Table 16–3). **Glucagon** and **epinephrine** act within minutes to elevate blood glucose, while the counterregulatory effects of **cortisol** and **growth hormone** are not seen for several hours. Epinephrine, cortisol, and growth hormone all stimulate glucagon release while epinephrine inhibits insulin, thus maximally increasing the glucagon:insulin ratio. In addition, these three hormones act directly on the liver to increase hepatic glucose production and peripherally to stimulate lipolysis and inhibit insulin-sensitive glucose uptake. During severe stress, hyperglycemia may actually result from the combined effects of counterregulatory hormones.

Similar but less marked effects occur in response to exercise when glucagon, catecholamines, and to a lesser extent cortisol help supply exercising muscle with glucose and fatty acids by increasing hepatic glucose output and lipolysis of fat stores, effects that are made possible by a lowering of insulin levels. Low insulin levels also allow muscles to utilize glycogen stores for energy.

19. In insulinopenic states, why are glucose loads not cleared, and why are substrates for hepatic gluconeogenesis and ketogenesis increased?
20. What is the effect of a protein meal on insulin versus glucagon secretion?
21. What is the difference in time course of action of the various counterregulatory hormones?

PATHOPHYSIOLOGY OF SELECTED ENDOCRINE PANCREATIC DISORDERS

DIABETES MELLITUS

Clinical Presentation

Diabetes mellitus is a heterogeneous disorder defined by the presence of **hyperglycemia.** Diagnostic criteria for diabetes include the presence of either a fasting glucose repeatedly greater than 140 mg/dL or a sustained (up to 2 hours) elevation in glucose (> 200 mg/dL) following an oral dose of 75 g of glucose (oral glucose tolerance test).

Hyperglycemia in all cases is due to a functional deficiency of insulin action. Deficient insulin action can be due to a decrease in insulin secretion by the B cell of the pancreas, a decreased response to insulin by target tissues **(insulin resistance),** or an increase in the counterregulatory hormones that oppose the effects of insulin. The relative contributions of each of these three factors not only form the basis of classification of this disorder into subtypes but also help to explain the characteristic clinical presentations of each subtype (Table 16–5).

Secondary diabetes, accounting for less than 5% of cases, is due to processes that inhibit insulin secretion by destroying the pancreas (eg, pancreatitis), specific inhibition of insulin secretion (eg, drug-induced diabetes), or increases in counterregulatory hormones (eg, Cushing's syndrome). Clinical presentations in these cases depend on the exact nature of the process and are not discussed here.

Table 16–5. Classification of diabetes mellitus.[1]

Primary diabetes mellitus (95%)
- Type I: Insulin-dependent diabetes mellitus (IDDM)
- Type II: Non-insulin-dependent diabetes mellitus (NIDDM)
- Gestational diabetes mellitus[2]

Secondary diabetes mellitus (5%)
- Destructive pancreatic disease
  - Chronic pancreatitis
  - Hemochromatosis (bronze diabetes)
  - Total pancreatectomy
- Endocrine diseases (high levels of insulin-antagonistic hormones)
  - Acromegaly (growth hormone)
  - Cushing's syndrome (cortisol)
  - Hyperthyroidism (thyroxine)
  - Pheochromocytoma (catecholamines)
  - Glucagonoma (glucagon)
- Drug-induced diabetes (including diuretics such as thiazides, furosemide; propranolol; antidepressants; phenothiazines)
- Stress diabetes[2]
- Miscellaneous genetic syndromes (increased incidence of diabetes)
  - Down's syndrome (trisomy 21; mongolism)
  - Turner's syndrome (45,XO)
  - Friedreich's ataxia
  - Klinefelter's syndrome (47,XXY)
  - Glycogen storage disease type I
  - Laurence-Moon-Biedl syndrome[3]
  - Refsum's syndrome[4]

[1] Modified and reproduced, with permission, from Chandrasoma P, Taylor CR: *Concise Pathology,* 2nd ed. Appleton & Lange, 1994.
[2] Gestational diabetes and stress diabetes probably represent patients with impaired glucose tolerance or with a genetic predisposition to diabetes who are decompensated by the physiologic changes of pregnancy or stress. The "diabetes" is often reversible, but such patients show a high incidence of diabetes in succeeding years.
[3] Retinitis pigmentosa, obesity, mental deficiency, skull defects with or without diabetes.
[4] Retinitis pigmentosa, polyneuropathy with or without diabetes.

Table 16–6. Some features distinguishing type I from type II diabetes mellitus.[1]

	Type I	Type II
Synonym	IDDM	NIDDM
Age at onset	Usually <30	Usually >40
Ketosis	Common	Rare
Body weight	Nonobese	Obese (80%)
Prevalence	0.2–0.3%	2–4%
Genetics		
HLA association	Yes	No
Monozygotic twin studies	30–50% concordance rate	90–100% concordance rate
Circulating islet cell antibodies	Yes	No
Associated with other autoimmune phenomena	Occasionally	No
Treatment with insulin	Always necessary	Usually not necessary
Complications	Frequent	Frequent
Insulin secretion	Severe deficiency	Variable: moderate deficiency to hyperinsulinemia
Insulin resistance	Occasional—with poor control or excessive insulin antibodies	Usual—due to receptor and postreceptor defects

[1] Reproduced, with permission, from Wyngaarden JB, Smith LH Jr, Bennett JC (editors): *Cecil Textbook of Medicine,* 19th ed. Saunders, 1992.

Over 90% of cases of diabetes are regarded as primary processes for which individuals have a genetic predisposition and are classified as either **type I (insulin-dependent diabetes mellitus, IDDM)** or **type II (non-insulin dependent diabetes mellitus [NIDDM])** (Tables 16–5 and 16–6). Type I diabetes mellitus is less common than type II, accounting for fewer than 10% of cases of primary diabetes. Type I diabetes is caused by autoimmune destruction of pancreatic B cells that leads to severe insulinopenia. The disease commonly affects individuals under age 30 (juvenile-onset diabetes), with peak incidence occurring at puberty. Although autoimmune destruction of the B cells does not occur acutely, clinical symptoms do. Patients present after only days or weeks of polyuria, polydipsia, and weight loss with markedly elevated serum glucose concentrations. **Ketone bodies** are also increased because of the marked lack of insulin, resulting in severe, life-threatening acidosis (diabetic ketoacidosis). Patients with type I diabetes require treatment with insulin.

Type II diabetes differs from type I in several distinct ways (Table 16–6): It is ten times more common, has a much stronger genetic component (Table 16–7), occurs most commonly in adults (adult-onset diabetes mellitus), and is associated with increased resistance to the effects of insulin at its sites of action as well as a decrease in insulin secretion by the pancreas. It is often (85% of cases) associated with obesity, an additional factor that increases insulin resistance. **Insulin resistance** is the hallmark of this disorder. Because these patients often have varying amounts of residual insulin secretion that prevent severe hyperglycemia or ketosis, they often are asymptomatic and are diagnosed long after the actual onset of disease by the discovery of an elevated fasting glucose on routine screening tests. Population screening surveys show that a remarkable 50% of cases of type II diabetes in the United States are undiagnosed. Once they are identified, these individuals can usually be managed with diet alone or with diet and medications (eg, sulfonylureas) that enhance endogenous insulin secretion and suppress insulin resistance. These patients therefore do not require insulin treatment for survival. However, some patients with type II diabetes are treated with insulin to achieve optimal glucose control.

Gestational diabetes mellitus occurs in 2–3% of pregnant women; may recur with subsequent pregnancies; and tends to resolve at parturition. It is asso-

Table 16–7. Incidence of diabetes mellitus in the United States.

	Type I (IDDM)	Type II (NIDDM)
In population	0.3–0.5%	2%
If proband with the disease is:		
Sibling	6%	38%[1]
Monozygotic twin	30–50%	90–100%
Parent	2–6%	33%[1]
Mother	2–3%	...
Father	5–6%	...

[1] Incidence of diabetes mellitus *or* abnormal glucose tolerance test.

ciated with a markedly increased risk—up to 50% in obese women—for the subsequent development of diabetes (Table 16–5). Because of its adverse effects on fetal outcome, gestational diabetes should be diagnosed or ruled out by routine screening with an oral glucose load at 24 weeks of gestation. Gestational diabetes usually occurs in the second half of gestation, precipitated by the increasing levels of hormones such as chorionic somatomammotropin, progesterone, cortisol, and prolactin that have counterregulatory anti-insulin effects.

Etiology

A. Type I Diabetes: Type I diabetes is caused by selective T lymphocyte-mediated autoimmune destruction of the B cells of the pancreatic islets. Macrophages are thought to be among the first inflammatory cells present in the islets. Later, the islets are infiltrated with activated, cytokine-secreting mononuclear cells. CD8 suppressor T lymphocytes comprise the majority of these cells and are thought to be the primary cell responsible for B cell destruction. CD4 helper T lymphocytes and B lymphocytes are also present in the islets. Autoimmune destruction of the B cell, a process that is thought to be mediated by cytokines, occurs gradually over several years until sufficient B cell mass is lost to cause symptoms of insulin deficiency. At the time of diagnosis, ongoing inflammation is present in some islets, while other islets are atrophic and consist only of glucagon-secreting A cells and somatostatin-secreting D cells.

Genetic susceptibility appears to play a much more important role in the development of type II than type I diabetes, as evidenced by a comparison of the concordance rates in monozygotic twins. Nonetheless, the risk for development of type I diabetes is clearly increased in first-degree relatives of individuals with type I diabetes (Table 16–7). Genetic susceptibility has been linked to the genes of the major histocompatibility complex (MHC) that encode class II human leukocyte antigens (HLA), molecules that are expressed on the surface of specific antigen-presenting cells such as macrophages. Class II molecules form a complex with processed foreign antigens or autoantigens which then activates CD4 T lymphocytes via interaction with the T cell receptor (Figure 16–7). Alleles at the class II HLA gene locus (known as the D locus) conferring risk for the development of diabetes vary with racial group and can be associated with amino acid substitutions in the antigen-binding domain of the encoded class II molecules. Identification of HLA haplotypes remains a research tool at this time.

Although B cell destruction is thought to be a cell-mediated and not a humoral process, **autoantibodies** are associated with the development of type I diabetes and have been used in research studies to predict disease onset. It is hypothesized that these antibodies serve as markers of immune destruction of the islets and may be directed against the B cell antigen that initiates the immune response. **Islet cell antibodies (ICA)** are measured by exposing serum to sections of pancreas, an assay that is commercially available but difficult to standardize. They are present in more than 50% of individuals at the time of diagnosis and are predictive of disease onset in both first-degree relatives and in the general population. Antibodies against insulin **(insulin autoantibody) [IAA]** are also present in 50% of newly diagnosed individuals. The combination of islet cell antibodies and insulin autoantibody is highly predictive for the development of type I diabetes (70% of first-degree relatives positive for both antibodies develop disease within 5 years). In addition to insulin, a number of other islet cell antigens have been identified. Among these, **glutamic acid decarboxylase (GAD)** has recently attracted the most attention since antibodies to this enzyme—which converts glutamate to GABA—are present early and are more highly predictive of disease than are islet cell antibodies or insulin autoantibodies.

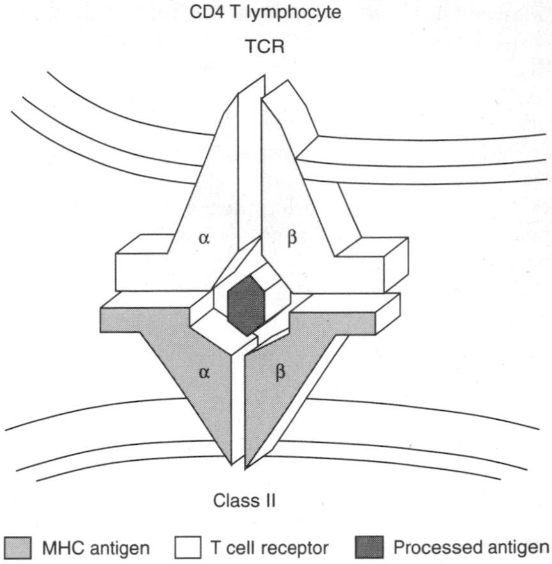

Figure 16–7. Presentation of processed antigen by HLA class II molecule to the T cell receptor. (Reproduced, with permission, from Muir A, Schatz DA, Maclaren NK: The pathogenesis, prediction, and prevention of insulin-dependent diabetes mellitus. Endocrinol Metab Clin North Am 1992;21:199.)

The low concordance rate for type I diabetes in twin studies suggests that environmental factors may also play a role in the development of type I diabetes. Evidence suggests that viral infections may precipitate disease, particularly in genetically susceptible individuals. It is hypothesized that an immune response to foreign antigens may incite B cell destruction if these foreign antigens have some homology with islet cell antigens **(molecular mimicry)**. For example, one identified islet cell antigen (GAD) shares homology with a coxsackievirus protein and another with bovine serum albumin, a protein present in cow's milk, whose consumption in early childhood may be associated with an increased incidence of type I diabetes.

In the development of diabetes, the appearance of islet cell antibodies is followed by progressive impairment of insulin release in response to glucose (Figure 16–8). These two criteria have been used with great success to identify first-degree relatives at risk for the development of diabetes with the ultimate goal of intervening to prevent the development of diabetes. However, since only 10% of individuals newly diagnosed with type I diabetes have a family history of diabetes, such screening methods will not identify the vast majority of individuals developing diabetes. Given the low incidence of type I diabetes in the population, current screening methods do not have sufficient sensitivity to identify most individuals at risk in the general population.

B. Type II Diabetes: Although type II diabetes is ten times more prevalent than type I diabetes and has a much stronger genetic predisposition, the specific molecular defect or defects causing type II diabetes remain largely unknown. While type I diabetes is caused by insulin deficiency, both defective insulin secretion and insulin resistance are present in type II diabetes and are required in the majority of cases for the disease to be clinically manifest. Individuals with type II diabetes secrete a decreased amount of insulin in response to glucose and have a characteristic decrease in the early release of insulin (first-phase insulin release). In addition, type II diabetics are resistant to the effects of insulin.

It is not known with certainty whether abnormal islet cell insulin release or insulin resistance is the primary lesion in type II diabetes. Several decades prior to the onset of clinical diabetes, both insulin resistance and high insulin levels are present. This has led researchers to hypothesize that **insulin resistance** could be the primary lesion, resulting in a compensatory increase in insulin secretion that ultimately cannot be maintained by the pancreas. When the pancreas becomes "exhausted" and cannot keep up with insulin demands, clinical diabetes results. Others have proposed that **hyperinsulinemia,** a primary B cell defect, could initiate the disease process. Elevated insulin levels down-regulate the number of insulin receptors, leading to insulin resistance and to

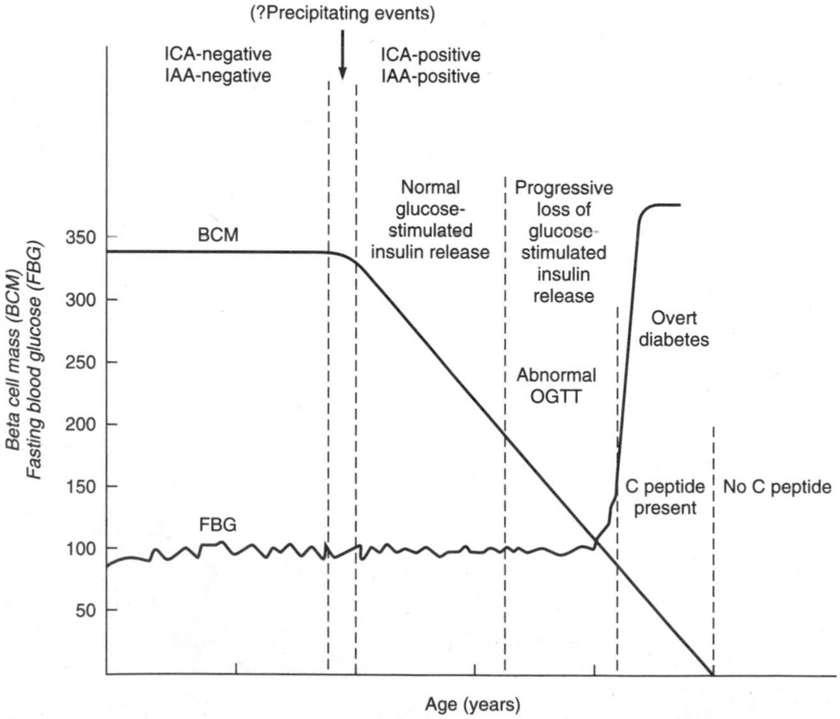

Figure 16–8. Stages in development of type I diabetes. (ICA, islet cell antibodies; IAA, insulin autoantibodies; OGTT, oral glucose tolerance test.) (Reproduced, with permission, from Wilson JD, Foster DW (editors): *Williams Textbook of Endocrinology*, 8th ed. Saunders, 1992.)

the eventual common pathway of B cell exhaustion. In this scenario, hyperinsulinemia is thought to be the expression of a "thrifty genotype" that offers a selective advantage to populations with inconstant food supplies but which leads to obesity and resultant increased insulin resistance in settings of abundant food. Others have proposed that **impaired early secretion of insulin** by islet cells in response to glucose (first-phase insulin release) may be the primary defect, resulting in hyperglycemia. Hyperglycemia and compensatory hyperinsulinemia could then contribute to the development of insulin resistance.

Candidate genes whose defective gene product could explain resistance to insulin action would include insulin itself, the insulin receptor, or other gene products responsible for the postreceptor effects of insulin. Reports of insulin resistance due to defects in insulin, such as mutations causing lack of processing of proinsulin to insulin, are rare. Proinsulin levels are elevated in many individuals with type II diabetes; the significance of this finding is unknown. Specific syndromes of severe insulin resistance distinct from type II diabetes that are caused either by **insulin receptor defects** (type A syndrome) or by **autoantibodies to the insulin receptor** (type B syndrome) have been identified. To date, however, there is no compelling evidence that defects in the insulin receptor are the primary lesion causing insulin resistance in type II diabetes. Therefore, insulin resistance is commonly thought to be due to a postreceptor defect. The defect could be in signaling intermediates distal to the insulin receptor kinases or the ultimate gene products reglated by insulin, such as glucose transporters or enzymes. For example, the gene for **GLUT 4,** the insulin-sensitive glucose transporter present in muscle and fat, has been studied as a possible candidate gene. Similarly, since muscle, the tissue responsible for the bulk of postprandial glucose disposal, appears to exhibit insulin resistance early in the prediabetic state owing to a defect in glycogen synthesis, the genes for enzymes responsible for glycogen synthesis—eg, **glycogen synthetase** or the phosphatases that activate this enzyme—are currently being studied as possible candidate genes.

Gene products capable of altering B cell insulin secretion are also being evaluated. Recently, a defect in the gene encoding glucokinase, the enzyme catalyzing the first step in glucose metabolism in the B cell, has been identified in a subset of type II diabetics **(maturity-onset diabetes of the young [MODY]).** Individuals with MODY have mild diabetes consistent with type II disease but are much younger than the average adult type II patient and inherit the disease in an autosomal dominant pattern. Glucokinase is thought to be the B cell glucose sensor. The potential role of alterations in glucokinase in type II diabetics is currently being studied. Another candidate gene product that may alter B cell function is the newly identified **islet amyloid polypeptide (IAPP; amylin),** which is cosecreted with insulin. Its physiologic role is not yet well understood, but amyloid deposits composed of IAPP occur in the islets of individuals with type II diabetes.

The majority of type II diabetics are obese. Obesity, particularly central abdominal obesity, increases insulin resistance. Obese nondiabetics have increased insulin levels and down-regulation of insulin receptors. Obese type II diabetics often have elevated insulin levels relative to nonobese controls. However, for a given level of glucose, insulin levels in obese type II diabetics are lower than those seen in obese controls. This suggests that type II diabetics have a relative insulin deficiency and cannot compensate for the increased insulin resistance caused by obesity. Obesity, therefore, plays a role in the development of type II diabetes. The importance of obesity in type II diabetes is underscored by the fact that weight loss in obese type II diabetics can ameliorate or even prevent the disorder.

22. What are three different mechanisms by which insulin action can be deficient, manifesting as diabetes mellitus?
23. What are three causes of secondary diabetes mellitus?
24. What are the key characteristics of type I and type II diabetes mellitus?
25. What is the role of heredity versus the environment in each of the two major types of diabetes mellitus?
26. What are two possible mechanism of insulin resistance in type II diabetes mellitus?
27. What is the role of obesity in type II diabetes mellitus?

Pathology & Pathogenesis

No matter what the origin, all types of diabetes result from a relative deficiency of insulin action. In addition, in both type I and type II diabetes, glucagon levels appear to be inappropriately high. This high **glucagon:insulin ratio** creates a state similar to that seen in fasting and results in a "super-fasting" milieu that is inappropriate for maintenance of normal fuel homeostasis (Table 16–4).

The resulting metabolic derangements depend on the degree of loss of insulin action. Adipose tissue is most sensitive to insulin action. Therefore, low insulin activity is capable of suppressing lipolysis and enhancing fat storage. Higher levels of insulin are required to oppose glucagon effects on the liver and block hepatic glucose output. In normal individuals, basal levels of insulin activity are capable of mediating these responses. However, the ability of muscle and other insulin-sensitive tissues to respond to a glucose load with insulin-mediated glucose uptake requires the stimulated secretion of insulin from the pancreas.

Mild deficiencies in insulin action are therefore manifested first by an inability of insulin-sensitive tissues to clear glucose loads. Clinically, this results in **postprandial hyperglycemia.** Such individuals, most commonly type II diabetics with residual insulin secretion but increased insulin resistance, will have abnormal oral glucose tolerance tests. However, fasting glucose levels remain normal since sufficient insulin action is present to counterbalance the glucagon-mediated hepatic glucose output that maintains them. When a further loss of insulin action occurs, glucagon's effects on the liver are not sufficiently counterbalanced. Individuals therefore have both postprandial and **fasting hyperglycemia.**

While type II diabetics usually have some degree of residual endogenous insulin action, type I diabetics have none. Therefore, untreated or inadequately treated type I diabetics manifest the most severe signs of insulin deficiency. In addition to fasting and postprandial hyperglycemia, they also develop **ketosis** since a marked lack of insulin allows maximal lipolysis of fat stores to supply substrates for unopposed glucagon stimulation of ketogenesis in the liver.

Fatty acids liberated from increased lipolysis, in addition to being metabolized by the liver into ketone bodies, can also be reesterified and packaged into VLDL. Furthermore, insulin deficiency causes a decrease in lipoprotein lipase, the enzyme responsible for hydrolysis of VLDL triglycerides in preparation for fatty acid storage in adipose tissue, thereby slowing VLDL clearance. Therefore, both type I and type II diabetics can have elevations in VLDL levels due both to an increase in VLDL production and a decrease in VLDL clearance.

Since insulin stimulates amino acid uptake and protein synthesis in muscle, the decrease in insulin action in diabetes results in decreased muscle protein synthesis. Marked insulinopenia, such as occurs in type I diabetics, can cause negative nitrogen balance and marked protein wasting. Amino acids not taken up by muscle are instead diverted to the liver where they are used to fuel gluconeogenesis.

In type I or type II diabetics, the superimposition of stress-induced counterregulatory hormones on what is already an insulinopenic state exacerbates the metabolic manifestations of deficient insulin action. The stress of infection, for example, can therefore induce diabetic ketoacidosis in both type I and some type II diabetics.

In addition to the metabolic derangements discussed above, diabetes causes other chronic complications that are responsible for the high morbidity and mortality rates associated with this disease. Diabetic complications are largely the result of vascular disease affecting both the microvasculature (retinopathy, nephropathy, and some types of neuropathy) and the macrovasculature (coronary artery disease, peripheral vascular disease).

Clinical Manifestations

A. Acute Complications

1. Hyperglycemia–When elevated glucose levels exceed the renal threshold for reabsorption of glucose, **glucosuria** results. This causes an osmotic diuresis manifested clinically by **polyuria,** including **nocturia.** Dehydration results, stimulating thirst that results in **polydipsia.** A significant loss of calories can result from glucosuria, since urinary glucose losses can exceed 75 g/d (75 g × 4 kcal/g = 300 kcal/d). **Polyphagia** results because of decreased activity of the satiety center in the hypothalamus. The three "polys" of diabetes—polyuria, polydipsia, and polyphagia—are common presenting symptoms in both type I and symptomatic type II patients. Weight loss can also occur due both to dehydration and loss of calories in the urine. Severe weight loss is most apt to occur in patients with severe insulinopenia (type I diabetes) and is due both to caloric loss and to muscle wasting. Increased protein catabolism also contributes to the growth failure seen in children with type I diabetes.

Elevated glucose levels raise plasma osmolality:

$$\frac{\text{Osmolality}}{(\text{mosm/L})} = 2[\text{Na}^+(\text{meq/L}) + \text{K}^+\,(\text{meq/L})] + \frac{\text{Glucose (mg/dL)}}{18} + \frac{\text{BUN (mg/dL)}}{2.8}$$

Changes in the water content of the lens of the eye in response to changes in osmolality can cause blurred vision.

In women, glucosuria can lead to an increased incidence of candidal vulvovaginitis. In some cases, this may be their only presenting symptom. In men, candidal balanitis (a similar infection of the glans penis) can occur.

2. Diabetic ketoacidosis–A profound loss of insulin activity leads not only to increased serum glucose levels due to increased hepatic glucose output and decreased glucose uptake by insulin-sensitive tissues but also to ketogenesis. In the absence of insulin, lipolysis is stimulated, providing fatty acids that are preferentially converted to ketone bodies in the liver by unopposed glucagon action. Typically, profound hyperglycemia and ketosis (diabetic ketoacidosis) occurs in type I diabetes, individuals who lack endogenous insulin. However, diabetic ketoacidosis can also occur in type II diabetes—particularly during infections, severe trauma, or other causes of stress that increase levels of counterregulatory hormones, thus producing a state of profound inhibition of insulin action.

Severe hyperglycemia with glucose levels reaching an average of 500 mg/dL can occur if compensation for the osmotic diuresis associated with hyperglycemia fails. Initially, when elevated glucose levels cause an increase in osmolality, a shift of water from the intracellular to the extracellular space and increased water intake stimulated by thirst help to maintain intravascular volume. If polyuria continues and these compensatory mechanisms cannot keep pace with fluid losses—particularly decreased intake due to the nausea and increased losses due to the vomiting that accompany ketoacidosis—the depletion of intravascular volume leads to decreased renal blood flow. The kidney's ability to excrete glucose is therefore reduced. Hypovolemia also stimulates counterregulatory hormones. Therefore, glucose levels rise acutely owing to increased glucose production stimulated by these hormones and decreased clearance by the kidney—the only source of glucose clearance in the absence of insulin-mediated glucose uptake.

In diabetic ketoacidosis, coma occurs in a minority of patients (10%). Hyperosmolality (not acidosis) is the cause of coma. Profound cellular dehydration occurs in response to the marked increase in plasma osmolality. A severe loss of intracellular fluid in the brain leads to coma. Coma occurs when the effective plasma osmolality reaches 340 mosm/L (normal: 280–295 mosm/L). Since urea is freely diffusible across cell membranes, BUN is not used to calculate the effective plasma osmolality:

$$\text{Effective osmolality} = 2[\text{Na}^+(\text{meq/L}) + \text{K}^+\,(\text{meq/L})] + \frac{\text{Glucose (mg/dL)}}{18}$$

The increase in **ketogenesis** caused by a severe lack of insulin action results in increased serum levels of ketones and ketonuria. Insulinopenia is also thought to decrease the ability of tissues to utilize ketones, thus contributing to the maintenance of ketosis. **Acetoacetate** and **β-hydroxybutyrate,** the chief ketone bodies produced by the liver, are strong organic acids and therefore cause metabolic acidosis, decreasing blood pH and serum bicarbonate (Figure 16–9). Respiration is stimulated in an attempt to compensate for the metabolic acidosis by reducing P_{CO_2}. When the pH is lower than 7.20, characteristic deep, rapid respirations occur **(Kussmaul breathing).** Although acetone is a minor product of ketogenesis (Figure 16–9), its fruity odor can be detected during diabetic ketoacidosis.

Sodium is lost in addition to water during the osmotic diuresis accompanying diabetic ketoacidosis. Therefore, total body sodium is depleted. Serum levels of sodium are usually low owing to the osmotic activity of the elevated glucose, which draws water into the extracellular space and in that way decreases the sodium concentration (sodium falls approximately 1.6 mmol/L for every 100 mg/dL increase in glucose).

Total body stores of potassium are also depleted by diuresis and vomiting. However, acidosis, insulinopenia, and elevated glucose levels cause a shift of potassium out of cells, thus maintaining normal or even elevated serum potassium levels until acidosis and hyperglycemia are corrected. With administration of insulin and correction of acidosis, serum potassium falls as potassium moves back into cells. Without treatment, potassium can fall to dangerously low levels, leading to potentially lethal cardiac arrhythmias. Therefore, potassium supplementation is routinely given in the treatment of diabetic ketoacidosis. Similarly, phosphate depletion accompanies diabetic ketoacidosis, though acidosis and insulinopenia can cause serum phosphorus levels to remain normal prior to treatment. Phosphate replacement is only provided in cases of extreme depletion given the risks of phosphate administration. (Intravenous phosphate may complex with calcium, resulting in hypocalcemia and calcium phosphate deposition in soft tissues.)

Marked **hypertriglyceridemia** frequently accompanies diabetic ketoacidosis because of the increased production and decreased clearance of VLDL that accompany insulin-deficient states. Increased production is due to the increased hepatic flux of fatty acids, which, in addition to fueling ketogenesis, can be repackaged and secreted as VLDL; decreased clearance is due to decreased lipoprotein lipase activity. Although serum sodium levels can be decreased owing to the osmotic effects of glucose, hypertriglyceridemia can interfere with some of the older procedures used to measure serum sodium. This causes pseudohyponatremia, ie, falsely low sodium values.

Nausea and vomiting often accompany diabetic ketoacidosis, contributing to further dehydration. Abdominal pain, present in 30% of patients, may be due to gastric stasis and distention. Amylase is fre-

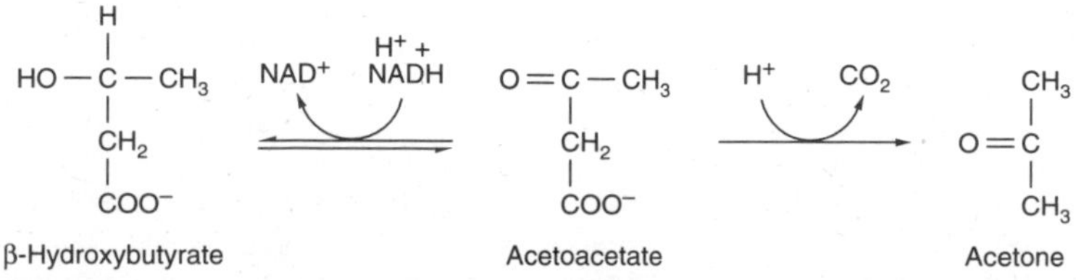

Figure 16–9. Interconversion of ketone bodies. (Reproduced, with permission, from Stryer L: *Biochemistry,* 3rd ed. Freeman, 1988.)

quently elevated (90% of cases), in part due to elevations of salivary amylase, but it is usually not associated with other symptoms of pancreatitis. Leukocytosis is frequently present and does not necessarily indicate the presence of infection. However, since infections can precipitate diabetic ketoacidosis in type I and type II diabetes, other manifestations of infection should be sought—such as fever, a finding that cannot be attributed to diabetic ketoacidosis.

Diabetic ketoacidosis is treated by replacement of water and electrolytes (NaCl) and administration of insulin. With fluid and electrolyte replacement, renal perfusion is increased, restoring renal clearance of elevated blood glucose; and counterregulatory hormone production is decreased, thus decreasing hepatic glucose production. Insulin administration also corrects hyperglycemia by restoring insulin-sensitive glucose uptake and inhibiting hepatic glucose output. Rehydration is a critical component of the treatment of hyperosmolality. If insulin is administered in the absence of fluid and electrolyte replacement, water will move from the extracellular space back into the cells with correction of hyperglycemia, leading to vascular collapse. Insulin administration is also required to inhibit further lipolysis, thus eliminating substrates for ketogenesis, and to inhibit hepatic ketogenesis, thereby correcting ketoacidosis.

During treatment of diabetic ketoacidosis, measured serum ketones may transiently rise instead of showing a steady decrease. This is an artifact due to the limitations of the nitroprusside test that is usually used to measure ketones in both serum and urine. Nitroprusside only detects acetoacetate and not β-hydroxybutyrate. During untreated diabetic ketoacidosis, accelerated fatty acid oxidation generates large quantities of NADH in the liver, which favors the formation of β-hydroxybutyrate over acetoacetate (Figure 16–9). With insulin treatment, fatty acid oxidation decreases and the redox potential of the liver shifts back in favor of acetoacetate formation. Therefore, while the absolute amount of hepatic ketone body production is decreasing with treatment of diabetic ketoacidosis, the relative amount of acetoacetate production is increasing, leading to a transient increase in measured serum ketones by the nitroprusside test.

3. Hyperosmolar coma–Severe hyperosmolar states in the absence of ketosis can occur in type II diabetes. These episodes are frequently precipitated by decreased fluid intake such as can occur during an intercurrent illness or in older debilitated patients who lack sufficient access to water and have abnormal renal function hindering the clearance of excessive glucose loads. The mechanisms underlying the development of hyperosmolality and **hyperosmolar coma** are the same as in diabetic ketoacidosis. However, since only minimal levels of insulin activity are required to suppress lipolysis, these individuals have sufficient insulin to prevent the ketogenesis that results from increased fatty acid flux. Because of the absence of ketoacidosis and its symptoms, patients often present later and therefore have more profound hyperglycemia and dehydration, with glucose levels ranging as high as 800–2400 mg/dL. Therefore, the effective osmolality exceeds 340 mosm/L more frequently in these patients than in those presenting with diabetic ketoacidosis, resulting in a higher incidence of coma.

Although ketosis is absent, mild ketonuria can be present if the patient has not been eating. Potassium losses are less severe than in diabetic ketoacidosis. Treatment is similar to that of diabetic ketoacidosis. Mortality is ten times higher than in diabetic ketoacidosis, because the type II diabetics who develop hyperosmolar nonketotic states are older and often have other serious precipitating or complicating illnesses. For example, myocardial infarction can precipitate hyperosmolar states, or it can result from the alterations in vascular blood flow and other stressors that accompany severe dehydration.

4. Hypoglycemia–Hypoglycemia is a complication of insulin treatment in both type I and type II diabetes, but it can also occur with oral hypoglycemic drug treatment. Hypoglycemia often occurs during exercise or with fasting, states that normally are characterized by slight elevations in counterregulatory hormones and depressed insulin levels. Low insulin levels in these conditions are permissive for the counterregulatory hormone-mediated mobilization of fuel substrates, increased hepatic glucose output, and inhibition of glucose disposal in insulin-sensitive tissues. Hypoglycemia is precipitated in diabetic patients in these circumstances by inappropriately large doses of insulin.

The acute response to hypoglycemia is mediated by the counterregulatory effects of glucagon and catecholamines (Table 16–8). Initial symptoms of hypoglycemia occur secondary to **catecholamine release** (shaking, sweating, palpitations). As glucose drops further, **neuroglycopenic symptoms** also occur from the direct effects of hypoglycemia on central nervous system function (confusion, coma). A characteristic set of symptoms (night sweats, nightmares, morning-headaches) also accompanies hypoglycemic episodes that occur during sleep (**nocturnal hypoglycemia**).

Type I diabetics are especially prone to hypoglycemia. After several years of diabetes, the glucagon response to hypoglycemia can become inadequate though the catecholamine response is still effective. If in later years the catecholamine response is lost as a consequence of autonomic neuropathy—a chronic complication of diabetes—these individuals will have no acute defense against hypoglycemia. Recurrent episodes of hypoglycemia are also thought to cause a decrease in the catecholamine response to hypoglycemia, thus increasing the risk of hypoglycemia in individuals who have already suffered from multiple episodes.

Table 16–8. Symptoms and signs of hypoglycemia.[1]

Secondary to catecholamine release (adrenergic)	
Sweating	Tremor
Shakiness	Hunger
Anxiety	Faintness
Palpitations	Tachycardia
Weakness	
Secondary to central nervous system dysfunction (neuroglycopenic)	
Confusion	Diplopia
Irritability	Inappropriate affect
Headaches	Motor incoordination
Abnormal behavior	Convulsion
Weakness	Coma
Nocturnal hypoglycemia (usually due to excessive insulin therapy; symptoms do not usually awaken the patient)	
Morning headaches	Difficulty in awakening
Lassitude	Psychologic changes
Night sweats	Restlessness during sleep
Nightmares	Loud respirations

[1] Reproduced, with permission, from Androli TE et al (editors): *Cecil Essentials of Medicine,* 3rd ed. Saunders, 1993.

Type I or type II patients with autonomic neuropathy who have a deficient catecholamine response to hypoglycemia and patients who are being treated with beta-adrenergic blockade for other conditions will not experience the catecholamine-mediated warning signs that precede neuroglycopenic symptoms (with the exception of sweating, which is preserved). Therefore, they are especially at risk for hypoglycemia.

Acute treatment of hypoglycemia in diabetic individuals consists of rapid oral or intravenous administration of glucose at the onset of warning symptoms, or the administration of glucagon intramuscularly. Rebound hyperglycemia can occur following hypoglycemia due to the actions of counterregulatory hormones **(Somogyi phenomenon),** an effect that can be aggravated by excessive glucose administration.

B. Chronic Complications: Over time, diabetes results in damage and dysfunction in multiple organ systems (Table 16–9). Vascular disease is a major cause of many of the sequelae of this disease. Both **microvascular disease** (retinopathy, nephropathy) and **macrovascular disease** (coronary artery disease, peripheral vascular disease) complications contribute to the high morbidity and mortality rates associated with diabetes. **Neuropathy** also causes increased morbidity, particularly by virtue of its role in the pathogenesis of foot ulcers.

Although type I and type II diabetics both suffer from the complete spectrum of diabetic complications, the incidence varies with each type. Macrovascular disease is the major cause of death in type II diabetes, while renal failure secondary to **nephropathy** is the most common cause in type I. Although blindness occurs in both types, proliferative changes in retinal vessels **(proliferative retinopathy)** are a major cause of blindness in type I while macular edema is the most important cause in type II diabetes. **Autonomic neuropathy,** one the manifestations of diabetic neuropathy, is more common in type I diabetics.

1. Role of glycemic control in preventing complications–There has been controversy for many years about whether the chronic complications of diabetes could be directly attributed to the effects of elevated glucose or to other genetic factors. This question has important implications for the treatment of diabetes, since a causative role for elevated glucose would suggest that normalization of glucose should be the goal of treatment **(tight or intensive diabetic control).** In 1993, publication of the results of the Diabetes Control and Complications Trial (DCCT) provided the first compelling evidence that intensive treatment could prevent both the development and the progression of retinopathy (50–80%); nephropathy, as measured by effects on proteinuria (40–50%); and neuropathy (60%). Although the study was not designed to test the effect of glycemic control on macrovascular disease, there was also some suggestion of a positive effect. While the DCCT did not include type II diabetics, it is generally now believed that microvascular complications in both type I and type II patients are related to the level of glycemia.

Three other interesting findings emerged from the study: (1) Despite best therapeutic efforts, complete normalization of blood glucose did not occur; (2) intensive treatment carried a threefold increased risk of hypoglycemia requiring assistance or resulting in seizures or coma; and (3) intensively treated patients experienced weight gain, a finding which underscores the anabolic effect of insulin.

While glycemic control clearly influences the occurrence of microvascular complications, genetic factors may also play a role. For example, evidence from a variety of studies suggests that approximately 20–40% of type I diabetics may be particularly susceptible to the development of severe microvascular complications. The reason for this increase is not known.

Table 16–9. Chronic complications of diabetes mellitus.[1]

Microvascular disease
Retinopathy
Nephropathy
Macrovascular disease
Coronary artery disease
Cerebrovascular disease
Peripheral vascular disease
Neuropathic
Peripheral symmetric polyneuropathy
Autonomic neuropathies
Mononeuropathies
Foot ulcers
Infections

[1] Reproduced, with permission, from Androli TE et al (editors): *Cecil Essentials of Medicine,* 3rd ed. Saunders, 1993.

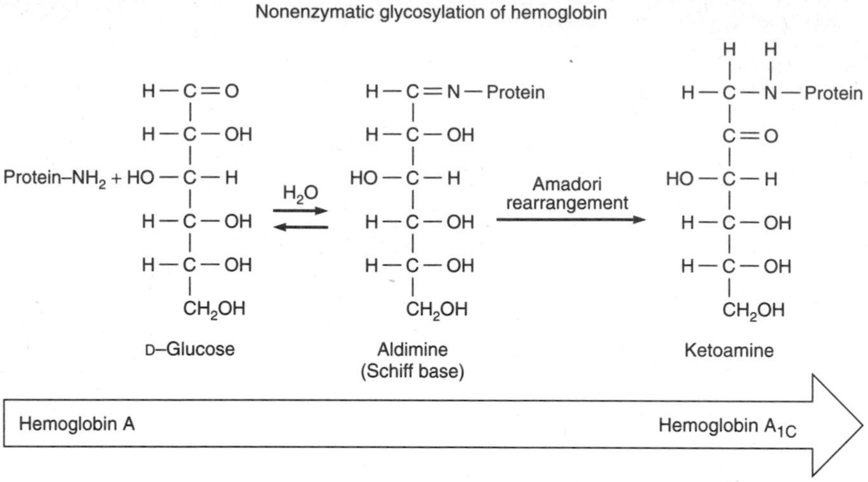

Figure 16–10. Amadori product. (Reproduced, with permission, from Wyngaarden JB, Smith LH Jr, Bennett JC [editors]: *Cecil Textbook of Medicine*, 19th ed. Saunders, 1992.)

2. Microvascular complications–Although microvascular complications are thought to be related to raised glucose levels, the pathogenesis of diabetic microvascular disease is not completely understood. Basement membranes in small vessels are thickened in diabetes and contain increased amounts of collagen and decreased amounts of proteoglycan, of which heparan sulfate is the major component.

One biochemical mechanism that has been proposed to account for the pathogenesis of microvascular lesions in diabetes is the formation of irreversibly glycated proteins called **advanced glycosylation end products (AGE).** When present in high concentrations, glucose can react nonenzymatically with amino groups in proteins to form an unstable intermediate, a Schiff base, that then undergoes an internal rearrangement to form a stable glycated protein, also known as an early glycosylation product **(Amadori product)** (Figure 16–10). Such a reaction accounts for the formation of **glycated HbA,** also known as **HbA$_{1c}$.** In diabetics, elevated glucose leads to increased glycation of HbA within red blood cells. Since red blood cells circulate for 120 days, measurement of HbA$_{1c}$ in diabetic patients serves as an index of glycemic control over the preceding 2–3 months. Early glycosylation products can undergo a further series of chemical reactions and rearrangements, leading to the formation of AGE, which are covalently and irreversibly linked by glucose-derived imidazole- and pyrrole-based cross-links (Figure 16–11). AGE can bind to the matrix components of the basement membrane. Both small and large vessels in diabetics show a continuous accumulation of plasma proteins. It is hypothesized that this may be due to the accumulation of AGE or to the capture by accumulated AGE of other normal plasma proteins, such as LDL. In addition, binding of AGE to specific receptors on macrophages causes the release of cytokines that can in turn affect the proliferation and function of vascular cells. AGE receptors are also present on endothelial cells.

Another biochemical pathway that has been extensively studied in diabetic nerve cells but which is also present in endothelial cells is the **polyol pathway** (Figure 16–12). Many cells contain aldose reductase, an enzyme that converts aldohexoses, such as glucose, to their respective alcohols (polyol pathway). Hyperglycemia provides increased substrate for this enzyme. The excess **sorbitol** produced from this reaction cannot exit the cell but instead is converted to fructose, a step that is rate-limiting. Therefore, sorbitol tends to accumulate in the cells in the presence of hyperglycemia. Sorbitol accumulation has been demonstrated in nerve and endothelial cells and in the lens of the eye, where it is associated with cataract formation. Sorbitol, perhaps through an increase in cell osmolality, is thought to decrease cellular myoinositol content. Hyperglycemia may also directly contribute to intracellular myoinositol depletion by inhibiting its uptake. Decreased myoinositol in turn alters inositol phosphate metabolism, ultimately leading to a protein kinase C-mediated decrease in cellular Na^+-K^+ ATPase activity. In nerve cells, these sorbitol-mediated effects are thought to be responsible for decreased nerve conduction. The effect of this pathway on vascular biology is not known.

a. Retinopathy–(Figure 16–13.) Diabetes is the leading cause of new blindness among United States adults. Diabetic retinopathy occurs in two distinct stages: nonproliferative and proliferative.

Nonproliferative retinopathy occurs frequently in both type I and type II diabetics. **Microaneurysms** of the retinal capillaries, appearing as tiny red dots, are the earliest clinically detectable sign of diabetic

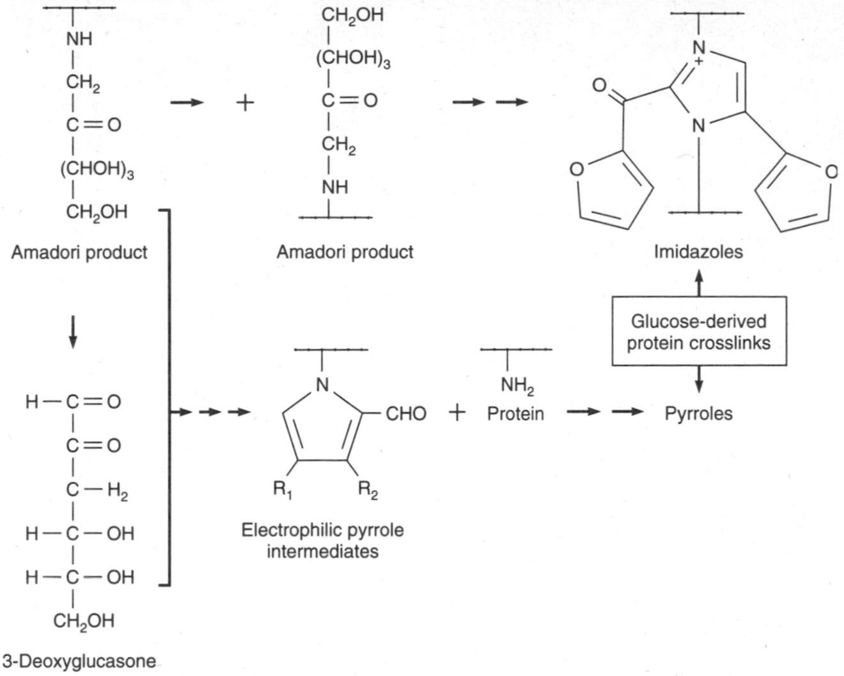

Figure 16–11. Formation of irreversible advanced glycosylation end products (AGE) from Amadori products. Through a complex series of chemical reactions, Amadori products can form families of imidazole-based and pyrrole-based glucose-derived cross-links. (Reproduced, with permission, from Kohler PO, Jordan RM [editors]: *Clinical Endocrinology.* Wiley, 1986.)

retinopathy **(background retinopathy).** These outpouchings in the capillary wall are thought to be related to loss of the pericytes that surround and support the capillary walls. Vascular permeability is increased. Fat that has leaked from excessively permeable capillary walls appears as shiny yellow spots with distinct borders **(hard exudates)** forming a ring around the area of leakage. The appearance of hard exudates in the area of the macula is often associated with macular edema, the most common cause of visual impairment in type II diabetes. As retinopathy progresses, signs of ischemia appear as background retinopathy worsens **(preproliferative stage).** Occlusion of capillaries and terminal arterioles causes areas of retinal ischemia that appear as hazy yellow areas with indistinct borders (**cotton wool spots** or **soft exudates**) due to the accumulation of axonoplasmic debris at areas of infarction. Retinal hemorrhages can also occur, and retinal veins develop segmental dilation.

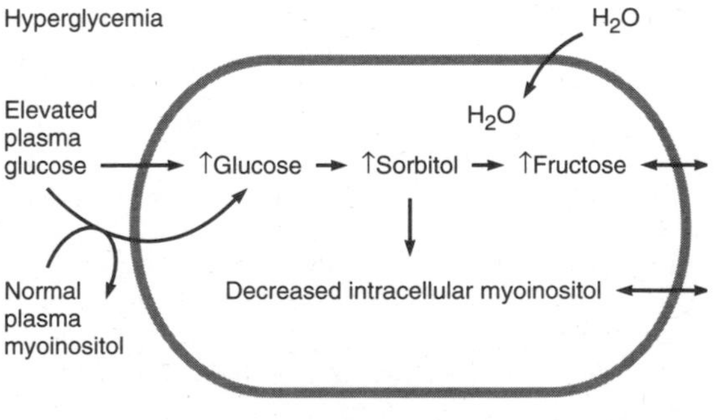

Figure 16–12. The sorbitol pathway. Hyperglycemia increases intracellular sorbitol, which in turn is associated with depletion of intracellular myoinositol levels. Hyperglycemia may also decrease myoinositol directly by inhibiting its uptake. (Modified and reproduced, with permission, from Wyngaarden JB, Smith LH Jr, Bennett JC [editors]: *Cecil Textbook of Medicine,* 19th ed. Saunders, 1992.) .

Retinopathy can progress to a second, more severe stage characterized by the proliferation of new vessels **(proliferative retinopathy). Neovascularization** is more prevalent in type I than in type II diabetes (60% versus 10% after 20 years) and is a major cause of blindness. It is hypothesized that retinal ischemia stimulates the release of growth-promoting factors, resulting in new vessel formation. However, these capillaries are abnormal, and traction between new fibrovascular networks and the vitreous can lead to **vitreous hemorrhage** or **retinal detachment,** two potential causes of blindness.

b. Nephropathy–In the United States, diabetes is the leading cause of end-stage renal disease requiring kidney dialysis or transplantation. Although end-stage renal disease occurs more frequently in type I than in type II diabetes (30% versus <10%), type II

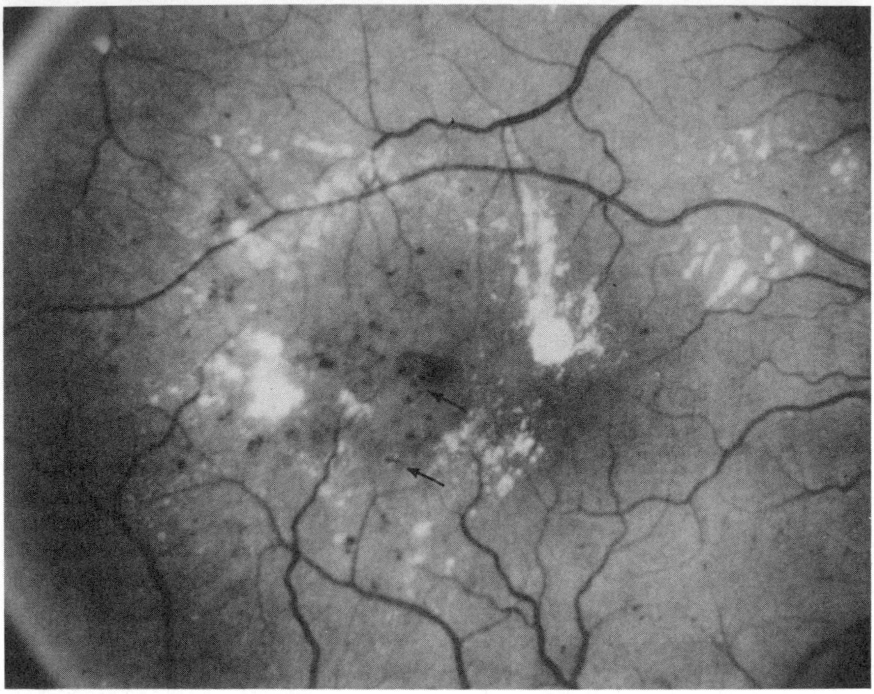

Figure 16–13. A hard caudate ring 1.5 disk diameters in diameter is centered 1.0 disk diameter superotemporal to the center of the macula in this right eye. Part of the ring is a plaque of hard exudate just above the center of the macula. Within the ring, many large microaneurysms can be seen, some with visible walls (arrows). They are slightly out of focus because the retina here is thickened (edematous) and the camera is focused on the surrounding retina. With stereoscopic viewing, retinal thickening was obvious and could be seen to extend into the center of the macula. (Courtesy of the ETDRS Research Group. Reproduced, with permission, from Davis MD: Diabetic retinopathy: A clinical overview. Diabetes Care 1992;15:1844.)

accounts for half of the diabetic population with end-stage renal disease because of its greater prevalence.

Diabetic nephropathy results primarily from disordered glomerular function. Histologic changes in glomeruli are indistinguishable in type I and type II diabetes and occur to some degree in the majority of individuals. Basement membranes of the glomerular capillaries are thickened and can obliterate the vessels; the mesangium surrounding the glomerular vessels is increased owing to the deposition of basement membrane-like material and can encroach on the glomerular vessels; and the afferent and efferent glomerular arteries are also sclerosed. (Figure 16–14). **Glomerulosclerosis** is usually diffuse, but in 50% of cases it is associated with nodular sclerosis. This nodular component, called **Kimmelstiel-Wilson nodules** after the investigators who first described the pathologic changes in diabetic kidneys, is pathognomonic for diabetes.

In type I diabetics, glomerular changes are preceded by a phase of **hyperfiltration** due to vasodilation of both the afferent and efferent glomerular arterioles, an effect perhaps mediated by two of the counterregulatory hormones, glucagon or growth hormone, or by hyperglycemia. It is unknown whether this early hyperfiltration phase occurs in type II diabetes. It has been proposed that the presence of atherosclerotic lesions in older type II diabetics may prevent hyperfiltration and thus account for the lower incidence of overt clinical nephropathy in these individuals.

Early in the course of the disease, the histologic changes in renal glomeruli are accompanied by **microalbuminuria,** a urinary loss of albumin that cannot be detected by routine clinical methods (Figure 16–15). Albuminuria is thought to be due to a decrease in the heparan sulfate content of the thickened glomerular capillary basement membrane. Heparan sulfate, a negatively charged proteoglycan, can inhibit the filtration of other negatively charged proteins, such as albumin, through the basement membrane; its loss therefore allows for increased albumin filtration.

If glomerular lesions worsen, **proteinuria** increases and overt nephropathy develops (Figure 16–15). Diabetic nephropathy is defined clinically by the presence of over 300–500 mg of urinary protein per day, an amount that can be detected by routine clinical methods. In diabetic nephropathy (unlike other renal diseases), proteinuria continues to increase as renal function decreases. Therefore,

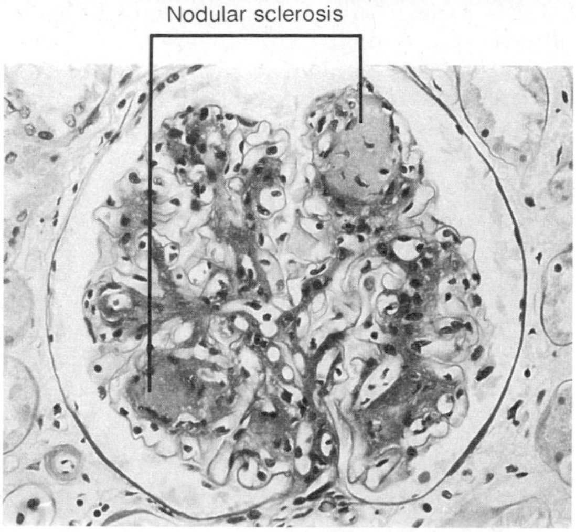

Figure 16–14. Diabetic retinopathy, showing nodular glomerulosclerosis (Kimmelstiel-Wilson disease). (Reproduced, with permission, from Chandrasoma P, Taylor CR: *Concise Pathology*, 2nd ed. Appleton & Lange, 1994.)

end-stage renal disease is preceded by massive, nephrotic-range proteinuria (> 4 g/d). The presence of hypertension speeds this process. While type II diabetics often already have hypertension at the time of diagnosis, type I patients usually do not develop hypertension until after the onset of nephropathy. In both cases, hypertension worsens as renal function deteriorates. Therefore, control of hypertension is critical in preventing the progression of diabetic nephropathy.

Retinopathy, a process that is also worsened by the presence of hypertension, usually precedes the development of nephropathy. Therefore, other causes of proteinuria should be considered in diabetic individuals who present with proteinuria in the absence of retinopathy.

3. Macrovascular complications–Atherosclerotic macrovascular disease occurs with increased frequency in diabetes, resulting in an increased incidence of myocardial infarction, stroke, and claudication and gangrene of the lower extremities. Although macrovascular disease accounts for significant morbidity and mortality in both types of diabetes, the effects of large vessel disease are particularly devastating in type II diabetes and are responsible for over 60% of deaths. The protective effect of gender is lost in women with diabetes; their risk of atherosclerosis is equal to that of men.

Reasons for the increased risk of **atherosclerosis** in diabetes are threefold: (1) The incidence of other known risk factors, such as hypertension and hyperlipidemia, is increased; (2) diabetes itself is an independent risk factor for atherosclerosis; and (3) diabetes appears to act synergistically with other known risk factors to markedly increase the risk of atherosclerosis. The elimination of other risk factors therefore can greatly reduce the risk of atherosclerosis in diabetes (Figure 16–16).

Hypertension occurs with increased frequency in type I and type II diabetes and is associated with an increase in total body extracellular sodium content, causing volume expansion and suppression of renin. Despite these similar findings, the epidemiology of hypertension in the two subtypes suggests that different pathophysiologic mechanisms may be operative.

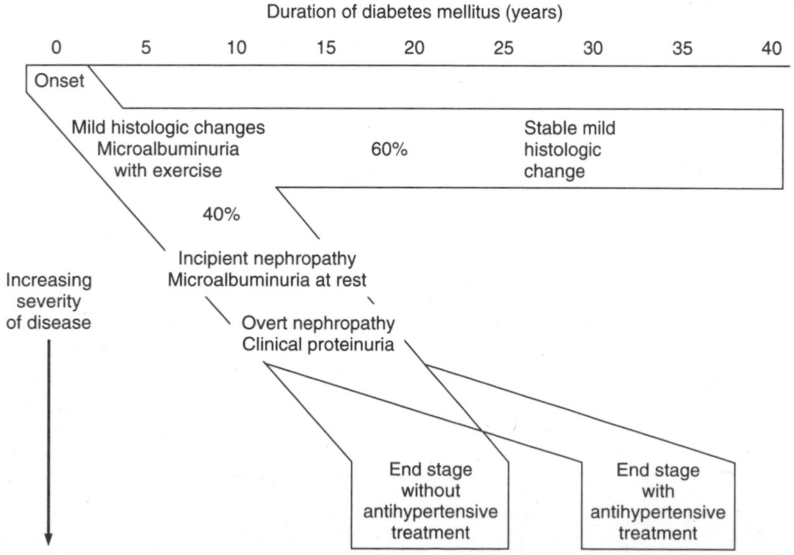

Figure 16–15. Development of renal failure in type I diabetes. (Reproduced, with permission, from Omachi R: The pathogenesis and prevention of diabetic nephropathy. West J Med 1986;145:222.)

In type I diabetes, hypertension usually occurs after the onset of nephropathy, when renal insufficiency impairs the ability to excrete water and solutes. In type II diabetes, hypertension is often present at the time of diagnosis in these older, obese, insulin-resistant individuals. It has been proposed that insulin resistance and hyperinsulinemia may play a central role both in diabetes and in hypertension. Insulin resistance and hyperinsulinemia have been reported in nondiabetics with essential hypertension. A cluster of metabolic abnormalities associated with an increased risk of cardiovascular disease in nondiabetic individuals—insulin resistance, hyperinsulinemia, glucose intolerance, hypertension, hypertriglyceridemia, and low levels of high-density lipoprotein (HDL)—has been called **syndrome X.** It is hypothesized that the metabolic abnormalities in syndrome X are caused by insulin resistance. Type II diabetes—with its overt hyperglycemia occurring in the setting of these same metabolic abnormalities—may lie at the extreme end of a continuum of metabolic derangements described by these signs.

The principal lipid abnormality in poorly controlled type I and type II diabetes is **hypertriglyceridemia,** which is due to increased VLDL. Hypertriglyceridemia, particularly in type II diabetes, can also be associated with decreased HDL cholesterol. LDL cholesterol may also be elevated both because of increased production (VLDL is catabolized to LDL) and decreased clearance (insulin deficiency may reduce LDL receptor activity). VLDL levels are increased because of insufficient insulin action in adipose tissue, resulting in decreased VLDL clearance due to decreased lipoprotein lipase activity and increased VLDL production due to increased fatty acid flux from adipose tissue to the liver (ie, increased lipolysis). Hypertriglyceridemia, low HDL cholesterol, and high LDL cholesterol are all risk factors for atherosclerosis. Insulin treatment usually corrects lipoprotein abnormalities in type I diabetes. In contrast, treatment of hyperglycemia often does not

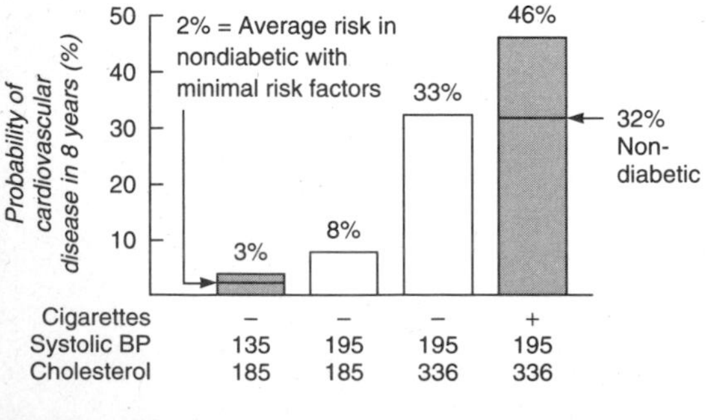

Figure 16–16. Relative importance of risk factors for coronary artery disease in a 40-year-old diabetic man. (Reproduced, with permission, from Siperstein MD: Diabetic microangiopathy, genetics, environment, and treatment. Am J Med 1988;85[Suppl 5A]:119.)

normalize lipid profiles in obese, insulin-resistant individuals with type II diabetes unless accompanied by weight reduction (ie, by a concomitant reduction in insulin resistance).

Possible reasons that diabetes may be an independent risk factor for atherosclerosis and may also act synergistically with other risk factors include the following: (1) alterations in lipoprotein composition in diabetes that make the particles more atherogenic (ie, increased small dense LDL, increased levels of Lp[a], enhanced oxidation and glycation of lipoproteins); (2) the occurrence of a relative procoagulant state in diabetes, including an increase in certain clotting factors and increased platelet aggregation; (3) proatherogenic alterations in the vessel walls caused either by the direct effects of hyperinsulinemia in type II diabetes or by boluses of exogenously administered insulin (versus hepatic first-pass clearance of endogenously secreted insulin) in type I diabetics. These include promotion of smooth muscle proliferation, alteration of vasomotor tone, and enhancement of foam cell formation (cholesterol-laden cells that characterize atherogenic lesions); and (4) proatherogenic alterations in the vessel walls caused by the direct effects of hyperglycemia, including deposition of glycated proteins, just as occurs in the microvasculature.

4. Neuropathy–(Table 16–10.) Neuropathy occurs commonly in both type I and type II diabetes and is a major cause of morbidity. Diabetic neuropathy can be divided into three major types: (1) a distal, primarily sensory, symmetric polyneuropathy that is by far the most common; (2) autonomic neuropathy, occurring frequently in individuals with distal polyneuropathy; and (3) the less common transient, asymmetric neuropathies involving specific nerves, nerve roots, or plexuses.

a. Symmetric distal polyneuropathy–Demyelination of peripheral nerves, which is a hallmark of diabetic polyneuropathy, affects distal nerves preferentially and is usually manifested clinically by a symmetric sensory loss in the distal lower extremities **(stocking distribution)** that is preceded by numbness, tingling, and paresthesias. These symptoms, which begin distally and move proximally, can also occur in the hands **(glove distribution).** Pathologic features of affected peripheral somatic nerves include demyelination and loss of nerve fibers with reduced axonal regeneration accompanied by microvascular lesions, including thickening of basement membranes. Activation of the polyol pathway in nerve cells is thought to play a major role in inducing symmetric distal polyneuropathy in diabetes. In addition, evidence suggests that the microvascular disease which accompanies these neural lesions may also contribute to nerve damage.

b. Autonomic neuropathy–Autonomic neuropathy often accompanies symmetric peripheral neuropathy, occurs more frequently in type I diabetes, and can affect all aspects of autonomic functioning, most notably those involving the cardiovascular, genitourinary, and gastrointestinal systems. Less information is available regarding the morphologic changes occurring in affected autonomic nerves, but similarities to somatic nerve alterations suggest a common pathogenesis.

Fixed, resting **tachycardia** and **orthostatic hypotension** are signs of cardiovascular involvement that can be easily ascertained on physical examination. Orthostatic hypotension can be quite severe. **Impotence** occurs in over 50% of diabetic men and is due both to neurogenic (parasympathetic control of penile vasodilation) and vascular factors. Sexual dysfunction in diabetic women has not been well studied. Loss of bladder sensation causes affected individuals to be unaware of bladder fullness, leading to overflow **incontinence** and an increased risk of urinary tract infections due to residual urine. Motor disturbances can occur throughout the gastrointestinal tract, resulting in delayed gastric emptying (gastroparesis), constipation, or diarrhea, perhaps due to the high somatostatin levels that are associated with insulin deficiency. Anhidrosis in the lower extremities can lead to excessive sweating in the upper body as a means of dissipating heat, including increased sweating in response to eating **(gustatory sweating).** Autonomic neuropathy can also result in decreased glucagon and epinephrine responses to hypoglycemia.

c. Mononeuropathy and mononeuropathy multiplex–The abrupt, usually painful onset of motor loss in isolated cranial or peripheral nerves (**mononeuropathy**) or in multiple isolated nerves (**mononeuropathy multiplex**) occurs less frequently than does symmetric polyneuropathy or autonomic neuropathy. Vascular occlusion and ischemia is thought to play a central role in the pathogenesis of these asymmetric focal neuropathies, which are usually of limited duration and occur more frequently in type II diabetics.

The third nerve is the most frequent cranial nerve involved, causing ipsilateral headache followed by ptosis and ophthalmoplegia with sparing of the pupil. Peripheral nerves are usually involved at sites of possible compression (eg, ulnar nerve at elbow; median nerve at the wrist).

Table 16–10. Classification of diabetic neuropathy.

1. Symmetric distal polyneuropathy (sensory ≫ motor)
2. Autonomic neuropathy
3. Asymmetric mononeuropathy or mononeuropathy multiplex (motor ≫ sensory)
   - Cranial nerves
     - Ocular (III ≫ VI > IV)
     - Bell's palsy (VII)
   - Peripheral nerves
     - Femoral
     - Obturator
     - Sciatic
     - Median
     - Ulnar

5. Diabetic foot ulcers:–Symmetric polyneuropathy, manifested on clinical examination by decreased vibratory and cutaneous pressure sensation and absence of ankle reflexes, is the leading cause of diabetic foot ulcers and is present in 75–90% of diabetics with foot ulcers. Diabetic foot ulcers often lead to **amputations** because of ischemia due to macrovascular disease (present in 30–40% of diabetics with foot ulcers) and to microvascular disease, infections due to alterations in neutrophil function and vascular insufficiency, and faulty wound healing due to unknown factors. The 3-year mortality rate for diabetics who have undergone amputations is 50%.

6. Infection–Neutrophil chemotaxis and phagocytosis are defective in poorly controlled diabetes. Cell-mediated immunity may also be abnormal. In addition, vascular lesions can hinder blood flow, preventing inflammatory cells from reaching wounds (eg, foot ulcers) or other possible sites of infection. Therefore, individuals with diabetes are more prone to develop infections and may have more severe infections. As a result, certain common infections (eg, **candidal infections, periodontal disease**) occur more frequently in diabetics. A number of unusual infections also are seen in diabetics, ie, **necrotizing papillitis; mucormycosis** of the nasal sinuses, invading the orbit and cranium; and **malignant otitis externa** caused by *Pseudomonas aeruginosa*).

28. How does type I diabetes mellitus result in negative nitrogen balance and protein wasting?
29. What are some acute clinical manifestations of diabetes mellitus?
30. Describe the pathophysiologic mechanisms at work in diabetic ketoacidosis?
31. What are some signs and symptoms observed in a patient in ketoacidosis?
32. Explain why ketones may appear to be increasing with appropriate treatment of ketoacidosis.
33. Explain why hyperosmolar coma without ketosis is a more common presentation than ketoacidosis in type II diabetes mellitus.
34. What are the clinical manifestations of iatrogenic hypoglycemia in patients with diabetes mellitus, and why do they develop?
35. What chronic complication of diabetes mellitus can exacerbate iatrogenic hypoglycemia?
36. What are the most common microvascular and macrovascular complications of long-standing diabetes mellitus, and what are their pathophysiologic mechanisms?
37. What were the major conclusions from the DCCT?
38. What are the proposed roles of nonenzymatic glycosylation and the polyol pathway in the development of complications of diabetes mellitus?

39. What are the characteristics of nonproliferative and proliferative retinopathy in diabetes mellitus?
40. What are the anatomic and physiologic changes observed during the progression of diabetic nephropathy?
41. Does nephropathy usually precede retinopathy in patients with diabetes mellitus?
42. Suggest three reasons for increased risk of atherosclerosis in diabetes mellitus.
43. What are the probable differences in the pathophysiology of hypertension in type I versus type II diabetes mellitus?
44. What three major types of neuropathy are observed in long-standing diabetes mellitus? What are the common signs and symptoms of each?
45. Which types of infections occur with increased frequency in patients with diabetes mellitus?

INSULINOMA

Clinical Presentation

The occurrence of fasting hypoglycemia in an otherwise healthy individual is usually due to an insulin-secreting tumor of the B cells of the islets of Langerhans (**insulinoma;** (Table 16–11). Although insulinoma is the most common islet cell tumor, it is still a rare disorder. Insulinomas occur most frequently in the fourth to seventh decades, though they can occur earlier, particularly when associated with multiple endocrine neoplasia type 1 (MEN 1), a neoplastic syndrome characterized by tumors of the parathyroids, pituitary, and endocrine pancreas (see Chapter 17). The diagnosis of hypoglycemia is based on Whipple's triad: (1) symptoms and signs of hypoglycemia, (2) an associated low plasma glucose level, and (3) reversibility of symptoms upon administration of glucose.

Etiology

In the great majority of cases, insulinomas are benign solitary lesions composed of whorls of insulin-secreting B cells. Multiple tumors, though infrequent (< 10%), are seen most often in patients with MEN 1. Fewer than 10% of the tumors are malignant, as determined by the presence of metastases.

Pathology & Pathogenesis

Inappropriately high levels of insulin in situations normally characterized by a lowering of insulin secretion (eg, fasting and exercise) result in hypoglycemia. Normally, in the postabsorptive and fasting state, insulin levels decline, leading to an increase in glucagon-stimulated hepatic glucose output and a decrease in insulin-mediated glucose disposal in the periphery which maintain normal serum glucose levels. With exercise, low insulin allows muscles to utilize glycogen; glucagon and other counterregulatory hormones to increase hepatic glucose output; and counterregulatory hormones to mobilize fatty acids for ketogenesis and fatty acid oxidation by muscle. With an insulinoma, insulin levels remain high during fasting or exercise. In this circumstance, glucagon-mediated hepatic glucose output is suppressed while insulin-mediated peripheral glucose uptake continues, and insulin stimulates hepatic fatty acid synthesis and peripheral fatty acid storage while suppressing fatty acid mobilization and hepatic ketogenesis. The result is fasting or exercise-induced hypoglycemia in the absence of ketosis.

Clinical Manifestations

Individuals with insulinomas often are symptomatic for years prior to diagnosis and self-treat with frequent food intake. Not all patients experience fasting hypoglycemia in the morning (only 30% of insulinoma patients develop hypoglycemia after a diagnostic 12-hour fast). Often they experience late afternoon hypoglycemia, particularly when precipitated by exercise. Since alcohol, like insulin, inhibits gluconeogenesis, alcohol ingestion can also precipitate symptoms. A high percentage of individuals with insulinoma experience neuroglycopenic as well as autonomic symptoms (Table 16–8). Confusion (80%), loss of consciousness (50%), and seizures (10%) often lead to misdiagnoses of psychiatric or neurologic disorders.

Fasting hypoglycemia can be due either to elevated insulin, as occurs in insulinoma, or to non-insulin-mediated effects such as loss of counterregulatory hormones (eg, loss of cortisol in Addison's disease), severe hepatic damage that prevents hepatic glucose production, loss of peripheral stores of substrates for hepatic glucose production (eg, cachexia), or some states of markedly increased glucose utilization (eg, sepsis, cancer). To distinguish **insulin-mediated** from **non-insulin-mediated fasting hypoglycemia,** patients suspected of having insulinoma are subjected to a diagnostic fast during which glucose, insulin, and C peptide levels are measured. Elevated insulin levels in the setting of hypoglycemia is diagnostic of an insulin-mediated cause of hypoglycemia.

Causes of insulin-mediated hypoglycemia other than insulinoma include **surreptitious injection of insulin** or ingestion of oral **hypoglycemic medications** or the presence of **insulin antibodies.** Binding of insulin to the antibodies prevents insulin action but still allows detection of insulin by most assays; release of insulin at an inappropriate time results in hypoglycemia. Surreptitious insulin administration can be ruled out by C peptide measurements. Since

Table 16–11. Syndromes associated with islet cell tumors.[1]

Tumor	Major Findings	Minor Findings	Other Hormones in Tumor or Plasma	Percent Malignancy	Hyperplasia	MEN Syndrome
Insulinoma	Adrenergic: palpitations, tremor, hunger, sweating Neuroglycopenic: confusion, seizures, transient focal deficit, coma	Ischemic cardiovascular disease, permanent neurologic deficits	Gastrin, glucagon, PP, somatostatin, GRH	10%	Occasional	10%
Gastrinoma	Peptic ulcers, enhanced acid secretion	Diarrhea, malabsorption, weight loss, dumping	ACTH, insulin, glucagon, VIP, 5-HIAA, MSH, somatostatin, calcitonin, PP	40–60%	10%	25%
VIPoma	Watery diarrhea, hypokalemia, hypochlorhydria	Hypercalcemia, hyperglycemia, weakness, hypomagnesemia	PHM, PP, prostaglandins(?), GRH, gastrin	40%	20%	Rare
Glucagonoma	Rash, diabetes, weight loss, anemia	Diarrhea, abdominal pain, thromboembolic disease	PP, VIP, 5-HIAA, gastrin, insulin	60%	Occasional	Occasional
Somatostatinoma	Diabetes, cholelithiasis, steatorrhea, malabsorption, weight loss	Indigestion, abdominal pain, anemia, diarrhea, ductal obstruction, hypoglycemia	ACTH, gastrin, calcitonin, PGE_2, glucagon, GRH, PP, VIP, 5-HIAA, substance P	66%	None reported	One case (MEN 3)
PPoma	None	Watery diarrhea, hypocalcemia, achlorhydria, abdominal pain, weight loss	Glucagon, insulin, somatostatin, VIP	40%	Occasional	25%

Key: ACTH = adrenocorticotropic hormone
GRH = growth hormone-releasing hormone
5-HIAA = 5-hydroxyindoleacetic acid
MEN = multiple endocrine neoplasia
MSH = melanocyte-stimulating hormone
PGE_2 = prostaglandin E_2
PHM = peptide histidine methionine
PP = pancreatic polypeptide
VIP = vasoactive intestinal polypeptide

[1] Reproduced, with permission, from Wyngaarden JB, Smith LH Jr, Bennett JC (editors): *Cecil Textbook of Medicine,* 19th ed. Saunders, 1992.

insulin and C peptide are cosecreted, insulinomas will cause elevations in both, while elevated levels of exogenous insulin will not be matched by elevations of C peptide in surreptitious injection of insulin. Similarly, insulin antibodies do not result in elevated C peptide levels. Since oral hypoglycemic medications stimulate endogenous insulin (and therefore C peptide) secretion, insulinoma and inappropriate ingestion of oral hypoglycemic agents can only be differentiated by measuring drug levels.

46. What are the common clinical manifestations of insulinoma?
47. How can surreptitious insulin injection be ruled out?

OTHER HORMONE-SECRETING PANCREATIC TUMORS

1. GLUCAGONOMA

Glucagonomas are usually diagnosed by the appearance of a characteristic rash in middle-aged individuals with mild diabetes mellitus (Table 16–11). Glucagon levels are usually increased tenfold rela-tive to normal values but can even be increased 100-fold.

Necrolytic migratory erythema begins as an erythematous rash on the face, abdomen, perineum, or lower extremities; it crusts over following the development of induration, with central blistering; and then it resolves, leaving an area of hyperpigmentation. These lesions may be the result of nutritional deficiency, such as the hypoaminoacidemia that occurs due to excessive glucagon stimulation of hepatic amino acid uptake and utilization as fuel for gluconeogenesis, rather than the direct effect of glucagon on the skin. Appearance of the rash is a late manifestation of the disease.

Diabetes mellitus or glucose intolerance is present in the vast majority of patients due to increased inappropriate glucagon stimulation of hepatic glucose output. Insulin levels are secondarily increased. Diabetes is therefore mild and is not accompanied by glucagon-stimulated ketosis, since sufficient insulin is present to suppress lipolysis, thus limiting potential substrates for ketogenesis.

Anemia and a variety of nonspecific gastrointestinal symptoms related to decreased intestinal motility also can accompany glucagonomas.

While these tumors are solitary and their growth is slow, they are usually large and have often metastasized by the time of diagnosis, making surgical resection difficult. Octreotide, the synthetic somatostatin analogue, can be used to ameliorate symptoms via its suppression of glucagon secretion.

2. SOMATOSTATINOMA

Somatostatinomas present with a variety of gastrointestinal symptoms in individuals with mild diabetes. However, these extremely rare tumors are almost uniformly found incidentally during operations for cholelithiasis or other abdominal complaints since the presenting symptoms are both nonspecific and commonplace in an adult population. Documentation of elevated somatostatin levels confirms the diagnosis.

A **classic triad** of symptoms frequently occurs with excessive somatostatin secretion: **diabetes mellitus,** due to its inhibition of insulin and glucagon secretion; **cholelithiasis,** due to its inhibition of gallbladder motility; and **steatorrhea,** due to its inhibition of pancreatic exocrine function. Hypochlorhydria, diarrhea, and anemia can also occur.

In type I and type II diabetes, the effects of insulin insufficiency are aggravated by the occurrence of elevated glucagon levels. In contrast, with somatostatinomas, both insulin and glucagon are suppressed. Therefore, the hyperglycemia resulting from insulinopenia is tempered by the absence of glucagon stimulation of hepatic glucose output. Although low insulin levels are permissive for lipolysis, glucagon deficiency prevents hepatic ketogenesis. The diabetes associated with somatostatinomas is therefore mild and not ketosis-prone.

While the majority of somatostatinomas occur in the pancreas, a significant number are found in the duodenum or jejunum. Like glucagonomas, somatostatinomas are often solitary and large and have frequently metastasized by the time of diagnosis.

48. What are the characteristic findings in a patient with glucagonoma?
49. What is the classic triad of findings in a patient with somatostatinoma?

REFERENCES

General

Unger RH, Orci L: Glucagon. In: *Diabetes Mellitus Theory and Practice,* 4th ed. Rifkin H, Porte D (editors). Elsevier, 1990.

Diabetes Mellitus

American Diabetes Association: Office guide to diagnosis and classification of diabetes mellitus and other categories of glucose intolerance. Diabetes Care 1993;16:4.

Bierman EL: Atherogenesis in diabetes. Arterioscler Thromb 1992;12:647.

Davis MD: Diabetic retinopathy: A clinical overview. Diabetes Care 1992:12:1844.

The Diabetes Control and Complications Trial Research Group: The effect of intensive treatment of diabetes on the development and progression of long-term complications in insulin-dependent diabetes mellitus. N Engl J Med 1993;329:86.

Dinneen S, Gerich J, Rizza R: Carbohydrate metabolism in non-insulin-dependent diabetes mellitus. N Engl J Med 1992;327:707.

Gerich JE et al: Hypoglycemia unawareness. Endocr Rev 1991;12:356.

Kolaczynski JW, Caro JF: Insulin-like growth factor-I therapy in diabetes: Physiologic basis, clinical benefits, and risks. Ann Intern Med 1994;120:47.

Mattock MB et al: Prospective study of microalbuminuria as predictor of mortality in NIDDM. Diabetes 1992;41:736.

Nathan DM: Long-term complications of diabetes mellitus. N Engl J Med 1993;328:1676.

Pyzdrowski KL et al: Preserved insulin secretion and insulin independence in recipients of islet autografts. N Engl J Med 1992;327:220.

Rossini AA et al: Immunopathogenesis of diabetes mellitus. Diabetes Reviews 1993;1:43.

Siperstein MD: Diabetic ketoacidosis and hyperosmolar coma. Endocrinol Metab Clin North Am 1992;21:415.

Skyler JS, Marks JB: Immune intervention in type I diabetes mellitus. Diabetes Reviews 1993;1:15.

Vinik AI et al: Diabetic neuropathies. Diabetes Care 1992;15:1926.

Insulinoma, Glucagonoma, and Somatostatinoma

Friesen SR: Tumors of the endocrine pancreas. N Engl J Med 1982;306:580.

Reichlin S: Somatostatin. (Two parts.) N Engl J Med 1983;309:1495,1556.

Service FJ et al: Functioning insulinoma: Incidence, recurrence, and long-term survival of patients. A 60 year study. Mayo Clin Proc 1991;66:771.

Unger RH, Orci L: Glucagon. In: *Diabetes Mellitus Theory and Practice*, 4th ed. Rifkin H, Porte D (editors). Elsevier, 1990.

Disorders of the Parathyroids & Calcium Metabolism

17

Dolores M. Shoback, MD, & Gordon J. Strewler, MD

This chapter presents a general overview of the key hormones involved in the regulation of calcium, phosphate, and bone mineral metabolism. These include **parathyroid hormone, vitamin D**—principally the 1,25-$(OH)_2$ vitamin D metabolite—and **calcitonin.** The cycle of bone remodeling is described as a basis for understanding normal mineral balance and the pathogenesis of mineral disorders and metabolic bone disease. The symptoms and signs caused by excess or deficiency of the calciotropic hormones are presented along with the natural histories of **primary hyperparathyroidism, hypercalcemia of malignancy,** different forms of **hypoparathyroidism,** and **medullary carcinoma of the thyroid.** Two of the most commonly encountered causes of osteopenia—**osteoporosis** and **osteomalacia**—are reviewed along with current theories of their pathogenesis.

NORMAL REGULATION OF CALCIUM METABOLISM

PARATHYROID GLANDS

Anatomy

Normal parathyroid glands each weigh about 30–40 mg and are grayish tan to yellow-gray in color. Each individual normally has four glands, so that the average total parathyroid tissue mass in the adult is about 120–160 mg.

The superior pair of parathyroid glands arises from the fourth branchial pouches. These glands are located near the point of intersection of the middle thyroid artery and the recurrent laryngeal nerve. The superior parathyroid glands may be attached to the thyroid capsule posteriorly or, rarely, embedded in the thyroid gland itself. Alternative locations include the tracheoesophageal groove and the retroesophageal space. The blood supply to the superior parathyroid glands is usually from the inferior thyroid artery or, in some cases, the superior thyroid artery.

The inferior parathyroid glands develop from the third branchial pouch, as does the thymus gland. These glands typically lie at or near the lower pole of the thyroid gland lateral to the trachea. The inferior glands receive their blood supply from the inferior thyroid arteries. The location of the inferior parathyroid glands is more variable. When there are ectopic glands, they are typically found in association with thymic remnants. A common site for ectopic glands is the anterior mediastinum. Less common ectopic locations are the carotid sheath, pericardium, and pharyngeal submucosa. About 10% of people have additional (supernumerary) parathyroid glands.

Histology

The parathyroid gland is composed of three different cell types: chief cells, clear cells, and oxyphil cells. Whether these cells serve specialized functions has not been established. **Chief cells** are thought to be responsible for the synthesis and secretion of **parathyroid hormone (PTH).** Histologically, chief cells are small (4–8 μm in diameter) with central nuclei. In their active state, they have a prominent endoplasmic reticulum and dense Golgi regions where PTH is synthesized and packaged for secretion. **Clear cells** are probably chief cells with an increased glycogen content. **Oxyphil cells** appear in the parathyroid glands after puberty. They are larger than chief cells (6–10 μm), and their number increases with age. It is not clear whether these cells secrete PTH and whether they are derived from chief cells.

The normal adult parathyroid gland contains fat. The relative contribution of fat to the glandular mass increases with age and may reach 60–70% of gland volume in the elderly. When the parathyroid gland undergoes hyperplasia or adenomatous changes, the component of the gland which is fat decreases dramatically.

Physiology

Approximately 99% of the total body calcium is found in the skeleton and teeth. The remaining calcium is in the extracellular fluids. Calcium in these fluids exists in three forms--as ionized, protein-bound, and complexed calcium. Approximately 45–50% of the total blood calcium is protein-bound, predominantly to albumin but also to globulins. A similar fraction is ionized. The remainder is complexed to organic ions such as citrate, phosphate, and bicarbonate. The ionized fraction of the serum calcium controls vital cellular functions such as muscle contraction, neuromuscular transmission, and blood clotting. The binding of calcium to albumin is pH-dependent, increasing with alkalosis and decreasing with acidosis. Thus, if the ionized calcium is low, acidosis tends to protect a subject from displaying the signs and symptoms of hypocalcemia. Conversely, alkalosis will predispose to symptomatic hypocalcemia.

Circulating levels of PTH can change within seconds after an alteration in serum calcium. PTH secretory rates are related to the serum ionized calcium by an inverse sigmoidal relationship (Figure 17–1). Low ionized calcium concentrations maximally stimulate secretion, while increases in calcium suppress the production and release of PTH. PTH secretion is exquisitely sensitive to very small changes in the calcium concentration, which have substantial effects on the rate of hormone synthesis and release.

A recently identified plasma membrane calcium receptor expressed by parathyroid cells detects changes in the extracellular calcium concentration. This receptor senses high calcium levels and couples to intracellular pathways that ultimately lead to inhibition of hormone secretion (Figure 17–2).

Chronic hypocalcemia is also a stimulus to the proliferation of parathyroid cells, which eventually results in glandular hyperplasia. The mechanism underlying this response to reduced calcium levels has not been clearly delineated.

PTH is produced in the parathyroid glands as a 115-amino-acid precursor molecule (preproPTH) which is successively cleaved within the cell to form the mature 84-amino-acid peptide PTH(1–84) (Figure 17–3). This form of the hormone is packaged into secretory granules and released into the circulation. PTH(1–84) is the biologically active form of PTH at target cells and has a very short half-life in vivo of approximately 10 minutes. PTH(1–84) is metabolized in the liver and other tissues to midregion and carboxyl terminal forms that are probably biologically inactive. These circulating fragments accumulate to very high levels in patients with renal failure, since the kidney is an important site for clearance of PTH from the body.

The assays most commonly used at present to assess PTH levels measure intact PTH(1–84). These are two-site immunoradiometric or immunochemiluminometric assays. They utilize antibodies directed against two different regions of the intact PTH(1–84) molecule (Figure 17–4). In the two-site assay, serum is incubated with the first antibody that is directed to the amino terminal portion of the molecule and which is also labeled. The second antibody, raised against the carboxyl terminal or the midregion of PTH [ie, PTH(39–84)] and conjugated to a bead, is

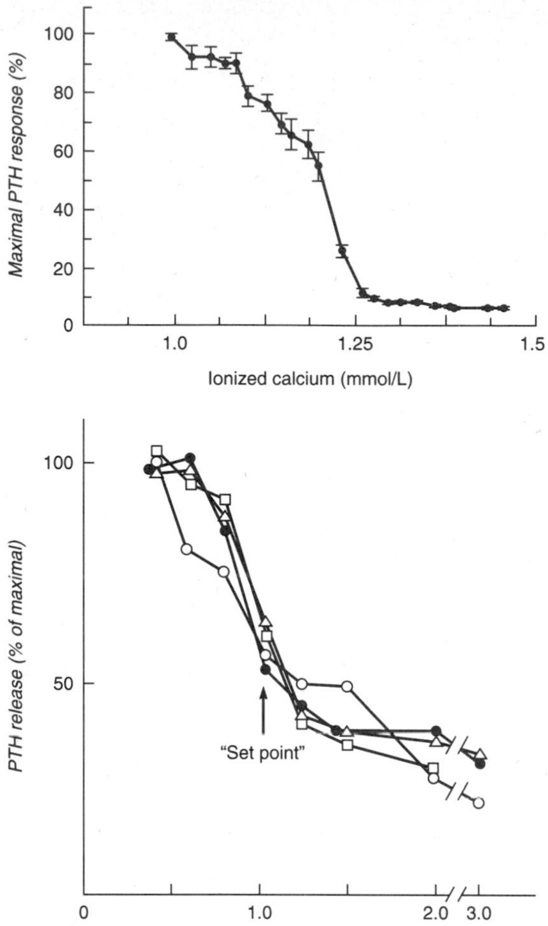

Figure 17–1. Inverse sigmoidal relationship between PTH release and the extracellular calcium concentration in human studies (upper panel) and in vitro in human parathyroid cells (bottom panel). Studies shown in the upper panel were performed by infusing calcium and the calcium chelator EDTA into normal subjects. Serum intact PTH was measured by a two-site immunoradiometric assay. In the lower panel, PTH was measured in the medium surrounding parathyroid cells in vitro by an assay for intact PTH. The midpoint between the maximal and minimal secretory rates is defined as the set-point for secretion. (Reproduced, with permission, from Brown E: Extracellular Ca^{2+} sensing, regulation of parathyroid cell function, and role of Ca^{2+} and other ions as extracellular [first] messengers. Physiol Rev 1991;71:371.)

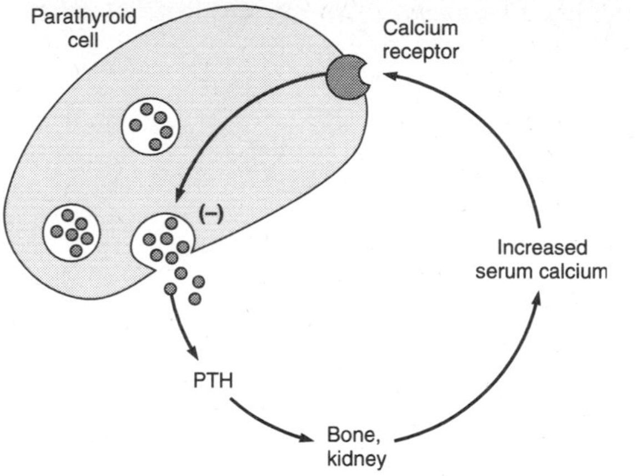

Figure 17–2. Sequence of events by which the calcium ion concentration is sensed by the parathyroid cell calcium receptor. Activation of this receptor is eventually linked through intracellular signal transduction pathways to the inhibition of PTH secretion. (Reproduced, with permission, from Taylor R: A new receptor for calcium ions. J NIH Res 1994:6:25.)

added in a second step. After the bead has been washed, the amount of bound label is determined by counting radioactivity or measuring luminescence. Only intact PTH(1–84) will be recognized by both antibodies, since it will be the only form of the peptide to have both immunodeterminants.

Many laboratories continue to perform more traditional midregion PTH assays, which typically detect those species of hormone containing amino acids 43–68 of the PTH molecule. This assay takes advantage of the higher levels of the midregion fragments due to their longer half-life. The concentration of these fragments provides a reasonable—albeit indirect—assessment of glandular secretion in clinical situations where renal function and thus PTH clearance are normal. Reduced clearance of midregion PTH fragments occurs when the glomerular filtration rate (GFR) declines below about 40 mL/min. Thus, in renal insufficiency, measurements of PTH using midregion assays do not accurately reflect glandular secretion. For this reason, uremic secondary hyperparathyroidism is best monitored by the use of the two-site assay for intact hormone, since there is no contribution to the PTH levels obtained with these assays when there is delayed clearance of hormone fragments.

Both midregion and intact PTH assays have been successfully employed to diagnose primary hyperparathyroidism and hypoparathyroidism (see below). In nonparathyroid hypercalcemia, one would predict that there should be little or no PTH immunoreactivity in the serum. Certain midregion PTH assays in the past, however, have yielded somewhat elevated (or at best nonsuppressed) PTH levels in patients with cancer and hypercalcemia. It has become clear, retrospectively, that these results were false positives. **Parathyroid hormone-related peptide (PTHrP),** which is responsible for hypercalcemia in most cancer patients, does not cross-react in PTH assays. False positives in patients with cancer and hypercalcemia do not occur with the current two-site assays for intact PTH. These assays, therefore, provide a clearer discrimination between non-PTH-mediated and PTH-mediated hypercalcemia in those clinical circumstances in which this distinction is most crucial.

Mechanism of Parathyroid Hormone Action

PTH and the recently identified PTHrP (described below) share the same receptor. The amino terminal portion of both peptides binds to PTH/PTHrP receptors, and this part of the molecule is also responsible for the activation of adenylyl cyclase and production of the second-messenger cAMP (Figure 17–5). Increasing evidence supports the idea that PTH/PTHrP receptors also couple to the stimulation of phospholipase C activity, leading to the generation of inositol trisphosphate and diacylglycerol (Figure 17–5). Activation of this signal transduction pathway induces intracellular calcium mobilization and protein kinase C activation in PTH- and PTHrP-responsive cells. The exact pathways responsible for specific actions of PTH in its target cells have not been firmly established.

Effects of Parathyroid Hormone

The serum ionized calcium and phosphate concentrations reflect the net transfer of these ions from bone, gastrointestinal tract, and glomerular filtrate. PTH and 1,25-$(OH)_2D$ play key roles in the regulation of calcium and phosphate balance (Figure 17–6). When the serum calcium falls, PTH is rapidly released and acts quickly to promote calcium reabsorption in the distal tubule and the medullary thick ascending limb of Henle's loop. PTH also stimulates the release of calcium from a rapidly exchangeable pool of bone calcium. These actions serve to restore serum calcium levels to normal.

The renal action of PTH is rapid, occurring within minutes after an increase in the hormone. The overall effect of PTH on the kidney, however, depends on several factors. When hypocalcemia is present and PTH is elevated, urinary calcium excretion is low. This reflects the full expression of the primary renal effect of PTH to enhance renal calcium reabsorption. When PTH levels are high in primary hyperparathyroidism, hypercalcemia results from increased mobilization of calcium from bone and enhanced intestinal calcium absorption. These events increase the delivery of calcium to the glomerular filtrate.

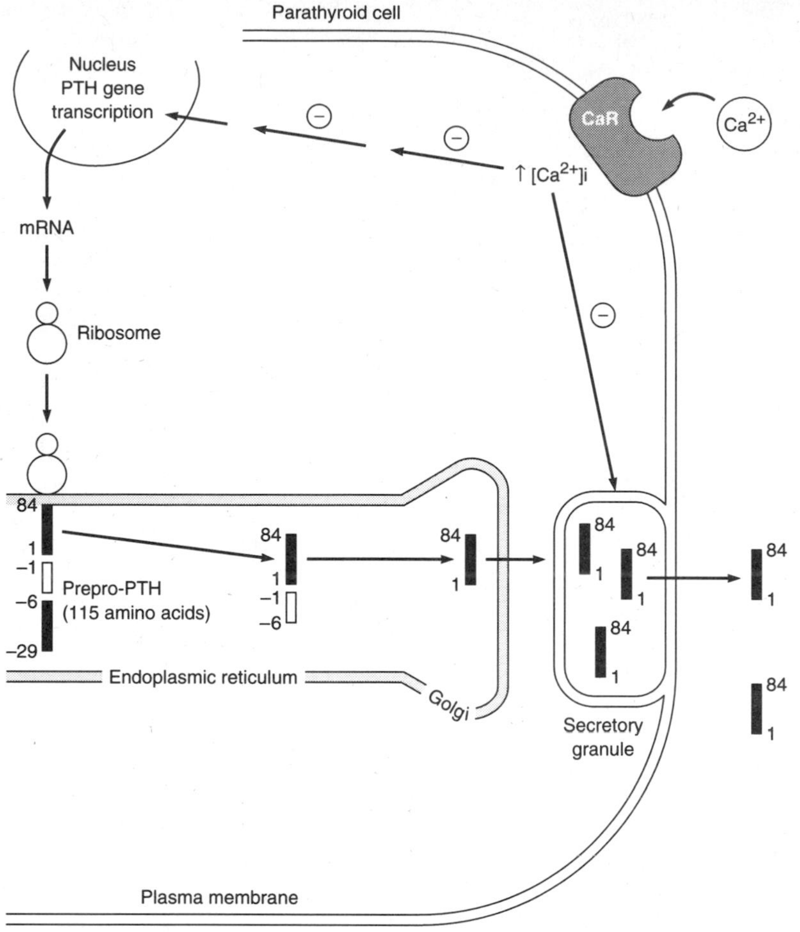

Figure 17–3. Biosynthetic events in the production of PTH within the parathyroid cell. PreproPTH gene is transcribed to its mRNA, which is translated on the ribosomes to preproPTH (amino acids –29 to +84). The pre- sequence is removed within the endoplasmic reticulum, yielding proPTH (–6 to +84). Mature PTH(1–84) released from the Golgi is packaged in secretory granules and released into the circulation in the presence of hypocalcemia. The calcium receptor is proposed to sense changes in extracellular calcium that affect both the release of PTH and the transcription of the preproPTH gene. (Modified and reproduced, with permission, from Habener JF et al: Biosynthesis of parathyroid hormone. Recent Prog Horm Res 1977;33:249.)

Because more calcium is filtered, more is excreted in the urine, despite the high PTH levels. If the filtered load of calcium is normal or low in a patient with primary hyperparathyroidism—because of a low dietary calcium intake or demineralized bone—urinary calcium excretion may be normal or even low. Thus, there may be considerable variability in calcium excretion among patients with hyperparathyroidism.

If kidney function is normal, chronic elevation in serum PTH increases renal 1,25-$(OH)_2D$ production. This steroid hormone stimulates both calcium and phosphate absorption across the small intestine (Figure 17–6). The effect requires at least 24 hours to develop fully and begin to restore normal calcium levels. Achievement of eucalcemia then leads to a downward readjustment in the PTH secretory rate. Any increase in 1,25-$(OH)_2D$ serves to inhibit further PTH synthesis.

The major effect of PTH on phosphate handling is to promote phosphate excretion by inhibition of sodium-dependent phosphate transport in the proximal and distal tubules. Serum phosphate levels do not alter PTH secretion rates directly. Hypophosphatemia enhances the conversion of 25-(OH)D to 1,25-$(OH)_2D$ in the kidney, which through its intestinal and renal effects promotes phosphate retention. Hyperphosphatemia inhibits 1,25-$(OH)_2D$ production (see below), lowers serum calcium by complexing it, and thus indirectly stimulates PTH secretion.

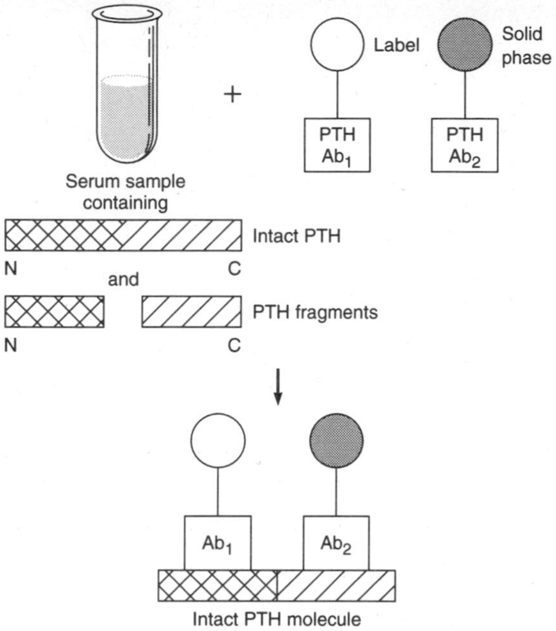

Figure 17–4. Schematic representation of the principle of the two-site assay for intact PTH. The label may be a luminescent probe or ^{125}I in the immunochemiluminometric or immunoradiometric assay, respectively. Two different region-specific antibodies are used (Ab_1 and Ab_2). Only the hormone species containing both immunodeterminants is counted in the assay.

PTH also increases urinary excretion of bicarbonate through its action on the proximal tubule. This can produce proximal renal tubular acidosis. These physiologic responses to PTH are the basis for the hypophosphatemia and hyperchloremic acidosis commonly observed in patients with hyperparathyroidism. Dehydration is also commonly seen in moderate to severe hypercalcemia of any origin. This is due to the effect of hypercalcemia on vasopressin action in the medullary thick ascending limb of the kidney. High calcium levels blunt the action of endogenous vasopressin on its receptor, and reabsorption of water is decreased.

In conjunction with 1,25-$(OH)_2D$, PTH increases bone resorption to restore normocalcemia (see below). PTH acts on bone in two steps. The first is to mobilize calcium and phosphate rapidly from a compartment in direct contact with extracellular fluids. The second step of calcium mobilization results from bone matrix dissolution and alterations in the bone remodeling process. The initial skeletal response to PTH occurs within 2–3 hours. Later effects require several hours to develop. In its initial action on bone, PTH enhances osteoclastic activity and thus bone resorption. Subsequently, PTH stimulates bone formation, since the processes of resorption and formation are coupled. In primary and secondary hyperparathyroidism, when PTH production rates are excessive, net bone loss may occur over time. This is thought to be due to the fact that although the processes of formation and resorption are coupled, they may not occur with 100% efficiency.

PARATHYROID HORMONE-RELATED PEPTIDE (PTHrP)

Parathyroid hormone-related peptide (PTHrP) is a 141-amino-acid peptide which is homologous with PTH at its amino terminal (Figure 17–7) and is recognized by PTH receptors. Consequently, PTHrP has effects on bone and kidney similar to those of PTH—it increases bone resorption, increases phosphate excretion, and decreases renal calcium excretion. PTHrP can be secreted by tumor cells and was originally identified as the cause of hypercalcemia of malignancy, a syndrome that can mimic primary hyperparathyroidism (see below).

Unlike PTH, which is exclusively the product of parathyroid cells, PTHrP is produced locally in many tissues and functions mainly as a tissue growth and differentiation factor at the local level. In the development of cartilage and bone, PTHrP stimulates the proliferation of chondrocytes and inhibits the miner-

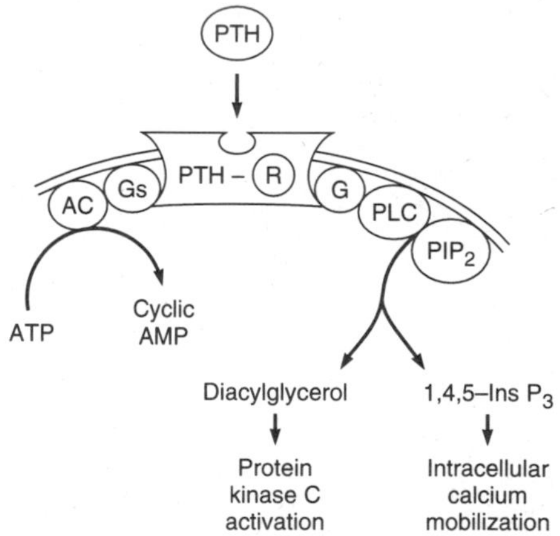

Figure 17–5. Signal transduction pathways activated by PTH binding to its receptor (PTH-R) in a target cell. PTH interacts with its receptor. This enhances GTP binding to the stimulatory G protein of adenylyl cyclase G_s, which activates the enzyme. cAMP is formed. PTH also increases G protein-dependent activation of phospholipase C (PLC), which catalyzes the breakdown of the membrane phospholipid phosphatidylinositol 4,5-bisphosphate (PIP_2). This produces the second messengers inositol trisphosphate (1,4,5-$InsP_3$) and diacylglycerol. 1,4,5-$InsP_3$ mobilizes intracellular calcium, and diacylglycerol activates protein kinase C.

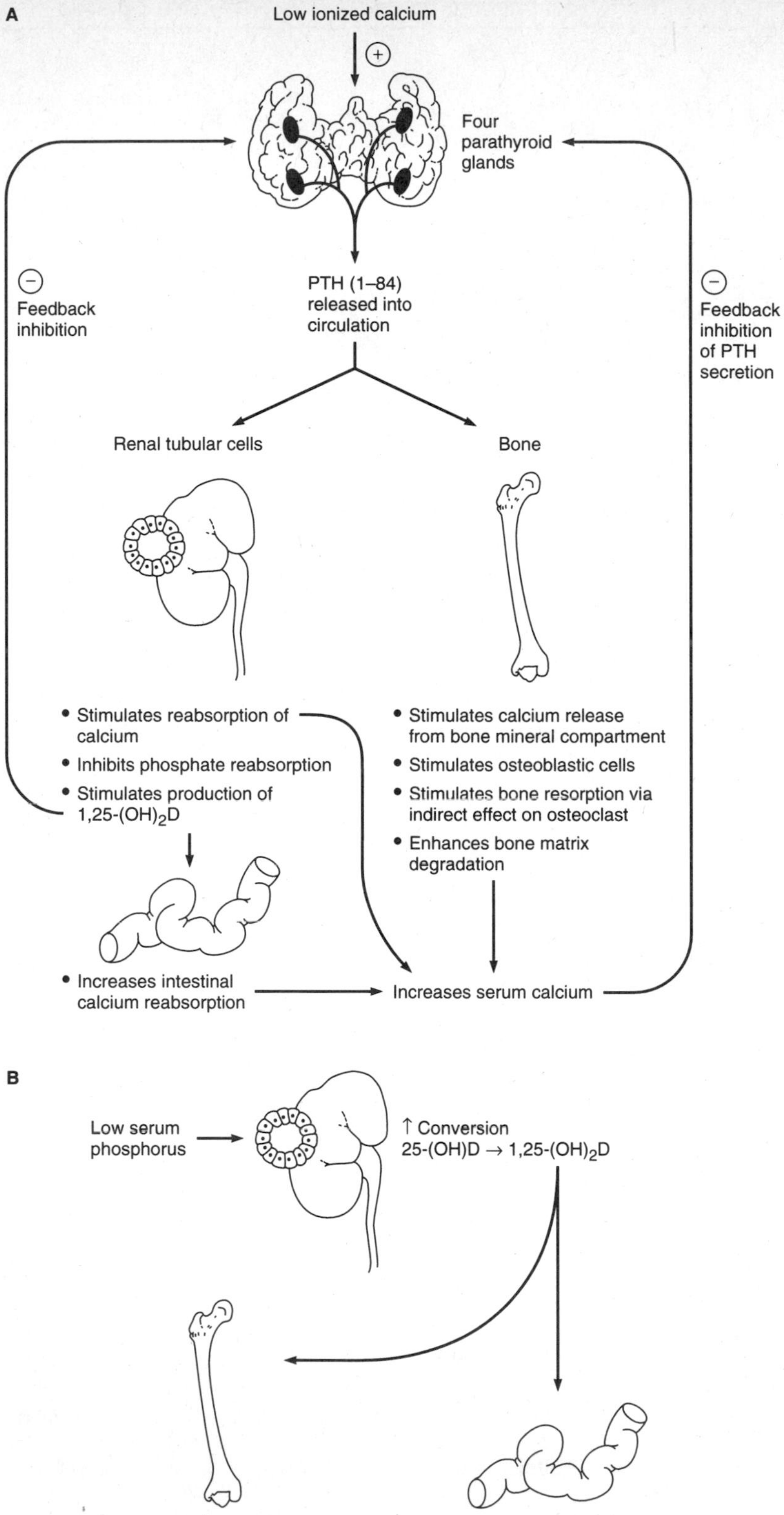

Figure 17–6. Main actions of PTH and 1,25-$(OH)_2D$ in the maintenance of calcium and phosphate homeostasis. (Modified and reproduced, with permission, from Chandrasoma P, Taylor CE: *Concise Pathology,* 2nd ed. Appleton & Lange, 1994.)

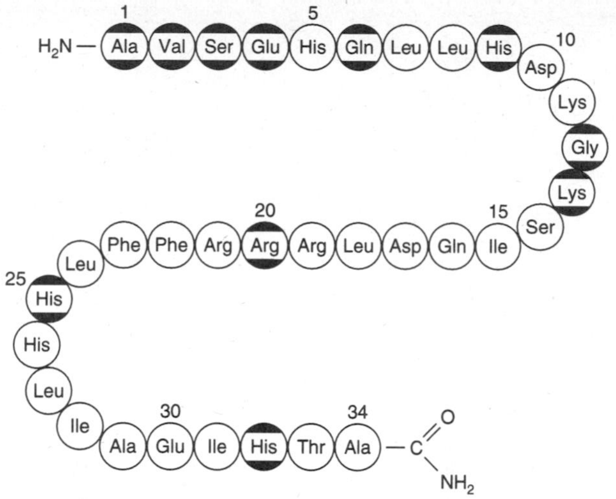

Figure 17–7. The amino acid sequence of PTHrP(1–34). Amino acids that are identical to those in PTH are shown with black borders. (Reproduced, with permission, from Felig P et al [editors]: *Endocrinology and Metabolism,* 3rd ed. McGraw-Hill, 1994.)

alization of cartilage. This is required for normal development. Embryos without PTHrP are nonviable, with multiple abnormalities of bone and cartilage. PTHrP also appears to regulate the normal development of skin, hair follicles, and breast. The list of normal functions of PTHrP is growing rapidly, and it is likely that ultimately it will be shown to regulate functions in many of the tissues in which it is expressed.

1. What is the cellular composition of the parathyroid gland?
2. How do serum albumin concentration and blood pH influence the distribution of calcium into ionized and protein-bound fractions?
3. What is the advantage of two-site immunoassays for PTH?
4. What are the actions of PTH and 1,25-$(OH)_2D$ on bone, kidney, and the gastrointestinal tract?
5. What is the role of PTHrP? How is its action similar to and different from that of PTH?

BONE

Bone has two compartments. On the outside is **cortical** or **compact** bone, which makes up 80% of the skeletal mass. In this dense tissue, the resident bone cells, called **osteocytes,** are deeply buried, communicating and receiving nutrients via a system of haversian canals. Because of the low ratio of surface to volume and the scarcity of osteocytes, cortical bone is remodeled only slowly.

Within the cortex lies the other compartment, **trabecular** or **cancellous** bone, which makes up 20% of skeletal mass. Trabecular bone consists of thin interconnected plates, the trabeculae, which are covered by bone cells. The spaces in this irregular honeycomb are filled with bone marrow—either red marrow, in which hematopoiesis is active, or white marrow, which is mainly fat. Because of its high surface-to-volume ratio and abundant cellular activity, trabecular bone is remodeled more rapidly than cortical bone. To understand the remodeling process, it is important to know something about bone cells.

The **osteoclast** is a multinucleated giant cell that is specialized for resorption of bone. Osteoclasts are terminally differentiated cells that arise continuously from hematopoietic precursors in the monocyte lineage and do not divide. In a process that requires hematopoietic growth factors such as macrophage colony-stimulating factor (M-CSF) and is accelerated by cytokines such as interleukin-6 and by the systemic calciotropic hormones PTH and vitamin D, osteoclast precursors gradually mature, acquire the capacity to produce osteoclast-specific enzymes, and finally fuse to produce the mature multinucleated cell.

To resorb bone, the motile osteoclast alights on a bone surface and seals off an area by forming an adhesive ring in which cellular integrins bind tightly to bone matrix proteins (Figure 17–8). Having isolated an area of bone surface, the osteoclast develops above the surface an elaborately invaginated plasma membrane structure called the **ruffled border.** The

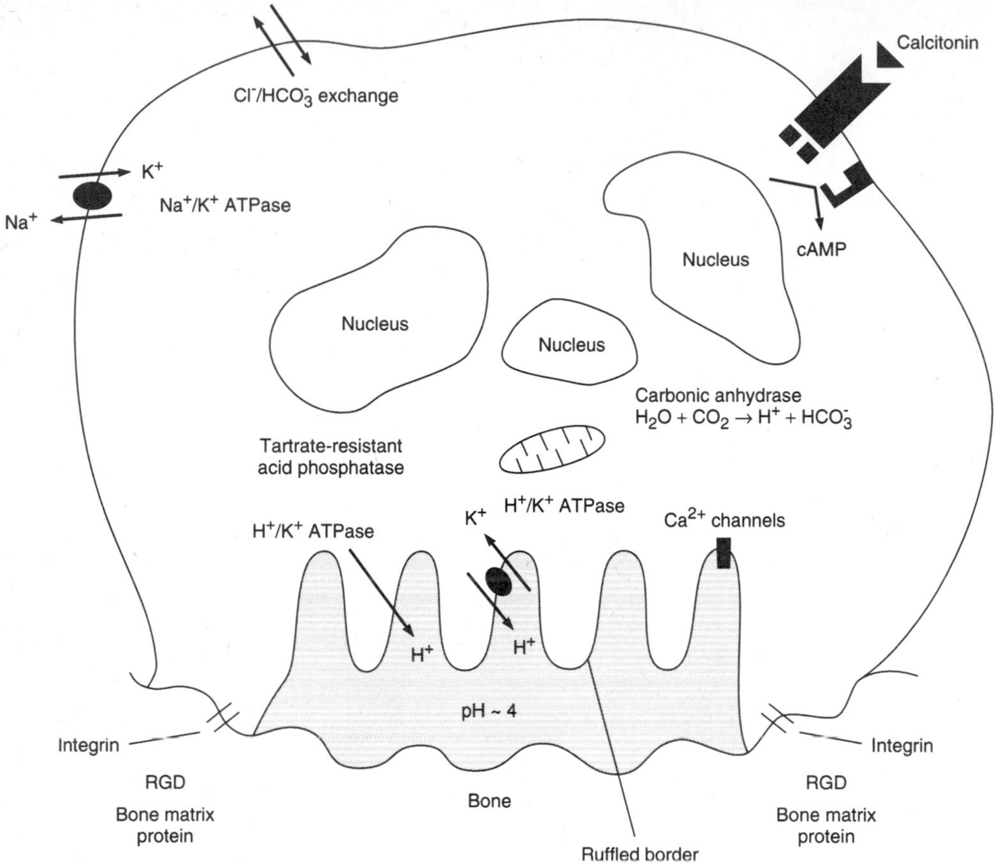

Figure 17–8. Schematic view of an active osteoclast. Calcitonin receptors, the ruffled border, and enzymes and channels involved in secretion of acid onto the bone surface are shown. Integrins are transmembrane-spanning receptors on osteoclasts which bind to determinants (RGD) in bone matrix proteins such as fibronectins. The integrins are responsible for the tight attachment of osteoclasts to the bone surface. (Reproduced, with permission, from Felig P et al [editors]: *Endocrinology and Metabolism,* 3rd ed. McGraw-Hill, 1994.)

ruffled border is a distinctive organelle, but it acts essentially as a huge lysosome, which dissolves bone mineral by secreting acid onto the isolated bone surface, and simultaneously breaks down the bone matrix by secretion of collagenase and catheptic proteases. The resulting collagen peptides have pyridinoline structures that can be assayed in urine as a measure of bone resorption rates. Bone resorption can be controlled in two ways: by regulating the formation of osteoclasts to change their number and by regulating the activity of the mature osteoclast. The mature osteoclast has receptors for calcitonin but does not appear to have PTH or 1,25-$(OH)_2$ vitamin D receptors.

The **osteoblast,** or bone-forming cell, arises from a mesenchymal precursor in the bone marrow stroma. When actively forming bone, the osteoblast is a tall, plump cell with an abundant Golgi apparatus. On active bone-forming surfaces, osteoblasts are found side by side, laying down bone matrix by secreting proteins and proteoglycans. The most important protein of bone matrix is type I collagen, which makes up 90% of bone matrix and is deposited in regular layers that serve as the main scaffold for deposition of minerals. There are many other constituents of bone matrix, including a protein called **osteocalcin** that is unique to bones and teeth and whose serum level is a clinical measure of the rate of bone formation. The **osteocyte** is a resident cell on the bone surface that may be regarded as a relatively inactive osteoblast.

Having laid down bone matrix, the osteoblast now mineralizes it, depositing hydroxyapatite crystals in an orderly array on the collagen layers to produce lamellar bone. The process of mineralization is poorly understood but requires an adequate supply of extracellular calcium and phosphate as well as the enzyme alkaline phosphatase, which is secreted in large amounts by active osteoblasts.

Bone remodeling occurs in an orderly cycle in

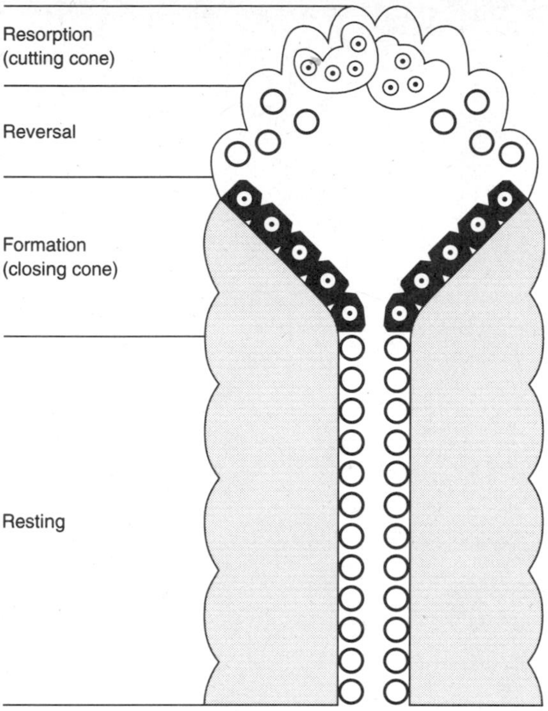

Figure 17–9. A cutting cone remodeling cortical bone. (Reproduced, with permission, from Felig P et al [editors]: *Endocrinology and Metabolism,* 3rd ed. McGraw-Hill, 1994.)

which old bone is first resorbed, and new bone then deposited. Cortical bone is remodeled from within by cutting cones (Figure 17–9), groups of osteoclasts that cut tunnels through the compact bone. They are followed by trailing osteoblasts, lining the tunnels and laying down a cylinder of new bone on their walls, so that the tunnels are progressively narrowed until all that remains are the tiny haversian canals, by which the cells that are left behind as resident osteocytes are fed.

In trabecular bone, the remodeling process occurs on the surface (Figure 17–10). Osteoclasts first excavate a pit, and the pit is then filled in with new bone by osteoblasts. In a normal adult, this cycle takes 200 days. At each remodeling site, bone resorption and new bone formation are ordinarily well coupled, so that in a state of zero net bone balance, the amount of new bone formed is precisely equivalent to the amount of old bone resorbed. This state of perfection is only briefly attained, however. Until the age of 20–30, we are consolidating the gains in bone growth that were achieved during adolescence. After age 30, we begin to lose bone slowly.

How osteoclasts and osteoblasts communicate to achieve the coupling that assures perfect (or near-perfect) bone balance is not fully known. It appears that the important signals are local, not systemic, but they have not been identified. The process of bone remodeling does not absolutely require systemic hormones except to ensure an adequate supply of calcium and phosphate. For example, bone is quite normal in patients with hypoparathyroidism. However, systemic hormones use the bone pool as a source of minerals for regulation of extracellular calcium homeostasis. Osteoblasts have receptors for PTH and 1,25-$(OH)_2$ vitamin D, but osteoclasts do not. Isolated osteoclasts do not respond to PTH or vitamin D except in the presence of osteoblasts. This coupling mechanism makes certain that when bone resorption is activated by PTH--eg, to provide calcium to correct hypocalcemia--bone formation will also increase, tending to replenish lost bone.

6. Describe the two compartments of bone.
7. How is bone resorption by osteoclasts controlled?
8. What is the role of osteoblasts in bone formation?
9. How are the actions of osteoblasts and osteoclasts coupled?

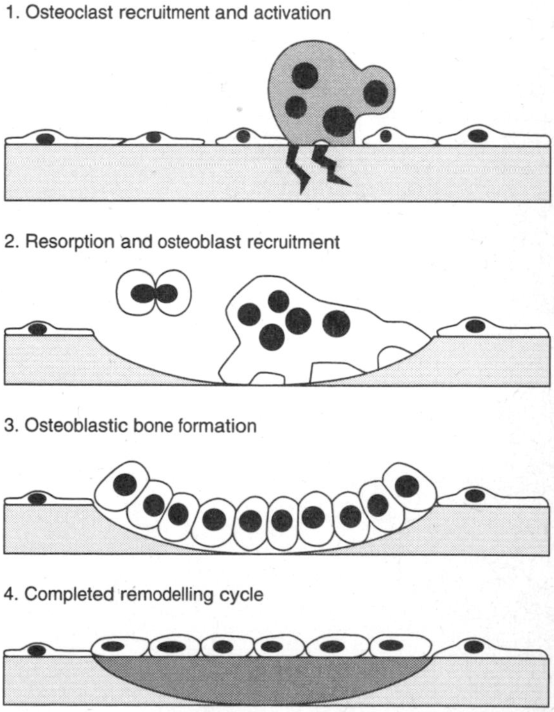

Figure 17–10. Sequential steps in remodeling of trabecular bone. (Reproduced, with permission, from Felig P et al [editors]: *Endocrinology and Metabolism,* 3rd ed. McGraw-Hill, 1994.)

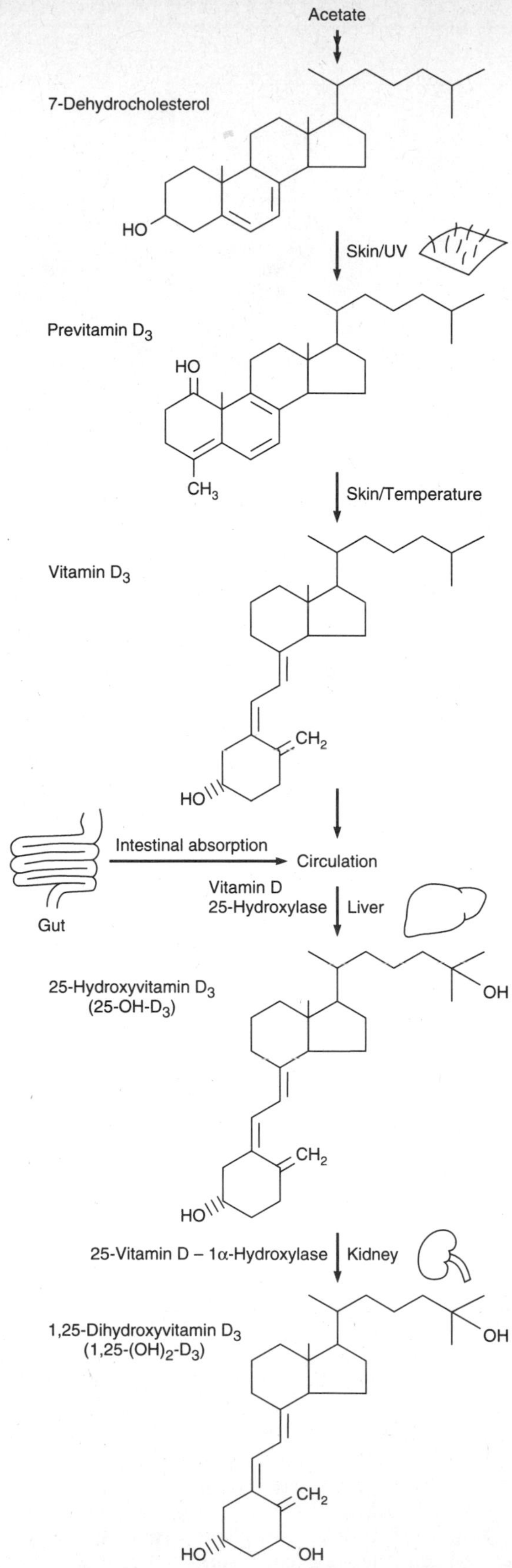

Figure 17–11. The formation and activation of vitamin D. (Reproduced, with permission, from Felig P et al [editors]: *Endocrinology and Metabolism,* 3rd ed. McGraw-Hill, 1994.)

VITAMIN D

Vitamin D is actually a hormone. With exposure to normal amounts of sunlight, we synthesize enough vitamin D in our skin to meet our needs. The only natural source of vitamin D in the diet is in the livers of meat-eating fish, who have simply stored vitamin D they ingested.

Physiology

Cholesterol in skin is metabolized to the vitamin D precursor 7-dehydrocholesterol, which is converted to vitamin D_3 (cholecalciferol) by a nonenzymatic process when skin is subjected to tanning wavelengths of ultraviolet light (Figure 17–11). This step involves breakage of the A ring of cholesterol to produce a sterol; hormones with an intact cholesterol nucleus (eg, estrogen) are called steroids.

Although cutaneous synthesis of vitamin D is often adequate for our needs, persons in northern climates may be borderline deficient in vitamin D at the end of the winter months, and the ill and infirm may not have adequate sunlight exposure. It is therefore recommended that the diet contain 400 IU of vitamin D per day (the RDA). In the United States, milk is supplemented with 400 IU of vitamin D per quart. Dietary supplements of vitamin D often consist of vitamin D_2 (ergocalciferol). Vitamin D_2 and vitamin D_3 are metabolized identically and are equipotent.

Vitamin D formed in the skin is a lipophilic substance that is transported to the liver bound to a specific vitamin D-binding protein. In the liver, vitamin D is hydroxylated to produce 25-hydroxyvitamin D [25-(OH)D] (Figure 17–11). This process, like cutaneous synthesis of vitamin D, is not closely regulated. 25-(OH)D is still rather lipophilic, and it is transported by the serum binding protein to fat stores, where it is the principal storage form of vitamin D. Therefore, the biochemical test for vitamin D deficiency is a measurement of the serum level of 25-(OH)D.

The final metabolic processing step in the synthesis of the active hormone takes place in the kidney. But unlike previous steps, the conversion of 25-(OH)D to 1,25-$(OH)_2$D in the renal cortex is tightly regulated. The synthesis of 1,25-$(OH)_2$D is increased by PTH, thus linking the formation of 1,25-$(OH)_2$D closely to PTH in the integrated control of calcium homeostasis. The production of 1,25-$(OH)_2$D is also stimulated by hypophosphatemia and probably by hypocalcemia. On the other hand, hypercalcemia, hyperphosphatemia, or an excess of 1,25-$(OH)_2$D will decrease the production of 1,25-$(OH)_2$D. The coordinated control by PTH, blood mineral levels, and the vitamin D supply is very efficient. Levels of 1,25-$(OH)_2$D vary little over an enormous range of vitamin D production rates but respond precisely to changes in the intake of calcium and phosphate within the normal range.

Vitamin D Action

The vitamin D receptor is a member of the steroid receptor superfamily of nuclear DNA-binding receptors. Upon ligand binding, the receptor attaches to enhancer sites in target genes and directly regulates their transcription. Thus, many of the effects of vitamin D involve new RNA and protein synthesis. However, the initial steps in stimulation of intestinal calcium transport may involve a nongenomic event. Although many vitamin D metabolites are recognized by the receptor, 1,25-$(OH)_2$D has an affinity approximately 1000-fold greater than that of 25-(OH)D.

The primary target organs for 1,25-$(OH)_2$D are intestine and bone. The most essential action of 1,25-$(OH)_2$D is to stimulate the intestinal transport of calcium. Although some calcium can be absorbed passively over a paracellular route, most calcium absorbed at typical levels of dietary intake is actively transported through the microvilli of intestinal epithelial cells in a process that is induced by 1,25-$(OH)_2$D. 1,25-$(OH)_2$D also induces the active transport of phosphate, but passive absorption dominates this process and the net effect of 1,25-$(OH)_2$D is small.

In bone, 1,25-$(OH)_2$D activates osteoblast synthetic activities and is necessary for normal mineralization of osteoid. However, the defect in mineralization that occurs in vitamin D deficiency may result in large part from decreased delivery of calcium and phosphate to sites of mineralization. 1,25-$(OH)_2$D also stimulates the osteoclast to resorb bone, releasing calcium to maintain extracellular calcium. This is an indirect effect of 1,25-$(OH)_2$D, probably involving stimulation of osteoblasts to release an osteoclast-activating substance.

Now consider a person who switches from a high normal to a low normal intake of calcium and phosphate—from 1200 mg to 300 mg per day of calcium (the equivalent of leaving three glasses of milk out of the diet). The net absorption of calcium falls sharply, causing a transient decrease in the serum calcium level. This activates a homeostatic response led by an increase in PTH. The increased PTH level stimulates the release of calcium from bone and the retention of calcium by the kidney. In addition, the increase in PTH, the fall in calcium, and the concomitant fall in the serum phosphate level (because of both decreased intake and PTH-induced phosphaturia) activate renal 1,25-$(OH)_2$D synthesis. 1,25-$(OH)_2$D increases the fraction of calcium that is absorbed, further increases calcium release from bone, and restores the serum calcium to normal.

10. How is vitamin D produced from cholesterol?
11. Where is vitamin D stored?
12. Where does the final step in activation of vitamin D take place, and how is it regulated?
13. What are the actions of vitamin D?

PARAFOLLICULAR CELLS (C CELLS)

Anatomy & Histology

C cells of the thyroid gland secrete the peptide hormone calcitonin. They constitute 0.1% or less of thyroid cell mass and are distributed in the central parts of the lateral lobes of the thyroid, especially between the upper and middle third of the lobes. C cells are neuroendocrine cells and are derived from the ultimobranchial body. This structure fuses with the thyroid to distribute C cells throughout the gland.

C cells are small spindle-shaped or polygonal cells. They contain abundant granules, mitochondria, and Golgi. They may be present as single cells or arranged in nests, cords, and sheets within the thyroid parenchyma. They are often found within thyroid follicles but are larger than follicular cells. They are identified by argyrophilia, metachromasia, and positive staining for calcitonin by immunoperoxidase methods.

Physiology

Calcitonin is a 32-amino-acid peptide hormone with a seven-membered amino terminal disulfide ring and carboxyl terminal prolineamide (Figure 17–12). Differential processing of the calcitonin gene can lead to the production of either calcitonin or calcitonin gene-related peptide. In C cells, the gene is transcribed so that calcitonin is the secreted product. In contrast, tissue-specific alternative splicing of the calcitonin gene in neurons leads to the production of calcitonin gene-related peptide. Although calcitonin gene-related peptide has cardiovascular and neurologic effects in pharmacologic doses, the function of the peptide in normal physiology is unknown. C cell tumors may release both peptides.

Hypercalcemia stimulates the release of calcitonin. The gastrointestinal hormones cholecystokinin and gastrin are also secretagogues for calcitonin. Substantial changes in serum calcium are normally required to modulate the release of calcitonin. It is not known whether small physiologic changes in serum calcium can elicit significant changes in calcitonin levels.

The assessment of calcitonin secretion in vivo is complicated by the presence in the circulation of oligomeric forms of the hormone as well as of the calcitonin monomer. In some radioimmunoassays, basal calcitonin levels are not detectable in normal people. Calcitonin rises to very high levels in patients with medullary carcinoma of the thyroid, and multiple forms of the hormone may circulate in these patients.

Actions of Calcitonin

Calcitonin interacts with receptors in kidney and bone. This interaction stimulates adenylyl cyclase activity and the generation of cAMP (as shown in Figure 17–5 for PTH). In the kidney, receptors for calcitonin are localized in the cortical ascending limb of Henle's loop, while in bone, calcitonin receptors are found on osteoclasts.

The main function of calcitonin is to lower serum calcium, and this hormone is rapidly released in response to hypercalcemia. Calcitonin inhibits osteoclastic bone resorption and rapidly blocks the release of calcium and phosphate from bone. The latter effect is apparent within minutes after the administration of calcitonin. This effect, along with the inhibition of resorption, ultimately leads to a fall in serum calcium and phosphate.

Calcitonin accomplishes its antiresorptive effect by acting directly on the osteoclast. Calcitonin blocks

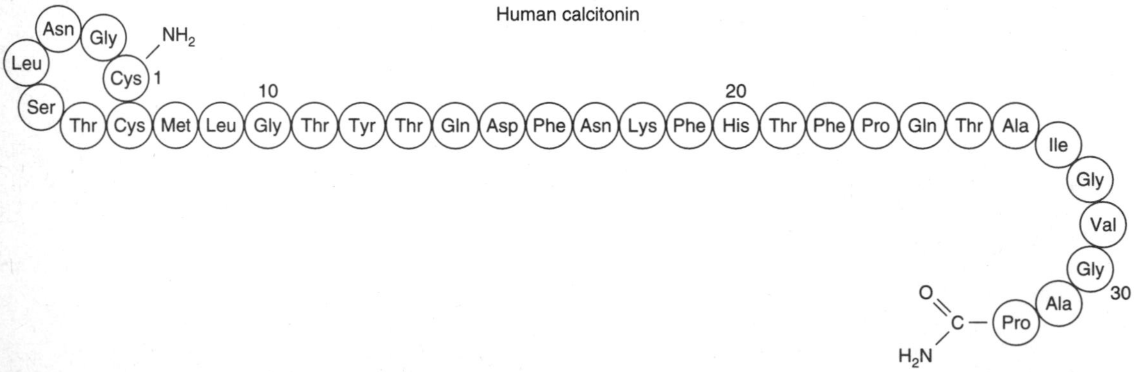

Figure 17–12. Amino acid sequence of human calcitonin, demonstrating its biochemical features, including an amino terminal disulfide bridge and carboxyl terminal prolineamide.

bone resorption induced by a variety of hormones, including PTH and vitamin D. The potency of calcitonin depends on the underlying rate of bone resorption. Calcitonin also has a modest effect on the kidney to produce mild phosphaturia. With prolonged administration of calcitonin, "escape" from its effects occurs.

The overall importance of calcitonin in the maintenance of calcium homeostasis is unclear. Serum calcium concentrations are normal in patients after thyroidectomy, which removes all functioning C cells.

14. What are the actions of calcitonin?
15. What is the effect of thyroidectomy (which also removes all calcitonin-secreting cells) on serum calcium?

PATHOPHYSIOLOGY OF SELECTED DISORDERS OF CALCIUM METABOLISM

PRIMARY & SECONDARY HYPERPARATHYROIDISM

Etiology

Primary hyperparathyroidism is due to excessive production and release of PTH by the parathyroid gland. The recognition of this disorder has increased substantially in the last 30 years as a result of the availability and routine performance of multichannel screening blood calcium analyses. The prevalence of hyperparathyroidism is approximately 1:1000 in the United States, and the incidence of the disease increases with age.

Primary hyperparathyroidism may be caused by any of the following: adenoma, carcinoma, or diffuse hyperplasia (Table 17–1). Chief cell adenomas are the most common cause, accounting for almost 85% of all cases. The vast majority of parathyroid adenomas occur sporadically and affect only a single gland.

Parathyroid hyperplasia classically refers to the enlargement or abnormalities of all four glands. In atypical forms of hyperplasia, only one gland may be enlarged, but the other three glands typically show at least slight microscopic abnormalities such as increased cellularity and reduced fat content. The distinction between hyperplasia and multiple adenomas may be very challenging to the pathologist, and all glands must be examined. The key characteristics for judging whether a gland is normal or not are its size, weight, and cellularity.

Table 17–1. Causes of primary hyperparathyroidism.

Solitary adenomas	80–85%
Hyperplasia	10%
Multiple adenomas	≈2%
Carcinoma	≈2–5%

Parathyroid hyperplasia may be part of the autosomal dominant **multiple endocrine neoplasia (MEN)** syndromes (Table 17–2). In patients with MEN 1, there is high penetrance of hyperparathyroidism, affecting as many as 95% of patients. When these glands are examined microscopically, there are usually abnormalities in all four glands. Recurrent hyperparathyroidism, even after initially successful surgery, is common in these patients. Hyperparathyroidism also occurs in MEN 2a and 2b, though at a much lower frequency in MEN 2a (≈20%) and rarely in MEN 2b. Familial hyperparathyroidism, without other features of MEN, characteristically involves all four glands. There is an increased risk of parathyroid cancer in these kindreds.

Parathyroid carcinoma is a rare malignancy, but the diagnosis should be considered in a patient with severe hypercalcemia and a palpable cervical mass. At surgery, cancers are firmer than adenomas and more likely to be attached to adjacent structures. It is sometimes difficult to distinguish parathyroid carcinomas from adenomas on histopathologic grounds. Vascular or capsular invasion by tumor cells is a good indicator of malignancy, but these features are not always present. In many cases, local recurrences or distant metastases to liver, lung, or bone are the clinical findings that support this diagnosis.

Table 17–2. Clinical features of multiple endocrine neoplasia syndromes.

MEN 1
- Benign parathyroid tumors (very common)
- Pancreatic tumors (benign or malignant)
  - Gastrinoma
  - Insulinoma
  - Glucagonoma, VIPoma (both rare)
- Pituitary tumors
  - Growth hormone-secreting
  - Prolactin-secreting
  - ACTH-secreting
- Other tumors: lipomas, carcinoids, adrenal and thyroid adenomas

MEN 2a
- Medullary carcinoma of the thyroid
- Pheochromocytoma (benign or malignant)
- Hyperparathyroidism

MEN 2b
- Medullary carcinoma of the thyroid
- Pheochromocytoma
- Mucosal neuromas, ganglioneuromas
- Marfanoid habitus
- Hyperparathyroidism (very rare)

Secondary hyperparathyroidism implies diffuse glandular hyperplasia due to a defect outside the parathyroids. Secondary hyperparathyroidism in patients with normal kidney function may be observed in patients with severe calcium and vitamin D deficiency states (see below). In patients with chronic renal failure, there are many causative factors that contribute to the often dramatic enlargement of the parathyroid glands. These include decreased 1,25-$(OH)_2D$ production, reduced intestinal calcium absorption, skeletal resistance to PTH, and renal phosphate retention. In most cases of secondary hyperparathyroidism, parathyroid hyperplasia regresses substantially with correction of the underlying abnormality.

Pathogenesis

PTH secretion in primary hyperparathyroidism is excessive, given the level of the serum calcium. At the cellular level, there is both increased cell mass and a secretory defect. The latter is characterized by reduced sensitivity of PTH secretion to suppression by the serum calcium concentration. This type of qualitative regulatory defect is more common than truly autonomous secretion. Thus, parathyroid glands from patients with primary hyperparathyroidism are typically enlarged and, in vitro, demonstrate a "shift to the right" in their calcium set-point for secretion (Figure 17–13). How these two potential defects interact in the pathogenesis of the disease remains to be fully elucidated.

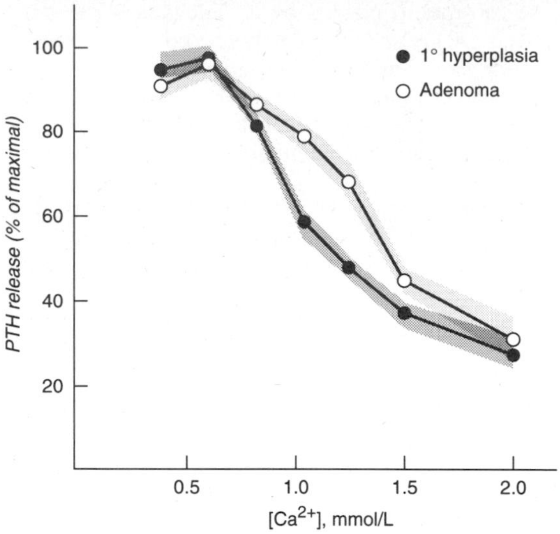

Figure 17–13. PTH secretion in vitro from human parathyroid cells from patients with parathyroid adenomas and hyperplasia. The set-point for secretion is the calcium concentration at which PTH release is suppressed by 50%. This is shifted to the right in the majority of parathyroid adenomas compared to normal tissues, in which the set-point is approximately 1.0 mmol/L ionized calcium. (Reproduced, with permission, from Brown EM et al: Dispersed cells prepared from human parathyroid glands: Distinct calcium sensitivity of adenomas vs primary hyperplasia. J Clin Endocrinol Metab 1978;46:267.)

The genetic defects responsible for primary hyperparathyroidism have received considerable attention. Genes that regulate the cell cycle are thought to be important in the pathogenesis of parathyroid tumors. The *PRAD 1* gene (*p*arathyroid *r*earrangement *ad*enoma), whose product is a D1 cyclin, has been implicated in parathyroid tumor development. Cyclins are cell cycle regulatory proteins. The *PRAD 1* gene is located on the long arm of chromosome 11, as is the gene encoding for PTH. Analysis of parathyroid tumor DNA suggests that a chromosome inversion event occurred which lead to the juxtaposition of the 5′-regulatory domain of the PTH gene upstream to the *PRAD 1* gene (Figure 17–14). Because regulatory sequences in the PTH gene are responsible for its cell-specific transcription, this inversion could lead to abnormally regulated transcription of the *PRAD 1* gene in a parathyroid cell-specific manner. Overproduction of the *PRAD 1* gene product, a cyclin, would enhance the proliferative potential of the cell bearing this inversion. Increased proliferation could lead to a clonal outgrowth of the original cell with the inversion. Approximately 5% of sporadic parathyroid adenomas are thought to be related to overexpression of the *PRAD 1* gene. *PRAD 1* has also been implicated in the pathogenesis of B cell lymphomas, breast and lung cancers, and squamous cell cancers of the head and neck.

The *MEN 1* gene has also been localized to the long arm of chromosome 11 and is postulated to encode for an as yet unidentified tumor-suppressor protein. Patients at risk for MEN 1 are thought to inherit an abnormal or inactivated *MEN 1* allele from one parent. This is a germ cell line defect and is present in all cells. During postnatal life, the other *MEN 1* allele in a parathyroid cell (for example) undergoes spontaneous mutation. If this second mutation confers a growth advantage to the descendant cells, there is clonal outgrowth of cells bearing the second mutation, and eventually a tumor results. The pathogenesis of hyperparathyroidism in either MEN 2a or MEN 2b is not established, but it is likely that the Ret protein, which plays an important role in the pathogenesis of the other endocrine tumors in these syndromes, plays a role (see below).

In approximately 25% of nonfamilial benign parathyroid adenomas, there is allelic loss of DNA from chromosome 11, which is where the putative *MEN 1* gene is mapped. While the *MEN 1* gene is a good candidate in the pathogenesis of benign

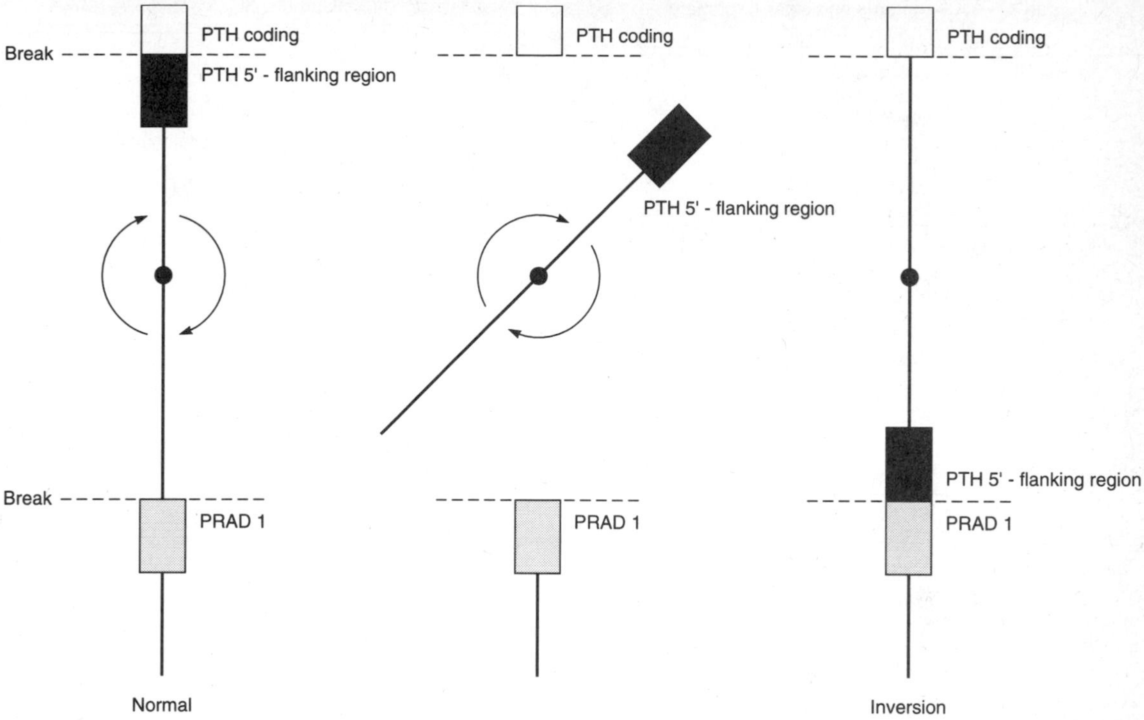

Figure 17–14. Proposed genetic rearrangement of chromosome 11 in a subset of sporadic parathyroid adenomas. An inversion of DNA sequence near the centromere of chromosome 11 places the 5′-regulatory region of the PTH gene (also on chromosome 11) adjacent to the *PRAD 1* gene, which is involved in cell cycle control. This places the *PRAD 1* gene under the control of PTH regulatory sequences, which would be predicted to be highly active in parathyroid cells. (Modified and reproduced, with permission, from Arnold A: Molecular genetics of parathyroid gland neoplasia. J Clin Endocrin Metabol 1993;77:1109.)

parathyroid tumors, there are probably other genes, such as the recently identified calcium sensor, that also play a role in this process.

Clinical Manifestations

Hyperparathyroidism may present in a variety of ways. Patients with this disease may be truly asymptomatic, and their diagnosis is made by screening laboratory tests. Other patients may have skeletal complications or nephrolithiasis. Because calcium affects the functioning of nearly every organ system, the symptoms and signs of hypercalcemia are protean (see Table 17–3). Depending on the nature of the complaints, the patient with primary hyperparathyroidism may be suspected of having a psychiatric disorder or even a malignancy.

Hyperparathyroidism is a chronic disorder in which long-standing PTH excess and hypercalcemia may produce increasing symptomatology, especially those related to renal stones and worsening osteopenia. Recurrent stones containing calcium phosphate or calcium oxalate occur in 10–15% of patients with primary hyperparathyroidism. Nephrolithiasis may be complicated by urinary outflow tract obstruction, infection, and progressive renal insufficiency. Patients with significant PTH excess may experience increased bone turnover and progressive loss of bone mineral. This is reflected in subperiosteal resorption, osteoporosis (particularly of cortical bone), and even pathologic fractures.

A sizable proportion of patients with primary hyperparathyroidism, however, are asymptomatic. These patients may experience no clinical deterioration if their hyperparathyroidism is followed and not treated surgically. Because it is difficult to identify these patients with certainty when the diagnosis of hyperparathyroidism is made, regular follow-up is mandatory. A minority of asymptomatic patients experience skeletal or renal deterioration, which is an indication for surgery.

Radiologic features of primary hyperparathyroidism are caused by the chronic effects of excess PTH on bone and kidney. These include subperiosteal resorption (evident most strikingly in the clavicles and distal phalanges), generalized osteopenia, and the characteristic but now rare

Table 17–3. Symptoms and signs of primary hyperparathyroidism.

Systemic	Weakness Easy fatigue Weight loss Anemia Anorexia Pruritus Ectopic calcifications
Neuropsychiatric	Depression Poor concentration Memory deficits Peripheral sensory neuropathy Motor neuropathy Proximal and generalized muscle weakness
Ocular	Band keratopathy
Cardiac	Shortened Q–T interval Hypertension
Renal	Stones Polyuria, polydipsia Metabolic acidosis Concentrating defects Nephrocalcinosis
Skeletal	Osteopenia Pathological fractures Brown tumors of bone Bone pain Gout Pseudogout Chondrocalcinosis Osteitis fibrosa cystica
Gastrointestinal	Peptic ulcer disease Pancreatitis Constipation Nausea Vomiting

Table 17–4. Differential diagnosis of hypercalcemia.

Primary hyperparathyroidism
Adenoma
Carcinoma
Hyperplasia
Familial (benign) hypocalciuric hypercalcemia
Malignancy-associated hypercalcemia
Solid tumors (majority with excess PTHrP production)
Multiple myeloma
Adult T cell leukemia and lymphoma
Other lymphomas
Thyrotoxicosis
Drugs
Thiazides
Lithium
Vitamin D or A intoxication
Granulomatous diseases
Sarcoidosis
Tuberculosis
Histoplasmosis (and other fungal diseases)
Milk-alkali syndrome
Adrenal insufficiency

brown tumors. Uncommonly, osteosclerosis may result from excessive PTH action on bone. Abdominal films may show nephrocalcinosis or nephrolithiasis.

The complete differential diagnosis of hypercalcemia should be considered in all patients with this abnormality (Table 17–4). Primary hyperparathyroidism accounts for most cases of hypercalcemia in the outpatient setting. The diagnosis of primary hyperparathyroidism is confirmed by at least two simultaneous measurements of calcium and immunoreactive PTH, preferably by an assay for intact PTH. An elevated or inappropriately normal PTH in the setting of hypercalcemia is the key feature in making the diagnosis of primary hyperparathyroidism (Table 17–5).

In the asymptomatic patient with elevated serum calcium and a normal or even mildly elevated PTH level, the possibility of familial hypocalciuric hypercalcemia must be considered. In this autosomal dominant disorder, patients have lifelong asymptomatic and usually mild hypercalcemia. They do not, however, suffer the consequences of end-organ dysfunction that is characteristic of hyperparathyroidism. This disorder is thought to be due to a defect in the membrane calcium ion sensing mechanism (ie, the calcium receptor). In the asymptomatic hypercalcemic patient, urinary calcium and creatinine excretion should be measured to rule out the possibility of familial hypocalciuric hypercalcemia. In familial hypocalciuric hypercalcemia, the urinary calcium levels are typically low and less than 100 mg/24 h (Table 17–5), or the calcium/creatinine clearance ratio is below 0.01.

In contrast to familial hypocalciuric hypercalcemia and other causes of hypercalcemia, urinary calcium levels vary from low to markedly elevated in patients with primary hyperparathyroidism. Although calcium excretion depends on the filtered load of calcium, urinary calcium in patients with primary hyperparathyroidism is lower—relative to the level of hypercalcemia—than in other hypercalcemic conditions. This is due to the distal tubular effect of PTH to enhance calcium reabsorption.

Patients with secondary hyperparathyroidism may have normal or subnormal calcium levels (see below). If renal function is normal, serum phosphate is also often reduced. Although serum PTH is elevated, the demineralized state of the bone and the chronic vitamin D deficiency combine to produce a low filtered load of calcium. Hence, urinary calcium excretion is often quite low. The 25-(OH)D level will also be low or undetectable in vitamin D deficiency states due to a variety of causes.

Table 17–5. Laboratory findings in hypercalcemia due to various causes.

	Serum Ca^{2+}	Serum PO_4^{3-}	Intact PTH	PTHrP	Urine Ca^{2+}
Primary hyperparathyroidism	↑	↓, N	↑	N, Und	N, ↑[1]
Malignancy-associated hypercalcemia	↑	↓, N	Und	↑[2]	↑
Familial (benign) hypocalciuric hypercalcemia	↑	N	N, ↑[3]	Und	↓

Key: N = normal; Und = undetectable
[1]Can also be low depending on the filtered load of calcium.
[2]In the 70–80% of patients with cancer and a humoral basis for hypercalcemia.
[3]Mild increases in PTH have been reported in some patients.

16. What is the most common cause of primary hyperparathyroidism?
17. What is the relationship of hyperparathyroidism to the multiple endocrine neoplasia (MEN) syndromes?
18. In what conditions does secondary hyperparathyroidism occur? By what symptoms and signs is it distinguished from primary hyperparathyroidism?
19. What are the common symptoms and signs of primary hyperparathyroidism?
20. How can primary hyperparathyroidism be distinguished from familial hypocalciuric hypercalcemia? What is the mechanism for this difference?

HYPERCALCEMIA OF MALIGNANCY

Etiology

Hypercalcemia occurs in approximately 10% of all malignancies. It is most commonly seen in solid tumors, particularly squamous cell carcinomas (lung, esophagus, etc), renal carcinoma, and breast carcinoma. Hypercalcemia occurs in over one-third of patients with multiple myeloma but is unusual in lymphomas and leukemias.

Pathogenesis

Solid tumors usually produce hypercalcemia by secreting PTHrP, whose properties have been described above. This is humoral hypercalcemia, which mimics primary hyperparathyroidism and results from a diffuse increase in bone resorption induced by high circulating levels of PTHrP and exacerbated by the effect of PTHrP to reduce renal excretion of calcium.

Multiple myeloma produces hypercalcemia by a different mechanism; myeloma cells induce local bone resorption or osteolysis in the bone marrow, probably by releasing cytokines with bone-resorbing activity, such as interleukin-1 and tumor necrosis factor. Rarely, lymphomas produce humoral hypercalcemia by secreting 1,25-$(OH)_2D$.

Finally, even though many hypercalcemic patients have bone metastases, these may not contribute directly to the pathogenesis of hypercalcemia.

Clinical Manifestations

Unlike patients with primary hyperparathyroidism, who often are minimally symptomatic, patients with hypercalcemia of malignancy are typically very ill. Hypercalcemia typically occurs in advanced malignancy—the average survival of hypercalcemic patients is only 6 weeks—and the tumor is almost invariably obvious. In addition, hypercalcemia is often severe and symptomatic, with nausea, vomiting, dehydration, confusion, or coma. Biochemically, malignancy-associated hypercalcemia is characterized by a decreased serum phosphate and a suppressed level of intact PTH (Table 17–5). With most solid tumors, the serum level of PTHrP is increased. These findings, together with the differences in clinical presentation, usually make the differentiation of this syndrome from primary hyperparathyroidism relatively easy.

21. What tumors commonly result in hypercalcemia?
22. What are the mechanisms by which a tumor may cause hypercalcemia?
23. What are the clinical symptoms and signs of hypercalcemia of malignancy?

HYPOPARATHYROIDISM & PSEUDOHYPOPARATHYROIDISM

Etiology

The total serum calcium measured in the clinical setting includes the contribution from ionized, protein-bound, and complexed forms of calcium. It should be recognized, however, that symptoms of

Table 17–6. Differential diagnosis of hypocalcemia.

Failure to secrete PTH
Hypoparathyroidism (see Table 17–7)
Resistance to PTH action
Pseudohypoparathyroidism (types 1a, 1b, 2)
Sepsis-associated hypocalcemia
Failure to secrete PTH and resistance to PTH action
Chronic magnesium depletion due to—
Diarrhea, malabsorption
Alcoholism
Drugs: aminoglycoside antibiotics, loop diuretics, cisplatin, amphotericin B
Parenteral nutrition
Primary renal wasting
Failure to produce 1,25-$(OH)_2D$
Vitamin D deficiency due to—
Nutritional causes
Liver disease
Cholestasis
Small intestinal disorders producing malabsorption
Renal failure
Vitamin D dependent rickets type 1 defective 1α-hydroxylase activity (very rare)
Tumor-induced osteomalacia
Resistance to 1,25-$(OH)_2D$ action
Vitamin D-dependent rickets type 2: defect in vitamin D receptor (rare)
Acute challenges to the homeostatic mechanisms
Pancreatitis (formation of calcium salts in retroperitoneal fat)
Drug-induced EDTA, citrate, plicamycin, bisphosphonates, phosphate, foscarnet
Liver transplantation (citrate is not metabolized, thereby increasing calcium citrate complexation and lowering ionized calcium)
Rhabdomyolysis
Hungry bone syndrome (increased deposition into demineralized bone)
Osteoblastic metastases (eg, breast or prostate cancer)
Tumor lysis syndrome (acute phosphate load released from tumor cells due to cytolytic therapy)

hypocalcemia occur only if the ionized fraction of calcium is reduced. Furthermore, only patients with low ionized calcium levels should be evaluated for the possibility of a hypocalcemic disorder.

A common cause of hypocalcemia measured in the clinical setting is hypoalbuminemia. A low serum albumin lowers only the protein-bound and not the ionized calcium. Thus, such patients need not be evaluated for mineral disorders. To determine whether a hypoalbuminemic patient has a low ionized calcium, this parameter can be measured directly. If this laboratory test is not readily available, a reasonable alternative is to correct the total serum calcium for the low serum albumin. This is done by adjusting the serum calcium upward by 0.8 mg/dL for each 1 g/dL reduction in serum albumin. This simple correction usually brings the adjusted serum calcium into the normal range.

The differential diagnosis of a low ionized calcium is lengthy (see Table 17–6). Hypocalcemia can result from reduced PTH secretion due to **hypoparathyroidism** or hypomagnesemia. It can be due to decreased end-organ responsiveness to PTH, despite adequate or even excessive levels of the hormone. This is termed **pseudohypoparathyroidism.**

All forms of hypoparathyroidism are uncommon (Table 17–7). Most cases are the result of inadvertent trauma to, removal of, or devascularization of the parathyroid glands during thyroid or parathyroid surgery. The incidence of postoperative hypoparathyroidism (range: 0.2–30%) depends on the extent of the antecedent surgery and the surgeon's skill in identifying normal parathyroid tissue and preserving its blood supply. Postoperative hypocalcemia may be transient or permanent. Some patients may also be left with diminished parathyroid reserve.

There are a variety of causes other than postsurgical complications which may produce an absolute or functional state of PTH deficiency (see Table 17–7). These include autoimmune glandular failure; magnesium depletion; autosomal dominant or recessive or X-linked hypoparathyroidism; and hypoparathyroidism due to iron overload or Wilson's disease. Rarely, there is congenital absence of the parathyroid glands **(DiGeorge syndrome),** which presents in infancy or childhood accompanied by a defect in cell-mediated immunity.

Two syndromes of **autoimmune polyglandular failure** have been recognized. Patients with type 1 polyglandular failure commonly have mucocutaneous candidiasis, Addison's disease (adrenal insufficiency), and hypoparathyroidism. These disorders typically present by the teens or early twenties (Figure 17–15). Autoantibodies to adrenal and parathyroid tissue are seen in the majority of these patients. Eventually, other endocrine glands may become involved (eg, the gonads, thyroid, and pancreas). Type 2 polyglandular failure syndrome **(Schmidt's syndrome)** is characterized by hypothyroidism and adrenal insufficiency and does not classically involve the parathyroid glands. Certain other rare congenital syndromes have hypoparathyroidism as one of their features (see Table 17–7).

Pathogenesis

The pathogenesis of hypoparathyroidism in most cases is straightforward. The mineral disturbance

Table 17–7. Causes of hypoparathyroidism.

Postsurgical
Autoimmune
Post-^{131}I therapy for Graves' disease or thyroid cancer
Secondary to iron overload, Wilson's disease
DiGeoge syndrome: autosomal recessive disorder with congenital absence of parathyroid glands and thymic dysgenesis or agenesis
Hereditary forms of hypoparathyroidism: autosomal dominant or recessive and X-linked recessive
Secondary to magnesium depletion
Tumor invasion (very rare)
Kearns-Sayre and Kenny syndromes
Hereditary nephrosis, nerve deafness, and hypoparathyroidism

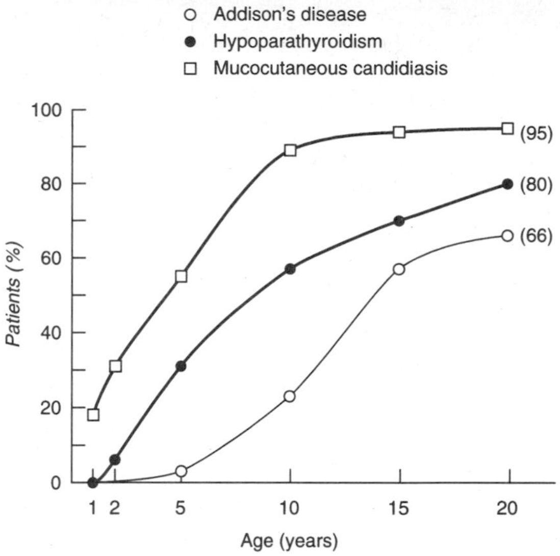

Figure 17–15. Cumulative incidence of three common manifestations of autoimmune polyglandular failure type 1 compared with age at onset in a cohort of 68 patients. (Data plotted from Ahonen P et al: Clinical variation of autoimmune polyendocrinopathy-candidiasis-ectodermal dystrophy [APECED] in a series of 68 patients. N Engl J Med 1990;26:1829.)

occurs because the amount of PTH released is inadequate to maintain normal serum calcium concentrations, and hypocalcemia results. Hyperphosphatemia is also observed in these patients because the proximal tubular effect of PTH to promote phosphate excretion is lost. Since PTH is required to stimulate the renal production of 1,25-$(OH)_2D$, levels of 1,25-$(OH)_2D$ are low in patients with hypoparathyroidism. Hyperphosphatemia further suppresses 1,25-$(OH)_2D$ synthesis. Low 1,25-$(OH)_2D$ levels lead to reduced intestinal calcium absorption. In the absence of adequate 1,25-$(OH)_2D$ and PTH, the mobilization of calcium from bone is abnormal. Since less PTH is available to act in the distal nephron, urinary calcium excretion may be high, especially in view of the hypocalcemia. A combination of these mechanisms contributes to the mineral disturbances seen in hypoparathyroid patients.

Magnesium depletion is a common cause of hypocalcemia. The pathogenesis of hypocalcemia in this clinical setting relates to a functional and reversible state of hypoparathyroidism. There is also decreased renal and skeletal responsiveness to PTH. Magnesium depletion may occur as a result of a variety of causes, including chronic alcoholism, diarrhea, and drugs such as loop diuretics, aminoglycoside antibiotics, amphotericin B, and cisplatin (Table 17–6). Magnesium is required to maintain normal PTH secretory responses. Once body magnesium stores are repleted, PTH levels rise appropriately in response to the hypocalcemia, and the mineral imbalance is corrected.

In **pseudohypoparathyroidism,** there are adequate levels of PTH in the circulation, but the ability of target tissues (kidney and bone) to respond to the hormone is subnormal. In type 1 pseudohypoparathyroidism, the ability of PTH to generate an increase in the second-messenger cAMP is reduced. In some patients, this is due to a deficiency in the cellular content of the alpha subunit of the stimulatory G protein (Gs-α) which couples the PTH receptor to the adenylyl cyclase enzyme (type 1a). In other patients with pseudohypoparathyroidism, Gs-α protein levels are normal, and another as yet unknown component in the PTH receptor–G protein–adenylyl cyclase complex is defective (type 1b). In patients with type 2 pseudohypoparathyroidism, urinary cAMP is normal, but the phosphaturic response to infused PTH is reduced. The pathogenesis of this more rare form of PTH resistance remains obscure.

Clinical Manifestations

The signs and symptoms of hypocalcemia are similar regardless of the underlying cause for the disturbance (see Table 17–8). Patients may be asymptomatic or may have latent or overt tetany. **Tetany** is defined as spontaneous tonic muscular contractions. Painful carpal spasms and laryngeal stridor are striking manifestations of tetany. Latent tetany may be demonstrated by testing for Chvostek's and Trousseau's signs. **Chvostek's sign** is elicited by

Table 17–8. Symptoms and signs of hypocalcemia.

Systemic	Confusion Weakness Mental retardation Behavioral changes
Neuromuscular	Paresthesias Psychosis Seizures Carpopedal spasms Chvostek's and Trousseau's signs Depression Muscle cramping Parkinsonism Irritability Basal ganglia calcifications
Cardiac	Prolonged Q–T interval T wave changes Congestive heart failure
Ocular	Cataracts
Dental	Enamel hypoplasia of teeth Defective root formation Failure of adult teeth to erupt
Respiratory	Laryngospasm Bronchospasm Stridor

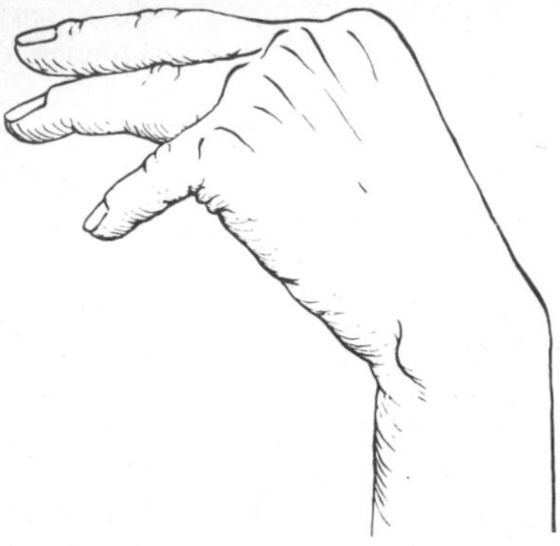

Figure 17–16. Position of fingers in carpal spasm due to hypocalcemic tetany. (Reproduced, with permission, from Ganong WF: *Review of Medical Physiology,* 16th ed. Appleton & Lange, 1993.)

tapping on the facial nerve anterior to the ear. Twitching of the ipsilateral facial muscles indicates a positive test. A positive **Trousseau sign** is demonstrated by inflating the sphygmomanometer above the systolic blood pressure for 3 minutes. In hypocalcemic individuals, painful carpal muscle contractions and spasms occur (Figure 17–16). If hypocalcemia is severe and unrecognized, airway compromise, generalized seizures, and even death may occur.

Chronic hypocalcemia can produce intracranial calcifications that have a predilection for the basal ganglia. These may be detectable by CT scanning or MRI or in some cases by plain skull radiographs. Chronic hypocalcemia may also enhance calcification of the lens and the formation of cataracts.

In addition to the symptoms and signs of hypocalcemia, patients with pseudohypoparathyroidism type 1a may have a constellation of features collectively known as **Albright's hereditary osteodystrophy.** These include short stature, obesity, mental retardation, brachycephaly, shortened fourth and fifth metacarpal and metatarsal bones, and subcutaneous ossifications. How these phenotypic features are related to the underlying molecular defect has not yet been explained.

In considering the differential diagnosis of hypocalcemia, one must be guided by the clinical setting. A positive family history can be very important in supporting a diagnosis of pseudohypoparathyroidism, autoimmune polyglandular failure, or other hereditary forms of hypoparathyroidism. The patient with hypocalcemia, hyperphosphatemia, and a normal serum creatinine most likely has hypoparathyroidism. A history of neck surgery or radiation should be sought. Clearly, there may be a long latent period before symptomatic hypocalcemia presents, even in postsurgical hypoparathyroidism. The physical examination can be helpful if it is directed toward identifying signs of hypocalcemia, stigmas of Albright's hereditary osteodystrophy, or other features of autoimmune polyglandular failure (eg, vitiligo, mucocutaneous candidiasis). Patients with pseudohypoparathyroidism and Albright's hereditary osteodystrophy often have other endocrine abnormalities such as primary hypothyroidism or gonadal failure.

In the differential diagnosis of disorders that present with hypocalcemia, laboratory findings are extremely useful (Table 17–9). Serum phosphate is often (not invariably) elevated in hypoparathyroidism and pseudohypoparathyroidism. In magnesium depletion, serum phosphate is usually normal. In secondary hyperparathyroidism not due to renal failure, serum phosphate is typically low. Serum PTH levels are crucial in determining the cause of hypocalcemia. PTH is classically elevated in untreated pseudohypoparathyroidism but not in hypoparathyroidism or magnesium depletion. Intact PTH may be undetectable, low, or normal in patients with hypoparathyroidism depending on the parathyroid functional reserve. In patients with secondary hyperparathyroidism due to defects in the production or bioavailability of vitamin D, the clinical setting often suggests a problem with vitamin D (eg, regional enteritis, bowel resection, liver disease). The presence

Table 17–9. Laboratory findings in hypocalcemia.

	Serum Ca^{2+}	Serum PO_4^{3-}	Intact PTH	25-(OH)D	Urinary cAMP Response to PTH Infusion
Hypoparathyroidism	↓	↑, N	↓, N[1]	N	N
Pseudohypoparathyroidism	↓	↑, N	↑	N	↓
Magnesium depletion	↓	N	↓, N[1]	N	N
Secondary hyperparathyroidism[2]	↓	N, ↓	↑	↓	N

[1]May be normal, but inappropriate to level of serum calcium.
[2]Due to vitamin D deficiency, for example; urinary calcium excretion usually less than 50 mg/24 h.

of a low 25-(OH)D level and an increased PTH confirms this diagnosis.

Measurement of serum magnesium is the first step in ruling out magnesium depletion as the cause of hypocalcemia and should be part of the initial evaluation. If urinary magnesium is inappropriately high relative to the serum magnesium, renal magnesium wasting is present. PTH levels in this setting are typically low or normal. Normal PTH levels, however, are inappropriate in the presence of hypocalcemia.

The diagnosis of pseudohypoparathyroidism can be confirmed by infusing synthetic human PTH(1–34) and measuring urinary cAMP and phosphate responses. This maneuver is designed to prove that there is end-organ resistance to PTH and to determine whether the diagnosis is pseudohypoparathyroidism type 1 or type 2.

Hypoparathyroidism may vary in its severity and therefore in the need for therapy. In some patients with decreased parathyroid reserve, only situations of increased stress on the glands, such as pregnancy or lactation, induce hypocalcemia. In other patients, PTH deficiency is a chronic symptomatic disorder necessitating lifelong therapy with calcium supplements and vitamin D analogues. All patients so treated should have periodic monitoring of serum calcium, urinary calcium, and renal function. Patients with autoimmune hypoparathyroidism should also be examined regularly for the development of adrenal insufficiency, hypothyroidism, and diabetes mellitus as well as other complications of the type 1 polyglandular failure syndrome.

The clinical course of patients with pseudohypoparathyroidism is variable. Many patients require chronic treatment with calcium supplementation and vitamin D analogues. Others, however, undergo spontaneous remission of the mineral disorder, become normocalcemic, and can discontinue therapy for extended periods of time. It is not known why these remissions occur.

24. What are the causes of hypoparathyroidism?
25. What is the mechanism of pseudohypoparathyroidism?
26. What are the symptoms and signs of hypocalcemia?
27. How can laboratory studies be used to distinguish various causes of hypocalcemia?

MEDULLARY CARCINOMA OF THE THYROID

Etiology

Medullary carcinoma of the thyroid gland, a C cell neoplasm, accounts for only 5–10% of all thyroid malignancies. Approximately 80% are sporadic and 20% are familial, occurring in autosomal dominant MEN 2a and MEN 2b and in non-MEN syndromes. In sporadic cases, the tumor is usually unilateral. In hereditary forms, however, tumors are often bilateral and multifocal. The most common location for these tumors is at the junctions of the middle and upper lobes of the thyroid gland—sites of the greatest number of C cells.

Pathogenesis

The growth pattern of medullary carcinoma is slow but progressive, and local invasion of adjacent structures is not uncommon. The tumor spreads hematogenously, with metastases typically to lymph nodes, bone, and lung. The clinical progression of this cancer is variable. While there may be early metastases to cervical and mediastinal lymph nodes in as many as 50–70% of patients, the tumor still usually behaves in an indolent fashion. In a minority of cases, a more aggressive pattern of tumor growth has been noted. Early detection in high-risk individuals, such as those with a family history of medullary carcinoma or MEN 2a or 2b, is crucial to prevent advanced disease and distant metastases. Overall survival is estimated to be 80% at 5 years and 60% at 10 years.

Patients with MEN 2 develop medullary carcinoma at frequencies approaching 100%. C cell hyperplasia typically precedes the development of cancer. In MEN 2a and 2b, the thyroid lesions are malignant. In contrast, pheochromocytomas associated with either MEN 2a or MEN 2b are infrequently malignant. Hyperparathyroidism in MEN 2a, which is uncommon, is usually due to diffuse hyperplasia and not to a malignancy. Chronic hypercalcitoninemia as a result of the tumor may also contribute to the pathogenesis of parathyroid hyperplasia. Parathyroid hyperplasia is rarely seen in patients with either MEN 2b or sporadic medullary carcinoma.

Germline abnormalities on chromosome 10 have been linked to the three familial forms of medullary carcinoma. Recently, several investigators have identified mutations in the *RET* proto-oncogene, located in the pericentromeric region of chromosome 10, in familial medullary carcinoma, MEN 2a, and MEN 2b. The Ret protein is a membrane-spanning tyrosine kinase that is thought to function in signal transduction, but its exact role in the pathogenesis of medullary carcinoma is not yet clear.

Clinical Manifestations

Sporadic medullary carcinoma occurs with about equal frequency in males and females and is typically found in patients over 50 years of age. In MEN 2a or 2b, the tumor occurs at a much younger age, often in childhood. In fact, medullary carcinoma in a patient under age 40 should suggest that the patient may be an index case of familial medullary carcinoma or MEN 2a or 2b. Medullary carcinoma may present as a single nodule or as multiple thyroid nodules.

Patients with sporadic medullary carcinoma often have palpable cervical lymphadenopathy.

Since C cells are neuroendocrine cells, these tumors have the capacity to release calcitonin and other hormones such as prostaglandins, serotonin, adrenocorticotropin, somatostatin, and calcitonin gene-related peptide. Serotonin, calcitonin, or the prostaglandins have been implicated in the pathogenesis of the secretory diarrhea observed in approximately 20–30% of patients with medullary carcinoma. If diarrhea is present, this usually indicates a large tumor burden or metastatic disease. Patients may also have flushing, which has been ascribed to the production by the tumor of substance P or calcitonin gene-related peptide, both of which are vasodilators.

In a patient suspected of having medullary carcinoma, a radionuclide thyroid scan may demonstrate one or more cold nodules. These nodules are solid by ultrasound. Fine-needle aspiration biopsy will show the characteristic C cell lesion with positive immunostaining for calcitonin. Surprisingly, the diagnosis of medullary carcinoma is not suspected preoperatively in most cases and is made instead by frozen section at the time of surgery. The tumor has the propensity to contain large calcifications, which can be seen on x-rays of the neck. Bone metastases may be lytic or sclerotic in their appearance, and pulmonary metastases may be surrounded by fibrotic reactions.

The most important laboratory test in determining the presence and extent of medullary carcinoma is the calcitonin level. Circulating calcitonin levels are typically elevated in most patients, and serum levels correlate with tumor burden. In C cell hyperplasia, basal calcitonin may or may not be elevated. These patients will usually, however, demonstrate abnormal provocative testing. Intravenous calcium gluconate (2 mg/kg of elemental calcium) is injected over 1 minute, followed by pentagastrin (0.5 μg/kg) over 5 seconds. Provocative testing is based on the ability of calcium and the synthetic gastrin analogue pentagastrin to hyperstimulate calcitonin release in a patient with increased C cell mass, due either to hyperplasia or to carcinoma. A greater than twofold increase in serum calcitonin above the normal response is considered abnormal. These tests should be performed routinely in patients with a family history of MEN 2a or 2b or medullary carcinoma to allow early diagnosis of the tumor with the goal of surgical cure.

Serial calcitonin levels are a useful parameter for following therapeutic responses in patients with medullary carcinoma or for diagnosing a recurrence. Calcitonin levels usually reflect the extent of disease. If the tumor becomes less differentiated, calcitonin levels may no longer reflect tumor burden. Another useful tumor marker for medullary carcinoma is carcinoembryonic antigen (CEA). This antigen is frequently elevated in patients with medullary carcinoma and is present at all stages of the disease. Rapid increases in CEA predict a worse clinical course.

Surgery is the mainstay of therapy for patients with medullary thyroid carcinoma. Total thyroidectomy is advocated because the tumors are often multicentric. Patients may also receive radioactive iodine ablation of any residual thyroid tissue, since any C cells remaining may undergo malignant degeneration. Patients should be monitored indefinitely for recurrences, because these tumors may be so indolent. Since the newly diagnosed patient with medullary carcinoma may be an index case of a familial form of the disease, first-degree relatives should be examined carefully and screened with measurements of calcitonin levels.

Patients with MEN 2a or 2b—even in the absence of symptoms—should undergo screening tests for the possibility of pheochromocytoma prior to thyroid surgery. These tests include the determination of urinary catecholamines and their metabolites and adrenal CT scanning. These tumors may be clinically silent at the time medullary carcinoma is diagnosed, and they should be removed before thyroidectomy.

28. How can you make the diagnosis of medullary carcinoma of the thyroid?
29. What is the treatment for medullary carcinoma?
30. Which patients are at higher risk for medullary carcinoma?

OSTEOPOROSIS

Etiology

Osteoporosis is defined as loss of bone mineral. A slow loss of mineral from bone is a normal part of the aging process, commencing after age 30 (Figure 17–17). Thus, after age 30, the bone mass is determined by the level of peak bone mass that was attained and the subsequent rate of loss. Heredity is important in determining bone mass. It has long been recognized that blacks have greater peak bone mass than whites or Asians and are relatively protected from osteoporosis. It now appears that within a Caucasian population, more than half the variance in bone mass is genetically determined. However, a number of hormonal and environmental factors can reduce the genetically determined peak bone mass or hasten the loss of bone mineral and thus present important risk factors for osteoporosis (Table 17–10).

The most important etiologic factor in osteoporosis is sex steroid deficiency. The estrogen deficiency that occurs after menopause accelerates loss of bone; postmenopausal women consistently have lower bone mass than men and a higher incidence of osteoporotic fractures. With respect to bone, testosterone serves the same function in men as estrogen in

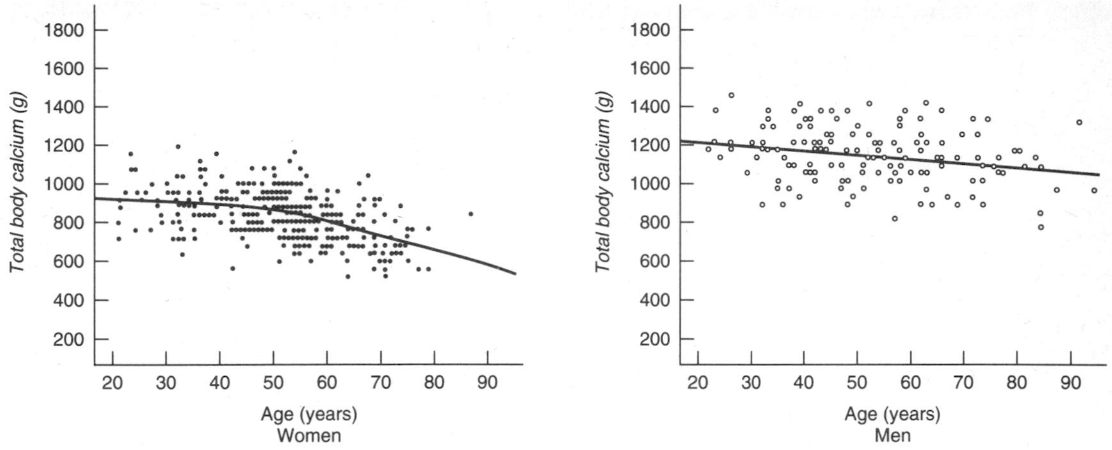

Figure 17–17. Total body calcium in women and men as a function of age. (Reproduced, with permission, from Aloia JF et al: A model for involutional bone loss. J Lab Clin Med 1985;106:630.)

women, and hypogonadal men also experience accelerated bone loss. Another important factor is the use of corticosteroids or endogenous cortisol excess in Cushing's syndrome. Glucocorticoid-induced osteoporosis is one of the most devastating complications of chronic therapy with these agents. Certain other medications, including thyroid hormone, anticonvulsants, and chronic heparin therapy, immobilization, alcohol abuse, and smoking, are also risk factors for osteoporosis. Diet is probably important as well. As discussed below, an adequate intake of calcium and vitamin D is necessary to build peak bone mass optimally and to minimize the rate of loss. Other dietary factors may also be important. Osteoporosis is most prevalent in Western societies, and it has been speculated that our high protein intake or related factors may predispose to osteoporosis, perhaps by enhancing urinary calcium losses.

Pathogenesis

Since bone remodeling involves the coupled resorption of bone by osteoclasts and the deposition of new bone by osteoblasts, bone loss could result from increased bone resorption, decreased bone formation, or a combination of the two. Postmenopausal osteoporosis is the consequence of accelerated bone resorption. The urinary excretion of calcium and of bone collagen metabolites such as hydroxyproline and pyridinoline cross-links increases, the serum PTH level is somewhat suppressed, and if bone is biopsied resorption surfaces are found to be increased. The bone formation rate is also increased, with an increase in serum alkaline phosphatase and in the serum level of the bone matrix protein osteocalcin, both reflecting increased osteoblastic activity. This high-turnover state is the direct result of estrogen deficiency and can be reversed by estrogen replacement therapy.

The accelerated phase of estrogen-deficient bone loss begins immediately after menopause (natural or surgical). It is most evident in trabecular bone, the compartment which is remodeled most rapidly. As much as 5–20% of spinal trabecular bone mineral is lost yearly in postmenopausal women, and osteoporotic fractures in early postmenopausal women are often in the spine, a site of trabecular bone. After 5–15 years, the rate of bone loss slows, so that after age 65 the rates are similar in women and men.

The cellular basis for the activation of bone resorption in estrogen- or androgen-deficient states is not fully understood. Osteoclasts have estrogen receptors and could respond directly to estrogen deficiency, but there is also evidence that osteoclast-stimulating cytokines such as interleukin-6 may be released from other bone cells in estrogen-deficient states.

The pathogenesis of age-related bone loss is less certain. It begins after age 30, is relatively slow, and occurs at a similar rate regardless of gender or race. It was once thought that elderly patients with osteoporosis ran the gamut from low-turnover states, characterized by markedly decreased osteoblastic activity, to high-turnover states that resemble the accelerated phase of postmenopausal bone loss. It now appears that only a few such individuals are truly in a low-turnover state. For example, serum osteocalcin levels remain elevated throughout the latter decades of life, suggesting that osteoblast activity is not absolutely diminished. It is probable, however, that the balance of cellular activity is altered, with a reduced

Table 17–10. Causes of osteoporosis.

Primary osteoporosis
Aging (senile or involutional)
Juvenile
Idiopathic (young adults)
Connective tissue diseases
Osteogenesis imperfecta
Homocystinuria
Ehlers-Danlos syndrome
Marfan's syndrome
Drug-induced
Corticosteroids
Alcohol
Thyroid hormone
Chronic heparin
Anticonvulsants
Hematologic
Multiple myeloma
Systemic mastocytosis
Immobilization
Endocrine
Hypogonadism
Hypercortisolism
Hyperthyroidism
Hyperparathyroidism
Gastrointestinal disorders
Subtotal gastrectomy
Malabsorption syndromes
Obstructive jaundice
Biliary cirrhosis

osteoblast response to continued bone resorption, so that resorption cavities are incompletely filled by new bone formation during the remodeling cycle.

One important factor in the pathogenesis of age-related bone loss (sometimes called senile osteoporosis) is a relative deficiency of dietary calcium and 1,25-$(OH)_2D$. The capacity of the intestine to absorb calcium is diminished in the aged. Because renal losses of calcium are obligatory, a decreased efficiency of calcium absorption means that dietary calcium intake must be increased to prevent negative calcium balance. However, the typical woman has reduced—not increased—her dietary intake of calcium. It is estimated that about 1200 mg/d of elemental calcium is required to maintain calcium balance in people over age 65 (Table 17–11). American women in this age group ingest 500–600 mg of calcium daily; the calcium intakes in men are higher. In addition, some of the aged are deficient in vitamin D, further impairing their ability to absorb calcium. Particularly in northern climates, where sunlight exposure is reduced in the winter months, borderline low levels of 25-(OH)D and mild secondary hyperparathyroidism are evident by the end of winter.

The PTH level increases with age. This may be an example of secondary hyperparathyroidism that results from the following sequence of events: The well known decrease in the mass of functioning renal tissue with age could lead to decreased renal synthesis of 1,25-$(OH)_2D$, which would directly release PTH secretion from its normal inhibition by 1,25-$(OH)_2D$. The reduced 1,25-$(OH)_2D$ level would also decrease calcium absorption, exacerbating an intrinsic inability of the aging intestine to absorb calcium normally. Secondary hyperparathyroidism would then result from the dual effects of 1,25-$(OH)_2D$ deficiency on the parathyroid gland and the intestine. In addition, the responsiveness of the parathyroid gland to inhibition by calcium is reduced with aging. The hyperparathyroidism of aging may thus result from the combined effects of age on the kidney, the intestine, and the parathyroid gland itself.

One thing that is clear is that provision of a dietary supplement together with adequate vitamin D will reduce the rate of age-related bone loss by at least 50%. This suggests that reduced calcium absorption and secondary hyperparathyroidism play significant roles in the pathogenesis of osteoporosis in the elderly. However, the loss of bone continues after calcium supplementation, albeit at a lower rate, and it is thus likely that intrinsic changes in bone remodeling—perhaps having to do with a reduced osteoblastic response to ongoing osteoclastic bone resorption—also contribute to senile osteoporosis.

In secondary osteoporosis associated with glucocorticoid administration or alcoholism, there is a marked reduction in bone formation rates and serum osteocalcin levels. It is likely that glucocorticoids produce a devastating osteoporotic syndrome because of the rapid loss of bone that results from frankly depressed bone formation in the face of normal or even increased bone resorption.

The form of secondary osteoporosis associated with immobilization is an example of a resorptive state with marked uncoupling of bone resorption and bone formation and is characterized by hypercalciuria and suppression of PTH. When individuals with a high preexisting state of bone remodeling are immobilized (eg, adolescents and patients with hyperthyroidism or Paget's disease), bone resorption may be accelerated enough to produce hypercalcemia.

Table 17–11. Calcium nutrition and osteoporosis.

Calcium requirements (to maintain balance)	
Children	800 mg daily
Adolescents	1200 mg daily
Adults	800 mg daily
Pregnant or lactating women	1200–1500 mg daily
Elderly (age >60)	1200–1500 mg daily
Calcium intake (avg in women age >65)	550 mg daily
Calcium sources:	
Dairy product-free diet	400 mg
Cow's milk (8 oz)	300 mg
Calcium carbonate (500 mg)	200 mg

Clinical Manifestations

Osteoporosis is asymptomatic until it produces fractures and deformity. Typical osteoporotic fractures occur in the spine, the hip, and the wrist (Colles' fracture). The vertebral bodies of the spine are predominantly trabecular bone, with a thin rim of cortex, and are thus prone to fracture relatively early in postmenopausal osteoporosis (Figure 17–18). The vertebral bodies may be crushed, resulting in loss of height, or may be wedged anteriorly, resulting in height loss and kyphosis. The dorsal kyphosis of elderly women ("dowager's hump'') results from anterior wedging of multiple thoracic vertebrae. Spinal fractures may be acute and painful or may occur gradually and be manifested only as kyphosis or loss of height.

The worst complication of osteoporosis is hip fracture. Hip fractures typically occur in the elderly, with a sharply rising incidence in both sexes after age 80, because bone loss in the hip, with its large mass of cortical bone, is slower than in the spine. The personal and social costs of hip fracture are enormous. One-third of American women who survive past age 80 will suffer a hip fracture. The acute mortality rate is approximately 20%, much of it resulting from the complications of immobilizing frail persons in a hospital bed, such as pulmonary embolus and pneumonia. About half of elderly people with a hip fracture will never walk freely again. The long-term costs of chronic care for these persons are a major social concern.

The diagnosis of osteoporosis is sometimes made radiologically, but in general x-rays are a poor diagnostic tool. A chest x-ray will miss 30–50% of cases of spinal osteoporosis, and if overpenetrated may lead to the diagnosis of osteoporosis in someone with a normal bone mass. The best way to diagnose osteoporosis is with a quantitative measurement of bone density. The preferred method at present is dual-energy x-ray absorptiometry (DXA), which uses a measurement of fractional absorption of photons from an x-ray source to quantitate bone mineral content. The technique is precise, rapid, and relatively inexpensive. It delivers a considerably lower radiation dose than a chest x-ray.

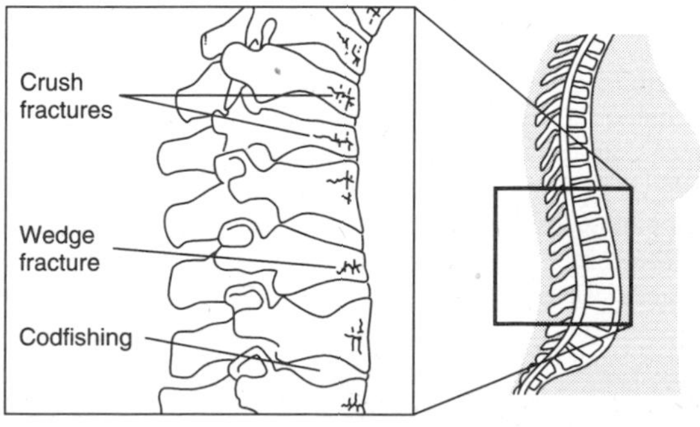

Figure 17–18. Types of vertebral osteoporotic fractures. (Reproduced, with permission, from Notelovitz M, Ware M: *Stand Tall: The Informed Women's Guide to Preventing Osteoporosis,* by Morris Notelovitz, M.D., and Marsha Ware. Illustration © 1982 by Triad Publishing Company.)

In an osteoporotic person, there are three risk factors for fracture: bone density, bone quality, and falls. The ability of bone density measurements to predict the likelihood of fractures has only recently been clarified. For every standard deviation below the mean bone density for age, there is a twofold to threefold increase in the risk of fracture. Thus, the risk of fracture is increased fourfold in someone at the lower limit of normal bone density for age (2 SD below the mean). Because bone loss is systemic, measurements at a single site (eg, the spine) are nearly as good a predictor of fracture at other sites (eg, the hip) as measurements at the site itself. Thus, measurements of bone density offer prognostic information in an asymptomatic individual with osteoporosis; of course, they also provide a means of assessing the efficacy of interventions.

Only a portion of the risk for fracture is captured by measurements of bone density because the mechanical strength of bone is also a function of bone quality--depending on the microarchitecture of a bone, its mechanical strength and its ability to withstand stress may be substantially different in two individuals with the same bone density. The assessment of bone quality is an active area of investigation.

Elderly persons with osteoporosis are unlikely to sustain a hip fracture unless they fall. Risk factors for falling include muscle weakness, impaired vision, impaired balance, sedative use, and environmental factors such as the necessity to climb stairs, negotiate loose carpeting, etc. Because we presently have a limited ability to intervene in osteoporosis with therapies that increase bone mass, strategies to prevent falls are an important part of the approach to the osteoporotic patient.

Most individuals at risk for osteoporosis benefit from calcium supplementation to a total intake about 1200–1500 mg/d. This can be accomplished with dairy products, the only rich dietary source of calcium, or with a calcium supplement such as calcium carbonate (Table 17–11). Vitamin D should be provided in approximately the multivitamin dose (400–800 IU). Calcium supplementation in younger individuals may increase peak bone mass and decrease premenopausal bone loss, but its optimal role in this age group has not been determined. Therapy of postmenopausal osteoporosis consists of estrogen replacement. A variety of other treatments for osteoporosis are under investigation, including other drugs to prevent bone resorption (calcitonin and bisphosphonates) and drugs to restore lost bone (synthetic PTH).

31. What is the relative importance of hereditary versus environmental or hormonal factors in contributing to osteoporosis?
32. What are the risk factors for osteoporosis?
33. What are the symptoms and signs of osteoporosis?
34. What are the risk factors for fracture in a patient with osteoporosis?
35. What treatment modalities can prevent bone loss or restore bone?

OSTEOMALACIA

Etiology

Osteomalacia is defined as a defect in the mineralization of bone. When it occurs in the young it also affects the mineralization of cartilage in the growth plate, a disorder called **rickets.** Osteomalacia can result from a deficiency of vitamin D, a deficiency of phosphate, an inherited deficiency in alkaline phosphatase (hypophosphatasia), or from agents that have adverse effects on bone (Table 17–12). Surprisingly, dietary calcium deficiency rarely produces osteomalacia, though a few cases have been reported.

Dietary vitamin D deficiency is rare in the United States because of adequate sunlight exposure and dietary supplementation with vitamin D in milk and other products. When vitamin D deficiency is encountered, it is usually the result of malabsorption of this fat-soluble vitamin. Severe rickets also occurs as part of two heritable disorders of vitamin D action, renal 1α-hydroxylase deficiency, in which vitamin D is not converted to $1,25\text{-}(OH)_2D$, and a vitamin D receptor defect.

Phosphate deficiency in osteomalacia is usually caused by heritable or acquired renal phosphate wasting. Osteomalacia has occasionally been seen in abusers of aluminum-containing antacids, which bind phosphate and prevent its absorption.

Pathogenesis

Vitamin D deficiency produces osteomalacia in stages. In the early stage, reduced calcium absorption produces secondary hyperparathyroidism, preventing hypocalcemia at the cost of increased renal phosphate excretion and hypophosphatemia. In later stages, hypocalcemia ensues and hypophosphatemia is progressive because of the combined effects of reduced absorption and the phosphaturic action of PTH. The poor delivery of minerals to bone (possibly coupled with the absence of direct effects of vitamin D on bone) impairs the mineralization of bone matrix, but osteoblasts actively form bone matrix. Thus, unmineralized matrix, or osteoid, accumulates at bone-forming surfaces.

Table 17–12. Causes of osteomalacia.

Vitamin D deficiency
Nutritional (rare)
Malabsorption
Hereditary vitamin D-dependent rickets
Type I (renal 1α-hydroxylase deficiency)
Type II (absent or defective vitamin D receptor)
Phosphate deficiency
Renal phosphate wasting
X-linked hypophosphatemia
Fanconi syndrome
Renal tubular acidosis (type II)
Oncogenic osteomalacia (acquired, associated with mesenchymal tumors)
Phosphate-binding antacids
Deficient alkaline phosphatase: hereditary hypophosphatasia
Toxic
Fluoride
Aluminum (chronic renal failure)
Etidronate disodium therapy
Phosphate-binding antacids
Chronic renal failure

Clinical Manifestations

Patients with vitamin D-deficient osteomalacia have bone pain, muscle weakness, and a waddling gait. Radiologically, they may have mild osteopenia, but the hallmark of the disorder is the pseudofracture--local bone resorption that has the appearance of a nondisplaced fracture, classically in the pubic rami, clavicles, or scapulas. In children with rickets, the leg bones are bowed (osteomalacia = "softening of bones''), the costochondral junctions are enlarged ("rachitic rosary''), and the growth plates are widened and irregular, reflecting the increase in unmineralized cartilage. Biochemically, the hallmarks of vitamin D-deficient osteomalacia are hypophosphatemia, hyperparathyroidism, variable hypocalcemia, and marked reductions in urinary calcium to less than 50 mg/d (Table 17–9). The 25-(OH)D level is reduced, indicative of decreased body stores of vitamin D. In vitamin D deficiency and other forms of osteomalacia, the alkaline phosphatase level is increased.

Although the disorder can be suspected strongly on clinical grounds and the biochemical changes summarized above are confirmatory, a firm diagnosis of osteomalacia requires either the radiologic appearance of rickets or pseudofractures or else bone biopsy. If bone is biopsied for quantitative histomorphometry, thickened osteoid seams and a reduction in the mineralization rate are found. Treatment with vitamin D or aggressive phosphate replacement in patients with renal phosphate wasting will reverse osteomalacia or heal rickets.

36. What are the causes of osteomalacia?
37. What are the two stages in which vitamin D deficiency produces osteomalacia?
38. What are the symptoms and signs of osteomalacia?

REFERENCES

General Bone and Mineral Metabolism and Vitamin D

Aurbach GD, Marx SJ, Spiegel AM: Parathyroid hormone, calcitonin, and the calciferols. In: *Williams Textbook of Endocrinology,* Wilson JD, Foster DW (editors). Saunders, 1992.

Johnson JA, Kumar R: Renal and intestinal calcium transport: Roles of vitamin D and vitamin D-dependent calcium binding proteins. Semin Nephrol 1994;14(2):119.

Pols HA, Birkenhager JC, van Leeuwen JP: Vitamin D analogues: From molecule to clinical application. Clin Endocrinol 1994;40:285.

Hyperparathyroidism

Arnold A: Molecular genetics of parathyroid gland neoplasia. J Clin Endocrinol Metab 1993;77:1108.

Deftos LJ, Parthemore JG, Stabile BE: Management of primary hyperparathyroidism. Annu Rev Med 1993; 44:19.

Delmez JA, Slatopolsky E: Clinical review 20: Recent advances in the pathogenesis and therapy of uremic secondary hyperparathyroidism. J Clin Endocrinol Metab 1991;72:735.

Heath H 3rd: Primary hyperparathyroidism: Recent advances in pathogenesis, diagnosis, and management. Adv Intern Med 1992;37:275.

Hypoparathyroidism

Ahonen P et al: Clinical variation of autoimmune polyendocrinopathy-candidiasis-ectodermal dystrophy (APECED) in a series of 68 patients. N Engl J Med 1990;322:1829.

Tohme JF, Bilezikian JP: Hypocalcemic emergencies. Endocrinol Metab Clin North Am 1993;22:363.

Medullary Carcinoma of the Thyroid

Barbot N: Pentagastrin stimulation test and early diagnosis of medullary thyroid carcinoma using an immunoradiometric assay of calcitonin: Comparison with genetic screening in hereditary medullary thyroid carcinoma. J Clin Endocrinol Metab 1994;78:114.

Gagel RF et al: Medullary thyroid carcinoma: Recent progress. J Clin Endocrinol Metab 1993;76:809.

Hofstra RM et al: A mutation in the RET proto-oncogene associated with multiple endocrine neoplasia type 2B and sporadic medullary thyroid carcinoma. Nature 1994;367:375.

Osteoporosis

Delmas PD: Biochemical markers of bone turnover: I. Theoretical considerations and clinical use in osteoporosis. Am J Med 1993;95(Suppl 5A):11S.

Heaney RP: Bone mass, nutrition, and other lifestyle factors. Am J Med 1993;95:29S.

Lang P et al: Osteoporosis: Current techniques and recent developments in quantitative bone densitometry. Radiol Clin North Am 1991;29:49.

Riggs BL, Melton LJ 3rd: The prevention and treatment of osteoporosis. N Engl J Med 1992;327:620.

Osteomalacia

Chines A, Pacifici R: Antacid and sucralfate-induced hypophosphatemic osteomalacia: A case report and review of the literature. Calcif Tissue Int 1990;47:291.

Diamond TH: Metabolic bone disease in primary biliary cirrhosis. J Gastroenterol Hepatol 1990;5:66.

Harvey JN, Gray C, Belchetz PE: Oncogenous osteomalacia and malignancy. Clin Endocrinol 1992;37:379.

Hutchison FN, Bell NH: Osteomalacia and rickets. Semin Nephrol 1992;12:127.

Hypercalcemia of Malignancy

Rosol TJ, Capen CC: Mechanisms of cancer-induced hypercalcemia. Lab Invest 1992;67:680.

Seymour JF, Gagel RF: Calcitriol: The major humoral mediator of hypercalcemia in Hodgkin's disease and non-Hodgkin's lymphomas. Blood 1993;82:1383.

Singer FR: Pathogenesis of hypercalcemia of malignancy. Semin Oncol 1991;18:4.

Strewler GJ, Nissenson RA: Hypercalcemia in malignancy. West J Med 1990;153:635.

18 Pituitary Disorders

Vishwanath R. Lingappa, MD, PhD

The pituitary gland, once viewed as the "master gland" regulating the endocrine system, is in fact a middle manager. Specific cells in the anterior pituitary gland are directed to secrete their hormones by specific hypothalamic peptides delivered via a specialized vascular connection from the hypothalamus to the pituitary. Disorders of the pituitary thus have important clinical implications for regulation of many different organ systems. This chapter will focus on four problems that reflect the diversity of pituitary disease: pituitary adenomas, panhypopituitarism, and disorders of deficiency or excess of vasopressin secretion.

NORMAL STRUCTURE & FUNCTION OF THE PITUITARY GLAND

The hypothalamus is a poorly demarcated region located in the floor and lateral walls of the third ventricle and comprising about 1% of the mass of the brain (Figures 18–1 and 18–2). It serves to integrate behavioral and homeostatic responses to vegetative stimuli. Neurons whose cell bodies lie in the hypothalamus perform these functions by secreting peptide hormones in response to changes in various parameters (eg, blood levels of glucocorticoids, estrogens, glucose, osmolality, volume, etc) monitored in particular hypothalamic nuclei (Table 18–1). Once secreted, the pituitary hormones travel via the bloodstream throughout the body and trigger the release of other hormones from particular endocrine glands. Endocrine hormones in turn have effects on target tissues that alter growth, reproduction, metabolism, and response to stress. The hierarchy of control involving higher brain centers, the hypothalamus, the anterior pituitary gland, endocrine organ, and target tissue is termed a neuroendocrine axis. A somewhat different neuroendocrine axis involves the posterior pituitary hormones.

ANATOMY, HISTOLOGY, & CELL BIOLOGY

The pituitary gland is composed of embryologically distinct anterior and posterior lobes (Figures 18–3 and 18–4). It is encased in a tough fibrous capsule, the sella turcica, connected to the hypothalamus at the base of the brain by a stalk (Figure 18–1). The intermediate lobe is rudimentary or absent in humans. Hypothalamic neurons project via that stalk to comprise the posterior pituitary (Figure 18–4). A specialized pituitary portal vascular supply carries blood directly from the hypothalamus to the anterior pituitary, where an anastomosing bed of capillaries bathes the cells of the anterior pituitary in blood rich in products secreted by neurons of the hypothalamus (Figure 18–5). An important feature of this direct connection of hypothalamus to anterior pituitary is that the concentration of releasing factors is sufficiently high to allow them to bind to their specific receptors on anterior pituitary cells despite relatively low affinities.

While most peptide factors secreted by the hypothalamus cause release of a pituitary hormone, some are inhibitory factors that block or diminish secretion of particular hormones. The anterior pituitary consists of cells each of which produces and secretes one of four families of hormones: proopiomelanocortin and adrenocorticotropin (ACTH), thyrotropin (TSH), growth hormone (GH) and prolactin (PRL), and the gonadotropins (LH and FSH).

The pituitary gland is bounded above by the optic chiasm and laterally by the cavernous sinus and the structures that traverse it (internal carotid artery, cranial nerves III, IV, V_1 and V_2 divisions of V, and VI).

1. Describe the levels of an anterior pituitary neuroendocrine feedback axis.
2. What structures surround the pituitary gland?
3. What roles do each of the four families of pituitary hormones play in regulation of normal physiology?
4. Where do the neurons whose axons comprise the substance of the posterior pituitary originate?

PHYSIOLOGY

1. ANTERIOR PITUITARY HORMONES

Broadly speaking, the hormones secreted by the hypothalamus and pituitary gland serve to ensure (1) that the brain has overall control of the action of the various endocrine glands which regulate the physiologic processes of growth, reproduction, metabolism, and response to stress; and (2) that the nervous and endocrine systems are themselves interconnected and appropriately regulated.

Proopiomelanocortin & ACTH

In response to a variety of indicators of stress, the hypothalamus releases corticotropin-releasing hormone (CRH), which triggers synthesis and intracellular transport of a large precursor protein termed proopiomelanocortin (POMC). During intracellular transport, POMC is processed by proteases to release smaller peptides, including a 39-amino-acid residue peptide, corticotropin (ACTH) (Figure 18–6). ACTH triggers synthesis and secretion of the corticosteroids from the adrenal cortex: glucocorticoids, androgens, and, to some extent, mineralocorticoids (see Chapter 13). These steroid hormones in turn have complex ef-

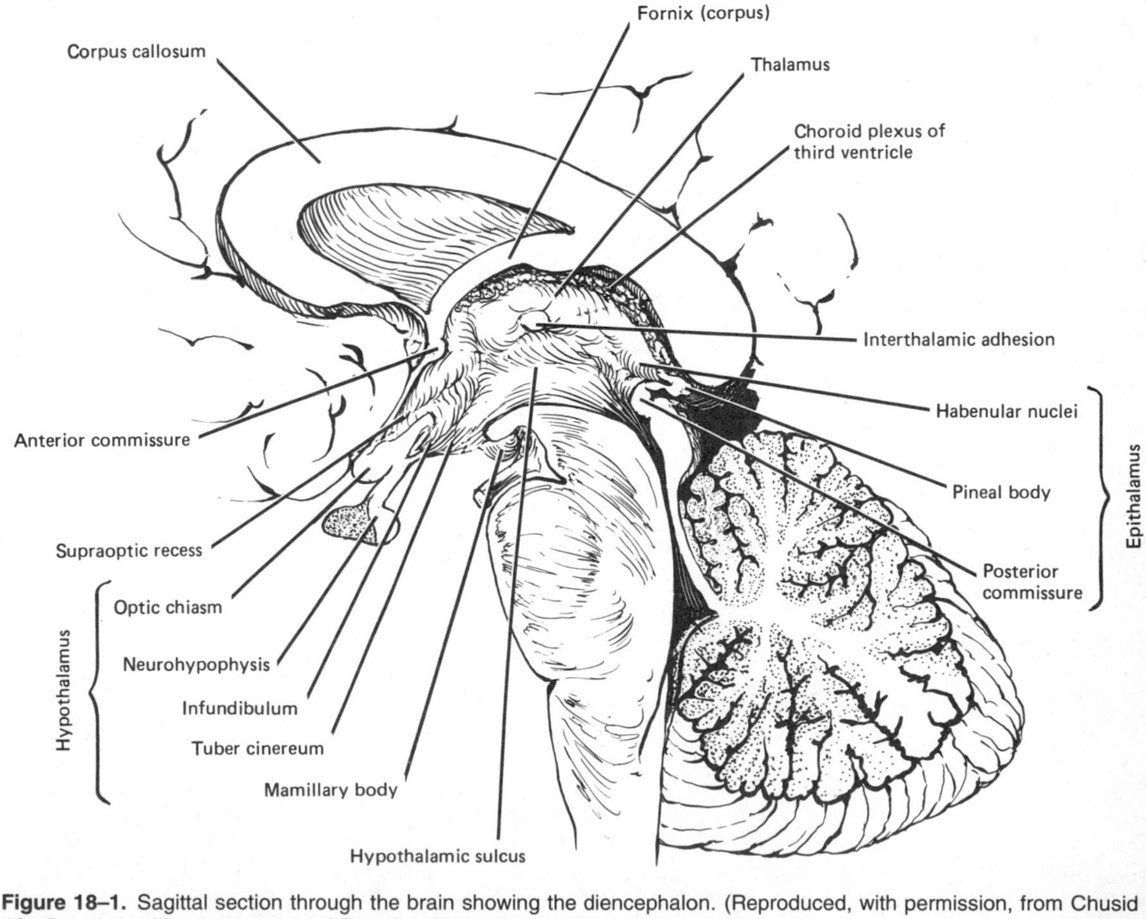

Figure 18–1. Sagittal section through the brain showing the diencephalon. (Reproduced, with permission, from Chusid JG: *Correlative Neuroanatomy and Functional Neurology,* 19th ed. Lange, 1985.)

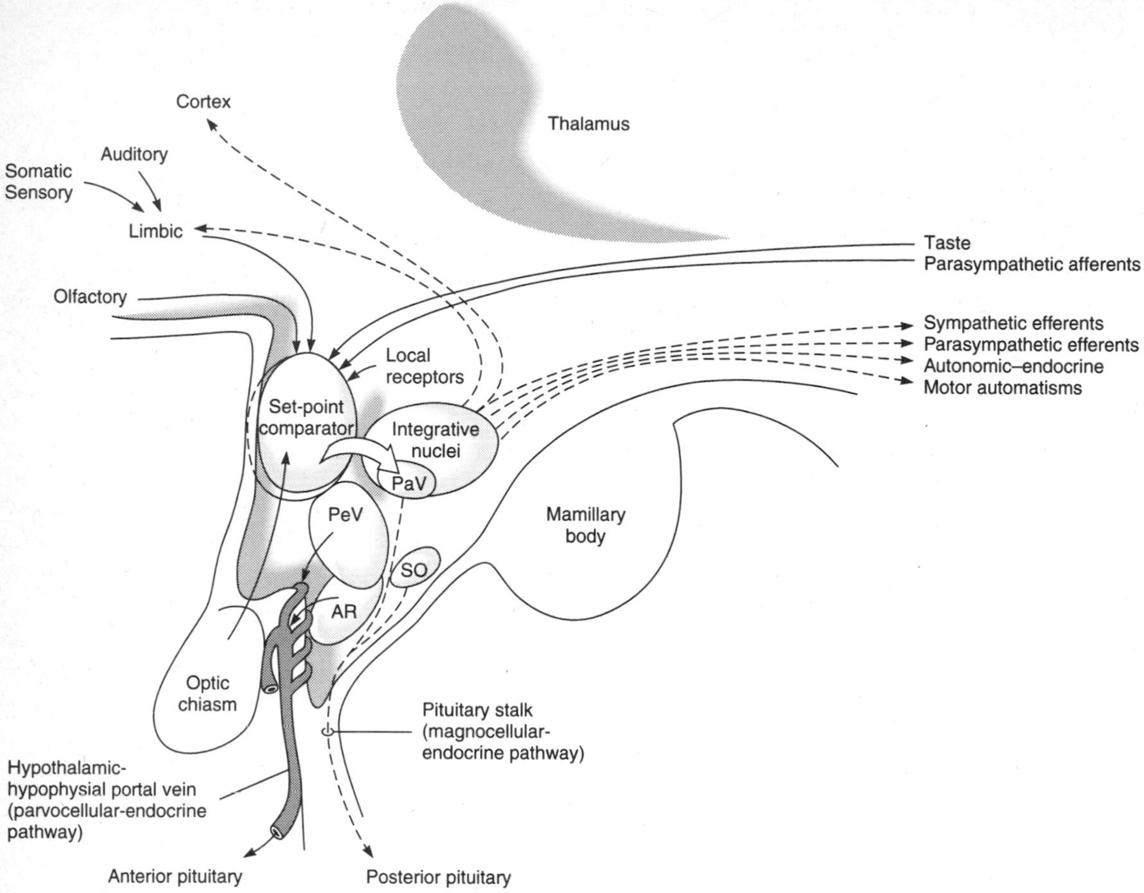

Figure 18–2. Functional organization of the hypothalamus. (Reproduced, with permission, from Saper CB: Hypothalamus. In: *Neurobiology of Disease.* Pearlman AL, Collins RC [editors]. Oxford Univ Press, 1990.)

Table 18–1. Functions of hypothalamic nuclei.[1]

Hypothalamic Region	Location and Description	Function
Periventricular zone	Most medial part of the hypothalamus; adjacent to third ventricle	Production of releasing factors for anterior pituitary hormones
Paraventricular and supraoptic nuclei	Medial zone (just lateral to periventricular zone)	Production of oxytocin and vasopressin stored in posterior pituitary
Medial preoptic nucleus, dorsomedial, ventromedial, premamillary, anterior and posterior hypothalamic nuclei	Medial zone	Controlling behavior for homeostasis
Medial forebrain bundle	Lateral zone tracts	Connect cells of the hypothalamic nuclei to both the brain stem and the forebrain
Anterior hypothalamic and preoptic areas	Anterior third of the hypothalamus	Integration of fluid and electrolyte, thermoregulatory, and nonendocrine reproductive functions
Tuberal region	Middle third of hypothalamus just posterior to the anterior area; gives rise to the pituitary stalk	Contain nuclei responsible for the endocrine and autonomic regulatory mechanisms and integration of energy, metabolic, and reproductive responses
Posterior, lateral, and premamillary nuclei	Posterior third of the hypothalamus	Involved in thermoregulatory and emergency response integration

[1]Reproduced, with permission, from Saper CB: Hypothalamus. In: *Neurobiology of Disease.* Pearlman AL, Collins RC (editors). Oxford Univ Press, 1990.

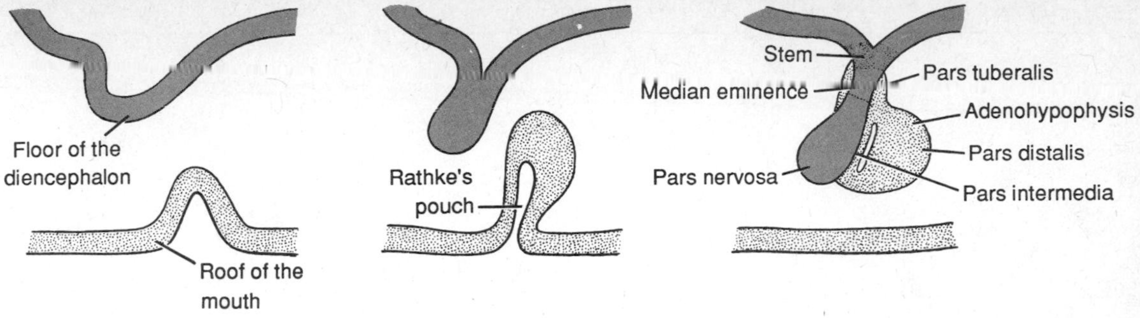

Figure 18–3. Diagram of the development of the adenohypophysis and neurohypophysis. The ectoderm of the roof of the mouth and its derivatives is shown stippled (lower portion). The upper portion shows the neural ectoderm from the floor of the diencephalon. (Reproduced, with permission, from Junqueira LC, Carneiro J, Kelley RO: *Basic Histology,* 7th ed. Appleton & Lange, 1992.)

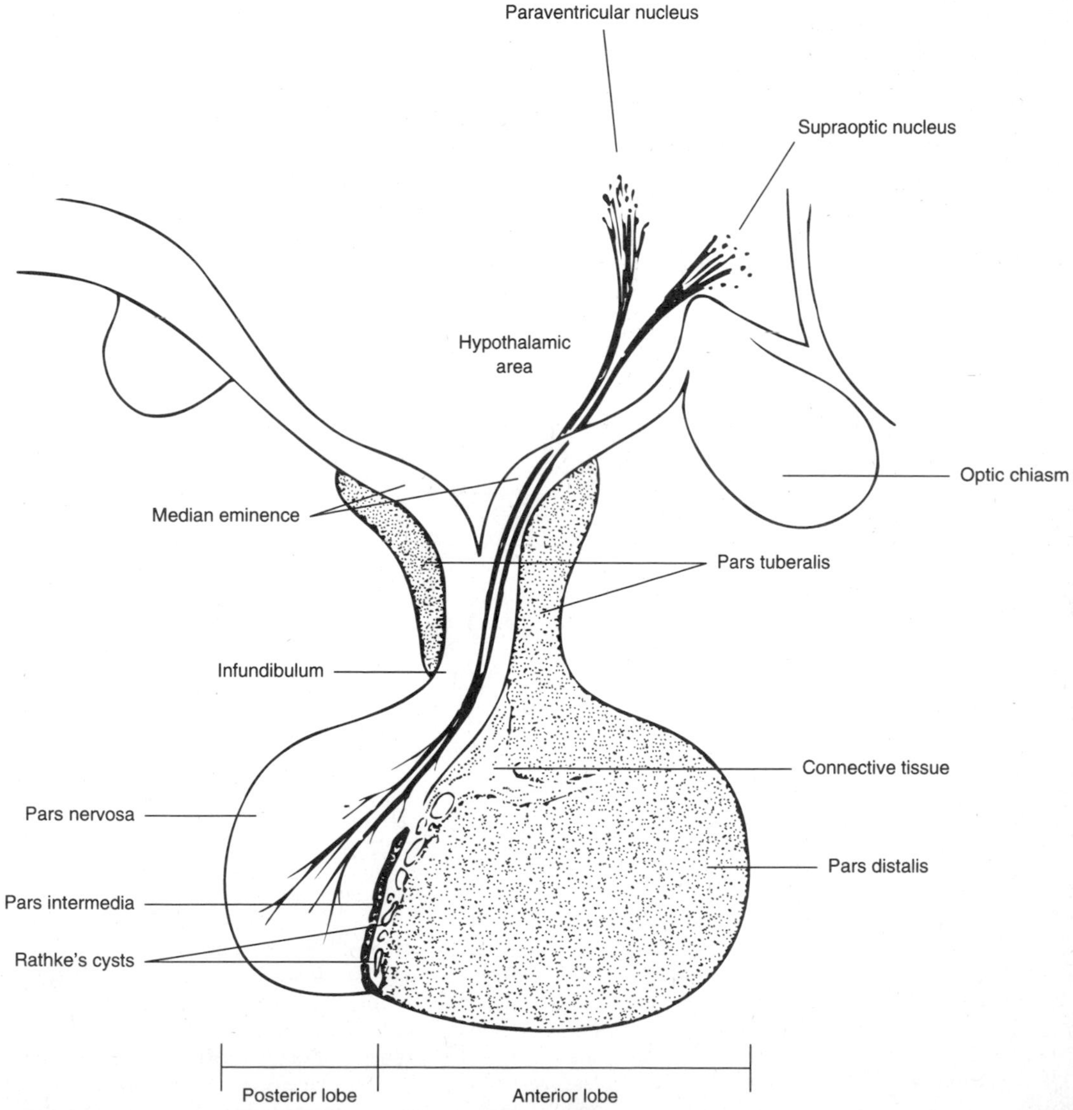

Figure 18–4. The component parts of the pituitary and their relationship to the hypothalamus. The pars tuberalis, pars distalis, and pars intermedia form the adenohypophysis. The infundibulum and pars nervosa form the neurohypophysis. (Modified, redrawn, and reproduced, with permission, from the *Ciba Collection of Medical Illustrations,* by Frank H. Netter, MD.)

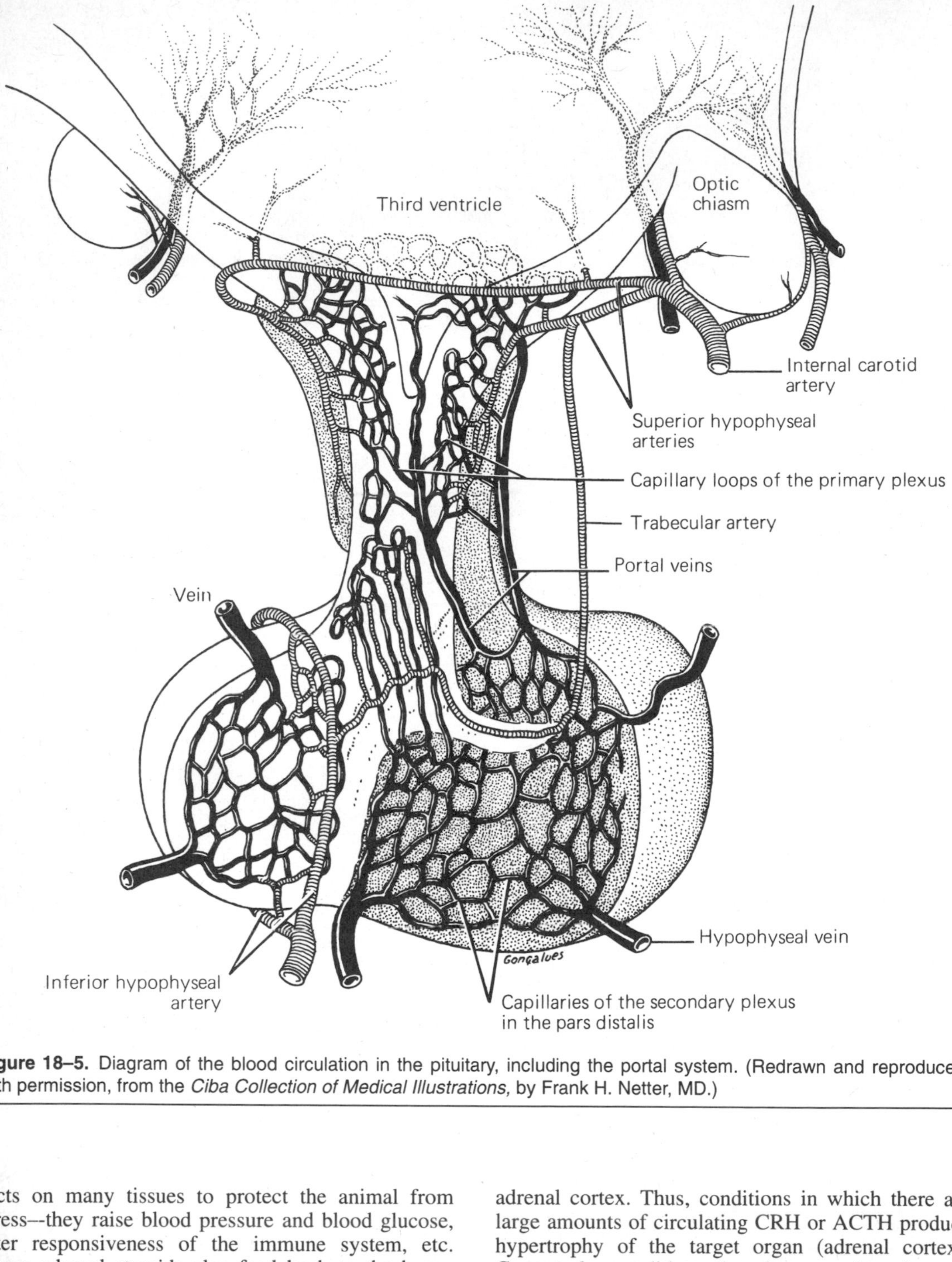

Figure 18–5. Diagram of the blood circulation in the pituitary, including the portal system. (Redrawn and reproduced, with permission, from the *Ciba Collection of Medical Illustrations,* by Frank H. Netter, MD.)

fects on many tissues to protect the animal from stress—they raise blood pressure and blood glucose, alter responsiveness of the immune system, etc. These adrenal steroids also feed back to the hypothalamus and inhibit CRH secretion and POMC and ACTH secretion. In the absence of unusual stress, there is a daily diurnal rhythm of CRH, ACTH, and adrenal steroid release.

In addition to stimulating synthesis and secretion of corticosteroids, ACTH stimulates growth of the glucocorticoid and androgen-secreting layers of the adrenal cortex. Thus, conditions in which there are large amounts of circulating CRH or ACTH produce hypertrophy of the target organ (adrenal cortex). Conversely, conditions that down-regulate the axis (eg, oral glucocorticoids) result in atrophy of the adrenal cortex because they reduce ACTH secretion to less than its normal diurnal levels (Chapter 13). However, ACTH has little or no effect on the growth of mineralocorticoid-secreting tissues of the adrenal cortex despite the fact that it does trigger, to some extent, release of mineralocorticoids.

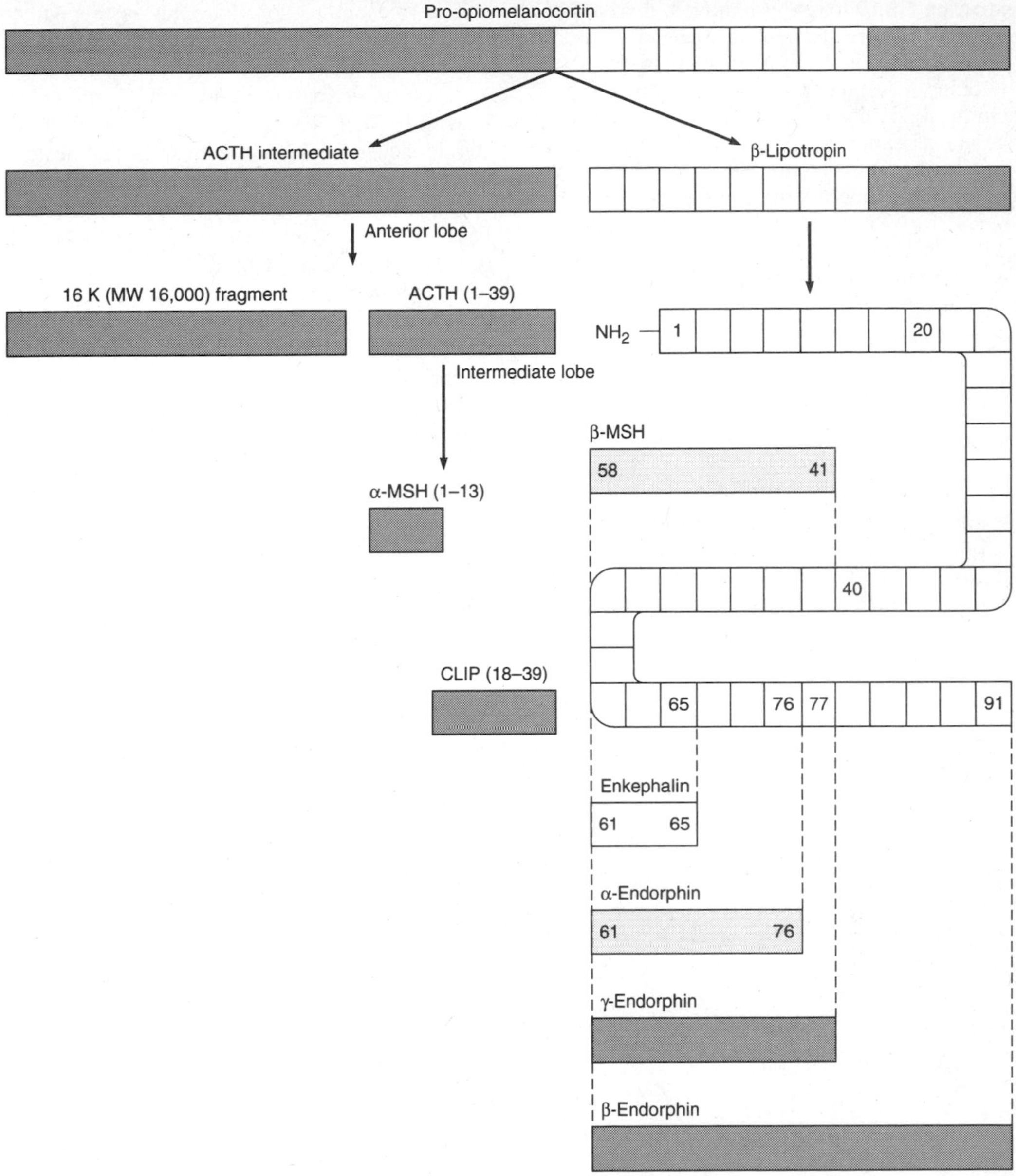

Figure 18–6. Processing of proopiomelanocortin in the anterior pituitary. (Reproduced, with permission, from Speroff L, Glass RH, Kase NG: *Clinical Gynecologic Endocrinology and Infertility,* 5th ed. Williams & Wilkins, 1994.)

Thyrotropin (TSH)

Thyrotropin is released from specific cells in the pituitary upon stimulation by thyrotropin-releasing hormone (TRH) from the hypothalamus. TSH in turn travels via the systemic bloodstream to the thyroid gland, where it stimulates synthesis and secretion of thyroid hormones, thyroxine and triiodothyronine. Thyroid hormone has effects on nearly every tissue in the body but especially the cardiovascular, respiratory, skeletal, and central nervous systems. Thyroid hormone is critical at key points in development, and its deficiency has effects—such as severe mental retardation and short stature—that are not reversible by subsequent thyroid hormone administration (Chapter 12).

Thyroxine undergoes an important metabolic modification in peripheral tissues, ie, removal of one of the four covalently attached iodine molecules.

Depending on which iodine is removed, thyroid hormone activity is increased tenfold (removal of an iodine in the 5′ position of thyroxine to form triiodothyronine [T_3]) or abolished (removal of an iodine in the 5 position to form reverse T_3). In severe illness, patients can have depressed T_4 and T_3 levels, with increased conversion to other thyroid hormone metabolites. This appears to be a physiologic response and does not require thyroid hormone replacement therapy. Besides its target tissue effects, thyroid hormone feeds back onto the pituitary and hypothalamus to inhibit secretion of TSH and TRH. TSH also triggers growth of thyroid tissue, resulting in goiter under conditions of chronic TSH stimulation (see Chapter 12).

Gonadotropins

LH and FSH are two-subunit glycoprotein hormones released by specific cells of the anterior pituitary termed gonadotrophs. The alpha subunits of LH and FSH (and TSH) are identical, while the beta subunits differ from each other and are responsible for the biologic differences between these hormones.

The role of the gonadotropins is to regulate the reproductive system's neuroendocrine axis. Thus, a releasing factor from the hypothalamus termed gonadotropin-releasing hormone (GnRH) stimulates LH and FSH secretion, which stimulates steroidogenesis within the ovaries and testes. The steroids produced by the ovaries (estrogens) and by the testes (testosterone) inhibit GnRH, LH, and FSH production and have target tissue effects on developing follicles within the ovary itself, on the uterus (controlling the menstrual cycle), on breast development, on spermatogenesis, and on many other tissues and physiologic processes (see Chapters 19 and 20).

As is the case with all neuroendocrine axes, the simple feedback loop is complicated by other inputs (eg, from the central nervous system) that modify responsiveness (Chapter 5). A notable feature for many hypothalamic releasing factors—but particularly GnRH—is that secretion occurs in pulsatile fashion and that changes in the rate and amplitude of secretion result in altered pituitary responsiveness due to

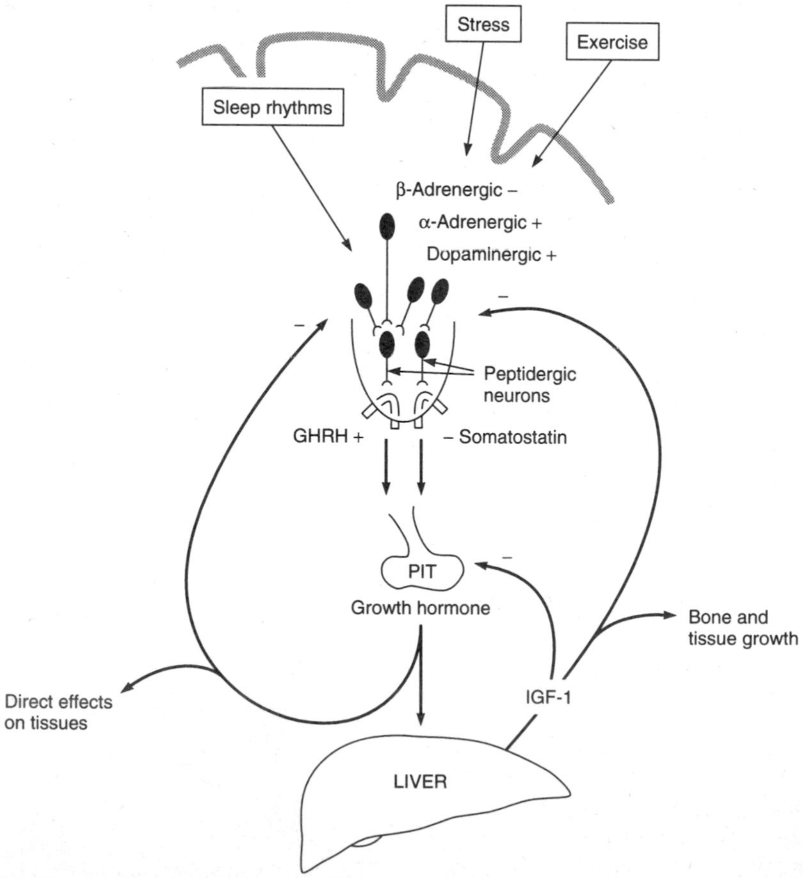

Figure 18–7. Schematic diagram of the hypothalamic control of growth hormone secretion. (Modified from Reichlin S: Neuroendocrinology. In: *Williams Textbook of Endocrinology,* 7th ed. Wilson JD, Foster DW [editors]. Saunders, 1985.)

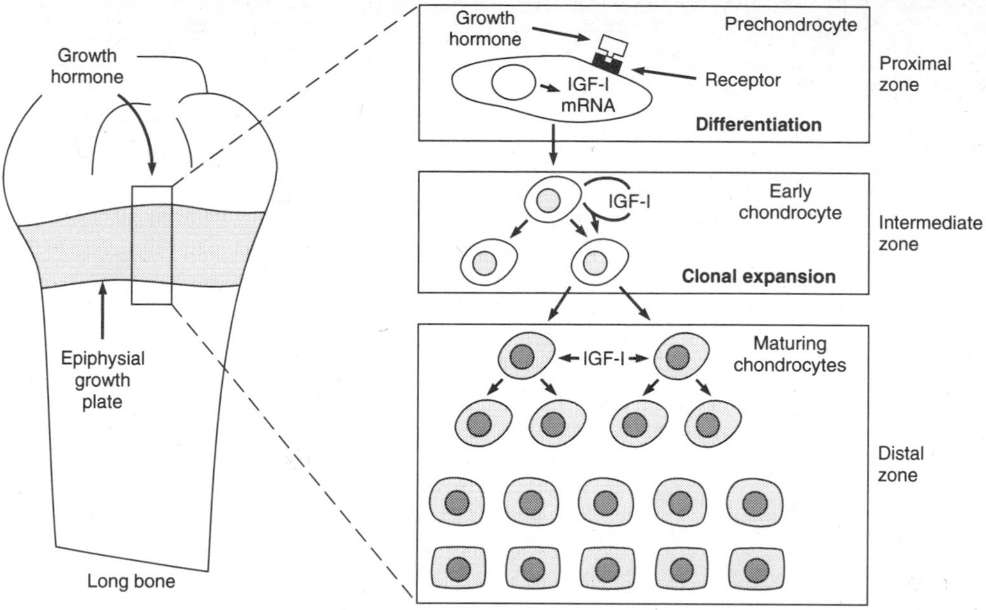

Figure 18–8. Growth hormone acts directly at the epiphysial plate to stimulate linear growth. Growth hormone stimulates differentiation of prechondrocytes into early chondrocytes, which then secrete IGF-1. In turn, IGF-1 stimulates clonal expansion and maturation of chondrocytes. (Modified by Thorner MO et al: The anterior pituitary. In: *Williams Textbook of Endocrinology,* 8th ed. Saunders, 1992; and from Isakson OPG et al: Direct action of growth hormone. In: *Basic and Clinical Aspects of Growth Hormone.* Plenum, 1988.)

down- or up-regulation of the receptors for the hypothalamic releasing factors found on the surface of the pituitary cells.

Growth Hormone & Prolactin

Growth hormone and prolactin are structurally related single polypeptides with quite different spectrums of action.

A. Growth Hormone: Growth hormone (GH), secreted in response to hypothalamic growth hormone-releasing hormone (GHRH) and somatostatin (Figure 8–7), triggers growth-promoting effects in a wide range of tissues. GH has direct actions (eg, stimulating the growth of cartilage) as well as indirect ones (eg, via insulin-like growth factor-1 [IGF-1], a polypeptide secreted by the liver and other tissues (Figures 18–8 and 18–9). IGF-1 has insulin-like effects of promoting fuel storage in various tissues. IGF-1 in turn inhibits GHRH and GH secretion. As in the other neuroendocrine feedback axes, the central nervous system and other factors can significantly influence the simple axis (Figure 18–7; Table 18–2).

Many of the direct actions of GH appear to have a "counter-regulatory" character in that they raise blood glucose levels and antagonize the action of insulin. In contrast, the indirect actions of GH via IGF-1 are insulin-like. This apparent contradiction makes sense when you consider that promoting growth requires first raising blood levels of substrates and then using them for synthesis and growth (Figure 18–9). To do the latter without the former would simply make the individual hypoglycemic without promoting long-term growth.

B. Prolactin: The primary role of prolactin in humans is to stimulate breast development and milk synthesis. It is discussed in greater detail in Chapter 19. Prolactin secretion is regulated by the neurotransmitter do-pamine from the hypothalamus rather than by a peptide. Furthermore, dopamine acts to inhibit rather than to stimulate prolactin secretion. Pathologic processes that result in separation of the pituitary gland from the hypothalamus cause loss of all pituitary hormones (**panhypopituitarism** from lack of the hypothalamic releasing hormones)—except prolactin. Instead, prolactin secretion is increased because separation from the hypothalmus removes the source of dopamine that normally controls prolactin secretion by inhibition.

2. POSTERIOR PITUITARY HORMONES

Vasopressin & Oxytocin

These peptide hormones vasopressin and oxytocin are synthesized in the supraoptic and paraventricular nuclei of the hypothalamus. The axons of the neurons

Table 18–2. Factors influencing normal growth hormone secretion.[1]

Factor	Augmented Secretion	Inhibited Secretion
Neurogenic	Stage III and stage IV sleep Stress (traumatic, surgical, inflammatory, psychic) Alpha-adrenergic agonists Beta-adrenergic antagonists Dopamine agonists Acetylcholine agonists	REM sleep Alpha-adrenergic antagonists Beta-adrenergic agonists Acetylcholine antagonists
Metabolic	Hypoglycemia Fasting Falling fatty acid level Amino acids Uncontrolled diabetes mellitus Uremia Hepatic cirrhosis	Hyperglycemia Rising fatty acid level Obesity
Hormonal	GHRH Low insulin-like growth factor level Estrogens Glucagon Arginine vasopressin	Somatostatin High insulin-like growth factor level Hypothyroidism High glucocorticoid levels

[1]Reproduced, with permission, from Thorner MO et al: The anterior pituitary. In: *Williams Textbook of Endocrinology,* 8th ed. Wilson JD, Foster DW Jr (editors). Saunders, 1992.

in these nuclei extend to form the posterior pituitary, where these peptide hormones are stored. Thus there is no need for a separate set of hypothalamic releasing factors to trigger vasopressin or oxytocin release.

A. Vasopressin: In response to physiologic stimuli (eg, a small increase in blood osmolality), the hypothalamic "osmostat" responds by triggering the subjective sense of thirst and at the same time the release of vasopressin. Vasopressin increases the number of active water channels in the renal collecting tubule, allowing conservation of free water that would otherwise be lost in the urine, thus increasing the concentration of the urine. Conservation of free water and stimulation of thirst have the net effect of correcting the small change in blood osmolality. While the minute-to-minute role of vasopressin is to maintain blood osmolality, its secretion is increased by large decreases in intravascular volume.

Vasopressin can bind to at least two classes of receptors. One of these classes of vasopressin receptors (V_1) is of lower affinity and is found on smooth muscle. Its major effect is to trigger vasoconstriction. The other class of receptors (V_2) is of higher affinity and is found in the distal nephron. Its major action is to mediate vasopressin's effects on osmolality. Because of its V_2-mediated actions, vasopressin is also known as **antidiuretic hormone (ADH).** The combination of vasoconstriction and water retention can be understood as a way of ensuring that perfusion of critical organs is maintained in the face of major intravascular volume deficits—even if the volume and osmolar composition of the perfusing blood is not ideal. The relationship between osmotic forces, volume, and vasopressin secretion is illustrated in Figure 18–10).

B. Oxytocin: Like vasopressin, this peptide is stored in nerve terminals of hypothalamic neurons that extend directly to the posterior pituitary. It plays an important role in smooth muscle contraction both

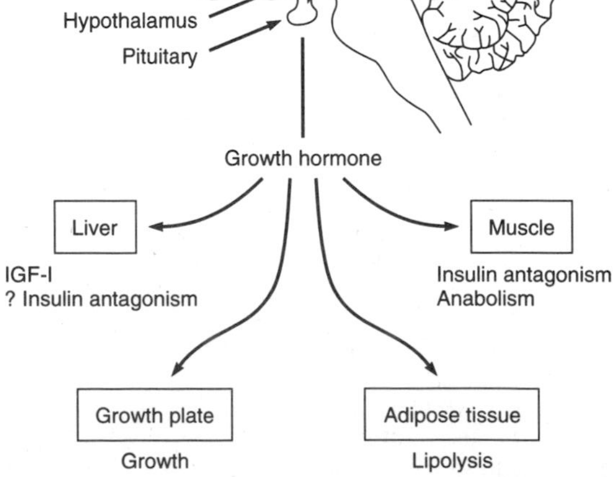

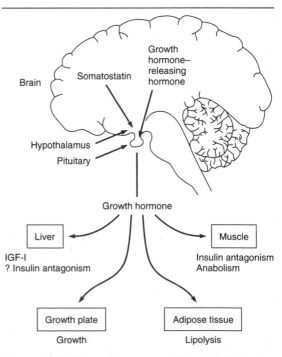

Figure 18–9. Schematic representation of multiple sites of GH action. (Reproduced, with permission, from Thorner MO et al: The anterior pituitary. In: *Williams Textbook of Endocrinology,* 8th ed. Wilson JD, Foster DW [editors]. Saunders, 1992.)

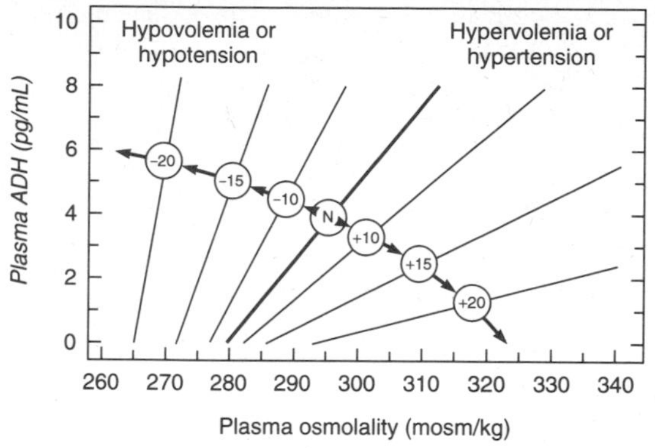

Figure 18–10. The influence of hemodynamic status on the osmoregulation of vasopressin in otherwise healthy humans. The numbers in the center circles refer to the percentage change in volume or pressure: N refers to the normovolemic normotensive subject. Note that the hemodynamic status affects both the slope of the relationship between the plasma vasopressin and osmolality and the osmotic threshold for vasopressin release. (Adapted from Robertson GL, Shelton RL, Athar S: The osmoregulation of vasopressin. Kidney Int 1976;10:25. Adapted by Rose BD in: *Clinical Physiology of Acid-Base and Electrolyte Disorders,* 3rd ed. McGraw-Hill, 1989. Reprinted by permission from *Kidney International.*)

5. How do neuroendocrine feedback loops of the anterior and posterior pituitary differ?
6. How can two polypeptide hormones whose mature forms have no sequence in common be derived from the same precursor?
7. Describe the distinguishing features of each pituitary neurendocrine feedback axis.
8. What is the significance of receptor down-regulation for hypothalamic control of pituitary function?

on a minute-to-minute basis during breast feeding and in contraction of the uterus during parturition.

PHYSIOLOGY OF THE PITUITARY GLAND

An understanding of the neuroendocrine feedback loops is important for proper clinical assessment and treatment of specific pituitary disorders. As a general rule, a partial or complete lesion at any given step of a neuroendocrine feedback loop (with the brain defined as the top step and the end-organ or target tissue as the bottom step) results in a correspondingly partial or complete loss in secretion of hormones at all lower steps and elevation of hormones at all higher steps (Figure 18–11). This makes sense since the lower steps are no longer being stimulated and the higher steps are therefore no longer receiving feedback inhibition. Similarly, an excess of hormone secreted at a given step of the axis results in suppression at all higher steps in the axis and an excess of hormone secreted at all lower steps of the feedback loop—for precisely the opposite reasons.

However, in assessing neuroendocrine feedback loops, simple measurement of hormone levels can be misleading for any of several reasons:

(1) Hypothalamic hormones are extremely short-lived and may not be detectable in the peripheral circulation even if they were present in high concentration in the pituitary portal circulation.

(2) Secretion by hypothalamic and pituitary cells is in some cases pulsatile (eg, GnRH and the gonadotropins) and in other cases episodic (eg, GHRH and GH). A random blood sample taken during a "peak" or "valley" in the time course of secretion will not reflect the underlying dynamic process averaged over time. Thus, a more reliable approach in assessing the neuroendocrine axis is to perform a challenge test: Administration of a stimulus to hormone secretion results in a measurable burst of its release into the bloodstream—unless there is a lesion of that gland.

(3) Some systems (in particular gonadotrophs) are quite sensitive to the particular *pattern* of stimulation they receive. Not only do they not respond if they do not receive enough stimulation; if given too much stimulation, they display down-regulation of receptors with a concomitant shutdown of secretion. This is an important consideration in management of disorders of reproductive function in women.

(4) In the higher steps of most neuroendocrine feedback loops, a large quantity of a given hormone for a long period of time not only stimulates secretion of the hormone at the lower steps but also causes hypertrophy or hyperplasia of the cells that secrete

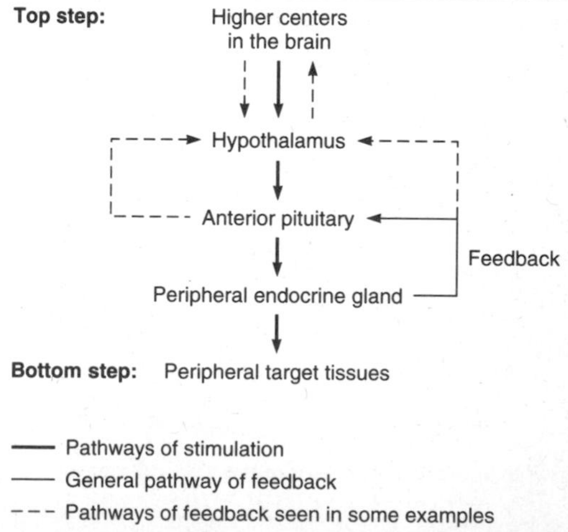

Figure 18–11. Idealized neuroendocrine feedback loop.

the lower-step hormones. Thus, for example, a woman found to have an enlarged pituitary does not-necessarily have a tumor needing surgery--she may simply be pregnant (with physiologic stimulation of the pituitary resulting in its hypertrophy).

(5) Conversely, prolonged excess of an end product or of a neuroendocrine axis results not only in feedback inhibition of the higher steps in the axis but in atrophy of the secretory cells at those higher steps as well. As a result of the latter phenomenon, return of the higher steps in an axis to "normal'' function after a period of excessive stimulation of an end organ—with concomitant feedback inhibition at the higher level--may take a long time. This is a classic problem seen in patients receiving protracted courses of exogenous glucocorticoids (adrenal steroids) (see Chapter 13).

9. What are some pitfalls in assessing features of neuroendocrine feedback loops?

PATHOPHYSIOLOGY OF SELECTED PITUITARY DISEASES

PITUITARY ADENOMA

An adenoma is a benign tumor of epithelial cell origin. Pituitary adenomas are of particular significance (1) because the pituitary is in an enclosed space with very limited capacity to accommodate an expanding mass; and (2) because they may arise in cells that secrete hormones, giving rise to hormone overproduction syndromes.

Clinical Presentation

Patients with adenomas or other tumors of the pituitary come to medical attention either with symptoms and signs related to an expanding intracranial mass (headaches, vision changes, etc; Table 18–3) or with manifestations of excess or deficiency of one or more pituitary hormones. Hormone deficiency results from destruction of the normal pituitary by the expanding adenoma. Hormone excess occurs when the adenoma secretes a particular hormone. **Microadenomas** (< 10 mm) are more likely to present with complaints related to hormone excess, since they are small and grow slowly. Conversely, whether or not they secrete hormones, **macroadenomas** (> 10 mm) can impinge on the optic chiasm above the sella turcica or the cavernous sinuses laterally.

Etiology

Any cell type in the pituitary gland can undergo hyperplasia or give rise to a tumor. Whether the patient with a pituitary tumor presents with a mass effect or symptoms referable to pituitary hormones depends on the size, growth rate, and secretory characteristics of the tumor. Which (if any) hormones the tumor secretes is generally a reflection of the cell type from which the tumor originated. **Gigantism** or **acromegaly** is due to oversecretion of

Table 18–3. Pituitary adenoma: Clinical effects.[1]

A. Mass Effects (Large Adenomas)	B. Excessive Hormone Secretion (Only Manifestation in Small Adenomas)
Usually nonfunctioning or growth hormone producing ↓	30%: Prolactin → galactorrhea
Destruction of normal pituitary cells → Hypopituitarism, diabetes insipidus Expansion of sella turcica → Visible on x-ray	25%: Growth hormone → Gigantism (child) → Acromegaly (adult)
Suprasellar extension through diaphragma sella ↓	10%: Corticotropin (ACTH) → Cushing's disease
Compression of optic chiasm or nerves → Visual field defects	5%: Thyrotropin (TSH) → hyperthyroidism, goiter
Compression of hypothalamus → Diabetes insipidus	Gonadotropins (LH, FSH) → amenorrhea, impotence, infertility
Interference with outflow of CSF from third ventricle → Raised intracranial pressure → Hydrocephalus	30%: No excessive hormone secretion
Compression of ventricles → Headache	
Cranial nerve compression (rare)	
May invade brain ("invasive adenoma"), paranasal sinuses, cavernous sinus	

[1]Reproduced, with permission, from Chandrasoma P, Taylor CR: *Concise Pathology,* 2nd ed. Appleton & Lange, 1994.

growth hormone. **Cushing's disease** is a syndrome of glucocorticoid excess due to oversecretion of ACTH. TSH and LH- or FSH-secreting tumors are rare. **Galactorrhea** occurs in prolactin-secreting tumors.

Pathophysiology

Most pituitary adenomas are clonal in origin: A single cell with altered growth control and feedback regulation gives rise to the adenoma. In a number of cases of pituitary adenomas, a point mutation has occurred in the alpha subunit of a cytosolic GTP-binding protein (G_s) that normally regulates growth-stimulatory signal transduction. As a result of this mutation, the G protein is "on" much longer. This is functionally analogous to the G protein activation that causes cholera. In the case of cholera, the G protein controls fluid secretion into the gut lumen, and G protein activation is due to a cholera toxin-mediated posttranslational modification of genetically normal G proteins. Thus, the disease is cured when the cholera bacterium is eliminated and the individual modified G protein polypeptides are degraded and replaced by newly synthesized G protein molecules. In the case of pituitary adenomas, the alteration is at the genetic level, and all cells of that clone thus need to be destroyed to eradicate the aberrant G protein.

Clinical Manifestations

Clinical manifestations related to mass effects are summarized in Figure 18–12. Bitemporal hemianopia is the classic visual field defect in a patient with an expanding pituitary mass (see Figure 18–13). It occurs because the crossing fibers of the optic tract, which lie directly above the pituitary gland and therefore are impinged on by an expanding mass, innervate the part of the retina responsible for temporal vision. However, in practice, a wide variety of visual field defects can actually be seen, reflecting the unpredictable nature of the direction and extent of tumor growth as well as anatomic variability. The clinical manifestations of hormone excess are discussed under specific syndromes below.

Regardless of whether a pituitary tumor is producing hormones or not, infarction of or hemorrhage into the expanding mass can destroy the normal pituitary gland, leaving the patient without pituitary hormones. The resulting clinical manifestations are considered below in the discussion of panhypopituitarism.

A. Prolactinoma: Hyperprolactinemia is the most common anterior pituitary disorder and has many causes (Table 18–4), including prolactin-secreting adenomas (prolactinomas). Prolactinomas are the most common pituitary adenomas, found in approximately one-fourth of all patients who come to autopsy. Most of these individuals had no symptoms from microadenomas and died of unrelated causes.

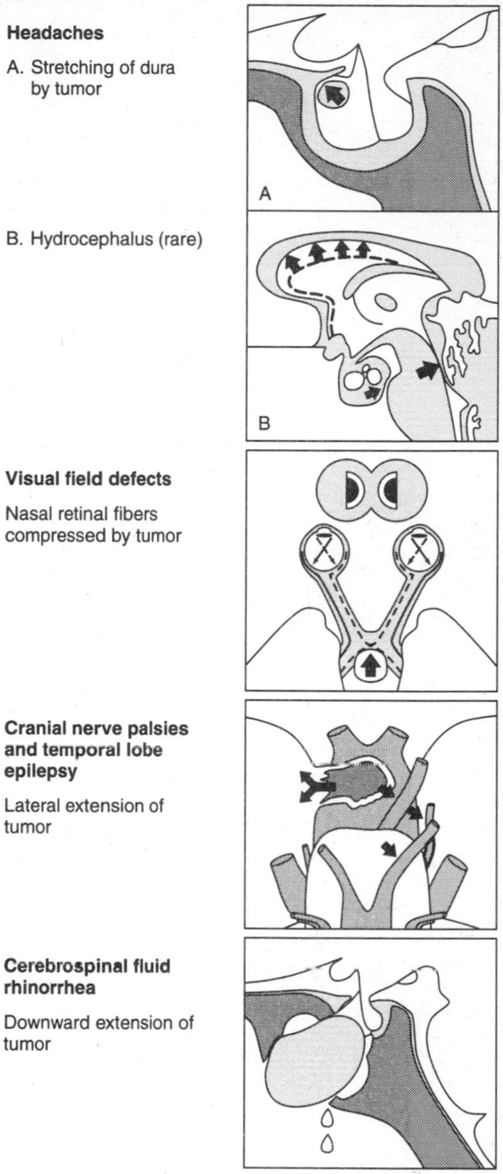

Figure 18–12. Various symptoms of pituitary tumor. Headaches are rarely caused by hydrocephalus. Visual field defects caused by extension of the tumor are plotted with the Goldmann perimeter. (From Wass JAH: Hypopituitarism. In: *Clinical Endocrinology: An Illustrated Text.* Gower, 1987.)

Patients with macroadenomas generally present with mass effect symptoms (Table 18–3) while those with microadenomas may develop symptoms related to hormonal effects, either due to the direct actions of prolactin (galactorrhea in 30–80% of women and up to one-third of men) or to prolactin's indirect effect of suppressing gonadal function (by decreasing

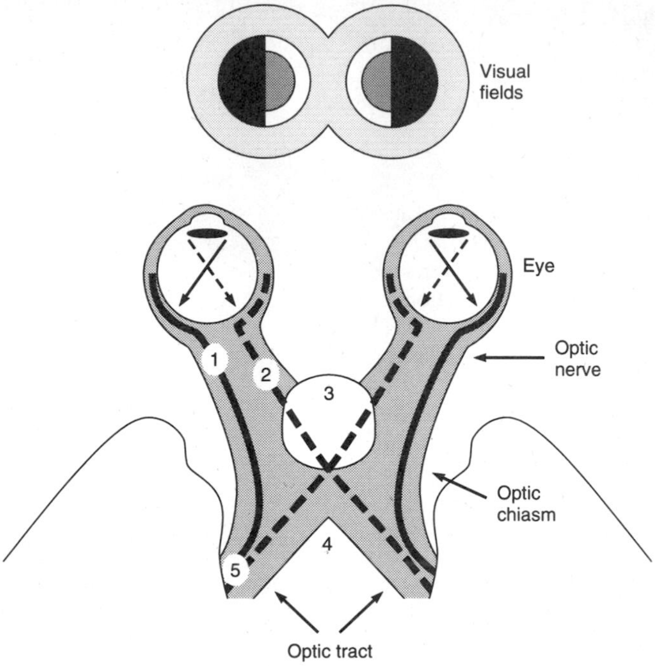

Figure 18–13. The most common visual field defect, bitemporal hemianopia (black areas of visual field), is caused by compression of the posterior aspect of the chiasm (4) from below. Visual disturbances resulting from compression of the optic nerves, chiasm, and tracts are listed below. The site of the lesion is indicated by the numbers.

Pattern	Visual Field and Acuity	Anatomic Correlate
1. Optic neuropathy	Normal contralateral field; decreased central acuity	Post-fixed chiasm or anterior extension
2. Junctional syndrome	Contralateral superotemporal field cut; decreased acuity	Junction of Willebrand knee
3. Bitemporal	Superior bitemporal desaturation; normal acuity	Inferior fibers cross first
4. Bitemporal scotoma	Relative central bitemporal defect; normal acuity	Relative macular involvement related to posterior compression
5. Tract	Homonymous hemianopia; normal acuity	Pre-fixed chiasm or posterior extension

(Figure modified from Wass JH: Hypopituitarism. In: *Clinical Endocrinology: An Illustrated Text.* Gower, 1987. Table from Newman SA: Advances in diagnosis and treatment of pituitary tumors. Reprinted with permission from Int Ophthalmol Clin 1986;26:285.)

GnRH secretion and perhaps by blocking gonadotropin actions at the ovary and testis). The resulting reproductive dysfunction presents variably: amenorrhea, irregular menses, or menses with infertility in women and decreased libido and partial or complete impotence or infertility in men.

Decreased bone density is another common consequence of hyperprolactinemia—due both to hypogonadism and perhaps also to poorly understood direct effects of prolactin on bone.

B. Growth Hormone-Secreting Adenoma: GH-secreting tumors give rise to the syndromes of **gigantism** or **acromegaly** depending on whether they develop before or after closure of the epiphyses. Clinical findings in gigantism and acromegaly are summarized in Tables 18–5 and 18–6 and reflect a combination of the insulin-like effects of the hormone, promoting visceromegaly, and the counterregulatory effects, promoting glucose intolerance.

10. What is a pituitary adenoma?
11. What brings patients with pituitary adenomas to medical attention?
12. What are the most common forms of pituitary adenoma?
13. How does a pituitary adenoma develop?

PANHYPOPITUITARISM

Panhypopituitarism is the syndrome resulting from partial or complete loss of the hormones secreted by the pituitary gland.

Table 18–4. Causes of hyperprolactinemia.[1]

Hypothalamic disease
Tumor, eg, metastases, craniopharyngioma, germinoma, cyst, glioma, hamartoma
Infiltrative disease, eg, sarcoidosis, tuberculosis, histiocytosis X, granuloma
Pseudotumor cerebri
Cranial radiation
Pituitary disease
Prolactinoma
Acromegaly
Cushing's disease
Pituitary stalk section
Empty sella syndrome
Other tumors, eg, metastases, nonfunctioning adenoma, gonadotroph adenoma, meningioma
Intrasellar germinoma
Infiltrative disease, eg, sarcoidosis, giant cell granuloma, tuberculosis
Drugs
Dopamine receptor antagonists, eg, chlorpromazine, fluphenazine, haloperidol, perphenazine, promazine, domperidone, metoclopramide, sulpiride
Other drugs
Antihypertensives, eg, methyldopa, reserpine, verapamil
Estrogens
Opioids
Cimetidine
Primary hypothyroidism
Chronic renal failure
Cirrhosis
Neurogenic, eg, breast manipulation, chest wall lesions, spinal cord lesions
Stress, eg, physical, psychologic
Idiopathic

[1]Reproduced, with permission, from Thorner MO et al: The anterior pituitary. In: *Williams Textbook of Endocrinology,* 8th ed. Wilson JD, Foster DW Jr (editors). Saunders, 1992.

Clinical Presentation

Patients with panhypopituitarism present with a variable complex of symptoms referable to the loss of one or more pituitary hormones depending on the extent and duration of disease.

In some cases panhypopituitarism is of sudden onset (eg, due to pituitary infarction or trauma). These patients may rapidly develop two potentially life-threatening situations as a consequence of loss of ACTH and vasopressin. First, since the patient is unable to mount a stress response due to lack of ACTH-stimulated glucocorticoid secretion, even relatively mild stress may be lethal. Second, a patient unable to maintain water intake will be unable to compensate for the massive diuresis associated with vasopressin deficiency **(diabetes insipidus).** Thus, the patient will quickly become comatose as a result of profound water loss and the complications of dehydration and hypernatremia.

In other cases, pituitary insufficiency develops more insidiously (eg, due to progressive destructionof the pituitary gland by a nonsecreting tumor or subsequent to pituitary radiation therapy). In many of these slowly developing cases of panhypopituitarism, the patient comes to medical attention with complaints related to reproductive functions (amenorrhea in women or infertility or impotence in men) due to LH and FSH deficiency. Other patients have nonspecific complaints (eg, lethargy or altered bowel habits), perhaps related to the gradual development of hypothyroidism (due to TSH deficiency). Panhypopituitarism may be unmasked only when the patient does poorly during some other unrelated medical emergency because of inability to mount a protective stress response due to ACTH and consequent glucocorticoid deficiency.

Etiology

Panhypopituitarism of sudden onset is usually due to traumatic disruption of the pituitary stalk, infarction and hemorrhage into a pituitary tumor, or ischemic destruction of the pituitary following systemic hypotension (eg, **Sheehan's syndrome** or postpartum hypopituitarism following massive blood loss in childbirth). A number of rare genetic causes have also been reported (Table 18–7). Gradual acquired hypopituitarism is most often due to extension of pituitary tumors or occurs as a complication of radiation therapy for brain tumors.

Pathophysiology

The biochemical hallmark of hypopituitarism is low levels of pituitary hormones in the face of low end-organ products of one or more components of the neuroendocrine axes involving the pituitary. By contrast, primary end-organ failure results in high levels of the relevant pituitary hormones.

Another biochemical difference between primary end-organ failure and end-organ failure secondary to hypopituitarism is that not all end-organ functions are equally controlled by the pituitary. In the case of the adrenal cortex, for example, mineralocorticoid secretion is only partly under the control of ACTH.

Both of the biochemical distinctions between primary end-organ failure and pituitary failure have important clinical implications. For example, hyperpigmentation occurs in primary adrenal insufficiency because melanocyte-stimulating hormone (MSH) is, like ACTH, a by-product of proopiomelanocortin precursor processing; its over production does not occur in adrenal insufficiency secondary to pituitary or hypothalamic disease. Similarly, the symptoms of adrenal insufficiency secondary to pituitary disease may be more subtle than in the case of primary adrenal failure, since a significant fraction of mineralocorticoid production is largely preserved even in the absence of ACTH (Chapter 13).

In the case of trauma and pituitary stalk transection, it is notable that hypopituitarism in general and vasopressin deficiency in particular may improve over time as edema diminishes and some degree of integrity of the pituitary stalk with its connection to the hypothalamus is reestablished. Sometimes how-

Table 18–5. Effects of growth hormone excess.[1]

Location	Symptoms	Signs
General	Fatigue Increased sweating Heat intolerance Weight gain Possible increased malignancy risk	Glucose intolerance Hypertriglyceridemia
Skin and subcutaneous tissue	Enlarging hands, feet Coarsening facial features Oily skin Hypertrichosis	Moist, warm, fleshy, doughy handshake Skin tags Acanthosis nigricans Increased heel pad
Head	Headaches	Parotid enlargement Frontal bossing
Eyes	Decreased vision	Visual field defects
Ears		Otoscope speculum cannot be inserted
Nose, throat, paranasal sinuses	Sinus congestion Increased tongue size Malocclusion Voice change	Enlarged furrowed tongue Tooth marks on tongue Widely spaced teeth Prognathism
Neck		Goiter Obstructive sleep apnea due to visceromegaly
Cardiorespiratory system	Congestive heart failure	Hypertension Cardiomegaly Left ventricular hypertrophy
Genitourinary system	Decreased libido Impotence Oligomenorrhea Infertility Renal colic	Urolithiasis
Neurologic system	Paresthesias Hypersomnolence	Carpal tunnel syndrome Nerve root compression due to bone and cartilage growth
Muscles	Weakness	Proximal myopathy
Skeletal system	Joint pains (shoulders, back, knees)	Osteoarthritis Increased 1,25-$(OH)_2D_3$ due to increased 1α-hydroxylase, resulting in increased Ca^{2+} absorption from gut and excretion in urine, increased bone density and turnover

[1]Reproduced, with permission, from Daniels GH, Norton IB: Neuroendocrine regulation and diseases of the anterior pituitary and hypothalamus. In: *Harrison's Principles of Internal Medicine,* 12th ed. McGraw-Hill, 1991.

ever, these symptoms and signs may worsen over time as the few residual intact cells or connections are lost.

Clinical Manifestations

The symptoms and signs of hypopituitarism depend on the extent and duration of specific pituitary hormone deficiencies and the patient's overall clinical status. Thus, a relative deficiency of vasopressin can be compensated for by increasing water intake; adrenal insufficiency may not be manifest until the patient needs to mount a stress response. Hypothyroidism may become manifest gradually over months because of the relatively long half-life and large reservoir of thyroid hormone normally available in the gland.

The clinical manifestations of hypopituitarism are those of the end-organ deficiency syndromes. Most important are adrenal insufficiency, hypothyroidism, and diabetes insipidus. Less crucial but often the most sensitive clue to the presence of pituitary disease are amenorrhea in women and infertility or impotence in men.

14. What are the most common causes of panhypopituitarism?
15. How do patients with panhypopituitarism come to medical attention?
16. How would you determine what replacement therapy is required for a patient with panhypopituitarism?

Table 18–6. Clinical and laboratory findings in 57 patients with acromegaly.[1]

Finding	%
Recent acral growth	100
Arthralgias	72
Excessive sweating	91
Weakness	88
Malocclusion	68
New skin tags	58
Hypertension (> 150/90)	37
Carpal tunnel syndrome	44
Fasting blood glucose > 6 mmol/L	30
Abnormal glucose tolerance test (blood glucose > 6.1 mmol/L [> 110 mg/dL])	68
Heel pad thickness > 22 mm	91
Serum prolactin > 25 μg/L	16
Serum phosphorus > 1.5 mmol/L (> 4.5 mg/dL)	48
Sella volume > 1300 mm^3	96
Serum T_4 < 53 nmol/L (< 3 ng/mL)	0[2]
Serum testosterone (men) < 10 nmol/L (<3 ng/mL)	23
8:00 AM serum cortisol < 200 nmol/L (<8 μg/dL)	4

[1]Modified and reproduced, with permission, from Clemmons DR et al: Evaluation of acromegaly by radioimmunoassay of somatomedin-C. N Engl J Med 1979;301:1138.
[2]Eleven patients were receiving T_4 replacement at the time of the study.

Table 18–8. Causes of central and nephrogenic diabetes insipidus.[1]

Central diabetes insipidus
- Hereditary, familial (autosomal dominant)
- Acquired
  - Idiopathic
  - Traumatic or postsurgical
  - Neoplastic disease: craniopharyngioma, lymphoma, meningioma, metastatic carcinoma
  - Ischemic or hypoxic disorder: Sheehan's syndrome, aneurysms, cardiopulmonary arrest, aortocoronary bypass, shock, brain death
  - Granulomatous disease: sarcoidosis, histiocytosis X
  - Infections: viral encephalitis, bacterial meningitis
  - Autoimmune disorder

Nephrogenic diabetes insipidus
- Hereditary, familial (X-linked)
- Acquired
  - Hypokalemia
  - Hypercalcemia
  - Postrenal obstruction
  - Drugs: lithium, demeclocycline, methoxyflurane
  - Sickle cell trait or disease
  - Amyloidosis
  - Pregnancy

[1]Modified and reproduced, with permission, from Reeves BW, Andreoli TE: The posterior pituitary and water metabolism. In: *Williams Textbook of Endocrinology,* 8th ed. Wilson JD, Foster DW Jr (editors). Saunders, 1992.

DIABETES INSIPIDUS

Diabetes insipidus is a syndrome of polyuria resulting from the inability to concentrate urine and therefore to conserve water as a result of lack of vasopressin action.

Clinical Presentation

The initial clinical presentation of diabetes insipidus is polyuria that persists in the face of circumstances which would normally lead to diminished urine output (eg, dehydration), accompanied by thirst. No further symptoms develop if the patient is able to maintain a water intake commensurate with water loss. The volume of urine produced in the total absence of vasopressin may reach 10–20 L/d. Thus, should the patient's ability to maintain this degree of fluid intake be compromised (eg, by whatever accident or process led to the development of diabetes insipidus in the first place), dehydration can develop and rapidly progress to coma.

Etiology

Diabetes insipidus can be due to diseases of the central nervous system **(central diabetes insipidus),** affecting the synthesis or secretion of vasopressin, or to disease of the kidney **(nephrogenic diabetes insipidus),** with loss of the kidney's ability to respond to circulating vasopressin by retaining water (Table 18–8). In both central and mephrogenic diabetes insipidus, urine is hypotonic. The most common central causes are accidental head trauma, intracranial tumor, and the post-intracranial surgery state. Less common causes are listed in Table 18–8. Nephrogenic diabetes insipidus may be familial or due to renal damage from a variety of drugs (Table 18–8). Diabetes insipidus-like syndromes may result from mineralocorticoid excess, pregnancy, and other causes. True nephrogenic diabetes insipidus must be distinguished from an osmotic (and hence vasopressin-resistant) diuresis. Likewise, washout of the medullary interstitial osmotic gradient (which is

Table 18–7. Causes of hypopituitarism.[1]

Ischemic necrosis of the pituitary
- Postpartum necrosis (Sheehan's syndrome)
- Head injury
- Vascular disease, commonly associated with diabetes mellitus

Neoplasms involving the sella turcica
- Nonfunctioning adenoma
- Craniopharyngioma
- Suprasellar chordoma
- Histiocytosis X (eosinophilic granuloma; Hand-Schüller-Christian disease)

Intrasellar cysts

Chronic inflammatory lesions
- Tuberculosis, syphilis, sarcoidosis

Infiltrative diseases
- Amyloidosis
- Hemochromatosis
- Mucopolysaccharidoses

Congenital pituitary dwarfism
- Laron type: normal proportions and intelligence but delayed sexual development
- Fröhlich type: obese with stunted growth, mental retardation, and abnormal sexual development

[1]Reproduced, with permission, from Chandrasoma P, Taylor CR: *Concise Pathology,* 2nd ed. Appleton & Lange, 1994.

necessary for the concentration of urine) may occur with prolonged diuresis due to any cause and may be confused with true diabetes insipidus. In both cases (osmotic diarrhea and medullary washout), the urine is hypertonic or isotonic rather than hypotonic.

Pathophysiology

A. Central Diabetes Insipidus: Central diabetes insipidus can be either permanent or transient, reflecting the natural history of the underlying disorder (Table 18–8). Only about 15% of the vasopressin-secreting cells of the hypothalamus need to be intact to maintain fluid balance under normal conditions. Simple destruction of the posterior pituitary does not cause sufficient neuronal loss to result in permanent diabetes insipidus. Rather, destruction of the hypothalamus or the higher supraoptic-hypophysial tract must also occur.

A more common finding is transient disease resulting from acute injury with neuronal shock and edema (eg, postinfarction or posttrauma), leading to cessation of vasopressin secretion with subsequent resumption of sufficient vasopressin secretion to resolve symptoms, either due to neuronal recovery or resolution of edema with reestablishment of hypothalamic-pituitary neurovascular integrity.

B. Nephrogenic Diabetes Insipidus: Familial nephrogenic diabetes insipidus appears to be the result of a generalized defect in the V_2 class of vasopressin receptors. Actions of vasopressin mediated by the V_1 class of receptors are unimpaired.

Drug-induced nephrogenic diabetes insipidus appears to result from a sensitivity of the vasopressin receptor to lithium, fluoride, and other salts. This occurs in about 12–30% of patients treated with these drugs. It is reversible upon termination of exposure to the offending drug (Tablc 18–8).

C. Mineralocorticoid Excess: In the case of mild hypernatremia associated with mineralocorticoid excess, it appears that chronic hypervolemia due to mineralocorticoid-induced sodium retention results in resetting of the osmotic threshold for vasopressin release. Correction of the volume overload with diuretics is sufficient to reset the osmostat and correct the hypernatremia.

D. Pregnancy: Diabetes insipidus is a rare complication of pregnancy and can have both central and nephrogenic features in that setting. It appears to be due to excessive vasopressinase in plasma. This enzyme, which selectively degrades vasopressin, is presumably released from the placenta. Normally, its level falls after delivery. The pathophysiology of excessive vasopressinase release is unclear. A hallmark of this entity is that it is reversed by administration of the vasopressin analogue desmopressin acetate, which is resistant to degradation by the enzyme.

Table 18–9. Major causes of hypernatremia.[1]

Impaired thirst
Coma
Essential hypernatremia
Excessive water losses
Renal
Central diabetes insipidus
Nephrogenic diabetes insipidus
Impaired medullary hypertonicity
Extrarenal
Sweating
Osmotic diarrhea
Burns
Solute diuresis
Glucose
Diabetic ketoacidosis
Nonketotic hyperosmolar coma
Other
Mannitol administration
Glycerol administration
Sodium excess
Administration of hypertonic NaCl
Administration of hypertonic $NaHCO_3$

[1]Modified and reproduced, with permission, from Reeves BW, Andreoli TE: The posterior pituitary and water metabolism. In: *Williams Textbook of Endocrinology,* 8th ed. Wilson JD, Foster DW Jr (editors). Saunders, 1992.

Clinical Manifestations

Diabetes insipidus must be distinguished from other causes of polyuria and hypernatremia (Table 18–9). The hallmark of diabetes insipidus is dilute urine in the face of hypernatremia. Dipstick testing of the urine for glucose distinguishes diabetes mellitus. Conditions in which **osmotic diuresis** is responsible for polyuria can be distinguished from diabetes insipidus by their high urine osmolality. **Primary polydipsia** (drinking too much water) is distinguished by the presence of hyponatremia, whereas in diabetes insipidus the serum sodium should be normal or elevated. In primary polydipsia, uncontrolled water ingestion drives the polyuria, whereas in diabetes insipidus, hypertonicity stimulates thirst.

Distinguishing central from nephrogenic diabetes insipidus depends ultimately on a determination of responsiveness to injected vasopressin, with a dramatic decrease in urine volume and increase in urine osmolality in the former and little or no change in the latter. Conversely, in central diabetes insipidus, circulating vasopressin levels are low for a given plasma osmolality while in nephrogenic diabetes insipidus they are high.

Polyuria in diabetes insipidus results from an inability to conserve water in the distal nephron due to lack of vasopressin-dependent water channels. These channels, which reside within vesicles just under the renal tubular cell surface, are inserted into the apical plasma membrane in response to vasopressin stimulation and allow conservation of water. Up to 13% of the volume of the glomerular filtrate can be reclaimed in this manner.

In diabetes insipidus of either central or nephrogenic origin, if the patient is unable to maintain sufficient water intake to offset polyuria, dehydration with consequent hypernatremia develops. Hypernatremia leads to a number of neurologic manifestations, including progressive obtundation (decreased responsiveness to verbal and physical stimuli), myoclonus, seizures, focal deficits, and coma. These neurologic manifestations result from cell shrinkage and volume loss due to osmotic forces, sometimes complicated by intracranial hemorrhage due to stretching and rupture of small blood vessels. Barring structural changes such as those leading to hemorrhage, the neurologic consequences of hypernatremia are reversible upon resolution of the underlying metabolic disorder.

The time course of hypernatremia is an important variable in the development of neurologic symptoms in that over time, neurons generate "idiogenic osmoles," ie, amino acids and other metabolites that serve to raise intracellular osmolality to the level in the blood and thereby minimize fluid shifts out of the cells of the brain. Thus, the more slowly hypernatremia develops, the less the likelihood of neurologic complications due to fluid shifts in the brain or of a vascular catastrophe.

17. What clues would suggest diabetes insipidus in a new patient?
18. How would you make a definitive diagnosis of diabetes insipidus?
19. What are the pathophysiologic differences between central and nephrogenic diabetes insipidus?

Table 18–10. The hypotonic syndromes.[1]

Excessive water ingestion
Decreased water excretion
Decreased solute delivery to diluting segments
Starvation
Beer potomania
Vasopressin excess
Syndrome of inappropriate antidiuretic hormone
Drug-induced vasopressin secretion
Vasopressin excess with decreased distal solute delivery
Congestive heart failure
Cirrhosis of the liver
Nephrotic syndrome
Cortisol deficiency
Hypothyroidism
Diuretic use
Renal failure

[1]Modified and reproduced, with permission, from Reeves BW, Andreoli TE: The posterior pituitary and water metabolism. In: *Williams Textbook of Endocrinology,* 8th ed. Wilson JD, Foster DW Jr (editors). Saunders, 1992.

Table 18–11. Causes of SIADH.[1]

Tumors
Bronchial carcinoma (particularly small-cell type)
Other carcinomas: duodenum, pancreas, bladder, ureter, prostate
Leukemia, lymphoma
Thymoma, sarcoma
Central nervous system disorders
Mass lesions: tumors, abscess, hematoma
Infections: encephalitis, meningitis
Cerebrovascular accident
Senile cerebral atrophy
Hydrocephalus
Trauma
Delirium tremens
Acute psychosis
Demyelinating and degenerative disease
Inflammatory disease
Pulmonary disorders
Infections: tuberculosis, pneumonia, abscess
Acute respiratory failure
Positive pressure ventilation
Drugs
Vasopressin, desmopressin acetate
Chlorpropamide
Clofibrate
Carbamazepine
Others: vincristine, vinblastine, tricyclic antidepressants, phenothiazines
Idiopathic
Diagnosis of exclusion

[1]Reproduced, with permission, from Chauvreau ME: Pathology of posterior pituitary. In: *Pathophysiologic Foundations of Critical Care.* Pinsky MR, Dhainaut JA (editors). Williams & Wilkins, 1993.

SYNDROME OF INAPPROPRIATE VASOPRESSIN SECRETION (SIADH)

The syndrome of inappropriate ADH (vasopressin) secretion (SIADH) is one of several causes of a hypotonic state (Table 18–10). SIADH is due to the secretion of vasopressin in excess of what is appropriate for hyperosmolality or intravascular volume depletion.

Clinical Presentation

The cardinal clinical presentation of SIADH is hyponatremia without edema. Depending on the rapidity of onset and the severity, the neurologic consequences of hyponatremia include confusion, lethargy and weakness, myoclonus, asterixis, generalized seizures, and coma.

Etiology

A variety of vasopressin-secreting tumors, central nervous system disorders, pulmonary disorders, and drugs have been associated with SIADH (Table 18–11). Several metabolic disorders can produce hyponatremia and must be investigated and ruled out before the diagnosis of true SIADH is made. In particular, adrenal insufficiency and hypothyroidism are often associated with hyponatremia. In these condi-

Table 18–12. Causes of pseudohyponatremia.[1]

Elevated plasma osmolality
Hyperglycemia
Mannitol administration
Glycerol administration
Normal plasma osmolality
Hyperproteinemia (eg, multiple myeloma)
Hyperlipidemia
Prostate surgery, with use of irrigant fluid containing glycine or sorbitol

[1]Modified and reproduced, with permission, from Reeves BW, Andreoli TE: The posterior pituitary and water metabolism. In: *Williams Textbook of Endocrinology,* 8th ed. Wilson JD, Foster DW Jr (editors). Saunders, 1992.

tions, sodium deficiency and subsequent volume depletion trigger vasopressin secretion.

Pathophysiology

The serum sodium level is normally determined by the balance of water intake, renal solute delivery (a necessary step in water excretion), and vasopressin-mediated distal renal tubular water retention. Disorders in any one of these features of normal sodium balance—or factors controlling them—can result in hyponatremia. Hyponatremia occurs when the magnitude of the disorder exceeds the capacity of homeostatic mechanisms to compensate for dysfunction. Thus, simple excess water ingestion is generally compensated for by renal water diuresis. The exceptions are (1) when water ingestion is extreme (greater than the approximately 18 L daily that can be excreted via the kidney) or (2) when renal solute delivery is limited (eg, in salt depletion), thereby limiting the ability of the kidney to excrete free water.

In hypoadrenal states, renal sodium loss due to lack of aldosterone has two consequences. First, diminished renal solute delivery impairs the ability of the kidney to excrete a water load—in the case where ingestion of water exceeds nonrenal water loss. Second, volume depletion as a consequence of renal sodium loss results in an appropriate stimulus for vasopressin secretion.

In hypothyroidism, both renal solute delivery and function of the osmostat to which vasopressin secretion is coupled appear to be impaired, resulting in hyponatremia.

True causes of hyponatremia, including SIADH, must also be distinguished from so-called pseudohyponatremia. **Pseudohyponatremia** occurs in two groups of conditions (Table 18–12). First, there are those in which infusion of hyperosmolar solutions (eg, glucose) pulls water out of cells, thereby diluting the sodium. The key feature of these conditions is hyponatremia without hypoosmolality. Secondly, pseudohyponatremia occurs when the nonaqueous fraction of plasma is larger than normal. Sodium only equilibrates with—and is regulated in—the aqueous fraction of plasma, and calculations of serum sodium concentration typically correct for total plasma volume since the nonaqueous fraction of plasma volume is normally negligible. In those relatively rare conditions where the nonaqueous fraction is significant (eg, severe hyperlipidemic states, multiple myeloma, and other conditions with higher than normal serum lipid or protein concentrations), the calculated sodium concentration will therefore be misleadingly low.

The pathophysiologic mechanisms behind most cases of SIADH are not well understood. It has been proposed that baroreceptor input from the lung is impaired in those pulmonary disorders that result in SIADH. Central nervous system lesions causing SIADH are presumed to interrupt the vasopressin-inhibiting neural pathways. Regardless of the mechanism, in most cases the hyponatremia of SIADH is partially limited by secretion of atrial natriuretic peptide. Thus, severe hyponatremia develops only when water intake is relatively increased, and edema formation is rare. The simplest therapy is restriction of free water intake and, in the case of central nervous system or pulmonary lesions, treatment of the underlying disease.

Clinical Manifestations

The clinical manifestations of SIADH are in part determined by the nature and course of any underlying disorder (eg, central nervous system or pulmonary disease), by the severity of hyponatremia, and by the rapidity with which hyponatremia develops. Regardless of its cause, SIADH can have neurologic manifestations, including confusion, asterixis, myoclonus, generalized seizures, and coma. These occur as a result of osmotic fluid shifts and resulting brain edema and elevated intracranial pressures, with brain swelling limited by the size of the skull. Physiologic mechanisms to counter this swelling include depletion of intracellular osmoles—especially potassium ions. The more rapid the progression of hyponatremia, the more likely it is that brain edema and increased intracranial pressure will develop and that the neurologic complications and herniation will lead to permanent damage. However, even when hyponatremia develops slowly, it can in extreme cases (eg, serum sodium < 110 meq/L) result in seizures and altered mental status. **Central pontine myelinolysis** can develop and cause permanent neurologic damage in patients whose hyponatremia is corrected too rapidly.

20. What conditions are associated with SIADH?
21. How would you distinguish SIADH from other causes of hyponatremia?
22. What are the neurologic consequences of SIADH, and how may they be prevented?

REFERENCES

General

Chandrasoma P, Taylor CE: *Concise Pathology,* 2nd ed. Appleton & Lange, 1994.

Chauveau ME: Pathology of posterior pituitary. In: *Pathophysiologic Foundations of Critical Care.* Pinsky MR, Dhainaut JA (editors). Williams & Wilkins, 1993.

Reeves WB, Andreoli TE: The posterior pituitary and water metabolism. In: *Williams Textbook of Endocrinology,* 8th ed. Wilson JD, Foster DW (editors). Saunders, 1992.

Thorner MO et al: The anterior pituitary. In: *Williams Textbook of Endocrinology,* 8th ed. Wilson JD, Foster DW (editors). Saunders, 1992.

Pituitary Adenoma

Abboud CF, Laws ER Jr: Diagnosis of pituitary tumors. Endocrinol Metab Clin North Am 1988;17:241.

Landis CA et al: GTPase inhibiting mutations activate the alpha chain of Gs and stimulate adenylyl cyclase in human pituitary tumors. Nature 1989;340:692.

Diabetes Insipidus and SIADH

Vokes TJ, Robertson GL: Disorders of antidiuretic hormone. Endocrinol Metab Clin North Am 1988; 17:281.

19 Disorders of the Female Reproductive Tract

Vishwanath R. Lingappa, MD, PhD

Disorders of the female reproductive system occur either as a result of disease involving one of the reproductive organs (ovaries, uterus, uterine [fallopian] tubes, vagina, breast) or involving organs whose functions affect reproductive organs (eg, brain, hypothalamus, pituitary, thyroid, adrenals, kidney, liver). Many female reproductive system disorders present during the reproductive years as **altered menstruation** or as **infertility.**

Disorders of reproductive function that are a consequence of disease in other systems (eg, hypothyroidism) are typically painless. Intrinsic disease of the reproductive organs can present either with or without pain. Pain may not occur until disease is far-advanced depending upon the location and anatomic features of reproductive organs. Some of these organs are deep and relatively inaccessible (eg, the ovaries) while others contain large amounts of adipose tissue (eg, the breast) or have a paucity of sensory nerve endings (eg, the ovary, the uterine tubes). These features contribute significantly, for example, to the high mortality rates and the high incidence of widespread metastases often associated with certain female reproductive system cancers. The widespread availability of the Papanicolaou smear as an early diagnostic test dramatically reduced the mortality rate of cervical cancer. However, the mortality rate from ovarian cancer has remained high.

The reproductive system and its hormones are involved in other functions besides reproduction, including maintenance and health of various tissues. Thus, besides menstrual disorders and infertility, the consequences of disorders of reproductive function can include **osteoporosis** (loss of bone mass), atrophy and inflammation of estrogen-deprived tissues (atrophic vaginitis), an increased risk of some forms of cancer, and unique variants of systemic disorders. The latter include gestational diabetes, and the hypertensive syndrome of **preeclampsia-eclampsia.**

1. How do female reproductive system disorders present during the reproductive years?
2. To what might you ascribe the *lack* of reduction in mortality rate from ovarian cancer in contrast to cervical cancer?
3. What are some consequences of reproductive system dysfunction?

NORMAL STRUCTURE & FUNCTION OF THE FEMALE REPRODUCTIVE TRACT

ANATOMY

The two **ovaries** house **oocytes** and produce estrogen and progesterone when appropriately stimulated. The ovaries contain thousands of **follicles**—oocytes with surrounding granulosa cells, which are steroid-producing cells that nourish and maintain the developing oocyte—embedded in a steroid-producing matrix of thecal cells. The ovary produces a wide range of endocrine and paracrine products besides steroids, which are likely to be important in follicular maturation and coordination of events in reproduction. However, currently the paracrine actions remain poorly understood (Table 19–1).

The **uterus** is a muscular pelvic organ with a hormone-responsive endometrial lining into which implantation of a fertilized egg occurs (Figure 19–1). Menstrual bleeding is the culmination of monthly cycles of endometrial growth, development, and sloughing in response to changes in blood levels of estrogen and progesterone (Figure 19–2). Besides

Table 19–1. Endocrine and paracrine products of the ovary.[1]

Protein	Compartment	Regulatory Factors
Inhibin	Granulosa, theca, corpus luteum	FSH, EGF, IGF-1, GnRH, VIP, TGF
Activin	Granulosa	FSH
Müllerian-inhibiting substance	Granulosa, cumulus oophorus	LH, FSH
Follistatin	Follicles	LH, FSH
Relaxin	Corpus luteum, theca	n.d.
	Placenta, uterus	?PRL, LH, oxytocin, PGs
Oocyte meiosis inhibitor	Follicular fluid	n.d.
Follicle regulatory protein	Follicular fluid, granulosa, luteal	FSH, GnRH
Plasminogen activator	Granulosa	n.d.
Extracellular membrane proteins	Granulosa, follicular fluid	FSH, GnRH
Insulin-like growth factor-1	Granulosa	LH, FSH, GH, EGF, TGF, PDGF, estrogen
Epidermal growth factor-like	Granulosa, theca	Gonadotropins
Transforming growth factor-α	Theca, interstitial	FSH
Basic fibroblast growth factor	Corpus luteum	n.d.
Transforming growth factor-β	Theca, interstitial, granulosa	Fibronectin, FSH, TGF-β
Platelet-derived growth factor	Granulosa	n.d.
Nerve growth factor	Ovary	n.d.
Proopiomelanocortin	Corpus luteum, interstitial, luteal, granulosa	n.d.
Enkephalin	Ovary	n.d.
Dynorphin	Ovary	n.d.
Gonadotropin-releasing hormone-like	Ovary, follicular fluid, ?granulosa	n.d.
Oxytocin	Corpus luteum, granulosa	LH, FSH, $PGF_{2\alpha}$
Vasopressin	Ovary, follicular fluid	n.d.
Renin	Follicular fluid, theca, luteal	LH, FSH
Angiotensin II	Follicular fluid	n.d.
Atrial natriuretic factor	Corpus luteum, ovary, follicular fluid	n.d.
Luteinization inhibitor and luteinization stimulator	Follicular fluid	n.d.
Gonadotropin surge-inhibiting factor	Granulosa	n.d.
Luteinizing hormone receptor-binding inhibitor	Corpus luteum	n.d.
Neuropeptide Y, calcitonin gene-related peptide, substance P, peptide histidine methionine, somatostatin	Nerve fibers	n.d.
Vasoactive intestinal peptide	Nerve fibers	n.d.
c-mos	Oocytes	Developmental

Key: EGF = epidermal growth factor; FSH = follicle-stimulating hormone; GH = growth hormone; GnRH = gonadotropin-releasing hormone; IGF = insulin-like growth factor; LH = luteinizing hormone; n.d. = not determined; PDGF = platelet-derived growth factor; PG = prostaglandin; PGF = prostaglandin F; PRL = prolactin; TGF = transforming growth factor; VIP = vasoactive intestinal peptide.

[1]Modified and reproduced, with permission, from Ackland JF et al: Nonsteroidal signals originating in the gonads. Physiol Rev 1992;72:731.

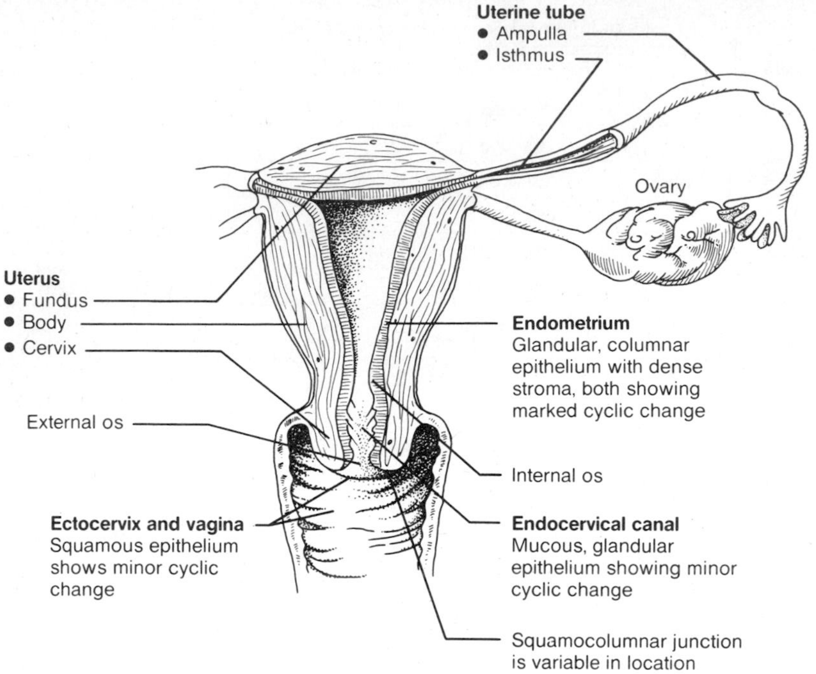

Figure 19–1. Anatomic landmarks of the uterus and adjacent organs. (Reproduced, with permission, from Chandrasoma P, Taylor CE: *Concise Pathology,* 2nd ed. Appleton & Lange, 1994.)

proliferation and maturation, the role of the endometrium includes production of a wide variety of endocrine and paracrine products (Table 19–2). Beneath the endometrium is a muscle layer termed the myometrium whose contraction is necessary to expel the fetus at parturition.

The **uterine tubes** connect the uterine lining, peritoneal space, and ovaries. The **vagina** is the muscular tube connecting the vulva with the uterine cervix (Figure 19–1).

The **breasts** produce, store, and eject milk upon appropriate hormonal and physical stimulation (Figure 19–3).

SEXUAL DIFFERENTIATION & MATURATION OF ESTROGEN-DEPENDENT TISSUES

Embryonic Sexual Differentiation

Normal human somatic cells have 46 chromosomes, including two sex chromosomes. In the case of females, both sex chromosomes are X chromosomes; males have one X and one Y chromosome. This distribution determines the **chromosomal sex** of an individual.

A gene on the Y chromosome determines whether the individual will develop male gonads (testes). In the absence of the influence of this Y chromosome gene, the individual will develop female gonads (ovaries). The presence of testes versus ovaries, a consequence of chromosomal sex, determines the **gonadal sex** of the individual.

In the weeks of embryonic development that follow germ cell migration, secretions of the male gonads (müllerian inhibitory substance, testosterone, and dihydrotestosterone) determine development of male internal and external genitalia. In the absence of these secretions, female internal and external genitalia develop. Thus, the male represents the induced phenotype. No ovarian secretions are necessary for expression of the female phenotype. This development constitutes the phenotypic sex of the individual. The development of **phenotypic sex** involves events during embryogenesis as well as events during puberty.

Before the eighth week of gestation, the sex of the embryo cannot be recognized. Appropriately, this period is termed the **indifferent phase** of sexual development. The embryo acquires a dual genital duct system within the primitive kidney. The first to form is the wolffian duct. Subsequently, the müllerian duct

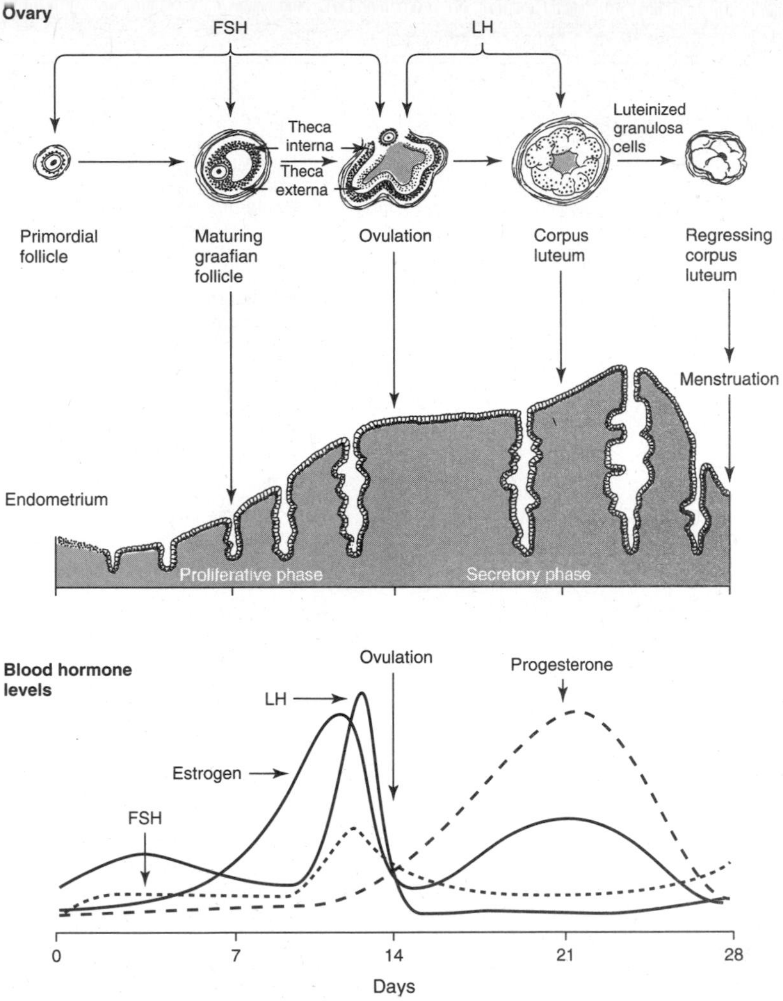

Figure 19–2. Changes in the ovary, endometrium, and blood hormone levels during the menstrual cycle. (Reproduced, with permission, from Chandrasoma P, Taylor CR: *Concise Pathology,* 2nd ed. Appleton & Lange, 1994.)

forms, dependent on prior wolffian duct development. These two duct systems have different embryologic derivations. After 8 weeks of gestation, the müllerian ducts regress in the male as a result of the production of **müllerian inhibitory substance** by Sertoli cells of the fetal testes, and the wolffian duct gives rise to the prostate, epididymis, and seminal vesicles. In the female, the internal reproductive organs are formed from the müllerian ducts, while the wolffian structures degenerate. External genitalia of both males and females develop from common embryologic structures under different hormonal influences. Thus, exposure to androgens results in virilization of the external genitalia of female embryos, whereas androgen failure results in defective male development (Figure 19–4).

The embryonic germ cells originate in the endoderm of the yolk sac, allantois, and hindgut of the embryo. By week 5–6 of gestation, they migrate to the genital ridge and multiply. By 24 weeks of gestation, there are about 7 million oogonia in the primitive ovaries. They continue to multiply, but most die around this time, so that only about 1 million primary oocytes are left at birth. This decreases to about 400,000 by puberty. The surviving oogonia are arrested at the prophase of meiosis. Completion of the first division of meiosis does not occur until the time of ovulation. Only about 400 of these oocytes actually mature and are released by ovulation in a

Table 19–2. Endocrine and paracrine products of the endometrium.[1]

Lipids	Cytokines	Peptides
Prostaglandins Thromboxanes Leukotrienes	Interleukin-1α Interleukin-1β Interleukin-6 Interferon-γ Colony-stimulating factor-1	Prolactin Relaxin Renin Endorphin Epidermal growth factor Insulin-like growth factors (IGFs) Fibroblast growth factor Platelet-derived growth factor Transforming growth factor IGF binding proteins Corticotropin-releasing hormone Fibronectin Tumor necrosis factor Parathyroid hormone-like peptide

[1]Reproduced, with permission, from Speroff L, Glass RH, Kase NG: *Clinical Gynecologic Endocrinology and Infertility,* 5th ed. Williams & Wilkins, 1994.

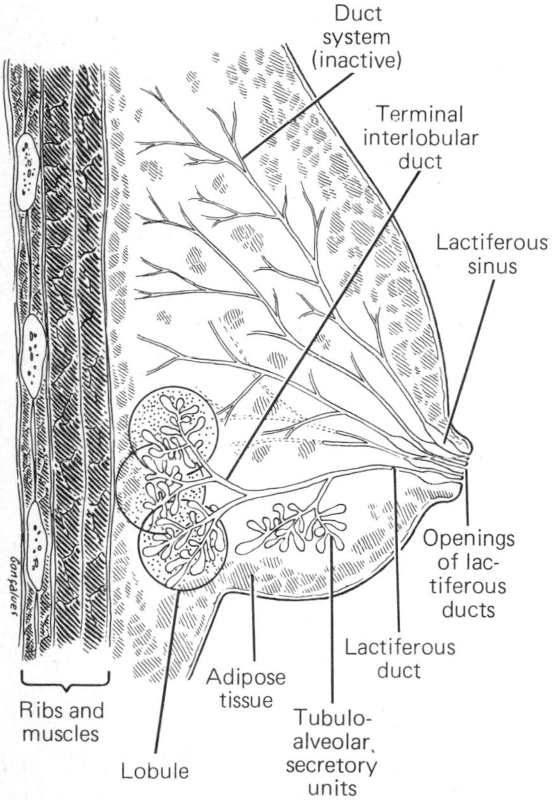

Figure 19–3. Schematic drawing of female breast showing the mammary glands with ducts that open in the nipple. The outlines of the lobules do not exist in vivo but are shown for instructional purposes. The stippling indicates the loose intralobular connective tissue. (Reproduced, with permission, from Junqueira LC, Carneiro J, Kelley RO: *Basic Histology,* 7th ed. Appleton & Lange, 1992.)

woman's lifetime; the others die at various stages of development.

Puberty

The secondary sexual characteristics develop at puberty (when maturation of the capacity for adult reproductive function occurs). Poorly understood changes occur in the brain and hypothalamus with the onset of puberty, resulting in the establishment first of sleep-dependent and later of truly pulsatile release of gonadotropin-releasing hormone from the hypothalamus. Prior to about age 10 in girls, gonadotropin secretion is at low levels and does not display a pulsatile character. The change sets pulsatile release of GnRH in motion and initiates the cyclic maturation and atresia of cohorts of follicles and the corresponding cyclic changes in estrogen and progesterone levels. The cyclic changes in estrogen and progesterone levels allow estrogen-dependent tissues to complete their maturation and manifest cyclic changes corresponding to the systemic hormonal environment. The appearance of the first menstrual period is termed the **menarche.**

Estrogen-Dependent Tissues

The major estrogen-dependent tissues include the brain, the hypothalamus and pituitary, and the ovary as well as the epithelium in the uterus and uterine tubes, the breasts, and the vagina. The vagina is lined with a squamous epithelium. Under the influence of estrogen, the vaginal epithelium accumulates glycogen, which is deposited in the vaginal lumen as epithelial cells **desquamate** (slough). Fermentation of this glycogen to lactate by normal vaginal bacteria maintains a low pH barrier to pathogenic microorganisms. Although the vagina lacks glands, fluid can extravasate through the epithelium upon appropriate stimulation.

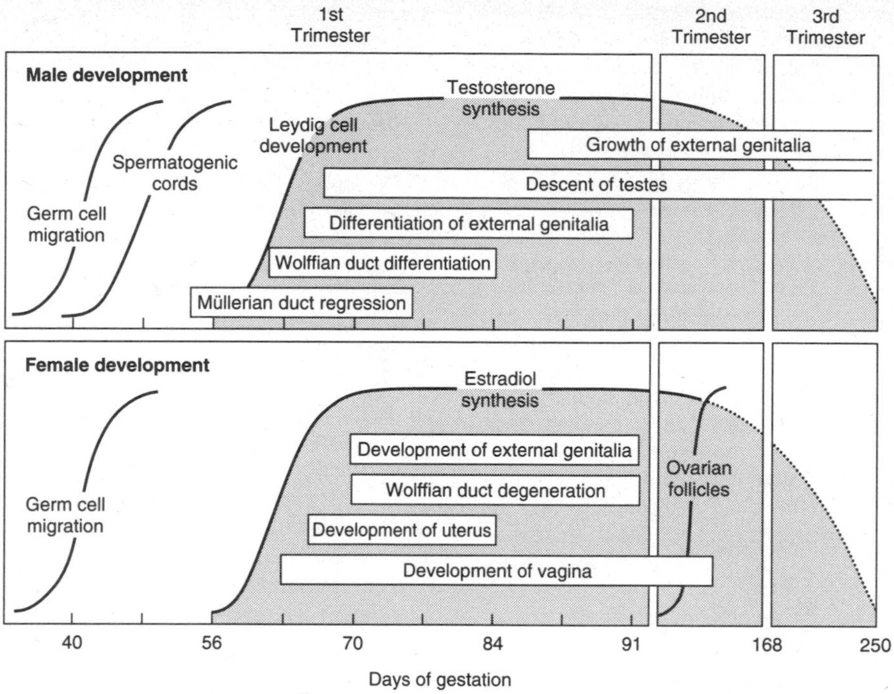

Figure 19–4. Timing of male and female human sexual differentiation. (Reproduced, with permission, from Griffin JE, Ojeda SR: *Textbook of Endocrine Physiology,* 2nd ed. Oxford Univ Press, 1992.)

4. What is the difference between the chromosomal, gonadal, and phenotypic sex of an individual?
5. Approximately what percentage of the total number of oocytes present in the ovaries of a female at birth complete their maturation and are released upon ovulation over the course of her reproductive life?
6. Describe some changes that occur in the female with onset of puberty.

The peptide **gonadotropin-releasing hormone (GnRH)** is secreted in a pulsatile manner from the hypothalamus into the pituitary portal circulation. Upon reaching the anterior pituitary, GnRH stimulates certain cells termed **gonadotrophs.** Gonadotrophs respond to GnRH by secreting two polypeptide hormones (gonadotropins) termed **luteinizing hormone (LH)** and **follicle-stimulating hormone (FSH).** The target tissues for LH and FSH are the ovaries, which respond in two general ways.

THE MENSTRUAL CYCLE

Normal female reproductive function involves a coordinated interaction of the hypothalamus, pituitary, ovary, and uterus under the influence of other organs such as the liver (which makes steroid-binding globulin), adrenals, and thyroid gland. The functional anatomy of the female reproductive system is best approached as a neuroendocrine feedback axis (Figure 19–5). The most striking feature of the female reproductive neuroendocrine axis is that its functions fluctuate on an approximately monthly cycle termed the **menstrual cycle** (Figure 19–2).

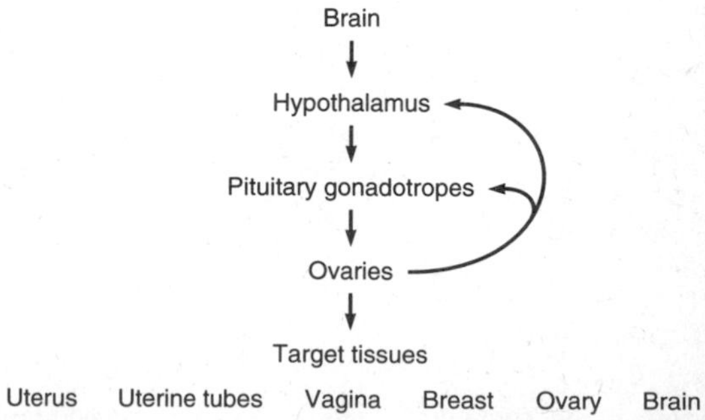

Figure 19–5. Female reproductive neuroendocrine feedback axis.

One ovarian response to gonadotropins—in particular to FSH—is maturation of oocytes (Figure 19–6). Under the influence of FSH, a cohort of follicles starts to mature. Normally, only one follicle in this cohort survives to complete the process, culminating in release of a fertilizable egg **(ovulation).** The other activated follicles succumb during the course of maturation to a process of degeneration and death termed **atresia.**

A second ovarian response to LH and FSH is synthesis, modification, and secretion of steroid hormones (Figure 19–7A). Steroid hormone production by the ovary occurs in two phases. Early in each ovarian cycle, the major steroids secreted are androgens and estrogens. Androgens made in the thecal cells diffuse into the follicles, where they are converted (by enzymatic reaction termed animatization) into estrogens in the granulosa cells. Over the first half of the cycle, termed the **follicular phase,** the level of estrogens rises. At the very end of the follicular phase, which lasts for 12–18 days, progesterone secretion begins. A midcycle surge of LH and FSH secretion, followed by ovulation, marks the end of the follicular phase. At ovulation, the mature follicle ruptures through the wall of the ovary, releasing the egg, which enters one of the uterine tubes and travels toward the endometrium. Fertilization, if it occurs, takes place along this path.

After release of the egg, what is left of the follicle develops into a structure termed the **corpus luteum** whose steroid-synthesizing capacity shifts from the production of estrogens alone to both estrogen and progesterone. During the second half of the cycle, termed the **luteal phase,** estrogens and progesterone rise dramatically. The high levels of estrogen and progesterone promote maturation of the endometrium, which had proliferated in the follicular phase with straight glands and thin secretions. Under the influence of progesterone, the endometrium develops tortuous glands engorged with thick secretions (Figure 19–2; Figure 19–8A and 19–8B). By itself, the corpus luteum is able to sustain progesterone production for only a limited period of time. This is because the high levels of estrogen and progesterone rapidly inhibit LH secretion, on which the survival of the corpus luteum depends. The luteal phase lasts 14 days.

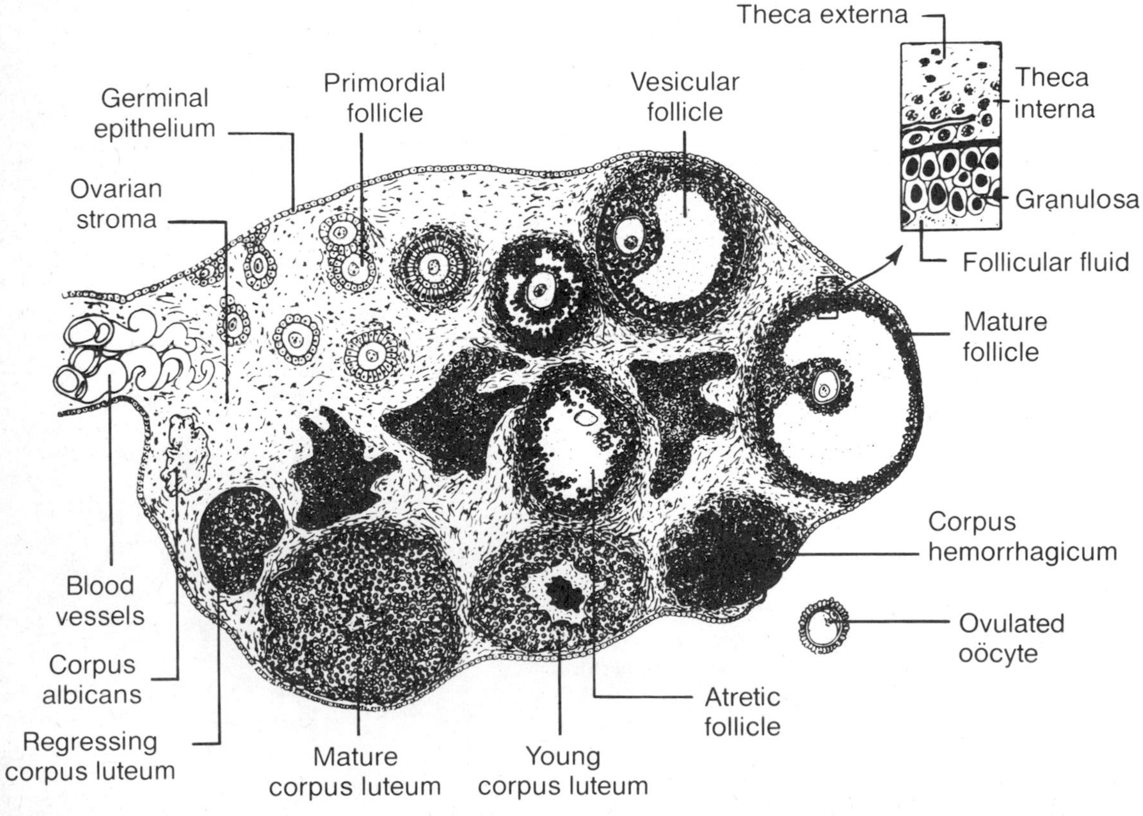

Figure 19–6. Diagram of mammalian ovary, showing the sequential development of a follicle and the formation of the corpus luteum. An atretic follicle is shown in the center, and the structure of the mature follicle is detailed at the upper right. (Reproduced, with permission, from Gorbman A, Bern H: *Textbook of Comparative Endocrinology.* Wiley, 1962.)

During that time, if fertilization and implantation have occurred, the developing placenta produces an LH-like hormone termed **human chorionic gonadotropin (hCG).** Unlike LH secretion by the gonadotrophs of the anterior pituitary, placental secretion of hCG is not inhibited by the high levels of estrogen and progesterone. hCG maintains the corpus luteum for a period of 8–10 weeks until the full progesterone-producing capacity of the placenta has developed. At that point, hCG levels fall and the placenta becomes the major producer of progesterone, working in concert with both mother and fetus to maintain the pregnancy (Figure 19–7B).

In the absence of fertilization and implantation, the corpus luteum degenerates as the LH level falls, and the levels of estrogen and progesterone decrease dramatically. The end of the menstrual cycle is marked by sloughing of the endometrium, which can no longer be maintained in the absence of estrogen (Figure 19–7A). The onset of menstruation marks the nadir of estrogen and progesterone levels, ending the preceding cycle and initiating maturation of a cohort of new follicles for the next cycle.

The ovarian steroid hormones have a wide range of effects on their target tissues, including (1) paracrine effects in the ovary itself; (2) feedback (inhibitory) effects on the brain, hypothalamus, and pituitary; and (3) feed-forward (stimulatory) effects on the end-organ target tissues of the axis: uterus, breast, vagina, uterine tubes.

The developing dominant follicle secretes many other products besides steroids, and many of these products act in a paracrine manner (Table 19–1).

Ovarian products drive not only the cyclic changes that occur in the ovary but also the cyclic changes in the end-organ target tissues. The transition from follicular to luteal phases of the cycle corresponds to the optimum environment in the uterus and uterine tubes for sperm and egg transport. Subsequently, the endometrial changes of the luteal phase are optimal for implantation and render the endometrium inhospitable for sperm transport to the uterine tube.

When perfectly coordinated with each other, the cyclic changes in structure during the course of the menstrual cycle allow the reproductive organs to perform different functions at different points in the cycle to optimize the chances for successful reproduction. When these mechanisms malfunction, the result may be infertility, altered menstrual bleeding, amenorrhea, or even cancer.

PHYSIOLOGY OF OVARIAN STEROIDS & CONTRACEPTION

Like the adrenal gland, the ovary is a massive steroid factory. The ovary secretes three types of steroids: **progestins,** containing 21 carbons; **androgens,** containing 19 carbons; and **estrogens,** containing 18 carbons. Outside of the ovary it is possible to convert the 19-carbon androgens to 18-carbon estrogens, but not the reverse. Steroid synthesis occurs by conversion from cholesterol in a series of biochemical reactions catalyzed by enzymes in the mitochondrial membrane and in the endoplasmic reticulum (see Chapter 13). Generally, the rate-limiting step in steroid production is side chain cleavage of cholesterol within the mitochondrion to generate the basic steroid nucleus that is further modified in the endoplasmic reticulum to generate the various steroids. Because steroids are synthesized by a cascade of enzyme reactions in various pathways, a block in one step (eg, due to a congenital enzyme defect or inhibition by certain drugs) can result in lack of synthesis of one steroid and "spillover" of precursors into another. Conversely, induction of new enzyme activities can convert progestins to androgens or androgens to estrogens.

The major mechanism of steroid hormone action involves diffusion across the plasma membrane, binding of the steroid to receptor proteins in the cytoplasm or nucleus, and activation of transcription of certain genes by binding of the steroid-receptor complex to specific regions of DNA. In this way the pattern of gene expression is changed in complex ways in the various steroid-responsive tissues (ie, those which contain steroid receptors).

While steroids are physiologic modulators of tissue phenotype through gene expression, modern medicine often uses them as pharmacologic agents. When used in this manner, certain steroid-mediated effects are viewed as desirable while others are considered undesirable "side effects." One of the common desirable pharmacologic uses of the ovarian steroids is contraception. Undesirable side effects include immediate consequences such as nausea and an increased risk of thrombosis and long-term consequences such as an increased risk of certain cancers.

Birth control pills are a pharmacologic means of inducing infertility by disrupting the precise timing of hormone-directed events necessary for reproduction. Formulations include estrogens alone, progestins alone, and combinations of estrogens and progestins. Most preparations of estrogen and progesterone block the LH/FSH surge at midcycle, thereby preventing ovulation. However, their contraceptive actions also include effects on other estrogen- and progesterone-sensitive tissues, such as inducing changes in cervical mucus and the endometrial lining that are unfavorable to sperm transport and implantation. Over the years, the amount of estrogen contained in birth control pills has been decreased and progestins have been added with considerable mitigation of unpleasant and dangerous side effects.

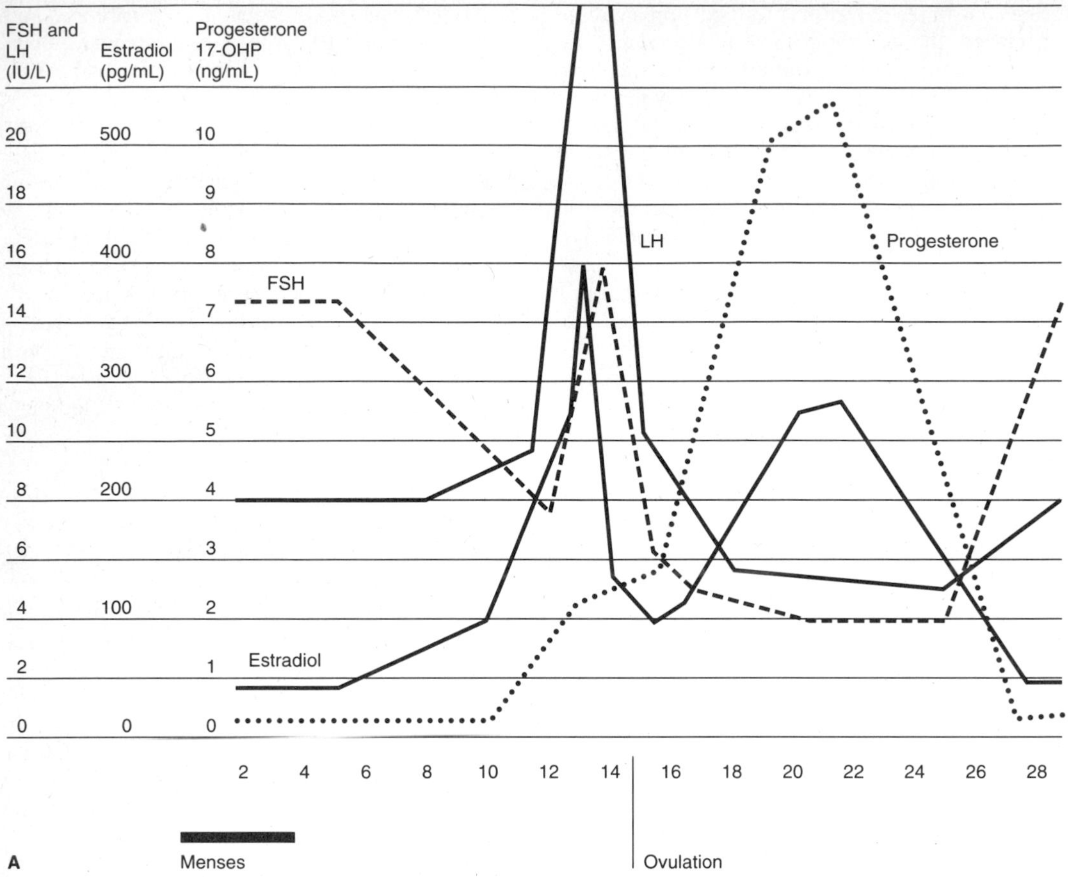

Figure 19–7. A. Steroid production during the menstrual cycle, Glass RH, Kase NG: (Reproduced, with permission, from Speroff L. *Clinical Gynecologic Endocrinology and Infertility,* 5th ed. Williams & Wilkins, 1994.)

7. What are the target tissues for GnRH? For gonadotropins? For ovarian steroids?
8. Why is pulsatile secretion of GnRH important?
9. What are some specialized features of GnRH action?
10. What are the specific effects of gonadotropins on the ovary?
11. How does the structure of the uterus differ in the midfollicular versus the late luteal stages, and for what reproduction-related events is each stage optimized?
12. What products are made by a granulosa cell in the dominant follicle over the course of its lifetime?
13. What steroids are synthesized by the ovary, and which can be generated outside of the ovary?

PREGNANCY

Prerequisites for a Successful Pregnancy

A number of changes must occur in reproductive and other organs for establishment and successful completion of a pregnancy. Fertilization requires not only successful ovulation but also effective transport of viable sperm into the uterine tube. This in turn is dependent on characteristics of the surface of the endometrium described above (Figures 19–2 and 19–8).

The uterine tubes allow the mature egg released upon ovulation to be captured and transported into the uterus, during which time fertilization may occur. If properly implanted in the wall of the uterus, the embryo will develop a placenta to support fetal growth and development. If fertilization or proper implantation does not occur, the endometrium is sloughed, only to regrow in response to the estrogen produced by the ovary during the next menstrual cycle (Figure 19–2).

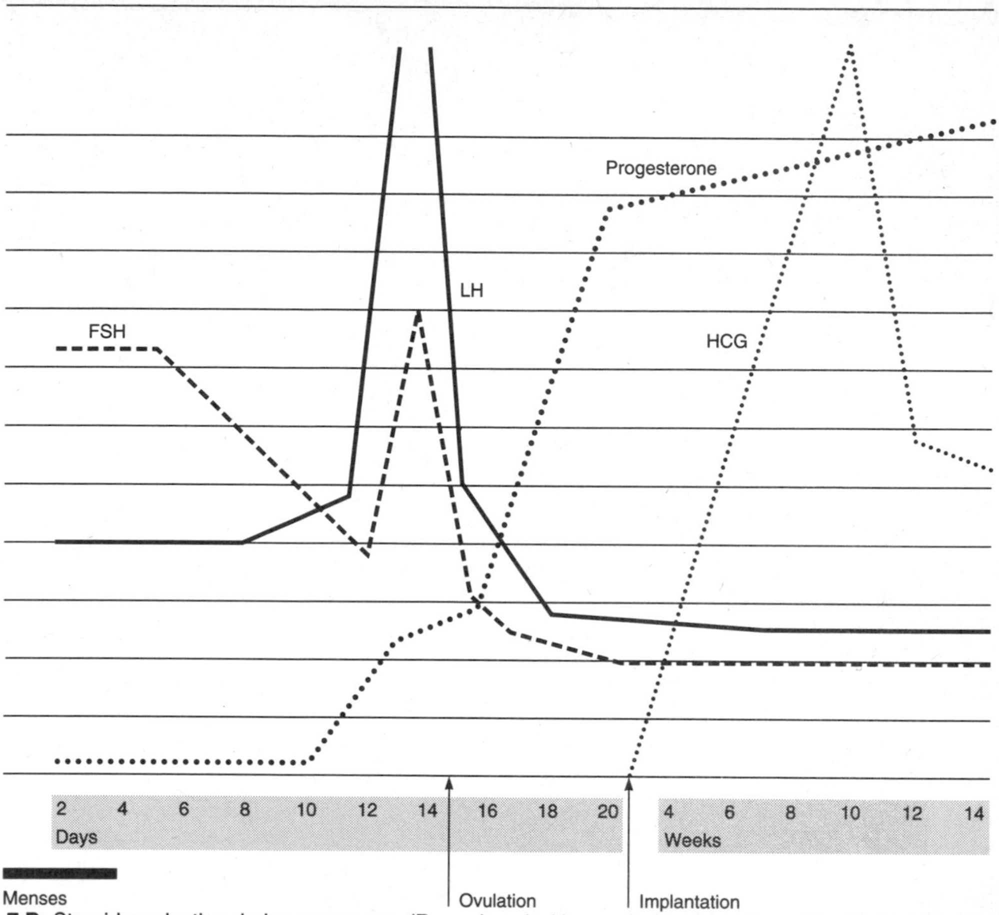

Figure 19–7 B: Steroid production during pregnancy. (Reproduced with permission, from Speroff L. *Clinical Gynecologic Endocrinology and Infertility*, 5th ed. Williams & Wilkins, 1994.)

The placenta is composed of three layers: the cytotrophoblast, the syncytiotrophoblast, and the decidual layer (Figure 19–9). The first two are derived from the embryo, the third from the maternal endometrium. The placenta allows close apposition of maternal and fetal circulations for exchange of nutrients, oxygen, and other substances. Moreover, the placenta develops the capacity to secrete a variety of important products, including hCG, progesterone, and a growth hormone-like protein termed **human chorionic somatomammotropin (hCS),** also known as **human placental lactogen (hPL)** (Table 19–3).

Placental hCG serves to maintain stimulation to the corpus luteum for progesterone secretion and hence to maintain the high levels of progesterone necessary for successful pregnancy. hCG production continues until the placenta has fully developed, a period of approximately 8–10 weeks, after which the corpus luteum atrophies, perhaps due to down-regulation of receptors by the high levels of hCG. By then, the mature placenta, working in concert with both the mother (who supplies the cholesterol) and the developing fetus, has developed the capacity to produce progesterone directly. During most of pregnancy, the fetus provides the placenta with androgens, which are used to make estrogens by the maternal compartment (Figure 19–10). This reflects the action of a special zone in the fetal adrenal cortex engaged in androgen production. Toward the end of pregnancy, the onset of ACTH secretion by the fetal pituitary triggers the fetal adrenal to produce cortisol rather than androgen. This switch may play a role in triggering onset of labor.

In addition to the changes in organs with pregnancy-specific functions, a number of physiologic changes occur in other maternal organ systems. These include increased blood volume (increased by more than 40% by the middle of the third trimester), increased total body water (increased by 6–8 L), and increased cardiac output due both to increased stroke volume (increased by 30%) as well as heart rate (increased by 15%). A striking increase in minute ventilation (increased by 50% over nonpregnant) without any change in respiratory rate is observed as a result

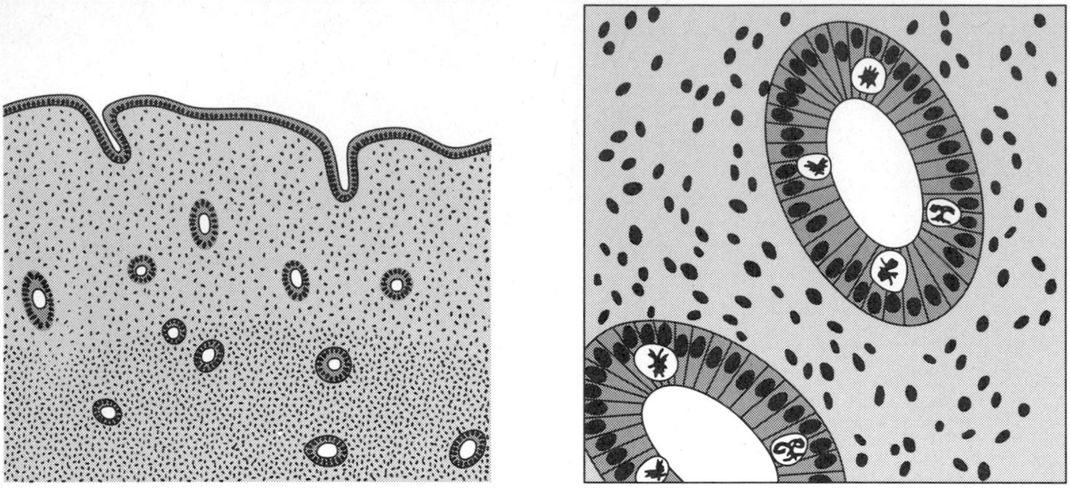

A. Early proliferative

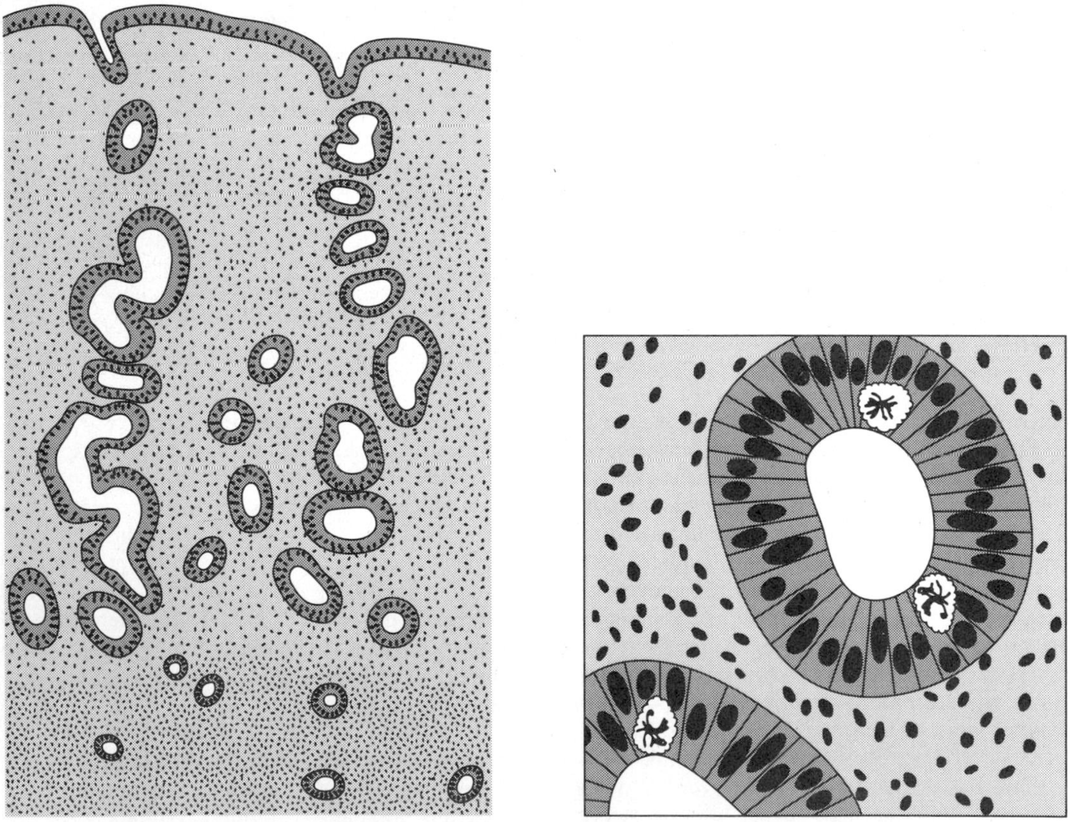

B. Late proliferative

Figure 19–8. Proliferative versus secretory endometrium (left, low power; right, high power). **A:** In the early proliferative phase, glands are narrow and tubular, lined by low columnar epithelial cells. Mitoses are prominent. **B:** In the late proliferative phase, the endometrium grows from 0.5 mm to 3.5–5.0 mm in height, and there is an increase in microvillous and ciliated cells. Lymphocytes and macrophages are diffusely distributed in the stroma. (Continued.)

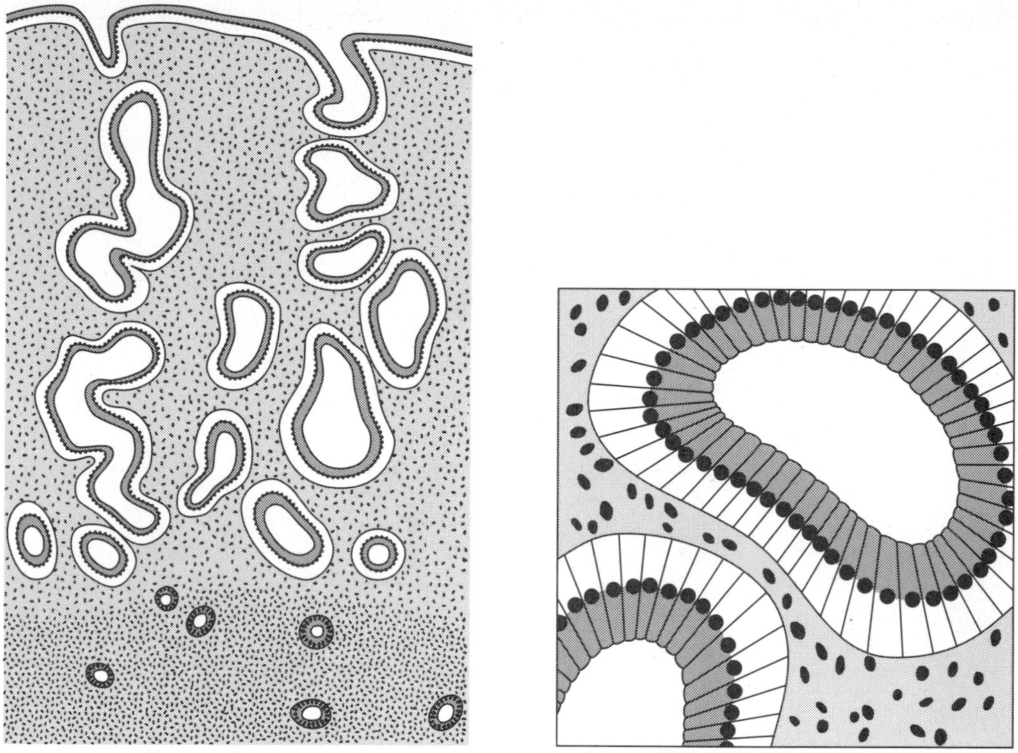

C. Early secretory

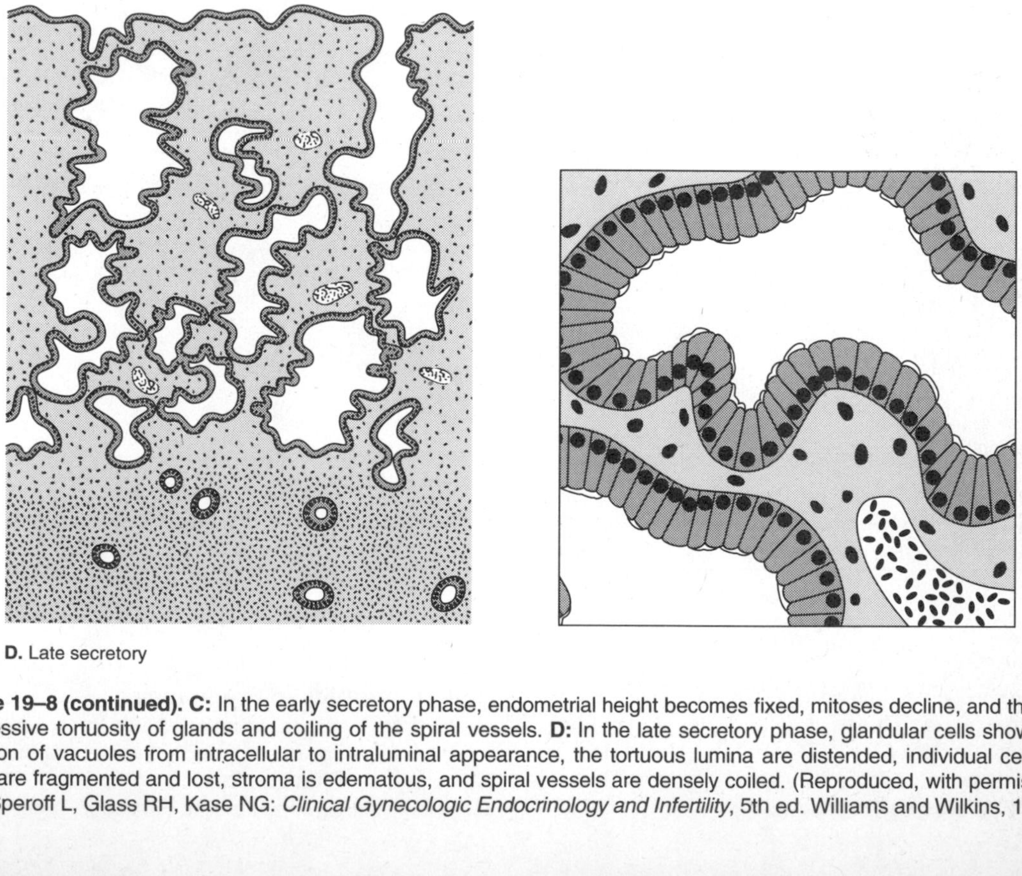

D. Late secretory

Figure 19–8 (continued). C: In the early secretory phase, endometrial height becomes fixed, mitoses decline, and there is progressive tortuosity of glands and coiling of the spiral vessels. **D:** In the late secretory phase, glandular cells show progression of vacuoles from intracellular to intraluminal appearance, the tortuous lumina are distended, individual cell surfaces are fragmented and lost, stroma is edematous, and spiral vessels are densely coiled. (Reproduced, with permission, from Speroff L, Glass RH, Kase NG: *Clinical Gynecologic Endocrinology and Infertility*, 5th ed. Williams and Wilkins, 1994.)

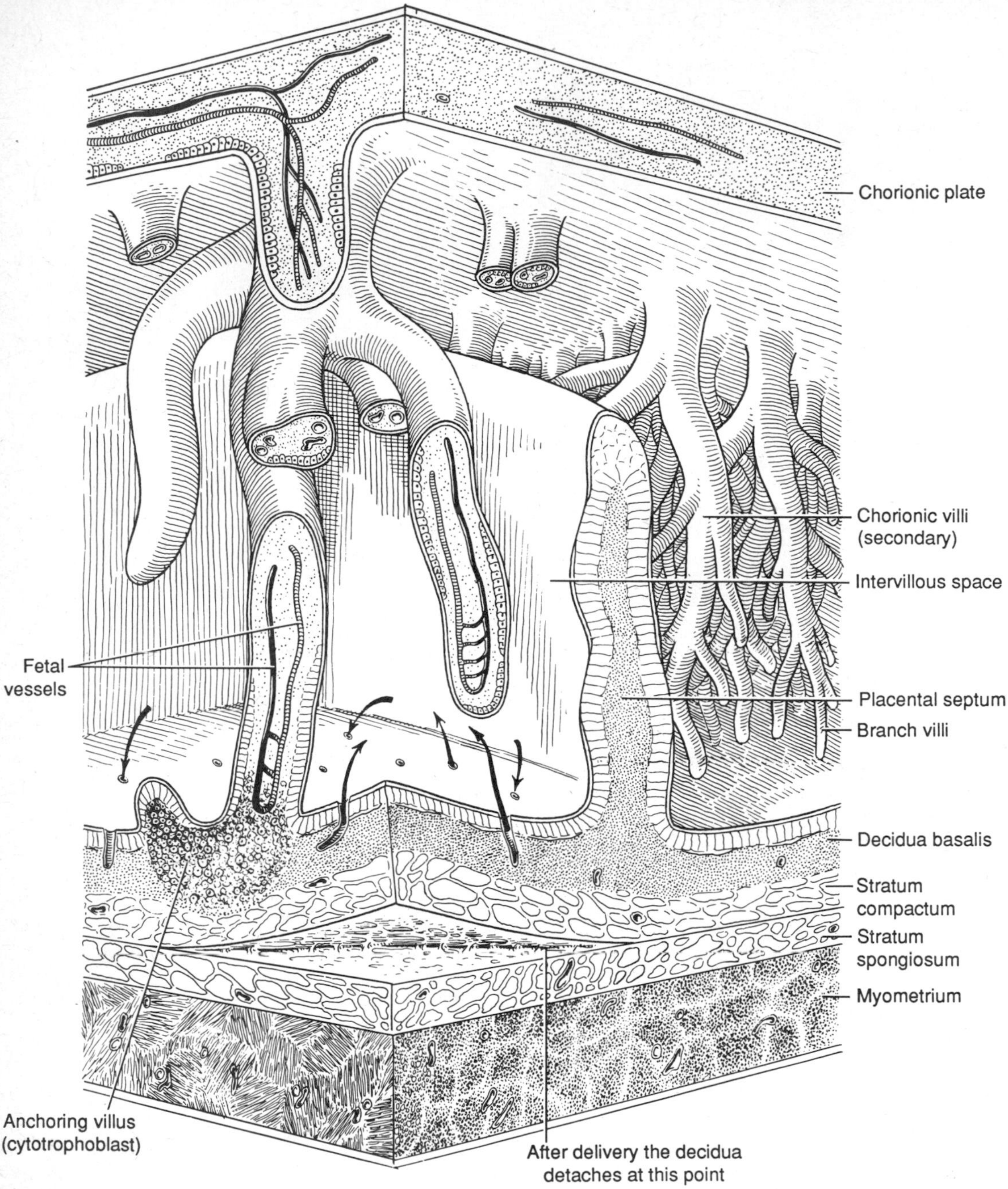

Figure 19–9. Placental anatomy. (Reproduced, with permission, from Copenhaver WM, Kelly DE, Wood RL: *Bailey's Textbook of Histology,* 17th ed. Williams & Wilkins, 1978.)

of increased tidal volume (see Chapter 7). Dramatic increases in renal blood flow and glomerular filtration rate (increased by 40%) are also seen. Most of these effects are related in complex ways to the effects of steroids in pregnancy.

Role of Steroids in Pregnancy

The precise role of various steroids in pregnancy is incompletely understood. The demonstrated and proposed roles of progesterone in pregnancy include (1) promotion of implantation; (2) suppression of the

Table 19–3. Endocrine and paracrine products in pregnancy[1]

Fetal Compartment	Placental Compartment	Maternal Compartment
Alpha-fetoprotein	Hypothalamic-like hormones GnRH CRH TRH Somatostatin Pituitary-like hormones hCG hCS hGH hCT ACTH Growth factors IGF-1 Epidermal growth factor Platelet-derived growth factor Fibroblast growth factor Transforming growth factor-β Inhibin Activin Cytokines Interleukin-1 Interleukin-6 Colony-stimulating factor Other Opioids Prorenin Pregnancy-specific β-glycoprotein Pregnancy-associated plasma protein A	Decidual proteins Prolactin Relaxin IGFBP-1 Interleukin-1 Colony-stimulating factor-1 Progesterone-associated endometrial protein Corpus luteum proteins Relaxin Prorenin

[1]Reproduced, with permission, from Speroff L, Glass RH, Kase NG: *Clinical Gynecologic Endocrinology and Infertility,* 5th ed. Williams & Wilkins, 1994.

maternal immune response to fetal antigens, thus preventing rejection of the fetus; (3) provision of substrate for manufacture by the fetal adrenal of glucocorticoids and mineralocorticoids; (4) maintenance of uterine quiescence through gestation; and (5) a role in parturition.

Human Chorionic Somatomammotropin & Fuel Homeostasis in Pregnancy

Another example of fetal-placental-maternal interactions is seen in the actions of hCS (Figures 19–11A and 19–11B). This "counterregulatory" hormone—ie, a hormone whose actions oppose those of insulin—appears to serve as a defense against fetal hypoglycemia. From a metabolic standpoint, pregnancy is a form of "accelerated starvation" characterized by fasting hypoglycemia, as fuel substrates produced by the mother are used by the growing fetus. hCS produced by the placenta in response to hypoglycemia serves to increase lipolysis, thereby raising maternal free fatty acid levels and ultimately blood glucose and ketone levels. This "diabetogenic" role of hCS is a major additional burden on the maternal compartment and contributes to the tendency for diabetes mellitus to emerge in susceptible individuals during pregnancy. Normally, glucose is the major fuel source for the fetus. However, in the event of glucose deprivation, ketones provide a ready emergency fuel supply (as they do in starvation) for both the mother and—via the placenta—for the fetus.

14. How is the corpus luteum maintained until the placenta has developed adequately?
15. What are some possible roles of steroids during pregnancy?
16. Why is new-onset diabetes mellitus a common complication of pregnancy?

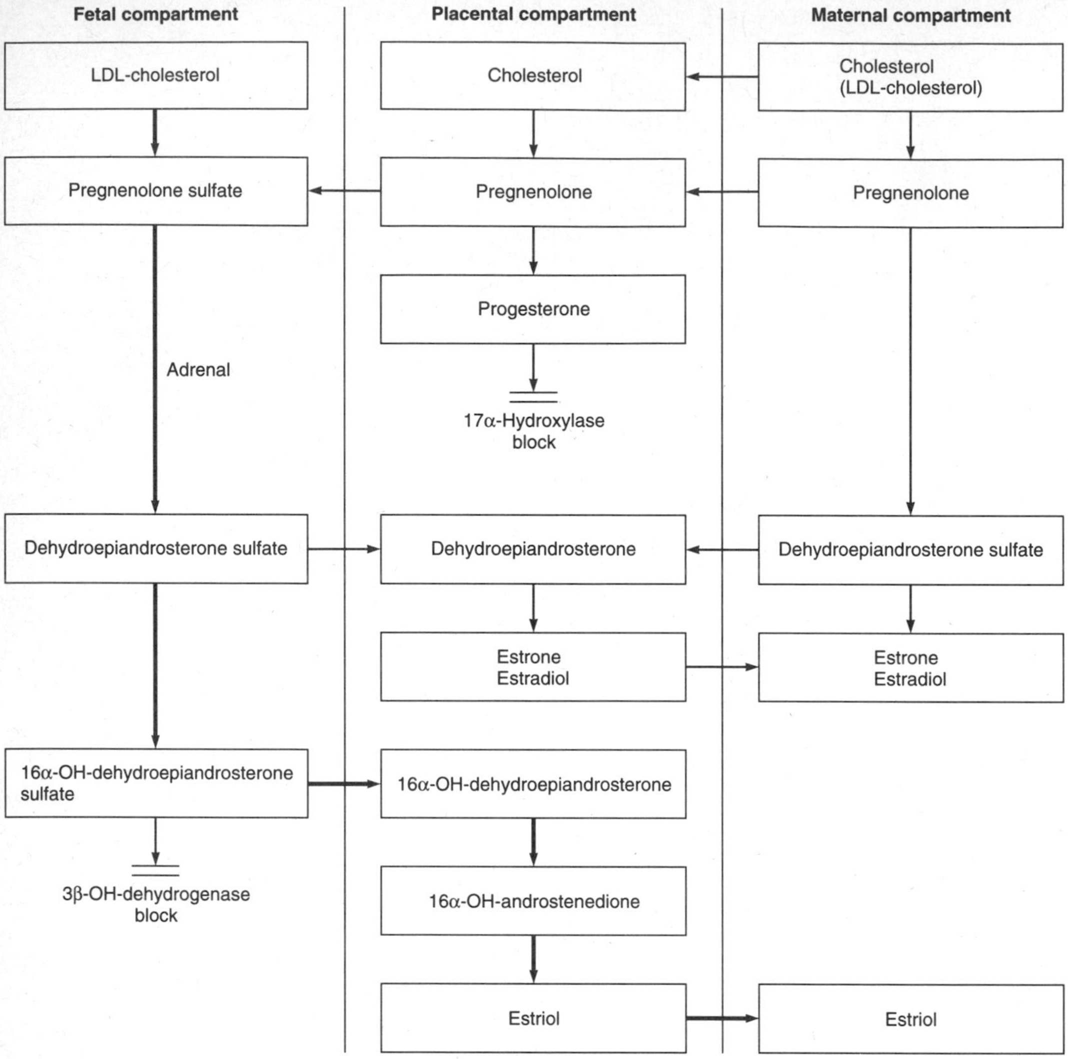

Figure 19–10. Fetal-placental-maternal cooperation in steroidogenesis. (Reproduced, with permission, from Speroff L et al: Regulation of the menstrual cycle. In: *Clinical Gynecologic Endocrinology and Infertility,* 5th ed. Williams & Wilkins, 1994.)

LACTATION

Breast Structure & Development

The mature adult female breast consists of a cluster of 15–25 lactiferous ducts, each emerging independently at the nipple (Figure 19–3). The rudiments for breast development are established during embryonic development. During puberty, rising estrogen levels stimulate breast growth as one of a number of female secondary sexual characteristics. Finally, during pregnancy, the hormones progesterone, prolactin, and chorionic somatomammotropin play a dominant role in stimulating breast growth and the capacity for milk synthesis. However, the presence of high levels of estrogen and progesterone during pregnancy block actual milk synthesis. Subsequent to delivery, with the fall in estrogen and progesterone levels, this block is removed. Both the pubertal and pregnant phases of breast growth require the permissive influence of glucocorticoids, thyroxine, and insulin for full development, and their actions are potentiated by estrogen and progesterone.

Breast growth involves both proliferation and branching of lactiferous ducts as well as accumulation of adipose and connective tissue. In the mature breast, each terminal lactiferous duct drains clusters

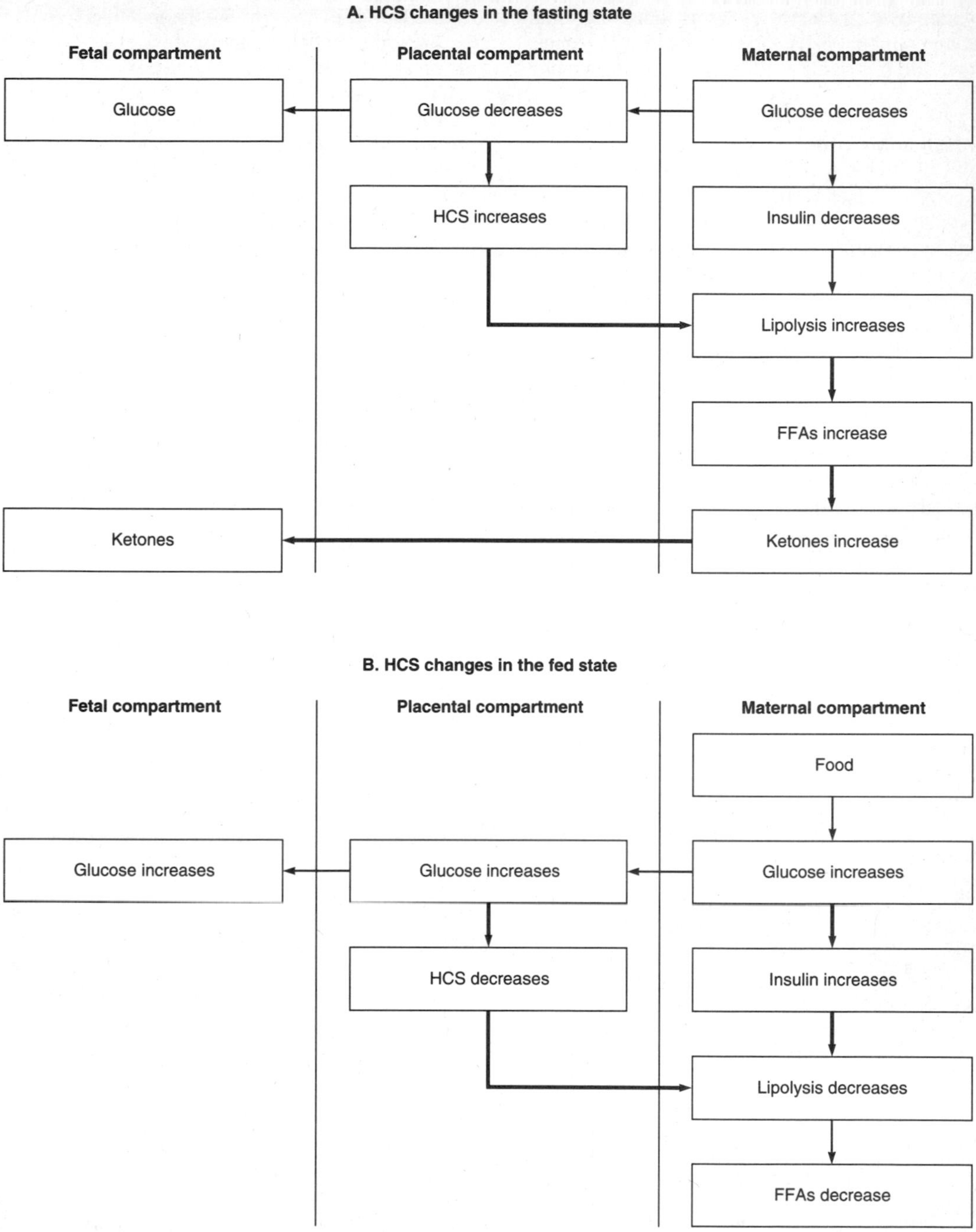

Figure 19–11. Fetal-placental-maternal cooperation in fuel homeostasis. (Reproduced, with permission, from Speroff L, Glass RH, Kase NG: *Clinical Gynecologic Endocrinology and Infertility,* 5th ed. Williams & Wilkins, 1994.)

of tubulo-alveolar secretory units lined by milk-secreting epithelial cells and is suspended in connective and adipose tissue well populated with lymphocytes.

Initiation & Maintenance of Milk Synthesis & Secretion

Although prolactin stimulates breast growth and milk synthesis, actual lactation, ie, milk release, is inhibited by the high levels of estrogen and progesterone prior to birth. After delivery of the placenta, estrogen and progesterone levels fall dramatically, removing this block. Maintenance of milk secretion requires the joint action of both anterior and posterior pituitary factors as well as of infant and mother (Figures 19–12). Suckling suppresses dopamine levels in the hypothalamus, thereby maintaining high levels of prolactin necessary for milk synthesis. At the same time, suckling (as well as other stimuli such as the baby's cry, etc) triggers an afferent sensory neural arc that stimulates synthesis, transport, and secretion of oxytocin involved in contraction of mammary myoepithelial cells.

Toward the end of pregnancy, there is an increase in the IgA-secreting lymphocyte population in the vasculature and connective tissue of the breast. These lymphocytes secrete IgA into the local bloodstream, from which it is taken up by the mammary epithelial cells. By the process of transcytosis, IgA crosses the mammary epithelial cell to be deposited into the luminal secretion (milk). This mechanism is responsible for conferring passive immunity on the newborn. Indeed, the earliest mammary gland secretion after birth, termed colostrum, has a particularly high immunoglobulin content.

The high level of prolactin maintained during lactation also has a contraceptive effect, primarily by inhibition of pulsatile secretion of GnRH. The precise mechanism is not known but may involve a short feedback loop by which prolactin elevates dopamine levels which in turn elevate endogenous opioids to inhibit GnRH secretion. There may also be effects of prolactin directly on the ovary which contribute to lactational amenorrhea and anovulation. However, it should be noted that this contraceptive influence is only moderate and of low reliability.

17. Which hormones are involved in breast development?
18. Why is milk rarely secreted prior to parturition?
19. What is the probable mechanism of lactational amenorrhea?

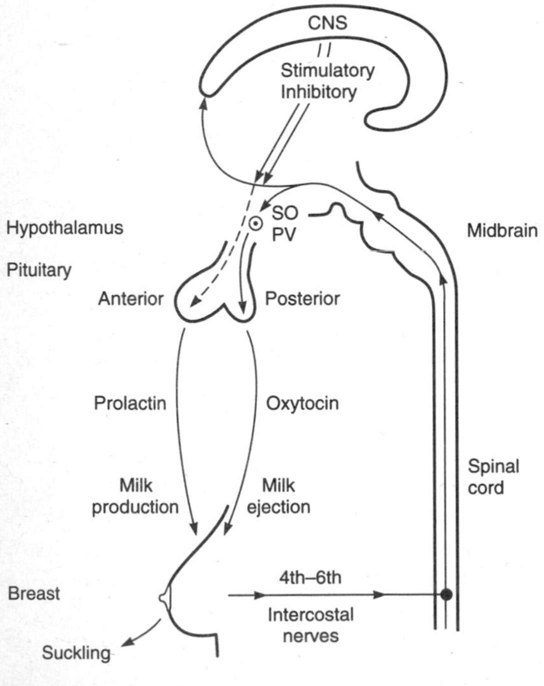

Figure 19–12. The role of anterior and posterior pituitary factors in milk synthesis and secretion. (SO, supraoptic nucleus; PV, paraventricular nucleus.) (Reproduced, with permission, from Rebar RW: The breast and physiology of lactation. In: *Maternal-Fetal Medicine: Principles and Practice.* Creasy RK, Resnick R [editors]. Saunders, 1984.)

MENOPAUSE

Menopause is the point in a woman's life when, as a result of exhaustion of the supply of functioning follicles within the ovary, menstrual cycles cease. After approximately age 40, even before menopause actually occurs, reproductive function starts to diminish. This is manifested as a decreased frequency of ovulation and atrophy of the reproductive organs. During this time, culminating in menopause, GnRH-stimulated LH and FSH secretion does not result in as much estrogen secretion as in earlier reproductive years because of the relative paucity of follicles. Hence the cyclic changes in estrogen-dependent tissues diminish and estrogen-dependent tissues atrophy as a consequence of estrogen deficiency. This period of diminished reproductive function approaching menopause is termed the **climacteric period.**

During the climacteric transition from a cyclic high-estrogen state to the low estrogen postmenopausal state, **vasomotor symptoms** such as hot flushes, sweating, and chills as well as psychologic symptoms such as irritability, tension, anxiety, and depression can be observed. Later, after the menopause, other more insidious changes occur. In addition to atrophy of estrogen-dependent tissues such as the vaginal epithelium, these include a gradual loss in bone density termed **osteoporosis.** Since lack of estrogen also results in an inability to inhibit gonadotropin secretion in a negative-feedback fashion, LH and FSH levels are typically very high in the postmenopausal woman.

A significant degree of androgen production from thecal cells of the residual ovarian stroma continues even in the absence of follicles. Even in postmenopausal women, ovarian and adrenal androgens can be aromatized into estrogens by adipose tissue and hair follicles. The significance of peripheral aromatization in relation to severity of symptoms of menopause may vary in different individuals.

20. What are the symptoms of menopause?
21. What is the source of the estrogen found in the bloodstream of postmenopausal women not on estrogen replacement therapy?
22. How do LH and FSH levels compare before puberty versus during the reproductive years versus after the menopause?

OVERVIEW OF FEMALE REPRODUCTIVE TRACT DISORDERS

Many female reproductive disorders can be traced back to a particular level of the neuroendocrine feedback axis and thus can be categorized as resulting from central (pituitary, hypothalamus, or higher brain centers with influence over the hypothalamus), or end organ (ovarian or uterine) dysfunction.

DISORDERS OF CENTRAL-HYPOTHALAMIC-PITUITARY FUNCTION

Any change in the precise rate and amplitude of GnRH secretion by the hypothalamus can result in altered pituitary responsiveness (eg, down-regulation of GnRH receptors or altered gonadotropin secretion). The alteration in pituitary function in turn results in altered ovarian function (eg, inadequate steroidogenesis with or without anovulation) and altered target tissue response (eg, menstrual abnormalities). Because many central (eg, psychic stress) and peripheral (eg, body fat content) inputs affecting pulsatile GnRH release are integrated in the hypothalamus, amenorrhea due to altered GnRH release is extremely common.

DISORDERS OF THE OVARY

Proper ovarian function involves responsiveness to gonadotropins, intrinsic viability of follicles, and a host of paracrine interactions within and between individual follicles. The polycystic ovary syndrome is an example of ovarian dysfunction due to a self-perpetuating cycle of altered feedback relationships and altered ovarian structure (see below). Polycystic ovary syndrome is manifested by anovulation, hirsutism, infertility, and either abnormal uterine bleeding or amenorrhea.

DISORDERS OF THE UTERUS & UTERINE TUBES & VAGINA

Since normal menstrual bleeding is most directly a function of the growth state of the uterine endometrium, disorders of the uterus, including myomas (fibroids), benign tumors of the underlying myometrium, and cancer of the endometrium itself, often present with abnormal vaginal bleeding.

Pelvic infections can produce adhesions and scarring of the uterus or uterine tubes that result in chronic pain and infertility.

Estrogen deficiency in postmenopausal women may present as dryness, irritation, and inflammation of estrogen-dependent tissues, including the vagina, with increased susceptibility to infection.

DISORDERS OF PREGNANCY

The normal events of pregnancy set the stage for a wide array of localized and systemic disorders:

(1) Abnormalities in the process of implantation appear to set in motion events leading to preeclampsia-eclampsia (see below).

(2) Inadequacy of the normal events of pregnancy (eg, insufficient steroidogenesis by the placenta) are believed to contribute to spontaneous abortions and premature labor.

(3) Genetic predispositions to disease that might otherwise remain latent for decades may manifest first—often transiently—during pregnancy. A good example is the genetic predisposition to development of diabetes mellitus. As discussed above, pregnancy is a counter-regulatory state, with elevation of multiple blood glucose-elevating hormones, especially hCS. Because of these counter-regulatory features of pregnancy, blood glucose control in pregnant diabetics (pregestational diabetes mellitus) is more difficult. Many patients without known diabetes mellitus first develop the disease during pregnancy (gestational diabetes mellitus). Gestational diabetes mellitus is six to ten times more common than pregestational diabetes mellitus and involves 2–5% of all

pregnancies in the United States. Many individuals who go on to manifest type II (non-insulin-dependent) diabetes mellitus later in life first manifest the disease during pregnancy.

Poor control of blood glucose during pregnancy has prominent effects on the mother, on the course of the pregnancy, and on the fetus. Retinopathy and nephropathy may first appear in the mother with known diabetes during pregnancy, though the long-term severity of the mother's disease is probably not altered by pregnancy. There is a higher incidence of acute complications of diabetes, including ketoacidosis, hypoglycemia, and infections during pregnancy. Patients with gestational and pregestational diabetes mellitus are at greater risk for preeclampsia-eclampsia. Because a long-term consequence of diabetes mellitus is small blood vessel damage, it has been proposed that preeclampsia-eclampsia in these patients results from endothelial cell injury as a consequence of ischemia. Poor glucose control also increases the rate and risk of cesarean section with associated anesthetic and surgical morbidity.

The effects of poor glucose control on the fetus are even more profound. Congenital anomalies and **macrosomia** (large body size) are increased, as are unexplained fetal deaths and spontaneous abortions. Macrosomia in turn increases the risk of complications of birth trauma and of cesarean section. High maternal blood glucose triggers increased fetal insulin secretion and therefore results in a larger fetus. As the fetus becomes larger, the risk of fetopelvic disproportion increases. Fetopelvic disproportion contributes to inability to deliver vaginally, therefore requiring cesarean section. Neonatal hypoglycemia, hypocalcemia, polycythemia, and hyperbilirubinemia also occur.

(4) The high levels of steroids and other products in the pregnant state can lead to a range of other serious medical complications. Thus, pregnancy is paradoxically associated with both hemorrhage and thrombosis. Both are related to the special functions of the placenta and its adaptations in the course of mammalian evolution.

Separation of the placenta from the wall of the uterus at birth poses a threat of massive, life-threatening hemorrhage given the intimate apposition of the placenta and the maternal blood supply. Perhaps as an adaptation to reduce this risk, a hypercoagulable state occurs in pregnancy. Physiologically, this increased tendency to coagulation and decreased activity of the fibrinolytic system serves to control postpartum hemorrhage. Pathologically, these same factors pose a risk of inappropriate thrombosis and disseminated intravascular coagulation. It has been calculated that the risk of thrombophlebitis is increased nearly 50 times in the first month postpartum compared with before pregnancy. The risk of thromboembolism in pregnancy increases with age, the presence of hypertension, bed rest, and delivery by cesarean section. Table 19–4 indicates some of the diverse ways in which pregnancy may predispose to inappropriate coagulation. When thrombosis does occur, therapy is complicated by the fact that the standard treatment with warfarin is contraindicated due to the risks of teratogenicity in early pregnancy and of fetal hemorrhage in the third trimester. Thus, pregnant patients with thrombosis are placed on subcutaneous heparin injection therapy.

One—but not the only—facet of the increased risk for thrombosis associated with pregnancy is the high-estrogen state. Thus, an increased risk of thrombosis is also seen in pharmacologic estrogen use as in oral contraceptives. The observation of enhanced cardiovascular mortality with birth control pills is probably due to these thrombogenic effects. The use of new low-dose estrogen combination pills reduces but may not eliminate this risk. Progestins have also been implicated.

Threatened Abortion & Placental Disorders

At least 15% of all pregnancies terminate spontaneously as a result of genetic or environmental factors prior to the period when extrauterine life is possible (about 20 weeks of gestation and 500 g of body weight). Abortion is threatened when painless uterine bleeding occurs with a closed, uneffaced cervix. Heavy bleeding, pain, and dilation of the internal os are signs of inevitable abortion. In patients presenting with these symptoms, abortion must be distinguished from ectopic pregnancy, which typically is associated with more severe abdominal pain, and from hydatidiform mole. The differential diagnosis relies on the rate of rise of serum β-hCG on serial determinations and on the findings on ultrasound.

Third-trimester bleeding is typically associated with **placenta previa** (implantation of trophoblastic tissue on the lower uterine segment obstructing all or

Table 19–4. Factors predisposing to thrombosis in pregnancy.

Factor	Mechanism
Estrogen effects	Alterations in blood flow resulting in increased stasis
	Increased blood viscosity due to impaired erythrocyte deformability
	Activation of coagulation due to elevated factors I (fibrinogen), VII, VIII, IX, X, and XII and decreased antithrombin III
Nonestrogen effect	Depressed fibrinolytic activity

part of the internal cervical os) or **placental abruption** (premature separation of a normally implanted placenta after more than 20 weeks of gestation).

Women who have had multiple prior pregnancies are at increased risk of placenta previa, which is believed to be due to scar tissue formation from previous implantations. Placental abruption is due to hemorrhage into the decidual plate secondary to vascular rupture and is associated with hypertension, smoking, and multiple pregnancies, all of which would be expected to affect the condition of the placental vasculature. Hemorrhage can be massive and life-threatening.

Trophoblastic Malignancies

Molar pregnancies are abnormal growths due to trophoblastic proliferation **(hydatidiform mole),** and rarely coexistent with a fetus **(partial mole).** The incidence in the USA is approximately 1:1500 pregnancies, but in certain areas of Asia it is as high as 1:125 pregnancies. The tissue in complete moles has higher malignant potential and is purely of paternal origin, while that of partial moles is usually benign and may simply contain an excess of paternal chromosomes. Most moles present with vaginal bleeding and are diagnosed during evaluation of threatened abortion by the lack of a fetus and the presence of trophoblastic tissue by ultrasound. Particularly severe nausea of pregnancy, a uterus larger than expected for gestational age, and an extremely elevated hCG level are suggestive but not diagnostic of molar pregnancy.

The complications of hydatidiform mole include high risks of (1) **choriocarcinoma,** a highly malignant, trophoblastic neoplasm with high potential for metastasis, especially to lung and brain; (2) hyperthyroidism with added risk of thyroid storm during induction of anesthesia; and (3) severe hemorrhage or trophoblastic tissue pulmonary embolism during suction curettage procedure to remove the molar products. Approximately 5% of women with hydatidiform mole subsequently develop choriocarcinoma. The serum β-hCG can be used as a sensitive test to detect the continued presence of malignant tissue. The exquisite sensitivity of choriocarcinoma to chemotherapy has made it a readily curable malignancy if detected early. The extremely high levels of β-hCG that occur with molar pregnancy and choriocarcinoma can result in cross-activation of the TSH receptor and trigger hyperthyroidism in some patients.

DISORDERS OF THE BREAST

Intrinsic disorders of the breast are either malignant (breast cancer) or benign (eg, fibrocystic disease). Breast disease can also occur as a result of the effects of other disorders or drug therapy, as in galactorrhea in women or gynecomastia in men. In females the breast, like the uterus and other estrogen- and progesterone-responsive tissues, displays cyclic changes in concert with alterations in the level of ovarian steroids through the menstrual cycle. Subtle imbalances in the relative levels of estrogen and progesterone have been considered a possible basis not only for endometrial dysfunction (infertility due to inadequate luteal phase progesterone support of the secretory endometrium) but also for so-called **benign breast disease** as well. This term refers to abnormalities ranging from normal premenstrual breast tenderness relieved with menstruation at one extreme to so-called fibrocystic disease at the other. In fibrocystic disease, there are both fibrosis and cysts in association with mammary epithelial hyperplasia. Normal breast tissue may have either fibrosis or cysts but not epithelial cell hyperplasia. True fibrocystic disease with epithelial cell hyperplasia is a risk factor for breast cancer in much the same way that endometrial hyperplasia due to unopposed estrogen action is a risk factor for endometrial cancer.

23. What are some central causes of menstrual disorders?
24. Are fibrocystic changes a risk factor for breast cancer?
25. Why might you expect some patients with choriocarcinoma to develop hyperthyroidism?

DISORDERS OF SEXUAL DIFFERENTIATION

Under certain circumstances, aberrations can occur during embryogenesis that alter the normal course of events in chromosomal, gonadal, or phenotypic sexual development. An example of an aberration in chromosomal sex is **Turner's syndrome** (45,X). Individuals with Turner's syndrome are phenotypic females with primary amenorrhea, absent secondary sexual characteristics, short stature, multiple congenital anomalies, and bilateral streak gonads.

An example of altered gonadal sex is the syndrome of pure **gonadal dysgenesis.** Affected individuals have bilateral streak gonads and an immature female phenotype, but unlike those with Turner's syndrome they are of normal height, have no associated somatic defects, and have a normal male or female karyotype.

Disorders of phenotypic sex include female and male **pseudohermaphroditism.** These syndromes result from exposure of female embryos to excessive androgens during sexual differentiation or from defects in androgen synthesis or tissue sensitivity in male embryos.

PATHOPHYSIOLOGY OF SELECTED FEMALE REPRODUCTIVE TRACT DISORDERS

MENSTRUAL DISORDERS

Disorders of the menstrual cycle involve either (1) **amenorrhea** (lack of menstrual bleeding), defined as primary amenorrhea, the failure of onset of menstrual periods by age 16, or secondary amenorrhea, the lack of menstrual periods for 6 months in a previously menstruating woman; (2) **dysmenorrhea** (pain) and other symptoms accompanying menstruation; or (3) **menorrhagia** or **metrorrhagia,** excessive or irregular vaginal bleeding (Table 19–5).

Etiology

A. Amenorrhea: The cause of amenorrhea can be traced to one of four broad categories of conditions (Table 19–6):

1. Normal physiologic processes such as pregnancy and menopause.

2. Disorders of the uterus or outflow tract such as destruction of the endometrium following excessive postpartum curettage, resulting in scarring and adhesion formation **(Asherman's syndrome).**

3. Disorders of the ovary such as gonadal failure due to a range of chromosomal, developmental, and structural abnormalities, autoimmune disorders, premature loss of follicles, and poorly understood syndromes in which ovaries with follicles are resistant to gonadotropin stimulation.

4. Disorders of the hypothalamus or pituitary resulting in either lack of or disordered GnRH secretion and as a consequence insufficient gonadotropin secretion to maintain ovarian steroid production. The causes of hypothalamic and pituitary dysfunction include prolactin-secreting tumors of the pituitary gland, hypothyroidism, excessive stress and exercise, and weight loss.

Within these categories, amenorrhea can have very diverse causes.

B. Dysmenorrhea: Dysmenorrhea is pain, typically cramping in character, lower abdominal in location, occurring in the days just before and during menstrual flow. Dysmenorrhea can occur as a primary disorder in the absence of identifiable pelvic disease or may be secondary to underlying pelvic disease, or as part of the premenstrual syndrome (Table 19–7).

C. Abnormal Vaginal Bleeding: Vaginal bleeding is abnormal if it occurs in childhood; if it occurs at the time of usual menses but is of longer duration than usual (metrorraghia); if it occurs at the time of usual menses but is heavier than usual (menorraghia); if it occurs between menstrual periods; or if it occurs after menopause in the absence of pharmacologic treatment with estrogen and progesterone. The categories of abnormal vaginal bleeding and some specific causes are set forth in Table 19–8.

Pathology & Pathogenesis

A. Amenorrhea: The pathogenesis of amenorrhea depends on the level of the neuroendocrine reproductive axis from which the disorder stems and, at each level of the axis, whether it is due to a structural problem at that level or due to a functional problem of hormonal control (Table 19–6). In a previously menstruating patient presenting with amenorrhea, it is important first to rule out pregnancy and then to assess thyroid function (serum TSH level) and pituitary function (serum prolactin level) before approaching the workup of amenorrhea compartment by compartment.

Table 19–5. Menstrual disorders.

Disorder	Defining Characteristic	Pathophysiologic Mechanism
Amenorrhea	No onset of menses by age 16 or no menstrual periods for 6 months after menstruation is established	Genetic disorders Disorders of brain, hypothalamus, pituitary, ovary, uterus, outflow tract Manifestations of endocrine disease (adrenal, thyroid)
Dysmenorrhea	Pain associated with menstrual flow	Altered prostaglandin physiology Ectopic endometrium Infection Inflammation Neoplasia
Irregular vaginal bleeding	Bleeding between periods or excessively heavy menstrual bleeding	Endometrial lesion (eg, cancer) Hormonal dysregulation

Table 19–6. Causes of amenorrhea.

Category	Common Causes	Pathophysiologic Mechanisms	How to Make a Diagnosis	Intervention
Normal physiologic processes	Pregnancy	Sustained high estrogen and progesterone	Serum β-hCG, history	Prenatal care
	Menopause	Lack of estrogen	Clinical diagnosis	Recommendations for osteoporosis prevention
Disorders of the uterus and outflow tract	Disorders of sexual development	Excessive androgen exposure	Physical examination	Surgical treatment
	Congenital anomalies (eg, imperforate hymen)		Physical examination	Surgical treatment
	Asherman's syndrome	Endometrial destruction, eg, by vigorous curettage	Lack of response to estrogen-progestin trial; direct visualization of endometrium	
Disorders of the ovary	Gonadal dysgenesis	Deletion of genetic material from the X chromosome	Karyotype	Remove streak gonads if Y chromosome is present in view of high risk of germ cell cancer
	Premature ovarian failure	Lack of viable follicles		
	Polycystic ovary disease	Altered intra-ovarian hormone relationships	Clinical diagnosis in patients with chronic anovulation and androgen excess	Decrease ovarian androgen secretion (wedge resection, oral contraceptives); increase FSH secretion
Disorders of the hypothalamus or pituitary	Stress, athletic endeavor, underweight	Altered GnRH pulses	Check serum TSH, PRL, gonadotropins	Replacement if deficient; search for tumor if excessive

Table 19–7. Categories of dysmenorrhea.

Categories	Etiology	Distinguishing Features
Primary	Prostaglandins	Lack of organic pelvic disease
Secondary		
Endometriosis	Ectopic endometrium, including intramyometrial endometrial tissue	Finding of endometrial tissue on laparoscopy
Pelvic inflammatory disease	Infection	Positive culture
Anatomic lesions (imperforate hymen, intrauterine adhesions, leiomyomas, polyps)	Congenital, inflammatory, or neoplastic	Findings on physical examination
Premenstrual syndrome (PMS)	Unknown	Association with emotional, behavioral, and other symptoms

Table 19–8. Causes of abnormal vaginal bleeding.

Childhood
Genital lesions
Vaginitis
Foreign body
Trauma
Tumors
Endocrine changes
Estrogen ingestion
Precocious puberty
Ovarian tumors
Adolescents and adults
Dysfunctional uterine bleeding
Estrogen breakthrough
Estrogen withdrawal
Diseases of the genital tract
Benign conditions
Uterine leiomyoma
Cervical polyp
Endometrial polyp
Genital laceration
Endometrial hyperplasia
Malignant diseases
Endometrial cancer
Cervical cancer
Vaginal cancer
Pregnancy
Ectopic pregnancy
Threatened abortion
Death of embryo
Other causes
Thyroid disease
von Willebrand's disease
Thrombocytopenia

[1]Reproduced, with permission, from Cowan BD, Morrison JC: Management of abnormal genital bleeding in girls and women. (Current Concepts.) N Engl J Med 1991;324:710.

1. Uterine disorders–Menstruation results from cyclic changes in the estrogen- and progesterone-sensitive endometrium. Thus, lack of an endometrium, or lack of cyclic estrogen-progesterone stimulation of the endometrium, results in amenorrhea. Most commonly this is an iatrogenic problem occurring after overly vigorous **curettage** (scraping of the endometrium) either for severe postpartum bleeding or dysfunctional uterine bleeding. Amenorrhea in such cases is due to scarring and destruction of the underlying stem cells from which the endometrium proliferates.

Renewed vaginal bleeding in an amenorrheic patient after a challenge with either progesterone alone or the sequential combination of estrogen and progesterone, followed by cessation of hormone therapy, suggests that the endometrium is intact. This response also indicates that the cause of amenorrhea lies elsewhere (ie, is due to something causing lack or insufficiency of cyclic estrogen and progesterone stimulation).

2. Ovarian failure–Amenorrhea due to ovarian failure can be either primary or secondary to dysfunction higher in the female neuroendocrine reproductive axis. Primary ovarian failure may occur as a result of genetic disorders (chromosomal aberrations) or premature loss of all follicles. The latter, excessive atresia, is due to structural abnormalities, which impede the normal paracrine interactions within the ovary (eg, thickening of the basement membrane between thecal and granulosa cells). Secondary ovarian failure results from lack of gonadotropin stimulation of otherwise normal ovaries, resulting in failure to produce the estrogen and progesterone needed for menstrual cycles.

a. Genetic causes–Genetic causes of ovarian failure include Turner's syndrome (abnormality in or absence of an X chromosome) and mosaicism (multiple cell lines of varying sex chromosome composition). Approximately 40% of patients who appear to have Turner's syndrome (short stature, webbed neck, shield chest, and hypergonadotropic hypoestrogenic amenorrhea) prove to be mosaics. The presence of any Y chromosome in the karyotype of these individuals carries a high risk of development of germ cell tumors and is an indication for surgery. Thus, a karyotype should be performed on any amenorrheic individual under the age of 30 with high FSH and LH levels.

b. Premature ovarian failure–Premature ovarian failure occurs when atresia of follicles is accelerated in an ovary of a woman of reproductive age. It presents with signs and symptoms of menopause due to estrogen deficiency at an inappropriately young age. LH and FSH levels are elevated. There is a lack of estrogen production and an absence of viable follicles. In some instances, premature ovarian failure is just one manifestation of an autoimmune polyglandular failure syndrome in which autoantibodies destroy a number of different tissues, including the ovary. These patients may also have associated hypothyroidism, adrenal insufficiency, or pernicious anemia (Chapter 9).

c. Chronic anovulation–Other patients are found to have adequate numbers of follicles that fail to mature and ovulate. This condition is known as **chronic anovulation** and is manifested as amenorrhea with intermittent bleeding between the expected time of menstrual periods (due to overgrowth of the endometrium). Left untreated, the high estrogen level places these women at increased risk for the development of endometrial and breast carcinomas. Among the causes of chronic anovulation is thyroid dysfunction (Table 19–9). Both hyperthyroidism and hypothyroidism can alter ovarian function and the metabolism of androgens and estrogens, resulting in a variety of menstrual disorders. Another cause of chronic anovulation is hyperprolactinemia. It has been proposed that progressively more severe hyperprolactinemia presents first as an inadequate luteal phase with recurrent abortion, then as anovulation with intermittent bleeding, and finally as amenorrhea.

d. Hormonal feedback disorders–Given the importance of hormone feedback in the menstrual cycle, it is not surprising that a prominent syndrome of

Table 19–9. Causes and mechanisms of chronic anovulation.

Causes	Mechanisms
Thyroid disease	
Hyperthyroidism	Increased estrogen clearance
Hypothyroidism	Decreased androgen clearance with resulting increased peripheral aromatization to estrogen
Hyperprolactinemia	Altered GnRH pulses
Obesity	Increased peripheral aromatization of androgens to estrogens Decreased steroid hormone-binding globulin, resulting in increased free estrogen and testosterone Increased insulin resistance, resulting in increased secretion of insulin which increases ovarian stromal production of androgens
Primary ovarian failure	Genetic disorders (eg, Turner's syndrome)
Secondary ovarian failure	Cytotoxic drugs Irradiation Autoimmune disorders

[1]Modified and reproduced, with permission, from Speroff L, Glass RH, Kase NG: *Clinical Gynecologic Endocrinology and Infertility,* 5th ed. Williams & Wilkins, 1994.

menstrual dysfunction is one in which key features of feedback are disordered. This condition, termed **polycystic ovary syndrome,** presents as hirsutism and infertility (Table 19–10). It affects 2–5% of women of reproductive age. Patients are often obese, and workup reveals elevated LH with exaggerated pulses, depressed FSH with few and small pulses, elevated plasma androgens, elevated plasma estrogens (estrone derived from peripheral aromatization of adrenal androgens but not estradiol generated by granulosa cell aromatase activity), anovulation (with associated amenorrhea, and estrogen-induced endometrial hyperplasia with breakthrough bleeding), and hyperinsulinemia with insulin resistance (Table 19–11).

The hyperinsulinemia is believed to be a key factor in development of the other abnormalities. Any cause of insulin resistance, including obesity and insulin receptor defects, results in hyperinsulinemia. This is because insulin resistance means that a higher blood insulin level is necessary to maintain (or, in a patient with overt diabetes mellitus, to at least try to maintain) a normal blood glucose. But as the blood insulin level rises, it has other actions besides its effects on fuel metabolism. For one, insulin results in a decreased hepatic synthesis of steroid hormone-binding globulin (SHBG) and insulin-like growth factor-1 (IGF-1) (Figure 19–13). A decrease in levels of these binding proteins results in an increase in free androgens, estrogens, and IGF-1.

Androgens worsen insulin resistance through effects on both the liver and the periphery and are a substrate for peripheral aromatization to further increase blood estrogens. Elevated estrogen levels at the wrong time in the menstrual cycle can inhibit the rise in FSH just before menses that is believed to be crucial to activating development of a new cohort of ovarian follicles. Elevated estrogen levels are also implicated in development of endometrial cancer and possibly breast cancer.

IGF-1 increases thecal androgen production in response to LH, contributing to the hyperandrogenemic state. At high enough levels, insulin also stimulates the IGF-1 receptor, further increasing thecal androgen production. The high androgens favor atresia of developing follicles and disruption of the feedback

Table 19–10. Manifestations of polycystic ovary syndrome.[1,2]

Hirsutism	95%
Large ovaries	95%
Infertility	75%
Amenorrhea	55%
Obesity	40%
Dysmenorrhea	28%
Persistent anovulation	20%

[1]Reproduced, with permission, from Beaulieu EE, Kelly PA (editors): *Hormones: From Molecules to Disease,* Champman & Hall, 1990.
[2]Percentages refer to proportion of patients with syndrome manifesting each symptom or sign.

Table 19–11. Clinical consequences of chronic anovulation.[1]

Infertility
Menstrual dysfunction (either amenorrhea or dysfunctional uterine bleeding)
Hirsutism and acne (androgen excess state)
Increased risk of endometrial cancer
Possible increased risk of breast cancer
Increased risk of cardiovascular disease
Increased risk of diabetes mellitus (hyperinsulinemia)

[1]Assembled from materials in Speroff L, Glass RH, Kase NG: *Clinical Gynecologic Endocrinology and Infertility,* 5th ed. Williams & Wilkins, 1994.

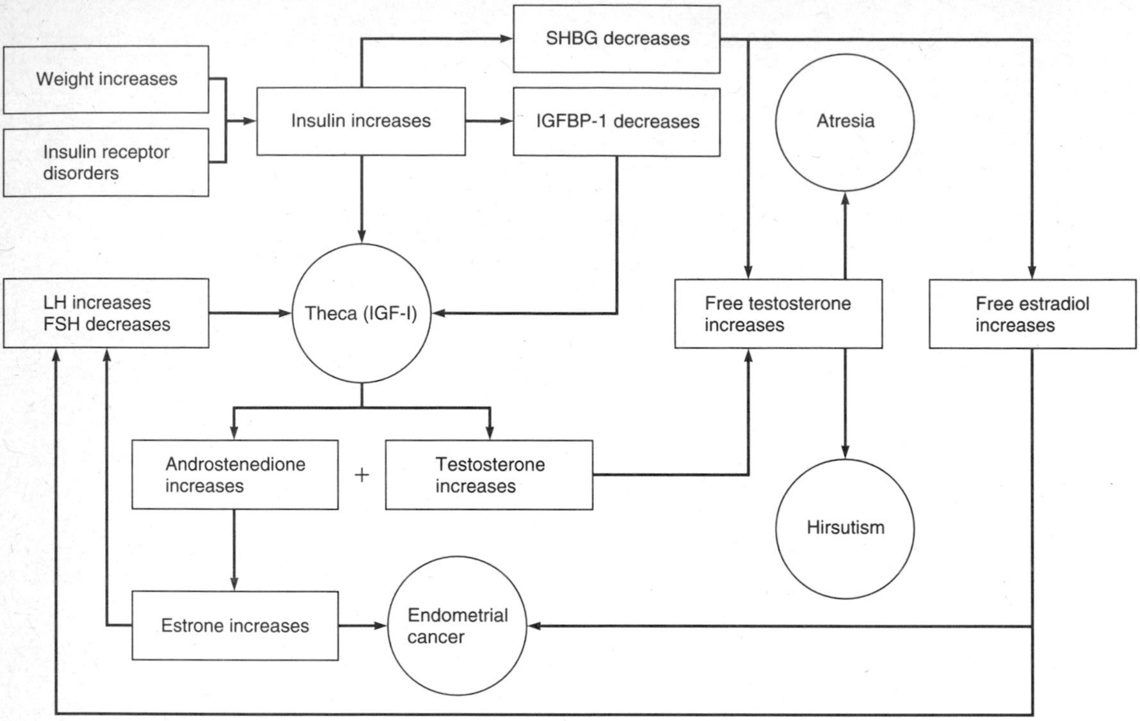

Figure 19–13. Pathogenesis of the various clinical manifestations of the polycystic ovary syndrome. (Reproduced, with permission, from Speroff L, Glass RH, Kase NG: *Clinical Gynecologic Endocrinology and Infertility,* 5th ed. Williams and Wilkins, 1994.

relationships that would normally result in selection of a dominant follicle for ovulation (Figure 19–13).

Events occurring in the brain, the ovary, and the bloodstream of these patients work together to constitute a vicious circle that maintains the aberrant feedback relationships.

In the brain (hypothalamus), GnRH pulses appear abnormal, perhaps as a result of chronic deprivation of progesterone due to persistent anovulation. FSH levels are diminished to the point that they are no longer sufficient to support the aromatase activity needed to complete follicular development. LH levels are high but lack the characteristic midcycle surge. As a result of excessive overall LH stimulation, there is thecal hypertrophy and androgen oversecretion by the ovary. Together these effects result in lack of ovarian follicular development, accelerated follicular atresia, and increased inhibin secretion.

The ovary develops a thickened fibrous capsule that itself may somehow contribute to maintenance of the abnormal feedback relationships. The high levels of androgens in the bloodstream are responsible for hirsutism. Furthermore, as a result of conversion of these androgens to estrogens by peripheral aromatase activity (eg, in fat and hair follicles, both of which are increased in these patients), exaggerated pituitary LH secretion, without a midcycle peak, is maintained. Patients with elevated androgens from totally different causes (eg, Cushing's disease and congenital adrenal hyperplasia), also display amenorrhea associated with polycystic ovaries, suggesting that the structural changes in the ovaries are secondary to the disordered feedback.

e. Pituitary and hypothalamic disorders– Trauma resulting in stalk transection with loss of hypothalamic-pituitary communication should be considered in patients with new-onset infertility with amenorrhea. So should vascular accidents, such as **Sheehan's syndrome** (postpartum hemorrhage causing hypotension and ischemic necrosis of the pituitary). Enlargement of the anterior pituitary during pregnancy (it approximately doubles in size, largely due to hypertrophy and hyperplasia of prolactin-secreting lactotrophs) may predispose to ischemia under conditions of hypotension.

f. Stress–Inputs from many different central pathways impinge on the mediobasal portion of the hypothalamus (including the arcuate nucleus) from which GnRH pulses originate. Thus, any of a wide range of factors that alter this pulsatile release of GnRH can influence female reproductive physiology. Some of the most prominent pathologic factors include a variety of forms of stress, including psychic stress, weight loss (decreased body fat), and vigorous exercise. Lack of menstrual periods due to a change in one of these factors is termed **hypothalamic amenorrhea.** It is a common cause of infertility and can be treated with pulsatile GnRH therapy, thereby reestablishing normal patterns of stimulation, receptormediated responsiveness, and feedback. Many different neurotransmitters affect GnRH secretion (opioids, dopaminergics, and norepinephrine) and thus a wide range of drugs that affect release or action of these neurotransmitters also have effects on GnRH secretion. This underscores the importance of a careful history in the workup of this common condition.

g. Indirect influences–In addition to factors that work directly on the GnRH-secreting neurons, indirect influences must be considered as well. Thus, primary hypothyroidism and primary or secondary hyperprolactinemia can result in altered GnRH pulse frequency and amplitude and therefore diminished gonadotropin secretion and secondary ovarian failure and amenorrhea.

Examples of conditions that result in secondary hyperprolactinemia include lactation, treatment with dopamine-blocking drugs, and stalk transection removing endogenous dopamine.

h. Amenorrhea associated with other functional or organic disorders–Finally, a number of complex syndromes are observed in which amenorrhea occurs in association with other findings. In patients with **anorexia nervosa,** distorted eating habits are associated with psychologic dysfunction, a distorted body image, weight loss, and a variety of medical problems including amenorrhea. Amenorrhea in these patients can occur even before onset of weight loss, implicating the psychiatric disorder rather than the stress of starvation as the cause.

26. Name four kinds of stress that can cause hypothalamic amenorrhea.
27. What are the consequences of untreated amenorrhea?

B. Dysmenorrhea: Primary dysmenorrhea is due to disordered or excessive prostaglandin production by the secretory endometrium of the uterus in the absence of a structural lesion. Prostaglandin $F_{2\alpha}$ ($PGF_{2\alpha}$) stimulates myometrial contractions of the nonpregnant uterus, while prostaglandins of the E series inhibit its contraction. It appears that patients with severe dysmenorrhea generally have excessive production of $PGF_{2\alpha}$ rather than increased sensitivity to this prostaglandin as a cause of excessive myometrial contraction. Excessive contractions of the myometrium result in ischemia of uterine muscle, which stimulates uterine pain fibers of the autonomic nervous system. As with any other cause of pain, anxiety, fear, and stress may lower the pain threshold and thereby exaggerate the prominence of these symptoms from one patient to another and over time in a given patient.

Among the secondary causes of dysmenorrhea is **endometriosis,** a disorder in which ectopic endometrial tissue responds cyclically to estrogen and progesterone (Table 19–7). This is a common disorder affecting 10–25% of women of reproductive age. The presenting symptoms of patients with endometriosis can range from pain and cramping during menstruation to adhesions with frank bowel obstruction in severe cases. Typical locations for ectopic endometrial tissue include the pelvic portion of the peritoneal space and ovaries. Establishment of endometrial tissue in these locations is believed to occur by either or both of two mechanisms: (1) by transport of sloughed endometrial tissue by retrograde menstruation through the uterine tubes; or (2) by metaplasia of undifferentiated celomic epithelial mesenchyme in the peritoneum, perhaps under the influence of growth factors present in retrograde menstrual efflux. A characteristic feature of endometriosis is amelioration after a pregnancy and after menopause. This observation provides a therapeutic rationale for the most common modes of medical therapy, which include birth control pills; synthetic androgens (danazol), which block the midcycle LH surge; and long-acting GnRH analogues that downregulate the reproductive neuroendocrine axis. It is unclear whether endometriosis causes infertility directly or simply as a consequence of resultant adhesions and scarring.

Other prominent causes of secondary dysmenorrhea are chronic pelvic infection or the adhesions resulting from prior pelvic infections and ectopic pregnancies. Infections of the pelvis typically present with abdominal and pelvic (cervical and adnexal) pain and with either fever, an elevated white blood cell count, or a positive endocervical culture. Common infectious agents include gonorrhea, anaerobic bacteria, and *Chlamydia.* Multiple organisms are usually involved. Aggressive antibiotic therapy is important in treating these infections to limit the damage to sensitive reproductive structures. Pelvic infections can develop into tubo-ovarian abscesses requiring surgical drainage.

Especially if untreated or inadequately treated, pelvic infections can result in scarring of the epithelial lining of the uterus or uterine tubes. Subsequently, these changes can impede transit of either the mature ovulated egg—or of sperms—through the uterine tube. If fertilization occurs with impeded transport of the fertilized egg out of the uterine tube, implantation into the lining of the tube can occur, resulting in an ectopic pregnancy. In this location, the embryo is not viable. Moreover, its growth results in rupture and potentially life-threatening hemorrhage unless surgically removed. Diagnosis is made by a failure of β-hCG to rise appropriately in the first several weeks of pregnancy and by ultrasonographic localization of the ectopic conceptus.

The symptoms of **premenstrual syndrome** (see below), with which dysmenorrhea is often associated, have been hypothesized to be due to escape of prostaglandins and their metabolites into the systemic circulation.

C. Abnormal Vaginal Bleeding: The pathogenesis of abnormal vaginal bleeding depends on the cause, as summarized and described in the following paragraphs.

1. Functional disorders–In these cases, depending on individual variables, the disorder results in altered amounts and timing of menstrual flow rather than a complete cessation of menses.

2. Structural lesions–Examples would be a benign or malignant tumor of the endometrium or myometrium, a foreign body, or a superimposed process (eg, pelvic infection). The most common cancers of the female genital tract involve the uterus. Two forms of uterine cancer are most prominent: endometrial and cervical. Cancer of the endometrium is generally believed to be a consequence of excessive or unopposed estrogen stimulation of this tissue, which normally proliferates in response to the cyclic presence of high estrogen levels. Unopposed estrogen stimulation can occur because of an ovarian disorder (eg, chronic anovulation); enhanced peripheral aromatization of adrenal androgens; or estrogen therapy (eg, postmenopausal replacement for prevention of osteoporosis) without a progestin. Endometrial cancer is largely a peri- and postmenopausal disease, with only 5% of cases occurring during the reproductive years. Endometrial cancer spreads by direct involvement of lymphatics with distant metastases to the lung, brain, skeleton, and abdominal organs. Patients with endometrial cancer typically present with abnormal vaginal bleeding. As with ovarian cancer, ascites, bowel obstruction, and associated pleural effusions occur in widespread disease.

In cancer of the uterine cervix, the pathophysiologic process is quite different. The major epidemiologic risk factors appear to be multiple sexual partners and onset of intercourse before age 20. Infection with human papillomavirus (HPV), herpesvirus type 2, and other sexually transmitted diseases predisposes to development of cervical cancer. HPV infection is found in approximately 25% of cases of severe cervical dysplasia (carcinoma in situ). Condylomas (viral warts), which are caused by HPV, are often seen adjacent to areas of severe dysplasia on pathologic specimens. Likewise, mutagens in sperm have been suspected of contributing to cervical dysplasia.

Unlike other female reproductive organ cancers, cervical cancer can be readily detected by the Papanicolaou smear. As a result, there has been a dramatic decrease in the mortality rate associated with cervical cancer over the last 4 decades. A Papanicolaou smear allows detection of both preneoplastic changes and cancer itself prior to metastasis, at which point it can be cured. If untreated, cervical cancer spreads directly into the pelvis, with death often occurring through hemorrhage, infection, or renal failure secondary to ureteral obstruction.

3. Systemic conditions with altered coagulation. Normal blood clotting involves both coagulation factors and platelets. Thus, disorders affecting the production, quality, and survival of either clotting factors or platelets can cause abnormal vaginal bleeding (Table 19–12).

28. What are effective medical therapies for endometriosis, and how do they work?
29. What factors predispose to cervical cancer?

Clinical Manifestations

A. Amenorrhea: The clinical signs and symptoms that accompany amenorrhea depend on its category (Table 19–6). In genetic disorders and disorders of sexual development, various degrees of delayed puberty, such as lack of breast development and absence of pubic hair, may accompany amenorrhea. In outflow tract disorders (eg, imperforate hymen), pain from occult menstruation occurs on a cyclic basis. Generally, disorders of the uterus and of the hypothalamic-pituitary axis that result in amenorrhea are painless. Ovarian failure resulting in amenorrhea is often preceded by symptoms referable to altered estrogen and progesterone production. These include hot flushes and other vasomotor symptoms and emotional lability and irritability.

The most common complication in the nonpregnant patient with amenorrhea is infertility. Additional complications depend on the specific cause of lack of

Table 19–12. Disorders of coagulation.[1]

Disorders resulting in thrombocytopenia
Suppressed platelet production
Splenic sequestration
Accelerated platelet destruction
Nonimmunologic (eg, prosthetic valves)
Immunologic
Viral and bacterial infections
Drugs
Autoimmune mechanisms (eg, idiopathic thrombocytopenic purpura)
Disorders resulting in clotting factor deficiency
Congenital disorders of coagulation
Acquired disorders of coagulation
Vitamin K deficiency
Liver disease
Disseminated intravascular coagulation

[1]Assembled from materials in Handin RI: Disorders of the platelet and vessel wall. In: *Harrison's Principles of Internal Medicine,* 12th ed. Wilson JD et al (editors). McGraw-Hill, 1991.

menstruation. Osteoporosis is the major long-term complication of inadequate estrogen stimulation. Inadequate estrogen can also be associated with thinning of estrogen-dependent epithelia, such as that of the vagina, resulting in atrophic vaginitis. The vaginitis responds to topical estrogen creams. In the case of inadequate progesterone production, typically associated with irregular vaginal bleeding but also seen in some cases of amenorrhea, the risk of endometrial cancer is greatly increased. Endometrial cancer is the most common cancer of the female genital tract, with 34,000 new cases annually in the United States. Risk factors for endometrial cancer include late meno-pause, nulliparity, obesity, hypertension, and diabetes mellitus.

B. Dysmenorrhea: Dysmenorrhea may be accompanied by a variable constellation of symptoms including sweating, weakness and fatigue, insomnia, nausea, vomiting, diarrhea, back pain, headache (including both migraine and tension headaches; see Chapter 5), dizziness, and even syncope.

In the **premenstrual syndrome,** dysmenorrhea is accompanied by additional symptoms including a sensation of bloating, weight gain, edema of the hands and feet, breast tenderness, acne, anxiety, aggression, mood swings, irritability, food cravings, and change in libido. An initial approach should be to encourage changes in lifestyle if indicated by the history (eg, more sleep, exercise, improved diet, less tobacco, alcohol, and caffeine). Approximately half of patients with premenstrual syndrome are not responsive to such measures and may benefit from monthly pharmacotherapy with prostaglandin synthesis inhibitors.

C. Abnormal Vaginal Bleeding: The signs and symptoms that accompany abnormal vaginal bleeding vary with the cause. In children, vulvovaginitis is the most frequent disorder, accompanied by a mucopurulent discharge that may become bloody with mucosal erosion. Other prominent causes, including foreign objects and tumors, can be assessed by physical examination. In adolescents and adults, dysfunctional uterine bleeding is most common, but other causes may be considered, including pregnancy (assessed by serial serum β-hCG determinations and ultrasound examination), trauma (by history and physical examination), cancer (by hysteroscopy), and systemic disorders such as a hemorrhagic diathesis (by prothrombin and partial thromboplastin time determinations) and thyroid disease (by serum TSH, total and free T_4 determinations). In postmenopausal women, one-fifth of cases of vaginal bleeding prove to be endometrial cancer.

INFERTILITY

The infertile patient presents with a history of at least 1 year of unprotected regular sexual intercourse without conception. Inability to become pregnant must be distinguished from inability to carry the pregnancy to term.

Etiology

In approximately 30% of cases, the cause of infertility is due to factors involving the male (eg, inadequate sperm count) (see Chapter 20). About 40% of cases of female infertility are due to ovulatory failure, about 40% due to endometrial or tubal disease, about 10% due to rarer causes (eg, thyroid disease or hyperprolactinemia), and about 10% remain undefined after full workup (Table 19–13).

Pathology & Pathogenesis

A. Ovulatory Causes: Infertility can result from disorders of the hypothalamus or pituitary, resulting in inadequate gonadotropic stimulation of the ovary; or from ovarian disorders, resulting either in inadequate secretory products or failure to ovulate; or from both types of disorders. The most common ovarian disorders are age-related and can involve both the oocytes themselves and the secretory products of the ovary.

There is accelerated loss of follicles with the approach of menopause. Loss of all follicles from the ovaries (ie, ovarian failure) results in permanent anovulation and menopause. With the approach of ovarian failure, FSH levels tend to rise, reflecting inadequate production of inhibin. In principle, this could result either from an inadequate number of follicles, diminished competence of the remaining follicles, diminished steroidogenesis by the aging ovary, or some combination of these factors. Regardless of the specific reason, the net effect is a shortened follicular phase and is associated with increased rates of infertility. Treatment with clomiphene citrate, a weak estrogen antagonist, is a means of diminishing negative feedback and thereby further increasing go-

Table 19–13. Causes of female infertility.[1,2]

Cause	Incidence in Patients With Infertility
Ovulatory failure	40%
Tubal or pelvic pathology	40%
Thick mucus	
Scarring and adhesions (from pelvic inflammatory disease, chronic infection, tubal surgery, ectopic pregnancy, or ruptured appendix)	
Miscellaneous	10%
Thyroid disease	
Pituitary disease (hyperprolactinemia)	
Unexplained	10%

[1]Modified and reproduced, with permission, from Speroff L, Glass RH, Case NG: *Clinical Gynecologic Endocrinology and Infertility,* 5th ed. Williams & Wilkins, 1994.
[2]In infertile couples, problems in the male account for 30% of the total.

nadotropin stimulation of the ovary. In some cases this appears to result in ovulation, perhaps due to prolongation of the follicular phase.

In some cases, infertility is due to a shortened or inadequate luteal phase manifested as an inadequate quantity or duration of progesterone production. One possible mechanism is excess estrogen in the follicular phase. Estrogen elevates $PGF_{2\alpha}$, which antagonizes the effect of LH, thereby decreasing progesterone production by the corpus luteum and shortening the luteal phase. This mechanism has a clinical correlation in the efficacy of postcoital high-dose estrogen as a contraceptive. The technique is effective only in the week subsequent to coitus, because hCG production upon implantation overcomes the antagonism of LH action caused by the elevated $PGF_{2\alpha}$.

Treatment with progesterone, either directly or indirectly by clomiphene or gonadotropin stimulation, can correct infertility due to a shortened luteal phase.

B. Tubal and Pelvic Causes: Given normal follicles and reproductive neuroendocrine axis function, the major cause of infertility is abnormality of the endometrium and uterine tubes. Prior or ongoing pelvic infections, with scarring and adhesions or inflammation, can result in failure of sperm or egg transport, failure of implantation or implantation in an inappropriate location (ectopic pregnancy). Since, on average, sperms are viable for only about 24 hours after insemination and a freshly released mature egg is only viable for about 12 hours, any impediment to transport of either sperm or egg or of implantation of a fertilized egg can greatly diminish the likelihood of pregnancy.

Endometriosis, with cyclic proliferation and sloughing of ectopic endometrial tissue, resulting in inflammation, scarring, and adhesions, should be suspected when infertility is associated with dysmenorrhea.

C. Other Causes of Female Infertility: Most of the less common causes of infertility can be grouped into those that affect the production of GnRH by the hypothalamus or its effect on the pituitary (eg, thyroid disease and hyperprolactinemia) and those that affect ovarian feedback (eg, hyperandrogenism and the polycystic ovary syndrome).

30. What are the most common causes of infertility in couples?
31. How do postcoital high-dose estrogens work as a contraceptive?
32. What feature of the history suggests a tubal or uterine cause of infertility?

PREECLAMPSIA-ECLAMPSIA

Pregnancy is associated with a host of medical complications whose principles of clinical management are grounded in the underlying physiology of pregnancy and the pathophysiology of the particular disorder. The syndrome of preeclampsia-eclampsia, characterized by hypertension, proteinuria, and edema, is chosen for focus for several reasons: First, because preeclampsia-eclampsia is the most important cause of maternal death in the USA and much of Western Europe; second, because it illustrates how pathophysiologic mechanisms in pregnancy may be far more complex—and the clinical consequences far more serious—than would have been expected from a simple consideration of each of the presenting symptoms in isolation; and third, because recent advances have significantly altered current thinking about the pathogenesis of this disorder.

Clinical Presentation

Hypertension is the most common medical complication of pregnancy and can be of two general forms. First, patients who may or may not have a history of elevated blood pressure may develop asymptomatic essential hypertension, typically early in pregnancy. A distinguishing feature of essential hypertension of pregnancy is that even slight overtreatment, which would be inconsequential in the nonpregnant state, may result in placental insufficiency and fetal distress. In this case, the placental insufficiency is due to underperfusion. The major complication of untreated essential hypertension in pregnancy, which typically appears before the 20th week of gestation, is the risk of placental damage and insufficiency and an increased risk of fetal distress later in gestation. Placental insufficiency in untreated essential hypertension results from loss of placental capacity due to small vessel infarction and hemorrhage.

A second, far more ominous syndrome of hypertension known as preeclampsia-eclampsia occurs in approximately 5% of pregnancies in the United States. Preeclampsia-eclampsia is associated with proteinuria (> 3 g/24 h) and edema and results in a cascade of changes that in its most dramatic form leads to hemorrhage, seizures, renal failure, disseminated intravascular coagulation (DIC), and death. Table 19–14 summarizes the symptoms and signs of preeclampsia-eclampsia.

Etiology

The underlying causes of both essential hypertension and preeclampsia-eclampsia remain unknown. However, important progress has been made in understanding the cause of preeclampsia-eclampsia. It has been suggested that preeclampsia-eclampsia is a disorder of endothelial cell function caused by faulty implantation (see below). As such, it is likely to be fundamentally different from essential hypertension.

Table 19–14. Symptoms and signs of preeclampsia-eclampsia.

Maternal syndrome
Pregnancy-induced hypertension
Excessive weight gain (>1 kg/wk)
Generalized edema
Ascites
Hyperuricemia
Proteinuria
Hypocalciuria
Increased plasma von Willebrand factor concentration
Increased plasma cellular fibronectin
Reduced plasma antithrombin III concentration
Thrombocytopenia
Increased packed cell volume
Increased serum liver enzyme levels
Fetal syndrome
Intrauterine growth retardation
Intrauterine hypoxemia

[1]Reproduced, with permission, from Roberts JM, Redman CWG: Preeclampsia: More than pregnancy-induced hypertension. Lancet 1993;341:1447.

Table 19–15. Complications of preeclampsia-eclampsia.[1]

Cerebral hemorrhage
Cortical blindness
Retinal detachment
HELLP syndrome (hemolysis, elevated liver enzymes, low platelets)
Hepatic rupture
Disseminated intravascular coagulation (DIC)
Pulmonary edema
Laryngeal edema
Acute renal cortical necrosis
Acute renal tubular necrosis
Abruptio placentae
Intrauterine fetal asphyxia and death

[1]Reproduced, with permission, from Roberts JM, Redman CWG: Pre-eclampsia: More than pregnancy-induced hypertension. Lancet 1993;341:1447.

Strongly suggestive of this etiologic distinction is the occurrence of a variant of preeclampsia-eclampsia, known as the HELLP syndrome (hemolysis, elevated liver enzymes, low platelets), in which hypertension is not present.

Pathology & Pathogenesis

The placenta in both essential hypertension of pregnancy and preeclampsia shows signs of premature aging, including degeneration, hyaline deposition, calcification, and congestion. In preeclampsia, the maternal half of the placenta shows hemorrhage and necrosis with thrombosis of spiral arteries and infarcts.

Predisposing factors for the development of preeclampsia include first pregnancies, multiple pregnancies, excess amniotic fluid, preexisting diabetes or hypertension, hydatidiform mole, malnutrition, and a family history of preeclampsia.

Normally, the blood vessels of the uterine wall at the site of implantation undergo striking morphologic changes such as increase in diameter of the spiral arteries and loss of their muscular and elastic components. These changes facilitate placental perfusion. This is believed to be related to an increase in production of the strong vasodilator prostacyclin and a concomitant decrease in the vasoconstrictor thromboxanes. For unknown (perhaps immune-mediated) reasons, these early changes of implantation do not occur—or at least not fully—in patients who develop preeclampsia-eclampsia. As a result, a condition of relative placental ischemia is established, with release of as yet unknown factors that damage vascular endothelium at first locally, within the placenta, and later throughout the body.

Endothelial damage has two important pathophysiologic consequences. First, the balance between vasodilation and vasoconstriction is altered, specifically by diminished production of vasodilatory products such as prostacyclin, increased production of vasoconstrictive thromboxane, and production of new vasoconstrictive products such as platelet-derived growth factor. As a result there is increased vasoconstriction of small blood vessels, with hypoperfusion and ischemia of downstream tissues and systemic hypertension. Second, the endothelial cell barrier between platelets and the collagen of basement membranes is breached.

As a result of these changes, additional events are set in motion including increased platelet aggregation, activation of the clotting cascade, and production of vasoactive substances causing capillary leak. This results in further tissue hypoperfusion, edema formation, and proteinuria, the hallmarks of preeclampsia-eclampsia. Because these processes result in further vascular endothelial damage, a vicious circle is established. Delivery of the fetus terminates the sequence of pathologic events by removing the ischemic placenta, the presumed source of the unknown products causing systemic endothelial damage.

Untreated, preeclampsia can proceed to eclampsia, a condition characterized by maternal seizures due to cerebral ischemia and petechial hemorrhage; hepatic periportal necrosis, congestion, and hemorrhage; and renal changes, including glomerular endothelial cell swelling, mesangial proliferation, and marked narrowing of glomerular capillary lumens. The renal cortex displays significant cortical ischemia that may progress to frank necrosis. Endothelial thickening, hemorrhage, and edema may occur in other tissues along with DIC (Table 19–15).

Clinical Manifestations

The clinical manifestations of preeclampsia-eclampsia fall on a continuum in which hypertension is the earliest manifestation, typically after the 20th week of gestation, followed by edema, proteinuria, muscle twitching, generalized tonic muscle contraction, seizures, and DIC (Table 19–14). Early delivery of the fetus appears to be a definitive cure for this syndrome, which otherwise carries a high mortality rate.

Unless prevented by early delivery, the risks of preeclampsia-eclampsia to the fetus are a consequence of placental deterioration and insufficiency, resulting in intrauterine growth retardation and hypoxia. The risks to the mother include development of malignant hypertension, placental abruption with serious hemorrhage, cerebrovascular accidents, renal failure, seizures and death (Table 19–15).

The pathophysiology of preeclampsia appears to be quite similar to that of thrombotic thrombocytopenic purpura and the hemolytic uremic syndrome. In those conditions, similar morphologic and biochemical changes consistent with endothelial cell dysfunction are observed, including diminished prostacyclin activity and increased thromboxane synthesis.

33. What are the hallmarks of preeclampsia-eclampsia?
34. What are the risks to the fetus of untreated maternal hypertension?
35. What other disorders in nonpregnant individuals have features in common with preeclampsia-eclampsia?

REFERENCES

General

Baulieu EE, Kelly PA (editors): *Hormones: From Molecules to Disease.* Chapman & Hall, 1990.

Ben-Rafael Z, Orvieto R: Cytokines: Involvement in reproduction. Fertil Steril 1992;58:1093.

Chandrasoma P, Taylor CR: *Concise Pathology.* Appleton & Lange, 1991.

Wilson JR, Carrington ER (editors): *Obstetrics and Gynecology,* 9th ed. Mosby Year Book, 1991.

Amenorrhea

Cowan BD, Morrison JC: Management of abnormal genital bleeding in girls and women. N Engl J Med 1991;324:1710.

Infertility

Speroff L, Glass RH, Kase NG: *Clinical Gynecologic Endocrinology and Infertility,* 5th ed. Williams & Wilkins, 1994.

Preeclampsia-Eclampsia

Roberts JM, Redman CWG: Pre-eclampsia: More than pregnancy-induced hypertension. Lancet 1993;341:1447.

Schafer AI: The hypercoagulable states. Ann Intern Med 1985;102;814.

Disorders of the Male Reproductive Tract

20

Stephen J. McPhee, MD

The male reproductive tract has two major functions: (1) the production of androgenic hormones needed for embryonic differentiation of male external and internal genitalia, development of male secondary sexual characteristics at puberty, and maintenance of libido and potency during adult life; and (2) the production of approximately 30 million spermatozoa per day during male reproductive life (from puberty to death). Both of these functions are interrelated, and both require an intact hypothalamic-pituitary-testicular axis. Thus, disorders of the hypothalamus, pituitary, testes, or accessory glands may result in abnormalities of androgen production (producing hypogonadism) or sperm production (producing infertility). In addition, testicular androgens play an important role in the development of prostatic adenomas and hyperplasia in older men. This chapter considers two common disorders of the male reproductive tract: male infertility and benign prostatic hyperplasia.

NORMAL STRUCTURE & FUNCTION OF THE MALE REPRODUCTIVE TRACT

ANATOMY & HISTOLOGY

The male reproductive tract is composed of the testes, genital ducts, accessory glands, and penis (Figure 20–1).

The **testes** are the two primary sex glands of the male. They are normally ovoid in shape, measuring about 4.5 × 3 × 2.5 cm in size. The testes have two functions: (1) to manufacture the male reproductive cells, the **spermatozoa;** and (2) to produce the androgenic hormones, **testosterone** and **dihydrotestosterone.** Anatomically, the testes are composed of loops of convoluted tubules, called **seminiferous tubules** (Figure 20–2). The spermatozoa are produced from primitive germ cells along the seminiferous tubule walls, deep in folds of cytoplasm of the **Sertoli cells,** in a process known as **spermatogenesis.** Between the tubules are the nests of **interstitial (Leydig) cells,** which manufacture testosterone and dihydrotestosterone and secrete them into the bloodstream.

The testes are found in the scrotum, which serves both to envelop and protect the testes and to maintain the testicular temperature at approximately 1.5–2 °C (2.7–3.6 °F) below abdominal temperature. Testicular spermatogenesis is sensitive to body temperature, occurring optimally at the lower temperature and being diminished or abolished at higher temperatures.

The genital ducts include the **epididymis** and **vas deferens.** Both ends of each seminiferous tubule loop drain into the head of the epididymis. The spermatozoa move from the seminiferous tubule to the epididymis, then into the vas deferens. During ejaculation, the sperm enter the urethra through the ejaculatory ducts located in the body of the prostate.

The accessory glands include the **seminal vesicles, Cowper's bulbourethral glands, urethral glands,** and **prostate** (Figure 20–3). These glands produce secretions that help to nourish and transport the spermatozoa to the outside.

The **prostate** is a muscular gland, roughly triangular in shape, situated in the pelvis at the posterior and inferior surface of the bladder, close to the rectum. It surrounds the upper (prostatic) urethra (Figure 20–3). The prostate has an anterior, middle, posterior and two lateral lobes. A shallow median posterior groove, readily palpated on digital rectal examination, separates the lateral lobes. Histologically, the prostate is a compound tubuloalveolar gland with a stroma composed of smooth muscle. The function of the prostate gland is to secrete **prostatic fluid,** a cloudy, alkaline fluid that is a major component of **semen,** the fluid that is ejaculated at orgasm.

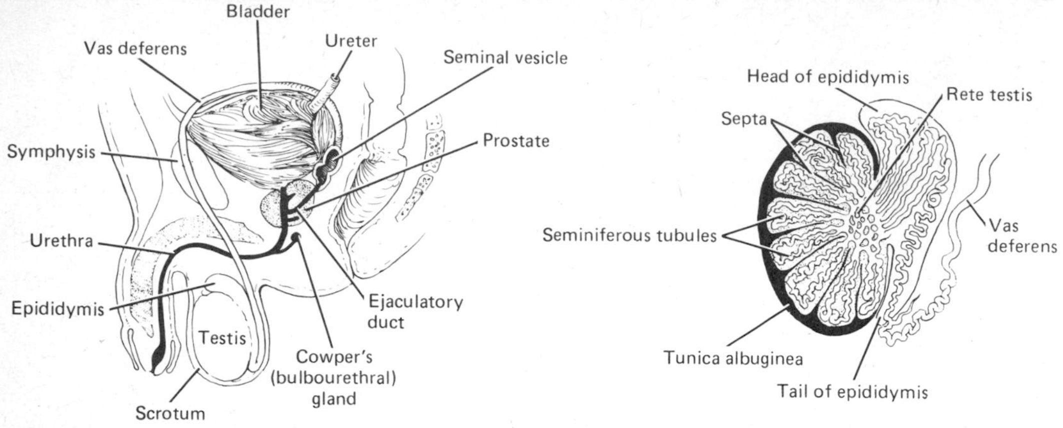

Figure 20–1. Anatomy of male reproductive system (left) and duct system of testis (right). (Reproduced, with permission, from Ganong WF: *Review of Medical Physiology,* 16th ed. Appleton & Lange, 1993.)

PHYSIOLOGY

Androgen Synthesis, Protein Binding & Metabolism

The testes secrete two steroid hormones that are essential to male reproductive function: testosterone and dihydrotestosterone. The pathways for testicular androgen biosynthesis are illustrated in Figure 20–4.

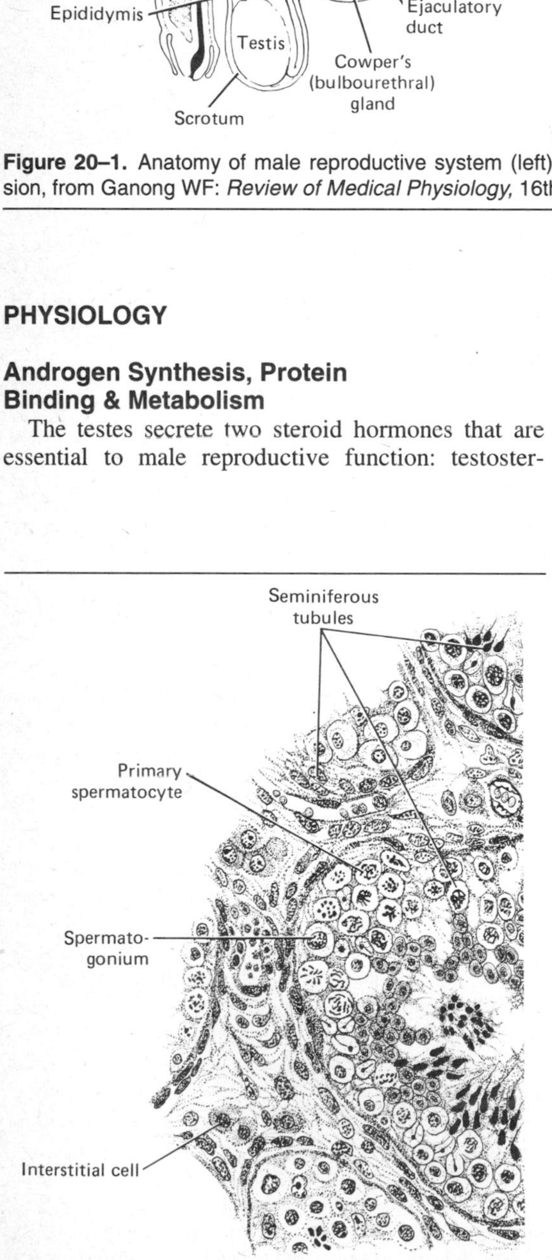

Figure 20–2. Schematic section of testis. (Reproduced, with permission, from Ganong WF: *Review of Medical Physiology,* 16th ed. Appleton & Lange, 1993.)

Testosterone, a C19 steroid, is synthesized from cholesterol by the interstitial (Leydig) cells of the testes and from androstenedione secreted by the adrenal cortex. In normal adult males, the testosterone secretion rate is 4–9 mg/d (13.9–31.2 nmol/d). In the blood, testosterone exists in both protein-bound and free (unbound) states. Ninety-eight percent of the testosterone in plasma is protein-bound: About 60% is bound to a beta-globulin called **sex-hormone binding globulin (SHBG)** (or gonadal steroid-binding globulin), and about 38% is bound to albumin. SHBG is similar in structure to, but not identical to, the androgen-binding protein secreted by the Sertoli cells (see below). SHBG is synthesized in the liver, and its gene is located on chromosome 17. Serum concentrations of SHBG are increased by hyperthyroidism, cirrhosis, and administration of various drugs, including estrogens, tamoxifen, phenytoin, and thyroid hormone, and decreased by hypothyroidism, obesity, acromegaly, and administration of exogenous androgens, glucocorticoids, or growth hormone. About 2% of the circulating testosterone is unbound and can enter cells to exert its metabolic action. In addition, some protein-bound testosterone can dissociate from its binding protein to enter the cells of target tissues. The normal plasma testosterone level for the adult male (including both free and bound testosterone) is 300–1100 ng/dL (10.4–38.2 nmol/L) (Table 20–1). The plasma testosterone level declines somewhat with age, as illustrated in Figure 20–5. The normal plasma free testosterone is 50–210 ng/dL (1.7–7.28 nmol/L).

Dihydrotestosterone (DHT) is derived both from

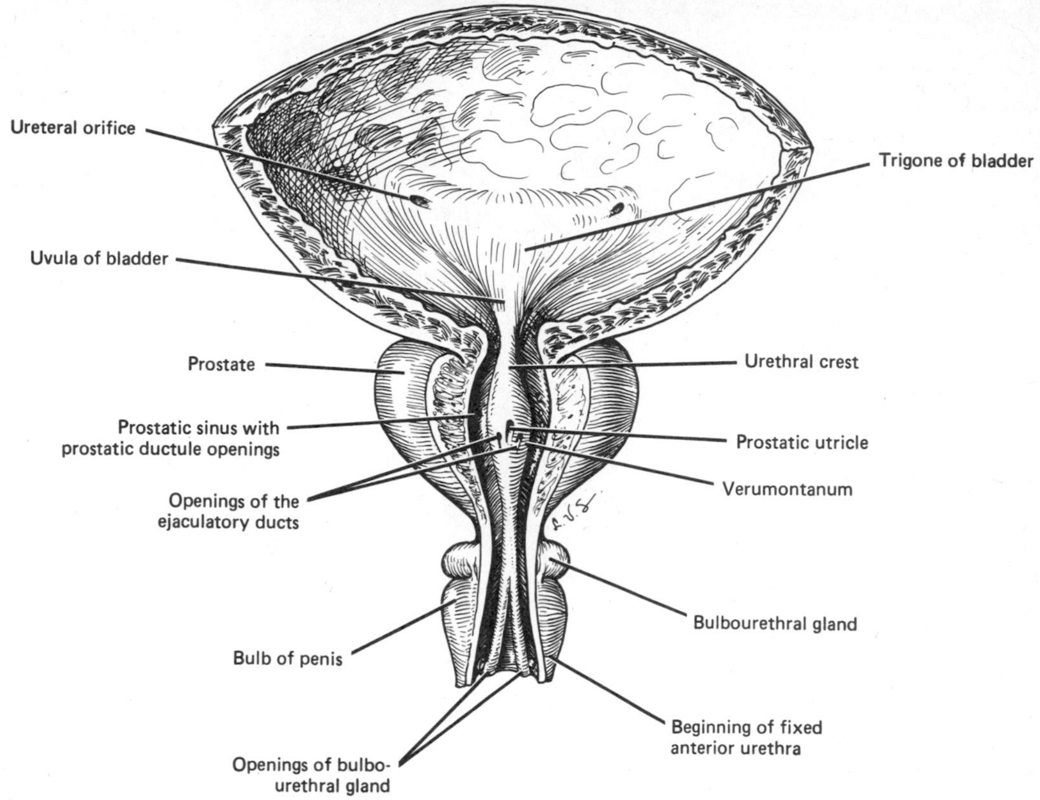

Figure 20–3. Anatomic relationships of the prostate. (Reproduced, with permission, from Lindner HH: *Clinical Anatomy.* Appleton & Lange, 1989.)

direct secretion by the testes (about 20%) and from conversion in peripheral tissues of testosterone and other androgen (and estrogen) precursors secreted by the testes and adrenals (about 80%). DHT circulates in the bloodstream. The normal plasma DHT level for the adult male is 27–75 ng/dL (0.9–2.6 nmol/L) (Table 20–1).

Regulation of Androgen Secretion & Control of Testicular Function

The endocrine mechanisms controlling male reproduction are diagrammed in Figure 20–6. The pituitary controls both testosterone production and spermatogenesis through the production of two gonadotropic hormones, **luteinizing hormone (LH)** and **follicle-stimulating hormone (FSH).** LH stimulates the testicular interstitial (Leydig) cells to produce testosterone. FSH acts on the testicular Sertoli cells to facilitate spermatogenesis. The normal ranges for plasma LH and FSH levels are given in Table 20–1.

A. Hypothalamic-Pituitary-Testicular (Leydig Cell) Axis: The hypothalamus controls the pituitary production of gonadotropins through secretion of a decapeptide, **gonadotropin-releasing hormone (GnRH).** The hypothalamus releases GnRH in a pulsatile fashion every 90–120 minutes into the portal circulation connecting the hypothalamus and anterior pituitary. When GnRH binds to the gonadotropes in the anterior pituitary, it stimulates release of LH and, to a lesser extent, FSH into the general circulation. In the testes, LH binds to specific membrane receptors on the Leydig cells. This binding causes activation of adenylyl cyclase and generation of cAMP, which in turn results in secretion of androgens.

As depicted in Figure 20–6, hormone production by the testes exerts a negative feedback influence on the hypothalamus and pituitary. Both the hypothalamus and the pituitary have androgen and estrogen receptors. Experimentally, administration of androgens such as DHT reduces LH pulse frequency, and administration of estrogens such as estradiol reduces LH pulse amplitude. In vivo, testosterone inhibits LH secretion directly by acting on the anterior pituitary and indirectly by inhibiting the secretion of GnRH from the hypothalamus. Estradiol, derived from the aromatization of testosterone (Figure 20–4), also exerts a major inhibitory effect on the hypothalamus.

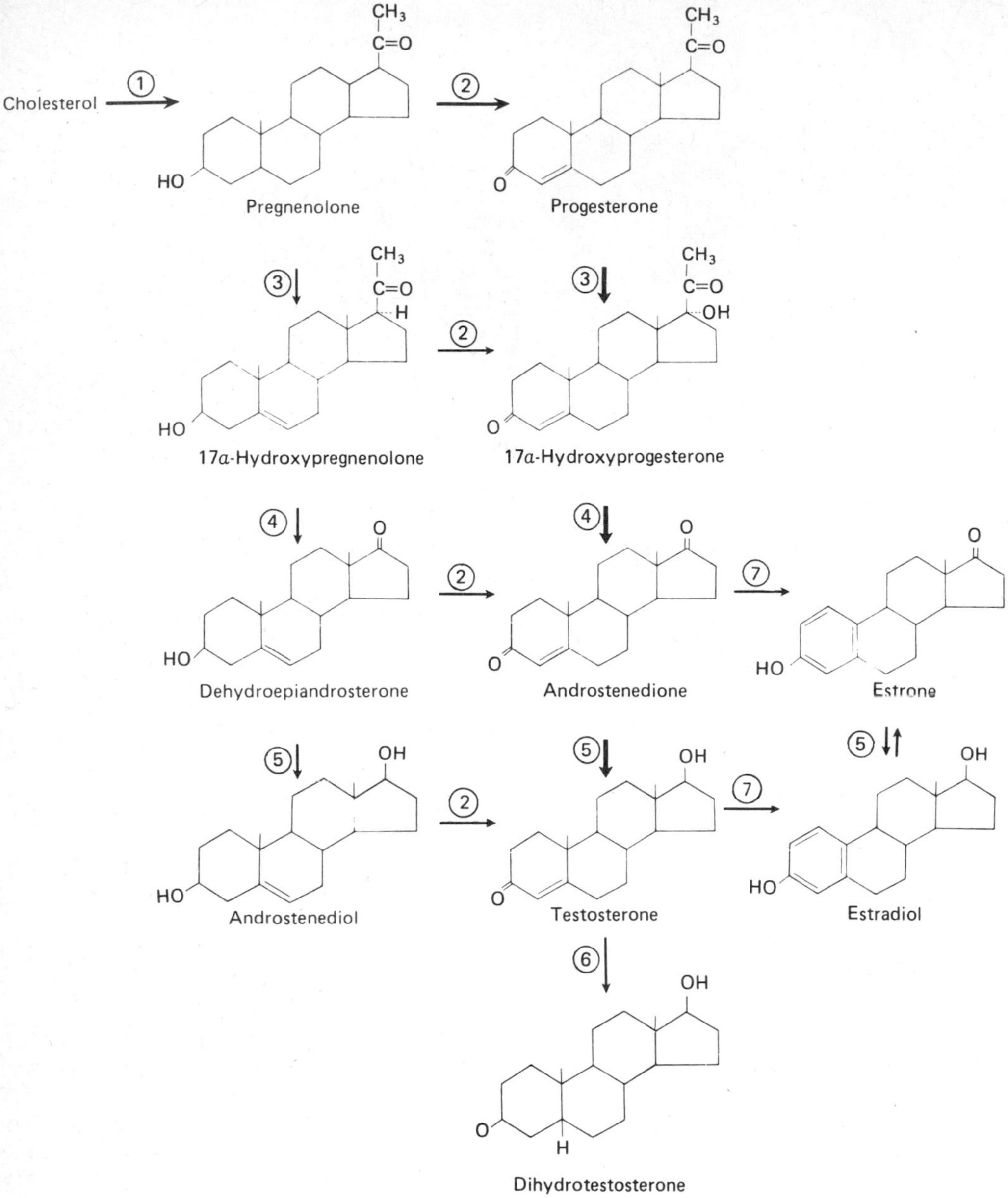

Figure 20–4. Biosynthesis and metabolism of testosterone. Heavy arrows indicate major pathways. (Circled numbers represent enzymes as follows: ①, 20,22-desmolase (P-450scc); ②, 3β-hydroxysteroid dehydrogenase and δ^5, δ^4-isomerase; ③, 17-hydroxylase (P-450c17); ④, 17,20-desmolase (P-450c17); ⑤, 17-ketoreductase; ⑥, 5α-reductase; ⑦, aromatase.) (Reproduced, with permission, from Greenspan FS, Baxter JD: *Basic and Clinical Endocrinology,* 4th ed. Appleton & Lange, 1994.)

B. Hypothalamic-Pituitary-Testicular (Seminiferous Tubule) Axis: Stimulation of the pituitary gonadotropes by GnRH also causes them to secrete FSH into the systemic circulation. In the testes, FSH acts on the Sertoli cells to produce **testicular fluid,** which helps to transport spermatozoa to the epididymis, and to promote synthesis and secretion of two proteins, androgen-binding protein and inhibin. **Androgen-binding protein** binds to testosterone and transports it into the lumen of the seminiferous tubules. In so doing, it guarantees a high local concentration of testosterone in the tubular fluid, which is necessary for normal spermatogenesis by the Sertoli cells. **Inhibin** acts directly on the anterior pituitary to inhibit FSH secretion without affecting LH release (figure 20–6). At least two forms of in-

Table 20–1. Normal plasma levels for pituitary and gonadal hormones in men.[1]

Hormone	Conventional Units	SI Units
Testosterone	300–1100 ng/dL	10.4–38.2 nmol/L
Free testosterone	50–210 pg/mL	1.7–7.28 pmol/L
Dihydrotestosterone	27–75 ng/dL	0.9–2.6 nmol/L
Androstenedione	50–200 ng/dL	1.7–6.9 nmol/L
Estradiol	15–40 pg/mL	55–150 pmol/L
Estrone	15–65 pg/mL	55.5–240 pmol/L
FSH	2–15 mIU/mL	2–15 IU/L
LH	2–15 mIU/mL	2–15 IU/L
Prolactin	4–18 ng/mL	4–18 μg/L

[1]Modified and reproduced, with permission, from Greenspan FS, Baxter JD: *Basic and Clinical Endocrinology*, 4th ed. Appleton & Lange, 1994.

hibin have been identified, and three genes have been found to direct its synthesis. Inhibin is probably the major physiologic regulator of pituitary FSH secretion along with the gonadal steroids testosterone, DHT, and estradiol.

Mechanism of Androgen Action

Testosterone acts much like other steroid hormones. When it leaves the circulation, it rapidly crosses the cell membrane (Figure 20–7). In the cytoplasm of most androgen target cells, testosterone is then converted to the more potent DHT by 5α-reductase. Both testosterone and DHT bind to an intracytoplasmic receptor protein (labeled R_c in Figure 20–7) that is distinct from both androgen-binding protein and SHBG. The gene encoding this protein is located on the X chromosome. Although DHT binds to the same intracellular receptor as testosterone, the DHT-

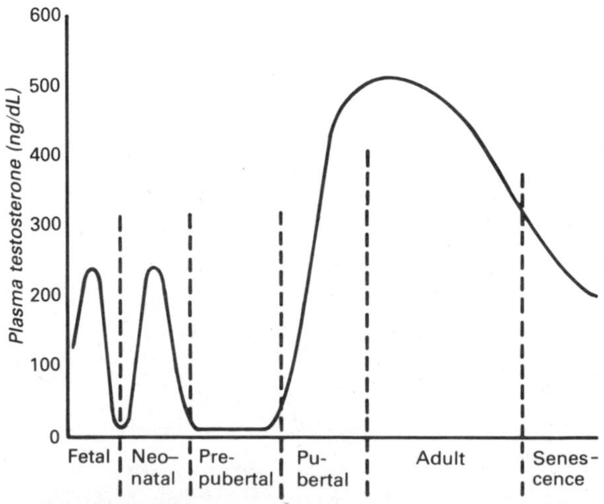

Figure 20–5. Plasma testosterone levels at various ages in males. (Reproduced, with permission, from Ganong WF: *Review of Medical Physiology,* 16th ed. Appleton & Lange, 1993.)

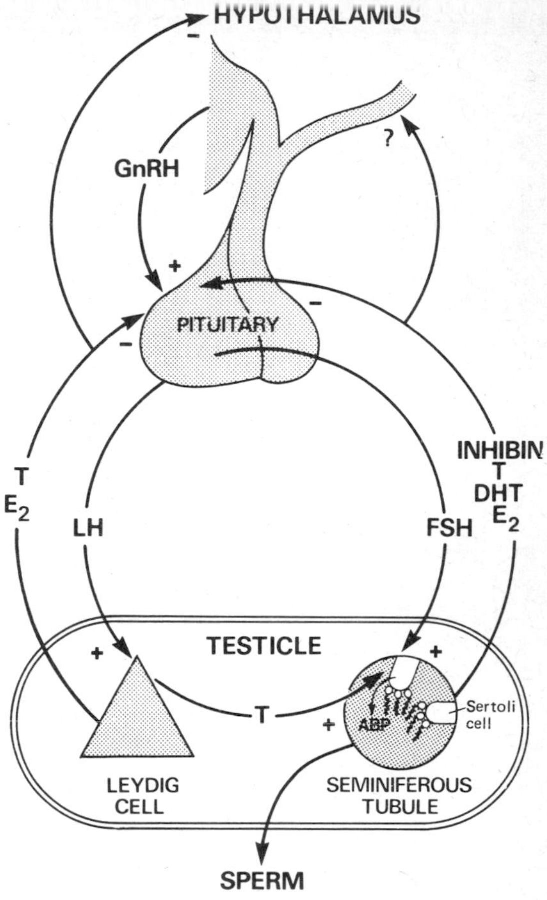

Figure 20–6. Endocrine control of male reproductive system. (GnRH, gonadotropin-releasing hormone; T, testosterone; E_2, estradiol; DHT, dihydrotestosterone.) (Reproduced, with permission, from Greenspan FS, Baxter JD: *Basic and Clinical Endocrinology,* 4th ed. Appleton & Lange, 1994.)

receptor complexes are more stable than the testosterone-receptor complexes. Thus, DHT formation serves to amplify the action of testosterone in target tissues.

The testosterone- or DHT-receptor protein complex then traverses the nuclear membrane, where it undergoes transformation (to T-R_n or DHT-R_n in Figure 20–7), enabling it to bind to DNA in the nuclear chromatin. The binding of the hormone-receptor complex to the nuclear chromatin results in synthesis of messenger RNA (mRNA). The mRNA is then transported to the cytoplasm, where it facilitates transcription of various genes, permitting synthesis of new proteins responsible for androgenic effects.

Effects of Androgens

In general, androgens act to promote growth and development, to promote spermatogenesis (see

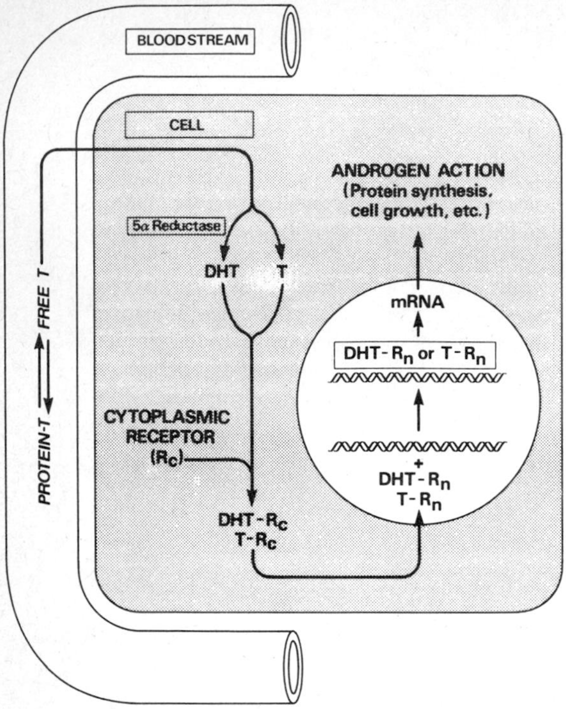

Figure 20–7. Mechanism of androgen action. (T, testosterone; DHT, dihydrotestosterone; R_n, nuclear receptor; mRNA, messenger RNA; R_c, cytoplasmic receptor.) (Reproduced, with permission, from Greenspan FS, Baxter JD: *Basic and Clinical Endocrinology,* 4th ed. Appleton & Lange, 1994.)

above), to develop and maintain the male secondary sex characteristics, and to inhibit pituitary secretion of LH. Their **anabolic effects** are mediated by an increase in the rate of synthesis and a decrease in the rate of breakdown of proteins.

In the fetus, androgens are necessary for normal differentiation and development of the internal and external male genitalia. During puberty, the androgens are needed for normal growth of the male genital structures, including the scrotum, epididymis, vas deferens, seminal vesicles, prostate, and penis. During adolescence, androgens cause rapid growth of skeletal muscle and bone. Androgenic stimulation of the epiphysial cartilaginous plates initially causes rapid growth of the skeleton but eventually causes the epiphyses to fuse to the long bones, ultimately stopping further growth. Androgens are also responsible for development of the secondary sex characteristics summarized in Table 20–2. During adult life, androgens are necessary for normal male reproductive function. Androgens also stimulate erythropoiesis.

1. What is the difference between the temperature in the scrotum and core body temperature?
2. In what conditions does the serum concentration of sex hormone-binding globulin (SHBG) increase?
3. In what conditions does it decrease?
4. What are the two testicular androgenic steroids, and what is their source?
5. How much of blood dihydrotestosterone is derived from peripheral conversion of testosterone?
6. How is testosterone secretion regulated?
7. Since there is only a single androgen receptor, how do you account for testosterone and dihydrotestosterone having different effects?
8. What are the effects of androgens?

PATHOPHYSIOLOGY OF SELECTED MALE REPRODUCTIVE TRACT DISORDERS

MALE INFERTILITY

Infertility—defined as the failure to conceive after 6–12 months of regular sexual intercourse without contraception—affects about 15–20% of married couples. About one-third of cases are due to male,

Table 20–2. Pubertal development of male secondary sex characteristics.[1]

External genitalia	Penis increases in length and width; scrotum becomes pigmented and rugose
Internal genitalia	Seminal vesicles enlarge and secrete
Larynx	Larynx enlarges, vocal cords increase in length and thickness, voice deepens
Hair	Beard appears; scalp hairline recedes anterolaterally; pubic hair appears with male pattern (triangle with apex up); axillary, chest, and perianal hair appears
Musculoskeletal	Shoulders broaden; skeletal muscles enlarge
Skin	Sebaceous gland secretions increase and thicken
Mental	More aggressive, active attitude appears; libido develops

[1]Reproduced, with permission, from Ganong WF: *Review of Medical Physiology,* 15th ed. Appleton & Lange, 1991.

Table 20–3. Etiology of male infertility.

Pretesticular	Testicular	Posttesticular

Hypothalamic-pituitary disorders
  Panhypopituitarism
  Gonadotropin deficiency
    Isolated LH deficiency (fertile eunuch)
    Biologically inactive LH
    Combined LH and FSH deficiency (eg, Kallmann's syndrome)
    Prader-Willi syndrome
    Laurence-Moon-Biedl syndrome
    Cerebellar ataxia
  Pituitary tumors (eg, prolactinoma)
  Systemic illness (eg, cirrhosis, uremia)
Androgen insensitivity (eg, androgen receptor deficiency, testicular feminization syndrome)
Thyroid disorders (eg, hyperthyroidism, hypothyroidism)
Adrenal disorders (eg, adrenal insufficiency, congenital adrenal hyperplasia)
Drugs (eg, phenytoin, androgens)
	Varicocele
	Trauma
	  Testicular torsion
	  Orchiopexy
	Infection
	  Mumps orchitis
	Drugs and toxins
	  Medications (eg, sulfasalazine, cimetidine, nitrofurantoin, cyclophosphamide, chlorambucil, vincristine, methotrexate, procarbazine)
	  Ingestants (eg, alcohol, marijuana)
	  Environmental exposures (eg, pesticides, radiation, thermal exposure)
	Chromosomal abnormalities (eg, Klinefelter's syndrome [XXY seminiferous tubule dysgenesis])
	Developmental abnormalities
	  Cryptorchidism
	  Congenital absence of vas deferens, seminal vesicles
	  Immotile cilia syndrome
	  Bilateral anorchia (vanishing testes syndrome)
	  Leydig cell aplasia
	  Noonan's syndrome (male Turner's syndrome)
	  Myotonic dystrophy
	  Defective androgen biosynthesis (eg, 5α-reductase deficiency)
		Ductular obstruction, scarring
		  Pelvic, retroperitoneal, inguinal, or scrotal surgery (eg, retroperitoneal lymphadenectomy, herniorrhaphy, Y-V plasty, transurethral resection of prostate)
		  Genital tract infections (eg, venereal disease, prostatitis, tuberculosis)
		  Cystic fibrosis
		Retrograde ejaculation (eg, diabetic autonomic neuropathy, postsurgical, medications)
		Antibodies to sperm or seminal plasma
		Developmental abnormalities
		  Penile anatomic defects (eg, hypospadias, epispadias, chordee)
		  Congenital ductal absence or obstruction
		Poor coital technique
		Sexual dysfunction, impotence
		Idiopathic

one-third to female, and one-third to combined male-female reproductive tract disorders.

Etiology

Table 20–3 lists the most common causes of male infertility. They can be classified into one of three etiologic categories:

A. Pretesticular Causes: These include endocrine disorders: hypothalamic or, more commonly, pituitary disorders—in which failure of gonadotropic hormone production leads to testicular failure **(hypogonadotropic hypogonadism)—** androgen insensitivity states, thyroid disorders, and adrenal disorders. In addition, some medications (eg, phenytoin) may lower FSH levels.

B. Testicular Causes: Varicocele, trauma, infection, drugs and toxins (including medications, ingestants, and environmental exposures), chromosomal abnormalities, and developmental abnormalities may be responsible for male factor infertility (Table 20–3). **Testicular atrophy** can result in end-organ failure and infertility. Conditions associated with testicular atrophy are listed in Table 20–4.

C. Posttesticular Causes: The most common posttesticular problem is bilateral obstruction to the outflow of spermatozoa, resulting in absence of sperm in semen **(azoospermia).** Obstruction is responsible for up to 50% of cases of male infertility

Table 20–4. Causes of testicular atrophy.[1]

Trauma
Testicular torsion
Hypopituitarism
Cryptorchidism
Klinefelter's syndrome (47,XXY)
Alcoholism and cirrhosis
Infection, eg, mumps orchitis, gonococcal epididymitis
Malnutrition and cachexia
Radiation
Obstruction to outflow of semen
Aging
Drugs, eg, estrogen therapy for prostate cancer

[1]Reproduced, with permission, from Chandrasoma P, Taylor CR: *Concise Pathology,* 2nd ed. Appleton & Lange, 1994.

and may be surgically correctable. The diagnosis is established by vasography, in which radiographic dye is used to visualize the vas deferens and to localize the obstruction, and by testicular biopsy, which demonstrates normal spermatogenesis. Other conditions producing posttesticular causes of infertility include retrograde ejaculation (often resulting from diabetic neuropathy), absence of seminal emission (often from radical pelvic or retroperitoneal surgery, producing damage to sympathetic nerves), antibodies to sperm or seminal plasma, developmental anomalies, sexual dysfunction, and poor coital technique (failure to deposit semen in the vagina during sexual intercourse).

Pathology

Testicular biopsy specimens may show any of several lesions involving the entire testes or only portions. The most common lesion is **"maturation arrest,"** defined as failure to complete spermatogenesis beyond a particular stage. There can be early or late arrest patterns, with cessation of development at either the primary spermatocyte or the spermatogonial stage of the spermatogenic cycle. The second most common and least severe lesion is **"hypospermatogenesis,"** in which all stages of spermatogenesis are present but there is a reduction in the number of germinal epithelial cells per seminiferous tubule. Peritubular fibrosis may be present. **"Germ cell aplasia"** is a more severe lesion characterized by complete absence of germ cells, with only Sertoli cells lining the seminiferous tubules ("Sertoli-cell-only" syndrome). The most severe lesion (eg, in Klinefelter's syndrome) is hyalinization, fibrosis, and sclerosis of the tubules. These findings usually indicate irreversible damage.

Pathogenesis

For conception to occur, the following conditions must be met: (1) The testes must have normal spermatogenesis; (2) the spermatozoa must complete their maturation; (3) the ducts for sperm transport must be patent; (4) the prostate and seminal vesicles must supply adequate amounts of seminal fluid; (5) the coital technique must enable the male partner to deposit his semen near the female's cervix; (6) the spermatozoa must be able to penetrate the cervical mucus and reach the uterine tubes; and (7) the spermatozoa must undergo capacitation and the acrosome reaction, fuse with the oolemma, and be incorporated into the ooplasm. Any defect in this pathway can result in infertility.

Failure of gonadotropic hormone production (hypogonadotropic hypogonadism) produces defective spermatogenesis. This defect can be overcome by gonadotropin therapy with chorionic gonadotropin. Hypogonadism refers to primary gonadal (end-organ) failure and is indicated by elevated serum FSH and LH levels due to the absence of negative feedback effects of testosterone and DHT on the pituitary and hypothalamus.

An elevated serum prolactin (PRL) level can inhibit the normal release of pituitary gonadotropins, probably through an effect on the hypothalamus (eg, patients with elevated prolactin levels have been found to have a reduced LH pulse frequency). Thus, a serum PRL measurement should be obtained in any patient with hypogonadotropic hypogonadism. If an elevated PRL level is found, the patient should be evaluated by radiographic imaging of the sella turcica to exclude a prolactinoma or other pituitary tumor. Other causes of hyperprolactinemia are discussed in Chapter 18.

Other endocrine disorders such as hyperthyroidism, hypothyroidism, adrenal insufficiency, and congenital adrenal hyperplasia are found in about 4% of men evaluated for infertility. Both hyperthyroidism and hypothyroidism can alter spermatogenesis. Hyperthyroidism affects both pituitary and testicular function by altering steroid hormone metabolism. In hyperthyroidism, there is increased conversion of androgens to estrogens which in turn leads to inappropriate feedback and consequent alterations in secretion of LH and FSH. In hypothyroidism, infertility results from enhanced release of prolactin (TRH simulates prolactin release). Similarly, primary adrenal insufficiency causes a reversible elevation of the serum prolactin level.

Testicular disorders, including cryptorchidism (undescended testes), adult seminiferous tubule failure, and sex chromosome abnormalities, are found in about 15% of infertile men.

Varicoceles are varicose enlargement of the veins of the spermatic cord. They are very common, being found in 8–20% of men in the general population and in 25–40% of patients with otherwise unexplained infertility. It is hypothesized that varicoceles may lead to oligospermia by increasing testicular temperature (see below). The incidence of varicoceles is much lower in men who have never fathered a child (primary male factor infertility) than in currently infertile men who were able to father a child in the past (secondary male factor infertility) (35% versus 81%). This finding suggests that varicoceles may cause a progressive decline in fertility and that prior fertility in men with varicoceles does not confer resistance to the varicocele-induced impairment of spermatogenesis. Prophylactic surgery remains controversial, but most clinicians would recommend surgical ligation of the incompetent spermatic veins in an infertile male with oligospermia. Of men so treated, about 50–75% will show improvement in semen quality, and 30–40% will initiate a pregnancy.

Chemotherapy or radiation therapy for malignancies may also impair spermatogenesis by their direct cytotoxic effects on the germ cells. For example, more than 80% of men who are cured of testicular cancer are infertile. The infertility is usually multifactorial, secondary to the chemotherapeutic agents, retroperitoneal lymph node dissection, and radiation therapy these patients receive.

A variety of drugs and environmental toxins may interfere with spermatogenesis, either directly or indirectly through alterations in the endocrine system. Recreational drugs (marijuana, alcohol) and medications (sulfasalazine, cimetidine, antimetabolites, phenytoin, monoamine oxidase inhibitors, and nitrofurantoin) have all been reported to interfere with spermatogenesis. Exogenous androgens and anabolic steroids can depress gonadotropin secretion. Discontinuation of these agents may restore sperm concentrations in semen to normal.

Men who are born with undescended testes **(cryptorchidism)** have poorer semen quality than normal men regardless of the timing of corrective orchiopexy (fixation of the testes in the scrotum by sutures). Approximately 30% of men with unilateral cryptorchidism and 50% with bilateral cryptorchidism will have low sperm counts. Experimental studies in animals have shown that there is a temperature differential between the abdomen and the scrotum of 1.5–2 °C (2.7–3.6 °F) and that the increase in testicular temperature in cryptorchidism can result in depression of spermatogenesis.

Other defects in spermatogenesis—eg, those produced by chromosomal abnormalities or associated with the immotile cilia syndrome—are not correctable.

Genital tract infections can impair fertility. Mumps orchitis can cause testicular atrophy, presumably as a consequence of inflammation, swelling, and pressure necrosis. Among men who develop mumps after onset of puberty, approximately 13% develop unilateral orchitis and 65% bilateral orchitis. Acute gonococcal epididymitis, chronic epididymo-orchitis, tuberculosis, or bacterial prostatitis can produce scarring and obstruction of the epididymis, vas deferens, or ejaculatory ducts and thus impair fertility. Prior venereal disease may also be associated with urethral strictures. Epididymovasostomy to relieve epididymal obstruction, vasovasotomy to correct localized obstruction of the vas deferens, and transurethral resection of the ejaculatory ducts or urethral stricture have all been associated with increases in ejaculate volume, sperm density and motility, and pregnancy rates.

Retrograde ejaculation of semen into the urinary bladder may occur with autonomic neuropathy (eg, from diabetes mellitus), with disruption of the internal bladder sphincter (eg, from corrective Y-V plasty of the bladder neck during childhood or from transurethral resection of the prostate), with disruption or dysfunction of sympathetic nerves (eg, following radical pelvic or retroperitoneal surgery), or with certain medications.

The role of antibodies to sperm (or to seminal plasma) in producing infertility remains controversial. A variety of autoimmune disorders can result in production of antisperm antibodies by the female partner. Such antibodies in the female genital tract can lead to agglutination or immobilization of sperm and can be responsible for failure of sperm to penetrate the ovum. However, this mechanism probably rarely causes infertility. Factors that cause antisperm antibody production by the male partner include vasectomy, ejaculatory duct obstruction, infection, varicocele, cryptorchidism, and testicular trauma, torsion, or cancer. Antisperm antibodies can be measured in serum or semen by a variety of techniques.

Infertility can also occur in patients with anatomic defects of the penis, such as **hypospadias** (urethral opening on the penile under surface), **epispadias** (urethral opening on the penile dorsal surface), and **chordee** (painful erection with penile curvature due to nondistensibility of one corpus cavernosum). These abnormalities may lead to an improper placement of the ejaculate in the vagina.

Poor coital technique and improper timing of intercourse can interfere with fertility. Too frequent masturbation in the periovulatory period can deplete the sperm reserve, particularly in an oligospermic male. Several commonly used lubricants (eg, K-Y Jelly, Surgilube, Keri Lotion, and even saliva) can be spermatotoxic, causing a deterioration in sperm motility.

Finally, sexual dysfunction can be responsible for male factor infertility. Male sexual dysfunction can be categorized into several problem areas. **Impotence** is defined as the consistent inability to maintain an erect penis with sufficient rigidity to allow sexual intercourse **(loss of erections).** Such erectile dysfunction may be the result of arterial, venous, neurogenic, or psychogenic causes. Impotence should be clearly distinguished from problems with libido, ejaculation, and orgasm. A **loss of libido** (sexual desire) may be the direct consequence of androgen deficiency, whether on the basis of hypothalamic, pituitary, or testicular disease. **Loss of emission** (lack of seminal fluid during ejaculation) may result from retrograde ejaculation (as noted above) or from androgen deficiency (which decreases prostatic and seminal vesicle secretions). **Premature ejaculation** is usually an anxiety-related disorder. **Loss of orgasm** is usually of psychologic origin.

9. What are the categories of infertility? Name several specific causes for each category.
10. From the perspective of the male reproductive system, what are the steps that must occur for conception?
11. What drugs commonly interfere with spermatogenesis?
12. What are the categories of impotence?

Clinical Manifestations

A. Symptoms and Signs: Infertility is often the only complaint. However, depending on the cause of the infertility, there may be other symptoms and signs. For example, with hypogonadotropic hypogonadism, there may be decreased libido and potency, emotional instability, fatigue, decreased mental concentration, and vasomotor instability (palpitations, hot flushes, diaphoresis). If hypogonadism occurs before onset of puberty, there may be other signs of androgen deficiency, such as decreased body hair, gynecomastia, and eunuchoid proportions (narrow shoulders, little muscle development). Galactorrhea in a male strongly suggests an anterior pituitary prolactinoma. Neurologic or ophthalmologic abnormalities suggest suprasellar extension of a pituitary tumor, and profuse polyuria consistent with diabetes insipidus suggests destruction of the posterior pituitary. Anosmia and a history of delayed sexual maturation are key features of **Kallmann's syndrome,** with associated hypogonadotropic hypogonadism. In Kallmann's syndrome, isolated gonadotropin deficiency is associated with aplasia of the olfactory cortex. During embryonic life, GnRH-producing neurons fail to migrate from the olfactory area to the medial basal hypothalamus. Affected patients may have undescended testes, gynecomastia, and obesity in addition to delays in reaching adult height and in sexual maturation during puberty. On the other hand, a history of precocious puberty suggests congenital adrenal hyperplasia. Patients with the immotile cilia syndrome have associated mucociliary transport defects in the lower airways that result in chronic obstructive pulmonary disease.

Physical examination of the male genitalia is very important in diagnosis of infertility. Testicular atrophy is diagnosed when the physical examination finds the testes to be smaller than the normal 4.5 × 3 × 2.5 cm. Careful palpation of the spermatic cord may reveal a varicocele, palpable as a boggy intrascrotal mass. Elicited increase in intra-abdominal pressure (eg, by Valsalva's maneuver: forced expiratory effort against a closed airway) will sometimes produce a palpable impulse in the mass. Varicoceles are more easily detected if the patient is examined in the standing position. They are more common on the left side. Infections of the epididymis may be associated with epididymal induration, irregularity, and cystic changes. There may be absence of the vas deferens or nodularity along its course suggestive of obstruction. An enlarged, boggy, or tender prostate suggests prostatitis. Finally, the penis must be carefully inspected for abnormal position of the urethral opening or abnormal penile angulation or curvature. The penile shaft should be palpated for fibrosis suggestive of Peyronie's disease, a disorder in which deposition of fibrous tissue around the corpus cavernosum of the penis causes deformity and painful erections.

B. Laboratory Tests and Evaluation: Figure 20–8 outlines an approach to the diagnosis of male

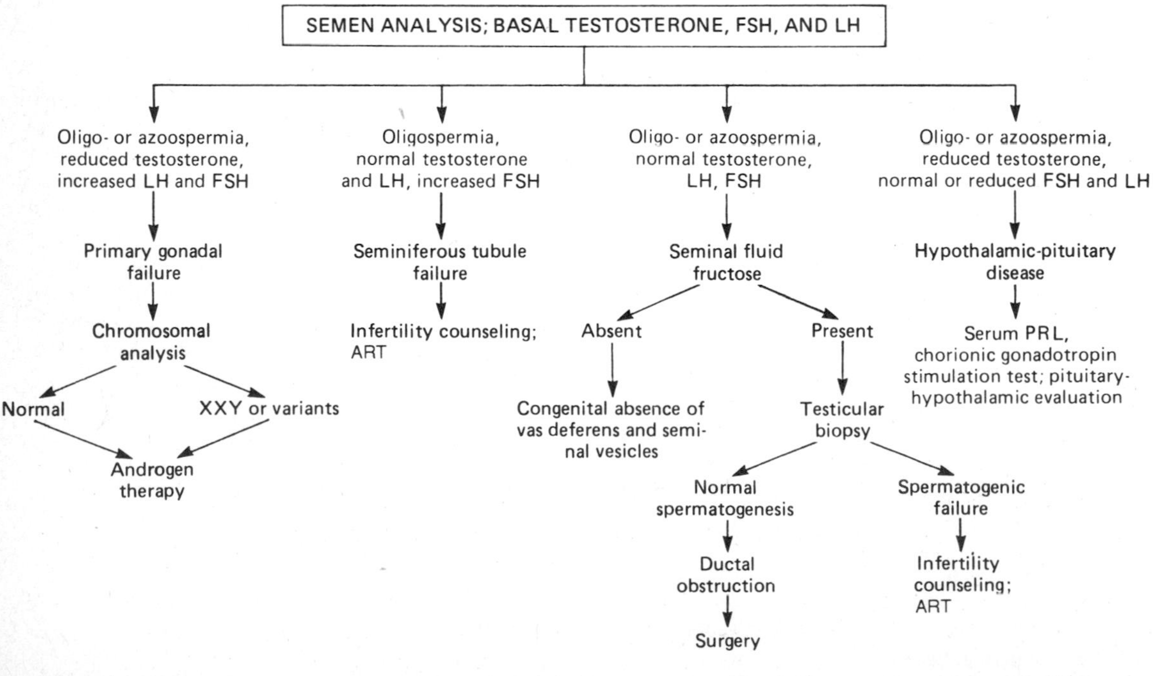

Figure 20–8. Approach to diagnosis of male infertility. (Reproduced, with permission, from Greenspan FS, Baxter JD: *Basic and Clinical Endocrinology,* 4th ed. Appleton & Lange, 1994.)

infertility. Determination of serum levels of testosterone, FSH, and LH and performance of semen analysis allow the clinician to classify patients as having either primary or secondary gonadal failure. Patients with primary gonadal failure have an abnormal semen analysis, low or low normal testosterone levels, and elevated FSH or LH levels. Those with secondary gonadal failure have an abnormal semen analysis, low serum testosterone level, and low or inappropriately normal FSH or LH levels.

Semen analysis involves examination of semen collected by masturbation (using a special plastic condom) after 72 hours of sexual abstinence. The analysis entails determination of the volume, sperm count, sperm motility, and sperm morphology. The reference standards for semen analysis are presented in Table 20–5. The average volume of ejaculate is 2.5–5 mL after 72 hours without intercourse. Volumes less than 1.5 mL may result in inadequate buffering of vaginal acidity to enable sperm survival and are usually caused by either retrograde ejaculation or androgen deficiency. There are normally about 100 million sperm per milliliter of semen. Both **azoospermia** (absence of sperm) and **oligospermia** (usually defined as < 20 million sperm per milliliter of semen) result in infertility. Men with poor sperm production frequently have poorly functioning sperm as well. Normal sperm motility and morphology are defined as at least 60% motile sperm and more than 60% with normal morphology. Abnormal motility may result from infection or antisperm antibodies. Abnormal morphology may be the result of varicocele, infection, or exposure to a toxin. Fructose is produced in the seminal vesicles, and its absence in the semen implies obstruction of the ejaculatory ducts. **Leukospermia** (excessive numbers of leukocytes in the semen) may adversely affect sperm movement and fertilization ability.

Several functional assays of spermatozoa are now available to assess the ability of the sperm to reach and penetrate the ova. The **postcoital test** assesses sperm interaction with cervical mucus. It is performed by examining the cervical mucus for the presence of viable sperm within a few hours after intercourse. The test is best conducted during the preovulatory phase of the menstrual cycle when cervical mucus is least viscous. The test is considered normal if there are at least 10–20 sperm per high power field and most of them demonstrate forward motility. Causes of an abnormal test include the presence of antibodies to sperm or seminal plasma in the cervical mucus or semen, anatomic abnormalities, poor coital technique, abnormal semen (demonstrable on semen analysis), and improper timing of the test.

In the **sperm penetration assay,** the infertile man's sperm are processed, allowed to capacitate, and then incubated with hamster oocytes that have had the zona pellucida removed enzymatically to allow penetration. Results are reported as either the percentage of ova that have been penetrated (normal is 10–30%) or as the number of sperm penetrations per ovum (normal is more than five).

The **hemizona assay** assesses the fertilizing capability of sperm using the zona pellucida from a nonfertilizable, nonliving human oocyte. The zona is divided in half. One half is incubated with the infertile man's sperm, while the other half is incubated with sperm from a known fertile donor. The number of sperm penetrations is compared and expressed as a ratio.

High resolution **transrectal ultrasonography** can be used to evaluate the seminal vesicles for dysplasia or obstruction; the ejaculatory ducts for scarring, cysts, or calcifications; and the prostate for calcifications. **Venography** is occasionally useful to demonstrate testicular venous reflux in a man with a suspected varicocele when the physical examination is difficult or in a man with a suspected recurrence following surgical repair. Finally, **testicular biopsy** is useful in azoospermic (and sometimes oligospermic) men to distinguish intrinsic testicular abnormalities from ductal obstruction.

Table 20–5. Normal values for semen analysis.[1]

Characteristic	Reference Standard
Ejaculate volume	1.5–5.0 mL
Sperm count	>20 million/mL
Sperm motility	>60%
Sperm morphology	>60% normal
Sperm forward progression	>2 (scale 0–4)
Sperm agglutination	Absent
Leukospermia	Absent
Hyperviscosity	Absent

[1]Reproduced, with permission, from Fisch H, Lipshultz LI: Diagnosing male factors of infertility. Arch Pathol Lab Med 1992;116:398.

BENIGN PROSTATIC HYPERPLASIA

Benign prostatic hyperplasia is a common age-related disorder, occurring in up to 50% of men between 40 and 60 years of age and 95% of men over age 70. Most men are asymptomatic, but clinical symptoms and signs occur in 5–10% of men over age 60, and a small number require surgery to relieve symptoms.

Etiology

The cause of benign prostatic hyperplasia is unknown. However, aging and hormonal factors are both clearly important. Age-related increases in prostate size are evident at autopsy, and the development of symptoms is age-related. Prostatic androgen

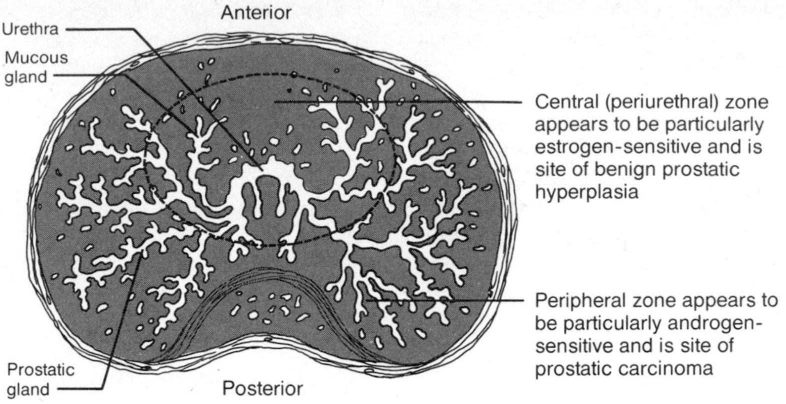

Figure 20–9. Structure of the prostate. (Reproduced, with permission, from Chandrasoma P, Taylor CE: *Concise Pathology,* 2nd ed. Appleton & Lange, 1994.)

levels, particularly dihydrotestosterone (DHT) levels, play an important role in development of the disorder. These factors are discussed below.

Pathology

The normal prostate is composed of both stromal (smooth muscle) and epithelial (glandular) elements. Each of these elements—alone or in combination—can give rise to hyperplastic nodules and ultimately the symptoms of benign prostatic hyperplasia. Pathologically, the hyperplastic gland is enlarged, with a firm, rubbery consistency. While small nodules are often present throughout the gland, benign prostatic hyperplasia arises most commonly in the periurethral and transition zones of the gland (Figure 20–9). With advancing age, there is an increase in the overall size of the transition zone as well as an increase in the number—and later the size—of nodules. The urethra is compressed and has a slit-like appearance.

Histologically, benign prostatic hyperplasia is a true hyperplastic process since studies document an increase in prostatic cell number. The prostatic nodules are composed of both hyperplastic glands and hyperplastic stromal muscle. Most periurethral nodules are stromal in character, but transition zone nodules are most often glandular tissue. The glands become larger than normal, with stromal muscle between the proliferative glands. The cellular proliferation leads to a tight packing of glands within a given area. There is an increase in the height of the lining epithelium, and the epithelium often shows papillary projections (Figure 20–10). There is also some hypertrophy of individual epithelial cells.

In men with benign prostatic hyperplasia, the bladder shows both detrusor smooth muscle hypertrophy and trabeculation associated with an increase in collagen deposition.

Pathogenesis

While the actual cause of benign prostatic hyperplasia is undefined, several factors are known to be involved in the pathogenesis. These include age-related prostatic growth, prostatic capsule, androgenic hormones and their receptors, prostatic smooth muscle and adrenergic receptors, and detrusor responses. Other factors that may be important in pathogenesis include stromal-epithelial interactions and growth factors (including basic and alpha fibroblastic growth factors, transforming growth factors, and epidermal growth factor).

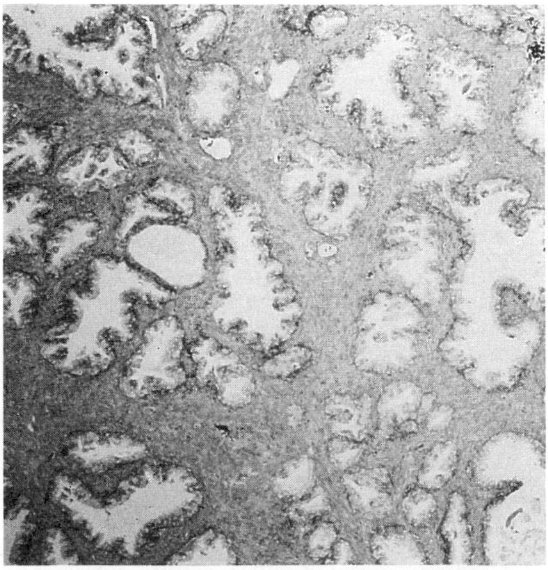

Figure 20–10. Benign prostatic hyperplasia. (Reproduced, with permission, from Chandrasoma P, Taylor CE: *Concise Pathology,* 2nd ed. Appleton & Lange, 1994.)

A. Age-Related Prostatic Growth: The size of the prostate does not always correlate with the degree of obstruction. The amount of periurethral and transition zone tissue may relate more to the degree of obstruction than the overall prostate size. However, the idea that the clinical symptoms of benign prostatic hyperplasia are due simply to a mass-related increase in urethral resistance is probably too simplistic. Instead, some of its symptoms may be due to obstruction-induced detrusor dysfunction and neural alterations in the bladder and prostate.

B. Prostatic Capsule: The presence of a capsule around the prostate is thought to play a role in development of obstructive symptoms. Besides man, the dog is the only animal known to develop benign prostatic hyperplasia. However, the canine prostate lacks a capsule, and dogs do not develop obstructive symptoms. In men, the capsule presumably causes the "pressure'' created by the expanded periurethral-transition zone tissue to be transmitted to the urethra, leading to an increase in urethral resistance. Surgical incision of the prostatic capsule or removal of the obstructing portion of the prostate--whether by transurethral resection or by open prostatectomy--is effective in relieving symptoms.

C. Hormonal Regulation of Prostatic Growth: Development of benign prostatic hyperplasia requires testicular androgens as well as aging. There are several lines of evidence for this relationship. First, men who are castrated before puberty or who have disorders of impaired androgen production or action do not develop benign prostatic hyperplasia. Second, the prostate—unlike other androgen-dependent organs—maintains its ability to respond to androgens throughout life. Androgens are required for normal cell proliferation and differentiation in the prostate. They may also actively inhibit cell turnover and death. Finally, androgen deprivation at various levels of the hypothalamic-pituitary-testicular axis can reduce prostate size and improve obstructive symptoms (Table 20–6).

While androgenic hormones are clearly required for the development of benign prostatic hyperplasia, testosterone is not the major androgen in the prostate. Instead, 80–90% of prostatic testosterone is converted to the more active metabolite dihydrotestosterone (DHT) by 5α-reductase. High levels of this enzyme are found in prostatic epithelial cells. DHT levels are the same in hyperplastic and normal glands. However, prostatic levels of DHT remain high with aging despite the fact that peripheral levels of testosterone decrease.

Suppression of androgens leads to reduction in prostate size and relief of symptoms of bladder outlet obstruction. A variety of antiandrogen treatment approaches have been successful, including gonadotropin-releasing hormone (GnRH) agonists (nafarelin, leuprolide, buserelin), androgen receptor inhibitors (cyproterone acetate, flutamide), progestogens, and 5α-reductase inhibitors (finasteride) (Figure 20–11). Most of these agents are associated with intolerable adverse effects, such as impotence, flushing, and loss of libido (Table 20–6). However, the 5α-reductase inhibitor finasteride has been shown to induce significant decreases in the size of the prostate as a whole and in the size of the periurethral zone. Finasteride has fewer adverse side effects, but it must be given for at least 6–12 months to have a beneficial effect and must be continued indefinitely thereafter.

Androgen receptor levels remain high with aging, thus maintaining the mechanism for androgen-dependent cell growth. Nuclear androgen receptor levels have been found to be higher in prostatic tissue from men with benign prostatic hyperplasia than in that from normal controls. The regulation of androgen receptor expression in benign prostatic hyperplasia is now being studied at the transcriptional level.

Finally, androgens are not the only important hormones contributing to the development of benign prostatic hyperplasia. Estrogens appear to be involved in induction of the androgen receptor. Serum

Table 20–6. Androgen ablation and blockade for benign prostatic hyperplasia.[1]

Agent	Action	Effects
Leuprolide, buserelin, nafarelin (GnRH agonists)	Inhibit pituitary luteinizing hormone secretion; decrease testosterone and dihydrotestosterone.	Impotence, loss of libido; hot flashes, gynecomastia.
Megestrol acetate, hydroxyprogesterone caproate (progestational agents)	Inhibit pituitary LH secretion; decrease testosterone and dihydrotestosterone.	Impotence, loss of libido.
Flutamide (antiandrogen)	Androgen receptor inhibition.	Gynecomastia, diarrhea; libido maintained.
Finasteride (5α-reductase inhibitor)	Decreases dihydrotestosterone.	Libido maintained.

[1]Reproduced, with permission, from Tierney LM Jr, McPhee SJ, Papadakis MA (editors): *Current Medical Diagnosis & Treatment 1995.* Appleton & Lange, 1995.

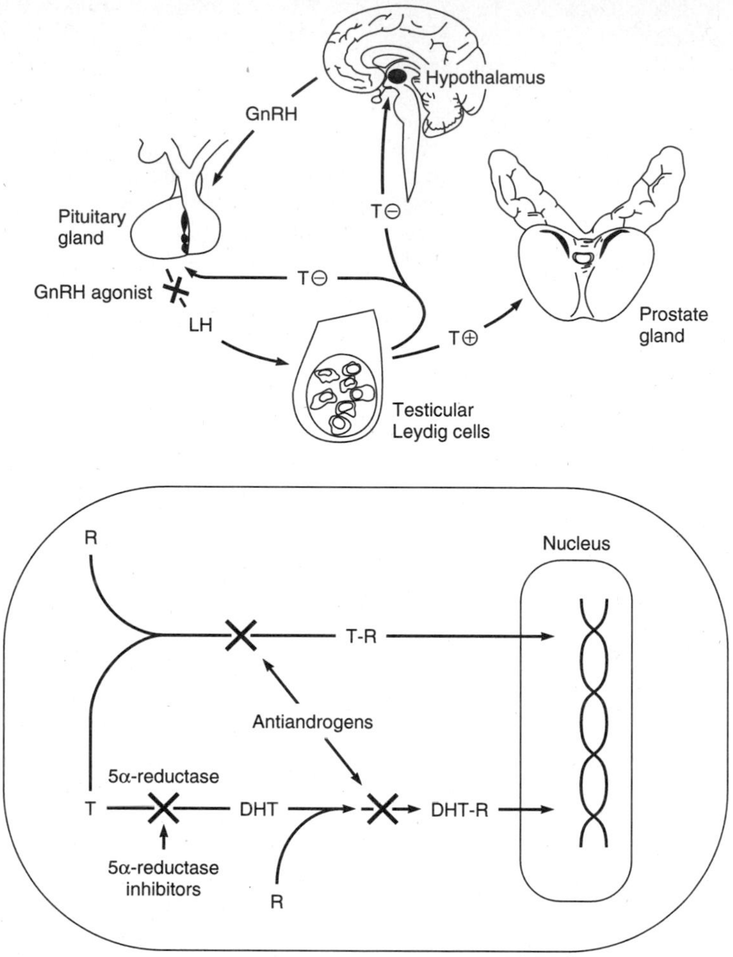

Figure 20–11. Site of action of gonadotropin-releasing hormone (GnRH) (or luteinizing hormone-releasing hormone [LHRH]) agonists, antiandrogens, and 5α-reductase inhibitors. (Adapted, with permission, from Oesterling JE: Endocrine therapies for symptomatic benign prostatic hyperplasia. Urology 1994,43[2 Suppl]:7.)

estrogen levels increase in men with age—absolutely or relative to testosterone level. Age-related increases in estrogens may thus increase androgen receptor expression in the prostate, leading to increases in cell growth (or decreases in cell death). Intraprostatic levels of estrogen are increased in men with benign prostatic hyperplasia. Studies of prostatic specimen tissue have documented an accumulation of DHT, estradiol, and estrone that correlates with patient age. The results show a dramatic increase of the estrogen:androgen ratio with increasing age, particularly in the stroma of prostatic tissue.

Estrogens may be causally linked to the onset of benign prostatic hyperplasia and may have an important supportive role in its maintenance. Antiestrogen therapy with atamestane, a newly developed aromatase inhibitor, has been investigated as treatment for men with benign prostatic hyperplasia (Figure 20–12). With atamestane treatment, serum estrogen levels and intraprostatic estrogen concentrations decrease markedly, mean prostatic volume decreases significantly, and hyperplasia-related symptoms improve considerably.

D. Prostatic Smooth Muscle and Adrenergic Receptors: Prostatic smooth muscle represents a significant proportion of the gland. Undoubtedly, both resting and dynamic prostatic smooth muscle tone play a major role in the pathophysiology of benign prostatic hyperplasia. Smooth muscle cells in the prostate—at the bladder neck and in the prostatic capsule—are richly populated with alpha-adrenergic receptors. Contraction of the prostate and bladder neck are mediated by α_1-adrenergic receptors. Stimulation of these receptors results in a dynamic increase in prostatic urethral resistance. Alpha$_1$-adrenergic receptor blockade clearly diminishes this response and has been found to improve symptoms, urinary flow rates, and residual urine volumes in patients with benign prostatic hyperplasia within 2–4 weeks after start of therapy. The selective α_1-

Table 20–7. Alpha receptor blockade for benign prostatic hyperplasia.

Agent	Site and Mechanism of Action	Side Effects
Phenoxybenzamine	Pre- and postsynaptic α_1 and α_2 blockade	Hypotension
Prazosin Terazosin Doxazosin Alfuzosin Tamsulosin	Postsynaptic α_1 blockade	Hypotension (especially postural hypotension leading to syncope)

blockers prazosin, terazosin, and alfuzosin, have been extensively studied and found to be effective; doxazosin and tamsulosin are newer agents that are currently under investigation (Table 20–7). Because the bladder's smooth muscle cells do not contain a significant number of α_1 receptors, alpha-blocker therapy can selectively diminish urethral resistance without affecting detrusor smooth muscle contractility.

Recent studies have suggested that the α_1 receptors involved in the contraction of prostate smooth muscle appear to be α_{1C} receptors. Development of subtype-selective α_{1C} antagonists is under way.

E. Bladder Response to Obstruction: Many of the clinical symptoms of benign prostatic hyperplasia are related to obstruction-induced changes in bladder function rather than to outflow obstruction per se. Thus, onc-third of men continue to have significant voiding problems even after surgical relief of obstruction. Obstruction-induced changes in bladder function are of two basic types. First, there are changes that lead to **detrusor instability.** These are clinically manifested by frequency and urgency. Second, there are changes that lead to **decreased detrusor contractility.** These are clinically manifested by symptoms of decreased force of the urinary stream, hesitancy, intermittency, increased residual urine, and, in a minority of cases, **detrusor failure.**

The bladder's response to obstruction is largely an adaptive one (Figure 20–13). The initial response is the development of detrusor smooth muscle hypertrophy. It is hypothesized that this increase in muscle mass, although an adaptive response to increased intravesical pressure and one that maintains urinary outflow, is associated with significant intra- and extracellular changes in smooth muscle cells that predispose to detrusor instability. In experimental animal models, unrelieved obstruction results in significant increases in detrusor extracellular matrix (collagen).

In addition to obstruction-induced changes in the smooth muscle cells and extracellular matrix of the bladder, there is increasing evidence that chronic obstruction in patients with untreated benign prostatic hyperplasia may alter neural responses as well, occasionally predisposing to detrusor failure.

Traditional therapies for symptoms associated with bladder obstruction have been directed toward relief of bladder outflow resistance. New treatments of obstructive detrusor instability have been suggested using drugs that are autonomically active (such as α_1 antagonists) and drugs that stabilize muscle cell membranes (such as anticholinergic agents).

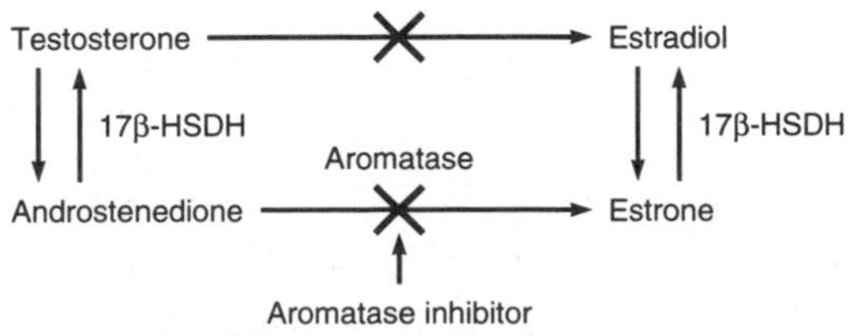

Figure 20–12. Site of action of aromatase inhibitors. (17β-HSDH, 17β-hydroxysteroid dehydrogenase). (Adapted, with permission, from Oesterling JE: Endocrine therapies for symptomatic benign prostatic hyperplasia. Urology 1994,43 [2 Suppl]:7.)

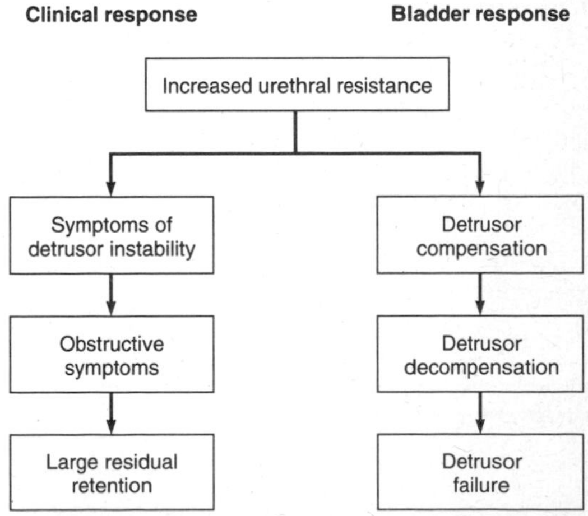

Figure 20–13. Schematic of natural history of benign prostatic hyperplasia. (Adapted, with permission, from McConnell JD: The pathophysiology of benign prostatic hyperplasia. J Androl 1991,11:356.)

The effects of chronic obstruction on the bladder are still not well understood. Future studies must examine the importance of changes in receptor density, affinity and distribution, and agonist release and degradation that occur during chronic obstruction and the ultrastructural and physiologic changes that occur with relief of obstruction.

Clinical Manifestations

A. Symptoms and Signs: Obstruction to urinary outflow and bladder dysfunction are responsible for the major symptoms and signs of benign prostatic hyperplasia. Prostatic enlargement may cause either acute or chronic urinary retention. With **acute urinary retention,** there is painful dilation of the bladder, with inability to void. Acute urinary retention is often precipitated by swelling of the prostate caused by infarction of a nodule or by certain medications. With **chronic urinary retention,** there are both obstructive and irritative voiding symptoms.

Obstructive symptoms result from distortion and narrowing of the bladder neck and prostatic urethra, leading to incomplete emptying of the bladder. Obstructive symptoms include difficulty in initiating urination, decreased force and caliber of the urinary stream, intermittency of the urinary stream, urinary hesitancy, and dribbling. **Irritative symptoms** occur as a consequence of bladder dysfunction and include urinary frequency, nocturia, and urgency. The patient commonly complains of difficulty initiating urination and decreased flow, causing a decreased caliber and force of the urinary stream.

Complications of the chronic bladder dilation include hypertrophy of the bladder wall musculature and development of diverticula; urinary tract infection of the stagnant bladder urine; hematuria, particularly with infarction of a prostatic nodule; and chronic renal failure and azotemia from bilateral hydroureter and hydronephrosis.

Digital rectal examination may reveal either focal or diffuse enlargement of the prostate. However, the size of the prostate as estimated by digital rectal examination does not correlate well with either the symptoms or signs of benign prostatic hyperplasia or the need for treatment. Examination of the lower abdomen may reveal a distended bladder, consistent with urinary retention, which may occur silently in the absence of severe symptoms.

B. Laboratory Tests and Evaluation: Laboratory tests performed to evaluate patients with benign prostatic hyperplasia include BUN and serum creatinine to exclude renal failure and urinalysis and urine culture to exclude urinary tract infection. **Intravenous pyelography (IVP)** is usually not performed in patients with normal findings on these simple laboratory tests. Instead, it is generally reserved for patients with hematuria or suspected hydronephrosis. When an IVP is done in men with benign prostatic hyperplasia, it typically shows elevation of the bladder base by the enlarged prostate; trabeculation, thickening, and diverticula of the bladder wall; elevation of the ureters; and poor emptying of the bladder. Uncommonly, the IVP shows hydronephrosis. The most useful technique for assessing the significance of benign prostatic hyperplasia is **urodynamic evaluation** with **uroflowmetry.** In this test, the patient voids and the maximal urinary flow rate is recorded. If the peak flow rate is less than 10 mL/s, the patient is considered to have significant bladder outlet obstruction. However, the patient must void at least 150 mL for the measurement to be considered reliable. **Cystourethroscopy** is usually reserved for patients who have hematuria that remains unexplained despite an IVP, or preoperatively for patients who require transurethral resection of the prostate.

13. Which is the major androgen controlling prostate size?
14. What are some of the different modalities by which androgens can be suppressed in order to decrease prostate size and obtain at least temporary relief of obstructive symptoms?
15. What are the effects of antiestrogen treatment on males with benign prostatic hyperplasia?
16. What is the role of (α_1-adrenergic receptors in benign prostatic hyperplasia?
17. What are some bladder changes that occur in patients with benign prostatic hyperplasia?
18. What are some symptoms and signs of benign prostatic hyperplasia?
19. How is the diagnosis of benign prostatic hyperplasia made?

REFERENCES

General

Chandrasoma P, Taylor CE: *Concise Pathology,* 2nd ed. Appleton & Lange, 1994.

Ganong WF: *Review of Medical Physiology,* 17th ed. Appleton & Lange, 1993.

Greenspan FS, Baxter JD: *Basic and Clinical Endocrinology,* 4th ed. Appleton & Lange, 1994.

McClure RD: Male infertility. In: *Smith's General Urology,* 13th ed. Tanagho EA, McAninch JW (editors). Appleton & Lange, 1992.

Male Infertility

Gangi GR, Nagler HM: Clinical evaluation of the subfertile male. Infertil Reprod Med Clin North Am 1992;3:299.

Guay AT et al: Possible hypothalamic impotence. Male counterpart to hypothalamic amenorrhea? Urology 1991;38:317.

Honig SC et al: Reassessment of male-factor infertility, including the varicocele, sperm penetration assay, semen analysis, and in vitro fertilization. Curr Opin Obstet Gynecol 1993;5:245.

Jarow JP, Sanzone JJ: Risk factors for male partner antisperm antibodies. J Urol 1992;148:1805.

Meacham RB et al: Evaluation and treatment of ejaculatory duct obstruction in the infertile male. Fertil Steril 1993;59:393.

NIH Consensus Development Conference: Impotence. NIH Consensus Statement, 1992, Dec 7–9,10:1–33.

Overstreet JW et al: Semen evaluation. Infertil Reprod Med Clin North Am 1992;3:329.

Swerdloff RS: Infertility in the male. Ann Intern Med 1985;103:906.

Benign Prostatic Hyperplasia

Algaba F: Pathophysiology of benign prostatic hyperplasia. Eur Urol 1994;25(Suppl 1):3.

Jonler M et al: Benign prostatic hyperplasia. Current pharmacological treatment. Drugs 1994;47:66.

Krieg M et al: Effect of aging on endogenous level of 5α-dihydrotestosterone, testosterone, estradiol, and estrone in epithelium and stroma of normal and hyperplastic human prostate. J Clin Endocrinol Metab 1993;77:375.

Lepor H et al: The alpha-adrenoreceptor subtype mediating the tension of human prostatic smooth muscle. Prostate 1993;22:301.

McConnell JD: The pathophysiology of benign prostatic hyperplasia. J Androl 1991;12:356.

McConnell JD et al: Benign prostatic hyperplasia: Diagnosis and treatment. Agency for Health Care Policy and Research. Clinical Practice Guideline. Quick Reference Guide for Clinicians, 1994 (Feb);8:1.

Oesterling JE: Endocrine therapies for symptomatic benign prostatic hyperplasia. Urology 1994;43(2 Suppl):7.

Tempany CM et al: The influence of finasteride on the volume of the peripheral and periurethral zones of the prostate in men with benign prostatic hyperplasia. Prostate 1993;22:39.

Index

NOTE: Page numbers in bold face type indicate a major discussion. A *t* following a page number indicates tabular material and an *i* following a page number indicates an illustration. Drugs are listed under their generic names. When a drug trade name is listed, the reader is referred to the generic name.